CLOHERTY AND STARK'S
MANUAL OF NEONATAL CARE

Eighth Edition

Eric C. Eichenwald, MD
Thomas Frederick McNair Scott Professor of Pediatrics
Perelman School of Medicine
University of Pennsylvania
Chief, Division of Neonatology
Children's Hospital of Philadelphia
Philadelphia, Pennsylvania

Anne R. Hansen, MD, MPH
Associate Professor
Department of Pediatrics
Harvard Medical School
Medical Director, Neonatal Intensive Care Unit
Boston Children's Hospital
Boston, Massachusetts

Camilia R. Martin, MD, MS
Assistant Professor
Department of Pediatrics
Harvard Medical School
Associate Director, Neonatal Intensive Care Unit and Director of
Cross Disciplinary Partnerships
Department of Neonatology and Division of Translational Research
Beth Israel Deaconess Medical Center
Boston, Massachusetts

Ann R. Stark, MD
Professor of Pediatrics
Vanderbilt University School of Medicine
Director, Neonatal-Perinatal Medicine Fellowship Program
Director, Fellowship Programs, Department of Pediatrics
Monroe Carell Jr. Children's Hospital at Vanderbilt
Nashville, Tennessee

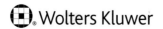

Philadelphia · Baltimore · New York · London
Buenos Aires · Hong Kong · Sydney · Tokyo

Acquisitions Editor: Rebecca Gaertner
Product Development Editor: Ashley Fischer
Editorial Assistant: Brian Convery
Marketing Manager: Rachel Mante Leung
Production Project Manager: Priscilla Crater
Design Coordinator: Teresa Mallon
Manufacturing Coordinator: Beth Welsh
Prepress Vendor: Absolute Service, Inc.

Eighth edition

Library of Congress Cataloging-in-Publication Data

Names: Eichenwald, Eric C., editor. | Hansen, Anne R., editor. | Martin,
   Camilia, editor. | Stark, Ann R., editor.
Title: Cloherty and Stark's manual of neonatal care / editors, Eric C.
   Eichenwald, Anne R. Hansen, Camilia R. Martin, Ann R. Stark.
Other titles: Manual of neonatal care
Description: Eighth edition. | Philadelphia : Wolters Kluwer, [2017] |
   Preceded by Manual of neonatal care / editors, John P. Cloherty ... [et
   al.]. 7th ed. c2012. | Includes bibliographical references and index.
Identifiers: LCCN 2016031579 | ISBN 9781496343611
Subjects: | MESH: Infant, Newborn, Diseases | Intensive Care, Neonatal |
   Neonatology—methods | Handbooks
Classification: LCC RJ251 | NLM WS 39 | DDC 618.92/.01—dc23 LC record available at
https://lccn.loc.gov/2016031579

CCS0120

We dedicate this edition

to former editor and inspiration for the Manual:
John P. Cloherty

to our spouses: Caryn, Jonathan, Brad, and Peter

to our children: Zachary, Taylor, Connor, Laura, Jonah,
Gregory, Linnea, Kathryn, Oliver, Julian, and Nathalie

to our grandchildren: Abe and Sascha

and to the many babies and parents we have cared for.

Contributors

Elisa Abdulhayoglu, MD, MS, FAAP
Instructor
Department of Pediatrics
Harvard Medical School
Staff Neonatologist
Brigham and Women's Hospital
Boston, Massachusetts
Chief of Neonatology
Newton-Wellesley Hospital
Newton, Massachusetts

Steven A. Abrams, MD
Professor
Department of Pediatrics
*Dell Medical School at the University of
Texas at Austin*
Austin, Texas

Diane M. Anderson, PhD, RD
Associate Professor
Department of Pediatrics
Baylor College of Medicine
Neonatal Nutritionist
Texas Children's Hospital
Houston, Texas

Theresa M. Andrews, RN, CCRN

Asimenia I. Angelidou, MD, PhD
Clinical Fellow
Division of Neonatal-Perinatal Medicine
Boston Children's Hospital
Boston, Massachusetts

John H. Arnold, MD
Professor of Anesthesia
Department of Anesthesia
Harvard Medical School
Senior Associate Anesthesia & Critical Care
Boston Children's Hospital
Boston, Massachusetts

Carlos A. Bacino, MD, FACMG
Professor
Vice-Chair Clinical Affairs
*Department of Molecular and Human
Genetics*
Baylor College of Medicine
Director
Pediatric Clinical Genetics Service
Texas Children's Hospital
Houston, Texas

Mandy Brown Belfort, MD, MPH
Assistant Professor
Department of Pediatric Newborn Medicine
Brigham and Women's Hospital
Boston, Massachusetts

John Benjamin, MD, MPH
Assistant Professor of Pediatrics
Division of Neonatology
*Monroe Carell Jr. Children's Hospital at
Vanderbilt*
Vanderbilt University Medical Center
Nashville, Tennessee

Jennifer Bentley, AuD
Audiologist
Department of Neonatology
Beth Israel Deaconess Medical Center
Boston, Massachusetts

Ann M. Bergin, MB, MRCP (UK), ScM
Assistant Professor
Department of Neurology
Boston Children's Hospital
Boston, Massachusetts

Vinod K. Bhutani, MD
Professor of Pediatrics (Neonatology)
Stanford University School of Medicine
Stanford, California

John P. Breinholt, MD
Associate Professor of Pediatrics
Director
Division of Pediatric Cardiology
Department of Pediatrics
University of Texas Health Science Center
* at Houston*
Children's Memorial Hermann Hospital
Houston, Texas

Heather H. Burris, MD, MPH
Attending Neonatologist
Beth Israel Deaconess Medical Center
Assistant Professor of Pediatrics
Assistant Professor of Obstetrics and
* Reproductive Biology*
Harvard Medical School
Assistant Professor
Department of Environmental Health
Harvard T.H. Chan School of Public Health
Boston, Massachusetts

Denise Casey, MS, RN, CCRN, CPNP
Clinical Nurse Specialist
Neonatal Intensive Care Unit
Boston Children's Hospital
Boston, Massachusetts

Yee-Ming Chan, MD, PhD
Associate in Medicine
Department of Medicine, Division of
* Endocrinology*
Boston Children's Hospital
Assistant Professor of Pediatrics
Harvard Medical School
Boston, Massachusetts

Kimberlee E. Chatson, MD
Assistant Professor
Boston Children's Hospital
Boston, Massachusetts;
Associate Medical Director
Winchester Hospital
Winchester, Massachusetts

Helen A. Christou, MD
Assistant Professor of Pediatrics
Harvard Medical School
Brigham and Women's Hospital
Boston Children's Hospital
Boston, Massachusetts

Javier A. Couto, BS
Research Fellow
Department of Plastic and Oral Surgery
Boston Children's Hospital
Boston, Massachusetts

Stacy E. Croteau, MD, MMS
Attending Physician
Division of Hematology/Oncology
Boston Children's Hospital
Boston, Massachusetts

Christy L. Cummings, MD
Assistant Professor of Pediatrics
Harvard Medical School
Ethics Associate
Division of Newborn Medicine Research
Boston Children's Hospital
Boston, Massachusetts

Emöke Deschmann, MD, MMSc
Attending Neonatologist
Instructor of Pediatrics
Department of Neonatology
Karolinska University Hospital
Stockholm, Sweden

Elizabeth G. Doherty, MD
Assistant Professor of Pediatrics
Harvard Medical School
Newborn Medicine
Boston Children's Hospital
Boston, Massachusetts

Christine Domonoske, PharmD
Neonatal Clinical Specialist
Department of Pharmacy Services
Children's Memorial Hermann Hospital
Houston, Texas

Caryn E. Douma, MS, RN, IBCLC
Director, CMHH Quality and Patient
* Safety, Palliative Care*
Children's Memorial Hermann Hospital
Houston, Texas

Stephanie Dukhovny, MD
Assistant Professor
Department of Obstetrics and Gynecology
Division of Maternal Fetal Medicine
Oregon Health & Science University
Portland, Oregon

Andrea F. Duncan, MD, MSClinRes
Associate Professor
Department of Pediatrics
Division of Neonatology
McGovern Medical School
University of Texas Health Science Center
* at Houston*
Houston, Texas

Eric C. Eichenwald, MD
Thomas Frederick McNair Scott Professor
* of Pediatrics*
Perelman School of Medicine
University of Pennsylvania
Chief, Division of Neonatology
Children's Hospital of Philadelphia
Philadelphia, Pennsylvania

Ayman W. El-Hattab, MD, FAAP,
FACMG
Consultant
Division of Clinical Genetics and Metabolic
* Disorders*
Pediatric Department
Tawam Hospital
Al-Ain, United Arab Emirates

Steven J. Fishman, MD
Professor of Surgery
Harvard Medical School
President, Physicians' Organization
Senior Vice-President, Access and Business
* Services*
Stuart and Jane Weitzman Family Chair
Vice-Chair of Surgery, Clinical Operations
Co-Director, Vascular Anomalies Center
Boston Children's Hospital
Boston, Massachusetts

Terri Gorman, MD
Brigham and Women's Hospital
Boston, Massachusetts

Arin K. Greene, MD, MMSC
Associate Professor of Surgery
Harvard Medical School
Department of Plastic Surgery
Boston Children's Hospital
Boston, Massachusetts

Mary Lucia P. Gregory, MD, MMSc
Assistant Professor of Pediatrics
Division of Neonatology
Monroe Carell Jr. Children's Hospital at
* Vanderbilt*
Nashville, Tennessee

Munish Gupta, MD, MMSc
Instructor in Pediatrics
Harvard Medical School
Beth Israel Deaconess Medical Center
Boston, Massachusetts

Susan Guttentag, MD
Julia Carell Stadler Professor of Pediatrics
Vanderbilt University School of Medicine
Director
Mildred Stahlman Division of Neonatology
Monroe Carell Jr. Children's Hospital at
* Vanderbilt*
Nashville, Tennessee

Anne R. Hansen, MD, MPH
Associate Professor
Department of Pediatrics
Harvard Medical School
Medical Director, Neonatal Intensive Care Unit
Boston Children's Hospital
Boston, Massachusetts

Gloria Heresi, MD
Professor, Pediatric Infectious Diseases
McGovern Medical School
UTHealth
Houston, Texas

Frank Hernandez, MD
Harvard Medical School
Boston, Massachusetts

Heather Y. Highsmith, MD
Fellow
Pediatric Infectious Diseases
Baylor College of Medicine
Texas Children's Hospital
Houston, Texas

Galit Holzmann-Pazgal, MD
Associate Professor
Department of Pediatric Infectious Diseases
University of Texas Health Science Center
* at Houston*
Houston, Texas

Nancy Hurst, PhD, RN, IBCLC
Assistant Professor
Department of Pediatrics
Baylor College of Medicine
Director
Lactation/Milk Bank Services
Texas Children's Hospital
Houston, Texas

Lise Johnson, MD
Assistant Professor of Pediatrics
Harvard Medical School
Department of Pediatric Newborn
* Medicine*
Brigham and Women's Hospital
Boston, Massachusetts

Patrick Jones, MD, MA
Assistant Professor of Pediatrics
Division of Neonatal-Perinatal Medicine
McGovern Medical School
University of Texas Health Science Center
* at Houston*
Houston, Texas

James R. Kasser, MD
Catharina Ormandy Professor of
* Orthopaedic Surgery*
Harvard Medical School
Orthopaedic Surgeon-in-Chief
Department of Orthopaedic Surgery
Boston Children's Hospital
Boston, Massachusetts

Amir M. Khan, MD
Professor of Pediatrics
McGovern Medical School
University of Texas Health Science Center
* at Houston*
Houston, Texas

Monica E. Kleinman, MD
Associate Professor of Anesthesia (Pediatrics)
Department of Anesthesiology, Perioperative
* and Pain Medicine*
Division of Critical Care Medicine
Harvard Medical School
Boston Children's Hospital
Boston, Massachusetts

Aimee Knorr, MD
Instructor in Pediatrics
Department of Pediatrics
Harvard Medical School
Assistant in Medicine
Associate Director
Infant Follow-up Program
Division of Newborn Medicine
Boston Children's Hospital
Boston, Massachusetts

Michelle A. LaBrecque, MSN, RN, CCRN
Clinical Nurse Specialist
Neonatal Intensive Care Unit
Boston Children's Hospital
Boston, Massachusetts

Heena K. Lee, MD, MPH
Instructor
Department of Pediatrics
Harvard Medical School
Attending Pediatrician
Department of Neonatology
Beth Israel Deaconess Medical Center
Boston, Massachusetts

Kristen T. Leeman, MD
Instructor in Pediatrics
Harvard Medical School
Physician in Medicine
Division of Newborn Medicine
Boston Children's Hospital
Boston, Massachusetts

Aviva Lee-Parritz, MD
Chair and Associate Professor
Boston University School of Medicine
Chief
Department of Obstetrics and Gynecology
Boston Medical Center
Boston, Massachusetts

Suzanne Lopez, MD
Associate Professor of Pediatrics
Department of Pediatrics
Division of Neonatology
Director
Neonatal-Perinatal Medicine Fellowship Program
McGovern Medical School
University of Texas Health Science Center at Houston
Houston, Texas

Melinda Markham, MD
Assistant Professor
Department of Pediatrics
Division of Neonatology
Vanderbilt University Medical Center
Nashville, Tennessee

Camilia R. Martin, MD, MS
Assistant Professor
Department of Pediatrics
Harvard Medical School
Associate Director
Neonatal Intensive Care Unit
Director
Cross Disciplinary Partnerships
Department of Neonatology and Division of Translational Research
Beth Israel Deaconess Medical Center
Boston, Massachusetts

Christopher C. McPherson, PharmD
Instructor
Department of Pediatrics
Harvard Medical School
Clinical Pharmacist
Department of Pediatric Newborn Medicine
Brigham and Women's Hospital
Boston, Massachusetts

Kenneth J. Moise Jr, MD
Professor
Department of Obstetrics, Gynecology and
  Reproductive Sciences
Professor of Pediatric Surgery
McGovern Medical School
University of Texas Health Science Center
  at Houston
Co-Director
The Fetal Center
Children's Memorial Hermann Hospital
Houston, Texas

Haendel Muñoz, MD
Pediatric Nephrologist
Pediatric Nephrology
Providence Sacred Heart Children's Hospital
Spokane, Washington

Elizabeth Oh, MD
Instructor
Department of Pediatrics
Harvard Medical School
Attending Pediatrician
Department of Neonatology
Beth Israel Deaconess Medical Center
Boston, Massachusetts

Deirdre O'Reilly, MD, MPH
Instructor in Pediatrics
Harvard Medical School
Department of Newborn Medicine
Boston Children's Hospital
Boston, Massachusetts

Lu-Ann Papile, MD
Professor Emerita
Department of Pediatrics
Division of Neonatal-Perinatal Medicine
University of New Mexico Health Sciences
  Center
Albuquerque, New Mexico

Richard B. Parad, MD, MPH
Associate Professor
Department of Pediatrics
Harvard Medical School
Assistant in Medicine
Department of Newborn Medicine
Brigham and Women's Hospital
Boston, Massachusetts

Stephen W. Patrick, MD, MPH, MS
Assistant Professor of Pediatrics and
  Health Policy
Division of Neonatology
Vanderbilt University School of Medicine
Nashville, Tennessee

Norma Pérez, MD
Assistant Professor of Pediatrics
McGovern Medical School
University of Texas Health Science Center
Houston, Texas

Sallie R. Permar, MD, PhD
Associate Professor of Pediatrics, Immunology,
  and Molecular Genetics and Microbiology
Duke University School of Medicine
Durham, North Carolina

Frank X. Placencia, MD
Assistant Professor
Department of Pediatrics
Section of Neonatology
Center for Medical Ethics and Health Policy
Baylor College of Medicine
Texas Children's Hospital
Houston, Texas

Erin J. Plosa, MD
Assistant Professor of Pediatrics
Department of Pediatrics
Division of Neonatology
Vanderbilt University School of Medicine
Nashville, Tennessee

Brenda B. Poindexter, MD, MS
Professor of Pediatrics
Department of Pediatrics
University of Cincinnati
Director
Clinical and Translational Research,
Perinatal Institute
Cincinnati Children's Hospital Medical Center
Cincinnati, Ohio

Muralidhar H. Premkumar, MBBS, MRCPCH
Assistant Professor
Department of Pediatrics
Baylor College of Medicine
Division of Neonatology
Texas Children's Hospital
Houston, Texas

Karen M. Puopolo, MD, PhD
Associate Professor of Clinical Pediatrics
University of Pennsylvania Perelman School of Medicine
Chief
Section on Newborn Pediatrics
Pennsylvania Hospital
Medical Director
CHOP Newborn Care at Pennsylvania Hospital
Philadelphia, Pennsylvania

Lawrence M. Rhein, MD, MPH
Associate Professor of Pediatrics
Divisions of Newborn Medicine and Pediatric Pulmonology
University of Massachusetts School of Medicine
Worcester, Massachusetts

Steven A. Ringer, MD, PhD
Associate Professor
Geisel School of Medicine at Dartmouth College
Hanover, New Hampshire

Joshua A. Samuels, MD, MPH
Professor, Pediatrics and Internal Medicine
UTHealth McGovern Medical School at Houston
Children's Memorial Hermann Hospital
Houston, Texas

Arnold J. Sansevere, MD
Assistant in Neurology
Department of Neurology
Division of Epilepsy
Boston Children's Hospital
Boston, Massachusetts

Matthew Saxonhouse, MD
Associate Professor
UNC School of Medicine Charlotte Campus
Assistant Professor
Division of Neonatology
Levine Children's Hospital
Charlotte, North Carolina

Bahaeddine Sibai, MD
Professor of Obstetrics and Gynecology
McGovern Medical School
University of Texas Health Science Center
Houston, Texas

Steven R. Sloan, MD, PhD
Associate Professor
Department of Laboratory Medicine
Harvard Medical School
Boston Children's Hospital
Boston, Massachusetts

Martha Sola-Visner, MD
Associate Professor
Division of Newborn Medicine
Harvard Medical School
Boston Children's Hospital
Boston, Massachusetts

Katherine A. Sparger, MD
Instructor in Pediatrics
Department of Pediatrics
Harvard Medical School
Associate Program Director
Massachusetts General Hospital for Children
Pediatric Residency Program; Neonatologist
Department of Pediatrics
Massachusetts General Hospital
Boston, Massachusetts

Vincent C. Smith, MD, MPH
Assistant Professor
Harvard Medical School
Associate Director
Neonatal Intensive Care Unit
Beth Israel Deaconess Medical Center
Boston, Massachusetts

Janet S. Soul, MDCM, FRCPC
Associate Professor of Neurology
Harvard Medical School
Director
Fetal-Neonatal Neurology Program
Boston Children's Hospital
Boston, Massachusetts

Carol Turnage Spruill, MSN, CNS, CPHQ
Clinical Nurse Specialist
Women, Infants and Children University of Texas Medical Branch
Galveston, Texas

Ann R. Stark, MD
Professor of Pediatrics
Vanderbilt University School of Medicine
Director
Neonatal-Perinatal Medicine Fellowship Program
Director
Fellowship Programs
Department of Pediatrics
Monroe Carell Jr. Children's Hospital at Vanderbilt
Nashville, Tennessee

Jeffrey R. Starke, MD
Professor of Pediatrics
Baylor College of Medicine
Houston, Texas

Jane E. Stewart, MD
Assistant Professor
Department of Pediatrics
Harvard Medical School
Associate Director
Department of Neonatology
Beth Israel Deaconess Medical Center
Boston, Massachusetts

V. Reid Sutton, MD
Professor
Department of Molecular and Human Genetics
Baylor College of Medicine
Texas Children's Hospital
Houston, Texas

Jonathan M. Swartz, MD
Instructor in Pediatrics
Department of Medicine
Division of Endocrinology
Boston Children's Hospital
Boston, Massachusetts

Rita D. Swinford, MD
Associate Professor
Department of Pediatrics
McGovern Medical School
University of Texas Health Science Center at Houston
Houston, Texas

Deborah K. VanderVeen, MD
Associate Professor
Department of Ophthalmology
Boston Children's Hospital
Harvard Medical School
Boston, Massachusetts

Linda J. Van Marter

Cristina Wallace

Benjamin Warf, MD
Associate Professor of Neurosurgery
Harvard Medical School
Director of Neonatal and Congenital
* Neurosurgery*
Boston Children's Hospital
Boston, Massachusetts

Ari J. Wassner, MD
Instructor
Department of Pediatrics
Harvard Medical School
Associate Director
Thyroid Program
Division of Endocrinology
Boston Children's Hospital
Boston, Massachusetts

Jörn-Hendrik Weitkamp, MD, FAAP
Associate Professor
Department of Pediatrics
Vanderbilt University Medical Center
Nashville, Tennessee

Louise E. Wilkins-Haug, MD, PhD
Professor
Harvard Medical School
Division Director, Maternal-Fetal Medicine
* and Reproductive Genetics*
Department of Obstetrics, Gynecology and
* Reproductive Medicine*
Brigham and Women's Hospital
Boston, Massachusetts

Gerhard K. Wolf, MD, PhD
Ludwig Maximilians University Munich
Children's Hospital Traunstein
Germany

Preface

This edition of the *Manual of Neonatal Care* has been completely updated and extensively revised to reflect the changes in fetal, perinatal, and neonatal care that have occurred since the seventh edition. In addition, we welcome Camilia R. Martin from Harvard as a new editor and collaborator.

In the *Manual*, we describe our current and practical approaches to evaluation and management of conditions encountered in the fetus and the newborn, as practiced in high-volume clinical services that include contemporary prenatal and postnatal care of infants with routine as well as complex medical and surgical problems. Although we base our practice on the best available evidence, we recognize that many areas of controversy exist, that there is often more than one approach to a problem, and that our knowledge continues to grow.

Our commitment to values, including clinical excellence, multidisciplinary collaboration, teamwork, and family-centered care, is evident throughout the book. Support of families is reflected in our chapters on breastfeeding, developmental care, bereavement, and decision making and ethical dilemmas. To help guide our readers, we have added a section of key points to each chapter.

We acknowledge the efforts of many individuals to advance the care of newborns and recognize, in particular, our teachers, colleagues, and trainees at Harvard, where the editors all trained in newborn medicine and practiced in the neonatal intensive care units (NICUs). We are indebted to Clement Smith and Nicholas M. Nelson for their insights into newborn physiology and to Stewart Clifford, William D. Cochran, John Hubbell, and Manning Sears for their contributions to the care of infants at the Boston Lying-In Hospital and all the former and current leaders of the Newborn Medicine Program at Harvard.

This would have been an impossible task without the administrative assistance of Ashley Park. We also thank Ashley Fisher of Wolters Kluwer for her invaluable help and patience.

We dedicate this book to Dr. Mary Ellen Avery for her contributions to the care of infants all over the world and to the personal support and advice she has provided to so many, including the editors. We also dedicate this book to our founding editor, Dr. John P. Cloherty, whose collaboration with current editor Dr. Ann R. Stark led to the first edition more than three decades ago, and is acknowledged in the revised title of this edition. Finally, we gratefully acknowledge the nurses, residents, fellows, parents, and babies who provide the inspiration for and measure the usefulness of the information contained in this volume.

Eric C. Eichenwald, MD
Anne R. Hansen, MD, MPH
Camilia R. Martin, MD, MS
Ann R. Stark, MD

Contents

General Newborn Condition

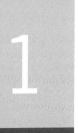

1

Fetal Assessment and Prenatal Diagnosis

Stephanie Dukhovny and Louise E. Wilkins-Haug

KEY POINTS

- Several different methods for prenatal diagnosis of fetal disease are currently available to the clinician.
- Fetal size and growth rate abnormalities may have significant implications for perinatal prognosis and care.
- Methods to assess fetal well-being prenatally and perinatally are central to obstetrical practice.

I. **GESTATIONAL AGE ASSESSMENT** is important to both the obstetrician and pediatrician and must be made with a reasonable degree of precision. Elective obstetric interventions such as chorionic villus sampling (CVS) and amniocentesis must be timed appropriately. When premature delivery is inevitable, gestational age is important with regard to prognosis, the management of labor and delivery, and the initial neonatal treatment plan.

A. **The clinical estimate** of gestational age is usually made on the basis of the first day of the last menstrual period (LMP). Accompanied by physical examination, auscultation of fetal heart sounds and maternal perception of fetal movement can also be helpful.

B. **Ultrasound** is the most accurate method for estimating gestational age. During the first trimester, fetal crown-rump length (CRL) can be an accurate predictor of gestational age. At <8 weeks and 6 days if the CRL and the LMP are >5 days different, the ultrasound is the best estimate for gestational age. From 9 0/7 to 15 6/7 weeks, CRL estimation of gestational age is expected to be within 7 days of the true gestational age. After 14 weeks, measurements of the biparietal diameter (BPD), the head circumference (HC), abdominal circumference (AC), and the fetal femur length best estimate gestational age. Strict criteria for measuring the cross-sectional images through the fetal head ensure accuracy. Nonetheless, owing to normal biologic variability, the accuracy of gestational age estimated by biometry decreases with increasing gestational age. For measurements made at 16 to 21 6/7 weeks of gestation, the variation is up to 10 days; at 22 to 27 6/7 weeks, the variation is up to 14 days; and at 28 weeks and beyond, the variation can be up to 21 days.

II. **PRENATAL DIAGNOSIS OF FETAL DISEASE** continues to improve. The genetic or developmental basis for many disorders is emerging, along with increased test accuracy. Two types of tests are available: screening tests and diagnostic procedures. Screening tests, such as a sample of the mother's blood or an ultrasound, are noninvasive but relatively nonspecific. A positive screening test, concerning family history, or an ultrasonic examination that suggests anomalies or aneuploidy may lead patient and physician to consider a diagnostic procedure. Diagnostic procedures, which necessitate obtaining a sample of fetal material, pose a small risk to both mother and fetus but can confirm or rule out the disorder in question.

A. **Screening by maternal serum analysis** during pregnancy individualizes a woman's risk of carrying a fetus with a neural tube defect (NTD) or an aneuploidy such as trisomy 21 (Down syndrome) or trisomy 18 (Edward syndrome).

1. **Maternal serum α-fetoprotein (MSAFP)** measurement between 15 and 22 weeks' gestation screens for NTDs. MSAFP elevated above 2.5 multiples of the median for gestation age occurs in 70% to 85% of fetuses with open spina bifida and 95% of fetuses with anencephaly. In half of the women with elevated levels, ultrasonic examination reveals another cause, most commonly an error in gestational age estimate. Ultrasonography that incorporates cranial or intracranial signs such as changes in head shape (lemon sign) or deformation of the cerebellum (banana sign) that are secondary to the NTD increase the sensitivity of ultrasound for the visual detection of open spinal defects.

2. **Second-trimester aneuploidy screening: MSAFP/quad panel.** Low levels of MSAFP are associated with chromosomal abnormalities. Altered levels of human chorionic gonadotropin (hCG), unconjugated estriol (uE3), and inhibin are also associated with fetal chromosomal abnormalities. On average, in a pregnancy with a fetus with trisomy 21, hCG and inhibin levels are higher than expected and uE3 levels are decreased. A serum panel in combination with maternal age can estimate the risk of trisomy 21 for an individual woman. For women <35 years, 5% will have a positive serum screen, but the majority (98%) will not have a fetus with aneuploidy. Only 80% of fetuses with trisomy 21 will have a "positive" quad screen (MSAFP, hCG, uE3, inhibin). Trisomy 18 is typically signaled by low levels of all markers.

3. **First-trimester serum screening.** Maternal levels of two analytes, pregnancy-associated plasma protein-A (PAPP-A) and hCG (either free or total), are altered in pregnancies with an aneuploid conception, especially trisomy 21. Similar to second-trimester serum screening, these values can individualize a woman's risk of pregnancy complicated by aneuploidy. However, these tests need to be drawn early in pregnancy (optimally at 9 to 10 weeks) and, even if abnormal, detect less than half of the fetuses with trisomy 21.

4. **First-trimester nuchal lucency screening.** Ultrasonographic assessment of the fluid collected at the nape of the fetal neck is a sensitive marker for aneuploidy. With attention to optimization of image and quality control, studies indicate a 70% to 80% detection of aneuploidy

in pregnancies with an enlarged nuchal lucency on ultrasonography. In addition, some fetuses with structural abnormalities such as cardiac defects will also have an enlarged nuchal lucency.

5. **Combined first-trimester screening.** Combining the two first-trimester maternal serum markers (PAPP-A and β-hCG) and the nuchal lucency measurements in addition to the maternal age detects 80% of trisomy 21 fetuses with a low screen positive rate (5% in women <35 years). This combined first-trimester screening provides women with a highly sensitive risk assessment in the first trimester.

6. **Combined first- and second-trimester screening for trisomy 21.** Various approaches have been developed to further increase the sensitivity of screening for trisomy 21 while retaining a low screen positive rate. These approaches differ primarily by whether they disclose the results of their first trimester results.

   a. Integrated screening. This is a nondisclosure approach that achieves the highest detection of trisomy 21 (97%) at a low screen positive rate (2%). It involves a first-trimester ultrasound and maternal serum screening in both the first and second trimester before the results are released.

   b. Sequential screening. Two types of sequential screening tools exist. Both are disclosure tests, which means that they release those results indicating a high risk of trisomy 21 in the first trimester but then go on to either further screen the entire remaining population in the second trimester (stepwise sequential) or only a subgroup of women felt to be in a medium-risk zone (contingent sequential). With contingent sequential screening, patients can be classified as high risk, medium risk, or low risk for Down syndrome in the first trimester. Low-risk patients do not return for further screening as their risk of a fetus with Down syndrome is low. When the two types of sequential tests are compared, they have similar overall screen positive rates of 2% to 3%, and both have sensitivities of >90% for trisomy 21 (stepwise, 95%; contingent, 93%)

7. **Cell-free fetal DNA screening for aneuploidy.** Newer technology has allowed analysis of cell-free fetal DNA from maternal serum in order to detect trisomies 13, 18, and sex chromosomal aneuploidies. The fetal DNA detected in maternal serum is placental in origin, can be detected as early as 9 weeks, and can be tested throughout the entire pregnancy. A number of laboratories have commercially available tests; all of which report a high sensitivity and specificity for trisomies 21 and 18. Sensitivity for trisomy 21 is reported at 99.3% and specificity at 99.8%. For trisomy 18, sensitivity is 97.4% and specificity is 99.8%. Sensitivity is lower for trisomy 13 (91%) with a specificity of 99.6%. Importantly, the positive predictive value (PPV) is lower for younger women secondary to the lower prevalence of aneuploidy in this population. For example, for trisomy 21, the PPV is 33% for women <25 years, in comparison to 87% for women >40 years. It is also important to note that cell-free fetal DNA targets specific aneuploidies and will ultimately miss abnormalities in other chromosomes and those with a mosaic karyotype. These abnormalities may have been detected by traditional screening methods. One study estimates up to 17% of significant chromosome abnormalities may go undetected with the use

of cell-free fetal DNA screening alone. For these reasons, cell-free fetal DNA screening for aneuploidy is not recommended for the general obstetric population and currently is recommended for women considered high risk for aneuploidy, including women who are >35 years old, have a history of a fetus or newborn with aneuploidy, carriers of a balanced translocation, or have a positive traditional screening test. Cell-free fetal DNA is considered a screening test, and any positive cell-free fetal DNA result should be followed up with a diagnostic test (CVS or amniocentesis) for confirmation of the diagnosis. Cell-free fetal DNA is also known as noninvasive prenatal testing (NIPT) despite that, as mentioned earlier, this test is considered a screening test and is not diagnostic.

8. Use of ultrasound following serum screening for aneuploidy

a. Second-trimester ultrasound targeted for the detection of aneuploidy has also been successful as a screening tool. Application of second-trimester ultrasound that is targeted to screen for aneuploidy can decrease the *a priori* maternal age risk of Down syndrome by 50% to 60% as well as the risk conveyed by serum screening. Second-trimester ultrasound following first-trimester screening for aneuploidy has likewise been shown to have value in decreasing the risk assessment for trisomy 21.

B. In women with a **positive family history of genetic disease**, a positive screening test, or at-risk ultrasonographic features, diagnostic tests are considered. When an invasive diagnostic test is performed for a structural abnormality detected on ultrasound, a chromosomal microarray is indicated, which will detect aneuploidy as well as smaller chromosomal deletions and duplications. If an invasive test is performed secondary to a positive screening test, either a chromosomal microarray or a karyotype can be offered. When a significant malformation or a genetic disease is diagnosed prenatally, the information gives the obstetrician and pediatrician time to educate parents, discuss options, and establish an initial neonatal treatment plan before the infant is delivered. In some cases, treatment may be initiated *in utero*.

1. **CVS.** Under ultrasonic guidance, a sample of placental tissue is obtained through a catheter placed either transcervically or transabdominally. Performed at or after 10 weeks' gestation, CVS provides the earliest possible detection of a genetically abnormal fetus through analysis of trophoblast cells. Transabdominal CVS can also be used as late as the third trimester when amniotic fluid is not available or fetal blood sampling cannot be performed. Technical improvements in ultrasonographic imaging and in the CVS procedure have brought the pregnancy loss rate very close to the loss rate after second-trimester amniocentesis, 0.5% to 1.0%. The possible complications of amniocentesis and CVS are similar. CVS, if performed before 10 weeks of gestation, can be associated with an increased risk of fetal limb-reduction defects and oromandibular malformations.

a. Direct preparations of rapidly dividing cytotrophoblasts can be prepared, making a full karyotype analysis available in 2 days. Although direct preparations minimize maternal cell contamination, most centers also analyze cultured trophoblast cells, which are embryologically closer to the fetus. This procedure takes an additional 8 to 12 days.

b. In approximately 2% of CVS samples, a mosaic diagnosis is made, which indicates that both karyotypically normal and abnormal cells are identified in the same sample. Because CVS-acquired cells reflect placental constitution, in these cases, amniocentesis is typically performed as a follow-up study to analyze fetal cells. Approximately one-third of CVS mosaicisms are confirmed in the fetus through amniocentesis.

2. **Amniocentesis.** Amniotic fluid is removed from around the fetus through a needle guided by ultrasonic images. The removed amniotic fluid ($\sim$20 mL) is replaced by the fetus within 24 hours. Amniocentesis can technically be performed as early as 10 to 14 weeks' gestation, although early amniocentesis (<13 weeks) is associated with a pregnancy loss rate of 1% to 2% and an increased incidence of clubfoot. Loss of the pregnancy following an ultrasonography-guided second-trimester amniocentesis (16 to 20 weeks) occurs in 0.5% to 1.0% cases in most centers, so they are usually performed in the second trimester.

a. Amniotic fluid can be analyzed for a number of compounds, including alpha-fetoprotein (AFP), acetylcholinesterase (AChE), bilirubin, and pulmonary surfactant. Increased levels of AFP along with the presence of AChE identify NTDs with >98% sensitivity when the fluid sample is not contaminated by fetal blood. AFP levels are also elevated when the fetus has abdominal wall defects, congenital nephrosis, or intestinal atresias. Several biochemical tests of the amniotic fluid are available to assess fetal lung maturity.

b. Fetal cells can be extracted from the fluid sample and analyzed for chromosomal and genetic makeup.

i. Among second-trimester amniocenteses, 73% of clinically significant karyotype abnormalities relate to one of five chromosomes: 13, 18, 21, X, or Y. These can be rapidly detected using fluorescent *in situ* hybridization (FISH), with sensitivities in the 90% range.

ii. **DNA analysis** is diagnostic for an increasing number of diseases.

a) Increasingly, **direct DNA methodologies** can be used when the gene sequence producing the disease in question is known. Disorders secondary to deletion of DNA (e.g., α-thalassemia, Duchenne and Becker muscular dystrophy, cystic fibrosis, and growth hormone deficiency) can be detected by the altered size of DNA fragments produced following a polymerase chain reaction (PCR). Direct detection of a DNA mutation can also be accomplished by allele-specific oligonucleotide (ASO) analysis. If the PCR-amplified DNA is not altered in size by a deletion or insertion, recognition of a mutated DNA sequence can occur by hybridization with the known mutant allele. Rapid advances in molecular technologies have provided many new opportunities for mutation identification which are now applicable to fetal DNA.

iii. **DNA sequencing** for many genetic disorders has revealed that a multitude of different mutations within a gene can result in the same clinical disease. For example, cystic fibrosis can result from >1,000 different mutations. Therefore, for any specific disease, prenatal diagnosis by DNA testing may require parental as well as fetal DNA.

3. **Percutaneous umbilical blood sampling (PUBS)** is performed under ultrasonic guidance from the second trimester until term. PUBS can provide diagnostic samples for cytogenetic, hematologic, immunologic, or DNA studies; it can also provide access for treatment *in utero*. An anterior placenta facilitates obtaining a sample close to the cord insertion site at the placenta. Fetal sedation is usually not needed. PUBS has a 1% to 2% risk of fetal loss along with complications that can lead to a preterm delivery in another 5%.

4. **Preimplantation biopsy or preimplantation genetic diagnosis (PGD).** During an *in vitro* fertilization process, early in gestation (at the eight-cell stage in humans), prior to transfer, one or two cells can be removed without known harm to the embryo. PGD is useful for a wide range of autosomal recessive, dominant, and X-linked molecular diagnoses. For couples at risk, testing allows for identification of embryos that carry the disorder in question, and transfer of unaffected embryos can occur. In women who are at risk for X-linked recessive disorders, determination of XX-containing embryos by FISH can enable transfer of only female embryos. Similarly, women at increased risk for a chromosomally abnormal conception can benefit from preimplantation biopsy. When one member of a couple carries a balanced translocation, only those embryos that screen negative for the chromosome abnormality in question are transferred. When more cells are needed for molecular diagnoses, biopsy on day 5 is considered. An alternative approach is analysis of the second polar body, which contains the same genetic material as the ovum. Preimplantation genetic screening (PGS) to assess preimplantation embryos for aneuploidy is not currently considered to provide reproductive advantage to women of advanced maternal age or poor reproductive histories.

5. **Cell-free fetal DNA in the maternal circulation.** Development of a noninvasive method of prenatal diagnosis for single-gene disorders would be ideal because it would eliminate the potential procedure-related loss of a normal pregnancy. Although fetal cells in the maternal circulation can be separated and analyzed, the limited numbers preclude using this technique on a clinical basis. Cell-free fetal DNA techniques are available commercially for identification of fetal Rh status for women at risk for isoimmunization. Additionally, proof of principle studies have demonstrated this technique for identification of fetuses at risk for single-gene disorders as well but currently are only performed on a research basis.

III. **FETAL SIZE AND GROWTH-RATE ABNORMALITIES** may have significant implications for perinatal prognosis and care (see Chapter 7). Appropriate fetal assessment is important in establishing a diagnosis and a perinatal treatment plan.

A. **Fetal growth restriction (FGR)** may be due to conditions in the fetal environment (e.g., chronic deficiencies in oxygen or nutrients or both) or to problems intrinsic to the fetus. It is important to identify constitutionally normal fetuses whose growth is impaired so that appropriate care can begin as soon as possible. Because their risk of mortality is increased severalfold before and during labor, FGR fetuses may need preterm intervention for best survival rates. Once delivered, these newborns are at increased risk for immediate complications including hypoglycemia and pulmonary hemorrhage, so they should be delivered at an appropriately equipped facility.

Intrinsic causes of FGR include chromosomal abnormalities (such as trisomies, microdeletions, or duplications), congenital malformations, and congenital infections (e.g., cytomegalovirus, toxoplasmosis, varicella, or rubella). Prenatal diagnosis of malformed or infected fetuses is important so that appropriate interventions can be made. Prenatal genetic assessment should be considered if FGR is <3% before 24 weeks or when structural anomalies or soft markers for aneuploidy are present. Investigation by cell-free DNA versus a karyotype/microarray or DNA diagnostic studies is individualized to the specific findings of the case. Prior knowledge that a fetus has a malformation (e.g., anencephaly) or chromosomal abnormality (e.g., trisomy 18) that limits life allows the parents to be counseled before birth of the child and may influence the management of labor and delivery.

1. **Definition of FGR.** There is no universal agreement on the definition of FGR. Strictly speaking, any fetus that does not reach his or her intrauterine growth potential is included. Typically, fetuses weighing <10th percentile for gestational age are classified as FGR; however, many of these fetuses are normal and at the lower end of the growth spectrum (i.e., "constitutionally small").

2. **Diagnosis of FGR.** Maternal clinical exam detects about two-thirds of cases and incorrectly diagnoses it about 50% of the time. Ultrasonography improves the sensitivity and specificity to >80%. FGR may be diagnosed with a single scan when a fetus <10th percentile demonstrates corroborative signs of a compromised intrauterine environment such as oligohydramnios, an elevated head–abdomen ratio in the absence of central nervous system pathology or abnormal Doppler velocimetry in the umbilical cord. Serial scans documenting absent or poor intrauterine growth regardless of the weight percentile also indicate FGR. From the large Prospective Observational Trial to Optimize Pediatric Health Trial in Intrauterine Growth Restriction (PORTO) study, the greatest risk for morbidity/mortality was among those fetuses below the 3% for estimated fetal weight with abnormal umbilical Doppler perfusion and delayed serial growth trajectory. The use of composite growth profiles derived from a variety of ultrasound measurements and repeated serially to identify individual restriction of fetal growth potential remains controversial.

B. **Macrosomia.** Macrosomic fetuses (>4,000 g) are at increased risk for shoulder dystocia and traumatic birth injury. Conditions such as maternal diabetes, postterm pregnancy, genetic overgrowth syndromes, and maternal obesity are associated with an increased incidence of macrosomia. Unfortunately, efforts to use a variety of measurements and formulas have met with only modest success in predicting the condition.

IV. **FUNCTIONAL MATURITY OF THE LUNGS** is one of the most critical variables in determining neonatal survival in the otherwise normal fetus. Currently, however, assessment of fetal maturity is reserved for the infrequent event of semi-elective births before 39 weeks. A number of tests can be performed on amniotic fluid specifically to determine pulmonary maturity (see Chapter 33).

V. ASSESSMENT OF FETAL WELL-BEING.
Acute compromise is detected by studies that assess fetal function. Some are used antepartum, whereas others are used to monitor the fetus during labor.

A. **Antepartum tests** generally rely on biophysical studies, which require a certain degree of fetal neurophysiologic maturity. The following tests are not used until the third trimester; fetuses may not respond appropriately earlier in gestation.

1. **Fetal movement monitoring** is the simplest method of fetal assessment. Fetuses normally have a sleep–wake cycle, and mothers generally perceive a diurnal variation in fetal activity. Active periods average 30 to 40 minutes. Periods of inactivity >1 hour are unusual in a healthy fetus and should alert the physician to the possibility of fetal compromise. A "count to 10" method by the mother is the only approach to fetal movement which has been validated and then evaluated as a screening test. The same time of day is chosen, fetal movements are noted with the expectation of 10 fetal movements achieved within 2 hours. The average time to 10 movements is 20 minutes (±18). Lack of attaining 10 movements prompts evaluation. However, although a mother's perception of decreased fetal movement should always elicit further surveillance, the specifics of fetal movement quantification remain to be further established.

2. The **nonstress test (NST)** is a reliable means of fetal evaluation. It is simple to perform, relatively quick, and noninvasive, with neither discomfort nor risk to mother or fetus.

   The NST is based on the principle that fetal activity results in a reflex acceleration in heart rate. The required fetal maturity is typically reached by approximately 32 weeks of gestation. Absence of these accelerations in a fetus who previously demonstrated them may indicate that hypoxia has sufficiently depressed the central nervous system to inactivate the cardiac reflex. Testing reflexes the current fetal state and cannot predict future events or precisely the neonatal outcome.

   The test is performed by monitoring fetal heart rate (FHR) either through a Doppler ultrasonographic device or through skin-surface electrodes on the maternal abdomen. Uterine activity is simultaneously recorded through a tocodynamometer, palpation by trained test personnel, or the patient's report. The test result may be reactive, nonreactive, or inadequate. The criteria for a reactive test are as follows: (i) heart rate between 110 and 160 bpm, (ii) normal beat-to-beat variability (5 bpm), and (iii) two accelerations of at least 15 bpm lasting for not <15 seconds each within a 20-minute period. A nonreactive test is defined as less than two accelerations in 40 minutes. If an adequate fetal heart tracing cannot be obtained for any reason, the test is considered inadequate.

   Statistics show that a reactive result is reassuring, with the risk of fetal demise within the week following the test at approximately 3 in 1,000. Negative predictive values for stillbirth within 1 week of reactive NSTs are 99.8%. A nonreactive test is generally repeated later the same day or is followed by another test of fetal well-being. The frequency with which NST should be performed is not established. The NST is commonly obtained on a weekly basis, although increased testing (two times per week to daily testing) is recommended for high-risk conditions.

3. The **contraction stress test (CST)** may be used as a backup or confirmatory test when the NST is nonreactive or inadequate, although with multiple other modalities for fetal surveillance, CST is now used less commonly.

   The CST is based on the idea that uterine contractions can compromise an unhealthy fetus. The pressure generated during contractions can briefly reduce or eliminate perfusion of the intervillous space. A healthy fetoplacental unit has sufficient reserve to tolerate this short reduction in oxygen supply. Under pathologic conditions, however, respiratory reserve may be so compromised that the reduction in oxygen results in fetal hypoxia. Under hypoxic conditions, the FHR slows in a characteristic way relative to the contraction. FHR begins to decelerate 15 to 30 seconds after onset of the contraction, reaches its nadir after the peak of the contraction, and does not return to baseline until after the contraction ends. This heart rate pattern is known as a *late deceleration* because of its relationship to the uterine contraction. Synonyms are type 2 deceleration or deceleration of uteroplacental insufficiency.

   Similar to the NST, the CST monitors FHR and uterine contractions. A CST is considered completed if uterine contractions have spontaneously occurred within 30 minutes, lasted 40 to 60 seconds each, and occurred at a frequency of three within a 10-minute interval. If no spontaneous contractions occur, they can be induced with intravenous oxytocin, in which case the test is called an *oxytocin challenge* test.

   A CST is positive if late decelerations are consistently seen in association with contractions. A CST is negative if at least three contractions of at least 40 seconds each occur within a 10-minute period without associated late decelerations. A CST is suspicious if there are occasional or inconsistent late decelerations. If contractions occur more frequently than every 2 minutes or last longer than 90 seconds, the study is considered a hyperstimulated test and cannot be interpreted. An unsatisfactory test is one in which contractions cannot be stimulated or a satisfactory FHR tracing cannot be obtained.

   A negative CST is even more reassuring than a reactive NST, with the chance of fetal demise within a week of a negative CST being approximately 0.4 per 1,000. If a positive CST follows a nonreactive NST, however, the risk of stillbirth is 88 per 1,000, and the risk of neonatal mortality is also 88 per 1,000. Statistically, about one-third of patients with a positive CST will require cesarean section for persistent late decelerations in labor.

4. The **biophysical profile** combines an NST with other parameters determined by real-time ultrasonic examination. A score of 0 or 2 is assigned for the absence or presence of each of the following: a reactive NST, adequate amniotic fluid volume (vertical fluid pocket >2 cm), fetal breathing movements, fetal activity, and normal fetal musculoskeletal tone. A modified BPP can assess both acute (NST) and chronic stress (amniotic fluid volumes). The total score determines the course

of action. Reassuring tests (8 to 10) are repeated at weekly intervals, whereas less reassuring results (4 to 6) are repeated later the same day. Very low scores (0 to 2) generally prompt delivery. The likelihood that a fetus will die *in utero* within 1 week of a reassuring test is approximately the same as that for a negative CST, which is approximately 0.6 to 0.7 per 1,000. Similarly, the negative predictive value for a stillbirth within 1 week of a reassuring BPP, modified BPP, and negative CST is >99.9%.

5. Doppler ultrasonography of **fetal umbilical artery blood flow** is a noninvasive technique to assess downstream (placental) resistance. Poorly functioning placentas with extensive vasospasm or infarction have an increased resistance to flow that is particularly noticeable in fetal diastole. Umbilical artery Doppler flow velocimetry is the primary surveillance tool for pregnancies with FGR and utilizes the peak systolic frequency shift (S) and the end-diastolic frequency shift (D). The PORTO study recently established the association of increased morbidity/mortality as occurring primarily among those FGR newborns with abnormal umbilical Doppler studies (pulsatility index >95th percentile or absent/reversed end-diastolic flow). Analyses of placental histology with abnormal umbilical Doppler flow have suggested loss of 70% function is reflected with absent/reversed umbilical Doppler readings. The two commonly used indices of flow are the systolic:diastolic ratio (S/D) and the resistance index (S-D/S). Umbilical artery Doppler velocimetry measurements have been shown to improve perinatal outcome only in pregnancies with a presumptive diagnosis of FGR and should not be used as a screening test in the general obstetric population. The use of umbilical artery Doppler velocimetry measurements, in conjunction with other tests of fetal well-being, can reduce the perinatal mortality in FGR by almost 40%. Doppler measurements of the **middle cerebral artery** can also be used in the assessment of the fetus that is at risk for either FGR or anemia. Further evidence of the progression of uteroplacental insufficiency can be revealed by ultrasound assessment of the ductus venous. Absent or even reversal of the normally forward end-diastolic flow through this vessel is considered a terminal finding. Clinical use remains controversial as the potential benefits of prolonging preterm gestation once abnormal ductus venous flow suggests extreme uteroplacental compromise have not been supported in all studies.

6. **Indications for fetal surveillance.** Pregnancies with ongoing increased risk for stillbirth (chronic hypertension, pregestational diabetes, poorly controlled gestational diabetes, growth restriction, advanced maternal age, increased maternal body mass, or vascular disease) or new risk (decreased fetal movement, abdominal trauma, vaginal bleeding) are candidates for fetal surveillance. Most fetal surveillance are begun at 32 weeks although in the setting of FGR, in particular, initiation prior to 32 weeks is often undertaken. The frequency of monitoring is typically weekly, although in high-risk conditions or those in which the mother's condition is changing, monitoring will often occur more frequently.

B. **Intrapartum assessment of fetal well-being** is important in the management of labor.

   1. **Continuous electronic fetal monitoring** is widely used despite the fact that its role in reducing perinatal mortality has been questioned and it does not lower rates of neurologic injury relative to auscultation by trained personnel. It has, however, increased the incidence of operative delivery. When used, the monitors simultaneously record FHR and uterine activity for ongoing evaluation. Either continuous or intermittent monitoring is acceptable for low-risk patients.

      a. The **FHR** can be monitored in one of three ways. The noninvasive methods are ultrasonic monitoring and surface-electrode monitoring from the maternal abdomen. The most accurate but invasive method is to place a small electrode into the skin of the fetal presenting part to record the fetal electrocardiogram directly. Placement requires rupture of the fetal membranes. When the electrode is properly placed, it is associated with a very low risk of fetal injury. Approximately 4% of monitored babies develop a mild infection at the electrode site, and most respond to local cleansing.

      b. Uterine activity can also be recorded either indirectly or directly. A tocodynamometer can be strapped to the maternal abdomen to record the timing and duration of contractions as well as crude relative intensity. When a more precise evaluation is needed, an intrauterine pressure catheter can be inserted following rupture of the fetal membranes to directly and quantitatively record contraction pressure. Invasive monitoring is associated with an increased incidence of chorioamnionitis and postpartum maternal infection.

      c. Parameters of the fetal monitoring record that are evaluated include the following:

         i. Baseline heart rate is normally between 110 and 160 bpm. The baseline must be apparent for a minimum of 2 minutes in any 10-minute segment and does not include episodic changes, periods of marked FHR variability, or segments of baseline that differ by >25 bpm. Baseline fetal bradycardia, defined as an FHR <110 bpm, may result from congenital heart block associated with congenital heart malformation or maternal systemic lupus erythematosus. Baseline tachycardia, defined as an FHR >160 bpm, may result from a maternal fever, infection, stimulant medications or drugs, and hyperthyroidism. Fetal dysrhythmias are typically associated with FHR >200 bpm. In isolation, tachycardia is poorly predictive of fetal hypoxemia or acidosis unless accompanied by reduced beat-to-beat variability or recurrent decelerations.

         ii. Beat-to-beat variability is recorded from a calculation of each RR interval. The autonomic nervous system of a healthy, awake term fetus constantly varies the heart rate from beat to beat by approximately 5 to 25 bpm. Reduced beat-to-beat variability may result from depression of the fetal central nervous system due to fetal immaturity, hypoxia, fetal sleep, or specific maternal medications such as narcotics, sedatives, β-blockers, and intravenous magnesium sulfate.

    iii. Accelerations of the FHR are reassuring, as they are during an NST.

    iv. Decelerations of the FHR may be benign or indicative of fetal compromise depending on their characteristic shape and timing in relation to uterine contractions.

        a) Early decelerations are symmetric in shape and closely mirror uterine contractions in time of onset, duration, and termination. They are benign and usually accompany good beat-to-beat variability. These decelerations are more commonly seen in active labor when the fetal head is compressed in the pelvis, resulting in a parasympathetic effect.

        b) Late decelerations are visually apparent decreases in the FHR in association with uterine contractions. The onset, nadir, and recovery of the deceleration occur after the beginning, peak, and end of the contraction, respectively. A fall in the heart rate of only 10 to 20 bpm below baseline (even if still within the range of 110 to160 bpm) is significant. Late decelerations are the result of uteroplacental insufficiency and possible fetal hypoxia. As the uteroplacental insufficiency/hypoxia worsens, (i) beat-to-beat variability will be reduced and then lost, (ii) decelerations will last longer, (iii) they will begin sooner following the onset of a contraction, (iv) they will take longer to return to baseline, and (v) the rate to which the fetal heart slows will be lower. Repetitive late decelerations demand action.

        c) Variable decelerations vary in their shape and in their timing relative to contractions. Usually, they result from fetal umbilical cord compression. Variable decelerations are a cause for concern if they are severe (down to a rate of 60 bpm or lasting for 60 seconds or longer, or both), associated with poor beat-to-beat variability, or mixed with late decelerations. Umbilical cord compression secondary to a low amniotic fluid volume (oligohydramnios) may be alleviated by amnioinfusion of saline into the uterine cavity during labor.

2. National Institute of Child Health and Diseases classification of intrapartum FHR monitoring

  a. Endorsed by the American College of Obstetricians and Gynecologists, a three-tiered classification of intrapartum monitoring was introduced in 2008 to promote a systematic interpretation and response to the subjective nature of fetal monitor interpretations. Category I tracings are considered reflexive of a fetus with a normal acid–base status but require repeated review. Category III tracings require prompt intervention, and if unresolved quickly, then delivery. For category II tracings, various precipitating factors may be addressed, and if unsuccessful, then delivery is recommended (see Table 1.1).

3. A **fetal scalp blood sample for blood gas** analysis may be obtained to confirm or dismiss suspicion of fetal hypoxia. An intrapartum scalp pH >7.20 with a base deficit <6 mmol/L is normal. However, these kits are no longer manufactured in the United States. Many obstetric units have replaced fetal scalp blood sampling with noninvasive techniques to assess fetal status. FHR accelerations in response to mechanical

Table 1.1. Classification of Intrapartum Monitoring

Category I	Tracings meeting these criteria are predictive of normal fetal acid–base balance at the time of observation.	All of the criteria must be present: ■ Baseline rate: 110–160 bpm ■ Moderate baseline FHR variability ■ No late or variable decelerations ■ Early decelerations may be present or absent. ■ Accelerations may be present or absent.
Category II	FHR tracing does not meet criteria for either category I or III and is considered indeterminate.	

Category III	■ Category III tracings are predictive of abnormal fetal acid–base status at the time of observation.
	■ Prompt evaluation is indicated and intervention indicated.
		Either 1 or 2 is present:
		1. Absent baseline FHR variability and any of the following:
		  ■ Recurrent late decelerations
		  ■ Recurrent variable decelerations
		  ■ Bradycardia
		2. Sinusoidal pattern

FHR, fetal heart rate.		

stimulation of the fetal scalp (gently nudging the presenting vertex with the examiner's finger or an Allis clamp) or to vibroacoustic stimulation are reassuring.

Suggested Readings

Aagaard-Tillery KM, Malone FD, Nyberg DA, et al. Role of second-trimester genetic sonography after Down syndrome screening. *Obstet Gynecol* 2009;114(6): 1189–1196.

Alfirevic Z, Devane D, Gyte GM. Continuous cardiotocography (CTG) as a form of electronic fetal monitoring (EFM) for fetal assessment during labour. *Cochrane Database Syst Rev* 2006;(3):CD006066.

Alfirevic Z, Gosden CM, Neilson JP. Chorion villus sampling versus amniocentesis for prenatal diagnosis. *Cochrane Database Syst Rev* 2000;(2):CD000055.

American College of Obstetricians and Gynecologists. ACOG Practice Bulletin No. 12: intrauterine growth restriction. *Obstet Gynecol* 2000;95(1).

American College of Obstetricians and Gynecologists. ACOG Practice Bulletin No. 106: intrapartum fetal heart rate monitoring: nomenclature, interpretation, and general management principles. *Obstet Gynecol* 2009;114(1):192–202.

Antsaklis A, Papantoniou N, Xygakis A, et al. Genetic amniocentesis in women 20–34 years old: associated risks. *Prenat Diagn* 2000;20(3):247–250.

Ball RH, Caughey AB, Malone FD, et al. First- and second-trimester evaluation of risk for Down syndrome. *Obstet Gynecol* 2007;110(1):10–17.

Lees CC, Marlow N, van Wassenaer-Leemhuis A, et al. 2 year neurodevelopmental and intermediate perinatal outcomes in infants with very preterm fetal growth restriction (TRUFFLE): a randomized trial. *Lancet* 2015; 385(9983):2162–2172.

Malone FD, Canick JA, Ball RH, et al. First-trimester or second-trimester screening, or both, for Down's syndrome. *N Engl J Med* 2005;353(19):2001–2011.

Moore TR, Piacquadio K. A prospective evaluation of fetal movement screening to reduce the incidence of antepartum fetal death. *Am J Obstet Gynecol* 1989;160(5, Pt 1):1075–1080.

Nicolaides KH, Brizot ML, Snijders RJ. Fetal nuchal translucency: ultrasound screening for fetal trisomy in the first trimester of pregnancy. *Br J Obstet Gynaecol* 1994;101(9):782–786.

Pandya PP, Brizot ML, Kuhn P, et al. First-trimester fetal nuchal translucency thickness and risk for trisomies. *Obstet Gynecol* 1994;84(3):420–423.

Platt LD, Greene N, Johnson A, et al. Sequential pathways of testing after first-trimester screening for trisomy 21. *Obstet Gynecol* 2004;104(4):661–666.

Unterscheider J, Daly S, Geary MP, et al. Optimizing the definition of intrauterine growth restriction: the multicenter prospective PORTO Study. *Am J Obstet Gynecol* 2013;208(4):290.e1–290.e6.

2 | Maternal Diabetes Mellitus

Aviva Lee-Parritz

KEY POINTS

- With appropriate management of pregnant women with diabetes, women with good glycemic control and minimal microvascular disease can expect pregnancy outcomes comparable to the general population.
- Women with type 1 and type 2 diabetes are at significantly increased risk for hypertensive disorders, such as preeclampsia, which is potentially deleterious to both maternal and fetal well-being.
- Route of delivery of a fetus affected by maternal diabetes is determined by ultrasonography-estimated fetal weight, maternal and fetal conditions, and previous obstetric history.
- Preconception glucose control for women with pregestational diabetes can reduce the risk of congenital anomalies to near that of the general population.
- Strict glycemic control can reduce fetal macrosomia in both pregestational and gestational diabetes. Targeting postmeal glycemia is more effective than solely premeal measurement to reduce fetal overgrowth.
- Women with pregestational diabetes and microvascular disease are at risk for indicated preterm delivery due to worsening maternal or fetal status.
- Tight intrapartum glucose control is important to reduce fetal oxidative stress and neonatal hypoglycemia.
- Women with pregestational diabetes may have reduced glycemic profiles and insulin requirements postpartum, especially in women breastfeeding.

I. **DIABETES AND PREGNANCY OUTCOME.** Improved management of diabetes mellitus and advances in obstetrics have reduced the incidence of adverse perinatal outcome in pregnancies complicated by diabetes mellitus. With appropriate management, women with good glycemic control and minimal microvascular disease can expect pregnancy outcomes comparable to the general population. Women with advanced microvascular disease, such as hypertension, nephropathy, and retinopathy, have a 25% risk of preterm delivery because of worsening maternal condition or preeclampsia. Pregnancy does not have a significant impact on the progression of diabetes. In women who begin pregnancy with microvascular disease, diabetes often worsens, but in most, the disease return to baseline. Preconception glucose control may reduce the rate of complications to as low as that seen in the general population.

II. DIABETES IN PREGNANCY

A. General principles

1. Diabetes that antedates the pregnancy can be associated with adverse fetal and maternal outcomes. The most important complication is diabetic embryopathy resulting in congenital anomalies. Congenital anomalies are associated with 50% of perinatal deaths among women with diabetes compared to 25% among nondiabetic women. The risk of congenital anomalies is related to the glycemic profile at the time of conception. The most common types of anomalies include cardiac malformations and neural tube defects. Women with type 1 and type 2 diabetes are at significantly increased risk for hypertensive disorders, such as preeclampsia, which is potentially deleterious to both maternal and fetal well-being. Gestational diabetes mellitus (GDM) is defined as carbohydrate intolerance of variable severity first diagnosed during pregnancy, and it affects 6% to 8% of pregnancies.

2. **Epidemiology of gestational diabetes.** Approximately 3% to 5% of patients with GDM actually have underlying type 1 or type 2 diabetes, but pregnancy is the first opportunity for testing. Risk factors for GDM include advanced maternal age, multifetal gestation, increased body mass index, and strong family history of diabetes. Certain ethnic groups, such as Native Americans, Southeast Asians, and African Americans, have an increased risk of developing GDM.

3. **Physiology unique to women with diabetes antedating pregnancy.** In the first half of pregnancy, as a result of nausea and vomiting, **hypoglycemia** can be as much of a problem as **hyperglycemia**. Hypoglycemia, followed by hyperglycemia from counter-regulatory hormones, may complicate glucose control. Maternal hyperglycemia leads to fetal hyperglycemia and fetal hyperinsulinemia, which results in fetal overgrowth. Gastroparesis from long-standing diabetes may be a factor as well. There does not appear to be a direct relationship between hypoglycemia alone and adverse perinatal outcome. Throughout pregnancy, **insulin requirements** increase because of the increasing production of placental hormones that antagonize the action of insulin. This is most prominent in the mid-third trimester and requires intensive blood glucose monitoring and frequent adjustment of medications to control blood glucose.

B. Complications of type 1 and type 2 diabetes during pregnancy

1. **Ketoacidosis** is an uncommon complication during pregnancy. However, ketoacidosis carries a 50% risk of fetal death, especially if it occurs before the third trimester. Ketoacidosis can be present in the setting of even mild hyperglycemia (200 mg/dL) and should be excluded in every patient with type 1 diabetes who presents with hyperglycemia and symptoms such as nausea, vomiting, or abdominal pain.

2. **Stillbirth** remains an uncommon complication of diabetes in pregnancy. It is most often associated with poor glycemic control, fetal anomalies, severe vasculopathy, and intrauterine growth restriction (IUGR) as well as severe preeclampsia. Shoulder dystocia that cannot be resolved can also result in fetal death.

3. **Polyhydramnios** is not an uncommon finding in pregnancies complicated by diabetes. It may be secondary to osmotic diuresis from fetal hyperglycemia. Careful ultrasonographic examination is required to rule out structural anomalies, such as esophageal atresia, as an etiology, when polyhydramnios is present.

4. **Severe maternal vasculopathy**, especially nephropathy and hypertension, is associated with uteroplacental insufficiency, which can result in IUGR, fetal intolerance of labor, and neonatal complications.

III. MANAGEMENT OF DIABETES DURING PREGNANCY

A. **General principles for type 1 or type 2 diabetes.** Management of type 1 or type 2 diabetes during pregnancy begins before conception. Tight glucose control is paramount during the periconceptional period and throughout pregnancy. Optimal glucose control requires coordinated care between endocrinologists, maternal–fetal medicine specialists, diabetes nurse educators, and nutritionists. Preconception glycemic control has been shown to decrease the risk of congenital anomalies to close to that of the general population. However, <30% of pregnancies are planned. Physicians should discuss pregnancy planning or recommend contraception for all diabetic women of childbearing age until glycemic control is optimized.

B. **General principles for gestational diabetes.** In the United States, most women are screened for GDM between 24 and 28 weeks' gestation by a 50-g, 1-hour glucose challenge. A positive result of a blood glucose ≥140 mg/dL is followed by a diagnostic 100-g, 3-hour oral glucose tolerance test (GTT). A positive test is defined as two or more elevated values on the GTT. There is a current movement to move to a single diagnostic test, consisting of a 75-g, 2-hour GTT, a method that is used uniformly outside of the United States. Uncontrolled pregestational and gestational diabetes can lead to fetal macrosomia and concomitant risk of fetal injury at delivery. GDM shares many features with type 2 diabetes. Women diagnosed with GDM have a 60% lifetime risk of developing overt type 2 diabetes.

1. **Testing (first trimester) for type 1 and type 2 diabetes**
   a. **Measurement of glycosylated hemoglobin** in the first trimester can give a risk assessment for congenital anomalies by reflecting ambient glucose concentrations during the period of organogenesis.
   b. **Accurate dating of the pregnancy** is obtained by ultrasonography.
   c. **Ophthalmologic examination** is mandatory because retinopathy may progress because of the rapid normalization of glucose concentration in the first trimester. Women with retinopathy need periodic examinations throughout pregnancy, and they are candidates for laser photocoagulation as indicated.

d. Renal function is assessed by either a spot protein/creatinine ratio or spot urine microalbumin, followed by a 24-hour urine collection for protein excretion and creatinine clearance if abnormal. Serum creatinine should also be assessed in patients with long-standing pregestational diabetes. Because the incidence of preeclampsia is significantly elevated in women with diabetes, identification of baseline proteinuria can impact the diagnosis of preeclampsia later in pregnancy.

e. Thyroid function should be evaluated.

f. Nuchal translucency and serum screening for aneuploidy. Although diabetes in and of itself is not a risk factor for aneuploidy, this is part of routine pregnancy care. Nuchal translucency assessment is particularly important because an abnormal measurement is also associated with structural abnormalities, the risk of which is increased in this group of patients.

2. **Testing (second trimester) for type 1 and type 2 diabetes**
   a. Maternal serum screening for neural tube defects is performed between 15 and 19 weeks' gestation. Women with diabetes have a 10-fold increased risk of neural tube defects compared to the general population.
   b. All patients undergo a thorough **ultrasonographic survey**, including fetal echocardiography for structural anomalies.
   c. Women older than 35 years of age or with other risk factors for fetal aneuploidy are offered **noninvasive prenatal testing or karyotyping via chorionic villus sampling or amniocentesis**.

3. **Testing (third trimester) for type 1 and type 2 diabetes, GDM**
   a. Ultrasonographic examinations are performed monthly through the third trimester for fetal growth measurement.
   b. Weekly or twice-weekly fetal surveillance using nonstress testing or biophysical profiles are implemented between 28 and 32 weeks' gestation, depending on glycemic control and other complications.

C. **Treatment for all types of glucose intolerance**
   Strict **diabetic control** is achieved with nutritional modification, exercise and medications, with the traditional goals of fasting glucose concentration <95 mg/dL and postprandial values <140 mg/dL for 1 hour and 120 mg/dL for 2 hours. Recent data have suggested that in pregnant women, euglycemia may be even lower, with fasting glucose levels in the 60 mg/dL range and postmeal glucose levels <105 mg/dL. Insulin therapy has the longest record of accomplishment of perinatal safety. It has been demonstrated that human insulin analogs do not cross the placenta. More recently, the oral hypoglycemic agents such as glyburide and metformin have been shown to be as effective as insulin in the management of GDM and may be applied to women with pregestational diabetes.

IV. MANAGEMENT OF LABOR AND DELIVERY FOR WOMEN WITH DIABETES

A. **General principles. The risk of spontaneous preterm labor is not increased in patients with diabetes**, although the risk of iatrogenic preterm delivery is increased for patients with microvascular disease as a result of IUGR, nonreassuring fetal testing, and maternal hypertension. Antenatal corticosteroids for induction of fetal lung maturity (FLM) should be employed for the usual obstetric indications. Corticosteroids can cause temporary hyperglycemia; therefore, patients may need to be managed with continuous intravenous (IV) insulin infusions until the effect of the steroids wear off. **Delivery is planned** for 39 to 40 weeks, unless other pregnancy complications dictate earlier delivery. Elective delivery after 39 weeks does not require FLM testing. Indicated delivery before 39 weeks' gestation should be carried out without FLM testing. **Route of delivery** is determined by ultrasonography-estimated fetal weight, maternal and fetal conditions, and previous obstetric history. The ultrasonography-estimated weight at which an elective cesarean delivery is recommended is a controversial issue, with the American College of Obstetricians and Gynecologists recommending discussion of cesarean delivery at an estimated fetal weight of >4,500 g due to the increased risk of shoulder dystocia.

B. **Treatment. Blood glucose concentration** is tightly controlled during labor and delivery. If an induction of labor is planned, patients are instructed to take one-half of their usual basal insulin on the morning of induction. During spontaneous or induced labor, blood glucose concentration is measured every 1 to 2 hours. Blood glucose concentration higher than 120 to 140 mg/dL is treated with an infusion of IV short-acting insulin. IV insulin is very short acting, allowing for quick response to changes in glucose concentration. Active labor may also be associated with hypoglycemia because the contracting uterus uses circulating metabolic fuels. **Continuous fetal monitoring** is mandatory during labor. Cesarean delivery is performed for obstetric indications. The risk of cesarean section for obstetric complications is approximately 50%. Patients with **advanced microvascular disease** are at increased risk for cesarean delivery because of the increased incidence of IUGR, preeclampsia, and nonreassuring fetal status. A history of retinopathy that has been treated in the past is not necessarily an indication for cesarean delivery. Patients with active proliferative retinopathy that is unstable or active hemorrhage may benefit from elective cesarean delivery. **Postpartum**, patients are at increased risk for hypoglycemia, especially in the postoperative setting with minimal oral intake. Patients with pregestational diabetes may also experience a "honeymoon" period immediately after delivery, with greatly reduced insulin requirements that can last up to several days. Lactation is also associated with significant glucose utilization and potential hypoglycemia especially in the immediate postpartum period. For women with type 2 diabetes, the use of metformin and glyburide are compatible with breastfeeding.

Suggested Readings

American College of Obstetricians and Gynecologists. ACOG Practice Bulletin. Clinical management guidelines for obstetricians–gynecologists. Number 60, March 2005. Pregestational diabetes mellitus. *Obstet Gynecol* 2005;105(3):675–685.

American College of Obstetricians and Gynecologists. Practice Bulletin No. 137: gestational diabetes mellitus. *Ostet Gynecol* 2013;122(2, Pt 1):406–416.

Crowther CA, Hiller JE, Moss JR, et al. Effect of treatment of gestational diabetes mellitus on pregnancy outcomes. *N Engl J Med* 2005;352(24):2477–2486.

de Veciana M, Major CA, Morgan MA, et al. Postprandial versus preprandial blood glucose monitoring in women with gestational diabetes mellitus requiring insulin therapy. *N Engl J Med* 1995;333(19):1237–1241.

Kitzmiller JL, Gavin LA, Gin GD, et al. Preconception care of diabetes. Glycemic control prevents congenital anomalies. *JAMA* 1991;265:731–736.

Landon MB, Langer O, Gabbe SG, et al. Fetal surveillance in pregnancies complicated by insulin-dependent diabetes mellitus. *Am J Obstet Gynecol* 1992;167:617–621.

Landon MB, Spong CY, Thom E, et al. A multicenter, randomized trial of treatment for mild gestational diabetes. *N Engl J Med* 2009;361(14):1339–1348.

Langer O, Conway DL, Berkus MD, et al. A comparison of glyburide and insulin in women with gestational diabetes mellitus. *N Engl J Med* 2000;343(16):1134–1138.

Metzger BE, Lowe LP, Dyer AR, et al. Hyperglycemia and adverse pregnancy outcomes. *N Engl J Med* 2008;358(19):1991–2002.

Miller EM, Hare JW, Cloherty JP, et al. Elevated maternal hemoglobin A1c in early pregnancy and major anomalies in infants of diabetic mothers. *N Engl J Med* 1981;304:1331–1334.

Moore LE, Clokey D, Rappaport VJ, et al. Metformin compared with glyburide in gestational diabetes: a randomized controlled trial. *Obstet Gynecol* 2010;115(1):55–59.

Naylor CD, Sermer M, Chen E, et al. Cesarean delivery in relation to birth weight and gestational glucose tolerance: pathophysiology or practice style? Toronto Trihospital Gestational Diabetes Investigators. *JAMA* 1996;275(15):1165–1170.

Parretti E, Mecacci F, Papini M, et al. Third-trimester maternal glucose levels from diurnal profiles in nondiabetic pregnancies: correlation with sonographic parameters of fetal growth. *Diabetes Care* 2001;24(8):1319–1323.

Philipps AF, Porte PJ, Stabinsky S, et al. Effects of chronic fetal hyperglycemia upon oxygen consumption in the ovine uterus and conceptus. *J Clin Invest* 1984;74(1):279–286.

Starikov R, Bohrer J, Goh W, et al. Hemoglobin A1c in pregestational diabetic gravidas and the risk of congenital heart disease in the fetus. *Pediatr Cardiol* 2013;34(7):1716–1722.

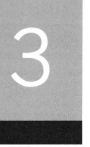

3

Preeclampsia and Related Conditions

Bahaeddine Sibai and Cristina Wallace

KEY POINTS

- Hypertensive disorders in pregnancy are a major cause of maternal morbidity and mortality, accounting for 15% to 20% of maternal deaths worldwide.
- The definitive treatment for preeclampsia is delivery. However, the severity of disease, dilatation/effacement of the maternal cervix, gestational age at diagnosis, and pulmonary maturity of the fetus all influence obstetric management.
- Because of the risks of rapid deterioration, patients with preeclampsia with severe features should be hospitalized after diagnosis at a center with adequate maternal and neonatal resources as well as readily available staff to provide close monitoring and care.
- Elevated blood pressure during pregnancy is associated with an increased risk of developing cardiovascular disease, chronic kidney disease, and diabetes mellitus later in life.

I. CATEGORIES OF PREGNANCY-ASSOCIATED HYPERTENSIVE DISORDERS

A. **Chronic hypertension.** Hypertension preceding pregnancy or first diagnosed before 20 weeks' gestation

B. **Chronic hypertension with superimposed preeclampsia.** Worsening hypertension and new-onset proteinuria, in addition to possible concurrent thrombocytopenia, or transaminase derangements after the 20th week of pregnancy in a woman with known chronic hypertension. It can be further subdivided into with or without severe features.

C. **Gestational hypertension.** Hypertension without proteinuria and without symptoms or abnormal laboratory tests after 20 weeks' gestation (Table 3.1)

D. **Preeclampsia.** Blood pressures >140 mm Hg systolic or 90 mm Hg diastolic with proteinuria after 20 weeks' gestation. It can be further subdivided into with or without severe features.

E. **Eclampsia.** Generalized tonic–clonic seizure activity in a pregnant woman with no prior history of a seizure disorder

F. **Hemolysis, elevated liver enzymes, and low platelets syndrome.** Clinical findings consistent with hemolysis, elevated liver function tests, and thrombocytopenia

Table 3.1. Diagnosis of Preeclampsia versus Gestational Hypertension

Recommendation	Gestational Hypertension	Preeclampsia
HTN >20 weeks	Yes	Yes
Previously normotensive	Yes	Yes
SBP: 140–159 mm Hg	Yes	Yes
DBP: 90–109 mm Hg	Yes	Yes
Persistent for 4 hours	Yes	Yes
Presence of symptoms	No	No
Normal blood tests	Yes	Yes
Proteinuria: ≥300 mg/24 hours Protein/creatinine ratio ≥0.3 Urine dip stick ≥1+	No	Yes

HTN, hypertension; SBP, systolic blood pressure; DBP, diastolic blood pressure.

II. **INCIDENCE AND EPIDEMIOLOGY.** Hypertensive disorders in pregnancy are a major cause of maternal morbidity and mortality, accounting for 15% to 20% of maternal deaths worldwide. In the United States, hypertensive disorders are the second leading cause of maternal mortality after thrombotic/hemorrhagic complications. Beyond 20 weeks' gestation, preeclampsia complicates 5% to 8% of pregnancies, and preeclampsia with severe features complicates <1% of pregnancies. Eclampsia itself is much less frequent, occurring in 0.1% of pregnancies. Several risk factors have been identified, as outlined in Table 3.2.

Preeclampsia has been called the "disease of theories," and many **etiologies** have been proposed. What is clear, however, is that it is a condition of dysfunction within the maternal endothelium. Increased levels of the soluble receptors *sFLT1* and *endoglin* within the maternal circulation for vascular endothelial growth factor (VEGF) and transforming growth factor-β (TGF-β), respectively, may be associated with preeclamptic pathology. Higher circulating levels of these soluble receptors reduce the bioavailable levels of VEGF, placental growth factor (PlGF), and TGF-β, resulting in endothelial dysfunction within the maternal circulatory system. This dysfunction can manifest as both increased arterial tone (hypertension) and increased capillary leak (edema/proteinuria/pulmonary congestion). It is unclear what insult prompts the initial increase in sFLT1 and endoglin in some women versus others. One suggestion has been that abnormal trophoblastic invasion of both the maternal decidual arteries with an accompanying abnormal maternal immune response is at the root of this condition. This abnormal placentation is believed to lead to a reduction in placental perfusion and relative placental ischemia. Both sFLT1 and endoglin are proangiogenic proteins and may represent a placental

Table 3.2. Risk Factors for Hypertensive Disorders
Risk Factors
Nulliparity
Age >40 years
Obesity
Preeclampsia in previous pregnancy
Family history of preeclampsia
Preexisting chronic hypertension
Chronic renal disease
History of thrombophilia
Diabetes (type 1 or type 2)
Multifetal pregnancy
Systemic lupus erythematosus
In vitro fertilization
Molar pregnancy
Fetal hydrops
Source: From the American College of Obstetricians and Gynecologists. Hypertension in pregnancy. http://www.acog.org/Resources-And-Publications/Task-Force-and-Work-Group-Reports/Hypertension-in-Pregnancy. Accessed May 28, 2016; and Moussa H, Arian S, Sibai B. Management of hypertensive disorders in pregnancy. *Womens Health (Lond Engl)* 2014;10(4):385–404.

compensatory response. Recent work has, however, called the implied causality of this hypothesis into question; in early pregnancy, when placental formation is most active, sFLT1 and P1GF levels have failed to reliably predict the occurrence of preeclampsia.

III. DIAGNOSIS. The classic presentation which defines preeclampsia is hypertension and proteinuria after 20 weeks' gestation. Some patients will also have nondependent edema, but this is no longer a part of the diagnostic criteria for preeclampsia. The clinical spectrum of preeclampsia ranges from mild to severe. Most patients have a nonsevere form of the disease that develops late in the third trimester (Fig. 3.1).

A. Criteria for the diagnosis of preeclampsia without severe features

1. **Hypertension** defined as a blood pressure elevation to 140 mm Hg systolic or 90 mm Hg diastolic over two measurements at least 4 hours apart.

Preeclampsia with Severe Features

GHTN-preeclampsia and any one of the following:

➢ SBP ≥160 mm Hg or DBP ≥110 mm Hg
  • *Two BP values 4 hours apart on bed rest*
  • *Once if antihypertensives are used*
➢ Persistent cerebral/visual disturbances
➢ Pulmonary edema
➢ Severe persistent RUQ/epigastric pain unresponsive to Rx
➢ Low platelets <100,000
➢ Elevated liver enzymes (>2 times upper normal)
➢ Serum creatinine >1.1 mg/dL

Figure 3.1. Diagnosis of preeclampsia with severe features. GHTN, gestational hypertension; SBP, systolic blood pressure; DBP, diastolic blood pressure; BP, blood pressure; RUQ, right upper quadrant; Rx, reaction.

Measurements should be taken in the sitting position at the level of the heart, and the proper cuff size needs to be ensured.

2. **Proteinuria** defined as at least 300 mg of protein in a 24-hour period or protein to creatinine ratio ≥0.3 mg/mg.

B. **Criteria for the diagnosis of preeclampsia with severe features**
Of note, you do not need every criteria listed here to make a diagnosis.

1. **Blood pressure** >160 mm Hg systolic or 110 mm Hg diastolic with the diagnostic readings taken twice at least 4 hours apart or severe hypertension can be verified within minutes to aid in administering antihypertensive therapy.

2. **Symptoms suggestive of end-organ dysfunction.** New visual disturbances such as scotomata, diplopia, blindness, or persistent severe headache. Other symptoms such as severe persistent right upper quadrant pain or severe epigastric pain not responsive to medications and not attributed to another medical cause are suggestive of preeclampsia with severe features.

3. **Pulmonary edema**

4. **Renal insufficiency** is defined as serum creatinine >1.1 mg/dL.

5. **Thrombocytopenia** is defined as a platelet count of <100,000.

6. **Hepatocellular dysfunction.** Elevated transaminases (to twice upper limit of normal concentration)

C. **HELLP syndrome** stands for hemolysis, elevated liver enzymes, and low platelets. It represents an alternative presentation of preeclampsia and reflects systemic end-organ damage. HELLP syndrome may appear without either hypertension or proteinuria.

IV. **COMPLICATIONS.** Complications of preeclampsia result in a maternal mortality rate of 3 per 100,000 live births in the United States. Maternal morbidity may include central nervous system complications (e.g., seizures, intracerebral hemorrhage, and blindness), disseminated intravascular coagulation (DIC), hepatic failure or rupture, pulmonary edema, and *abruptio placentae* leading to maternal hemorrhage and/or acute renal failure. Fetal mortality markedly increases severity of disease process. Fetal morbidity may include intrauterine fetal growth restriction, fetal acidemia, and complications from prematurity.

V. CONSIDERATIONS IN MANAGEMENT

A. **The definitive treatment for preeclampsia is delivery.** However, the severity of disease, dilatation/effacement of the maternal cervix, gestational age at diagnosis, and pulmonary maturity of the fetus all influence obstetric management. Delivery is usually indicated if there is nonreassuring fetal testing in a viable fetus or if the maternal status becomes unstable regardless of either gestational age or fetal maturity.

B. **Delivery should be considered** for all patients at ≥37 weeks with any degree of gestational hypertension or preeclampsia.

C. Pregnancies may continue for patients with **preterm gestation and preeclampsia without severe features/gestational hypertension**, with close observation as outlined in section VI until 37 weeks' gestation or some other ominous development such as the progression to preeclampsia with severe features, nonreassuring fetal testing, or maternal instability.

D. **If the patient has preeclampsia with severe features, treatment varies based on the severity of the patient's disease and the gestational age.** If the patient is >34 weeks, the recommendation by the American College of Obstetricians and Gynecologists (ACOG) is delivery. Prior to 34 weeks, three management options include delivery immediately, betamethasone then delivery, and expectant management. The timing of delivery is discussed in further detail in section VII.

E. **Expectant management entails hospitalization and frequent maternal and fetal surveillance.** This should only be undertaken in carefully selected patients after an initial period of observation to ensure stability of the pregnant woman. Monitoring of these patients includes daily maternal–fetal testing, routine vital signs, and monitoring for symptoms of preeclampsia. Patients may even be given oral antihypertensive drugs to bring their blood pressure down. Women with uncontrolled hypertension despite maximum doses of antihypertensive medications, thrombocytopenia, hepatocellular dysfunction, pulmonary edema, compromised renal function, or persistent headache or visual changes are not candidates for expectant management.

F. **The mode of delivery does not need to be a cesarean section.** A number of factors have to be assessed including the fetal position, maternal status, gestational age, cervical status, and fetal condition. At earlier gestational ages, a trial of labor induction is not contraindicated in patients with preeclampsia with severe features; however, the success rate is low. The managing team must balance the risks of progression of the disease against the time required to induce labor.

VI. CLINICAL MANAGEMENT OF PREECLAMPSIA WITHOUT SEVERE FEATURES

A. **Antepartum management.** Conservative management of preeclampsia without severe features generally consists of daily assessment by the maternal symptoms and fetal movement by the women, biweekly blood pressure checks, and weekly assessment of platelet counts and liver enzymes. It is recommended that strict bed rest and salt restriction not be prescribed in these women.

1. **Fetal evaluation**

   a. An initial ultrasound should be performed at the time of diagnosis to rule out intrauterine fetal growth restriction and/or oligohydramnios. A nonstress test (NST) or biophysical profile may also be performed as indicated.

   b. Ultrasonography every 3 weeks for growth is recommended. Twice-weekly NSTs with amniotic fluid index measurements are recommended. The frequency of these tests can be changed based on the findings noted during the evaluations.

   c. Any **change in maternal status** should prompt evaluation of fetal status.

   d. Fetal indications for delivery include nonreassuring fetal testing. If severe growth restriction and/or oligohydramnios is noted, then further assessment of the fetus is recommended with umbilical artery Doppler studies.

2. **Maternal evaluation**

   a. Women should be **evaluated for signs and symptoms** of preeclampsia with severe features.

   b. Initial laboratory evaluation includes platelet count, transaminases, hemoglobin/hematocrit, creatinine, and urine protein-to-creatinine ratio.

   c. If criteria for preeclampsia with severe features are not met, laboratory studies should be performed at weekly intervals to assess for worsening disease.

   d. Maternal indications for delivery include a gestational age $\geq$37 weeks; thrombocytopenia ($<$100,000); progressive deterioration in hepatic or renal function; placental abruption; and persistent severe headaches, visual changes, or epigastric pain.

   e. Antihypertensive agents are not routinely given because they have not been shown to improve the outcome in cases of preeclampsia without severe features.

   f. When early delivery is indicated, it is our practice that vaginal delivery is preferred. Cesarean delivery should be reserved for cases with nonreassuring fetal testing, when further fetal evaluation is not possible, or when a rapidly deteriorating maternal condition mandates expeditious delivery (e.g., HELLP syndrome with decreasing platelet counts, abruption).

B. **Intrapartum management of preeclampsia**

1. **Magnesium sulfate** is not routinely recommended for women with preeclampsia without severe features or gestational hypertension unless

symptoms of worsening disease are noted such as systolic blood pressure >160 mm Hg, diastolic blood pressure >110 mm Hg, or maternal symptoms noted.

2. **Antihypertensive therapy** is not recommended unless the systolic blood pressure is >160 mm Hg or the diastolic blood pressure is >110 mm Hg.

3. **Continuous electronic fetal monitoring** is recommended given the potential for placental dysfunction in the preeclamptic setting. Monitoring should be established during the initial evaluation, induction of labor, and labor itself. Continuous monitoring is not recommended during intervals of prolonged expectant management. Patterns that suggest fetal compromise include persistent tachycardia, minimal or absent fetal heart rate variability, and recurrent variable or late decelerations not responsive to standard resuscitative measures.

4. Patients may be safely administered **epidural anesthesia** if the platelet count is >70,000 and there is no evidence of DIC. Consideration should be given for early epidural catheter placement when the platelet count is reasonable and there is concern that it is decreasing. Any anesthesia should be administered by properly trained personnel experienced in the care of women with preeclampsia given the hemodynamic changes associated with the condition. Adequate preload should be ensured to minimize the risk of hypotension.

5. **Invasive central monitoring** of the mother is rarely indicated, even in the setting of preeclampsia with severe features.

C. **Postpartum management.** The mother's condition may worsen immediately after delivery. However, signs and symptoms usually begin to resolve within 24 to 48 hours postpartum, and in most women, it usually resolves within 1 or 2 weeks.

VII. MANAGEMENT OF PREECLAMPSIA WITH SEVERE FEATURES (Fig. 3.2)

A. **Timing of delivery**

1. If <23 weeks' or >**34 weeks' gestation**, delivery is indicated.

2. Prior to 34 weeks, **expectant management** can be attempted unless there is evidence of eclampsia, pulmonary edema, DIC, uncontrollable severe hypertension, nonviable fetus, abnormal fetal test results, placental abruption, or intrapartum fetal demise. In those situations, the goal is to stabilize the mother and then deliver. If the patient has evidence of persistent symptoms, HELLP, partial HELLP, fetal growth restriction with severe oligohydramnios (largest vertical pocket <2 cm) or reversed end-diastolic flow on umbilical artery Doppler studies, labor, or significant renal dysfunction, the goal is to administer betamethasone for fetal lung maturity and plan on delivery after 48 hours. If the patient does not meet any of the criteria for delivery, expectant management is recommended until 34 weeks or delivery can be performed sooner if the patient develops evidence of worsening disease. Two randomized trials performed in the United States compared immediate delivery

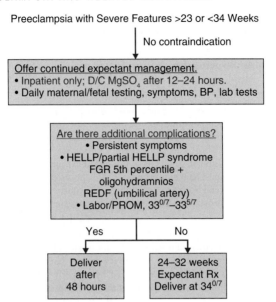

Figure 3.2. Management of preterm preeclampsia with severe features. D/C, discontinue; MgSO$_4$, magnesium sulfate; BP, blood pressure; HELLP, hemolysis, elevated liver enzymes, and low platelets; FGR, fetal growth restriction; REDF, reversed end diastolic flow; PROM, premature rupture of membrane; Rx, reaction.

versus expectant management in mothers with preeclampsia with severe features. These trials showed that expectant management led to prolongation of pregnancy by about 7 days with a significant reduction in total neonatal complications from 75% to 33%. The disadvantage of expectant management is that preeclampsia with severe features can lead to acute and long-term complications for the patient including the progressive deterioration of the maternal and fetal condition.

3. Because of the risks of rapid deterioration, patients with preeclampsia with severe features should be hospitalized after diagnosis at a center with adequate maternal and neonatal resources as well as readily available staff to provide close monitoring and care.

B. **Intrapartum management**

1. Magnesium sulfate (6 g intravenous [IV] load followed by 2 g/hour infusion) is used as seizure prophylaxis. It is started when the decision to proceed with delivery is made and is continued for at least 24 hours postpartum. Magnesium sulfate has been shown to be the agent of choice for seizure prophylaxis in randomized double-blind comparisons against both placebo and conventional antiepileptics. In patients with myasthenia gravis or hypocalcemia, magnesium sulfate

is contraindicated and should not be given. Because magnesium sulfate is excreted from the kidneys, urine output should be carefully monitored. Signs and symptoms of maternal toxicity include loss of deep tendon reflexes, somnolence, respiratory depression, cardiac arrhythmia, and in extreme cases, cardiovascular collapse.

2. Careful monitoring of fluid balance is critical because preeclampsia is associated with endothelial dysfunction leading to decreased intravascular volume, pulmonary edema, and oliguria. A serum magnesium level should be considered if reduced renal function is suspected while magnesium sulfate is being administered. In addition, if the patient has evidence of reduced kidney function, that is, serum creatinine >1.1 mg/dL, magnesium sulfate maintenance dose can be started at 1 g/hour after the initial bolus. If the patient's creatinine is >2.5 mg/dL, a maintenance dose may not be necessary.

3. Continuous fetal heart rate monitoring is recommended. Reduced fetal heart rate variability may also result from maternal administration of magnesium sulfate.

4. Severe hypertension may be controlled with agents including IV hydralazine, IV labetalol, or oral nifedipine. Sodium nitroprusside should be avoided before delivery because of potential fetal cyanide toxicity. It is important to avoid large or abrupt reductions in blood pressure because decreased intravascular volume and poor uteroplacental perfusion can lead to acute placental insufficiency and a resulting loss of reassurance regarding fetal well-being.

C. **Postpartum management**

1. Because postpartum eclamptic seizures generally occur within the first 48 hours and usually within the first 24 hours after delivery, magnesium sulfate prophylaxis is continued for at least 24 hours. Close monitoring of fluid balance is continued. While on magnesium sulfate, the patient's blood pressure is monitored closely, urine output, lung evaluation, and deep tendon reflexes for evidence of magnesium sulfate toxicity.

2. Hypertension >150 mm Hg systolic or 100 mg Hg diastolic on at least two occasions 4 to 6 hours apart needs to be treated in the postpartum period with antihypertensive therapy. Some patients, although sufficiently stable for discharge, may require antihypertensive medications for up to 8 weeks after delivery.

3. Typically, blood pressures tend to decrease within the first 48 hours after delivery and increase 3 to 6 days later. It is recommended to monitor patients' blood pressures closely for 72 hours after delivery, preferably in the hospital, and then to have the patient return to clinic 7 to 10 days after delivery again to reassess blood pressure. If the patient develops symptoms of preeclampsia in the interim, he or she should be assessed again sooner.

4. Nonsteroidal anti-inflammatory agents generally should be avoided in the postpartum period in patients with severe hypertension and in those with superimposed preeclampsia. These medications can increase blood pressure and increase sodium retention.

VIII. MANAGEMENT OF ECLAMPSIA

A. Approximately half of **eclamptic seizures** occur before delivery, 20% occur during delivery, and another 30% occur in the postpartum period. Although there is no clear constellation of symptoms that will accurately predict which patients will have an eclamptic seizure, headache is a frequently reported heralding symptom, but most preeclamptic women with headaches do not develop seizures.

B. **Basic principles of maternal resuscitation** should be followed in the initial management of an eclamptic seizure: airway protection, oxygen supplementation, left lateral displacement to prevent uterine compression of vena cava, intravenous access, and blood pressure control.

C. Magnesium sulfate should be initiated for **prevention of recurrent seizures**. Ten percent of women with eclamptic seizures will have a recurrent seizure after initiation of magnesium sulfate.

D. A **transient fetal bradycardia** is usually seen during the seizure followed by a **transient fetal tachycardia** with loss of variability. Ideally, the fetus should be resuscitated *in utero*.

E. **Eclampsia is an indication for delivery but not necessarily an indication for cesarean delivery.** No intervention should be initiated until maternal stability is ensured and the seizure is over. Because of the risk of DIC, coagulation parameters should be assessed and appropriate blood products should be available if necessary.

F. A **neurologic exam** should be performed once the patient recovers from the seizure. If the seizure is atypical or any neurologic deficit persists, **brain imaging** is indicated.

G. If a patient has recurrent seizures while on magnesium sulfate, a reloading dose of 2 g of magnesium sulfate can be given one or two times. If seizures persist after two additional boluses of magnesium sulfate, consideration should be given to adding IV lorazepam.

IX. RECURRENCE RISK.
Patients who have a history of preeclampsia are at increased risk for hypertensive disease in a subsequent pregnancy. Recurrence risk is as high as 40% in women with preeclampsia before 32 weeks of gestation, as opposed to 10% or less in women with preeclampsia near term. Severe disease and eclampsia are also associated with recurrence. Racial differences exist, with African American women having higher recurrence rates. The recurrence rate for HELLP syndrome is approximately 5%.

X. RISK OF CHRONIC HYPERTENSION.
Elevated blood pressure during pregnancy, regardless of type and even without known risk factors, can be indicative of a high risk of cardiovascular disease, chronic kidney disease, and diabetes mellitus later in life. In addition, women with recurrent preeclampsia, women with early-onset preeclampsia, and multiparas with a diagnosis of preeclampsia (even if not recurrent) may be at an even higher risk than those with just gestational hypertension. Given this high risk of future morbidity, the ACOG Task Force on Hypertension in Pregnancy recommends that women with a

history of preeclampsia delivered prior to 37 weeks or who have had recurrent preeclampsia be screened annually for blood pressure, lipids, fasting blood glucose, and body mass index.

XI. INNOVATIONS AND PROPOSED TREATMENTS

A. Several analytic assays based on sFLT1 and PIGF protein levels and soluble endoglin early in the second trimester are currently under evaluation. The ultimate clinical utility of these analytes has yet to be determined. Some newer studies show that these biomarkers in combination with uterine artery Dopplers may be predictive of early-onset preeclampsia. In addition, randomized trials are ongoing to evaluate several modalities to prolong gestation during expectant management of early onset preeclampsia.

B. **Low-dose aspirin** is recommended for women with a medical history of preeclampsia <34 weeks or preeclampsia in more than one previous pregnancy. The recommended dose is between 60 and 80 mg, and it should be started late in the first trimester.

C. Although earlier studies suggested that **antenatal calcium supplementation** may reduce the incidence of hypertensive disorders of pregnancy, a large National Institutes of Health–sponsored placebo-controlled trial did not show any benefit when given to healthy nulliparous women. This is especially true in populations like the United States where calcium intake is adequate.

D. Recent enthusiasm for antioxidant therapy has also been dulled after a well-executed trial found vitamin E supplementation during pregnancy to be associated with an increased risk of adverse outcome compared with placebo.

XII. IMPLICATIONS FOR THE NEWBORN

A. Infants born to mothers with preeclampsia with severe features or superimposed preeclampsia may show evidence of **IUGR** and are frequently delivered prematurely. They may tolerate labor poorly and therefore require resuscitation.

B. **Medications used ante- or intrapartum** may affect the fetus.

   1. **Short-term sequelae of hypermagnesemia**, such as hypotonia and respiratory depression, are sometimes seen. Long-term maternal administration of magnesium sulfate has rarely been associated with neonatal parathyroid abnormalities or other abnormalities of calcium homeostasis

   2. **Antihypertensive medications**, including calcium channel blockers, may have fetal effects, including hypotension in the infant. Antihypertensive medications and magnesium sulfate generally are not contraindications to breastfeeding.

   3. **Low-dose aspirin therapy** does not appear to increase the incidence of intracranial hemorrhage, asymptomatic bruising, bleeding from circumcision sites, or persistent pulmonary hypertension.

4. Approximately one-third of infants born to mothers with early-onset preeclampsia with severe features have **decreased platelet counts at birth**, but the counts generally increase rapidly to normal levels. Approximately 40% to 50% of newborns have neutropenia that generally resolves before 3 days of age. These infants may be at increased risk for neonatal infection.

Suggested Readings

Altman D, Carroli G, Duley L, et al. Do women with pre-eclampsia, and their babies, benefit from magnesium sulphate? The Magpie Trial: a randomized placebo controlled trial. *Lancet* 2002:359:1877–1890.

American College of Obstetricians and Gynecologists. Hypertension in pregnancy. http://www.acog.org/Resources-And-Publications/Task-Force-and-Work-Group-Reports/Hypertension-in-Pregnancy. Accessed May 28, 2016.

Levine RJ, Maynard SE, Qian C, et al. Circulating angiogenic factors and the risk of preeclampsia. *N Engl J Med* 2004;350:672–683.

Männistö T, Mendola P, Vääräsmäki M, et al. Elevated blood pressure in pregnancy and subsequent chronic disease risk. *Circulation* 2013;127(6):681–690.

Markham KB, Funai EF. Pregnancy-related hypertension. In: Creasy RK, Resnik R, Iams JD, et al., eds. *Creasy & Resnik's Maternal-Fetal Medicine: Principles and Practice.* 7th ed, Philadelphia, PA: WB Saunders; 2014:756–784.

Moussa H, Arian S, Sibai B. Management of hypertensive disorders in pregnancy. *Womens Health (Lond Engl)* 2014;10(4):385–404.

Sibai BM, Barton JR. Expectant management of severe preeclampsia remote from term: patient selection, treatment, and delivery indication. *Am J Obstet Gynecol* 2007;196(6):514.e1–514.e9.

4

Resuscitation in the Delivery Room

Steven A. Ringer

KEY POINTS

- Anticipation is key to ensuring that adequate preparations have been made for a neonate likely to require resuscitation at birth.
- The primary goal in neonatal resuscitation must be to ensure an adequate airway and respiration
- Thermal control should be of paramount concern and additional steps taken to ensure that the infant temperature remains normal during transition.

I. **GENERAL PRINCIPLES.** A person skilled in basic neonatal resuscitation, whose primary responsibility is the newly born baby, should be present at every birth. Delivery of all high-risk infants should be ideally attended by personnel who possess the skills required to perform a complete resuscitation.

The highest standard of care requires the following: (i) knowledge of perinatal physiology and principles of resuscitation, (ii) mastery of the technical skills required, and (iii) a clear understanding of the roles of other team members and coordination among team members. This allows anticipation of each person's reactions in a specific instance and helps ensure that care is timely and comprehensive. Completion of the Newborn Resuscitation Program (NRP) of the American Academy of Pediatrics/American Heart Association by every caregiver helps ensure a consistent approach to resuscitations and team-based training. NRP provides an approach to resuscitation that is successful in a very high percentage of cases and aids clinicians in more rapidly identifying those unusual cases in which specialized interventions may be required.

A. **Perinatal physiology.** Resuscitation efforts at delivery are designed to help the newborn make the respiratory and circulatory transitions that must be accomplished immediately after birth: The lungs expand, fetal lung fluid is cleared, effective air exchange is established, and the right-to-left circulatory shunts terminate. The critical period for these physiologic changes is during the first several breaths, which result in lung expansion and elevation of the partial pressure of oxygen (PO_2) in both the alveoli and the arterial circulation. Elevation of the PO_2 from the fetal level of approximately 25 mm Hg to values of 50 to 70 mm Hg is associated with (i) decrease in pulmonary vascular resistance, (ii) decrease in right-to-left shunting through the ductus arteriosus, (iii) increase in venous return to the left atrium, (iv) rise in left atrial pressure, and (v) cessation of right-to-left shunt through the foramen ovale. The end result is conversion from fetal to transitional to neonatal circulatory pattern. Adequate systemic arterial oxygenation results from perfusion of well-expanded, well-ventilated lungs and adequate circulation.

Conditions at delivery may compromise the fetus's ability to make the necessary transitions. Alterations in tissue perfusion and oxygenation ultimately result in depression of cardiac function, but human fetuses initially respond to hypoxia by becoming apneic. Even a relatively brief period of oxygen deprivation may result in this **primary apnea**. Rapid recovery from this state is generally accomplished with appropriate stimulation and oxygen exposure. If the period of hypoxia continues, the fetus will irregularly gasp and lapse into **secondary apnea**. This state may occur remote from birth or in the peripartum period. Infants born during this period require resuscitation with assisted ventilation and oxygen (see section III.B).

B. **Timing of cord clamping.** The following discussion focuses on infants who require some measure of resuscitation after birth. For the majority of infants, no additional steps are needed beyond drying and provision of warmth and initial stimulation. If the infant is breathing spontaneously at birth, the cord should not be clamped and divided until at least 30 to 60 seconds have passed. The infant should be placed on the maternal chest or abdomen, be dried, and kept warm.

For those infants who require resuscitation beyond the initial steps because of inadequate or absent respiratory effort, the cord should be clamped and divided shortly after birth. Ongoing studies continue to evaluate the feasibility and effectiveness of providing resuscitation with the umbilical circulation still intact.

C. **Goals of resuscitation** are the following:

1. **Minimizing immediate heat loss** by drying and providing warmth, thereby decreasing oxygen consumption by the neonate

2. **Establishing normal respiration and lung expansion** by clearing the upper airway and using positive-pressure ventilation if necessary

3. **Increasing arterial PO$_2$** by providing adequate alveolar ventilation. The **routine** use of added oxygen is not warranted, but this therapy may be necessary in some situations.

4. **Supporting adequate cardiac output**

II. **PREPARATION.** Anticipation is key to ensuring that adequate preparations have been made for a neonate likely to require resuscitation at birth. It is estimated that as many as 10% of neonates require some assistance at birth for normal transition, whereas <1% require extensive resuscitative measures.

A. **Perinatal conditions associated with high-risk deliveries.** Ideally, the obstetrician should notify the pediatrician well in advance of the actual birth. The pediatrician may then review the obstetric history and events leading to the high-risk delivery and prepare for the specific problems that may be anticipated. If time permits, the problems should be discussed with the parent(s). The following antepartum and intrapartum events warrant the presence of a resuscitation team at delivery.

1. **Evidence of nonreassuring fetal status**

   a. Category III fetal tracing including either sinusoidal pattern or absent fetal heart rate (FHR) variability and any of the following: late decelerations, recurrent variable decelerations, or bradycardia

   b. History of an acute perinatal event (e.g., placental abruption, cord prolapse or abnormal fetal testing, or a scalp pH of 7.20 or less)

   c. History of decreased fetal movement, diminution in growth, or abnormalities of umbilical vessel Doppler flow studies

2. **Evidence of fetal disease or potentially serious conditions** (see Chapter 1)

   a. Meconium staining of the amniotic fluid and/or other evidence of possible fetal compromise (see Chapter 35)

   b. Prematurity ($<$37 weeks), postmaturity ($>$42 weeks), anticipated low birth weight ($<$2.0 kg), or high birth weight ($>$4.5 kg)

   c. Major congenital anomalies diagnosed prenatally

   d. Hydrops fetalis

   e. Multiple gestation (see Chapter 11)

3. **Labor and delivery conditions**

   a. Significant vaginal bleeding

   b. Abnormal fetal presentation

   c. Prolonged or unusual labor

   d. Concern about a possible shoulder dystocia

B. The following conditions do not require a pediatric team to be present, but personnel should be available for assessment and triage.

1. **Neonatal conditions**

   a. Unexpected congenital anomalies

   b. Respiratory distress

   c. Unanticipated neonatal depression, for example, Apgar score of $<$6 at 5 minutes

2. **Maternal conditions**

   a. Signs of maternal infection

      i. Maternal fever

      ii. Membranes ruptured for $>$24 hours

      iii. Foul-smelling amniotic fluid

      iv. History of sexually transmitted disease

   b. Maternal illness or other conditions

      i. Diabetes mellitus

      ii. Rh or other isoimmunization without evidence of hydrops fetalis

      iii. Chronic hypertension or pregnancy-induced hypertension

      iv. Renal, endocrine, pulmonary, or cardiac disease

      v. Alcohol or other substance abuse

   c. Mode of delivery

   In the absence of other antenatal risk factors, delivery via cesarean section done using regional anesthesia at $>$37 to 39 weeks' gestation does not increase the likelihood of a baby requiring endotracheal (ET) intubation, compared to vaginal delivery at term.

C. **Necessary equipment** must be present and operating properly. Each delivery room should be equipped with the following:

1. **Radiant warmer** with procedure table or bed. The warmer should be turned on and checked before delivery. For a very low birth weight (VLBW) infant, additional warming techniques should be available, which might include prewarming the delivery room to 26°C, plastic wrap for covering the baby, or the use of an exothermic mattress. When used in combination, care should be taken to avoid hyperthermia.

2. **A blended oxygen source (adjustable between 21% and 100%)** with adjustable flowmeter and adequate length of tubing. A humidifier and heater may be desirable.

3. **Pulse oximeter** available for use when oxygen therapy is anticipated.

4. Flow-inflating **bag** with adjustable pop-off valve or self-inflating bag with reservoir. The bag must be appropriately sized for neonates (generally about 750 mL) and capable of delivering 100% oxygen.

5. **Face mask(s)** of appropriate size for the anticipated infant

6. **A bulb syringe** for suctioning

7. **Stethoscope** with infant- or premature-sized head

8. **Equipped emergency box or cart**
   a. Laryngoscope with no. 0 and no. 1 blades. For extremely low birth weight infants, a no. 00 blade may be preferred.
   b. Extra batteries
   c. Uniform diameter ET tubes (2.5-, 3.0-, and 3.5-mm internal diameters), two of each
   d. Drugs, including epinephrine (1:10,000), and NaCl 0.9% (normal saline). Sodium bicarbonate (0.50 mEq/mL) and naloxone are rarely useful and are not part of usual resuscitation algorithm.
   e. Umbilical catheterization tray with 3.5 and 5 French catheters
   f. Syringes (1.0, 3.0, 5.0, 10.0, and 20.0 mL), needles (18 to 25G), T-connectors, and stopcocks

9. Transport incubator with battery-operated heat source and portable-blended oxygen supply should be available if delivery room is not close to the nursery.

10. Pulse oximetry is recommended when oxygen is being administered and/or positive-pressure ventilation is used more than for a few breaths. It can be applied immediately after birth and successfully used to provide information on oxygen saturation and heart rate. It may take around 60 to 90 seconds to obtain an accurate reading; pulse oximetry may fail if cardiac output is low.

11. Electrocardiography can be used if there is a question about the heart rate. Leads can be quickly applied and the heart rate determined within about 30 seconds. Caregivers must be aware of the possibility that pulseless electrical activity may occur in the depressed newborn.

12. End-tidal CO_2 monitor/indicator to confirm ET tube position after intubation.

D. Preparation of equipment. Upon arrival in the delivery room, check that the transport incubator is plugged in and warm and has a full oxygen tank. The specialist should introduce himself or herself to the obstetrician and anesthesiologist, the mother (if she is awake), and the father (if he is present). While the history or an update is obtained, the following should be done:

1. Ensure that the radiant warmer is on and that dry, warm blankets are available.

2. Turn on the oxygen source or air–oxygen blend and adjust the flow to 5 to 8 L/min. Adjust the oxygen concentration to the desired initial level.

3. Test the flow-inflating bag (if used) for pop-off control and adequate flow. Be sure the proper-sized mask is present.

4. Make sure the laryngoscope light is bright and has an appropriate blade for the anticipated baby (no. 1 for full-term neonates, no. 0 for premature neonates, no. 00 for extremely low birth weight neonates).

5. Set out an appropriate ET tube for the expected birth weight (3.5 mm for full-term infants, 3.0 mm for premature infants >1,250 g, and 2.5 mm for smaller infants). The NRP recommends a 4.0-mm tube for larger babies, but this is rarely necessary. For all babies, the tube should be 13 cm long. An intubation stylet may be used if the tip is kept at least 0.5 cm from the distal end of the ET tube.

6. If the clinical situation suggests that extensive resuscitation may be needed, the following actions may be required:
   a. Set up an umbilical catheterization tray for venous catheterization.
   b. Draw up 1:10,000 epinephrine and isotonic saline for catheter flush solution and volume replacement.
   c. Check that other potentially necessary drugs are present and ready for administration.

E. Universal precautions. Exposure to blood or other body fluids is inevitable in the delivery room. Universal precautions must be practiced by wearing caps, goggles or glasses, gloves, and impervious gowns until the cord is cut and the newborn is dried and wrapped.

III. DURING DELIVERY. The team should be aware of the type and duration of anesthesia, extent of maternal bleeding, and newly recognized problems such as a nuchal cord or meconium in the amniotic fluid.

A. Immediately following delivery, begin a process of evaluation, decision, and action (resuscitation)

1. Place the newborn on the warming table.

2. Dry the infant completely and discard the wet linens, including those on which the infant is lying. Drying should be thorough but gentle, avoid vigorous rubbing or attempts to clean all blood or vernix from the baby. Ensure that the infant remains warm. Extremely small infants may require extra warming techniques such as wrapping the body and extremities in a plastic wrap or bag or the use of an exothermic mattress.

3. Place the infant with head in midline position, with slight neck extension.

4. Suction the mouth, oropharynx, and nares thoroughly with a suction bulb if there is obvious obstruction or the baby requires positive-pressure ventilation. Deep pharyngeal stimulation with a suction catheter may cause arrhythmias that are probably of vagal origin and should be avoided. If meconium-stained amniotic fluid is present, be vigilant for the increased possibility of upper airway obstruction and have equipment for suctioning available (see section IV.A and Chapter 35).

B. Assessment of the need for supplemental oxygen. In the normal fetal environment, oxygen saturation levels are well below those necessary during extrauterine life. These levels do not completely rise to the normal postnatal range for about 10 minutes after birth, and oxygen saturation levels of 70% to 80% are normal for several minutes. During this time, the baby may appear cyanotic, although clinical assessment of cyanosis has been shown to be an unreliable indicator of actual oxyhemoglobin saturation. However, either insufficient or excessive oxygenation can be harmful to the newborn.

1. Pulse oximetry. Several studies have examined the change in oxygen saturation levels in the minutes following birth and have defined percentile ranges for uncompromised babies born at full term. The best defined data have been obtained using readings made at a "preductal" site (i.e., the right upper extremity) in order to avoid the potentially confounding effect of shunting during the transition to an adult-type circulation. Probes specifically designed for neonates can provide reliable readings within 1 to 2 minutes or less; however, oxygen saturation measurements may be unreliable when cardiac output and skin perfusion are poor. It is recommended that oximetry be available for use in the delivery room so that it will be available when

a. Resuscitation can be anticipated, as noted earlier.

b. Positive-pressure ventilation is used for more than a few breaths.

c. Cyanosis is persistent despite interventions.

d. Supplemental oxygen is administered.

C. The concentration of oxygen used to begin resuscitation remains an area of debate. Several trials have shown that survival is improved when resuscitation is initiated with room air compared with 100% oxygen in full-term infants, although there are no studies evaluating other oxygen concentrations. Studies of preterm infants have shown that the use of air or a minimally increased concentration of a blended air–oxygen mixture as the initial gas resulted in an appropriate rise in oxygen saturation levels after birth. Once assisted ventilation or supplemental oxygen use is begun, the oxygen concentration should be adjusted so that the measured preductal oxygen saturation value lies within a specified minute-specific reference range (Table 4.1) as advocated by the NRP. The best available reference is the interquartile range of saturations measured in healthy term babies following vaginal birth at sea level. Different ranges have not been determined for preterm babies or those born via cesarean or vaginal routes.

Because when using these guidelines, the administered oxygen concentration is guided by the measured oxygen saturation, the choice of initial concentration is discretionary, but a uniform approach makes sense.

Table 4.1. Target Preductal SPO$_2$ during the First 10 Minutes after Birth

1 minute	60%–65%
2 minute	65%–70%
3 minute	70%–75%
4 minute	75%–80%
5 minute	80%–85%
10 minute	85%–95%

We use **room air** as the initial concentration for term babies and **21% to 30% oxygen** for premature babies <32 weeks' gestation.

1. Air should be used if blended oxygen is not available.

2. Oxygen concentration should be increased to 100% if bradycardia (heart rate <60 bpm) does not improve after 90 seconds of resuscitation while employing a lower oxygen concentration.

D. **Sequence of intervention.** Although Apgar scores (Table 4.2) are assigned at 1 and 5 minutes, resuscitative efforts should begin during the initial neonatal stabilization period. The NRP recommends that at the time of birth, the baby should be assessed by posing three basic questions: (i) Is it a term gestation? (ii) Does the baby have good muscle tone? (iii) Is the baby crying or breathing? If the answer to any of these questions is "no," the initial steps of resuscitation should commence. In the newly born infant, essentially all

Table 4.2. Apgar Scoring System

	Score		
Sign	**0**	**1**	**2**
Heart rate	Absent	<100 bpm	>100 bpm
Respiratory effort	Absent	Slow (irregular)	Good crying
Muscle tone	Limp	Some flexion of extremities	Active motion
Reflex irritability	No response	Grimace	Cough or sneeze
Color	Blue, pale	Pink body, blue extremities	All pink

Source: Adapted from Apgar V. A proposal for a new method of evaluation of the newborn infant. *Curr Res Anesth Analg* 1953;32:260–267.

resuscitation problems within the initial postnatal period occur as a result of inadequate respiratory effort or some obstruction to the airway. Therefore, the initial focus must be on ensuring an adequate airway and adequate breathing.

First, assess whether the infant is **breathing spontaneously**. Next, assess whether the **heart rate is >100 bpm**. Finally, evaluate whether the **infant's overall color is pink** (acrocyanosis is normal) or whether the oxygen saturation level is appropriate (see Table 4.1). If any of these three characteristics is abnormal, take immediate steps to correct the deficiency and reevaluate every 15 to 30 seconds until all characteristics are present and stable. In this way, adequate support will be given while overly vigorous interventions are avoided when newborns are making adequate progress on their own. This approach will help avoid complications such as laryngospasm and cardiac arrhythmias from excessive suctioning or pneumothorax from injudicious bagging. Some interventions are required in specific circumstances.

1. **Infant breathes spontaneously, heart rate is >100 bpm, and color is judged to be becoming pink (Apgar score of 8 to 10).** Under these circumstances, there is no need or indication for directly measuring oxygen saturation. This situation is found in >90% of all term newborns, with a median time to first breath of approximately 10 seconds. Following (or during) warming, drying, positioning, and any necessary oropharyngeal suctioning, the infant should be assessed. If respirations, heart rate, and color are normal, this initial assessment can be done while the infant is placed on mother's chest.

   Some newborns do not immediately establish spontaneous respiration but will rapidly respond to tactile stimulation, including vigorous flicking of the soles of the feet or rubbing the back (e.g., cases of **primary apnea**). More vigorous or other techniques of stimulation have no therapeutic value and are potentially harmful. If breathing does not start after **two** attempts at tactile stimulation, the baby should be considered to be in **secondary apnea**, and respiratory support should be initiated. It is better to overdiagnose secondary apnea in this situation than to continue attempts at stimulation that are not successful.

2. **Infant breathes spontaneously, heart rate is >100 bpm, but the overall color appears cyanotic (Apgar score of 5 to 7).** This situation is not uncommon and may follow primary apnea. A pulse oximeter should be placed on right upper extremity (usually the hand) as soon as possible after birth. If the measured levels are below the range in Table 4.1 at a specific time after birth, blended blow-by oxygen should be administered beginning with about 30% at a rate of 5 L/min by mask or by tubing held approximately 1 cm from the face. If the saturation improves, the oxygen concentration should be adjusted or gradually withdrawn as indicated to maintain saturation levels in the reference range.

   The early initiation of continuous positive airway pressure (CPAP) to a preterm infant who is spontaneously breathing but exhibiting respiratory distress in the delivery room is strongly advocated. In studies of infants born at <29 weeks' gestation, CPAP begun shortly after birth was equally as effective in preventing death or oxygen requirement at 36 weeks' postmenstrual age compared with initial intubation and mechanical ventilation. Early CPAP use reduced the need for intubation, mechanical ventilation, and exogenous surfactant administration but was associated in one study with a higher incidence of pneumothorax. In spontaneously breathing preterm infants with respiratory distress, use of CPAP in the delivery room is a reasonable alternative to intubation and mechanical ventilation. Using a pressure-regulated means of administration, such as a T-piece resuscitator or ventilator, is preferable. Although individual institutions have preferences regarding CPAP delivery device, there is no evidence that one means of administration is superior.

3. **The infant is apneic despite tactile stimulation or has a heart rate of <100 bpm despite apparent respiratory effort (Apgar score of 3 to 4).** This represents **secondary apnea** and requires treatment with bag-and-mask ventilation. When starting this intervention, call for assistance if your team is not already present.

A bag of approximately 750 mL volume should be connected to an air–oxygen blend (initial concentration depending on gestational age as in section III.C.) at a rate of 5 to 8 L/min and to a mask of appropriate size. The mask should cover the chin and nose but leave eyes uncovered. After positioning the newborn's head in the midline with slight extension, the initial breath should be delivered at a peak pressure that is adequate to produce appropriate chest rise; often, 20 cm H_2O is effective, but 30 to 40 cm H_2O may be needed in the term infant. This will establish functional residual capacity, and subsequent inflations will be effective at lower inspiratory pressures.

The inspiratory pressures for subsequent breaths should be adjusted to ensure that there is adequate but not excessive chest rise. In infants with normal lungs, this inspiratory pressure is usually no >15 to 20 cm H_2O. In infants with known or suspected disease causing decreased pulmonary compliance, continued inspiratory pressures in excess of 20 cm H_2O may be required. If no chest rise can be achieved despite apparently adequate pressure and no evidence of a mechanical obstruction, intubation should be considered. Especially in premature infants, every effort should be made to use the minimal pressures necessary for chest rise and the maintenance of normal oxygen saturation levels. A rate of 40 to 60 breaths per minute should be used, and the infant should be reassessed in 15 to 30 seconds. It is usually preferable to aim for a rate closer to 40 bpm, as many resuscitators deliver less adequate breaths at higher rates. Support should be continued until respirations are spontaneous, and the heart rate is >100 bpm, but effectiveness can also be gauged by improvements in oxygen saturation and tone before spontaneous respirations are established.

Such moderately depressed infants will be acidotic but generally able to correct this respiratory acidosis spontaneously after respiration is established. This process may take up to several hours, but unless the pH remains <7.25, acidosis does not need further treatment.

a. If positive-pressure ventilation is continued beyond a few breaths, and especially if the infant is intubated, the use of a T-piece resuscitator (Neopuff Infant T-Piece Resuscitator, Fisher & Paykel Inc, Irvine, CA) enhances the ability to provide consistent pressure-regulated breaths. This is a manually triggered, pressure-limited, and manually cycled device that is pneumatically powered by a flowmeter. It offers greater control over manual ventilation by delivering breaths of reproducible size (peak and end-expiratory pressures) and a simplified method to control delivered breath rate.

b. Laryngeal masks are easy to insert and are effective for ventilating newborns >2,000 g. They should be considered when bag-and-mask ventilation is not effective and intubation is unsuccessful or no skilled intubator is immediately available. The current models of laryngeal masks are not useful for tracheal suctioning and have not been studied as a means of administering intratracheal medications.

4. **The infant is apneic, and the heart rate is <100 bpm despite 30 seconds of assisted ventilation (Apgar score of 0 to 2).** If the heart rate is >60 bpm, positive-pressure ventilation should be continued, and the heart rate rechecked in 30 seconds. It is appropriate to carefully assess the effectiveness of support during this time using the following steps.

a. Adequacy of ventilation is the most important and should be assessed by observing chest wall motion at the cephalad portions of the thorax and listening for equal breath sounds laterally over the right and left hemithoraces at the midaxillary lines. The infant should be ventilated at 40 to 60 breaths per minute using the minimum pressure that will move the chest and produce audible breath sounds. Infants with respiratory distress syndrome, pulmonary hypoplasia, or ascites may require higher pressures. The equipment should be checked, and the presence of a good seal between the mask and the infant's face should be quickly ascertained. At the same time, the position of the infant's head should be checked and returned as needed to midline and slight extension. The airway should be cleared as needed.

b. Increase the oxygen concentration to 100% for infants of any gestational age if the resuscitation was started using an air–oxygen blend.

Continue bag-and-mask ventilation and reassess in 15 to 30 seconds. The most important measure of ventilation adequacy is infant response. If, despite good air entry, the heart rate fails to increase and color/oxygen saturation remains poor, intubation should be considered. Air leak (e.g., pneumothorax) should be ruled out (see Chapter 38).

c. Intubation is absolutely indicated only when a diaphragmatic hernia or similar anomaly is suspected or known to exist. The use of an alternate airway is recommended when bag-and-mask ventilation is ineffective, when chest compressions are administered and when an ET tube is needed for emergency administration of drugs, or when the infant requires transportation for more than a short distance after stabilization. Even in these situations, effective ventilation with a bag and mask may be done for long periods, and it is preferred over repeated unsuccessful attempts at intubation or attempts by unsupervised personnel unfamiliar with the procedure. If only inexperienced personnel are available, a laryngeal mask should be considered if an alternate airway is required.

Intubation should be accomplished rapidly by a skilled person. If inadequate ventilation was the sole cause of the bradycardia, successful intubation will result in an increase in heart rate to >100 bpm and a rapid improvement in oxygen saturation. Detection of expiratory carbon dioxide by a colorimetric detector is an effective means of confirming appropriate tube positioning, especially in the smallest infants.

The key to successful intubation is to correctly position the infant and laryngoscope and to know the anatomic landmarks. If the baby's chin, sternum, and umbilicus are all lined up in a single plane and if, after insertion into the infant's mouth, the laryngoscope handle and blade are aligned in that plane and lifted vertically at approximately a 60-degree angle to the baby's chest, only one of four anatomic landmarks will be visible to the intubator: From cephalad to caudad, these include the posterior tongue, the vallecula and epiglottis, the larynx (trachea and vocal cords), or the esophagus. The successful intubator will view the laryngoscope tip and a landmark and should then know whether the landmark being observed is cephalad or caudad to the larynx. The intubator can adjust the position of the blade by several millimeters and locate the vocal cords. The ET tube can then be inserted under direct visualization (see Chapter 69).

d. Circulation. If, after intubation and 30 seconds of ventilation with 100% oxygen, the heart rate remains <60 bpm, **cardiac massage** should be instituted. The best technique is to encircle the chest with both hands, placing the thumbs together over the lower third of the sternum, with the fingers wrapped around and supporting the back. If the infant is intubated, this can be done effectively while standing at the head of the bed next to the person performing ventilation and encircling the chest with the thumbs pointing toward the infant's feet. This approach ensures that other caregivers can access the infant for assessment and/or placement of an umbilical catheter. Alternatively, one can stand at the side of the infant and encircle the chest with both hands, a configuration that is "upside down" from the first method. In either method, compress the sternum about one-third the diameter of the chest at a rate of 90 times per minute in a ratio of three compressions for each breath. Positive-pressure ventilation should be continued at a rate of 30 breaths per minute, interspersed in the period following every third compression. Determine effectiveness of compressions by palpating the femoral, brachial, or umbilical cord pulse.

Periodically (every 45 to 60 seconds), one can briefly suspend both ventilation and compression as heart rate is assessed, but frequent interruptions of compressions will compromise maintenance of systemic and coronary perfusion. If the rate is >60 bpm, chest compression should be discontinued and ventilation continued until respiration is spontaneous. If no improvement is noted, compression and ventilation should be continued.

Infants requiring ventilatory and circulatory support are markedly depressed and require immediate, vigorous resuscitation. This will require at least three trained people working together.

e. Medications. If, despite adequate ventilation with 100% oxygen and chest compressions, a heart rate of >60 bpm has not been achieved by 1 to 2 minutes after delivery, medications such as chronotropic and inotropic agents should be given to support the myocardium, ensure adequate fluid status, and in some situations to correct acidosis. (See Table 4.3 for drugs, indications, and dosages.) Medications provide substrate and stimulation for the heart so that it can support circulation of oxygen and

Table 4.3. Neonatal Resuscitation

Drug/Therapy	Dose/kg	Weight (kg)	Volume IV (mL)	Volume IT (mL)	Method	Indication
Epinephrine 1:10,000 0.1 mg/mL	0.01–0.03 mg/kg IV 0.03–0.10 mg/kg IT	1 2 3 4	0.2 0.4 0.6 0.8	0.6 1.2 1.8 2.4	Give IV push or IT push. The current IT doses do not require dilution or flushing with saline. Do not give into an artery; **do not mix** with bicarbonate; repeat in 5 min PRN.	Asystole or severe bradycardia
Volume expanders Normal saline 5% albumin plasma Whole blood	— 0.1–0.2 mg/kg	1 2 3 4	10 mL 20 mL 30 mL 40 mL		Give IV over 5–10 minutes. Slower in premature infants	Hypotension because of intravascular volume loss (see Chapter 40)
Naloxone (Narcan) 0.4 mg/mL	0.1–0.2 mg/kg	1 2 3 4	0.25–0.50 0.50–1.00 0.75–1.50 1.0–2.0		Give IV push, IM, SQ, or IT; repeat PRN 3 times if no response; **if material narcotic addiction is suspected, do not give;** do not mix with bicarbonate (see Chapter 12).	Narcotic depression

	Dose				
Dopamine	30/60/90 mg/100 mL of solution	—	—	Give as continuous infusion	Hypotension because of poor cardiac output (see Chapter 40)
Cardioversion/ defibrillation (see Chapter 41)	1 to 4 J/kg increase 50% each time	—	—	—	Ventricular fibrillation, ventricular tachycardia
ET tube (see Chapter 66)	—	<1,000 g 1,000–2,000 g 2,000–4,000 g >4,000 g	—	Internal diameter (mm) 2.5 uncuffed 3.0 uncuffed 3.5 uncuffed 3.5–4.0 uncuffed	Distance of tip of ET tube 7 cm (for nasal) 8 cm (intubation) 9 cm (add 2 cm) 10 cm
Laryngoscope blades (see Chapter 69)		<2,000 g >2,000 g	—		0 (straight) 1 (straight)

IV, intravenous; IT, intratracheal; PRN, as needed; IM, intramuscular; SQ, subcutaneous; ET, endotracheal.

nutrients to the brain. For rapid calculations, use 1, 2, or 3 kg as the estimate of birth weight.

  i. The most accessible intravenous (IV) route for neonatal adminis-
     tration of medications is catheterization of the umbilical vein (see
     Chapter 69), which can be done rapidly and aseptically. Although
     the saline-filled catheter can be advanced into the inferior vena
     cava (i.e., 8 to 10 cm), in 60% to 70% of neonates, the cath-
     eter may become wedged in an undesirable or dangerous location
     (e.g., hepatic, portal, or pulmonary vein). Therefore, the catheter
     should only be advanced approximately 2 to 3 cm past the ab-
     dominal wall (4 to 5 cm total in a term neonate), just to the point
     of easy blood return, to a position that is safest for injection of
     drugs. In this position, the catheter tip will be in or just below the
     ductus venosus. It is important to flush all medications through
     the catheter because there is no flow through the vessel after cord
     separation.

 ii. **Drug therapy** as an adjunct to oxygen is to support the myo-
     cardium and correct acidosis. Continuing bradycardia is an
     indication for **epinephrine** administration, once effective venti-
     lation has been established. Epinephrine is a powerful adrenergic
     agonist and works in both adults and neonates by inducing an
     intense vasoconstriction and improved coronary (and cerebral)
     artery perfusion. The recommended dose is extrapolated from
     the apparently efficacious dose in adults and is based on both
     measured responses and empiric experience. The IV dose of 0.1
     to 0.3 mL/kg (up to 1.0 mL) of a 1:10,000 epinephrine solution
     should ideally be given through the umbilical venous catheter and
     flushed into the central circulation. This dose may be repeated
     every 3 to 5 minutes if necessary, and there is no apparent benefit
     to higher doses.

     When access to central circulation is difficult or delayed,
     epinephrine may be delivered through an ET tube for transpul-
     monary absorption, although a positive effect of this therapy has
     only been shown in animals at doses much higher than those
     currently recommended. This route of administration may be
     considered while IV access is being established, using doses of 0.5
     to 1.0 mL/kg of 1:10,000 dilution (0.05 to 0.10 mg/kg). These
     larger doses need not be diluted to increase the total volume. If
     two doses of epinephrine do not produce improvement, addi-
     tional doses may be given, but one should consider other causes
     for continuing depression.

iii. **Volume expansion.** If ventilation and oxygenation have been
     established but blood pressure is still low or the peripheral perfu-
     sion is poor, volume expansion may be indicated. In most in-
     stances, the use of 10 mL/kg of normal saline is effective, but in
     specific cases, the use of emergency whole blood may be a bet-
     ter choice (see section IV.B). Additional indications for volume
     expansion include evidence of acute bleeding or poor response
     to resuscitative efforts. Volume expansion should be carried out

cautiously in newborns in whom hypotension may be caused by asphyxial myocardial damage rather than hypovolemia. It is important to use the appropriate gestational age– and birth weight–related blood pressure norms to determine volume status (see Chapter 40).

In most situations, there is no value to the administration of bicarbonate or other buffers during immediate resuscitation. Because there are potential risks as well as benefits for all medications (see Table 4.3), drug administration through the umbilical vein should be reserved for those newborns in whom bradycardia persists despite adequate oxygen delivery and ventilation, only after establishment of an adequate airway. Once an adequate airway has been established, adequate ventilation achieved, and the heart rate exceeds 100 bpm, the infant should be moved to the neonatal intensive care unit (NICU), where physical examination, determination of vital signs, and test results including a chest radiograph will help to more clearly identify needs for specific interventions.

iv. **Reversal of narcotic depression is rarely necessary** during the primary steps of resuscitation and is not recommended. If the mother has received narcotic analgesia within a few hours of delivery, the newborn may manifest respiratory depression and require ongoing respiratory support until the drug effect abates.

IV. SPECIAL SITUATIONS

A. **Meconium aspiration** (see Chapter 35)

1. In the presence of any meconium staining of the amniotic fluid, the obstetrician should quickly assess the infant during the birth process for the presence of secretions or copious amniotic fluid. **Routine suctioning** of all meconium-stained infants is not recommended, but in the presence of significant fluid or secretions, the mouth and pharynx should be aspirated with a bulb syringe after delivery of the head and before breathing begins.

2. The newborn should immediately be assessed to determine whether it is vigorous, as defined by strong respiratory effort, good muscle tone, and a heart rate >100 bpm. Infants who are vigorous should be treated as normal, despite the presence of meconium-stained fluid. If both the obstetric provider and the pediatric team in attendance agree that the infant is vigorous, it is not necessary to take the infant from his or her mother after birth.

   If the infant is not vigorous, appropriate resuscitative measures should be given. Routine tracheal suctioning is not recommended, but it is important to maintain vigilance for possible airway obstruction by thick secretions and to suction as necessary.

3. For infants at risk for meconium aspiration syndrome who show initial respiratory distress, oxygen saturation levels should be monitored and kept in the normal range by administering adequate supplemental oxygen.

B. **Shock.** Some newborns present with pallor and shock in the delivery room (see Chapters 40 and 43). Shock may result from significant intrapartum blood loss because of placental separation, fetal–maternal hemorrhage, avulsion of the umbilical cord from the placenta, vasa or placenta previa, incision through an anterior placenta at cesarean section, twin–twin transfusion, or rupture of an abdominal viscus (liver or spleen) during a difficult delivery. It may also result from vasodilation or loss of vascular tone because of septicemia or hypoxemia and acidosis. These newborns will be pale, tachycardic (>180 bpm), tachypneic, and hypotensive with poor capillary filling and weak pulses.

After starting respiratory support, immediate transfusion with O-negative packed red blood cells and administration of normal saline boluses may be necessary if acute blood loss is the underlying cause. A volume of 20 mL/kg can be given through an umbilical venous catheter. If clinical improvement is not seen, causes of further blood loss should be sought, and more vigorous blood and possible colloid replacement should be continued. It is important to remember that the hematocrit may be normal immediately after delivery if the blood loss occurred acutely during the intrapartum period.

Except in cases of massive acute blood loss, the emergent use of blood replacement is not necessary, and acute stabilization can be achieved with crystalloid solutions. Normal saline is the primary choice of replacement fluid. This allows time to obtain proper products from the blood bank, if blood replacement is subsequently needed.

Except in the most extreme emergency situation where no other therapeutic option exists, the use of autologous blood from the placenta is not recommended.

C. **Air leak.** If an infant fails to respond to resuscitation despite apparently effective ventilation, chest compressions, and medications, consider the possibility of air leak syndromes. Pneumothoraces (uni- or bilateral) and pneumopericardium should be ruled out by transillumination or diagnostic thoracentesis (see Chapter 38) and treated if present.

D. **Prematurity.** Premature infants require additional special care in the delivery room, including the use of oxygen–air mixtures and oximetry monitoring, and precautions such as plastic wraps or bags, and/or the use of exothermic mattresses to prevent heat loss because of thinner skin and an increased surface-area-to-body-weight ratio. Apnea secondary to respiratory insufficiency is more likely at lower gestational ages, and support should be provided. Surfactant-deficient lungs are poorly compliant, and higher ventilatory pressures may be needed for the first and subsequent breaths. Depending on the reason for premature birth, perinatal infection is more likely in premature infants, which increases their risk of perinatal depression.

V. APGAR SCORES. Evaluation and decisions regarding resuscitation measures should be guided by assessment of respiration, heart rate, and color/oxygen saturation. This said, Apgar scores are conventionally assigned after birth and recorded in the newborn's chart. The Apgar score consists of the total points assigned to five objective signs in the newborn. Each sign is evaluated and given a score of 0, 1, or 2. Total scores at 1 and 5 minutes after birth are usually noted.

If the 5-minute score is 6 or less, the score is then noted at successive 5-minute intervals until it is >6 (see Table 4.2). A score of 10 indicates an infant in perfect condition; this is quite unusual because most babies have some degree of acrocyanosis. The scoring, if done properly, yields the following information:

A. **One-minute Apgar score.** This score generally correlates with umbilical cord blood pH and is an index of intrapartum depression. It does not correlate with outcome. Babies with a score of 0 to 4 have been shown to have a significantly lower pH, higher partial pressure of carbon dioxide ($PaCO_2$), and lower buffer base than those with Apgar scores >7. In the VLBW infant, a low Apgar score may not indicate severe depression. As many as 50% of infants with gestational ages of 25 to 26 weeks and Apgar scores of 0 to 3 have a cord pH of >7.25. Therefore, a VLBW infant with a low Apgar score cannot be assumed to be severely depressed. Nonetheless, such infants should be resuscitated actively and will usually respond more promptly and to less invasive measures than newborns whose low Apgar scores reflect acidemia.

B. **Apgar scores beyond 1 minute** are reflective of the infant's changing condition and the adequacy of resuscitative efforts. Persistence of low Apgar scores indicates need for further therapeutic efforts and usually the severity of the baby's underlying problem. In assessing the adequacy of resuscitation, the most common problem is inadequate pulmonary inflation and ventilation. It is important to verify a good seal with the mask, correct placement of the ET tube, and adequate peak inspiratory pressure applied to the bag if the Apgar score fails to improve as resuscitation proceeds.

The more prolonged the period of severe depression (i.e., Apgar score 3), the more likely is an abnormal long-term neurologic outcome. Nevertheless, many newborns with prolonged depression (>15 minutes) are normal in follow-up. Moreover, most infants with long-term motor abnormalities such as cerebral palsy have not had periods of neonatal depression after birth and have normal Apgar scores (see Chapter 55). Apgar scores were designed to monitor neonatal transition and the effectiveness of resuscitation, and their utility remains essentially limited to this important role. These scores are somewhat subjective, especially in the assessment of premature infants. The American Academy of Pediatrics is currently recommending an expanded Apgar score reporting form, which details both the numeric score as well as concurrent resuscitative interventions.

VI. **EVOLVING PRACTICES.** The practice of neonatal resuscitation continues to evolve with the availability of new devices and enhanced understanding of the best approach to resuscitation.

A. **End-tidal or expiratory CO_2 detectors** are already widely used to aid in confirming appropriate ET tube placement in the trachea. These devices may also have utility during bag-and-mask ventilation in helping to identify airway obstruction. Whether they may help ensure that appropriate ventilation is being offered or to assess return of spontaneous circulation has not yet been determined.

B. **Induced therapeutic hypothermia** is the standard therapy for infants born at ≥36 weeks' gestation who manifest moderate to severe hypoxic-ischemic encephalopathy. Most protocols include initiation of therapy within 6 hours of birth, but it is currently unknown whether earlier initiation may increase effectiveness or whether later initiation has any value. More mildly affected infants may benefit from this therapy under certain circumstances, but this remains under study. The role for passive cooling similarly requires more complete evaluation, but it does make sense to avoid active warming of an infant for whom this therapy is being considered while taking care to ensure that the infant's temperature does not drop below about 33.5°C. Avoidance of maternal or neonatal **hyperthermia** is warranted and may prevent subtle neurologic injury (see Chapter 55).

C. **Withholding or withdrawing resuscitation.** Resuscitation at birth is indicated for those babies likely to have a high rate of survival and a low likelihood of severe morbidity, including those with a gestational age of ≥25 weeks. In those situations where survival is unlikely or associated morbidity is very high, the wishes of the parents as the best spokespeople for the newborn should guide decisions about initiating resuscitation (see Chapter 19).

If there are no signs of life in an infant after 10 minutes of aggressive resuscitative efforts, with no evidence for other causes of newborn compromise, discontinuation of resuscitation efforts may be appropriate. There are data which suggest that with the availability of therapeutic hypothermia in infants ≥36 weeks' gestation, the outcome in this circumstance may not be as uniformly dismal as previously thought, but the ability to generalize those results remains in question. In each case, the decision to stop resuscitation should be individualized, with consideration of the uncertainty about the duration of asystole and whether the resuscitation interventions have been optimized. It is also appropriate to assess the availability of advanced intensive care, including therapeutic hypothermia, the baby's gestational age, and any specific circumstances prior to birth related to the presumed etiology and timing of the perinatal events. If possible, an opportunity to understand parental wishes under these circumstances may be very helpful.

Suggested Readings

Burchfield DJ. Medication use in neonatal resuscitation. *Clin Perinatol* 1999;26: 683–691.

Chettri S, Adhisivam B, Bhat BV. Endotracheal suction for nonvigorous neonates born through meconium stained amniotic fluid: a randomized controlled trial. *J Pediatr* 2015;166(5):1208.e1–1213.e1.

Davis PG, Tan A, O'Donnell CP, et al. Resuscitation of newborn infants with 100% oxygen or air: a systemic review and meta-analysis. *Lancet* 2004;364: 1329–1333.

Dawson JA, Kamlin CO, Wong C, et al. Oxygen saturation and heart rate during delivery room resuscitation of infants <30 weeks' gestation with air or 100% oxygen. *Arch Dis Child Fetal Neonatal Ed* 2009;94:F87–F91.

Kasdorf E, Laptook A, Azzopardi D, et al. Improving infant outcome with a 10 min Apgar of 0. *Arch Dis Child Fetal Neonatal Ed* 2015;100(2):F102–F105.

Morley CJ, Davis PG, Doyle LW, et al. Nasal CPAP or intubation at birth for very preterm infants. *N Engl J Med* 2008;358:700–708.

Ostrea EM Jr, Odell GB. The influence of bicarbonate administration on blood pH in a "closed system": clinical implications. *J Pediatr* 1972;80:671–680.

Perlman JM, Risser R. Cardiopulmonary resuscitation in the delivery room. Associated clinical events. *Arch Pediatr Adolesc Med* 1995;149:20–25.

Saugstad OD. Resuscitation of newborn infants with room air or oxygen. *Semin Neonatol* 2001;6:233–239.

Saugstad OD, Rootwelt T, Aalen O. Resuscitation of asphyxiated newborn infants with room air or oxygen: an international controlled trial. *Pediatrics* 1998;102:e1.

Vain NE, Szyld EG, Prudent LM, et al. Oropharyngeal and nasopharyngeal suctioning of meconium-stained neonates before delivery of their shoulders: multicentre, randomised controlled trial: the Resair 2 study. *Lancet* 2004;364:597–602.

Weiner G, Zaichkin J, eds. *Textbook of Neonatal Resuscitation*. 7th ed. Dallas, TX: American Academy of Pediatrics and American Heart Association; 2016.

Nonimmune Hydrops Fetalis

Kenneth J. Moise Jr and Suzanne Lopez

KEY POINTS

- Hydrops fetalis has classically been defined as the presence of extracellular fluid in at least two fetal body compartments.
- With routine use of Rhesus (Rh) immune globulin for the prevention of Rh alloimmunization, 95% of hydrops cases are classified as nonimmune.
- Treatment focuses on the etiology of hydrops, although many cases remain idiopathic.
- Plans for neonatal resuscitation should account for the location and severity of extravascular fluid collections and assess the need for immediate drainage as part of the initial resuscitation.

I. **DEFINITION.** Hydrops fetalis has classically been defined as the presence of extracellular fluid in at least two fetal body compartments. These fluid collections include skin edema (>5-mm thickness), pericardial effusion, pleural effusions, and ascites; all are easily recognized on prenatal ultrasound (Figs. 5.1–5.4). Frequent additional findings included polyhydramnios (deepest vertical pocket of amniotic fluid of >8 cm or amniotic fluid index >24 cm) and placentomegaly (>4-cm thickness in the second trimester or >6-cm thickness in the third trimester).

II. **INCIDENCE.** The reported incidence of nonimmune hydrops fetalis (NIHF) varies between 1 in 1,700 and 3,700 pregnancies.

III. **ETIOLOGY** (Table 5.1). The advent of the widespread use of Rh immune globulin for the prevention of RhD alloimmunization has resulted in a shift in favor of nonimmune etiologies of fetal hydrops. In 1970, McAfee et al. reported that 82% of cases of fetal hydrops were related to red cell alloimmunization, whereas in one more recent series, 95% of cases of hydrops were classified as nonimmune. The etiology of NIHF is diverse. A systematic review of literature reports involving >10 cases was undertaken by Bellini et al. between 1997 and 2007. Fifty-one papers met the strict criteria of the authors and involved 5,437 patients. The authors found that cardiovascular malformations represented the most common etiology followed by idiopathic causes,

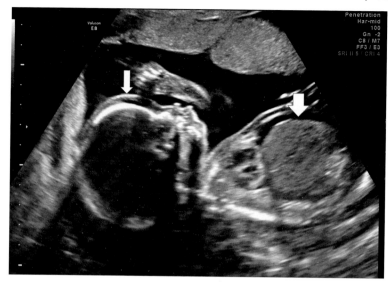

Figure 5.1. Scalp edema (*small arrow*) and ascites (*larger arrow*) in a case of nonimmune hydrops fetalis secondary to parvovirus at 22 weeks' gestation.

chromosomal abnormalities, and hematologic etiologies. A subsequent review by the same authors between 2007 and 2013 revealed an additional 24 papers involving 1,338 patients. A decreasing trend in chromosomal abnormalities, thoracic problems, urinary tract malformations, and twin–twin transfusion was noted between the two consecutive time periods while etiologies of lymphatic

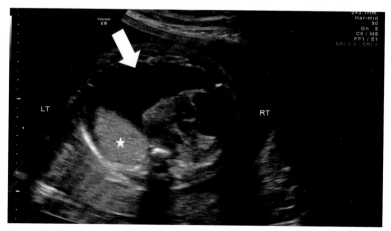

Figure 5.2. Large left-sided pleural effusion (*arrow*) in a fetus at 28 weeks' gestation with bronchopulmonary dysplasia (lesion indicated by *star*).

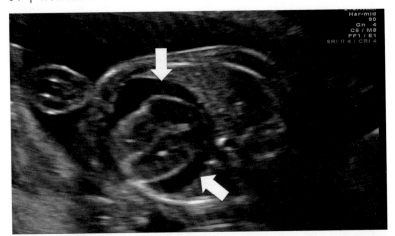

Figure 5.3. Pericardial effusion (between the *arrows*) in a recipient twin with severe twin–twin transfusion at 24 weeks' gestation.

dysplasia and gastrointestinal causes appear to have increased. The overall contributions of the various etiologies from the two series are noted in Table 5.1.

A recent systematic review addressed the issue of evaluation for lysosomal storage disease in cases of NIHF. In the 676 cases that were specifically evaluated for these conditions, the incidence was 5.2% of all cases tested and 17.5% of cases initially thought to be idiopathic. The three most common disorders were mucopolysaccharidosis type VII, Gaucher disease, and GM1 gangliosidosis.

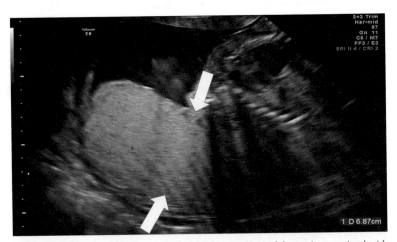

Figure 5.4. Placentomegaly (between the *arrows*) at 25 4/7 weeks' gestation associated with nonimmune hydrops fetalis in a fetus with an unbalanced atrioventricular canal and heterotaxy syndrome.

Table 5.1. Etiologies of Nonimmune Hydrops

Category	%	Typical Causes
Cardiovascular	21.4	Hypoplastic left heart, Ebstein anomaly, endocardial cushion defect, bradyarrhythmias/tachyarrhythmias
Idiopathic	18.2	—
Chromosomal	12.5	45 XO, trisomy 21, trisomy 18
Hematologic	10.1	α-Thalassemia, fetomaternal hemorrhage
Lymphatic dysplasia	7.5	Congenital lymphatic dysplasia
Infections	6.8	Parvovirus, CMV, adenovirus, enterovirus
Thoracic	5.3	CCAM, diaphragmatic hernia, extra-pulmonary sequestration, hydrothorax, chylothorax
Twin–twin transfusion	5.3	Donor/recipient fetus (more common)
Syndromic	4.6	Noonan syndrome
Miscellaneous	3.7	—
Urinary tract malformations	2.0	Urethral obstruction, prune belly syndrome
Inborn errors of metabolism	1.1	Lysosomal storage diseases
Extrathoracic tumors	0.7	Vascular tumors, teratomas, leukemia, hepatic tumors, neuroblastoma
Gastrointestinal	0.7	Meconium peritonitis, GI obstruction

CMV, cytomegalovirus; CCAM, congenital cystic adenomatoid malformation; GI, gastrointestinal.
Source: Modified from Bellini C, Domarini G, Paladini D, et al. Etiology of non-immune hydrops fetalis: an update. *Am J Med Genet* 2015;167A:1082–1088.

IV. **PATHOPHYSIOLOGY.** Because the etiology of NIHF is so diverse, few studies have addressed the pathophysiology of this condition. Lymphatic return of interstitial fluid to the vascular space is either inadequate or compromised. Anatomical obstruction is present in cases of Turner syndrome or lymphatic dysplasia, whereas a functional obstruction can occur due to elevated right atrial pressures noted in cases of severe fetal anemia (parvovirus) or tachyarrhythmias.

Certain cardiac malformations (Ebstein anomaly) or intrathoracic tumors (cystic adenomatoid malformation) are associated with increased venous pressure and a resultant increase in the production of interstitial fluid. Alternatively, vasculitis from infection (cytomegalovirus) can result in intravascular protein loss and enhanced interstitial fluid production.

In a series of 20 fetuses with NIHF, umbilical venous pressure was elevated at the time of cordocentesis in 65% of the cases. Correction of some of the lesions resulted in normalization of the venous pressure on subsequent measurement which was accompanied by resolution of the hydrops. These authors concluded that an elevated umbilical venous pressure signaled inadequate cardiac output as the cause of the NIHF. Normalization of the venous pressure after correction of the fetal condition invariably resulted in perinatal survival.

V. EVALUATION (Table 5.2).

The initial diagnosis of NIHF is often made at the time of a routine ultrasound examination (Fig. 5.5). At other times, the patient complains of a decrease in fetal movement or a rapid increase in weight gain or abdominal girth—signs of significant polyhydramnios.

A comprehensive ultrasound examination should be undertaken. Special emphasis should be placed on evaluation of cardiac structures and rhythm. If necessary, a fetal echocardiogram should be undertaken. The peak systolic velocity of the middle cerebral artery (MCA) should be measured as an elevated value of >1.5 multiples of the median corrected for gestational age has been associated with fetal anemia in cases of NIHF.

A careful maternal and reproductive history should then be undertaken. This should include queries regarding exposure to children with fifth disease ("slapped cheek" disease caused by parvovirus B19). Maternal symptoms that would indicate subsequent infection would include fever, arthralgia, and an exanthema on the upper body; however, as many as one-third of maternal infections are not accompanied by symptoms. A previous obstetrical history of stillbirth or a hydropic fetus should lead the investigator to contemplate lysosomal storage diseases. Similarly, a consanguineous relationship would also lead one to consider autosomal recessive diseases as the etiology. If the couple is of far Eastern descent, review of the maternal red cell mean corpuscular volume (MCV) (<82 = abnormal) should lead to an evaluation for α-thalassemia.

The next step in the diagnostic evaluation usually entails maternal venipuncture. Tests should include an antibody screen for anti–red cell antibodies, rapid test for syphilis, and a Kleihauer-Betke test or fetal cell stain by flow cytometry. Maternal serologies for toxoplasmosis, cytomegalovirus, and parvovirus are often ordered (toxoplasmosis, rubella, cytomegalovirus, and herpes simplex virus [TORCH] panel). Unfortunately, these tests can be nonspecifically elevated, and awaiting their result can lead to a significant delay in treatment.

Amniocentesis is warranted to complete the acute investigation. Samples should be sent for fluorescent *in situ* hybridization (FISH), computerized microarray, and polymerase chain reaction (PCR) testing for toxoplasmosis, cytomegalovirus, parvovirus, adenovirus, and enterovirus. Cultured amniocytes can be held in reserve and later sent to specific laboratories for lysosomal storage disease panels.

Table 5.2. Evaluation of Hydrops Fetalis

Prenatal Evaluation (Alive Fetus)	Prenatal Evaluation (Intrauterine Demise)
■ Maternal history* ■ Maternal blood type* ■ Fetal echocardiogram ■ Comprehensive obstetrical ultrasound ■ MCA Doppler* ■ Amniotic fluid analysis (viral PCR, karotype, FISH, CMA) ■ MRI	■ Autopsy (+ placenta) ■ Fetal DNA ■ Fibroblast culture ■ Skeletal survey ■ Immunohistochemical studies ■ Photographs ■ Frozen tissues
Postnatal Evaluation (Alive Newborn)	**Postnatal Evaluation (Neonatal Demise)**
■ Physical exam ■ Echocardiogram* ■ Ultrasound: head and abdomen ■ Chromosomes ■ Viral cultures ■ Blood gas* ■ Blood count* ■ Blood type + Coombs test* ■ Electrolytes ■ Urinalysis ■ Analysis of fluid (ascites, pleural effusion) ■ Liver functions ■ Radiographs	■ Autopsy (+ placenta) ■ Fetal DNA ■ Fibroblast culture ■ Skeletal survey ■ Immunohistochemical studies ■ Photographs ■ Frozen tissues

*Evaluations performed in immune hydrops fetalis.
MCA, middle cerebral artery; MRI, magnetic resonance imaging.
Source: Modified from Bellini C, Domarini G, Paladini D, et al. Etiology of non-immune hydrops fetalis: an update. *Am J Med Genet* 2015;167A:1082–1088.

VI. **PRENATAL TREATMENT.** A limited number of cases of NIHF can be treated in utero; however, these cases are based on an accurate determination of the specific etiology (see Table 5.1).

A. **Parvovirus infection.** Parvovirus has been associated with profound fetal anemia and hydrops fetalis when maternal infection occurs prior to 20 weeks' gestation (see Chapter 48). In one series of 1,019 pregnant women with seroconversion, the risk for fetal hydrops was 3.9%. The MCA Doppler can be used in an analogous fashion to confirm the anemia when there is an elevated peak systolic velocity of >1.5 multiples of the median. Although maternal serology (positive immunoglobulin M [IgM] or new presence of

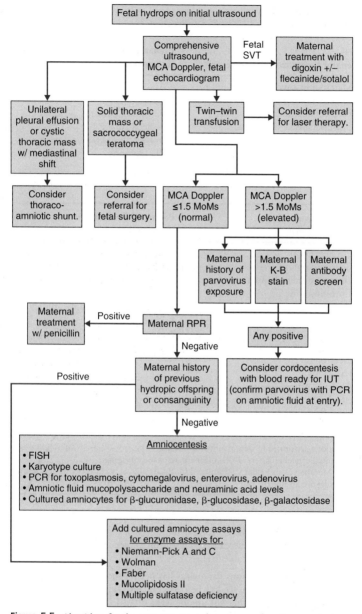

Figure 5.5. Algorithm for the management and treatment of nonimmune hydrops fetalis. MCA, middle cerebral artery; SVT, supraventricular tachycardia; MoM, multiples of median; K-B, Kleihauer-Betke; RPR, rapid plasma reagin; IUT, intrauterine transfusion; PCR, polymerase chain reaction; FISH, fluorescent *in situ* hybridization.

an IgG antibody in a patient that was previously seronegative) can be used to confirm cases, amniocentesis for PCR determination of parvovirus can usually be diagnostic in 24 to 48 hours. In one series, intrauterine transfusion (IUT) of packed red cells was associated with survival in approximately 85% of cases, whereas those cases with hydrops that were observed universally had a fatal outcome. IUTs have also proven successful in cases of fetal hydrops secondary to fetomaternal hemorrhage. If a recurrent decline in fetal hematocrit is detected due to a persistent fetomaternal bleed, abandonment of additional transfusions may be warranted. Fetal α-thalassemia with Bart's hemoglobin and NIHF has been treated with serial IUTs. Continued transfusion therapy, chelation, and eventual bone marrow transplant are required after birth due to abnormal hemoglobin production in these cases.

B. **Other infections.** Other treatable bacterial, parasitic, and viral infections associated with NIHF include syphilis, toxoplasmosis, and adenovirus. Fetal infection with syphilis that results in NIHF can reverse with maternal treatment with penicillin; however, the overall prognosis due to cerebral complications remains high. NIHF related to fetal toxoplasmosis has resolved after maternal administration of pyrimethamine, sulfadiazine, and folinic acid with good short-term neurologic outcome. Adenovirus can cause fetal myocarditis with resulting hydrops. Maternal administration of digoxin has been successful in increasing fetal myocardial function resulting in resolution of the hydrops.

C. **Cardiac arrhythmias.** Both fetal bradyarrhythmias and tachyarrhythmias have been associated with fetal hydrops. Ventricular rates of <50 bpm due to structural cardiac lesions or inflammation secondary to maternal anti-Ro antibodies are not amenable to therapy. The administration of maternal betamimetics has not been successful at increasing the fetal heart rate. Attempts at direct fetal pacing have also failed. Both fetal atrial flutter and supraventricular tachycardia are associated with NIHF. Maternal administration of digoxin followed by the addition of flecainide or sotalol is usually successful in converting these to a sinus rhythm with subsequent resolution of NIHF.

D. **Fetal lung lesions.** Unilateral pleural effusions (typically a chylothorax) or a large, predominantly congenital cystic adenomatoid malformation (CCAM) of the fetal lung represent space-occupying lesions that can shift the mediastinum to the opposite side of the fetal chest. These lesions can therefore cause an obstruction to venous return as well as decreased cardiac output and subsequent development of NIHF. In both lesions, thoracoamniotic shunt placement under ultrasound guidance has been successful in decreasing the size of the lesion resulting in a return of the mediastinum to its midline position. Hydrops will usually resolve within several weeks. In solid CCAM lesions with mediastinal shift and NIHF, maternal steroid administration has resulted in resolution of the hydrops. In cases of bronchopulmonary sequestration with NIHF, needle-guided laser therapy to coagulate the arterial feeder vessel has resulted in resolution of the hydrops.

E. **Twin–twin transfusion.** The recipient twin can exhibit NIHF in cases of twin–twin transfusion in up to 7% of cases. Laser photocoagulation of the putative placental anastomoses can result in complete resolution of the NIHF with an 80% perinatal survival. Most cases of donor NIHF occur after successful laser therapy. These cases are thought to the result of the acute anemia that can occur during the laser procedure; they are transient and resolve spontaneously.

VII. MATERNAL COMPLICATIONS OF FETAL HYDROPS (see Table 5.3). Fetal hydrops is often associated with polyhydramnios leading to such maternal complications as supine hypotension syndrome, preterm labor, and preterm premature rupture of the membranes. If placental hydrops is significant, an additional life-threatening complication has been described—Ballantyne syndrome (also known as mirror syndrome, triple edema, and pseudotoxemia). First described in association with hydrops secondary to maternal Rh alloimmunization in 1892, many subsequent case descriptions have appeared in the literature secondary to NIHF due to a variety of etiologies. In a recent review of 56 cases published between 1956 and 2009, Braun et al. noted clinical and laboratory findings similar to preeclampsia (see Table 5.3). However, unlike preeclampsia where hemoconcentration secondary to a reduced intravascular volume is the rule, mirror syndrome appears to be routinely associated with an expanded intravascular volume. Maternal hematocrit and albumin are low with minimal or no loss of urinary protein. Although the pathophysiology is unknown, hyperplacentosis is thought to be central to the cause. Reversal of maternal symptoms has been reported with the resolution of fetal hydrops after in utero treatment. Severe maternal complications have been reported with pulmonary edema in 25% of cases; progression to eclampsia has also been reported. In these situations, delivery should be undertaken.

Table 5.3. Maternal Symptoms with Mirror Syndrome	
Symptom	**Frequency (%)**
Edema/weight gain	89.3
Hypertension	60.7
Anemia	46.4
Proteinuria	42.9
Elevated uric acid/creatinine	25.0
Elevated hepatic enzymes	19.6
Oliguria	16.1
Headache/visual disturbances	14.3

Source: Modified from Braun T, Brauer M, Fuchs I, et al. Mirror syndrome: a systematic review of fetal associated conditions, maternal presentation and perinatal outcome. *Fetal Diagn Ther* 2010;27:191–203.

VIII. DELIVERY CONSIDERATIONS. All efforts should be undertaken to determine the etiology of NIHF because in many instances, this will determine the chance for perinatal survival. The maternal condition should also be taken into account because early signs of mirror syndrome warrant consideration for delivery unless an etiology for the NIHF can be identified that can be treated with in utero therapy. Findings of trisomy 18 or severe Ebstein anomaly warrant consultation with the palliative care team because prolonged survival after birth is unlikely. In cases of idiopathic NIHF, perinatal mortality rates approach 50%. Collaborative consultation between maternal–fetal medicine (MFM) and neonatology is paramount.

IX. NEONATAL MANAGEMENT OF FETAL HYDROPS

A. **Predelivery consultation.** Predelivery outpatient prenatal consultation with neonatology, pediatric subspecialty services, and perinatal palliative care team should be considered at tertiary care centers with an MFM delivery service. Prenatal consultations include discussion of postdelivery care of the fetal condition with and without premature delivery, tour of neonatal intensive care unit, and opportunity address specific neonatal questions (resuscitation, hospitalization course, outcomes, and possible birth plan). Consultation discussions can be added to maternal records for communication between services and in the event of an emergent delivery at a later date. Institutions unable to provide the needed level of maternal or neonatal care should consider a predelivery maternal transfer to a tertiary care center if possible.

B. **Delivery room management.** Resuscitation team preparation should occur well before delivery when possible. Plans for resuscitation should account for the location, and severity of extravascular fluid collections and assess the need for immediate drainage as part of the initial resuscitation. Large pleural fluid collections or ascites may severely restrict ventilation of the lungs until adequately drained. Appropriate equipment and health care personnel with skills in ventilation and emergency procedures (endotracheal intubation, thoracentesis, paracentesis, thoracotomy tube placement, umbilical line placement) should be immediately available in the delivery room (Table 5.4). Associated fetal health issues may warrant other subspecialty presence (i.e., pediatric cardiology, pediatric anesthesia) for management (cardiac arrhythmia, pericardial effusion, abnormal airway) during resuscitation.

C. **Postdelivery management.** Management after delivery is focused on treating the hydrops etiology (if known) and measures to correct abnormalities associated with hydrops. Patients with heart failure frequently will suffer from respiratory failure, anemia, hypoproteinemia, metabolic acidosis, hypotension, oliguria, and pulmonary hypertension. Hemodynamic instability is common secondary to rapid fluid shifts secondary to extravascular fluid drainage and the presence of hypoalbuminemia and hypoproteinemia.

D. **Ventilatory management** can be complicated by pulmonary hypoplasia, reaccumulation of pleural fluid and/or ascites, and persistent pulmonary hypertension. Chest or peritoneal tube placement may be needed to evacuate reaccumulating fluid in the pleural and peritoneal space. Exogenous

Table 5.4. Suggested Hydrops Fetalis Resuscitation Equipment and Personnel

Equipment	Personnel
Three thoracentesis/paracentesis kits (one for each side of the chest and one for the abdomen)	Team leader (neonatologist)
One pericardiocentesis kit (prepare if known pericardial effusion)	A resuscitation team member for each anticipated procedure (minimum of four)
Two thoracotomy kits (available in the event of pneumothorax during resuscitation)	Nursing personnel for code drugs and recording (preferably two)
Umbilical catheter setup (one for emergent umbilical venous catheter)	Respiratory therapist
Normal saline for infusion (avoid 5% albumin)	Consider pediatric subspecialist for anticipated airway or medical stabilization.
Resuscitation medications: epinephrine (use dry weight at 50th percentile for gestational age)	
Type O, RhD negative blood crossmatched with mother if severe anemia is suspected	
Blood gas syringes	
Code medications and code sheet	

surfactant administration should be considered if the infant is premature or there is evidence of surfactant deficiency disease.

E. **Fluid management** should be based on a calculated "dry weight" of the patient (usually the 50th percentile for gestational age). Maintenance intravenous fluids should start at 40 to 60 mL/kg/day of 10% dextrose solution and adjusted for serum glucose levels. Frequent evaluation of serum electrolytes, urine, and fluid drainage composition along with total fluid intake and output are necessary for fluid management. Free water and salt intake should be restricted in the first few days because these patients have high extravascular salt and water content. Use of diuretics should be cautious and include frequent electrolyte monitoring.

F. **Hemodynamic management** may require use of inotropes to improve cardiac output. In addition to placement of central venous and arterial lines for monitoring and management, an echocardiogram should be obtained to evaluate ventricular function, cardiac filling, and pulmonary pressures.

Most hydropic infants are normovolemic, so care should be taken to not volume overload if there is evidence of cardiac failure.

G. **Hematology management** includes evaluation of hematocrit and clotting factors. Euvolemic partial exchange transfusion should be considered in the anemic heart failure patient (hematocrit <30%) to improve oxygen-carrying capacity and increase hematocrit.

Suggested Readings

American Academy of Pediatrics, American Heart Association. 2010 American Heart Association guidelines for cardiopulmonary resuscitation and emergency cardiovascular care. In: American Academy of Pediatrics, American Heart Association. *Neonatal Resuscitation Textbook*. 6th ed. Elk Grove Village, IL: American Academy of Pediatrics; 2011:303–320.

Barton JR, Thorpe EM Jr, Shaver DC, et al. Nonimmune hydrops fetalis associated with maternal infection with syphilis. *Am J Obstet Gynecol* 1992;167:56–58.

Bellini C, Domarini G, Paladini D, et al. Etiology of non-immune hydrops fetalis: an update. *Am J Med Genet* 2015;167A:1082–1088.

Braun T, Brauer M, Fuchs I, et al. Mirror syndrome: a systematic review of fetal associated conditions, maternal presentation and perinatal outcome. *Fetal Diagn Ther* 2010;27:191–203.

Carlton DB. Pathophysiology of edema. In: Polin RA, Fow WW, Abman AH, eds. *Fetal and Neonatal Physiology*. 4th ed. Philadelphia, PA: Elsevier; 2011:1451–1454.

Carpenter RJ Jr, Strasburger JF, Garson A Jr, et al. Fetal ventricular pacing for hydrops secondary to complete atrioventricular block. *J Am Coll Cardiol* 1986;8:1434–1436.

Laine GA, Allen SJ, Katz J, et al. Effect of systemic venous pressure elevation on lymph flow and lung edema formation. *J Appl Physiol (1985)* 1986;61:1634–1638.

Lindenburg IT, Smits-Wintjens VE, van Klink JM, et al. Long-term neurodevelopmental outcome after intrauterine transfusion for hemolytic disease of the fetus/newborn: the LOTUS study. *Am J Obstet Gynecol* 2012;206(2):141. e1–141.e8.

McAfee CAJ, Fortune DW, Beischer NA. Non-immunological hydrops fetalis. *J Obstet Gynaecol Br Commw* 1970;77:226–237.

Moïse AA, Gest AL, Weickmann PH, et al. Reduction in plasma protein does not affect body water content in fetal sheep. *Pediatr Res* 1991;29:623–626.

Skinner JR, Sharland G. Detection and management of life threatening arrhythmias in the perinatal period. *Early Hum Dev* 2008;84:161–172.

6 Birth Trauma
Elisa Abdulhayoglu

KEY POINTS

- Birth injury is defined by the National Vital Statistics Report as "an impairment of the infant's body function or structure due to adverse influences that occurred at birth."
- When fetal size, immaturity, or malpresentation complicate delivery, the normal intrapartum compressions, contortions, and forces can lead to injury in the newborn.
- A newborn at risk for birth injury should have a thorough examination, including a detailed neurologic evaluation.
- The birth injury rate has been decreasing steadily in the past decade.
- Injury may occur antenatally, intrapartum, or during resuscitative efforts.
- Not all birth injury is avoidable.
- Risk factors: fetal size and/or malpresentation, prematurity, instrumented delivery, maternal factors
- Long-term prognosis for most birth injuries is resolution without permanent injury.

I. **BACKGROUND.** Birth injury is defined by the National Vital Statistics Report as "an impairment of the infant's body function or structure due to adverse influences that occurred at birth." Injury may occur antenatally, intrapartum, or during resuscitation and may be avoidable or unavoidable.

   A. **Incidence.** The birth trauma and injury rate fell from 2.6 per 1,000 live births in 2004 to 1.9 per 1,000 live births in 2012.

   B. **Risk factors.** When fetal size, immaturity, or malpresentation complicate delivery, the normal intrapartum compressions, contortions, and forces can lead to injury in the newborn. Obstetrical instrumentation may increase the mechanical forces, amplifying or inducing a birth injury. Breech presentation carries the greatest risk of injury; however, cesarean delivery without labor does not prevent all birth injuries. The following factors may contribute to an increased risk of birth injury:

   1. Primiparity

   2. Small maternal stature

   3. Maternal pelvic anomalies

   4. Prolonged or unusually rapid labor

5. Oligohydramnios

6. Malpresentation of the fetus

7. Use of midforceps or vacuum extraction

8. Versions and extraction

9. Very low birth weight or extreme prematurity

10. Fetal macrosomia or large fetal head

11. Fetal anomalies

12. Maternal obesity—body mass index >40 kg/m^2

C. **Evaluation.** A newborn at risk for birth injury should have a thorough examination, including a detailed neurologic evaluation. Newborns who require resuscitation after birth should be evaluated because occult injury may be present. Particular attention should be paid to symmetry of structure and function, cranial nerves, range of motion of individual joints, and integrity of the scalp and skin.

II. TYPES OF BIRTH TRAUMA

A. **Head and neck injuries**

1. **Injuries associated with intrapartum fetal monitoring.** Placement of an electrode on the fetal scalp or presenting part for fetal heart monitoring occasionally causes superficial abrasions or lacerations. These injuries require minimal local treatment, if any. Facial or ocular trauma may result from a malpositioned electrode. Abscesses rarely form at the electrode site.

2. **Extracranial hemorrhage**
   a. **Caput succedaneum**
      i. **Caput succedaneum** is a commonly occurring subcutaneous, extraperiosteal fluid collection that is occasionally hemorrhagic. It has poorly defined margins and can extend over the midline and across suture lines. It typically extends over the presenting portion of the scalp and is usually associated with molding.
      ii. The lesion usually resolves spontaneously without sequelae over the first several days after birth. It rarely causes significant blood loss or jaundice. There are rare reports of scalp necrosis with scarring.
      iii. **Vacuum caput** is a caput succedaneum with margins well demarcated by the vacuum cup.
   b. **Cephalohematoma**
      i. A **cephalohematoma** is a subperiosteal collection of blood resulting from rupture of the superficial veins between the skull and periosteum. The lesion is always confined by suture lines. It may occur in as many as 2.0% of all live births. It is more commonly seen in instrumented deliveries.
      ii. An extensive cephalohematoma can result in significant hyperbilirubinemia. Hemorrhage is rarely serious enough to necessitate blood transfusion. Infection is also a rare complication and usually

occurs in association with septicemia and meningitis. Skull fractures have been associated with 5% of cephalohematomas. Head magnetic resonance imaging (MRI) should be obtained if neurologic symptoms are present. Most cephalohematomas resolve within 8 weeks. Occasionally, they calcify and persist for several months or years.

  iii. Management is limited to observation in most cases. Incision and aspiration of a cephalohematoma may introduce infection and is contraindicated. Anemia or hyperbilirubinemia should be treated as needed.

c. Subgaleal hematoma

  i. Subgaleal hematoma is hemorrhage under the aponeurosis of the scalp. It is more often seen after vacuum- or forceps-assisted deliveries.

  ii. Because the subgaleal or subaponeurotic space extends from the orbital ridges to the nape of the neck and laterally to the ears, the hemorrhage can spread across the entire calvarium.

  iii. The initial presentation typically includes pallor, poor tone, and a fluctuant swelling on the scalp. The hematoma may grow slowly or increase rapidly and result in shock. With progressive spread, the ears may be displaced anteriorly and periorbital swelling can occur. Ecchymosis of the scalp may develop. The blood is resorbed slowly, and swelling gradually resolves. The morbidity may be significant in infants with severe hemorrhage who require intensive care for this lesion. The mortality rate can range from 12% to 14%. Death is attributed to significant volume loss, resulting in hypovolemic shock and coagulopathy.

  iv. There is no specific therapy. The infant must be observed closely for signs of hypovolemia, and blood volume should be maintained as needed with transfusions. Phototherapy should be provided for hyperbilirubinemia. An investigation for a bleeding disorder should be considered. Surgical drainage should be considered only for unremitting clinical deterioration. A subgaleal hematoma associated with skin abrasions may become infected; it should be treated with antibiotics and may need drainage.

3. Intracranial hemorrhage (see Chapter 54)

4. Skull fracture

  a. Skull fractures may be either linear, usually involving the parietal bone, or depressed, involving the parietal or frontal bones. The latter are often associated with forceps use. Occipital bone fractures are most often associated with breech deliveries.

  b. Most infants with linear or depressed skull fractures are asymptomatic unless there is an associated intracranial hemorrhage (e.g., subdural or subarachnoid hemorrhage). Occipital osteodiastasis is a separation of the basal and squamous portions of the occipital bone that often results in cerebellar contusion and significant hemorrhage. It may be a lethal complication in breech deliveries. A linear fracture that is associated with a dural tear may lead to herniation of the meninges and brain, with development of a leptomeningeal cyst.

c. Uncomplicated linear fractures usually require no therapy. The diagnosis is made by a radiograph of the skull. Head MRI should be obtained if intracranial injury is suspected or if neurologic symptoms develop. Depressed skull fractures require neurosurgical evaluation. Some may be elevated using closed techniques. Comminuted or large skull fractures associated with neurologic findings need immediate neurosurgical evaluation. If leakage of cerebrospinal fluid from the nares or ears is noted, antibiotic therapy should be started and neurosurgical consultation obtained. Follow-up imaging should be performed at 8 to 12 weeks to evaluate possible leptomeningeal cyst formation.

5. **Facial or mandibular fractures**
   a. Facial fractures can be caused by numerous forces including natural passage through the birth canal, forceps use, or delivery of the head in breech presentation.
   b. Fractures of the mandible, maxilla, and lacrimal bones warrant immediate attention. They may present as facial asymmetry with ecchymoses, edema, and crepitance or respiratory distress with poor feeding. Untreated fractures can lead to facial deformities with subsequent malocclusion and mastication difficulties. Treatment should begin promptly because maxillar and lacrimal fractures begin to heal within 7 to 10 days, and mandibular fractures start to repair at 10 to 14 days. Treated fractures usually heal without complication.
   c. Airway patency should be closely monitored. A plastic surgeon or otorhinolaryngologist should be consulted and appropriate radiographic studies obtained. Head computed tomography (CT) scan or MRI may be necessary to evaluate for retro-orbital or cribriform plate disruption. Antibiotics should be administered for fractures involving the sinuses or middle ear.

6. **Nasal injuries**
   a. Nasal fracture and dislocation may occur during the birth process. The most frequent nasal injury is dislocation of the nasal cartilage, which may result from pressure applied by the maternal symphysis pubis or sacral promontory. The reported prevalence of dislocation is <1%.
   b. Infants with significant nasal trauma may develop respiratory distress. Similar to facial fractures, nasal fractures begin to heal in 7 to 10 days and must be treated promptly. Rapid healing usually occurs once treatment is initiated. If treatment is delayed, deformities are common.
   c. A misshapen nose may appear dislocated. To differentiate dislocation from a temporary deformation, compress the tip of the nose. With septal dislocation, the nares collapse and the deviated septum is more apparent. With a misshapen nose, no nasal deviation occurs. Nasal edema from repeated suctioning may mimic partial obstruction. Patency can be assessed with a cotton wisp under the nares. Management involves protection of the airway and otorhinolaryngology consultation.
   d. If nasal dislocations are left untreated, there is an increased risk of long-term septal deformity.

7. Ocular injuries

a. Retinal and subconjunctival hemorrhages are commonly seen after vaginal delivery. They result from increased venous congestion and pressure during delivery. Malpositioned forceps can result in ocular and periorbital injury including hyphema, vitreous hemorrhage, lacerations, orbital fracture, lacrimal duct or gland injury, and disruption of Descemet's membrane of the cornea (which can lead to astigmatism and amblyopia). Significant ocular trauma occurs in <0.5% of all deliveries.

b. Retinal hemorrhages usually resolve within 1 to 5 days. Subconjunctival hemorrhages resorb within 1 to 2 weeks. No long-term complications usually occur. For other ocular injuries, prompt diagnosis and treatment are necessary to ensure a good long-term outcome.

c. Management. Prompt ophthalmologic consultation should be obtained.

8. Ear injuries

a. Ears are susceptible to injury, particularly with forceps application. More significant injuries occur with fetal malposition. Abrasions, hematomas, and lacerations may develop.

b. Abrasions generally heal well with local care. Hematomas of the pinna may lead to the development of a "cauliflower" ear. Lacerations may result in perichondritis. Temporal bone injury can lead to middle and inner ear complications, such as hemotympanum and ossicular disarticulation.

c. Hematomas of the pinna should be drained to prevent clot organization and development of cauliflower ear. If the cartilage and temporal bone are involved, an otolaryngologist should be consulted. Antibiotic therapy may be required.

9. Sternocleidomastoid (SCM) injury

a. SCM injury is also referred to as congenital or muscular torticollis. The etiology is uncertain. The most likely cause is a muscle compartment syndrome resulting from intrauterine positioning. Torticollis can also arise during delivery as the muscle is hyperextended and ruptured, with development of a hematoma and subsequent fibrosis and shortening.

b. Torticollis may present at birth with a palpable 1- to 2-cm mass in the SCM region and head tilt to the side of the lesion. More often, it is noted at 1 to 4 weeks of age. Facial asymmetry may be present along with hemihypoplasia on the side of the lesion. Prompt treatment may lessen or correct the torticollis.

c. Other conditions may mimic congenital torticollis and should be ruled out. These include cervical vertebral anomalies, hemangioma, lymphangioma, and teratoma.

d. Treatment is initially conservative. Stretching of the involved muscle should begin promptly and be performed several times per day. Recovery typically occurs within 3 to 4 months in approximately 80% of cases. Surgery is needed if torticollis persists after 6 months of physical therapy.

e. In up to 10% of patients with congenital torticollis, congenital hip dysplasia may be present. A careful hip examination is warranted with further evaluation as indicated.

10. **Pharyngeal injury**

a. Minor submucosal pharyngeal injuries can occur with postpartum bulb suctioning. More serious injury, such as perforation into the mediastinal or pleural cavity, may result from nasogastric or endotracheal tube placement. Affected infants may have copious secretions and difficulty swallowing, and it may be difficult to advance a nasogastric tube.

b. Mild submucosal injuries typically heal without complication. More extensive trauma requires prompt diagnosis and treatment for complete resolution.

c. The diagnosis of a retropharyngeal tear is made radiographically using water-soluble contrast material. Infants are treated with broad-spectrum antibiotics, and oral feedings are usually withheld for 2 weeks. The contrast study may be repeated to confirm healing before feeding is restarted. Infants with pleural effusions may require chest tube placement. Surgical consultation is obtained if the leak persists or the perforation is large.

B. **Cranial nerve, spinal cord, and peripheral nerve injuries**

1. **Cranial nerve injuries**

   a. **Facial nerve injury (cranial nerve VII)**

      i. Injury to the facial nerve is the most common peripheral nerve injury in neonates, occurring in up to 1% of live births. The exact incidence is unknown, as many cases are subtle and resolve readily. The etiology includes compression of the facial nerve by forceps (particularly midforceps), pressure on the nerve secondary to the fetal face lying against the maternal sacral promontory, or, rarely, from pressure of a uterine mass (e.g., fibroid).

      ii. Facial nerve injury results in asymmetric crying facies.

         a) **Central facial nerve injury** occurs less frequently than peripheral nerve injury. Paralysis is limited to the lower half to two-thirds of the contralateral side, which is smooth with no nasolabial fold present. The corner of the mouth droops. Movement of the forehead and eyelid is unaffected.

         b) **Peripheral injury** involves the entire side of face and is consistent with a lower motor neuron injury. The nasolabial fold is flattened and the mouth droops on the affected side. The infant is unable to wrinkle the forehead and close the eye completely. The tongue is not involved.

         c) **Peripheral nerve branch injury** results in paralysis that is limited to only one group of facial muscles: the forehead, eyelid, or mouth.

      iii. Differential diagnosis includes Möbius syndrome (nuclear agenesis), intracranial hemorrhage, congenital hypoplasia of the depressor anguli oris muscle, and congenital absence of facial muscles or nerve branches.

      iv. The prognosis of acquired facial nerve injury is excellent, with recovery usually complete by 3 weeks. Initial management is directed at prevention of corneal injuries by using artificial tears and protecting the open eye by patching. Electromyography may be helpful to predict recovery or potential residual effects. Full recovery is most likely.

b. Recurrent laryngeal nerve injury

 i. Unilateral abductor paralysis may be caused by recurrent laryngeal injury secondary to excessive traction on the fetal head during breech delivery or lateral traction on the head with forceps. The left recurrent laryngeal nerve is involved more often because of its longer course. Bilateral recurrent laryngeal nerve injury can be caused by trauma but is usually due to hypoxia or brainstem hemorrhage.

 ii. A neonate with unilateral abductor paralysis is often asymptomatic at rest but has hoarseness and inspiratory stridor with crying. Unilateral injury is occasionally associated with hypoglossal nerve injury and presents with difficulty with feedings and secretions. Bilateral paralysis usually results in stridor, severe respiratory distress, and cyanosis.

 iii. Differential diagnosis of symptoms similar to unilateral injury includes congenital laryngeal malformations. Particularly with bilateral paralysis, intrinsic central nervous system (CNS) malformations must be ruled out, including Chiari malformation and hydrocephalus. If there is no history of birth trauma, cardiovascular anomalies and mediastinal masses should be considered.

 iv. The diagnosis can be made using direct or flexible fiberoptic laryngoscopy. A modified barium swallow and speech pathology consultation may be helpful to optimize feeding. Unilateral injury usually resolves by 6 weeks of age without intervention and treatment. Bilateral paralysis has a variable prognosis; tracheostomy may be required.

2. Spinal cord injuries

a. Vaginal delivery of an infant with a hyperextended head or neck, breech delivery, and severe shoulder dystocia are risk factors for spinal cord injury. However, significant spinal cord injuries are rare with a prevalence rate of <0.2 per 10,000 live births. Injuries include spinal epidural hematomas, vertebral artery injuries, traumatic cervical hematomyelia, spinal artery occlusion, and transection of the cord.

b. Spinal cord injury presents in four ways:

 i. Some infants with severe high cervical or brainstem injury present as stillborn or in poor condition at birth, with respiratory depression, shock, and hypothermia. Death generally occurs within hours of birth.

 ii. Infants with an upper or midcervical injury present with central respiratory depression. They have lower extremity paralysis, absent deep tendon reflexes and sensation in the lower half of the body, urinary retention, and constipation. Bilateral brachial plexus injury may be present.

 iii. Injury at the seventh cervical vertebra or lower may be reversible. However, permanent neurologic complications may result, including muscle atrophy, contractures, bony deformities, and constant micturition.

 iv. Partial spinal injury or spinal artery occlusions may result in subtle neurologic signs and spasticity.

c. Differential diagnosis includes amyotonia congenita, myelodysplasia associated with spina bifida occulta, spinal cord tumors, and cerebral hypotonia.

d. The prognosis depends on the severity and location of the injury. If a spinal injury is suspected at birth, efforts should focus on resuscitation and prevention of further damage. The head, neck, and spine should be immobilized. Neurology and neurosurgical consultations should be obtained. Careful and repeated examinations are necessary to help predict long-term outcome. Cervical spine radiographs, CT scan, and MRI may be helpful.

3. **Cervical nerve root injuries**
   a. **Phrenic nerve injury (C3, C4, or C5)**
      i. Phrenic nerve damage leading to paralysis of the ipsilateral diaphragm may result from a stretch injury due to lateral hyperextension of the neck at birth. Risk factors include breech and difficult forceps deliveries. Injury to the nerve is thought to occur where it crosses the brachial plexus. Therefore, approximately 75% of patients also have brachial plexus injury. Occasionally, chest tube insertion or surgery injures this nerve.
      ii. Respiratory distress and cyanosis are often seen. Some infants present with persistent tachypnea and decreased breath sounds at the lung base. There may be decreased movement of the affected hemithorax. Chest radiographs may show elevation of the affected diaphragm, although this may not be apparent if the infant is on continuous positive airway pressure (CPAP) or mechanical ventilation. If the infant is breathing spontaneously and not on CPAP, increasing atelectasis may develop. The diagnosis is confirmed by ultrasonography or fluoroscopy that shows paradoxical (upward) movement of the diaphragm with inspiration.
      iii. Differential diagnosis includes cardiac, pulmonary, and other neurologic causes of respiratory distress. These can usually be evaluated by a careful examination and appropriate imaging. Congenital absence of the nerve is rare.
      iv. The initial treatment is supportive. CPAP or mechanical ventilation may be needed, with airway care to avoid atelectasis and pneumonia. Most infants recover in 1 to 3 months without permanent sequelae. Diaphragmatic plication is considered in refractory cases. Phrenic nerve pacing is possible for bilateral paralysis.
   b. **Brachial plexus injury**
      i. The incidence of brachial plexus injury is 1.5 per 1,000 live births in the United States. The cause is excessive traction on the head, neck, and arm during birth. Risk factors include macrosomia, shoulder dystocia, malpresentation, and instrumented deliveries. Injury usually involves the nerve root, especially where the roots come together to form the nerve trunks of the plexus.
      ii. Duchenne-Erb palsy involves the upper trunks (C5, C6, and occasionally C7) and is the most common type of brachial plexus injury, accounting for approximately 90% of cases. Total brachial

plexus palsy occurs in some cases and involves all roots from C5 to T1. Klumpke palsy involves C7/C8–T1 and is the least common.

  a) **Duchenne-Erb palsy.** The arm is typically adducted and internally rotated at the shoulder. There is extension and pronation at the elbow and flexion of the wrist and fingers in the characteristic "waiter's tip" posture. The deltoid, infraspinatus, biceps, supinator and brachioradialis muscles, and the extensors of the wrist and fingers may be weak or paralyzed. The Moro, biceps, and radial reflexes are absent on the affected side. The grasp reflex is intact. Sensation is variably affected. Diaphragm paralysis occurs in 5% of cases.

  b) **Total brachial plexus injury.** Accounts for approximately 10% of all cases. The entire arm is flaccid. All reflexes, including grasp and sensation, are absent. If sympathetic fibers are injured at T1, Horner syndrome may be seen.

  c) **Klumpke palsy.** The rarest of the palsies, accounting for <1% of brachial plexus injuries. The lower arm paralysis affects the intrinsic muscles of the hand and the long flexors of the wrist and fingers. The grasp reflex is absent. However, the biceps and radial reflexes are present. There is sensory impairment on the ulnar side of the forearm and hand. Because the first thoracic root is usually injured, its sympathetic fibers are damaged, leading to an ipsilateral Horner syndrome.

iii. **Differential diagnosis** includes a cerebral injury, which usually has other associated CNS symptoms. Injury of the clavicle, upper humerus, and lower cervical spine may mimic a brachial plexus injury.

iv. Radiographs of the shoulder and upper arm should be performed to rule out bony injury. The chest should be examined to detect diaphragm paralysis. Initial treatment is conservative. Physical therapy and passive range of motion exercises prevent contractures. These should be started at 7 to 10 days when the postinjury neuritis has resolved. "Statue of Liberty" splinting should be avoided, as contractures in the shoulder girdle may develop. Wrist and digit splints may be useful.

v. The prognosis for full recovery varies with the extent of injury. If the nerve roots are intact and not avulsed, the prognosis for full recovery is excellent (>90%). Notable clinical improvement in the first 2 weeks after birth indicates that normal or near-normal function will return. Most infants recover fully by 3 months of age. In those with slow recovery, electromyography and nerve-conduction studies may distinguish an avulsion from a stretch injury. Surgery has most commonly been recommended when there is a lack of biceps function at 3 months of age.

C. Bone injuries

1. **Clavicular fracture** is the most commonly injured bone during delivery, occurring in up to 2% newborns. Many clavicular fractures are not identified until after discharge from the hospital.

   a. These fractures are seen in vertex presentations with shoulder dystocia or in breech deliveries when the arms are extended. Macrosomia is a risk factor.

b. A greenstick or incomplete fracture may be asymptomatic at birth. The first clinical sign may be a callus at 7 to 10 days of age. Signs of a complete fracture include crepitus, palpable bony irregularity, and spasm of the SCM. The affected arm may have a pseudoparalysis because motion causes pain.

c. Differential diagnosis includes fracture of the humerus or a brachial plexus palsy.

d. A **clavicular fracture** is confirmed by radiograph. If the arm movement is decreased, the cervical spine, brachial plexus, and humerus should be assessed. Therapy should be directed at decreasing pain with analgesics. The infant's sleeve may be pinned to the shirt to limit movement until the callus begins to form. Complete healing is expected.

2. Long bone injuries
   a. Humeral fractures have a prevalence of 0.05 per 1,000 live births.
      i. Humeral fractures typically occur during a difficult delivery of the arms in the breech presentation and/or of the shoulders in vertex. Direct pressure on the humerus may also result in fracture.
      ii. A greenstick fracture may not be noted until the callus forms. The first sign is typically loss of spontaneous arm movement, followed by swelling and pain on passive motion. A complete fracture with displaced fragments presents as an obvious deformity. X-ray confirms the diagnosis.
      iii. Differential diagnosis includes clavicular fracture and brachial plexus injury.
      iv. The prognosis is excellent with complete healing expected. Pain should be treated with analgesics.
         a) A fractured humerus usually requires splinting for 2 weeks. Displaced fractures require closed reduction and casting. Radial nerve injury may be seen.
         b) Epiphyseal displacement occurs when the humeral epiphysis separates at the hypertrophied cartilaginous layer of the growth plate. Severe displacement may result in significant compromise of growth. The diagnosis can be confirmed by ultrasonography because the epiphysis is not ossified at birth. Therapy includes immobilization of the limb for 10 to 14 days.
   b. Femoral fractures have a prevalence of 0.17 per 1,000 live births.
      i. Femoral fractures usually follow a breech delivery. Infants with congenital hypotonia are at increased risk.
      ii. Physical examination usually reveals an obvious deformity of the thigh. In some cases, the injury may not be noted for a few days until swelling, decreased movement, or pain with palpation develops. The diagnosis is confirmed by x-ray.
      iii. Complete healing without limb shortening is expected.
         a) Fractures, even if unilateral, should be treated with splinting and immobilization using a spica cast or Pavlik harness.
         b) Femoral epiphyseal separation may be misinterpreted as developmental dysplasia of the hip because the epiphysis is not ossified at birth. Pain and tenderness with palpation are more likely with epiphyseal separation than dislocation. The diagnosis is

confirmed by ultrasonography. Therapy includes limb immobilization for 10 to 14 days and analgesics for pain.

D. Intra-abdominal injuries. Intra-abdominal birth trauma is uncommon.

1. Hepatic injury

a. The liver is the most commonly injured solid organ during birth. Macrosomia, hepatomegaly, and breech presentation are risk factors for hepatic hematoma and/or rupture. The etiology is thought to be direct pressure on the liver.

b. Subcapsular hematomas are generally not symptomatic at birth. Nonspecific signs of blood loss such as poor feeding, pallor, tachypnea, tachycardia, and onset of jaundice develop during the first 1 to 3 days after birth. Serial hematocrits may suggest blood loss. Rupture of the hematoma through the capsule results in discoloration of the abdominal wall and circulatory collapse with shock.

c. Differential diagnosis includes trauma to other intra-abdominal organs.

d. Management includes restoration of blood volume, correction of coagulation disturbances, and surgical consultation for probable laparotomy. Early diagnosis and correction of volume loss increase survival.

2. Splenic injury

a. Risk factors for splenic injury include macrosomia, breech delivery, and splenomegaly (e.g., congenital syphilis, erythroblastosis fetalis).

b. Signs are similar to hepatic rupture. A mass is sometimes palpable in the left upper quadrant, and the stomach bubble may be displaced medially on an abdominal radiograph.

c. Differential diagnosis includes injury to other abdominal organs.

d. Management includes volume replacement and correction of coagulation disorders. Surgical consultation should be obtained. Expectant management with close observation is appropriate if the bleeding has stopped and the patient has stabilized. If laparotomy is necessary, salvage of the spleen is attempted to minimize the risk of sepsis.

3. Adrenal hemorrhage

a. The relatively large size of the adrenal gland at birth may contribute to injury. Risk factors are breech presentation and macrosomia. Ninety percent of adrenal hemorrhages are unilateral; 75% occur on the right.

b. Findings on physical examination depend on the extent of hemorrhage. Classic signs include fever, flank mass, purpura, and pallor. Adrenal insufficiency may present with poor feeding, vomiting, irritability, listlessness, and shock. The diagnosis is made with abdominal ultrasound.

c. Differential diagnosis includes other abdominal trauma. If a flank mass is palpable, neuroblastoma and Wilms tumor should be considered.

d. Treatment includes blood volume replacement. Adrenal insufficiency may require steroid therapy. Extensive bleeding that requires surgical intervention is rare.

E. Soft tissue injuries

1. Petechiae and ecchymoses are commonly seen in newborns. The birth history, location of lesions, their early appearance without development of new lesions, and the absence of bleeding from other sites help differentiate petechiae and ecchymoses secondary to birth trauma from those caused by a vasculitis or coagulation disorder. If the etiology is uncertain, studies to rule out coagulopathies and infection should be performed. Most petechiae and ecchymoses resolve within 1 week. If bruising is excessive, jaundice and anemia may develop. Treatment is supportive.

2. **Lacerations and abrasions** may be secondary to scalp electrodes and fetal scalp blood sampling or injury during birth. Deep wounds (e.g., scalpel injuries during cesarean section) may require sutures. Infection is a risk, particularly with scalp lesions and an underlying caput succedaneum or hematoma. Treatment includes cleansing the wound and close observation.

3. **Subcutaneous fat necrosis** is not usually recognized at birth. It usually presents during the first 2 weeks after birth as sharply demarcated, irregularly shaped, firm, nonpitting subcutaneous plaques or nodules on the extremities, face, trunk, or buttocks. The injury may be colorless or have a deep-red or purple discoloration. Calcification may occur. No treatment is necessary. Lesions typically resolve completely over several weeks to months.

Suggested Readings

Agency for Healthcare Research and Quality. 2014 National Healthcare Quality and Disparities Report. http://www.ahrq.gov/research/findings/nhqrdr/2014chartbooks/healthyliving/hl-mch4.html. Accessed May 28, 2016.

Basha A, Amarin Z, Abu-Hassan F. Birth-associated long bone fractures. *Int J Gynaecol Obstet* 2013;123(2):127–130.

Borschel GH, Clarke HM. Obstetrical brachial plexus palsy. *Plast Reconstr Surg* 2009;124(1 Suppl):144e–155e.

Doumouchtsis SK, Arulkumaran S. Are all brachial plexus injuries caused by shoulder dystocia? *Obstet Gynecol Surv* 2009;64(9):615–623.

Doumouchtsis SK, Arulkumaran S. Head trauma after instrumental births. *Clin Perinatol* 2008;35:69–83.

Goetz E. Neonatal spinal cord injury after an uncomplicated vaginal delivery. *Pediatr Neurol* 2010;42:69–71.

Moczygemba CK, Paramsothy P, Meikle S, et al. Route of delivery and neonatal birth trauma. *Am J Obstet Gynecol* 2010;202:361.e1–361.e6.

Rosenberg AA. Traumatic birth injury. *NeoReviews* 2003;4(10):e270–e276.

Uhing MR. Management of birth injuries. *Clin Perinatol* 2005;32:19–38.

7

The High-Risk Newborn: Anticipation, Evaluation, Management, and Outcome

Vincent C. Smith

KEY POINTS

- Because certain maternal, placental, or fetal conditions are associated with high risk to newborns, providers must prepare to stabilize and manage these infants.
- To properly contextualize the risk, providers must understand the gestational age (GA) determination.
- Risk factors such as pre- and postterm birth, small for gestational age (SGA), and large for gestational age (LGA) all have associated clinical management challenges of which providers should be aware.
- The placenta should be saved in all cases of high-risk delivery.

I. **HIGH-RISK NEWBORNS** are often associated with certain maternal, placental, or fetal conditions; when one or more are present, nursery staff should be aware and prepared for possible difficulties. The placenta should be saved in all cases of high-risk delivery, including cases that involve transfer from the birth hospital because an elusive diagnosis such as toxoplasmosis may be made on the basis of placental pathology. The following factors are associated with high-risk newborns:

A. **Maternal characteristics and associated risk for fetus or neonate**

1. **Age at delivery**

a. **Over 40 years.** Chromosomal abnormalities, macrosomia, intrauterine growth retardation (IUGR), blood loss (abruption or previa)

b. **Under 16 years.** IUGR, preterm birth, child abuse/neglect (mother herself may be abused)

2. **Personal factors**

a. **Poverty.** Preterm birth, IUGR, infection

b. **Smoking.** Increased perinatal mortality, IUGR

c. **Drug/alcohol use.** IUGR, fetal alcohol syndrome, withdrawal syndrome, sudden infant death syndrome, child abuse/neglect

d. Poor diet. Ranges from mild IUGR to fetal demise with severe malnutrition

e. Trauma (acute, chronic). Fetal demise, abruptio placentae, preterm birth

3. **Medical conditions**
   a. Diabetes mellitus. Stillbirth, macrosomia/birth injury/IUGR in advanced stages with vascular insufficiency, respiratory distress syndrome (RDS), hypoglycemia, congenital anomalies (see Chapter 2)
   b. Thyroid disease. Goiter, hypothyroidism, hyperthyroidism (see Chapter 61)
   c. Renal disease. Stillbirth, IUGR, preterm birth
   d. Urinary tract infection. Preterm birth, sepsis
   e. Heart and/or lung disease. Stillbirth, IUGR, preterm birth
   f. Hypertension (chronic or pregnancy-related). Stillbirth, IUGR, preterm birth, asphyxia, polycythemia, thrombocytopenia, leukopenia
   g. Anemia. Stillbirth, IUGR, hydrops, preterm birth, asphyxia
   h. Isoimmunization (red cell antigens). Stillbirth, hydrops, anemia, jaundice
   i. Thrombocytopenia, including alloimmunization (platelet antigens). Stillbirth, bleeding including intracranial hemorrhage (ICH)

4. **Obstetric history**
   a. Past history of infant with preterm birth, jaundice, RDS, or anomalies. Same with current pregnancy
   b. Maternal medications (see Appendix A and B)
   c. Bleeding. Stillbirth, preterm birth, anemia
   d. Hyperthermia. Fetal demise, fetal anomalies
   e. Premature rupture of membranes. Infection/sepsis
   f. Toxoplasmosis, other, rubella, cytomegalovirus, and herpes simplex (TORCH) infections (see Chapter 48)

B. **Fetal characteristics and associated risk for fetus or neonate**

1. **Multiple gestation.** IUGR, twin–twin transfusion syndrome, preterm birth, asphyxia, birth trauma

2. **IUGR.** Fetal demise, genetic abnormalities, congenital anomalies, asphyxia, hypoglycemia, polycythemia

3. **LGA and/or macrosomia.** Congenital anomalies, birth trauma, hypoglycemia

4. **Abnormal fetal position/presentation.** Congenital anomalies, birth trauma, hemorrhage

5. **Abnormality of fetal heart rate or rhythm.** Congestive heart failure, heart block, hydrops, asphyxia

6. **Decreased activity.** Fetal demise, neurologic abnormalities, asphyxia

7. **Polyhydramnios.** Anencephaly, other central nervous system (CNS) disorders, neuromuscular disorders, problems with swallowing (e.g., esophageal atresia, agnathia, any mass in the mouth), chylothorax, diaphragmatic hernia, omphalocele, gastroschisis, trisomy, tumors, hydrops, isoimmunization, anemia, cardiac failure, intrauterine infection,

maternal diabetes or other etiologies of inability to concentrate urine, LGA, preterm delivery

   8. Oligohydramnios. Fetal demise, placental insufficiency, IUGR, renal agenesis, pulmonary hypoplasia, deformations, intrapartum distress, postterm delivery

C. **Conditions of labor and delivery and associated risk for fetus or neonate**

   1. Preterm delivery. RDS, other issues of preterm birth (see Chapter 13)

   2. Postterm delivery (occurring >2 weeks after term). Stillbirth, asphyxia, meconium aspiration (see section IV)

   3. Maternal fever. Infection/sepsis

   4. Maternal hypotension. Stillbirth, asphyxia

   5. Rapid labor. Birth trauma, ICH, retained fetal lung fluid/transient tachypnea

   6. Prolonged labor. Stillbirth, asphyxia, birth trauma

   7. Abnormal presentation. Birth trauma, asphyxia

   8. Uterine tetany. Asphyxia

   9. Meconium-stained amniotic fluid. Stillbirth, asphyxia, meconium aspiration syndrome, persistent pulmonary hypertension

   10. Prolapsed cord. Stillbirth, asphyxia

   11. Cesarean section. RDS, retained fetal lung fluid/transient tachypnea, blood loss

   12. Obstetric analgesia and anesthesia. Respiratory depression, hypotension

   13. Placental anomalies
      a. Small placenta. IUGR
      b. Large placenta. Hydrops, maternal diabetes, large infant
      c. Torn placenta and/or umbilical vessels. Blood loss, anemia
      d. Abnormal attachment of vessels to placenta. Blood loss, anemia

D. **Immediately evident neonatal conditions and associated risk for fetus or neonate**

   1. Preterm birth. RDS, other sequelae of preterm birth

   2. Low 5-minute Apgar score. Prolonged transition (especially respiratory)

   3. Low 10-minute Apgar score. Neurologic damage

   4. Pallor or shock. Blood loss

   5. Foul smell of amniotic fluid or membranes. Infection

   6. SGA (see section V)

   7. LGA (see section VI). Hypoglycemia, birth trauma, congenital anomalies

   8. Postmaturity syndrome (see section IV)

II. GA AND BIRTH WEIGHT CLASSIFICATION. Neonates should be classified by GA, if at all possible, as this generally correlates more closely with outcomes

than birth weight does. Birth weight becomes significant if neonate is either SGA or LGA.

A. GA classification

1. Assessment based on **obstetric information** is covered in Chapter 1. Note that GA estimates by first-trimester ultrasonography are accurate within 7 days. Second- and third-trimester ultrasounds are within approximately 11 to 14 and 21 days, respectively.

2. To **confirm or supplement** obstetric dating, the modified Dubowitz (Ballard) examination for newborns (Fig. 7.1) may be useful in GA estimation. There are limitations to this method, especially with use of the neuromuscular component in sick newborns.

3. **Infant classification by GA**

   a. Preterm are born at <37 completed weeks of gestation (258 days). Subgroups of preterm infant include the following:

      i. Extremely preterm infants are born <28 weeks (195 days).

      ii. Early preterm infants are born <34 weeks (237 days).

      iii. Late preterm infants are born between 34 0/7 and 36 6/7 weeks of gestation (238 to 258 days).

   b. Term infants are born between 37 0/7 and 41 6/7 weeks of gestation (259 to 293 days).

      i. Early term infants are subgroup of term infants born between 37 0/7 and 38 6/7 weeks of gestation (259 to 272 days).

   c. Postterm infants are born after 42 weeks of gestation (294 days) or more.

B. Birth weight classification. Although there is no universal agreement, the commonly accepted definitions are as follows:

1. **Normal birth weight (NBW).** From 2,500 to 4,000 g

2. **Low birth weight (LBW).** <2,500 g

   Note that, although most LBW infants are preterm, some are term but SGA. LBW infants can be further subclassified as follows:

   a. Very low birth weight (VLBW). <1,500 g

   b. Extremely low birth weight (ELBW). <1,000 g

III. PRETERM BIRTH. A preterm neonate is one who is born <37 weeks' gestation (as noted earlier).

A. Incidence. Approximately 10% of all births in the United States are preterm. In 2014, the National Center for Health Statistics officially completed the transition to a new method of quantifying GA, shifting from the previous practice of counting from last menstrual period (LMP) to using best obstetric estimate (OE) of gestation at delivery. The 2014 preterm birth rate was 9.57%, down slightly from 9.62% in 2013. The percentage of births delivered preterm has declined 8% since 2007 (from 10.44%), the first year for which national OE data are available for this measure (and differs from the LMP-based rate previously published). The rate of infants born early preterm (<34 weeks) was down slightly, from 2.79% to 2.75% for 2013 to 2014; this rate of early preterm births has declined 6% since 2007. The late preterm birth rate (34 to 36 weeks) was essentially stable at 6.82% in 2014; this rate of late preterm birth has declined 9% since 2007.

MATURATIONAL ASSESSMENT OF GESTATIONAL AGE (New Ballard Score)

NAME _____ SEX _____
HOSPITAL NO. _____ BIRTH WEIGHT _____
RACE _____ LENGTH _____
DATE/TIME OF BIRTH _____ HEAD CIRC. _____
DATE/TIME OF EXAM _____ EXAMINER _____
AGE WHEN EXAMINED _____
APGAR SCORE: 1 MINUTE _____ 5 MINUTES _____ 10 MINUTES _____

NEUROMUSCULAR MATURITY

NEUROMUSCULAR MATURITY SIGN	SCORE							RECORD SCORE HERE
	-1	0	1	2	3	4	5	
POSTURE								
SQUARE WINDOW (Wrist)	>90°	90°	60°	45°	30°	0°		
ARM RECOIL		180°	140°–180°	110°–140°	90°–110°	<90°		
POPLITEAL ANGLE	180°	160°	140°	120°	100°	90°	<90°	
SCARF SIGN								
HEEL TO EAR								

TOTAL NEUROMUSCULAR MATURITY SCORE

SCORE
Neuromuscular ____
Physical ____
Total ____

MATURITY RATING

SCORE	WEEKS
-10	20
-5	22
0	24
5	26
10	28
15	30
20	32
25	34
30	36
35	38
40	40
45	42
50	44

GESTATIONAL AGE (weeks)

By dates _____
By ultrasound _____
By exam _____

PHYSICAL MATURITY

PHYSICAL MATURITY SIGN	SCORE							RECORD SCORE HERE
	-1	0	1	2	3	4	5	
SKIN	sticky friable transparent	gelatinous red translucent	smooth pink visible veins	superficial peeling &/or rash, few veins	cracking pale areas rare veins	parchment deep cracking no vessels	leathery cracked wrinkled	
LANUGO	none	sparse	abundant	thinning	bald areas	mostly bald		
PLANTAR SURFACE	heel-toe 40–50 mm: -1 <40 mm: -2	>50 mm no crease	faint red marks	anterior transverse crease only	creases ant. 2/3	creases over entire sole		
BREAST	imperceptible	barely perceptible	flat areola no bud	stippled areola 1–2 mm bud	raised areola 3–4 mm bud	full areola 5–10 mm bud		
EYE / EAR	lids fused loosely: -1 tightly: -2	lids open pinna flat stays folded	sl. curved pinna; soft; slow recoil	well-curved pinna; soft but ready recoil	formed & firm instant recoil	thick cartilage ear shift		
GENITALS (Male)	scrotum flat, smooth	scrotum empty faint rugae	testes in upper canal rare rugae	testes descending few rugae	testes down good rugae	testes pendulous deep rugae		
GENITALS (Female)	clitoris prominent & labia flat	prominent clitoris & small labia minora	prominent clitoris & enlarging minora	majora & minora equally prominent	majora large minora small	majora cover clitoris & minora		

TOTAL PHYSICAL MATURITY SCORE

Figure 7.1. New Ballard score. (From Ballard JL, Khoury JC, Wedig K, et al. New Ballard Score, expanded to include extremely premature infants. *J Pediatr* 1991;119:417–423.)

B. Etiology is unknown in most cases. Preterm and/or LBW delivery is associated with the following conditions:

1. **Low socioeconomic status** (SES), whether measured by family income, educational level, geographic area/ZIP code, social class, and/or occupation

2. **Non-Hispanic black** women are more than three times as likely to deliver an extremely preterm infant (<28 weeks of gestation) compared with non-Hispanic white and Hispanic women. In 2014, the rate for non-Hispanic black women was 13.23% that, although significantly higher than that of non-Hispanic white and Hispanic women, has dropped from its peak of 18.3% in 2007. This disparity in very short gestation delivery by race/ethnicity contributes to the substantial black–white gap in infant mortality. Disparities persist even when SES is taken into account.

3. **Women younger than 16 or older than 35 years** are more likely to deliver preterm or LBW infants; the association with age is more significant in whites than in African Americans.

4. **Maternal activity** requiring long periods of standing or substantial amounts of physical stress may be associated with IUGR and preterm birth.

5. **Acute or chronic maternal illness** is associated with early delivery, whether onset of labor is spontaneous or, not infrequently, induced.

6. **Multiple-gestation births** frequently deliver preterm (57% of twins and 93% of triplets in the United States in 2013). In such births, the higher rate of neonatal mortality is primarily due to preterm birth.

7. **Prior poor birth outcome** is the single strongest predictor of poor birth outcome. A preterm first birth is the best predictor of a second preterm birth. One preterm birth increases the risk for a second fourfold.

8. **Obstetric factors** such as uterine malformations, uterine trauma, placenta previa, abruptio placentae, hypertensive disorders, preterm cervical shortening, previous cervical surgery, premature rupture of membranes, and chorioamnionitis also contribute to preterm birth.

9. **Fetal conditions** such as nonreassuring testing of fetal well-being (see Chapter 1), IUGR, or severe hydrops may require preterm delivery.

10. **Inadvertent early delivery** because of incorrect estimation of GA is increasingly uncommon using the OE method.

C. **Problems associated with preterm birth** are related to difficulty in extrauterine function due to immaturity of organ system.

   1. **Respiratory.** Preterm infants may experience the following:
      a. Perinatal depression in the delivery room due to hypoxic ischemia perinatal conditions (see Chapter 55)
      b. RDS due to surfactant deficiency and pulmonary immaturity (see Chapter 33)
      c. Apnea due to immaturity in mechanisms controlling breathing (see Chapter 31)
      d. Eventual development of chronic lung disease (CLD) of prematurity also referred to as bronchopulmonary dysplasia (see Chapter 34)

   2. **Neurologic.** Preterm infants have a higher risk of neurologic problems including the following:
      a. Perinatal depression (see Chapter 55)
      b. ICH (see Chapter 54)
      c. Periventricular leukomalacia (see Chapter 54)

3. **Cardiovascular.** Preterm infants may present with cardiovascular problems including the following:
   a. **Hypotension**
      i. Hypovolemia
      ii. Cardiac dysfunction
      iii. Sepsis-induced vasodilation
   b. **Patent ductus arteriosus** is common and may lead to pulmonary overcirculation and diastolic hypotension (see Chapter 41).

4. **Hematologic.** Conditions for which preterm infants are at higher risk include the following:
   a. **Anemia** (see Chapter 45)
   b. **Hyperbilirubinemia** (see Chapter 26)

5. **Nutritional.** Preterm infants require specific attention to the content, caloric density, volume, and route of feeding, including parental nutrition when indicated (see Chapter 21).

6. **Gastrointestinal.** Premature infants are at increased risk for necrotizing enterocolitis; formula feeding is an additional risk factor; a mother's own breast milk appears to be protective (see Chapter 27).

7. **Metabolic.** Problems, especially in glucose and calcium metabolism, are more common in preterm infants (see Chapters 24 and 25).

8. **Renal.** Immature kidneys are characterized by low glomerular filtration rate as well as an inability to process water, solute, and acid loads. Therefore, fluid and electrolyte management require close attention (see Chapters 23 and 28).

9. **Temperature regulation.** Preterm infants are especially susceptible to hypothermia; iatrogenic hyperthermia can also be a problem (see Chapter 15).

10. **Immunologic.** Because of deficiencies in both humoral and cellular response, preterm infants are at greater risk for infection than are term infants.

11. **Ophthalmologic.** Retinopathy of prematurity may develop in the immature retina of infants <32 weeks or with birth weight <1,500 g (see Chapter 67).

D. **Management of the preterm infant** (see Chapter 13)

1. **Immediate postnatal management**
   a. **Delivery** in an appropriately equipped and staffed hospital is preferable. Risks to the very premature or sick preterm infant are greatly increased by delays in initiating necessary specialized care.
   b. **Resuscitation and stabilization** require the immediate availability of qualified personnel and equipment. Resuscitation of the newborn at delivery should be in accordance with the American Academy of Pediatrics Neonatal Resuscitation Program (NRP). Anticipation and prevention are always preferred over reaction to problems already present. Adequate oxygen delivery and maintenance of proper temperature are immediate postnatal goals (see Chapter 4).

2. **Neonatal management**
   a. **Thermal regulation** should be directed toward achieving a neutral thermal zone; that is, environmental temperature sufficient to maintain body

temperature with minimal oxygen consumption. For the small preterm infant, this will require either an overhead radiant warmer (with the advantages of infant accessibility and rapid temperature response) or a closed incubator (with the advantages of diminished insensible water loss) (see Chapter 15).

b. Oxygen therapy and assisted ventilation (see Chapter 29)

c. Fluid and electrolyte therapy must account for relatively high insensible water loss while avoiding overhydration and maintaining normal glucose and plasma electrolyte concentrations (see Chapter 23).

d. Nutrition may be complicated by the inability of many preterm infants to tolerate enteral feedings, necessitating treatment with parenteral nutrition. When enteral feedings are tolerated, ineffective suck and swallow usually necessitate gavage feeding (see Chapter 21).

e. Hyperbilirubinemia, which is inevitable in less mature infants, can usually be managed effectively by careful monitoring of bilirubin levels and early use of phototherapy. In the most severe cases, exchange transfusion may be necessary (see Chapter 26).

f. Infection may be the precipitant of preterm delivery. If an infant displays signs or symptoms that could be attributed to infection, the infant should be carefully evaluated for sepsis (e.g., physical exam, +/− CBC, +/− blood culture). There should be a low threshold for starting broad-spectrum antibiotics (e.g., ampicillin and gentamicin) until sepsis can be ruled out. Consider antistaphylococcal antibiotics for VLBW infants who have a central venous catheter, have undergone multiple procedures, or have remained for long periods in the hospital and are at increased risk for nosocomial infection (see Chapters 48 and 49).

g. Patent ductus arteriosus in preterm infants with birth weight >1,000 g often requires only conservative management with fluid restriction (usually 110 to 130 mL/kg/day) and supportive care. Supportive care includes a neutral thermal environment, adequate oxygenation to minimize demands on left ventricular (LV) function, use of positive end-expiratory pressure (PEEP) to improve gas exchange in infants with respiratory compromise, and maintenance of the hematocrit at 35% to 40% to help increase pulmonary vascular resistance and reduce left-to-right shunting. In smaller infants, a prostaglandin antagonist such as indomethacin or ibuprofen may be necessary. In the most symptomatic infants or those for whom medical therapy is either contraindicated or fails to close the ductus, surgical ligation may be necessary (see Chapter 41).

h. Immunizations. Diphtheria, tetanus toxoids, and acellular pertussis (DTaP) vaccine; inactivated poliovirus vaccine (IPV); multivalent pneumococcal conjugate vaccine (PCV); and *Haemophilus influenzae* type b (Hib) vaccine are given in full doses to preterm infants on the basis of their chronologic age (i.e., weeks after birth). Although the majority of preterm infants develop protective levels of antibodies, overall they have reduced immune response to vaccines as compared to term infants and therefore develop the best protection if they receive a booster after 12 months. Hepatitis B (HepB) vaccine administration for medically stable preterm infants of hepatitis B surface antigen (HBsAg)-negative mothers may be given on a modified schedule. Respiratory syncytial virus (RSV) and influenza prophylaxis should be given as indicated. Special consideration should be given to the rotavirus vaccine (RV) because it is a live oral vaccine that is not typically given until neonatal intensive care unit (NICU) discharge with strict limitation on its administration. All Centers for Disease Control and Prevention (CDC) and Advisory Committee on Immunization Practices (ACIP) recommendations can be found at http://www.cdc.gov/vaccines (see Chapters 48 and 49).

E. **Survival of preterm infants.** For many reasons, survival statistics vary by institution as well as geographic region and country. Figures 7.2 and 7.3 show survival rates of VLBW preterm infants from nearly 1,000 centers around the globe that voluntarily submit data about the care and outcomes of high-risk newborn infants enrolled in the Vermont Oxford Network (VON) in 2014. The VON databases hold critical information on >2 million infants representing >63 million patient days.

F. **Long-term problems of preterm birth.** Preterm infants are vulnerable to a wide spectrum of morbidities. The risk of morbidity and mortality declines steadily with increasing GA.

  1. **Neurologic disability**
     a. **Major handicaps** (cerebral palsy, developmental delay)
     b. **Cognitive dysfunction** (language disorders, learning disability, hyperactivity, attention deficits, behavior disorders)

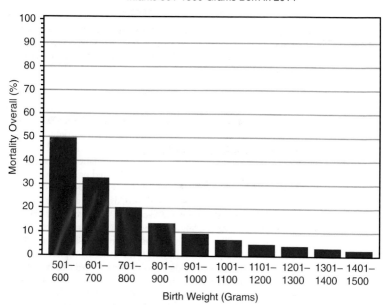

MORTALITY OVERALL BY BIRTH WEIGHT
Infants 501-1500 Grams Born in 2014

Figure 7.2. Mortality by birth weight. (From Vermont Oxford Network 2014 with permission of Erika M. Edwards, PhD, MPH, Editor of 2014 Very Low Birth Weight Database Summary. Vermont Oxford Network, 33 Kilburn Street, Burlington, VT 05401. E-mail: nightingale@vtoxford.org. Website: www.vtoxford.org.)

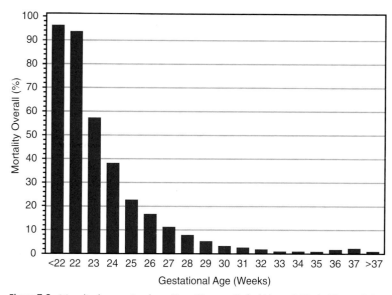

Figure 7.3. Mortality by gestational age. (From Vermont Oxford Network 2014 with permission of Erika M. Edwards, PhD, MPH, Editor of 2014 Very Low Birth Weight Database Summary. Vermont Oxford Network, 33 Kilburn Street, Burlington, VT 05401. E-mail: nightingale@ vtoxford.org. Website: www.vtoxford.org.)

    c. Sensory impairments (hearing loss, visual impairment) (see Chapters 67 and 68)

2. **Retinopathy of prematurity** (see Chapter 67)

3. **Chronic lung disease (CLD)** (see Chapter 34)

4. **Poor growth.** Preterm infants are at risk for a wide range of growth problems (see Chapter 21). Although it is imperative for clinicians to visually assess the size and growth rate of individual infants, there is considerable controversy on which growth charts to use, and thus there are several approaches to monitoring infant growth. Because extrauterine preterm infants grow at a different rate than their intrauterine fetal counterparts, some argue that a different measure may be needed to assess fetal growth than is used to follow longitudinal preterm infant growth. Although more accurate, the use of multiple growth charts can become confusing and complex. A simpler approach is to use the same growth curve to assess fetal growth (size at birth) and preterm infant longitudinal growth (Fig. 7.4). For example, the Fenton growth charts use a relatively recent and diverse cohort of infants who had accurate GA assessments, but they rely on data that is statistically smoothed between

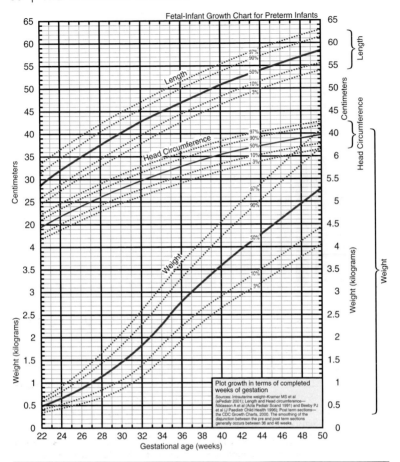

Figure 7.4. Fetal–infant growth chart for preterm infants (weight, head circumference, and length). SGA, small for gestational age; AGA, appropriate for gestational age; LGA, large for gestational age. (Reproduced with permission from Fenton TR; licensee BioMed Central Ltd. This is an open-access article: Verbatim copying and redistribution of this article are permitted in all media for any purpose, provided this notice is preserved along with the article's original URL. http://www.biomedcentral.com/1471-2431/3/13.)

36 and 46 weeks (see Fig. 7.4). This growth chart may not be appropriate for monitoring postnatal growth in infants >36 weeks' gestation. Using the simpler approach, one must recognize that the preterm infants are not likely to achieve the same growth rates as the fetuses of the same postmenstrual age used to generate the growth chart.

5. Increased rates of childhood illness and readmission to the hospital

IV. POSTTERM INFANTS

A. Definition. Approximately 6% (3% to 14%) of pregnancies extend beyond 42 weeks of gestation and are considered postterm. The rate of postterm pregnancies is heavily influenced by local obstetrical practices.

B. Etiology. Some cases of postterm pregnancy are the result of inaccurate dating of the pregnancy. In most cases, the cause of prolonged pregnancy is unknown. There is no association between maternal age or race and the incidence of postterm pregnancy. Risk factors for postterm pregnancies include the following:

1. Nulliparity

2. Previous postterm pregnancy

3. Obesity

4. Male fetus

5. Anencephaly. An intact fetal pituitary–adrenal axis appears to be necessary for the initiation of labor.

6. Trisomies 13 and 18

7. Seckel syndrome (bird-headed dwarfism)

C. Morbidities associated with postterm pregnancy include the presence of meconium-stained amniotic fluid, meconium aspiration, oligohydramnios, nonreassuring fetal heart rate tracing in labor, low Apgar scores, birth injury, fetal macrosomia, or fetal weight loss.

D. Postmaturity syndrome. Postterm infants have begun to lose weight but usually have normal length and head circumference. They may be classified as follows:

1. Stage 1
   a. Dry, cracked, peeling, loose, and wrinkled skin
   b. Malnourished appearance
   c. Decreased subcutaneous tissue
   d. Open-eyed and alert

2. Stage 2
   a. All features of stage 1
   b. Meconium staining of amniotic fluid (MSAF)
   c. Perinatal depression (in some cases)

3. Stage 3
   a. The findings in stages 1 and 2
   b. Meconium staining of cord and nails due to long-term exposure to MSAF
   c. A higher risk of fetal, intrapartum, or neonatal death

E. **Management**

1. **Antepartum management**

   a. Careful **estimation of true GA**, including ultrasonographic data

   b. **Antepartum assessments** by cervical examination and monitoring of fetal well-being (see Chapter 1) should be initiated between 41 and 42 weeks on at least a weekly basis. If fetal testing is not reassuring, delivery is usually initiated. In most instances, a patient is a candidate for induction of labor if the pregnancy is at >41 weeks of gestation and the condition of the cervix is favorable.

2. **Intrapartum management** involves use of fetal monitoring and preparation for possible perinatal depression and meconium aspiration.

3. **Postpartum management**

   a. **Evaluation for other conditions.** Infant conditions more frequently associated with postterm delivery include the following:

      i. Congenital anomalies

      ii. Perinatal depression

      iii. Persistent pulmonary hypertension

      iv. Meconium aspiration syndrome

      v. Hypoglycemia

      vi. Hypocalcemia

      vii. Polycythemia

   b. **Attention to proper nutritional support**

V. INFANTS WHO ARE SMALL FOR GESTATIONAL AGE OR INTRAUTERINE GROWTH RETARDATION (see Chapter 1)

A. **Definition.** Although many use the terms "small for gestational age" (SGA) and "intrauterine growth retardation" (IUGR) interchangeably, they refer to two subtly different populations. SGA describes a neonate whose birth weight or birth crown-heel length is <10th percentile for GA or <2 standard deviations (SDs) below the mean for the infant's GA (approximately the 3rd percentile for GA). IUGR describes diminished growth velocity in the fetus as documented by at least two intrauterine growth assessments (e.g., a fetus that is "falling off" its own growth curve). Babies who are constitutionally SGA are at overall lower risk compared to those who are IUGR due to some pathologic process. Numerous "normal birth curves" have been defined using studies of large infant populations (see Fig. 7.4); it should be noted that over the past 30 years, birth weight has increased in the general population. The etiology and management of SGA and IUGR fetuses overlaps considerably.

B. **Etiology.** Approximately one-third of LBW infants are also SGA/IUGR. There is an association between the following factors and SGA/IUGR infants:

1. **Maternal factors** include genetic size; demographics (age at the extremes of reproductive life, race/ethnicity, SES); nulliparity and grand multiparity status; underweight before pregnancy (e.g., malnutrition); uterine anomalies; chronic disease; factors interfering with placental flow and oxygenation (cardiovascular disease, renal disease, hypertension [chronic or pregnancy-induced]); sickle cell anemia; pulmonary disease; collagen-vascular disease; diabetes (classes D, E, F, and R);

autoimmune diseases; thrombotic disease (see Chapter 2); postterm delivery; high-altitude environment; exposure to teratogens including radiation; and alcohol, tobacco, or cocaine use.

2. **Placental and umbilical anatomical factors** include malformations (e.g., chorioangioma, infarction, circumvallate placenta, placental mosaicism, obliterative vasculopathy of the placental bed, vascular malformations, or velamentous umbilical cord insertion), infarction or focal lesions, abruption, suboptimal implantation site (e.g., low-lying placenta), previa, insufficient uteroplacental perfusion, and single umbilical artery.

3. **Fetal factors** include constitutional (normal, "genetically small"), malformations (e.g., abnormalities of CNS and skeletal system), chromosomal abnormality (<5% of SGA infants; more likely in the presence of malformation), congenital infection (i.e., rubella and cytomegalovirus [CMV]) (see Chapter 48), and multiple gestation.

C. **Management of Small for Gestational Age/Intrauterine Growth Retardation**

1. **Pregnancy** (see Chapter 1)

   a. Attempt to **determine the cause** of SGA/IUGR by searching for relevant factors (listed earlier) by history, laboratory, and ultrasonic examination. Treat any underlying cause (e.g., hypertension) when possible. Chronic fetal hypoxemia is encountered in about 30% of SGA/IUGR fetuses. Once the diagnosis is made, changes in obstetrical management may improve outcome.

   b. Monitor fetal well-being, including nonstress and oxytocin challenge testing, a biophysical profile, fetal movement counts, amniotic fluid volume evaluation, and serial ultrasonic examinations (see Chapter 1). Doppler evaluation of placental flow may be used to evaluate uteroplacental insufficiency.

   c. Consider the issue of **fetal lung maturity** if early delivery is contemplated (see Chapter 1).

2. **Delivery.** Early delivery is necessary if the risk to the fetus of remaining in utero is considered greater than the risks of preterm birth.

   a. Generally, **indications for delivery** are arrest of fetal growth and/or fetal distress, especially in the setting of pulmonary maturity near term.

   b. Acceleration of pulmonary maturity with glucocorticoids administered to the mother should be considered if amniotic fluid analyses suggest pulmonary immaturity or delivery is anticipated remote from term.

   c. If there is **poor placental blood flow**, the fetus may not tolerate labor and may require cesarean delivery.

   d. Infants with extreme SGA/IUGR are at **risk for perinatal problems** and often require specialized care in the first few days of life. Therefore, if possible, delivery should occur at a center with a NICU or special care nursery. The delivery team should be prepared to manage fetal distress, perinatal depression, meconium aspiration, hypoxia, hypoglycemia, and heat loss.

3. **Postpartum**

   a. If unknown, the etiology of SGA/IUGR should be investigated.

      i. Newborn examination. The infant should be evaluated for signs of any of the previously listed causes of poor fetal growth, especially chromosomal abnormalities, malformations, and congenital infection.

  a) Infants with growth restriction that affects the later part of pregnancy will have a relatively normal head circumference, some reduction in length, but a more profound reduction in weight. This is thought to be due to the redistribution of fetal blood flow preferentially to vital organs, mainly the brain; hence, the term "head-sparing IUGR." The Ponderal index ([cube root of birth weight in grams $\times$ 100]/[length in centimeters]) or the weigh-to-length ratio may be used to categorize growth-retarded infants into those with asymmetric growth retardation (low Ponderal index, weight for GA proportionately more affected than length) and symmetric growth retardation (normal Ponderal index, both weight and length affected). These infants may have little subcutaneous tissue, peeling loose skin, a wasted appearance, and meconium staining.

  b) Infants whose growth restriction began early in pregnancy will have proportionally small head circumference, length, and weight in contrast to IUGR that began later in pregnancy. These infants are sometimes referred to as *symmetrically IUGR* and their ponderal index may be normal. Symmetrical IUGR infants are more likely to have significant intrinsic fetal problems (e.g., chromosomal defects, malformations, and/or congenital infections acquired early in pregnancy).

  ii. Pathologic examination of the placenta for infarction, congenital infection, or other abnormalities may be helpful.

  iii. Because of potential for hearing loss associated with infection, it is reasonable to screen SGA/IUGR infants for CMV. Screening for other congenital infection is often part of routine testing with the newborn screen. Other **serologic screening** for congenital infection is generally not indicated unless history or examination is suggestive of infection.

b. SGA infants generally require **more calories per kilogram** than appropriate for gestational age (AGA) infants for "catch-up" growth; term SGA infants will often regulate their intake accordingly.

c. Potential complications related to SGA/IUGR

  i. Congenital anomalies
  ii. Perinatal depression
  iii. Meconium aspiration
  iv. Pulmonary hemorrhage
  v. Persistent pulmonary hypertension
  vi. Hypotension
  vii. Hypoglycemia from depletion of glycogen stores
  viii. Hypocalcemia
  ix. Hypothermia from depletion of subcutaneous fat
  x. Polycythemia
  xi. Neutropenia
  xii. Thrombocytopenia
  xiii. Dyslipidemia
  xiv. Acute tubular necrosis/renal insufficiency

D. Outcomes of SGA/IUGR infants. At the same birth weight, SGA/IUGR infants have a lower risk of neonatal death compared with preterm AGA infants. Compared to AGA infants of the same GA, SGA/IUGR infants have a higher incidence of neonatal morbidity and mortality. In general, SGA/IUGR infants and children (especially those from disadvantaged socioeconomic environments) are at higher risk for poor postnatal growth, neurologic impairment, delayed cognitive development, and poor academic achievement. Finally, some adults who were SGA/IUGR at birth appear to have a higher risk of coronary heart disease, hypertension, non–insulin-dependent diabetes, stroke, obstructive pulmonary disease, renal impairment, decreased reproductive function, as well as other health risks and growth-related psychosocial issues.

E. Management of subsequent pregnancies is important because SGA and IUGR will often reoccur. The mother should be cared for by personnel experienced in handling high-risk pregnancies. The health of mother and fetus should be assessed throughout pregnancy with ultrasonography and nonstress tests (see Chapter 1). Early delivery should be considered if fetal growth is poor.

VI. INFANTS WHO ARE LARGE FOR GESTATIONAL AGE (see Chapter 1)

A. Definition. As with SGA, there is no uniform definition of LGA, although most reports define it as 2 SDs above the mean for GA or >90th percentile.

B. Etiology

1. Constitutionally large infants (large parents)

2. Infants of diabetic mothers (e.g., classes A, B, and C)

3. Beckwith-Wiedemann and other overgrowth syndromes

4. Some postterm infants

C. Management

1. Look for evidence of birth trauma, including brachial plexus injury and perinatal depression (see Chapters 6 and 55).

2. Allow the infant to feed early and monitor the blood sugar level. Some LGA infants may develop hypoglycemia secondary to hyperinsulinism (especially infants of diabetic mothers, infants with Beckwith-Wiedemann syndrome, or infants with erythroblastosis) (see Chapters 2 and 24).

3. Consider polycythemia (see Chapter 46).

VII. CORD BLOOD BANKING. The following text is summarized from the American Academy of Pediatrics and American College of Obstetricians and Gynecologists 2007 (see Chapter 42).

A. Prospective parents may seek information regarding umbilical cord blood banking. Balanced and accurate information regarding the advantages and disadvantages of public versus private banking should be provided. Health care providers should dispense the following information:

1. There is clinical potential of hematopoietic stem cells found in cord blood.

2. Where logistically possible, collection and support of umbilical cord blood for public banking is encouraged.

3. The indications for autologous (self) transplantation are limited.

4. Private cord blood banking should be encouraged when there is knowledge of a family member, particularly a full sibling, with a current or potential medical condition (malignant or genetic) that could potentially benefit from cord blood transplantation.

5. Storing cord blood as "biological insurance" should be discouraged because there currently is no scientific data to support autologous (self) transplantation.

Suggested Readings

Alsafadi TR, Hashmi SM, Youssef HA, et al. Polycythemia in neonatal intensive care unit, risk factors, symptoms, pattern, and management controversy. *J Clin Neonatol* 2014;3(3):93–98.

American Academy of Pediatrics, American College of Obstetricians and Gynecologists. *Guidelines for Perinatal Care.* 7th ed. Elk Grove Village, IL: American Academy of Pediatrics; Washington, DC: American College of Obstetricians and Gynecologists; 2012.

American Academy of Pediatrics Committee on Infectious Diseases. Updated guidance for Palivizumab prophylaxis among infants and young children at increased risk of hospitalization for respiratory syncytial virus infection. *Pediatrics* 2014;134(2):e620–e638.

Dancis J, O'Connell JR, Holt LE Jr. A grid for recording the weight of premature infants. *J Pediatr* 1948;33:570–572.

Doherty L, Norwitz ER. Prolonged pregnancy: when should we intervene? *Curr Opin Obstet Gynecol* 2008;20(6):519–527.

Goldstein M, Merritt TA, Phillips R, et al. National Perinatal Association 2015 Respiratory Syncytial Virus (RSV) Prevention Guideline. *Neonatology Today* 2014;9(11):1–12. http://www.neonatologytoday.net/newsletters/nt-nov14.pdf. Accessed May 12, 2016.

Grisaru-Granovsky S, Reichman B, Lerner-Geva L, et al. Population-based trends in mortality and neonatal morbidities among singleton, very preterm, very low birth weight infants over 16 years. *Early Hum Dev* 2014;90:821–827.

Hamilton BE, Martin JA, Osterman MJ, et al. Births: preliminary data for 2014. *Natl Vital Stat Rep* 2015;64(6):1–19.

Horbar JD, Carpenter JH, Badger GJ, et al. Mortality and neonatal morbidity among infants 501 to 1500 grams from 2000 to 2009. *Pediatrics* 2012;129(6):1019–1026.

Kimberlin DW, Long SS, Brady MT, et al. *Redbook: 2015 Report of the Committee on Infectious Diseases.* 30th ed. Elk Grove Village, IL: American Academy of Pediatrics; 2015.

Mandruzzato G, Antsaklis A, Botet F, et al. Intrauterine restriction (IUGR). *J Perinat Med* 2008;36(4):277–281.

Olsen IE, Groveman SA, Lawson ML, et al. New intrauterine growth curves based on United States data. *Pediatrics* 2010;125:e214–e244.

Saenger P, Czernichow P, Hughes I, et al. Small for gestational age: short stature and beyond. *Endocr Rev* 2007;28(2):219–251.

Woythaler MA, McCormick MC, Smith VC. Late preterm infants have worse 24-month neurodevelopmental outcomes than term infants. *Pediatrics* 2011;127(3):e622–e629.

Vohr B. Long-term outcomes of moderately preterm, late preterm, and early term infants. *Clin Perinatol* 2013;40(4):739–751.

8 Assessment of the Newborn History and Physical Examination of the Newborn

Lise Johnson

KEY POINTS

- The initial examination of the newborn is an important opportunity to detect congenital anomalies and assess the infant's transition from fetal to extrauterine life.
- Routine pulse oximetry screening to detect critical congenital heart disease (CCHD) is recommended for all newborns, ideally between 24 and 48 hours of age.
- All expectant parents dream of the healthy child and worry about the possibility of abnormality or illness in their infant. Most newborns have normal physical examinations and smooth transitions from fetal to extrauterine life; this is a source of delight and reassurance to families.

I. **HISTORY.** The family, maternal, pregnancy, perinatal, and social history should be reviewed (Table 8.1).

II. **ROUTINE PHYSICAL EXAMINATION OF THE NEONATE.** Although no statistics are available, the first routine examination likely reveals more abnormalities than any other physical examination. Whenever possible, the examination should be performed in the presence of the parents to encourage them to ask questions regarding their newborn and allow for the shared observation of physical findings both normal and abnormal.

A. **General examination.** At the initial examination, attention should be directed to determine (i) whether any congenital anomalies are present; (ii) whether the infant has made a successful transition from fetal life to air breathing; (iii) to what extent gestation, labor, delivery, analgesics, or anesthetics have affected the neonate; and (iv) whether the infant has any signs of infection or metabolic disease.

1. The infant should be undressed for the examination, ideally in a well-lit room under warming lights to avoid hypothermia which occurs easily in the neonatal period.

Table 8.1. Important Aspects of Maternal and Perinatal History

Family History

Inherited diseases (e.g., metabolic disorders, bleeding disorders, hemoglobinopathies, cystic fibrosis, polycystic kidneys, sensorineural hearing loss, genetic disorders or syndromes)

Developmental disorders including autism spectrum disorders

Disorders requiring follow-up screening in family members (e.g., developmental dysplasia of the hip, vesicoureteral reflux, congenital cardiac anomalies, familial arrhythmias)

Maternal History

Age

Gravidity and parity

Infertility treatments required for pregnancy, including source of egg and sperm (donor or parent)

Prior pregnancy outcomes (terminations, spontaneous abortions, fetal demises, neonatal deaths, prematurity, postmaturity, malformations)

Blood type and blood group sensitizations

Chronic maternal illness (e.g., diabetes mellitus, hypertension, renal disease, cardiac disease, thyroid disease, systemic lupus erythematosus, myasthenia gravis)

Infectious disease screening in pregnancy (rubella immunity status; syphilis, gonorrhea, chlamydia, and HIV screening; hepatitis B surface antigen screening, group B *Streptococcus* [GBS] culture, varicella, cytomegalovirus, and toxoplasmosis testing, if performed; purified protein derivative [PPD] status and any past treatments; any recent infections or exposures)

Inherited disorder screening (e.g., hemoglobin electrophoresis, glucose-6-phosphate dehydrogenase [G6PD] deficiency screening, "Jewish panel" screening, cystic fibrosis mutation testing, fragile X testing)

Medications

Tobacco, alcohol, and illegal substance use

Pregnancy complications (e.g., gestational diabetes mellitus, preeclampsia, infections, bleeding, anemia, trauma, surgery, acute illnesses, preterm labor with or without use of tocolytics or glucocorticoids)

Fetal Testing

First- and/or second-trimester screens for aneuploidy (serum markers and ultrasonographic examination)

Second-trimester (approximately 18 weeks) fetal survey by ultrasound

(continued)

Table 8.1. Important Aspects of Maternal and Perinatal History *(Continued)*

Genetic testing, including preimplantation, chorionic villus sampling, amniocentesis genetic testing and cell free fetal DNA testing

Ultrasound monitoring of fetal well-being

Tests of fetal lung maturity

Intrapartum History

Gestational age at parturition and method of calculation (e.g., ultrasound, artificial insemination or *in vitro* fertilization, last menstrual period)

Presentation

Onset and duration of labor

Timing of rupture of membranes and appearance of amniotic fluid (volume, presence of meconium, blood)

Results of fetal monitoring

Fever

Medications, especially antibiotics, analgesics, anesthetics, and magnesium sulfate

Complications (e.g., excessive blood loss, chorioamnionitis, shoulder dystocia)

Method of delivery

Infant delivery room assessment including Apgar scores and any resuscitation measures required

Placental examination

Social History

Cultural background of family

Marital status of mother

Nature of involvement of father of baby

Household members

Custody of prior children

Maternal and paternal occupations

Identified social supports

Current social support service involvement

Past or current history of involvement of child protective agencies

Current or past history of domestic violence

2. Care providers should develop a consistent order to their physical examination, generally beginning with the cardiorespiratory system which is best assessed when the infant is quiet. If the infant being examined is fussy, a gloved finger to suck on may be offered. The opportunity to perform the eye examination should be seized whenever the infant is noted to be awake and alert.

B. Vital signs and measurements. Vital signs should be taken when the infant is quiet, if possible.

1. **Temperature.** Temperature in the neonate is usually measured in the axilla. Rectal temperature can be measured to confirm an abnormal axillary temperature, although they tend to correlate quite closely. Normal axillary temperature is between 36.5° and 37.4°C (97.7° and 99.3°F)

2. **Heart rate.** Normal heart rate in a newborn is between 95 and 160 bpm. Vagal slowing may be noted and appreciated as a reassuring sign. Some infants, particularly those born postdates, may have resting heart rates as low as 80 bpm. Good acceleration with stimulation should be verified in these infants. A normal blood pressure is reassuring that cardiac output is adequate in the setting of marked sinus bradycardia.

3. **Respiratory rate.** Normal respiratory rate in a newborn is between 30 and 60 breaths per minute. Periodic breathing is common in newborns; short pauses (usually 5 to 10 seconds) are considered normal. Apneic spells (defined as 20 seconds or longer) associated with cyanosis and/or bradycardia are not normal in term infants and deserve further evaluation (see Chapter 31).

4. **Blood pressure.** Blood pressure is not routinely measured in otherwise well newborns. When measurement of blood pressure is clinically indicated, care should be taken that the proper neonatal cuff size is chosen and the extremity used is documented in the blood pressure recording. A gradient between upper and lower extremity systolic pressure >10 mm Hg should be considered suspicious for coarctation or other anomalies of the aorta (see Chapter 41).

5. **Pulse oximetry.** Mild cyanosis can be easily overlooked in newborns, particularly those with darker skin pigmentation. Multiple studies over more than a decade have assessed the role of pulse oximetry to improve the detection of CCHD in neonates before hospital discharge. The results of these studies have led the U.S. Department of Health and Human Services and the American Academy of Pediatrics to recommend universal pulse oximetry screening in the newborn nursery. Recommended strategies include screening between 24 and 48 hours of age, ensuring staff are properly trained in pulse oximetry measurement, and using later generation pulse oximeters which are less sensitive to motion artifact. Criteria for a positive screening test that merits further clinical investigation for CCHD include (i) any oxygen saturation measure <90%; (ii) oxygen saturation <95% in the right hand and either foot on three measures, each separated by 1 hour; or (iii) there is a >3% absolute difference in oxygen saturation between the right hand and foot on three measures, each separated by 1 hour.

6. **Measurements.** All newborns should have their weight, length, and head circumference measured shortly after birth. These measurements

should be plotted on standard growth curves such that the newborn may be determined to be appropriate for gestational age (AGA), small for gestational age (SGA), or large for gestational age (LGA). SGA or LGA newborns may require further evaluation of both the etiology and sequelae of these conditions (see Chapter 7). Newborns with extensive molding and/or caput may require a repeat head circumference measurement a few days after birth.

C. Cardiorespiratory system

1. **Color.** The healthy newborn should have a reddish pink hue, except for the possible normal cyanosis of the hands and feet (acrocyanosis). Excessive paleness or ruddiness should prompt hematocrit measurement to detect relative anemia (hematocrit <42%) or polycythemia (hematocrit >65%), respectively (see Chapters 45 and 46).

2. **Respiratory pattern.** The majority of the neonatal respiratory examination may be performed visually without the use of a stethoscope. At rest, a newborn past initial transition should exhibit unlabored breathing without grunting (self-generated positive end-expiratory pressure [PEEP]), nasal flaring (decrease in airway resistance), or intercostal retractions (chest wall stabilization). Significant respiratory disease in the absence of tachypnea is rare unless the infant also has severe central nervous system depression. Rales, decreased breath sounds, decreased or displaced heart sounds, or asymmetry of breath sounds are occasionally found by auscultation in an asymptomatic infant and may reveal occult disease that should be confirmed by chest x-ray (e.g., pulmonary edema, neonatal pneumonia, pneumothorax, pneumomediastinum, dextrocardia).

3. **Heart.** The examiner should observe precordial activity, rate, rhythm, the quality and intensity of heart sounds, and the presence or absence of murmurs.

   a. It should be determined whether the heart is on the left or right side of the chest by palpation of the point of maximum impulse (PMI) and auscultation.

   b. Arrhythmias, most often due to premature atrial contractions, are occasionally heard on the routine newborn examination. An electrocardiogram (EKG) with rhythm strip should be obtained to identify the etiology of the arrhythmia and screen for evidence of structural disease.

   c. The heart sounds should be auscultated, with attention paid to the reassuring presence of a split second heart sound (evidence of the presence of two semilunar valves), detection of any gallops (an ominous finding that deserves further evaluation), and detection of ejection clicks which may indicate pulmonary or aortic valve stenosis or a bicuspid aortic valve.

   d. Murmurs in newborns can be misleading. Systolic murmurs are frequently heard transiently in neonates without significant structural heart disease, particularly as the ductus arteriosus is closing or in those with mild pulmonary branch stenosis. On the other hand, a newborn with serious, hemodynamically significant heart disease may have no murmur. Diastolic murmurs should always be considered abnormal. In an otherwise asymptomatic infant with a persistent or otherwise concerning murmur (e.g., loud, harsh, pansystolic, diastolic), investigation should include an EKG, pre- and postductal oxygen saturation measurement, and four extremity blood pressure measurement. A plain chest x-ray may also be considered. In consultation with a pediatric cardiologist, echocardiogram may also be obtained if available. Where echocardiography is not available, a hyperoxia test should be obtained to determine the presence of cyanotic heart disease and the potential need for institution of prostaglandin E1 (see Chapter 41).

e. Femoral pulses should be palpated, although, often, they are weak in the first day or two after birth. Femoral pulses are most easily appreciated if the infant is calm. If there is doubt about the femoral pulses by the time of discharge, the blood pressure in the upper and lower extremities should be measured to investigate the concern for coarctation of the aorta.

D. Thorax

1. The clavicles should be palpated. Crepitus or, less commonly, a "step off" may be appreciated in the presence of a clavicle fracture. Clavicle palpation should always be repeated on the discharge examination because some fractures may be more apparent on the second or third day of life. On follow-up examinations after hospital discharge, a healed clavicle fracture may leave a firm bump on the bone. No special care beyond gentle handling to avoid pain in the first neonatal days is required for clavicle fractures, which generally heal uneventfully and without sequelae. Undoubtedly, many fractured clavicles in the newborn period occur unnoticed.

2. The thorax should be inspected for shape and symmetry. One or more accessory nipples in the mammary line may be noted occasionally. Tiny periareolar skin tags which generally dry up and fall off in the first days of life may also be noted. Breast buds due to the influence of maternal hormones can normally be palpated in term newborns. Parents will sometimes need reassurance that the tip of the xiphoid process, which can be quite prominent in the newborn, is also a normal finding.

E. Abdomen. The abdominal examination of a newborn differs from that of older infants in that observation can again be used to greater advantage.

1. The anterior abdominal organs, particularly bowel, can sometimes be seen through the abdominal wall, especially in thin or premature infants. Diastasis rectus abdominis is frequently seen in neonates, most evident during crying. Asymmetry due to congenital anomalies or masses is often first appreciated by observation.

2. When palpating the abdomen, start with gentle pressure or stroking, moving from lower to upper quadrants to reveal edges of the liver or spleen. The normal liver edge may extend up to 2.5 cm below the right costal margin. The spleen is usually not palpable. Remember there may be situs inversus.

3. After the abdomen has been gently palpated, deep palpation is possible, not only because of the lack of developed musculature but also because there is no food and little air in the intestine. Kidneys may be palpated and abdominal masses may be appreciated, although the clinically meaningful yield of this portion of the examination may be low in the current age of fetal ultrasonography.

4. The umbilical stump should be inspected. The umbilical vein and one or two umbilical arteries should be identified. Discharge, odor, or periumbilical erythema should be noted, if present. Umbilical hernias are frequently seen in neonates and are generally benign and resolve spontaneously.

F. **Genitalia and rectum**

1. **Male**

   a. The **penis** almost invariably has marked phimosis. Stretched penile length <2.5 cm is abnormal and requires evaluation (see Chapter 63). If present, the degree of hypospadias should be noted as well as the presence and degree of chordee. Circumcision should be deferred to a urologist whenever hypospadias is identified.

   b. The **scrotum** is often quite large because it is an embryonic analog of the female labia and responds to maternal hormones. Hyperpigmentation of the scrotum should raise suspicion for one of the adrenogenital syndromes (see Chapter 63). The scrotum may also be enlarged due to the presence of a **hydrocele**, which can be identified as a transilluminating mass in either or both sides of the scrotum. Hydroceles are collections of peritoneal fluid in the scrotum due to patency of the processus vaginalis in fetal life. They are common and require no immediate action, although they should be monitored to ensure resolution in the first year of life. The **testes** should be palpated. The testes should be the same size and they should not appear blue (a sign of torsion) through the scrotal skin. Normal testicle size in a term newborn ranges from 1.6 cm (length) × 1.0 cm (width) up to 2.9 cm × 1.8 cm. Approximately 2% to 5% of term males will have an undescended testicle at birth, which should be followed for descent in the first months of life.

2. **Female**

   a. The **labia minora** and **labia majora** should be examined. The relative size of the labia majora and labia minora changes over the last weeks of gestation with labia minora receding in prominence as the fetus progresses to term. The labia majora of term newborn girls are frequently reddened and swollen due to the influence of maternal hormones, which are also responsible for a clear or white vaginal discharge in the first days of life. Occasionally, a small amount of blood (pseudomenses) accompanies the discharge after the first few days of life as maternal hormones in the neonate wane.

   b. The **vaginal introitus** should be examined and the hymen identified. The finding of an imperforate hymen, which can sometimes be difficult to distinguish from a paraurethral cyst, should prompt referral to a pediatric gynecologist for management. Hymeneal tags are commonly noted and their presence is of no clinical significance.

   c. The **clitoris**, which recedes in prominence with increasing gestational age, should be noted. Mean clitoral length in term infants ±1 *SD* is 4.0 ± 1.24 mm. Clitoral enlargement, particularly when there is accompanying hyperpigmentation, should raise suspicion for androgen excess (see Chapter 63).

3. The anus should be checked carefully for patency, position, and size. Occasionally, a large fistula is mistaken for a normal anus; upon closer examination, it may be noted that the fistula is positioned either anterior or posterior to the usual location of a normal anus.

G. **Skin.** There are numerous, mostly benign, skin findings commonly seen in newborns (see Chapter 65).

1. **Dryness**, sometimes accompanied by cracking or peeling of the skin, is common, especially in the postmature newborn.

2. **Milia**, which are inclusion cysts filled with keratinous debris, are tiny, discrete, often solitary, white papules commonly seen on the face and scalp. Milia resolve spontaneously in the first weeks to months of life.

3. **Sebaceous hyperplasia** appears as tiny yellowish white follicular papules most commonly clustered on the nose. These papules self-resolve in the first weeks of life.

4. **Erythema toxicum neonatorum** occurs in approximately half of full-term newborns. Classically, the lesions of erythema toxicum are yellowish papules on an erythematous base, prompting the name "flea bite" dermatitis. Presentations may range from a few scattered isolated lesions to extensive, sometimes confluent, areas of pustules or papules with surrounding erythema. When unroofed and scraped, the contents of the papules and pustules will contain eosinophils on Wright or Giemsa stain. Erythema toxicum most typically appears on the second or third day of life, waxes and wanes for a few days, and resolve within the first week of life.

5. **Nevus simplex or salmon patch** refers to a frequently seen capillary malformation located on the forehead (typically V-shaped), nape of the neck, eyelids, nose, and upper lip. Although most salmon patches on the face ("angel kisses") resolve in the first year or so, those on the nape of the neck ("stork bites") will sometimes persist.

6. **Transient pustular melanosis neonatorum (TPMN)**, most common in darker pigmented infants, consists of 2- to 10-mm fragile, neutrophil-containing pustules that spontaneously break, leaving a collarette of scales and underlying hyperpigmented macules which eventually (weeks to months) fade. Frequently, infants at birth will be found to have the hyperpigmented macules of TPMN with the pustular phase having presumably occurred *in utero*. TPMN may sometimes need to be distinguished from bacterial (usually staph) pustules which are generally larger than TPMN, yield positive cultures, and are not associated with the typical hyperpigmented macules.

7. **Dermal melanocytosis**, commonly seen in darker skinned and Asian individuals, consists of dermal collections of melanocytes that appear as varying size macules or patches of black, gray, or slate blue skin, most often on the buttocks, although many other locations are also possible. It is prudent to make note of dermal melanocytosis on the newborn examination so that there is no confusion in the future with traumatic bruises.

8. **Sucking blisters** are occasionally on the hand or forearm of a newborn at birth. They resolve without incident and should not be a cause for concern.

9. The presence of **jaundice** on examination in the first 24 hours of life is not normal and should prompt further evaluation. Some degree of jaundice after the first day of life is common (see Chapter 26).

H. Palpable **lymph nodes** are found in approximately one-third of normal neonates. They are usually <12 mm in diameter and are often found in the inguinal, cervical, and, occasionally, the axillary area. Excess lymphadenopathy should prompt further evaluation.

I. **Extremities, joints, and spine** (see Chapter 58)

1. **Extremities.** Anomalies of the digits, such as polydactyly (especially postaxial polydactyly which is sometimes familial), clinodactyly, or some degree of webbing or syndactyly are seen relatively frequently. Palmar creases should be examined. Approximately 4% of individuals have a single palmar crease on one hand. Bilateral single palmar creases are less common but need not prompt concern unless associated with other dysmorphic features. Because of fetal positioning, many newborns have forefoot adduction, tibial bowing, or even tibial torsion. Forefoot adduction, also known as metatarsus adductus, will often correct itself within weeks and may be followed expectantly with stretching exercises. Mild degrees of tibial bowing or torsion are also normal. Talipes equinovarus, or clubfoot, always requires orthopedic intervention which should be sought as soon as possible after birth (see Chapter 58).

2. **Joints.** All newborns should be examined for the presence of developmental dysplasia of the hips. Hip "clunks" can be sought by both the Barlow maneuver, which causes posterior dislocation of an unstable hip, and the Ortolani maneuver, which causes reduction of the dislocation. Hip "clicks," due to movement of the ligamentum teres in the acetabulum, are much more common than hip "clunks" and not a cause for concern.

3. **Spine.** The infant should be turned over and suspended face down with the examiner's hand supporting the chest. The back, especially the lower lumbar and sacral areas, should be examined. Special care should be taken to look for pilonidal sinus tracts, skin findings, or small soft midline swellings that might indicate a small meningocele or other anomaly (see Chapter 57). Simple, blind-ending midline sacral dimples, a common finding, need no further evaluation unless they meet high-risk criteria for spinal dysraphism including being deep, >0.5 cm, are located >2.5 cm from the anal verge, or are associated with other cutaneous markers.

J. **Head and neck**

1. **Head**

   a. Scalp. The scalp should be inspected for cuts, abrasions, or bruises from the birth process. Particular note should be made of puncture wounds from the application of fetal monitor leads because these may occasionally become infected and require further attention. Rarely, cutis aplasia congenita or a nevus sebaceous may also be identified.

   b. Swelling. Swelling should be noted and identified, distinguishing between **caput succedaneum**, **cephalohematomas**, and **subgaleal hemorrhage**. Caput succedaneum, often boggy in texture, is simply soft tissue swelling from the birth process. Caput is most commonly located occipitally, although it may also have a "sausage" shape in the parietal area, may cross suture lines, and most often resolves within a day or two. Cephalohematomas, more common in the setting of an instrumented vaginal birth and most often involving one of the parietal bones, are the result of subperiosteal bleeding and, thus, do not cross suture lines. Cephalohematomas may initially be obscured by overlying caput and become increasingly apparent over the first 3 to 4 days of life. They are typically more tense to palpation than caput and may take weeks to even months to fully resolve. Cephalohematomas are a source of excess bilirubin production, which may contribute to neonatal jaundice. Subgaleal hemorrhages, also associated with vacuum extractions but much rarer in incidence, result from bleeding underneath the aponeurosis of the occipitofrontalis muscle and, classically, result in very loose, soft swelling which may flow freely from the nape of the neck to the forehead. It may even be possible to generate a fluid wave across the swelling from a subgaleal hemorrhage. If a subgaleal hemorrhage is suspected, the newborn should be carefully monitored for possible hemodynamically significant bleeding within the hemorrhage.

c. Skull bones. The skull bones (occipital, parietal, and frontal) should be examined, and suture lines (sagittal, coronal, lambdoidal, and metopic) should be palpated. Mobility of the sutures will rule out craniosynostosis. Mobility can be appreciated by placing one's thumbs on opposite sides of the suture and then pushing in alternately while feeling for motion. Any molding of the skull bones, which resolves over the first days of life, should be noted. The skull should also be observed for deformational plagiocephaly and, when present, positioning instructions to aid in its resolution should be given. Occasionally, craniotabes may be found, with palpation of the skull bones (usually the parietal bones) resulting in an indenting similar to the effect of pressing on a ping pong ball. Craniotabes generally resolves in a matter of weeks with no further evaluation necessary if an isolated finding.

d. Fontanelles. The fontanelles should be palpated. As long as the head circumference is normal and there is motion of the suture lines, one need pay little attention to the size (large or small) of the fontanelles. Very large fontanelles reflect a delay in bone ossification and may be associated with hypothyroidism (see Chapter 61), trisomy syndromes, intrauterine malnutrition, hypophosphatasia, and osteogenesis imperfecta. Fontanelles should be soft, particularly when the infant is in an upright or sitting position. Tense or full fontanelles should raise concern for elevated intracranial pressure due to such causes as meningitis or acute intracranial bleeding.

2. **Eyes**

The eyes should be examined for the presence of scleral hemorrhages, icterus, conjunctival exudate, iris coloring, extraocular muscle movement, and pupillary size, equality, reactivity, and centering. The red reflex should be assessed and cataracts ruled out. Of note, cataracts may cause photophobia resulting in difficulty obtaining cooperation from the infant in maintaining his or her eyes open for the examination. Puffy eyelids sometimes make examination of the eyes impossible. If so, this fact should be noted so that the eyes will be examined on follow-up.

3. **Ears**

Note the size, shape, position, and presence of auditory canals as well as preauricular sinus, pits, or skin tags.

4. **Nose**

The nose should be inspected, noting any deformation from *in utero* position, patency of the nares, or evidence of septal injury.

5. **Mouth**

The mouth should be inspected for palatal clefts. **Epstein pearls** (small white inclusion cysts clustered about the midline at the juncture of the hard and soft palate) are a frequent and normal finding. Much less common findings include mucoceles of the oral mucosa, a sublingual ranula, alveolar cysts, and natal teeth. The lingual frenulum should also be inspected and any degree of ankyloglossia noted.

6. **Neck**

Because newborns have such short necks, the chin should be lifted to expose the neck for a thorough assessment. The neck should be checked for range of motion, goiter, and thyroglossal and branchial arch sinus tracts.

K. Neurologic examination. In approaching the neurologic examination of the neonate, the examiner must be at once humble and ambitious. On the one hand, severe neurologic anomalies may be inapparent on examination in the newborn. Also, good evidence of the prognostic significance of the neonatal neurologic examination is lacking. On the other hand, with a trained eye, a broad range of clinically relevant observations can be made of the newborn's neurologic system. Categorizing neurobehavioral observations into four systems—autonomic, motor, state, and responsiveness—allows the clinician to capture nuances of a newborn's competence or vulnerability, regulation or dysregulation, maturity or immaturity, as well as identify evidence of neurologic injury or impairment, if present.

1. Examination of the neonatal **autonomic system** includes evaluation of vital sign stability, neurocutaneous stability (pink color vs. mottling or cyanosis), gastrointestinal stability, and the presence or absence of jitteriness or myoclonic jerks. Marked jitteriness should be investigated for etiologies including hypoglycemia, hypocalcemia, hypomagnesemia, or withdrawal from *in utero* exposure to drugs including opiates, cocaine, tobacco, or selective serotonin reuptake inhibitor (SSRIs) (see Chapter 12). Sneezes, hiccups, and frequent yawns may also be considered subtle expressions of autonomic stress in the neonate and are very commonly seen in normal term infants. Many of the items on the Finnegan Neonatal Abstinence Score are signs and symptoms of autonomic dysregulation.

2. Assessment of the **motor system** begins with noting extremity and axial tone, particularly looking for asymmetries, such as those seen in brachial plexus injuries. An asymmetric grimace during crying may indicate injury to the seventh cranial nerve (especially if accompanied by incomplete ipsilateral eyelid closure) or congenital absence or hypoplasia of the depressor angularis oris muscle, a condition that becomes less noticeable over time. Self-regulatory motor activities such as hand-to-mouth efforts, tucking, bracing, grasping, or dysregulatory motor activities such as arching, flailing, hand splaying, should also be noted. The motor portion of the neurologic examination is completed by elicitation of the primitive reflexes including palmar and plantar grasp, Babinski, Moro response, root, suck, Galant, tonic neck reflex,

stepping, and placing and observation of the quality and quantity of the infant's motor activity.

3. The six behavioral states of the newborn are deep sleep, light sleep, drowsiness, quiet alertness, active alertness (or fussing), and crying. Aspects of the **state system** that can be observed include the clarity of the infant's states, the range of states displayed, the way in which the newborn moves between states, the ability to protect sleep from outside stimulation, and the quality of crying and ability to be consoled.

4. Finally, the newborn's **responsiveness** to the outside world can be observed. The ability to engage socially may be noted, including the ability to fix on and follow a face and voice. Response to inanimate stimuli such as the ability to fix on and follow a small, high-contrast object (such as a bright red ball) or respond to a sound such as a bell or rattle can also be observed.

L. **Summary.** All expectant parents hope for a healthy child and worry about the possibility of abnormality or illness in their infant. Whether the newborn examination is performed with the parents or alone in the nursery, the care provider should summarize the findings of the initial assessment for the parents. Most newborns have normal physical examinations and smooth transitions from fetal to extrauterine life; although perhaps mundane knowledge for care providers, this is a source of delight and reassurance to the family. When problems or abnormalities are uncovered in the initial newborn assessment, it is of critical importance that they are discussed clearly and sensitively with parents, including any plans for further evaluation, monitoring, or treatment.

Suggested Readings

Brazelton TB, Nugent JK. *Neonatal Behavioral Assessment Scale.* 4th ed. London, United Kingdom: Mac Keith Press; 2011.

Chou J. PediTools: clinical tools for pediatric providers. http://www.peditools.org/. Accessed May 16, 2016.

Eichenfeld LF, Frieden IJ, Esterly NB. *Neonatal Dermatology.* 2nd ed. Philadelphia, PA: WB Saunders; 2008.

Kemper AR, Mahle WT, Martin GR, et al. Strategies for implementing screening for critical congenital heart disease. *Pediatrics* 2011;128:e1259–e1267.

Mayfield SR, Bhatia J, Nakamura KT, et al. Temperature measurement in term and preterm neonates. *J Pediatr* 1984;104:271–275.

Nugent JK, Keefer CH, Minear S, et al. *Understanding Newborn Behavior and Early Relationships: The Newborn Behavioral Observations (NBO) System Handbook.* Baltimore, MD: Paul H. Brookes; 2007.

Stanford School of Medicine. Newborn Nursery at LPCH professional education. http://newborns.stanford.edu/RNMDEducation.html. Accessed May 16, 2016.

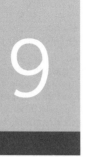

Care of the Well Newborn

Heena K. Lee and Elizabeth Oh

KEY POINTS

- Family-centered maternity care helps promote the initiation of breastfeeding and early bonding.
- Routine care of the well newborn includes important screening and prevention measures.
- The hospital stay of the mother and her newborn allows identification of early problems, ensures that the mother is prepared to care for the infant at home, and reduces the risk of readmission.

I. **ADMISSION TO THE NEWBORN NURSERY.** Healthy newborns may room-in with their mothers all or nearly all the time while they remain in the hospital. Every effort should be made to avoid separation of mother and infant especially during the first hour of life (the "golden hour") in order to promote immediate initiation of breastfeeding and early bonding through skin-to-skin contact. Delaying birth weight measurements is acceptable to allow the opportunity to breastfeed. These recommendations follow the global Baby-Friendly Initiative of the World Health Organization (WHO) and the United Nations Children's Fund (UNICEF) to strengthen maternity practices and improve exclusive breastfeeding. Family-centered maternity care, in which the nurse cares for the mother and baby together in the mother's room (couplet care), facilitates teaching and helps support this Baby-Friendly Initiative.

A. Criteria for admission to the normal newborn nursery or couplet care with the mother vary among hospitals. The minimum requirement typically is a well-appearing infant of at least 35 weeks' gestational age, although some nurseries may specify a minimum birth weight, for example, 2 kg.

B. Security in the nursery and mother's room is necessary to protect the safety of families and to prevent the abduction of newborns.

1. Many nurseries use electronic security systems to track newborns.

2. Identification (ID) bands with matching numbers are placed on the newborn, mother, and father/partner/support person as soon after birth as possible. Transport of infants between areas should not occur until ID banding has been confirmed.

3. All staff are required to wear a picture ID badge, and parents should be instructed to allow the infant to be taken only by someone wearing an appropriate ID badge.

II. TRANSITIONAL CARE

A. The transitional period is usually defined as the first 4 to 6 hours after birth. During this period, the infant's pulmonary vascular resistance decreases, blood flow to the lungs is greatly increased, overall oxygenation and perfusion improve, and the ductus arteriosus begins to constrict or close.

B. Interruption of normal transitioning, usually due to complications occurring in the peripartum period, will cause signs of distress in the newborn.

C. Common signs of disordered transitioning are the following:

1. Respiratory distress $+/-$ cyanosis

2. Poor perfusion

D. Transitional care of the newborn can take place in the mother's room or in the nursery.

1. Infants are evaluated for problems that may require a higher level of care, such as gross malformations and disorders of transition.

2. The infant should be evaluated every 30 to 60 minutes during this period. This evaluation includes the assessment of heart rate, respiratory rate, and temperature; assessment of color and tone; and observation for signs of withdrawal from maternal medications.

3. When disordered transitioning is suspected, a hemodynamically stable infant can be observed closely in the normal nursery setting for a brief period of time. Infants with persistent signs of disordered transitioning require transfer to a higher level of care.

III. ROUTINE CARE

A. Rooming-in should be encouraged during the infant's hospital stay. When possible, physical assessments, administration of medications, routine laboratory tests, and bathing should occur in the mother's room. For family-centered maternity care, nursing ratios should not exceed 1:4 mother–baby couplets.

1. Upon admission to the nursery, the infant's weight, head circumference, and length are recorded. On the basis of these measurements, the infant is classified as average for gestational age (AGA), small for gestational age (SGA), or large for gestational age (LGA) (see Chapter 7).

2. If the gestational age of the infant is uncertain, an assessment of gestational age can be performed using the expanded Ballard score (see Chapter 7).

B. The infant's temperature is stabilized with one of the following modalities:

1. Skin-to-skin contact with the mother

2. Open radiant warmer on servo control

C. Universal precautions should be used with all patient contact.

D. The first bath is given with warm tap water and nonmedicated soap after an axillary temperature $>97.5°F$ has been recorded.

E. There are several acceptable practices for umbilical cord care. Dry cord care is generally sufficient and has not been shown to increase infection rates in developed countries. However, antiseptics, such as alcohol or triple dye, or topical antibiotics can be considered if there is concern for infection. Keeping the cord dry also promotes earlier detachment of the umbilical stump.

IV. ROUTINE MEDICATIONS

A. All newborns should receive prophylaxis against gonococcal ophthalmia neonatorum within 1 to 2 hours of birth, regardless of the mode of delivery. Prophylaxis is administered as a single ribbon of 0.5% erythromycin ointment bilaterally in the conjunctival sac (see Chapter 49). Although 1% tetracycline ointment is equally effective, it is not available in the United States.

B. A single, intramuscular dose of 0.5 to 1 mg of vitamin K (phytonadione) should be given to all newborns before 6 hours of age to prevent vitamin K deficiency bleeding (VKDB). Currently available oral vitamin K preparations are not recommended because late VKDB (which occurs at 2 to 12 weeks of age) is best prevented by the administration of parenteral vitamin K (see Chapter 43).

C. Administration of the first dose of preservative-free, single-antigen hepatitis B vaccine is recommended for all infants during the newborn hospitalization, even if the mother's hepatitis B surface antigen (HBsAg) test is negative (see Chapter 48).

1. Hepatitis B vaccine is administered by 12 hours of age when the maternal HBsAg is positive or unknown. Infants of HBsAg-positive mothers also require hepatitis B immune globulin (see Chapter 48).

2. The vaccine is given after parental consent as a single intramuscular injection of 0.5 mL of either Recombivax HB (5 μg) (Merck & Co, Inc, Whitehouse Station, New Jersey) or Engerix-B (10 μg) (GlaxoSmithKline Biologicals, Rixensart, Belgium).

3. Parents must be given a vaccine information statement (VIS) at the time the vaccine is administered. Updated VIS, in English and in other languages, is available at http://www.cdc.gov/vaccines/hcp/vis.

V. SCREENING

A. Prenatal screening test results should be reviewed and documented on the infant's chart at the time of delivery. Maternal prenatal screening tests typically include the following:

1. Blood type, Rh, antibody screen

2. Hemoglobin or hematocrit

3. Rubella antibody

4. HBsAg

5. Serologic test for syphilis (Venereal Disease Research Laboratory [VDRL] or rapid plasmin reagin [RPR])

6. Group B *Streptococcus* (GBS) culture

7. Human immunodeficiency virus (HIV)

   8. Gonorrhea and *Chlamydia* cultures

   9. Glucose tolerance test

   10. Antenatal testing results, including multiple marker screenings, and ultrasonography results

   11. Cystic fibrosis carrier testing

B. Screening for neonatal sepsis risk

   1. All newborns should be screened for the risk of perinatally acquired GBS disease (see Chapter 49) as outlined by the Centers for Disease Control and Prevention. Risk factors for early-onset neonatal sepsis include maternal GBS colonization in the genitourinary or gastrointestinal tract, gestational age <37 weeks, inadequate GBS prophylaxis, maternal intrapartum temperature ≥100.4°F (38°C), rupture of membranes >18 hours, and signs of chorioamnionitis.

   2. Penicillin is the preferred intrapartum chemotherapeutic agent. Intravenous intrapartum administration of penicillin, ampicillin, or cefazolin (for penicillin-allergic women without history of anaphylaxis) ≥4 hours before delivery provides adequate neonatal prophylaxis. Penicillin-allergic women at high risk for anaphylaxis should receive clindamycin or vancomycin; erythromycin is no longer recommended.

   3. The latest guideline from 2010 can be found at http://www.cdc.gov/groupbstrep/guidelines.

C. Cord blood screening

   1. Cord blood may be saved up to 30 days, depending on blood bank policy.

   2. A blood type and direct Coombs test (also known as direct antiglobulin test or DAT) should be performed on any infant born to a mother who is Rh-negative, has a positive antibody screen, or who has had a previous infant with Coombs-positive hemolytic anemia.

   3. A blood type and DAT should be obtained on any infant if jaundice is noted within the first 24 hours of age or there is unexplained hyperbilirubinemia (see Chapter 26).

D. Glucose screening

   1. Infants should be fed early and frequently to prevent hypoglycemia.

   2. Infants of diabetic mothers (see Chapter 2), infants who are SGA or LGA, and preterm infants should be screened for hypoglycemia in the immediate neonatal period (see Chapter 24).

E. Newborn metabolic screening

   1. The American Academy of Pediatrics (AAP), March of Dimes, and American College of Medical Genetics recommend universal newborn screening for specific disorders for which there are demonstrated benefits of early detection and efficacious treatment of the condition being tested (see Chapter 60).

   2. In the United States, newborn screening programs are operated at the state level in all 50 states, the District of Columbia, Guam, Puerto Rico, and the U.S. Virgin Islands.

3. The U.S. Secretary of Health and Human Services has established the Recommended Uniform Screening Panel (RUSP), which lists the disorders that these state-based screening programs should universally include. Currently, the RUSP contains 32 core conditions and 26 secondary conditions, such as congenital hypothyroidism, phenylketonuria, galactosemia, hemoglobinopathies, cystic fibrosis, as well as amino acid, fatty acid, and organic acid disorders. An updated list of screened conditions in each state can be found at http://www.babysfirsttest.org.

4. Routine collection of the specimen is between 24 and 72 hours of life.

F. Bilirubin screening

1. Before discharge, all newborns should be screened for the risk of subsequent development of significant hyperbilirubinemia. A predischarge serum or transcutaneous bilirubin measurement combined with risk factor assessment best predicts subsequent hyperbilirubinemia requiring treatment. A total serum bilirubin measurement can be obtained at the time of the newborn metabolic screen.

2. Risk factors for developing significant hyperbilirubinemia include hemolytic disease, prematurity, glucose-6-phosphate dehydrogenase (G6PD) deficiency, ethnicity (especially East Asian), presence of cephalohematoma or significant bruising, exclusive breastfeeding with weight loss, and a sibling history of phototherapy treatment.

3. Jaundice during the first 24 hours of life is considered pathologic and warrants a total serum bilirubin level.

4. The bilirubin result should be plotted and interpreted on an hour-specific nomogram to determine the need for phototherapy (see Chapter 26).

5. Parents should be given verbal and written information about newborn jaundice.

G. Hearing screening

1. Routine screening for hearing loss in newborns is mandated in most states (see Chapter 68) as outlined by the AAP and The Joint Committee on Infant Hearing.

2. Verbal and written documentation of the hearing screen results should be provided to the parents with referral information when needed.

H. Critical congenital heart disease screening

1. In 2011, the U.S. Secretary of Health and Human Services recommended that screening for critical congenital heart disease (CCHD) using pulse oximetry be added to the uniform newborn screening panel. This has been endorsed by the AAP, the American Heart Association, and the American College of Cardiology Foundation (see Chapter 41).

2. CCHDs are congenital heart defects requiring surgery or catheter intervention within the first year of life. In combination with a physical examination, pulse oximetry has been demonstrated to increase the ability to identify certain CCHDs in newborns prior to discharge from the hospital and, in some newborns, before audible murmurs or other symptoms appear.

3. Pulse oximetry screening (of pre- and postductal oxygen saturations) is most likely to help diagnose the following seven CCHDs:

a. Hypoplastic left heart syndrome

b. Pulmonary atresia

c. Tetralogy of Fallot

d. Total anomalous pulmonary venous return

e. D-transposition of the great arteries

f. Tricuspid atresia

g. Truncus arteriosus

4. Other CCHDs that may not be detected as consistently with pulse oximetry include coarctation of the aorta, double-outlet right ventricle, Ebstein anomaly, interrupted aortic arch, single ventricle, and L-transposition of the great arteries.

5. A normal pulse oximetry reading does not rule out all congenital heart diseases. Conversely, a low pulse oximetry reading does not always signify congenital heart disease; it may reflect a newborn's transitional postnatal circulation or a noncardiac disorder, such as sepsis or pulmonary process (transient tachypnea of the newborn, meconium aspiration syndrome, pneumonia, pulmonary hypertension of the newborn, pneumothorax).

VI. ROUTINE ASSESSMENTS

A. The physician should perform a complete physical examination within 24 hours of birth.

B. Vital signs, including respiratory rate, heart rate, and axillary temperature, are recorded every 8 to 12 hours.

C. Each urine and stool output is recorded in the infant's chart. The first urination should occur by 24 hours of age. The first passage of meconium is expected by 48 hours of age. Delayed urination or stooling is cause for concern and must be investigated.

D. Weights are recorded in the infant's chart. Weight loss in excess of 10% to 12% of birth weight, although common, should be investigated especially for exclusively breastfed newborns. Lactation support is important to help determine further management inpatient and outpatient. If caloric intake is thought to be adequate, organic etiologies should be considered, such as infection, metabolic or thyroid disorders.

VII. FAMILY AND SOCIAL ISSUES

A. Sibling visitation is encouraged and is an important element of family-centered care. However, siblings with fever, signs of acute respiratory or gastrointestinal illness, or a history of recent exposure to communicable diseases, such as influenza or chicken pox, are discouraged from visiting.

B. Social service involvement is helpful in circumstances such as teenage mothers; lack of, or limited, prenatal care; history of domestic violence; maternal substance abuse; history of previous involvement with child protective services or similar agency.

VIII. FEEDINGS. The frequency, duration, and volume of each feed will depend on whether the infant is feeding breast milk or formula. Details about each feeding session should be recorded in the infant's medical record.

  A. Exclusive breastfeeding for the first 6 months of a newborn's life has long been the goal of the WHO, U.S. Department of Health and Human Services, AAP, and the American College of Obstetricians and Gynecologists.

   1. Mothers should initiate breastfeeding as soon as possible after delivery, preferably in the delivery room, and then feed on demand, 8 to 12 times per day during the newborn hospitalization (see Chapter 22).

   2. Consultation with a lactation specialist during the postpartum hospitalization is strongly recommended for all breastfeeding mothers.

  B. Standard 19 or 20 cal/oz, iron-containing infant formula is offered to infants for whom breastfeeding is contraindicated, or at the request of a mother who desires to formula-feed. Unless contraindicated by a strong family history, lactose-containing formulas with milk protein (whey and casein) can be given to all newborns.

   1. Formula-fed infants are fed at least every 3 to 4 hours.

   2. During the first few days of life, the well newborn should consume at least 0.5 to 1 oz per feed.

IX. NEWBORN CIRCUMCISION

  A. The AAP states that scientific evidence demonstrates potential medical benefits of newborn male circumcision; however, these data are not sufficient to recommend routine neonatal circumcision. Potential benefits are decreased incidence of urinary tract infection in the first year of life, decreased risk for the development of penile cancer, and decreased risk of acquiring sexually transmitted diseases, particularly HIV infection.

  B. Informed consent is obtained before performing the procedure. The potential risks and benefits of the procedure are explained to the parents.

   1. The overall complication rate for newborn circumcision is approximately 0.5%.

   2. The most common complication is bleeding (~0.1%) followed by infection. A family history of bleeding disorders, such as hemophilia or von Willebrand disease, needs to be explored with the parents when consent is obtained. Appropriate testing to exclude a bleeding disorder must be completed before the procedure if the family history is positive.

   3. The parents should understand that newborn circumcision is an elective procedure; the decision to have their son circumcised is voluntary and not medically necessary.

   4. Contraindications to circumcision in the immediate newborn period that may require further consultation include the following:
      a. Sick or unstable clinical status
      b. Premature infants. Circumcision should be delayed until infant is of adequate size to perform the procedure safely.

c. Diagnosis of a congenital bleeding disorder. Circumcision can be performed if the infant receives appropriate medical therapy before the procedure (i.e., infusion of factor VIII or IX).

d. Inconspicuous or "buried" penis

e. Anomalies of the penis, including hypospadias, ambiguity, chordee, or micropenis

f. Bilateral cryptorchidism. Circumcision should be delayed until cleared by a pediatric urologist.

C. Adequate analgesia must be provided for neonatal circumcision. If used, topical analgesia creams may cause a higher incidence of skin irritation in low birth weight infants compared with infants of normal weight. Therefore, penile nerve block techniques should be used in this group of newborns.

D. In addition to analgesia, other methods of comfort are provided to the infant during circumcision.

   1. Twenty-four percent sucrose on a pacifier, per nursery protocol, may be given as an adjunct to analgesia.

   2. The infant's upper extremities should be swaddled, and the infant placed on a padded circumcision board with restraints on the lower extremities only.

   3. Administration of acetaminophen before the procedure is not an effective adjunct to analgesia.

E. Circumcision in the newborn can be performed using one of three different methods:

   1. Gomco clamp

   2. Mogen clamp

   3. Plastibell device

F. Oral or written instructions explaining postcircumcision care should be given to all parents.

X. DISCHARGE PREPARATION

A. Parental education on routine newborn care should be initiated at birth and continued until discharge. Written information in addition to verbal instruction may be helpful, and in some cases, it is mandated. The following newborn issues should be reviewed at discharge:

   1. Adequacy of oral intake, particularly for breastfed infants. This includes a minimum of eight feeds per day; one wet diaper per day of age, constant at the sixth day of life; and at least one stool per day.

   2. Routine cord and skin care

   3. Routine postcircumcision care (when indicated)

   4. Signs of infant illness including fever, irritability, lethargy, or a poor feeding pattern

   5. Observation for neonatal jaundice

6. Safe sleep environment, such as supine positioning for sleep, using tight-fitting crib sheets, having no loose blankets or materials in the crib, and sleeping in proximity but not bed sharing

7. Appropriate installation and use of an infant car seat

8. Other infant safety matters, such as maintaining a smoke-free environment, checking smoke detectors, lowering the hot water temperature at home, and hand hygiene

B. Discharge readiness

1. Each mother–infant dyad should be evaluated to determine the optimal time of discharge.

2. The hospital stay of the mother and her newborn should be long enough to identify early problems and to ensure that she is able and prepared to care for the infant at home.

3. All efforts should be made to promote the simultaneous discharge of a mother and her infant.

C. The AAP recommends that the following minimum discharge criteria be met before any term newborn (37 0/7 to 41 6/7 weeks' gestation) is discharged from the hospital.

1. Clinical course and physical examination reveal no abnormalities that require continued hospitalization.

2. The infant's vital signs are documented to be within normal ranges (with appropriate physiologic variations) and stable for 12 hours preceding discharge.

3. The infant has urinated regularly and passed at least one stool spontaneously.

4. The infant has completed at least two successful feedings.

5. There is no excessive bleeding at the circumcision site for at least 2 hours.

6. The clinical significance of jaundice has been assessed and appropriate management and follow-up plans have been determined.

7. The infant has been adequately evaluated and monitored for sepsis based on maternal risk factors.

8. Maternal and infant laboratory tests have been reviewed.

9. The infant's initial hepatitis B vaccine has been administered.

10. The mother's vaccine status has been updated, including influenza (during the flu season) and tetanus toxoid, reduced diphtheria toxoid, acellular pertussis (Tdap).

11. Newborn metabolic, hearing, and CCHD screenings have been completed per hospital protocol and state regulations.

12. Parental competency to care for the newborn has been demonstrated.

13. Appropriate car safety seat has been obtained, and the parent has demonstrated proper infant positioning and use.

14. Family members or other support persons are available to mother and infant after discharge.

15. A physician-directed source of continuing health care (medical home) has been identified.

16. Family, environmental, and social risk factors have been assessed.

D. Late-preterm infants who are 35 0/7 to 36 6/7 weeks' gestation are often eligible for admission to the well newborn nursery or couplet care. However, they are at greater risk for morbidity and mortality than term infants and are more likely to encounter problems in the neonatal period such as jaundice, temperature instability, feeding difficulties, and respiratory distress. Late-preterm infants are usually not expected to meet the necessary competencies for discharge before 48 hours of age. AAP discharge criteria for late-preterm infants are similar to criteria developed for healthy term infants with the following additions:

1. Accurate gestational age has been determined.

2. A physician-directed medical home has been identified, and a follow-up visit has been arranged within 48 hours of discharge.

3. A formal evaluation of breastfeeding has been documented in the chart by trained caregivers at least twice daily since birth.

4. The infant has demonstrated 24 hours of successful feeding with the ability to coordinate sucking, swallowing, and breathing while feeding.

5. A feeding plan has been developed and is understood by the family.

6. The infant has passed a car safety seat test to observe for apnea, brady-cardia, or oxygen desaturation with results documented in the chart.

XI. FOLLOW-UP

A. For infants discharged before 48 hours of life, an appointment with a health care provider should be arranged within 48 hours of discharge. If early follow-up cannot be ensured, early discharge should be deferred.

B. For newborns discharged between 48 and 72 hours of age, outpatient follow-up should be within 2 to 3 days of discharge. Timing should be based on risk for subsequent hyperbilirubinemia, feeding issues, or other concerns.

C. The follow-up visit is designed to perform the following functions:

1. Establish a relationship with the medical home and verify the plan for health care maintenance.

2. Assess the infant's general state of health including weight, hydration, and degree of jaundice and identify any new problems.

3. Review feeding patterns; encourage and support breastfeeding.

4. Review adequacy of stool and urine patterns.

5. Provide referral for lactation support if feeding and elimination patterns are not reassuring.

6. Assess quality of mother–infant bonding.

7. Reinforce maternal or family education.

8. Review results of any outstanding laboratory tests.

9. Perform screening tests in accordance with state regulations.

10. Assess parental well-being and screen for maternal postpartum depression.

Suggested Readings

American Academy of Pediatrics Section on Breastfeeding. Breastfeeding and the use of human milk. *Pediatrics* 2012;129(3):e827–e841.

Benitz WE. Hospital stay for healthy term newborn infants. *Pediatrics* 2015;135(5):948–953.

Flaherman VJ, Schaefer EW, Kuzniewicz MW, et al. Early weight loss nomograms for exclusively breastfed newborns. *Pediatrics* 2015;135(1):e16–e23.

Verani JR, McGee L, Schrag SJ. Prevention of perinatal group B streptococcal disease: revised guidelines from CDC, 2010. *MMWR Recomm Rep* 2010;59(RR-10): 1–32. http://www.cdc.gov/groupbstrep/guidelines. Accessed May 17, 2016.

Warren JB, Phillipi CA. Care of the well newborn. *Pediatr Rev* 2012;33(1):4–18.

World Health Organization, United Nations Children's Fund. The baby-friendly hospital initiative. http://www.who.int/nutrition/topics/bfhi/en and http://www.babyfriendlyusa.org. Accessed May 17, 2016.

10 Genetic Issues Presenting in the Nursery

Carlos A. Bacino

KEY POINTS

- Approximately 1 in 20 newborns have a major birth defect.
- Evaluation includes a comprehensive medical/family history and physical examination.
- Testing should be targeted to a suspected etiology.

I. GENERAL PRINCIPLES

A. Approximately 4% to 5% of newborns have a major birth defect and require genetic evaluation. These birth defects or malformations can be sporadic or associated with other anomalies. Some children may have physical features consistent with a well-known syndrome, whereas others may have sporadic anomalies detected prenatally or postnatally. Other neonatal presentations include acidosis that occurs with some inborn errors of metabolism (IEM), unexplained seizures, extreme hypotonia, or feeding difficulties. Infants with ambiguous genitalia require a multidisciplinary evaluation involving clinicians from genetics, endocrinology, urology, pediatrics or neonatology, and psychology. A thorough clinical evaluation requires a detailed prenatal history, a family history, and a comprehensive clinical exam, often including anthropometric measurements.

B. Congenital anomalies are considered major or minor.

   1. **Major malformations** are structural abnormalities that have medical and cosmetic consequence. They may require surgical intervention. Examples include cleft palate and congenital heart disease such as tetralogy of Fallot.

   2. **Minor malformations** are anomalies with no medical or cosmetic significance. A single transverse palmar crease is an example, although most minor abnormalities are limited to the head and neck region. Minor anomalies may aid in the diagnosis or recognition of a specific syndrome. Infants with three or more minor malformations are at high risk for having a major malformation (20% to 25%) and/or a syndrome.

C. **Major and minor malformations are often part of patterns.**

1. A **syndrome** consists of a group of anomalies that are associated due to single or similar etiologies, with known or unknown cause, such as Down syndrome due to trisomy 21.

2. **Associations** are clusters of malformations that occur together more frequently than occur sporadically, such as VACTERL association (vertebral, anal, cardiac, tracheoesophageal fistula, renal, and limb—radial ray defects) where at least three anomalies are required for the diagnosis.

3. A **developmental field defect** consists of a group of anomalies resulting from defective development of a related group of cells (developmental field). In this case, the involved embryonic regions are usually spatially related but may not be contiguous in the infant. Holoprosencephaly affecting the forebrain and face is an example and secondary to an abnormality in a group of cells that form the rostral aspect of the prechordal mesoderm that will ultimately induce development of the forebrain and midface.

4. **Disruptions** are extrinsic events that occur during normal development. These events can compromise the fetal circulation and result in a major birth defect. An example of a disruption is amniotic bands that may result in amputation of digits or limbs.

5. **Deformations** can occur when physical forces act on previously formed structures. Examples of deformations include uterine crowding or oligohydramnios that results in plagiocephaly or clubfeet.

II. **INCIDENCE.** The Centers for Disease Control and Prevention (CDC) monitors rates of birth defects in the United States (http://www.cdc.gov/ncbddd/birthdefects/data.html). Approximately 1 of 33 children has a major birth defect. Infants with birth defects account for 20% of infant deaths.

III. **ETIOLOGY.** The etiology of approximately 50% of birth defects is unknown. Of the remainder, etiology is attributed as follows: 6% to 10% chromosomal, 3% to 7.5% single-gene Mendelian disorders, 20% to 30% multifactorial, and 4% to 5% environmental exposures. The development of more sensitive molecular technology is likely to establish etiology in more cases.

IV. **APPROACH TO THE INFANT WITH BIRTH DEFECTS**

A. A comprehensive history is an important step in evaluating an infant with a birth defect.

1. **Prenatal** history should include the following:
   a. Chronic maternal illnesses including diabetes (insulin- and non–insulin-dependent), seizures, hypertension, myotonic dystrophy, phenylketonuria, Graves disease (see Table 10.1 for prenatal exposures and effects).
   b. Drug exposures should include prescribed drugs, such as antihypertensives (angiotensin-converting enzyme inhibitors), seizure medications, antineoplastic agents (methotrexate), and illicit drugs (e.g., cocaine).

Table 10.1. Well-Recognized Human Teratogens

Exposure Type	Fetal Effect
Drugs	
Aminopterin/methotrexate	Growth restriction, clefting, syndactyly, skeletal defects, craniosynostosis, dysmorphic features
Retinoic acid	CNS defects, microtia, ID, conotruncal defects: VSD, ASD, TOF
Lithium	Ebstein anomaly
Propylthiouracil, iodine	Hypothyroidism
Warfarin	Skeletal anomalies, stippled epiphyses, nasal hypoplasia
ACE inhibitors	Skull defects, renal hypoplasia/agenesis
Alcohol	Fetal alcohol syndrome or alcohol-related neuro-developmental disorders
Thalidomide	Limb reduction defects
Valproic acid	Neural tube defects
Phenytoin	Dysmorphic features, nail hypoplasia, cleft lip and palate, ID, growth restriction
Diethylstilbestrol	Clear cell cervical cancer in female progeny
Cocaine	Vascular disruptions, CNS anomalies
Misoprostol (Cytotec)	Limb malformations, absent digits
Statins (HMG-CoA reductase inhibitor)	Limb defects, CNS abnormalities, congenital heart disease
Maternal conditions	
Maternal phenylketonuria	Microcephaly, ID
Myasthenia gravis	Neonatal myasthenia
Systemic lupus erythematosus	Cardiac conduction abnormalities
Diabetes	Neural tube defects, sacral agenesis, congenital heart disease, renal anomalies

(continued)

Table 10.1. Well-Recognized Human Teratogens *(Continued)*

Exposure Type	Fetal Effect
Other exposures	
Radiation	Miscarriage, growth restriction
Prolonged heat exposure	Microcephaly
Smoking	Growth restriction
Lead	Low birth weight, neurobehavioral and neuro-logic deficits
Mercury	CNS anomalies, neurobehavioral and neurologic deficits
Infections	
Varicella	Limb scars
Cytomegalovirus	Microcephaly, chorioretinitis, ID
Toxoplasmosis	Microcephaly, brain calcifications, ID
Rubella	Microcephaly, deafness, congenital heart disease, ID

CNS, central nervous system; ID, intellectual disability; VSD, ventricular septal defect; ASD, atrial septal defect; TOF, tetralogy of Fallot; ACE, angiotensin-converting enzyme

Other drugs that may result in birth defects include misoprostol (to in-duce abortions). Timing of the exposure is important. Teratogenic agents tend to have their maximum effect during the embryonal period, from the beginning of the fourth to the end of the seventh week postfertilization, with the exception of severe forms of holoprosencephaly when exposure may occur around or before 23 days (see Appendix B).

c. Infections and immunizations

d. Social history

e. Other exposures may include alcohol; physical agents such as x-rays, high temperature; chemical agents; tobacco (see Table 10.1).

f. Nutritional status

g. Fertility issues and use of reproductive assistance (e.g. history of mul-tiple miscarriages, *in vitro* fertilization [IVF] or medications to stimulate ovulation). Genetic disorders such as Beckwith-Wiedemann syndrome, Silver-Russell syndrome, and Angelman syndrome that can be caused by imprinting defects (epigenetic mutations) have been seen in children conceived by assisted reproductive technology using intracytoplasmic sperm injection (ICSI).

h. Multiple gestations (see Chapter 11)

i. Results of prenatal studies should be obtained including ultrasono-graphic and magnetic resonance imaging (MRI) and chromosome or microarray studies done on samples obtained by amniocentesis, chorionic villi sampling (CVS), or percutaneous umbilical blood sampling.

j. Results should be obtained from first- and second-trimester screening including triple and quad screens. First-trimester screening combines the use of nuchal translucency with serum levels of pregnancy-associated plasma protein A (PAPP-A) and human chorionic gonadotropin (hCG) measured as free beta subunit (β-hCG) or total hCG. The second-trimester screen includes alpha-fetoprotein (AFP), unconjugated estriol (uE3), free β-hCG for the triple screen, plus inhibin A, as part of the quad screen. A low maternal serum alpha-fetoprotein (MSAFP) level can be seen in trisomies 21, 18, and 13. A high MSAFP may be a sign of multiple gestation, open neural tube defect, abdominal wall defect, impending fetal death, congenital nephrosis, or epidermolysis bullosa. A high hCG can be seen with trisomy 21, whereas low hCG may occur with trisomies 18 and 13.

k. Noninvasive prenatal testing (NIPT) is slowly replacing the first- and second-trimester screens. This technique consists of the analysis of cell-free fetal DNA present in maternal serum. Many companies provide this analysis and mostly target the presence of common trisomies such as trisomy 21 (Down syndrome, sensitivity 99.3%) and trisomy 18 (sensitivity 97.4%). Sensitivity is lower for trisomy 13 (91.4%) and sex chromosome (91%). NIPT is used in high-risk situations such as advanced maternal age and abnormal ultrasound examinations. For low-risk presentations, conventional first- and or second-trimester screens are preferred. The American College of Obstetricians and Gynecologists recommends conventional screening methods as the most appropriate choice for first-line screening for most women in the general obstetric population.

l. Newer forms of NIPT include common microdeletions, e.g., 22q11.2 microdeletions (DiGeorge/velocardiofacial syndrome [VCFS]) and Wolf-Hirschhorn deletion.

m. Quality and frequency of fetal movements should be documented. Rapid and intense movements could be due to fetal seizures, whereas decreased movement can be seen with spinal muscular atrophy, Prader-Willi syndrome, and other congenital myopathies.

2. Family history should include the following questions:

a. Are there any previous children with multiple congenital anomalies?

b. What is the ethnicity of the parents? Some diseases are more prevalent in specific populations.

c. Is there consanguinity, or are the parents from the same geographic area? What is the population size of the parents' community? In cases of rare autosomal recessive disorders, the parents may be related.

d. Is there a history of infertility, multiple miscarriages, multiple congenital anomalies, neonatal deaths, or children with developmental delay? These can be secondary to a balanced chromosome rearrangement in one of the parents but unbalanced in the progeny.

3. Pre- and perinatal events should be evaluated:

a. What was the fetal presentation, and how and for how long was the head engaged? Was there fetal crowding, such as might occur with multiple gestation? Are there uterine abnormalities (e.g., septate uterus, myomatosis)? Various deformations, sagittal synostosis, and clubfeet can be caused by fetal constraints.

b. What was the growth pattern throughout gestation? Was there proportionate or disproportionate growth restriction?

c. What was the mode of delivery? Was there fetal distress or any events potentially leading to hypoxemia?

d. Placenta appearance: Is there evidence of placental infarcts? Is the umbilical cord normal? Inspection of the cord may reveal severe narrowing, clots, or knots.

4. **Neonatal events**

   a. What were the Apgar scores? Was resuscitation needed? Was intubation and ventilator assistance needed? Were there severe feeding difficulties necessitating parenteral nutrition or tube feedings? Were there neonatal seizures? Was there hypotonia or hypertonia?

B. **Physical examination**

1. **Anthropometric measurements.** The assessment of growth parameters is extremely valuable to determine growth patterns such as restriction, overgrowth, disproportion, or microcephaly. In addition, precise measurements of anatomic structures and landmarks can aid the diagnostic evaluation process. Examples are ear length, eye measurements for hypertelorism or hypotelorism (widely or closely spaced eyes), finger length, and internipple distance. Extensive reference tables for many of these measurements are available for children of all ages, including preterm infants starting at 27 weeks' gestation (see "Suggested Readings").

2. A thorough clinical evaluation is needed to document the presence of dysmorphic features: head shape (e.g., craniosynostosis, trigonocephaly, brachycephaly); ear shape (e.g., microtia, ear pits or tags) and positioning; midface hypoplasia, clefting, micrognathia, short neck; and limb anomalies (e.g., asymmetry, clinodactyly, brachydactyly, polydactyly). A good clinical description can aid the diagnosis as features can be matched to those in a database such as London Dysmorphology Database or Pictures of Standard Syndrome and Undiagnosed Malformations (POSSUM). Some physical findings can be obscured by aspects of clinical care such as endotracheal tube position and taping or intravenous armboard and tape over the limbs. In this case, the infant should be reexamined when these are no longer present.

3. Ancillary evaluations include a hearing screen (otoacoustic emissions testing) that is done typically before discharge from the nursery or neonatal intensive care unit (NICU) and an ophthalmologic evaluation.

C. **Laboratory studies**

1. Chromosome studies are typically performed on whole blood drawn into sodium heparin tubes. The T lymphocytes in the blood are stimulated with mitogens, cultured for 72 hours, placed on slides, and karyotyped through the help of banding techniques such as Giemsa trypsin G-banding (GTG). In extremely ill infants, those with immunosuppression, or who have low T-cell counts (as in DiGeorge syndrome), cell growth may be impaired and cell stimulation fails. In this case, it is preferable to perform a molecular-based assay such as array comparative

genomic hybridization (aCGH) (see following discussion). In the past, a punch skin biopsy would be performed to obtain chromosomes from skin fibroblasts, but this is no longer routinely done. The disadvantage of using skin fibroblasts is the delay of up to several weeks before a result is available. Chromosome studies on skin are reserved in some cases of suspected mosaicism. Chromosome studies can detect up to 5% of abnormalities. Tables 10.2 and 10.3 list the main clinical findings of the most common chromosome aneuploidies.

2. Fluorescent *in situ* hybridization (FISH) studies can be useful for the rapid detection of aneuploidies. These studies are done on unstimulated interphase cells, and the results are typically available in a few hours or overnight. Rapid FISH is used for evaluation in trisomies 13 and 18 and for sex chromosome testing in infants with ambiguous genitalia. More specific studies, such as FISH for SRY (the sex-determining region on the Y chromosome), require more time and are done on stimulated metaphase cells.

3. aCGH, also known as chromosome microarray, is a molecular technique that allows detection of DNA copy number losses (deletions) and copy number gains (duplications, triplications) of small genomic regions, sometimes even at the level of the exon. This study is based on the comparison of a known genome from a normal individual against the test sample and is often done with a matched sex control. Chromosome microarrays can detect 14% to 16% more abnormalities than conventional cytogenetic studies (regular karyotype). Disadvantages of microarray testing include failure to detect inversions, balanced chromosome translocations, and low-level mosaicism. Any loss or gain of genetic material must be confirmed by molecular techniques such as FISH, polymerase chain reaction (PCR), or multiplex ligation-dependent probe amplification (MLPA). Both parents must be studied after the confirmation to determine if one of them is a carrier and to aid with the interpretation of the finding(s) in case it is a polymorphic variant. Consultation with a cytogeneticist or clinical genetics specialist is essential to interpret abnormal array results. The most common microdeletion syndromes detected in newborns are described in Table 10.4.

4. DNA testing is mainly reserved for single-gene disorders. They are caused by inherited or new mutations and often transmitted in a Mendelian fashion, such as autosomal recessive, autosomal dominant, and/or X-linked disorders. Many of them can present in newborns as life-threatening disorders. These include spinal muscular atrophy; congenital adrenal hyperplasia (most commonly due to 21-hydroxylase deficiency); congenital myotonic dystrophy (only when inherited from an affected mother); osteogenesis imperfecta due to type I collagen mutations and other rare recessive forms (*CRTAP, LEPRE-1, PPIB*); holoprosencephaly due to mutations in *SHH* (accounts for 30% to 40%), *ZIC2, TGIF, SIX3, PTCH1, GLI2*; cystic fibrosis due to *CFTR* mutations; and autosomal recessive polycystic kidney disease. A number of IEM are Mendelian disorders. Other non–life-threatening single-gene disorders that can present in the newborn period include achondroplasia, due to FGR3 mutations, and nonsyndromic deafness, due to connexin 26 and connexin 30 mutations.

Table 10.2. Common Chromosome Anomalies (Aneuploidies)

	Trisomy 13	Trisomy 18	Trisomy 21	Turner Syndrome
Growth	Growth restriction	Growth restriction	Normal	Mild growth restriction
Craniofacial	Hypotelorism, cleft lip and palate, small malformed ears, colobomas, microphthalmia	Triangular facies, micrognathia, pointy rotated low set ears	Upslanting palpebral fissures, epicanthal folds, midface hypoplasia, small round ears, tongue thrusting	Frontal prominence, low posterior hairline
Neck	Short		Short, redundant skin	Short, webbed, pterygium, cystic hygroma
Central nervous system	Holoprosencephaly, microcephaly	Microcephaly	Microcephaly	Normal
Neurologic	Hypertonia, seizures, apnea	Hypertonia, apnea	Hypotonia	Normal tone, mild developmental delay
Heart	ASD, VSD	Multiple valvular anomalies	AV canal, VSD, ASD	Aortic coarctation
Abdominal	Multicystic kidneys, horseshoe kidneys, double ureters	Omphalocele, renal anomalies	Duodenal atresia, Hirschsprung disease	Horseshoe kidneys
Limbs	Polydactyly, nail dysplasia	Overlapping fingers, nail hypoplasia, rocker-bottom feet	Brachydactyly, 5th finger clinodactyly, single transverse palmar crease	Hand and feet lymphedema, deep-set nails
Skin	Scalp defects	Decreased subcutaneous tissue	Cutis marmorata	Multiple nevi

ASD, atrial septal defect; VSD, ventricular septal defect; AV, atrioventricular

Table 10.3. Other Common Chromosome Abnormalities

	Cri-du-chat Syndrome	Wolf-Hirschhorn Syndrome	1p36.3 Deletion Syndrome	Killian/Teschler–Nicola Syndrome (Pallister Mosaic Syndrome)
Chromosomal defect	Deletion of 5p15.2	Deletion of 4p16.3	Deletion of distal short arm of chromosome 1 (1p36.3)	Tetrasomy 12p; mosaicism for isochromosome 12p
Growth	Growth restriction	Growth restriction, FTT	Growth restriction, FTT	Normal or increased weight, later growth deceleration, macrocephaly
Craniofacial	Hypertelorism, round face, low-set ears, epicanthal folds, micrognathia	Hypertelorism, cleft palate, prominent glabella with Greek helmet warrior appearance	Thin horizontal eyebrows, midface hypoplasia, pointy chin, cleft lip/palate, large anterior fontanel	Hypertelorism, sparse hair on lateral frontal region, eyebrows and eyelashes, prominent forehead, chubby cheeks, thick lips, coarse features
Skin		Posterior scalp defects		Linear hyper and hypopigmented skin lesions
Central nervous System	Microcephaly	Microcephaly	Microcephaly	Polymicrogyria
Neurologic	High-pitched characteristic shrill cry (catlike), severe ID	Seizures that may improve with age, hypotonia, severe ID	Moderate-to-severe ID/absent speech, seizures	Seizures, hypotonia, contractures develop later, profound ID

(continued)

Table 10.3. Other Common Chromosome Abnormalities *(Continued)*

	Cri-du-chat Syndrome	Wolf-Hirschhorn Syndrome	1p36.3 Deletion Syndrome	Killian/Teschler–Nicola Syndrome (Pallister Mosaic Syndrome)
Heart		ASD, VSD	Cardiomyopathy	
Abdominal		Malrotation, absent gallbladder		Diaphragmatic hernia, imperforate anus
Limbs	Nail hypoplasia	Clubfeet, hyperconvex nails		Brachydactyly, broad digits
Genitourinary		Hypospadias, cryptorchidism, absent uterus		Hypospadias
Other			Sensorineural hearing loss	Mosaicism is often found in skin fibroblasts and rarely present in blood chromosomes.
Natural history	Severe ID, aggressive behavior, self-mutilation	Profound ID, major feeding difficulties sometimes require gastrostomy	Moderate to severe ID, seizures in 50% often improve, hearing loss leads to speech delays	Profound ID, no speech, seizures, joint contractures

FTT, failure to thrive; ID, intellectual disability; ASD, atrial septal defect; VSD, ventricular septal defect.

Table 10.4. Common Chromosome Microdeletions Ascertained in the Neonatal Period

	Prader-Willi Syndrome	DiGeorge Syndrome and Velocardiofacial Syndrome	Williams Syndrome	Miller-Dieker Syndrome
Chromosomal and genetic defect	15q11q13 deletion 70% UPD 20%–25% Imprinting center defect 5%	22q11.2 deletion	7q11.23 deletion	17p13.3 deletion
Critical gene(s) involved	SNRPN	TBX1	ELN (Elastin)	LIS-1
Growth	Normal birth weight, poor feeding, poor suck	Short stature	Short stature	IUGR
Craniofacial	Bitemporal narrowing, almond-shaped eyes	Prominent tubular nose, small ears, cleft palate, velopharyngeal incompetence (nasal regurgitation)	Supraorbital fullness, stellate pattern of the iris, long philtrum, everted lower lip	Microcephaly, bitemporal hollowing, furrow over mid-forehead, low-set ears
Abdomen		Absent/hypoplastic kidneys	Nephrocalcinosis, renal artery stenosis	Duodenal atresia, omphalocele
Central nervous system	Moderate-to-severe ID	Mild-to-moderate ID	Mild-to-moderate ID	Lissencephaly, agyria, pachygyria, heterotopias, absent corpus callosum, profound ID

(continued)

Table 10.4. Common Chromosome Microdeletions Ascertained in the Neonatal Period *(Continued)*

	Prader-Willi Syndrome	DiGeorge Syndrome and Velocardiofacial Syndrome	Williams Syndrome	Miller-Dieker Syndrome
Neurologic	Severe hypotonia in the first few weeks of life, poor feeding			Hypertonia, progressive spasticity, decerebrate posture, seizures
Heart	Normal	Conotruncal heart defects: VSD, ASD, tetralogy of Fallot, interrupted aortic arch	Supravalvular aortic stenosis,	Congenital heart defects
Limbs	Small hands and feet	Long digits	Normal	Normal
Skin	Lighter pigmentation than parents (in deletion cases)	Normal	Normal	Normal
Other		T-lymphocyte dysfunction: frequent infection	Hypercalcemia	
Natural history	Obesity and hyperphagia after 2–3 years	Normal life span	Normal life span	Death before age 2 years

UPD, uniparental disomy; IUGR, intrauterine growth restriction; ID, intellectual disability; VSD, ventricular septal defect; ASD, atrial septal defect.

5. Exome sequencing studies are performed in the clinical evaluation of children with multiple anomalies who had a normal chromosome microarray study. This test allows the sequencing of all the exons of the genome (20,000 genes approximately) in a single pass using next-generation sequencing, a technique that reads small stretches of DNA multiple times, making the results more robust. The exons code for proteins and are the best known components of the genes. Exome sequencing detects the etiology in approximately 26% in patients whose etiology was not detected by previous studies.

6. **Infection.** Toxoplasmosis, other, rubella, cytomegalovirus, herpes simplex (TORCH) infection may be suspected in children with microcephaly, cataracts, deafness (cytomegalovirus, rubella, toxoplasmosis), congenital heart disease (rubella). In that case, immunoglobulin G (IgG) and immunoglobulin M (IgM) antibodies or PCR-based testing should be ordered. Brain imaging studies and funduscopic exam could reveal brain calcifications and/or chorioretinitis. Parvovirus should be considered in cases of hydrops fetalis. The differential for nonimmune hydrops also includes several rare lysosomal storage disorders (see Chapter 60).

7. **Metabolic testing** for IEM is typically included in newborn screening programs. In most states, mandatory newborn screening is done initially between 24 and 48 hours of age. The March of Dimes and the American College of Medical Genetics and Genomics recommend 29 conditions for testing. Most of these conditions can be managed by medications and/or special diets, and treatment in many can be lifesaving. Additional metabolic studies considered for the diagnosis of IEM include acylcarnitine profile for fatty acid oxidation disorders, urine organic acids for organic acidemias, very long chain fatty acids for peroxisomal disorders (Zellweger syndrome), sterol panel (Smith-Lemli-Opitz syndrome associated with low 7-dehydrocholesterol levels), and plasma amino acids for aminoacidopathies (e.g., phenylketonuria, tyrosinemia, nonketotic hyperglycinemia), plasma ammonia, and urine orotic acid (urea cycle disorders). The anion gap should be measured in cases of acidosis; if the anion gap is increased, measure lactic acid in whole plasma from a free-flowing blood sample (ideally arterial) and measure organic acids in urine. It is important to note that many IEM will not manifest symptoms until the infant is receiving milk feedings (see Chapter 60).

D. Ancillary evaluations

1. Imaging studies
   a. **Ultrasonography:** brain imaging to detect major malformation and intracranial hemorrhage; abdominal ultrasound exam to detect major liver, kidney anomalies, presence and position of testicles/ovaries; and echocardiography to detect heart defects
   b. **Brain MRI**, to delineate brain anatomy in greater detail
   c. Magnetic resonance spectroscopy (MRS) in infants with lactic acidosis to evaluate for mitochondrial disorders
   d. Magnetic resonance angiography (MRA) in infants with vascular malformations and to rule out further involvement such as arteriovenous fistulas, hemangiomas

e. Skeletal survey in children with intrauterine growth restriction (IUGR), poor linear growth, and especially if disproportionate growth, to evaluate for skeletal dysplasias. If fractures are present, a survey can be valuable to evaluate for osteogenesis imperfecta.

E. Anatomic pathology

1. Muscle biopsy in children with severe hypotonia can be considered in conjunction with nerve biopsy to assess for disorders such as congenital muscular dystrophy, amyoplasia congenita, and hypomyelination syndromes. Sometimes, a muscle biopsy can be postponed until the infant is at least 6 months of age to gather better quality and more complete information.

2. Autopsy studies in stillbirths or infants who die in the neonatal period may provide a diagnosis and help with counseling and recurrence risks. Good documentation should be obtained and radiographs should be considered in addition to pathologic exam.

3. Placental pathology can be useful in infants with growth restriction. A sample of the placenta can also be submitted for genetic studies such as karyotyping.

F. Follow-up

1. Patients with birth defects require close follow-up evaluation after hospital discharge either to aid in the diagnosis or to educate the family. Because approximately 50% of patients born with multiple congenital anomalies have no known diagnosis, the follow-up may reveal new findings that will contribute to the final diagnosis. This will help predict the natural history and allow a proper assessment of the recurrence risk.

2. Infants suspected to be at risk for developmental delay should be referred for therapy services or early childhood intervention programs.

Suggested Readings

American College of Obstetricians and Gynecologists. ACOG Committee Opinion No. 640: cell free DNA screening for fetal aneuploidy. http://www.acog.org/Resources-And-Publications/Committee-Opinions/Committee-on-Genetics/Cell-free-DNA-Screening-for-Fetal-Aneuploidy. Accessed May 9, 2016.

GeneTests. http://www.ncbi.nlm.nih.gov/sites/GeneTests/?db=GeneTests. Accessed May 9, 2016.

Gripp KW, Slavotinek AM, Hall JG, et al. *Handbook of Physical Measurements*. 3rd ed. New York, NY: Oxford University Press; 2013.

Hennekam R, Allanson J, Krantz I. *Gorlin's Syndromes of the Head and Neck*. 5th ed. New York, NY: Oxford University Press; 2010.

Jones KL, Jones MC, Del Campo M. *Smith's Recognizable Patterns of Human Malformations*. 7th ed. Philadelphia, PA: Elsevier Saunders; 2013.

Online Mendelian Inheritance in Man. Up-to-date online catalogue of Mendelian genetic disorders and traits with a useful search engine for the identification of syndromes. http://omim.org/. Accessed May 9, 2016.

Multiple Births
Melinda Markham

I. CLASSIFICATION

A. **Zygosity.** Monozygotic (MZ) twins originate and develop from a single fertilized egg (zygote) as a result of division of the inner cell mass of the blastocyst. MZ twins are the same sex and genetically identical. Dizygotic (DZ) or fraternal twins originate and develop from two separately fertilized eggs. Triplets and higher order pregnancies (quadruplets, quintuplets, sextuplets, septuplets, etc.) can be multizygotic, MZ and identical, or rarely, a combination of both.

B. **Placenta and fetal membranes.** A major portion of the placenta and the fetal membranes originate from the zygote. The placenta consists of two parts: (i) a larger fetal part derived from the villous chorion and (ii) a smaller maternal part derived from the decidua basalis. The chorionic and amniotic sacs surround the fetus. The chorion begins to form at day 3 after fertilization, and the amnion begins to form between days 6 and 8. The two membranes eventually fuse to form the amniochorionic membrane.

1. MZ twins commonly have one placenta with one chorion and two amnions (**monochorionic diamniotic**) or rarely, one placenta with one chorion and one amnion (**monochorionic monoamniotic**).

2. If early splitting occurs before the formation of the chorion and amnion (days 0 to 3), MZ twins can have two placentas with two chorions and two amnions (**dichorionic diamniotic**).

3. DZ twins always have two placentas with two chorions and two amnions (dichorionic diamniotic); however, the two placentas and chorions may be fused.

II. EPIDEMIOLOGY

A. Incidence. The twin birth rate in 2013 was 33.7 per 1,000 live births, increased slightly from 2012. However, the rate of twin birth has been relatively stable over the past 10 years.

   1. The rate of MZ twinning has remained relatively constant (3.5 per 1,000 births).

   2. The rate of DZ twinning is approximately 1 in 100 births. This rate is influenced by several factors such as ethnicity and maternal age. The frequency of DZ twinning has a genetic tendency that is affected by the genotype of the mother and not that of the father. In the United States, approximately two-thirds of twins are DZ.

   3. The birth rate of triplet and higher order multiples peaked in 1998 at 194 per 100,000 live births. The rate declined to 111 per 100,000 live births in 2013. The rates for other higher order multiples (quadruplets and higher) fell to 85 per 100,000 in 2013 compared to peak rates in 1998.

B. Causative factors. Two main factors account for the increase in multiple births since the early 1990s: (i) increased use of fertility-enhancing therapies including assisted reproductive technologies (ARTs) such as *in vitro* fertilization (IVF), and non-ART therapies such as ovulation-inducing drugs and artificial insemination; and (ii) **older maternal age** at childbearing (peak at 35 to 39 years), which is associated with an increase in multiples.

III. ETIOLOGY

A. MZ pregnancies result from the splitting of a single egg between days 0 and 14 postfertilization. The type of placenta that forms depends on the day of embryo splitting.

   1. A **dichorionic diamniotic** placenta results when early splitting occurs at days 0 to 3 before chorion formation (which usually occurs about day 3) and before implantation. A **monochorionic diamniotic** placenta results when splitting occurs about days 4 to 7 at which time the blastocyst cavity has developed and the chorion has formed. Amnion formation occurs at days 6 to 8, and splitting of the egg after this time (days 8 to 13) results in a **monochorionic monoamniotic** placenta. The frequency of placentation types is 30% dichorionic diamniotic, 70% monochorionic diamniotic, and <1% monochorionic monoamniotic. At day 14 and thereafter, the primitive streak begins to form and late splitting of the embryo at this time results in **conjoined twins**.

   2. **DZ or multizygous pregnancies** result when more than one dominant follicle has matured during the same menstrual cycle and multiple ovulations occur. Increased levels of follicle stimulating hormone (FSH) in the mother have been associated with spontaneous DZ twinning. FSH levels increase with advanced maternal age (peak at age ~37 years). A familial tendency toward twinning has also been shown to be associated with increased levels of FSH.

IV. DIAGNOSIS. Multiple gestational sacs can be detected by ultrasonography as early as 5 weeks, and cardiac activity can be detected from more than one fetus at 6 weeks.

A. **Placentation.** First-trimester ultrasonography can best determine the chorionicity of a multiple gestation; chorionicity is more difficult to determine in the second trimester. From weeks 10 to 14, a fused dichorionic placenta may often be distinguished from a true monochorionic placenta by the presence of an internal dividing membrane or ridge at the placental surface (lambda sign). The dividing septum of a dichorionic placenta appears thicker and includes two amnions and two chorionic layers. In contrast, the dividing septum of a monochorionic placenta consists of two thin amnions. One placenta, same-sex fetuses, and absence of a dividing septum suggest monoamniotic twins, but absence of a dividing septum may also be due to septal disruption.

B. **Zygosity. DNA typing** can be used to determine zygosity in same-sex twins if this information is desired. Prenatally, DNA can be obtained by chorionic villus sampling (CVS) or amniocentesis. Postnatally, DNA typing should optimally be performed on umbilical cord tissue, buccal smear, or a skin biopsy specimen rather than blood. There is evidence that DZ twins, even in the absence of vascular connections, can also carry hematopoietic stem cells (HSCs) derived from their twin. HSCs are most likely transferred from one fetus to the other through maternal circulation.

C. **Pathologic examination of the placenta(s)** at birth is important in establishing and verifying chorionicity.

V. PRENATAL SCREENING AND DIAGNOSIS

A. **Zygosity** determines the degree of risk of chromosomal abnormalities in each fetus of a multiple gestation. The risk of aneuploidy in each fetus of an MZ pregnancy is the same as a singleton pregnancy, and except for rare cases of genetic discordancy, both fetuses are affected. In a DZ pregnancy, each twin has an independent risk of aneuploidy; thus, the pregnancy has twice the risk of having a chromosomal abnormality compared with a singleton.

B. **Second-trimester maternal serum screening** for women with multiples is limited because each fetus contributes variable levels of these serum markers. When levels are abnormal, it is difficult to identify which fetus is affected.

C. **First-trimester ultrasonography** to assess for **nuchal translucency** is a more sensitive and specific test to screen for chromosomal abnormalities. A **second-trimester ultrasonography exam** is important in surveying each fetus for **anatomic defects**. **Second-trimester amniocentesis** and **first-trimester CVS** can be safely performed on multiples and are both accurate diagnostic procedures for determining aneuploidy. Cell-free fetal DNA testing on maternal blood to evaluate most common chromosomal abnormalities is not valid in pregnancies with more than one fetus.

VI. MATERNAL COMPLICATIONS

A. **Gestational diabetes** has been shown in some studies to be more common in twin pregnancies.

B. **Spontaneous abortion** occurs in 8% to 36% of multiple pregnancies with reduction to a singleton pregnancy by the end of the first trimester ("**vanishing twin**"). Possible causes include abnormal implantation, early cardiovascular developmental defects, and chromosomal abnormalities. Before fetal viability, the management of the surviving co-twin in a dichorionic pregnancy includes expectant management, in addition to close surveillance for preterm labor, fetal well-being, and fetal growth. The management of a single fetal demise in a monochorionic twin pregnancy is more complicated. The surviving co-twin is at high risk for ischemic multiorgan and neurologic injury that is thought to be secondary to hypotension or thromboembolic events. Fetal imaging by ultrasonography or magnetic resonance imaging (MRI) may demonstrate neurologic injury but would not exclude a poor outcome if normal.

C. **Incompetent cervix** occurs in up to 14% of multiple gestations.

D. **Placental abruption** risk rises as the number of fetuses per pregnancy increases. In a large retrospective cohort study, the incidence of placental abruption was 6.2, 12.2, and 15.6 per 1,000 pregnancies in singletons, twins, and triplets, respectively.

E. **Preterm premature rupture of membranes** complicates 7% to 10% of twin pregnancies compared with 2% to 4% of singleton pregnancies. **Preterm labor and birth** occur in approximately 57% of twin pregnancies and in 90% of higher order multiple gestations.

F. **Pregnancy-induced hypertension (PIH) and preeclampsia** are 2.5 times more common in multifetal pregnancies compared with singleton pregnancies.

G. **Cesarean delivery.** Approximately 66% of patients with twins and 91% of patients with triplets have cesarean delivery. Breech position of one or more fetuses, cord prolapse, and placental abruption are factors that account for the increased frequency of cesarean deliveries for multiple gestations.

VII. FETAL AND NEONATAL COMPLICATIONS

A. **Prematurity and low birth weight.** The average duration of gestation is shorter in multifetal pregnancies and further shortens as the number of fetuses increases. The mean gestational age at birth is 36, 33, and 29 1/2 weeks, respectively, for twins, triplets, and quadruplets. The likelihood of a birth weight <1,500 g is 8 and 33 times greater in twins and triplets or higher order multiples, respectively, compared with singletons.

B. **Intrauterine growth restriction (IUGR).** Fetal growth is independent of the number of fetuses until approximately 30 weeks' gestation, after which growth of multiples gradually falls off compared with singletons. IUGR is defined as an estimated fetal weight (EFW) less than either the 3rd percentile for gestational age or an EFW <10th percentile for gestational age with evidence of fetal compromise. The mechanisms are likely uterine crowding, limitation of placental perfusion, anomalous umbilical cord insertion, infection, fetal anomalies, maternal complications (e.g., maternal hypertension), and monochorionicity. Monochorionic twins are more likely than dichorionic twins to be IUGR and have higher perinatal mortality.

C. **Fetal growth discordance** is typically defined as a difference in birth weight of more than 20% of the larger twin's weight. It can also be categorized as mild (<15%), moderate (15% to 30%), or severe (>30%). Risk factors for discordant growth include monochorionic placentation associated with velamentous cord insertion, placental dysfunction, preeclampsia, antepartum bleeding, twin-to-twin transfusion syndrome (TTTS), fetal infection, and fetal structural and chromosomal abnormalities. The smaller twin has an increased risk of fetal demise, perinatal death, and preterm birth. Five percent to 15% of twins and 30% of triplets have fetal growth discordance that is associated with a sixfold increase in perinatal morbidity and mortality.

D. **Intrauterine fetal demise (IUFD)** refers to fetal demise after 20 weeks' gestation but before delivery and is confirmed by ultrasonographic evidence of absent fetal cardiac activity. The death of one twin, which occurs in 9% of multiple pregnancies, is less common in the second and third trimesters. The risk of IUFD is 4 to 6 times greater in MZ pregnancies. Because almost all MZ twins have placental vascular connections with resulting shared circulations, there is a significant risk (20% to 40%) of neurologic injury (multicystic encephalomalacia) in the surviving co-twin as a result of associated severe hypotension or thromboembolic events upon death of the co-twin. Because their circulation is not shared, the death of one DZ twin usually has minimal adverse effect on the surviving co-twin. In this case, the co-twin is either completely resorbed if death occurs in the first trimester or is compressed between the amniotic sac of its co-twin and the uterine wall (fetus papyraceous). Other complications involving the surviving co-twin include stillbirth, preterm birth, placental abruption, and chorioamnionitis.

In the event of a demise of one monochorionic twin, immediate delivery of the surviving co-twin should be considered after fetal viability. However, this does not seem to change the outcome as neurologic injury is thought to occur at the time of the co-twin's death. Disseminated intravascular coagulopathy is a complication seen in 20% to 25% of women who retain a dead fetus for more than 3 weeks. Monitoring of maternal coagulation profiles is recommended and delivery within this time frame should be considered.

E. **Congenital malformations** occur in approximately 6% of twin pregnancies or 3% of individual twins. The risk in MZ twins is approximately 2.5-fold greater than in DZ twins or singletons. Structural defects specific to MZ twins include (i) early malformations that share a common origin with the twinning process, (ii) vascular disruption syndromes, and (iii) deformations.

1. **Early structural defects** include the following:
   a. Caudal malformations (sirenomelia, sacrococcygeal teratoma)
   b. Urologic malformations (cloacal or bladder exstrophy)
   c. The vertebral anomalies, anal atresia, cardiac, tracheoesophageal, renal, and limb defects (VACTERL) spectrum

d. Neural tube defects (anencephaly, encephalocele, or holoprosencephaly)

e. Defects of laterality (situs inversus, polysplenia, or asplenia)

2. Vascular disruption syndromes may occur early or late in gestation.

a. The presence of large anastomoses between two embryos early in development may cause unequal arterial perfusion resulting in **acardia**. One embryo receives only low-pressure blood flow through the umbilical artery and preferentially perfuses its lower extremities. Profound malformations can result ranging from complete amorphism to severe upper body abnormalities such as anencephaly, holoprosencephaly, rudimentary facial features and limbs, and absent thoracic or abdominal organs. The co-twin is usually well formed. Acardia is rare, occurring in 1% monoamniotic twin pregnancies and affecting 1 in 35,000 to 150,000 births. In acardiac twin pregnancies, the incidence of spontaneous abortion and prematurity is 20% and 60%, respectively. Perinatal mortality in the donor twin is 40%.

b. Vascular disruptions that occur later in gestation are due to embolic events or the exchange of tissue between twins through placental anastomoses. Late vascular disruptions often occur after the demise of one fetus. Resulting malformations include cutis aplasia, limb interruption, intestinal atresia, gastroschisis, anorchia or gonadal dysgenesis, hemifacial microsomia, Goldenhar syndrome (facio-auriculo-vertebral defects), or Poland sequence. Cranial abnormalities include porencephalic cysts, hydranencephaly, microcephaly, and hydrocephalus.

3. Deformations such as clubfoot, dislocated hips, and cranial synostosis are more frequent in multiple pregnancies as a result of overcrowding of the intrauterine environment.

4. Surveillance. Twin pregnancies should be evaluated for anomalies by fetal ultrasonography or more invasive procedures if indicated. Congenital anomalies are concordant only in a minority of cases, even in MZ twins. Whether assisted reproductive techniques result in an increased incidence in congenital birth defects is uncertain.

F. Chromosomal anomalies occur at a higher frequency in offspring of multiple gestations. **Advanced maternal age** contributes to the increased risk in chromosomal anomalies. The risk in MZ twins is equivalent to that of a singleton. The risk in DZ twins is independent for each fetus, so the risk of chromosomal abnormality in at least one DZ twin is twice that of a singleton fetus.

G. Conjoined twins result when incomplete embryonic division occurs late after day 14 postconception. At this time, differentiation of the chorion and amnion has occurred, and therefore, conjoined twins are seen only in monochorionic monoamniotic twins. Conjoined twins are rare and occur in approximately 1 in 50,000 to 100,000 births. The most common sites of fusion are the chest and/or abdomen. Survival is rare when there is cardiac or cerebral fusion. Serial ultrasonography can define the fetal anatomy and help determine management options. Polyhydramnios can affect as many as 50% of cases of conjoined twins and may require amnioreduction. Elective cesarean delivery close to term is recommended. Decisions regarding separation are complex and depend on anatomic factors, associated anomalies, and parental wishes. Fewer than 20% of conjoined twins survive.

H. TTS occurs only in monochorionic gestations.

1. The **pathophysiology** of TTTS is not completely understood, but placental vascular anastomoses, unequal placental sharing, and abnormal umbilical cord insertions are all necessary for TTTS to occur. Vascular connections occur in 85% of monochorionic placentas. These include superficial arterial-to-arterial (AA) and venous-to-venous (VV) anastomoses with bidirectional flow and deep interfetal artery-to-vein (AV) communications with unidirectional flow located in the placental cotyledons that are supplied by one fetus and drained by the other. The number and type of anastomoses affect whether the exchange of blood between the twins is balanced or unbalanced. TTTS results when there is limited bidirectional flow through AA or VV connections. AA connections are thought to be protective, associated with a ninefold reduction in the risk of developing chronic TTTS; AV anastomoses with unidirectional flow lead to shunting of blood from one twin to the other and are associated with worse perinatal outcome. **Ten percent to 20% of monochorionic placentas have sufficient circulatory imbalance to produce TTTS.** One fetus (**the donor**) slowly pumps blood into the co-twin's circulation (**the recipient**). Complications in the donor include anemia, hypovolemia and resultant activation of the renin-angiotensin-aldosterone system, growth restriction, brain ischemic lesions, renal hypoperfusion and insufficiency, oligohydramnios ("stuck twin"), lung hypoplasia, limb deformation, and high risk of fetal demise. Complications in the recipient include polycythemia, thrombosis, cerebral emboli, disseminated intravascular coagulation (DIC), polyhydramnios, progressive cardiomyopathy due to volume overload, and fetal hydrops.

2. Diagnosis is usually made between 17 and 26 weeks' gestation, but the process may occur as early as 13 weeks. Severe cases of TTTS have signs before 20 weeks' gestation and have a mortality rate in at least one fetus of 80% to 100% if left untreated. **Diagnostic criteria** for TTTS include monochorionicity, polyhydramnios in the sac of one twin (the recipient) and oligohydramnios in the sac of the other twin (the donor), umbilical cord size discrepancy, cardiac dysfunction in the polyhydramniotic twin, abnormal umbilical artery and/or ductus venosus Doppler velocimetry, and significant growth discordance (>20%). These findings are suggestive of TTTS, although not all are necessary for a diagnosis. Several staging systems have been used to classify disease severity and progression of disease, and provide criteria for escalation of care to a specialty referral center, and a framework to evaluate therapeutic trials. The most commonly used system is the Quintero staging system. This system is based on a series of ultrasonographic findings and does not include fetal echocardiographic findings. The extent to which fetal cardiovascular changes in the recipient twin correlate better with disease severity and predict outcome or disease progression requires further validation. Additional clinical trials are needed to evaluate other physiologic parameters (e.g., cardiac indices or markers of systemic hemodynamic alterations) that will improve prediction of disease severity, progression, and outcome.

3. **Fetal treatment** interventions depend on the gestational age and stage at the time TTTS is identified. Many pregnancies with stage I TTTS can be managed expectantly because more than 75% regress or remain stable with no invasive intervention, and perinatal survival is approximately 86%. Most cases are detected in the second trimester at more advanced stages. Most experts recommend fetoscopic laser photocoagulation of placental anastomoses for stages II to IV at <26 weeks' gestation, although data are limited. In the Eurofetus trial that included 142 women, laser treatment improved perinatal survival (76% vs. 56%) and decreased cystic periventricular leukomalacia (6% vs. 14%), and infants were more likely to have no neurologic complications at 6 months of age compared to serial amnioreduction. In a systematic Cochrane review, the two trials that compared amnioreduction to laser ablation found no difference in death. In follow-up at 6 years of age, no additional deaths occurred in the group of infants alive at 6 months. Normal neurologic evaluation was similar between groups (82% and 70% in the laser and amnioreduction groups, respectively, $P = .12$), but due to the increased survival at 6 months of age, more infants were alive without neurologic abnormality at 6 years of age in the laser group.

4. **Neonatal management** may include **resuscitation** at birth and need for continued ventilatory and cardiovascular support, rapid establishment of **intravascular access** for volume expansion to treat hypotension, correction of hypoglycemia, red blood cell transfusion to treat anemia, and **partial exchange transfusion** in the recipient to treat significant polycythemia. **Neuroimaging** should be performed to detect central nervous system (CNS) injury.

5. **Persistent pulmonary hypertension of the newborn (PPHN).** In a series of 73 consecutive twin pregnancies with TTTS, 4 of 135 (3%) liveborn twins had severe PPHN compared to 0 of 161 in a control group of monochorionic twins without TTTS. Factors that may contribute to the association of PPHN and TTTS in the recipient twin include increased preload, volume overload, polycythemia, increased pulmonary vascular resistance, and increased afterload due to vasoactive substances. Susceptibility of the donor twin may be related to IUGR or lower levels of specific amino acids such as arginine, a nitric oxide precursor that plays a role in decreasing pulmonary vascular resistance after birth (see Chapter 36).

I. **Velamentous cord insertion and vasa previa** occur 6 to 9 times more often in twins than singletons and even more in higher order gestations. Contributing factors may include placental crowding and abnormal blastocyst implantation. All types of placentation can be affected. With velamentous cord insertion, vessels are unprotected by Wharton jelly and are more prone to compression, thrombosis, or disruption, leading to fetal distress or hemorrhage (see Chapter 43).

J. The perinatal mortality in monochorionic monoamniotic twins is reported to be as high as 40% due to umbilical cord entanglements and compression, congenital anomalies, preterm birth, and IUGR. The risk of fetal loss increases with gestational age, so most monochorionic monoamniotic twins are delivered electively at 32 to 34 weeks.

VIII. OUTCOMES

A. **Neonatal mortality.** Twin birth is associated with an increased risk of neonatal mortality compared to singleton births at all gestational ages. In a retrospective cohort study of matched U.S. multiple birth and death data from 1995 to 2000 in infants without congenital anomalies, the perinatal mortality rate is greater in second-born twins compared to first-born (16.5 vs. 15.4 per 1,000 live births). The mortality increases threefold and fourfold for triplet and quadruplet births, respectively. As with singleton births, preterm birth contributes substantially to mortality. In addition, the risk of stillbirth in twin pregnancies increases with advancing gestational age, so delivery is typically considered at 37 to 38 weeks of gestation. Prematurity and low birth weight are the predominating factors that increase the rates of mortality and morbidity for multiple births. Assisted reproduction contributes to the increased incidence of multifetal pregnancies, and preterm birth is strongly correlated with the number of fetuses. Techniques that limit the number of reimplanted eggs or transferred embryos or selective reduction of higher order multiples may improve the likelihood of a successful outcome.

B. **Morbidity. Prematurity and growth restriction** are associated with increased risk of morbidities such as bronchopulmonary dysplasia, necrotizing enterocolitis, retinopathy of prematurity, and intraventricular hemorrhage (IVH) (see Chapters 27, 34, 54, and 67).

C. **Long-term morbidity** such as cerebral palsy (CP) and other neurologic handicaps affect more twins and higher order multiples than singletons. The risk of CP in multiples compared with singleton gestations is increased 5- to 10-fold. Twins account for 5% to 10% of all cases of CP in the United States. The prevalence of CP in twins is 7.4%, compared with 1% in singletons. The higher prevalence of CP in twins is primarily observed among larger twins, especially among same-sex pairs; the relative risk of CP in twins ≥2,500 g at birth compared to twins <2,500 g is 6.3 (95% confidence interval [CI], 2.0 to 20.1). Thus, the higher prevalence of CP among twins compared to singleton births is due to a greater frequency of prematurity and low birth weight in twins as well as a higher prevalence of CP among larger twin pairs. Death of a co-twin is considered an independent risk factor for CP in the surviving twin. Other risk factors for CP in twins include same-sex pairs, monochorionicity, severe birth weight discordance, TTTS, and artificial reproductive technology. Among extremely low birth weight (ELBW) infants, the frequency of CP is not significantly different between singletons and twins. In addition, the frequency of chronic lung disease and IVH are not significantly different between singletons and twins ≤28 weeks' gestation. Twins have a greater risk of learning disabilities even after controlling for CP and low birth weight.

D. **Impact of ART on outcomes.** In the United States, 19% of twin births and 32% of triplet or higher order births result from ART. Multiple reports note increased adverse maternal and perinatal outcomes associated with ART. However, the extent to which the increased frequency of multiple births following ART (~44% with ART vs. ~3% with natural conception) contribute to this risk requires further study. Recent population-based studies in the United States demonstrate an increased risk of adverse perinatal outcomes in twin versus singleton ART births and non-ART twins, including prematurity, low birth weight, and very low birth weight. The rates of cesarean delivery are also increased in ART twins. Although multiple gestation overall is associated with an increased risk of neurodevelopmental abnormalities, this risk is similar in spontaneously conceived and ART multiples and is independent of the type of assisted reproduction. Studies evaluating the increased risk of birth defects among ART births have been inconsistent. However, a number of studies have demonstrated up to a twofold increased risk of congenital anomalies among ART births following either IVF or intracytoplasmic sperm injection (ICSI). Cardiac, urogenital, as well as ocular birth defects have been reported with ART. In addition, rare imprinting disorders have been reported with ART including Beckwith-Wiedemann syndrome (BWS) and Angelman syndrome. However, larger prospective cohort studies are required to definitively relate these rare conditions to ART.

E. **Economic impact.** Health care costs associated with twins and higher order multiples are substantially greater than singleton infants. Costs are largely influenced by preterm birth and the contribution of ART to multiple birth rates.

F. **Social and family impact.** Caring for twins or higher order multiples contributes to increased marital strain, financial stress, parental anxiety, and depression and has a greater influence on the professional and social life of mothers of these infants, particularly first-time mothers, compared with mothers of singletons. Multiples are more likely to have medical complications (i.e., prematurity, congenital defects, IUGR) that result in prolonged hospital stays and contribute further to a family's emotional and financial stress. Social services, lactation support, and assistance from additional caregivers and family members can help parents cope with the increased amount of care required by multiples. Organizations of parents of multiples can provide advice and emotional support that can further help new parents of multiples cope.

Suggested Readings

Chauhan SP, Scardo JA, Hayes E, et al. Twins: prevalence, problems, and preterm births. *Am J Obstet Gynecol* 2010;203:305–315.

Khalek N, Johnson MP, Bebbington MW. Fetoscopic laser therapy for twin-to-twin transfusion syndrome. *Semin Pediatr Surg* 2013;22:18–23.

Simpson L. What you need to know when managing twins: 10 key facts. *Obstet Gynecol Clin North Am* 2015;42:225–239.

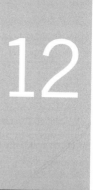

Maternal Drug Use, Infant Exposure, and Neonatal Abstinence Syndrome

Stephen W. Patrick

KEY POINTS

- An estimated 440,000 substance-exposed infants are born each year.
- Verbal screening for substance use should occur in every pregnancy.
- Opioid use in pregnancy is increasingly common and can result in drug withdrawal.
- Every birth hospital should have a protocol in place to screen, evaluate, and treat substance-exposed infants.
- An opioid (morphine or methadone) should be the first choice for opioid withdrawal if pharmacotherapy is required.

I. MATERNAL DRUG USE

A. **Use of illicit substances.** Data from the National Survey of Drug Use and Health (NSDUH) suggest that at least 5.4% of pregnant women use illicit drugs in pregnancy. Illicit drug use is highest among younger women, with the highest rate (14.6%) in 15- to 17-year-old girls. Overall, the rate of illicit drug use in pregnant women is nearly half that of the general population (11.4%), and women are less likely to use in the third trimester (2.4%). This suggests that, although illicit drug use in pregnancy is common, becoming pregnant may motivate some women to engage in treatment of substance use disorders. NSDUH reports the most common illicit drugs used as a percentage of the U.S. population >12 years old in the United States are marijuana (7.5%), psychotherapeutics used illicitly (2.5%), cocaine (0.6%), hallucinogens (0.5%), inhalants (0.2%), heroin (0.1%).

B. **Maternal use and misuse of legal substances.** The use of prescription medicines in pregnancy grew by nearly 70% over the last three decades. Pregnant women use an average of 1.8 prescription medications, and data on risk of fetal effects are limited for many. Prescribed medications include atypical antipsychotics (e.g., risperidone), antidepressants (e.g., sertraline), and opioid (e.g., hydrocodone). In addition, NSDUH reports high use by pregnant women of alcohol (9.4%) and cigarettes (15.4%). The Centers for Disease

Control and Prevention website Treating for Two (http://www.cdc.gov/pregnancy/meds/treatingfortwo/) provides information to support safer medication use in pregnancy.

II. DIAGNOSIS OF DRUG USE IN PREGNANCY.

A comprehensive medical and social history should be obtained from the mother with every newborn evaluation and should include use of illicit drugs, prescription drugs, tobacco, and alcohol. The American College of Obstetricians and Gynecologists recommends use of a validated screening tool for drug use such as the 4 Ps or CRAFFT (Table 12.1). This history can be augmented by communication with obstetric providers and, when available, the state's prescription drug monitoring program database.

Table 12.1. Clinical Screening Tools for Prenatal Substance Use and Abuse

4 P's

Parents: Did any of your parents have a problem with alcohol or other drug use?
Partner: Does your partner have a problem with alcohol or drug use?
Past: In the past, have you had difficulties in your life because of alcohol or other drugs, including prescription medications?
Present: In the past month have you drunk any alcohol or used other drugs?

Scoring: Any "yes" should trigger further questions.

Ewing H. A practical guide to intervention in health and social services with pregnant and postpartum addicts and alcoholics: theoretical framework, brief screening tool, key interview questions, and strategies for referral to recovery resources. Martinez (CA): The Born Free Project, Contra Costa County Department of Health Services; 1990.

CRAFFT—Substance Abuse Screen for Adolescents and Young Adults

C Have you ever ridden in a CAR driven by someone (including yourself) who was high or had been using alcohol or drugs?
R Do you ever use alcohol or drugs to RELAX, feel better about yourself, or fit in?
A Do you ever use alcohol or drugs while you are by yourself or ALONE?
F Do you ever FORGET things you did while using alcohol or drugs?
F Do your FAMILY or friends ever tell you that you should cut down on your drinking or drug use?
T Have you ever gotten in TROUBLE while you were using alcohol or drugs?

Scoring: Two or more positive items indicate the need for further assessment.

Center for Adolescent Substance Abuse Research, Children's Hospital Boston. The CRAFFT screening interview. Boston (MA): CeASAR; 2009. Available at: http://www.ceasar.org/CRAFFT/pdf/CRAFFT_English.pdf. Retrieved February 10, 2012. Copyright © Children's Hospital Boston, 2011. All rights reserved. Reproduced with permission from the Center for Adolescent Substance Abuse Research, CeASAR, Children's Hospital Boston, 617-355-5133, or www.ceasar.org.
Source: American College of Obstetricians and Gynecologists Committee Opinion No. 524: opioid abuse, dependence, and addition in pregnancy. *Obstet Gynecol* 2012;119(5):1070–1076.

A. Accurate information regarding illicit drug use may be difficult to obtain. Nonspecific maternal and infant associations with illicit drug use include the following:

1. Maternal
  a. Poor or no prenatal care
  b. Preterm labor
  c. Placental abruption
  d. Precipitous delivery

2. Infant
  a. Small for gestational age
  b. Intrauterine growth restriction
  c. Microcephaly
  d. Neonatal stroke

B. Diagnostic testing can be useful to supplement standardized verbal screening tools. Testing should be considered in infants with signs consistent with neonatal abstinence, severe intrauterine growth restriction without an identified etiology, intracranial hemorrhage or stroke, or placental abruption. It is important to know state, local, and institutional reporting requirements to child welfare agencies for positive test results as laws may be interpreted differently among jurisdictions.

1. Urine testing is a quick, noninvasive way to test for recent drug exposure in the neonate. For example, cocaine will appear in the urine up to 3 days after the most recent use, marijuana for 7 to 30 days, methamphetamine for 3 to 5 days, and opiates (including methadone) 3 to 5 days. Drugs administered during labor may cause difficulty in interpreting results.

2. Meconium testing provides information about drug use for a longer period in pregnancy. However, collection is time intensive for nursing staff, stools can be missed, and specimens can be contaminated.

3. Umbilical cord testing may provide similar data to meconium, although collection and storage of the umbilical cord at birth can be resource intensive.

C. Risk of infection. Illicit drug use increases the risk of infections in the pregnant woman and her infant, especially when associated with intravenous drug use or other high-risk behaviors (e.g., prostitution). The mother's HIV, hepatitis B, hepatitis C, and syphilis status should be determined, and the infant should be managed accordingly (see Chapters 48 and 51).

III. NONOPIOID SUBSTANCE EXPOSURE. Substance use in pregnancy may result in abnormal psychomotor behavior in the newborn that is consistent with toxicity or withdrawal, as summarized in Table 12.2.

IV. NEONATAL ABSTINENCE SYNDROME FOLLOWING OPIOID EXPOSURE IN PREGNANCY

A. Because of the high prevalence of opioid use during pregnancy, the American Academy of Pediatrics (AAP) recommends that all hospitals that care for infants at risk for withdrawal have policies in place for screening and

Table 12.2. Onset and Duration of Clinical Signs Consistent with Neonatal Withdrawal after Intrauterine Substance Exposure (Excluding Narcotics)

Drug	Signs	Onset of Signs	Duration of Signs[a]
Alcohol	Hyperactivity, crying, irritability, poor suck, tremors, seizures; onset of signs at birth, poor sleeping pattern, hyperphagia, diaphoresis	3–12 h	18 mo
Barbiturates	Irritability, severe tremors, hyperacusis, excessive crying, vasomotor instability, diarrhea, restlessness, increased tone, hyperphagia, vomiting, disturbed sleep; onset first 24 h of life or as late as 10–14 d of age	1–14 d	4–6 mo with prescription
Caffeine	Jitteriness, vomiting, bradycardia, tachypnea	At birth	1–7 d
Chlordiazepoxide	Irritability, tremors; signs may start at 21 d	Days–weeks	9 mo; 11/2 mo with prescription
Clomipramine	Hypothermia, cyanosis, tremors; onset 12 h of age		4 d with prescription
Diazepam	Hypotonia, poor suck, hypothermia, apnea, hypertonia, hyperreflexia, tremors, vomiting, hyperactivity, tachypnea (mother receiving multiple drug therapy)	Hours–weeks	8 mo; 10–66 d with prescription
Ethchlorvynol	Lethargy, jitteriness, hyperphagia, irritability, poor suck, hypotonia (mother receiving multiple drug therapy)		Possibly 10 d with prescription
Glutethimide	Increased tone, tremors, opisthotonos, high-pitched cry, hyperactivity, irritability, colic		6 mo

(continued)

Table 12.2. *(Continued)*

Drug	Signs	Onset of Signs	Duration of Signs[a]
Hydroxyzine	Tremors, irritability, hyper-activity, jitteriness, shrill cry, myoclonic jerks, hypotonia, increased respiratory and heart rates, feeding problems, clonic movements (mother receiving multiple drug therapy)		5 wk with prescription
Meprobamate	Irritability, tremors, poor sleep patterns, abdominal pain		9 mo; 3 mo with prescription
SSRIs	Crying, irritability, tremors, poor suck, feeding difficulty, hypertonia, tachypnea, sleep disturbance, hypoglycemia, seizures	Hours–days	1–4 wk

[a]Prescription indicates the infant was treated with pharmacologic agents, and the natural course of the signs may have been shortened.
Source: Hudak ML, Tan RC. Neonatal drug withdrawal. *Pediatrics* 2012;129:e540–e560.

treatment. Adherence to such protocols appears to impact clinical outcomes more than pharmacotherapy. Neonatal abstinence syndrome (NAS) can result from a variety of opioids including prescription opioids (e.g., hydrocodone), illicit opioids (e.g., heroin), or medication-assisted treatment (e.g., methadone). Although medication-assisted treatment increases an infant's risk of NAS, the infant's risk of being born preterm or low birth weight is less than with continued heroin use. As a result, the American College of Obstetrics and Gynecologists recommends medication-assisted treatment.

B. An infant's risk of drug withdrawal and its severity varies by opioid type and the presence of additional exposures. Methadone has the greatest risk, which becomes less with buprenorphine, followed by a long-acting opioid (MS Contin, morphine sulfate extended release), and then a short-acting opioid (hydrocodone). Adjunctive use of tobacco, selective serotonin reuptake inhibitors, atypical antipsychotics, and benzodiazepines increase the likelihood of NAS or make it more severe.

C. Timing of presentation. The initial presentation of NAS depends on when the drug was last used in pregnancy, infant metabolism, and half-life of the opioid used. In addition, for reasons that are uncertain, not all infants develop withdrawal. As a result, the AAP recommends that all opioid-exposed infants be observed in the hospital for signs of withdrawal for 4 to 7 days after birth.

D. Site of care. There is increasing evidence that processes of care that keep mother and infant together (e.g., rooming in), promote bonding, breast-feeding, and may reduce infant symptomatology and decrease NAS severity. Where possible, infants should not be separated from their mothers.

E. Assessment. Infants at risk for drug withdrawal should be assessed for drug withdrawal using an available scoring tool. We use the modified Finnegan Neonatal Abstinence Score Tool (NAST) (see Table 12.2). Scoring should begin soon after admission and continue every 3 to 4 hours, reflecting the preceding period and depending on the frequency of feedings, taking of vital signs, and provision of care. If infants appear hungry, we provide half of the feeding volume and then complete scoring. Infants are scored for a total of 4 days if pharmacologic intervention is not required. We continue to score infants who require pharmacologic therapy for the duration of therapy and for 48 to 72 hours after drug is discontinued to ensure that symptoms do not redevelop. We typically score infants who do not require pharmacologic intervention for a total of 4 days.

  1. Signs of withdrawal include the following:
    a. Central nervous system/neurologic excitability: tremors, irritability, increased wakefulness/sleep disturbance, frequent yawning and sneezing, high-pitched cry, increased muscle tone, hyperactive reflexes (e.g., Moro), seizures
    b. Gastrointestinal dysfunction: poor feeding, uncoordinated and constant sucking, vomiting, diarrhea, dehydration, and poor weight gain
    c. Autonomic signs: sweating, nasal stuffiness, fever/temperature instability, and mottling

F. Management. Infants with signs of withdrawal are treated based on NAST scores. Treatment begins with nonpharmacologic measures. Infants with severe withdrawal are treated with an opioid (morphine or methadone) as a first-line agent. Examples of treatment protocols using morphine (Vanderbilt University School of Medicine) and methadone (University of Michigan) are shown in the text and Figure 12.1.

  1. Nonpharmacologic interventions are implemented for NAST scores <8.
    a. Decrease stimulation by reducing lights, noise, and touch.
    b. Promote infant self-regulation by encouraging pacifier use, nonnutritive sucking, and swaddling.
    c. Room in with mother if possible.
    d. Encourage holding, especially skin-to-skin.
    e. Encourage breastfeeding.

  2. Pharmacologic interventions are implemented for NAST scores ≥8, whereas nonpharmacologic interventions are continued. Infants treated with an opioid should be on a cardiac and respiratory monitor, particularly in the initial period, to ensure there are no clinical signs of respiratory depression.
    a. We use morphine as the first-line drug, although methadone is an appropriate alternative. We use a dosing interval of 3 hours although, depending on feeding schedule, some infants benefit from alternative

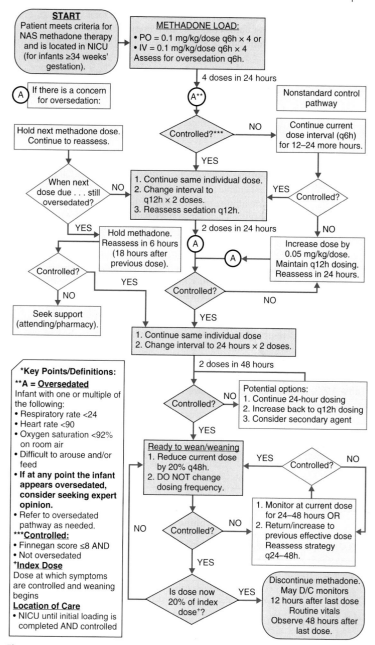

Figure 12.1. Neonatal abstinence syndrome treatment protocol used at University of Michigan (methadone for pharmacologic treatment). NICU, neonatal intensive care unit; PO, orally; IV, intravenous; D/C, discontinue.

dosing intervals to provide the same 24-hour total dose (e.g., a baby feeding every 4 hours could be dosed every 4 hours).

   i. Morphine dose is adjusted based on the NAST score as shown in Table 12.3.

   ii. One rescue dose of oral morphine 0.05 mg/kg is available for each infant until appropriate dosing changes are made. It may only be given once and must then be reordered by the clinician after reassessment of the maintenance dose. If scores are ≥8 following weaning, one rescue dose can be considered with return to the previous dose/dosing level. One rescue dose may be considered before adding clonidine.

b. Adjunct management

   i. We reevaluate infants who reach level 4 and continue to score ≥8 and consider addition of clonidine, as shown in Table 12.4.

   ii. If we are unable to wean morphine after 3 weeks of treatment, we consider adjunct management with oral phenobarbital.

c. Weaning begins when the average daily score is <8 without a single score of ≥14. Morphine is typically weaned by dose, not interval. If treatment includes clonidine, we wean the morphine first.

   i. If the NAST score remains <8 for 48 hours, we wean morphine by 10% of the maximum dose every 48 hours if the average score continues to remain <8. We consider a faster wean after 24 hours if the NAST score remains <8.

   ii. We discontinue morphine if the score remains <8 on 25% of the maximum morphine dose for 48 hours and continue to score for 48 to 72 hours. If the score is ≥8, we increase to the previous dose.

Table 12.3. Neonatal Abstinence Score Tool Score

Score	Action
≥8 for two to three times	Determine NAS level and dose.
<8	Continue same dose for 24–48 hours and then consider weaning.
8 for two times	Go to next higher level and dose.

Oral Morphine Dosing Tool		
NAS Level	**NAST Score**	**Morphine Dose (0.4 mg/mL)**
1	8–10	0.04 mg/kg/dose q3h
2	11–13	0.06 mg/kg/dose q3h
3	14–16	0.09 mg/kg/dose q3h
4	≥17	0.11 mg/kg/dose q3h

NAS, neonatal abstinence syndrome; NAST, Neonatal Abstinence Score Tool.

Table 12.4. Use of Clonidine as an Adjunct

Initial clonidine dose	1 µg/kg/dose PO every 6 hours
Dose titration	If scores continue ≥8 for two measurements and blood pressure is stable, increase dose to 2 µg/kg per dose every 6 hours.
	If scores remain elevated, consider dose increase to maximum of 3 µg/kg per dose every 6 hours.
Monitor	Monitor blood pressure every 6 hours during treatment to assess for hypotension; monitor for 48 hours after stopping to assess for rebound hypertension.
PO, orally.	

    iii. If the morphine has been weaned off and scores are ≥8, we consider one rescue dose and return to previous dose/dosing level.

    iv. Clonidine weaning depends on the maximum dose used and the volume of measurable doses. Assistance by a pharmacist in generating a weaning plan is helpful if available. We begin to wean clonidine when morphine has been discontinued for 24 to 48 hours, continue to wean every 48 hours if the NAST score remains <8, and discontinue at the final step if the score is <8 for 24 hours.

  3. Educational interventions

    a. Caregivers and families should be provided verbal and written education about NAS.

    b. Families should receive communication about the plan of care, a safety plan and referral to social service, and the appropriate state agency when indicated.

    c. The family should be engaged in the care of the infant, including infant scoring (Tables 12.5 and 12.6; Fig. 12.1).

V. BREASTFEEDING OF SUBSTANCE-EXPOSED INFANTS.

In addition to its advantages in nonexposed infants (see Chapter 22), breastfeeding of substance-exposed infants can enhance maternal/infant bonding and can reduce withdrawal severity and duration in infants with NAS.

  A. We encourage breastfeeding in the following circumstances:

    1. Mother is in treatment for substance abuse and allows newborn providers to discuss progress in treatment and plans for postpartum treatment with substance abuse provider.

    2. Substance abuse treatment provider endorses that mother has been able to achieve and maintain sobriety prenatally.

    3. Mother plans to continue in substance abuse treatment in the postpartum period.

Table 12.5. Neonatal Abstinence Scoring Tool

Date: _____

Signs & Symptoms	Time:												Comments
Central Nervous System Disturbances													
Excessive High-Pitched Cry	2												
Continuous High-Pitched Cry	3												
Sleeps <1 Hour After Feeding	3												
Sleeps <2 Hours After Feeding	2												
Sleeps <3 Hours After Feeding	1												
Hyperactive Moro Reflex	2												
Markedly Hyperactive Moro Reflex	3												
Mild Tremors: Disturbed	1												
Mod-Severe Tremors: Disturbed	2												
Mild Tremors: Undisturbed	3												
Mod-Severe Tremors: Undisturbed	4												
Increased Muscle Tone	2												

Excoriation (Specific Areas)	1															
Myoclonic Jerks	3															
Generalized Convulsions	5															
Metabolic/Vasomotor/Respiratory Disturbances																
Sweating	1															
Fever: 37.2–38.3 C	1															
Fever: 38.4 C and Higher	2															
Frequent Yawning (>3)	1															
Mottling	1															
Nasal Stuffiness	1															
Sneezing (>3)	1															
Nasal Flaring	2															
Resp. Rate >60/min	1															
Resp. Rate >60/min w/ Retractions	2															

(continued)

Table 12.5. Neonatal Abstinence Scoring Tool (Continued)

Signs & Symptoms	Time:									Comments
Gastrointestinal Disturbances										
Excessive Sucking	1									
Poor Feeding	2									
Regurgitation	2									
Projectile Vomiting	3									
Loose Stools	2									
Watery Stools	3									
Total Score:										
Initials of Scorer										

Signature: _____ Initials: _____ Date: _____ Time: _____

Source: Courtesy of Vanderbilt Children's Hospital.

Table 12.6. Definitions of Scoring Items on Neonatal Abstinence Scoring Tool

Scoring Item	Definition
Excessive high-pitched cry	Unable to self-console in 15 seconds or continuous up to 5 minutes despite intervention
Continuous high-pitched cry	Unable to self-console in 15 seconds or continuous >5 minutes despite intervention
Sleep	Based on longest period of sleep (light or deep) after feeding
Hyperactive Moro reflex	Elicit from a quiet infant; jitteriness that is rhythmic, symmetrical, and involuntary
Markedly hyperactive Moro reflex	Elicit from a quiet infant; jitteriness that is rhythmic, symmetrical, and involuntary AND clonus of hands/arms; may test at hands or feet if unclear (more than 8–10 beats)
Mild tremors when disturbed	Involuntary, rhythmical, and equal strength in hands or feet only while being handled
Moderate to severe tremors when disturbed	Involuntary, rhythmical, and equal strength in arms or legs while being handled
Mild tremors when undisturbed	Involuntary, rhythmical, and equal strength in hands or feet only while NOT being handled; should be assessed while unwrapped 15–30 seconds after touching the infant, not while sleeping
Moderate to severe tremors when undisturbed	Involuntary, rhythmical, and equal strength in arms or legs while NOT being handled; should be assessed while unwrapped 15–30 seconds after touching the infant, not while sleeping
Increased muscle tone	Perform pull-to-sit maneuver if tolerated; no head lag with total body rigidity. Do not test while asleep or crying.
Excoriation	Reddened areas from increased movement present at nose, chin, cheeks, elbows, knees, or toes. Do not score for reddened diaper area related to loose/frequent stools.
Myoclonic jerks	Involuntary twitching of face/extremities or jerking at extremities which is more pronounced than jitteriness of tremors

(continued)

Table 12.6. Definitions of Scoring Items on Neonatal Abstinence Scoring Tool *(Continued)*

Scoring Item	Definition
Generalized convulsions	Tonic seizures with extension or flexion of limb(s); does not stop with containment; may include few clonic beats and/or apnea
Sweating	Wetness at forehead, upper lip, or back of neck; do not score if related to the environment.
Fever <101°F	37.2°–38.3°C
Fever >101°F	38.4°C and higher
Frequent yawning	More than three to four times, individually or serially, over scoring interval/time period
Mottling	Pink and white marbled appearance present at chest, trunk, arms, or legs
Nasal stuffiness	With or without runny nose
Sneezing	More than three to four times, individually or serially, over scoring interval/time period
Excessive sucking	Rooting with more than three attempts noted to suck fist, hand, or pacifier before or after feeding
Poor feeding	Excessive sucking as above but infrequent or uncoordinated with feeding, or gulping with frequent rest periods to breath
Regurgitation	Effortless, not associated with burping; more than two episodes
Loose stools	Loose, curdy, seedy, or liquid without water ring
Watery stools	Soft, liquid, or hard with water ring

4. Mother has abstained from illicit drug use or illicit drug abuse for 90 days prior to delivery and demonstrates the ability to maintain sobriety in an outpatient setting as follows:

   a. Negative maternal urine toxicology testing at delivery except for prescribed medications

   b. Received consistent prenatal care

   c. No medical contraindication to breastfeeding (such as HIV)

   d. Not taking a psychiatric medication that is contraindicated during lactation

   e. Stable on methadone or buprenorphine (regardless of dose)

B. We discourage breastfeeding in the following circumstances:

1. Illicit drug use or licit substance misuse in the 30-day period prior to delivery. In some cases, breastfeeding may be permissible for mothers with illicit drug use in the previous 30 days if the mother is not currently using, has engaged in treatment and the provider team, including the infant's provider, and the mother's substance abuse treatment provider deem it appropriate.

2. Active substance use while not in substance abuse treatment or refusal to allow communication with substance abuse treatment provider

3. Positive maternal urine toxicology testing for drugs of abuse or misuse of licit drugs at delivery

4. No confirmed plans for postpartum substance abuse treatment or pediatric care

5. Erratic behavioral or other indicators of active drug use

6. No prenatal care

C. We evaluate for breastfeeding in the following circumstances:

1. Relapse to illicit substance use or licit substance misuse in the 90- to 30-day period prior to delivery but abstinent for the 30 days prior to delivery

2. Concomitant use of other prescription (i.e., psychotropic) medications

3. Sobriety obtained in an inpatient setting

4. Isolated marijuana use (or in conjunction with medication-assisted treatment): The literature to support breastfeeding in the context of marijuana use is limited; some data suggest long-term cognitive/developmental delays for exposed infants. We therefore inform the mother that the effects of marijuana use are not well understood and may cause cognitive/developmental delays in her infant. If the mother is aware of this risk and wishes to breastfeed, she is allowed and is encouraged to discontinue marijuana use.

VI. **DISCHARGE.** Clinical signs of NAS may last for months, and infants with NAS are two and a half times as likely as uncomplicated term infants to be readmitted to the hospital within 30 days of discharge. The following should be done to help ensure a safe discharge home:

A. Pediatrician follow-up within a few days of discharge

B. Home nurse visitation where available

C. Communication with child protective services when applicable

D. Referral to early intervention services

E. Parental education

1. Clinical signs of NAS

2. How to seek help

3. Relevant community resources

F. Ideally, infant care would be coordinated with maternal care (e.g., addiction medicine, obstetrics).

VII. **LONG-TERM OUTCOMES.** Data for long-term infant outcomes of substance use in pregnancy are limited but are summarized in Table 12.7.

Table 12.7. Short- and Long-Term Effects of Substance Use in Pregnancy

	Nicotine	Alcohol	Marijuana	Opiates	Cocaine	Methamphetamine
Short-term effects/birth outcome						
Fetal growth	Effect	Strong effect	No effect	Effect	Effect	Effect
Anomalies	No consensus on effect	Strong effect	No effect	No effect	No effect	No effect
Withdrawal	No effect	No effect	No effect	Strong effect	No effect	*
Neurobehavior	Effect	Effect	Effect	Effect	Effect	Effect
Long-term effects						
Growth	No consensus on effect	Strong effect	No effect	No effect	No consensus on effect	*
Behavior	Effect	Strong effect	Effect	Effect	Effect	*
Cognition	Effect	Strong effect	Effect	No consensus on effect	Effect	*
Language	Effect	Effect	No effect	*	Effect	*
Achievement	Effect	Strong effect	Effect	*	No consensus on effect	*

*Limited or no data available.
Source: Behnke M, Smith VC. Prenatal substance abuse: short- and long-term effects on the exposed fetus. *Pediatrics* 2013;131:e1009–e1024.

Suggested Readings

American College of Obstetricians and Gynecologists Committee on Health Care for Underserved Women. ACOG Committee Opinion No. 524: opioid abuse, dependence, and addiction in pregnancy. *Obstet Gynecol* 2012;119:1070–1076.

Behnke M, Smith VC. Prenatal substance abuse: short- and long-term effects on the exposed fetus. *Pediatrics* 2013;131:e1009–e1024.

Hudak ML, Tan RC. Neonatal drug withdrawal. *Pediatrics* 2012;129:e540–e560.

Jansson LM. ABM Clinical Protocol #21: guidelines for breastfeeding and the drug-dependent woman. *Breastfeed Med* 2009;4:225–228.

Patrick SW, Dudley J, Martin PR, et al. Prescription opioid epidemic and infant outcomes. *Pediatrics* 2015;135:842–850.

13 Care of the Extremely Low Birth Weight Infant

Steven A. Ringer

KEY POINTS

- If possible, extremely premature infants should be delivered in a facility with a high-risk obstetrical service and a level 3 or 4 neonatal intensive care unit (NICU).
- Uniformity of approach within an institution and a commitment to provide and evaluate care in a collaborative manner across professional disciplines may be the most important aspects of protocols for the care of extremely low birth weight (ELBW) infants.
- Careful attention to detail and frequent monitoring are the basic components of care of the ELBW infant because critical changes can occur rapidly.

I. **INTRODUCTION.** Extremely low birth weight (ELBW; birth weight <1,000 g) infants are a unique group of patients in the neonatal intensive care unit (NICU). Because these infants are so physiologically immature, they are extremely sensitive to small changes in respiratory management, blood pressure, fluid administration, nutrition, and virtually all other aspects of care. The optimal way to care for these infants continues to be determined by ongoing research. However, the most effective care based on currently available evidence is best ensured through the implementation of standardized protocols for the care of the ELBW infant within individual NICUs. One approach is outlined in Table 13.1. Uniformity of approach within an institution and a commitment to provide and evaluate care in a collaborative manner across professional disciplines may be the most important aspects of such protocols.

II. **PRENATAL CONSIDERATIONS.** If possible, extremely premature infants should be delivered in a facility with a high-risk obstetrical service and a level 3 or 4 NICU; the value of this practice in preventing mortality and morbidity in ELBW infants has been demonstrated in several studies. The safety of maternal transport must of course be weighed against the risks of infant transport (see Chapter 17). Prenatal administration of glucocorticoids to the mother, even if there is not time for a full course, reduces the risk of respiratory distress syndrome (RDS) and other sequelae of prematurity and is strongly recommended.

A. **Neonatology consultation.** If delivery of an extremely premature infant is threatened, a neonatologist should consult with the parents, preferably with

Table 13.1. Elements of a Protocol for Standardizing Care of the Extremely Low Birth Weight (ELBW) Infant

Prenatal consultation
Parental education
Determining parental wishes when viability is questionable
Defining limits of parental choice; need for caregiver–parent teamwork
Delivery room care
Define limits of resuscitative efforts
Respiratory support
Low tidal volume ventilation strategy
Prevention of heat and water loss
Early surfactant therapy
Ventilation strategy
Low tidal volume, short inspiratory time
Avoid hyperoxia and hypocapnia
Early surfactant therapy as indicated
Define indications for high-frequency ventilation
Fluids
Early use of humidified incubators to limit fluid and heat losses
Judicious use of fluid bolus therapy for hypotension
Careful monitoring of fluid and electrolyte status
Use of double-lumen umbilical venous catheters for fluid support
Nutrition
Initiation of parenteral nutrition shortly after birth
Early initiation of trophic feeding with maternal milk
Advancement of feeding density to provide adequate calories for healing and growth
(continued)

Table 13.1. Elements of a Protocol for Standardizing Care of the Extremely Low Birth Weight (ELBW) Infant *(Continued)*

Cardiovascular support
Maintenance of blood pressure within standard range
Use of dopamine for support as indicated
Corticosteroids for unresponsive hypotension
PDA
Avoidance of excess fluid administration
Consider medical therapy when hemodynamically significant PDA is present.
Consider surgical ligation after failed medical therapy.
Infection control
Scrupulous hand hygiene, use of bedside alcohol gels
Limiting blood drawing, skin punctures
Protocol for CVL insertion and care, minimize dwell time
Minimal entry into CVLs, no use of fluids prepared in NICU

PDA, patent ductus arteriosus; CVL, central venous line; NICU, newborn intensive care unit.

the obstetrician present. There are no reliable systems or prognostic scores that allow one to make **firm** predictions about a particular case, in part because outcome is also affected by variable practices and beliefs about aggressive resuscitation of these infants. The most useful current data is based on a study of ELBWs born in NICUs participating in the Eunice Shriver National Institute of Child Health and Human Development (NICHD) Neonatal Network. This study reported that survival free from neurodevelopmental disability for infants born between 22 and 25 weeks of gestation was dependent not only on completed weeks of gestation but also on (i) sex, (ii) birth weight, (iii) exposure to antenatal corticosteroids, and (iv) singleton or multiple gestation. Using these data, the NICHD developed a web-based tool to *estimate* the likelihood of survival with and without severe neurosensory disability (https://www.nichd.nih.gov/about/org/der/branches/ppb/programs/epbo/Pages/epbo_case.aspx). To use the tool, data are entered in each of the five categories (estimated gestational age and birth weight, sex, exposure to antenatal glucocorticoids, and singleton or multiple birth). The tool calculates outcome estimates for survival and survival with moderate or severe disabilities. It is helpful to use this estimator tool as a guide, tempered by the experience in the individual institution, during antenatal discussions with parents. A general approach to consultation is as follows:

1. **Survival.** To most parents, the impending delivery of an extremely premature infant is frightening, and their initial concern almost always focuses on the likelihood of infant survival. Recent studies have reported that survival is possible at gestational age as low as 22 weeks. The NICHD network reported survival rates of 6% at 22 completed weeks, 26% at 23 weeks, and 55% and 72% at 24 and 25 weeks, respectively. Other studies have reported even higher survival rates, even at 22 weeks. Assessments based solely on best obstetrical estimate of gestational age do not allow for the impact of other factors, whereas those based on birth weight (a more accurately determined parameter), don't fully account for the impact of growth restriction. The use of the NICHD estimator allows the consultant to estimate the impact and interaction between gestational maturity, weight, and the other identified critical factors. Although extremely helpful as a starting point, at least two important cautions should be considered in individual cases. First, birth weight has to be estimated for purposes of antenatal discussion, although reliable estimates are often available from ultrasonographic examinations, assuming a technically adequate examination can be performed. If this information is not known, gestational age estimates for appropriate for gestational age (AGA) fetuses can be roughly converted as follows: 600 g = 24 weeks; 750 g = 25 weeks; 850 g = 26 weeks; 1,000 g = 27 weeks. Second, there may be important additional information in individual cases that will significantly impact prognosis, such as the presence of anomalies, infection, chronic growth restriction, or evidence of deteriorating status before birth. Clinical experience must be used to guide interpretation of the impact of such factors.

2. For antenatal counseling, it may also be important to interpret published data in the light of local results. The best obstetrical estimate of gestational age may vary between institutions, and local practices and capabilities may significantly affect both mortality and morbidity in ELBW infants. Within individual institutions, practitioners tend to agree on the gestational age at which an infant has any hope of survival, and this can in effect make prognostication a self-fulfilling prophecy. In counseling, practitioners must avoid simply perpetuating local dogma but at the same time remain cognizant of the current institutional capabilities.

   In discussions with parents, it is important to attempt to reach a collaborative decision about what course of treatment would be best for their baby. We advocate attempting resuscitation of all newborns who are potentially viable, but recognize that the personal views of parents regarding what might be an acceptable outcome for their child will vary, and thereby impact decisions about offering resuscitation. Currently, we inform them that resuscitation at birth has been technically feasible at gestational age as low as about 22 weeks and a birth weight as low as about 500 g. In an individual case, the superimposition of medical problems other than prematurity may make survival extremely unlikely or impossible even at higher gestational ages. In counseling parents, we stress that within these parameters, delivery room resuscitation alone has a high (but not absolute) chance of success, but that this in no way guarantees survival beyond these early minutes. Studies show that decisions based on the apparent condition at birth are unreliable in terms of viability or long-term outcome. We also note that the initiation of intensive care in no way mandates that it be continued if it is later determined to be futile or very likely to result in a poor long-term outcome. We assure parents that initial resuscitation is always followed by frequent reassessment in the NICU and discussions with them and that intensive support may be appropriately withdrawn if the degree of immaturity results in no response to therapy or if catastrophic and irreversible complications occur. Parents are counseled that the period of highest vulnerability may last several weeks in infants of lowest gestational ages. Once all these components are discussed, a recommendation can be made regarding an approach to initial resuscitation.

If parents disagree with this recommendation, differences may be resolved by ensuring that they understand the medical information and that their views and concerns are understood as well as recognition of their central role in determining appropriate care for their child. Almost always, a consensus on a plan of care can be reached, but if an impasse continues, consultation from the institutional ethics service may be warranted (see Chapter 19).

3. **Morbidity.** Care decisions and parental expectations must be based not only on estimates of survival but also on information about likely short- and long-term prognosis. Before delivery, particular attention is paid to the problems that might appear at birth or shortly thereafter. We explain the risk of RDS and the potential need for ventilatory support. Increasingly, support includes continuous positive airway pressure (CPAP) alone, but mechanical ventilation, at least for a short period, is still required for a significant percentage of infants at the lowest gestational ages. Parents should also be informed of the likelihood of infection at birth depending on perinatal risk factors as well as any plan to screen for it and begin empiric antibiotic therapy while final culture results are pending.

4. **Potential morbidity.** During prenatal consultation, it is generally recommended to avoid giving parents detailed information on every potential sequela of extreme prematurity because they may be too overwhelmed to process extensive information during this time. We do specifically discuss those problems that are most likely to occur in many ELBW infants or will be screened for during hospitalization. These include apnea of prematurity, intraventricular hemorrhage (IVH), nosocomial sepsis (or evaluations for possible sepsis), and feeding difficulties as well as long-term sensory disabilities. We make a point of briefly discussing the risks of retinopathy of prematurity and subsequent visual deficits and the need for hearing screening and the potential for hearing loss. These complications are not diagnosed until late in the hospital course, but we find that giving parents some perspective on the entire hospitalization is helpful to them.

5. **Parents' desires.** In most instances, parents are the best surrogate decision makers for their child. We believe that, within each institution, there should be a uniform approach to parental demands for attempting or withholding resuscitation at very low gestational ages. The best practice is to formulate decisions in concert with parents, after providing them with clear, realistic, and factual information about the possibilities for success of therapy and its long-term outcome.

During the consultation, the neonatologist should try to understand parental wishes about resuscitative efforts and subsequent support especially when chances for infant survival are slim. When counseling parents around an expected birth at <24 weeks, we specifically offer them the choice of limiting delivery room interventions to those designed to ensure comfort alone if they feel that the prognosis appears too bleak for their child. We encourage them to voice their understanding of the planned approach and their expectations for their soon-to-be born child. We reassure them that the strength of their wishes does help guide caregivers in determining whether and how long to continue resuscitation attempts. Through this approach, the parents' role in decision making as well as the limitations of that role is clarified. In practice, parents' wishes about resuscitation are central to decision making when the gestational age is <24 completed weeks. At 25 weeks and above, in the absence of other factors, we very strongly advocate for attempting resuscitation and make this clear to parents.

III. **DELIVERY ROOM CARE.** The pediatric team should include an experienced pediatrician or neonatologist, particularly when the fetus is of <26 weeks' gestational age. The approach to resuscitation is similar to that in more mature infants (see Chapter 4). Special attention should be paid to the following:

A. **Warmth and drying.** The ELBW neonate is at particular risk for hypothermia. Better temperature control may be achieved with at least one of the following techniques: (i) immediately wrapping the undried baby's body and extremities in plastic wrap or a placing them in a plastic bag (we have had most success using a large sheet of plastic and quickly wrapping the baby in a swaddling fashion), (ii) the use of an exothermic mattress, (iii) ensuring that the delivery room temperature has been set at 26°C. Use of two modalities increases the likelihood of avoiding hypothermia. Care must be taken to avoid overheating the baby, especially when more than one of these modalities is employed.

B. **Respiratory support.** Most ELBW infants require some degree of ventilatory support because of pulmonary immaturity and limited respiratory muscle strength. Blended oxygen and air should be available to help avoid prolonged hyperoxia after the initial resuscitation, and it should be used in conjunction with pulse oximetry, using a probe placed on the right upper ("preductal") extremity. Studies have demonstrated that a blend of oxygen and air is preferable; it is recommended that resuscitation usually start with 21% to 30% oxygen and titrate the concentration titrated based on measured oxygen saturation. Oxygen saturation should be targeted as identified for all babies the first several minutes after birth (see Table 4.1), and thereafter oxygen concentration adjusted so as to keep the saturation level the same as that used during NICU care for all babies <32 weeks (suggested target of 90% to 95%). If the neonate cries vigorously at birth, room air or blow-by blended oxygen may be administered if required on the basis of the measured saturation and the infant observed for signs of distress.

Many of these infants will require some ventilatory support because of apnea or ineffective respiratory drive. If the infant is breathing spontaneously, albeit with distress, initial respiratory support can be provided by either positive pressure ventilation or CPAP. In studies comparing these modalities, there were no differences in survival or incidence of chronic lung disease with CPAP versus initial mechanical ventilation. We therefore favor using CPAP at 6 to 8 cm H_2O as initial support, although infants may require a breath or two with bag and mask before they breathe spontaneously. If the infant is not breathing spontaneously, positive pressure ventilation must be started using pressures adequate to produce chest rise; provision of adequate support will result in or maintain a normal heart rate. Judgment is required regarding ongoing support, depending on the baby's status and local practice patterns. If positive pressure ventilation is required, care should be taken to use the smallest tidal volumes and peak pressure possible while still adequately ventilating the infant. These infants usually require continued respiratory support and do benefit from early application of end-expiratory pressure; our practice is to provide this via endotracheal intubation and ventilation shortly after birth. Many centers employ a T-piece device (Neopuff Infant T-Piece Resuscitator, Fisher & Paykel Healthcare, Inc, Irvine, CA) instead of hand-bagging or giving CPAP via bag and mask because it ensures adequate and regulated positive end-expiratory pressure and regulated inflation pressures. Although commonly practiced in many institutions, administration of exogenous surfactant therapy before the first breath has not been proven to be more beneficial than administration after initial stabilization of the infant. Exogenous surfactant may be safely administered in the delivery room once correct endotracheal tube position has been confirmed clinically.

The pediatrician should assess the response to resuscitation and gauge the need for further interventions. If the infant fails to respond, the team should recheck that all support measures are being effectively administered. Support for apnea or poor respiratory effort must include intermittent inflating breaths or regulated nasal CPAP. CPAP delivered via face mask alone is not adequate support for an apneic baby, and a failure to respond to this limited intervention does not mean that the infant is too immature to be resuscitated. If, on the other hand, there is no positive response to resuscitation after a reasonable length of time, we consider limiting support to comfort measures alone. In all cases, communication with the parents should be maintained through a designated member of the care team

C. Care after resuscitation. Immediately after resuscitation, the plastic-wrapped infant should be placed in a prewarmed transport incubator for transfer to the NICU. Within practical limits, we encourage as much interaction between baby and the parents in the delivery room (while in the transport incubator) to enhance the beginning of parent–infant interaction. In the NICU, the infant is moved to an incubator/radiant warmer combination unit (Giraffe Bed, Ohmeda Medical, Madison, WI) where a complete assessment is done and treatment initiated. The infant's temperature should be rechecked at this time and closely monitored. As soon as possible, the unit is closed to function as an incubator for continued care. Humidity is maintained at 70% for the first week of life and 50% to 60% thereafter up to 32 weeks corrected gestation. In addition to reducing insensible fluid losses and thereby simplifying fluid therapy, the use of incubators aids in reducing unnecessary stimulation and noise experienced by the baby.

IV. CARE IN THE INTENSIVE CARE UNIT. Careful attention to detail and frequent monitoring are the basic components of care of the ELBW infant because critical changes can occur rapidly. Large fluid losses, balances between fluid intake and blood glucose levels, delicate pulmonary status, and the immaturity and increased sensitivity of several organ systems all require close monitoring. Monitoring itself, however, may pose increased risks because each laboratory test requires a significant percentage of the baby's total blood volume, tiny-caliber vessels may be hard to cannulate without several attempts, and limited skin integrity increases susceptibility to injury or infection. Issues in routine care that require special attention in ELBW infants include the following:

A. **Survival.** The first several days after birth, and in particular the first 24 to 48 hours, are the most critical for survival. Infants who require significant respiratory, cardiovascular, and/or fluid support are assessed continuously, and their chances for ongoing survival are evaluated as part of this process. If caregivers and the parents determine that death is imminent, continued treatment is futile, or treatment is likely to result in survival of a child with profound neurologic impairment, it is appropriate to recommend withdrawal of ventilator and other invasive support and redirection of care to comfort measures and support of the family.

B. **Respiratory support.** Most ELBW infants require initial respiratory support.

1. **CPAP.** In our population, a very large majority of ELBW infants have been exposed to antenatal corticosteroids, and respiratory support may be accomplished with CPAP alone. It is generally initiated at 6 cm H_2O pressure, and the pressure increased in 1 cm increments to a maximum of 8 cm, if the oxygen requirement exceeds 40%. One key to successful CPAP therapy and the prevention of atelectasis is to ensure that the CPAP is not interrupted, even briefly. There is no conclusive evidence that one mode of CPAP delivery is superior to another. If the oxygen requirement rises even after the maximal pressure has been reached, or if there is recurrent apnea, mechanical ventilation is indicated.

2. **Conventional ventilation.** We generally use conventional pressure-limited synchronized intermittent mandatory ventilation (SIMV), usually in a volume guarantee mode, as our primary mode of mechanical ventilation (see Chapter 29). The lowest possible tidal volume to provide adequate ventilation and oxygenation and a short inspiratory time should be used. Special effort should be made to avoid hyperoxia by targeting specific oxygen saturations. Several reports have demonstrated that oxygen saturation limits for babies <32 weeks' gestation who require supplemental oxygen should be lower than those used in more mature babies, in order to limit the number of hypoxia–hyperoxia

fluctuations and reduce the incidence and severity of retinopathy of prematurity. A recent report found that a target range of 85% to 89% decreased retinopathy but may be associated with an increase in mortality, compared to a range of 90% to 94%. We aim for a target range of 90% to 95%. We encourage close monitoring including observation to determine if oxygen saturation outside the range will correct without intervention, thereby decreasing the tendency for hypoxia–hyperoxia fluctuations. It is hypothesized that limiting hyperoxia may also reduce the incidence or severity of chronic lung disease. It is important as well to avoid hypocapnia, although the potential benefit of permissive hypercapnia as a ventilatory strategy remains a subject of debate.

3. **Surfactant therapy** (see Chapter 33). We administer surfactant to infants with RDS who are ventilated with a mean airway pressure of at least 7 cm H_2O and have an inspired oxygen concentration (FiO_2) of 0.3 or higher in the first 2 hours after birth. The first dose should be given as soon as possible after birth after intubation, preferably within the first hour, although with increased use of CPAP as initial therapy, the timing of surfactant therapy may be delayed. We have found that many treated infants can be rapidly transitioned to support with CPAP shortly after surfactant administration.

4. **High-frequency oscillatory ventilation (HFOV)** is used in infants who fail to improve after surfactant administration and require conventional ventilation at high mean airway pressures. For infants with an air leak syndrome, especially pulmonary interstitial emphysema (see Chapter 38), high-frequency jet ventilation may be the preferred mode of ventilation.

5. **Caffeine citrate** administered within the first 10 days after birth at standard doses (see Appendix A) has been associated with a reduced risk of developing bronchopulmonary dysplasia (BPD).

C. **Fluids and electrolytes** (see Chapters 23 and 28). Fluid requirements increase as gestational age decreases <28 weeks, owing to both an increased surface area–body weight ratio and immaturity of the skin. Renal immaturity may result in large losses of fluid and electrolytes that must be replaced. Early use of humidified incubators significantly reduces insensible fluid losses and therefore the total administered volume necessary to maintain fluid balance, especially when care interventions are coordinated to ensure that the incubator top is only rarely opened.

1. **Route of administration.** Whenever possible, double-lumen umbilical venous line should be placed shortly after birth, along with an umbilical arterial line for infants requiring higher levels of support or those with blood pressure instability. Arterial lines generally are maintained for a maximum of 7 to 10 days and then replaced by peripheral arterial lines if needed. Because of an increased risk of infection, the dwell time for umbilical venous catheters (UVC) in most cases is limited to 10 days. These are often replaced by percutaneously inserted central venous catheters (PICC) if continued long-term intravenous (IV) access is required.

2. **Rate of administration.** Table 13.2 presents initial rates of fluid administration for different gestational ages and birth weights when

Table 13.2. Fluid Administration Rates for the First 2 Days of Life for Infants on Radiant Warmers*

Birth Weight (g)	Gestational Age (week)	Fluid Rate (mL/kg/day)	Frequency of Electrolyte Testing
500–600	23	110–120	q6h
601–800	24	100–110	q8h
801–1,000	25–26	80–100	q12h

*Rates should be 20%–30% lower when a humidified incubator is used. Urine output and serum electrolytes should be closely monitored to determine the best rates.

humidified incubators are used. Weight, blood pressure, urine output, and serum electrolyte levels should be monitored frequently. Fluid rate is adjusted to avoid dehydration or hypernatremia. Serum electrolytes should generally be measured before the age of 12 hours (6 hours for infants <800 g) and repeat as often as every 6 hours until the levels are stable. By the second to third day, many infants have a marked diuresis and natriuresis and require continued frequent assessment and adjustment of fluids and electrolytes. Insensible water loss diminishes as the skin thickens and dries over the first few days of life.

3. **Fluid composition.** Initial IV fluids should consist of dextrose solution in a concentration sufficient to maintain serum glucose levels >45 to 50 mg/dL. Often, immature infants do not tolerate dextrose concentrations >10% at high fluid rates, so use of dextrose 7.5% or 5% solutions is frequently needed. Usually, a glucose administration rate of 4 to 10 mg/kg/minute is sufficient. If hyperglycemia results, lower dextrose concentrations should be administered; hypoosmolar solutions (dextrose <5%) should be avoided. If hyperglycemia persists at levels above 180 to 220 mg/dL with glycosuria, an insulin infusion at a dose of 0.05 to 0.1 unit/kg/hour may be required and adjusted as needed to maintain serum glucose levels at acceptable levels (see Chapter 24).

ELBW infants begin losing protein and develop negative nitrogen balance almost immediately after birth. To avoid this, we start parenteral nutrition immediately upon admission to the NICU for all infants with a birth weight <1,250 g, using a premixed stock solution of amino acids and trace elements in dextrose 5% to 7.5%. Multivitamin solutions are not included in this initial parenteral nutrition because of shelf-life issues but are added within 24 hours after delivery. No electrolytes are added to the initial solution other than the small amount of sodium phosphate needed to buffer the amino acids. The solution is designed so that the administration of 60 mL/kg/day (the maximum infusion rate used) provides 2 g of protein/kg/day. Additional fluid needs are met by the solutions described earlier. Customized parenteral nutrition, including lipid infusion, is begun as soon as it is available, generally within the first day.

4. **Skin care.** Immaturity of skin and susceptibility to damage requires close attention to maintenance of skin integrity (see Chapter 65). Topical emollients or petroleum-based products are not used except under extreme situations, but semipermeable coverings (Tegaderm and Vigilon) may be used over areas of skin breakdown.

D. Cardiovascular support

1. **Blood pressure.** There is disagreement over acceptable values for blood pressure in extremely premature infants and some suggestion that cerebral perfusion may be adversely affected at levels below a mean blood pressure of 30 mm Hg. In the absence of data demonstrating an impact on long-term neurologic outcome, we accept mean blood pressures of 26 to 28 mm Hg for infants of 24 to 26 weeks' gestational age in the transitional period after birth if the infant appears well perfused and has a normal heart rate. Early hypotension is more commonly due to altered vasoreactivity than hypovolemia, so therapy with fluid boluses are generally limited to 10 to 20 mL/kg, after which pressor support, initially with dopamine, is begun. Stress-dose hydrocortisone (1 mg/kg every 12 hours for two doses) may be useful in infants with hypotension refractory to this strategy (see Chapter 40).

   If the infant is breathing spontaneously at birth, cord clamping should be delayed until 30 to 60 seconds have elapsed. This practice has been shown to decrease the incidence of early hypotension in premature infants.

2. **Patent ductus arteriosus (PDA).** The incidence of symptomatic PDA is as high as 70% in infants with a birth weight <1,000 g. The natural timing of presentation has been accelerated by exogenous surfactant therapy so that a symptomatic PDA now commonly occurs between 24 and 48 hours after birth, manifested by an increasing need for ventilatory support or an increase in oxygen requirement. A murmur may be absent or difficult to hear, and the physical signs of increased pulses or an active precordium may be difficult to discern. Most importantly, it remains a matter of controversy whether a patent ductus is always harmful or requires treatment. Infants with a symptomatic PDA have a higher risk of BPD, but early closure does not decrease this risk. Recent studies suggest that a large percentage of PDAs will ultimately close spontaneously, and the risks of either medical or surgical therapy may have an adverse effect on both acute and long-term outcome. This suggests that some of the outcomes attributed to the PDA might be related to the impact of the therapies employed in an effort to close it. We thus remain vigilant for the presence of a PDA but delay pharmacologic therapy until an echocardiogram has been performed and the PDA is noted to be large (≥3 mm) or shown to be causing a diminution in left ventricular function and distal flow in the descending aorta. If initial medical therapy fails to eliminate the hemodynamic impact of the PDA, we administer a second course of pharmacologic therapy (indomethacin or ibuprofen). Prophylactic treatment with indomethacin has been demonstrated to reduce the incidence and severity of PDA and the need for subsequent ligation. However, it has not been shown to result in a change in long-term neurologic or respiratory outcome. Although it has

not become routine therapy, many centers continue to use prophylactic indomethacin. Surgical ligation is infrequently necessary and should only be considered if there is clear evidence of a significant left to right shunt after medical management.

E. Blood transfusions. These are often necessary in small infants because of large obligatory phlebotomy losses. Infants who weigh <1,000 g at birth and are moderately or severely ill may receive as many as eight or nine transfusions in the first few weeks of life. Donor exposure can be successfully limited by reducing laboratory testing to the minimum necessary level, employing strict uniform criteria for transfusion, and by identifying a specific unit of blood for each patient likely to need several transfusions (see Chapter 45). Each such unit can be split to provide as many as eight transfusions for a single patient over a period of 21 days with only a single donor exposure. Erythropoietin therapy in conjunction with adequate iron therapy will result in accelerated erythropoiesis, but it has not been shown to reduce the need for transfusion and is not routinely used in these patients.

F. Infection and infection control (see Chapter 49). In general, premature birth is associated with an increased incidence of early-onset sepsis, with an incidence of 1.5% in infants having birth weight <1,500 g. Group B *Streptococcus* (GBS) remains an important pathogen, but gram-negative organisms now account for most of early-onset sepsis in infants weighing <1,500 g. We almost always screen for infection immediately after birth in cases in which there are perinatal risk factors for infection and treat with prophylactic antibiotics (ampicillin and gentamicin) pending culture results. ELBW infants are particularly susceptible to hospital-acquired infections (occurring at >72 hours after birth), with about half due to coagulase-negative *Staphylococcus*. Mortality, as well as long-term morbidity, is higher among infants who develop these late-onset infections, particularly in those with gram-negative or fungal infections. Risk factors for late-onset infection include longer duration of mechanical ventilation, presence of central catheters, and parenteral nutrition support.

The risk of these late-onset infections (particularly central line–associated infections) can be decreased by improvements in care practices. Foremost among these is meticulous attention to hand hygiene. Alcohol-based gel for hand hygiene should be available at every bedside and prominently in other spots throughout the NICU. Periodic anonymous observation to monitor and report on hand hygiene practices before any caregiver–patient contact may help maintain compliance. In-line suctioning is used in respiratory circuits to minimize disruption, and every effort is made to minimize the duration of mechanical ventilation. We only use parenteral nutrition solutions that have been prepared under laminar flow and never alter them after preparation. The early introduction of feedings, preferably with human milk, minimizes the need for central lines and provides the benefits of milk-borne immune factors. When central lines are necessary, we have an observer monitor the PICC insertion technique and immediately identify deviation or omission from a standard checklist. Dedicated central line insertion teams are employed in many units and help standardize insertion techniques to reduce the risk of infection. After insertion, attention to scrupulous central line care to avoid line hub bacterial colonization also has been shown to reduce the risk of central line–associated bacterial infection. The need for the line should be reassessed daily to reduce line dwell time to a minimum. Minimal laboratory testing as allowed by the infant's condition and clustering blood draws whenever possible help reduce the number of skin punctures and reduce patient handling. These practices are part of a standardized protocol for skin care for all neonates born with weight of <1,000 g. Ideally, the establishment of a uniform NICU culture that rejects the idea that these infections are inevitable and fosters pride in care and cooperation has helped create an environment of blameless questioning between practitioners.

G. **Nutritional support** (see Chapter 21)

1. **Initial management.** In all infants who weigh <1,000 to 1,200 g at birth, parenteral nutrition is begun shortly after birth using a standard solution administered at a rate of 60 mL/kg/day (see section IV.C), resulting in protein administration of 2 g/kg/day. On subsequent days, customized parenteral solutions are formulated to increase the protein administration rate by 1 g/kg/day up to a maximum of 4 g/kg/day. Parenteral lipids are begun on day 2 and advanced each day to a maximum of 3 g/kg/day as allowed by triglyceride levels. Enteral feeding is begun as soon as the patient is clinically stable and is not receiving indomethacin or pressor therapy.

2. The safe initiation of enteral feeds begins with the introduction of small amounts of expressed breast milk (10 to 20 mL/kg/day), with the goal of priming the gut by inducing local factors necessary for normal function. In many units, donor breast milk is used for the highest risk infants if expressed breast milk is not available; in units without availability of donor breast milk, options include use of preterm formula or delay in initiation of enteral feedings for 3 to 4 days until expressed breast milk or colostrum is available. These small amounts of enteral feedings may be started even in the presence of an umbilical arterial line and continued for 3 to 5 days before advancement. A standardized approach to feeding advancement may reduce the risk of feeding intolerance or necrotizing enterocolitis (see Chapters 21 and 27). As feedings are advanced, signs of feeding intolerance such as abdominal distention, vomiting (which is rare), and increased gastric residuals should be monitored. It is important but often difficult to differentiate the characteristically poor gastrointestinal motility of ELBW infants from signs of a more serious gastrointestinal disorder such as necrotizing enterocolitis (see Chapter 27). At least two-thirds of ELBW infants have episodes of feeding intolerance that result in interruption of feeds, including small bilious gastric residuals as feeds are begun. Once successful tolerance of feedings is established at 90 to 100 mL/kg/day, caloric density is advanced to 24 cal/30 mL, and then the volume advanced to 150 to 160 mL/kg/day (see Chapter 21). This eliminates a drop in caloric intake as parenteral nutrition is weaned while feedings advance. Once tolerance of full feedings of 24 cal/30 mL is established, the density of feedings may be advanced if needed for adequate growth by 2 cal/30 mL/day up to a maximum of 30 cal/30 mL, although this higher caloric density is rarely required. Protein powder may be added to a total protein content of 4 g/kg/day because this promotes improved somatic and head growth over the first several weeks of life.

Many extremely small infants may benefit from restriction of total fluids to 130 to 140 mL/kg/day. This minimizes problems with fluid excess while still providing adequate caloric intake.

Suggested Readings

Brix N, Sellmer A, Jensen MS, et al. Predictors for an unsuccessful INtubation-SURfactant-Extubation procedure: a cohort study. *BMC Pediatr* 2014;14:155. doi:10.1186/1471-2431-14-155.

Carlo WA, Finer NN, Walsh MC, et al. Early CPAP versus surfactant in extremely preterm infants. *N Engl J Med* 2010;362:1970–1979.

Carlo WA, Finer NN, Walsh MC, et al. Target ranges of oxygen saturation in extremely preterm infants. *N Engl J Med* 2010;362:1959–1969.

Doglioni N, Cavallin F, Mardegan V, et al. Total body polyethylene wraps for preventing hypothermia in preterm infants: a randomized trial. *J Pediatr* 2014;165(2):261.e1–266.e1.

Horbar JD, Rogowski J, Plsek P, et al. Collaborative quality improvement for neonatal intensive care. NIC/Q Project Investigators of the Vermont Oxford Network. *Pediatrics* 2001;107:14–22.

Laughon MM, Simmons MA, Bose CL. Patency of the ductus arteriosus in the premature infant: is it pathologic? Should it be treated? *Curr Opin Pediatr* 2004;16:146–151.

Manley BJ, Dawson JA, Kamlin CO, et al. Clinical assessment of extremely premature infants in the delivery room is a poor predictor of survival. *Pediatrics* 2010;125:e559–e564.

Morley CJ, Davis PG, Doyle LW, et al. Nasal CPAP or intubation at birth for very preterm infants. *N Engl J Med* 2008;358:700–708.

Raju TNK, Mercer BM, Burchfield DJ, et al. Periviable birth: executive summary of a Joint Workshop by the Eunice Kennedy Shriver National Institute of Child Health and Human Development, Society for Maternal-Fetal Medicine, American Academy of Pediatrics, and American College of Obstetricians and Gynecologists. *J Perinatol* 2014;34:333–342.

Seri I. Management of hypotension and low systemic blood flow in the very low birth weight neonate during the first postnatal week. *J Perinatol* 2006;26(Suppl 1):S8–S13.

Stoll BJ, Hansen N, Fanaroff AA, et al. Late-onset sepsis in very low birth weight neonates: the experience of the NICHD Neonatal Research Network. *Pediatrics* 2002;110:285–291.

Tyson JE, Parikh NA, Langer J, et al. Intensive care for extreme prematurity—moving beyond gestational age. *N Engl J Med* 2008;358:1672–1681.

Vohra S, Roberts RS, Zhang B, et al. Heat loss prevention (HeLP) in the delivery room: a randomized controlled trial of polyethylene occlusive skin wrapping in very preterm infants. *J Pediatr* 2004;145:750–753.

Wood NS, Marlow N, Costeloe K, et al. Neurologic and developmental disability after extremely preterm birth. EPICure Study Group. *N Engl J Med* 2000;343:378–384.

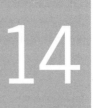

14 Developmentally Supportive Care

Lu-Ann Papile and Carol Turnage Spruill

KEY POINTS

- Infant cues form the basis for all handling and caregiving.
- Environments are modified to meet individual infants' requirements based on age, current abilities, and vulnerability.
- Parents are encouraged to provide care and nurturing for their infant in the neonatal intensive care unit (NICU).

I. **INTRODUCTION.** Individualized developmentally supportive care (IDSC) promotes a culture that respects the personhood of preterm and medically fragile term infants and optimizes the care and environment in which health care is delivered to this neurodevelopmentally vulnerable population. Implementing the principles of family-focused IDSC in a neonatal intensive care unit (NICU) environment facilitates family adaptation and may improve neurodevelopmental outcomes.

Preterm infants have a substantially higher incidence of cognitive, neuromotor, neurosensory, and feeding problems than infants born at full term. Fluctuations in the cerebral circulation that occur even during routine care and smaller than expected brain volumes at 36 to 40 weeks' postmenstrual age (PMA) may contribute to this increased morbidity. Changes in cerebral oxygenation and blood volume measured with near-infrared spectroscopy (NIRS) that occur during diaper changes with elevation of legs and buttocks, endotracheal tube (ET) suctioning, repositioning, routine physical assessment, and gavage feedings have been associated with early parenchymal brain abnormalities. IDSC helps to minimize these disturbances.

II. **ASSESSMENT.** Identification of an infant's stress responses and self-regulating behaviors at rest, as well as during routine care and procedures, is essential for the creation of care plans that support and promote optimal neurodevelopment (Table 14.1). Ideally, an infant's cues are continuously monitored and the care plan is modified as needed to lower stress and promote stability. Acutely ill term infants have responses to stress and pain similar to those of preterm infants; however, their cues are often easier to read because they have more mature behaviors.

A. **Stress responses.** A baseline profile of an infant's overall tolerance to various stimuli includes a combination of autonomic, motoric, state organizational behavior, and attentional/interactive signs of stress. Autonomic signs of stress include changes in color, heart rate, and respiratory patterns, as well

Table 14.1. Neurobehavioral Organization and Facilitation

System	Signs of Stress	Signs of Stability	Interventions
Autonomic			
Respiratory	Tachypnea, pauses, irregular breathing pattern, slow respirations, sighing, or gasping	Smooth, unlabored breathing; regular rate and pattern	Reduce light, noise, and activity at bedside (place pagers/phone on vibrate, lower conversation levels at bedside).
Color	Pale, mottled, red, dusky, or cyanotic	Stable, overall pink color	Use hand containment and pacifier during exams, procedures, or care.
			Slowly awaken with soft voice before touch including all procedures, exams, and care unless hearing impaired; use slow movement transitions.
Visceral	Several coughs, sneezes, yawns, hiccups, gagging, grunting and straining associated with defecation, spitting up	Visceral stability, smooth digestion, tolerates feeding	Pace feedings by infant's ability and cues in appropriately modified environment.
Autonomic-related motor patterns	Tremors, startles, twitches of face and/or body, extremities	Tremors, startles, twitching not observed	Gently reposition while containing extremities close to body if premature.
			Avoid sleep disruption.

(continued)

Table 14.1. Neurobehavioral Organization and Facilitation *(Continued)*

System	Signs of Stress	Signs of Stability	Interventions
			Position appropriately for neuromotor development and comfort; use nesting/boundaries or swaddling as needed to reduce tremors, startles.
			Manage pain appropriately.
Motor			
Tone	Either hypertonia or hypotonia; limp/flaccid body, extremities, and/or face; hyperflexion	Consistent, reliable tone for postmenstrual age (PMA); controlled or more control of movement, activity, and posture	Support rest periods/reduce sleep disruption, minimize stress, contain or swaddle.
Posture	Unable to maintain flexed, aligned, comfortable posture	Improved or well-maintained posture, with maturation posture sustainable without supportive aids	Provide boundaries, positioning aids, or swaddling for flexion, containment, alignment, and comfort as appropriate.
Level of activity	Frequent squirming, frantic flailing activity, or little to no movement	Activity consistent with environment, situation, and PMA	Intervene as needed for pain management, environmental modification, less stimulation; encourage skin-to-skin holding; containment.

State		
Sleep	Restless, facial twitching, movement, irregular respirations, fussing, grimacing, whimpers, or makes sounds; responsive to environment	Quiet, restful sleep periods; less body/facial movement; little response to environment	Comfortable and age-appropriate positioning for sleep with a quiet, dim environment and no interruptions except medical necessity Position with hands to face or mouth or so they can learn to achieve this on their own.
Awake	Low-level arousal with unfocused eyes; hyperalert expression of worry/panic; cry face or crying; actively avoids eye contact by averting gaze or closing eyes; irritability, prolonged awake periods; difficult to console or inconsolable	Alert, bright, shiny eyes with focused attention on an object or person; robust crying; calms quickly with intervention, consolable in 2–5 minutes	Encourage parent holding as desired either traditional or skin-to-skin. May be ready for brief eye contact around 30–32 weeks without displaying stress cues Support awake moments with PMA-appropriate activity based on stress and stability data for individual infant.
Self-regulation		
Motor	Little attempt to flex or tuck body, few attempts to push feet against boundaries, unable to maintain hands to face or mouth, sucking a pacifier may be more stressful than soothing	Strategies for self-regulation include foot bracing against boundaries or own feet/leg; hands grasped together; hand to mouth or face, grasping blanket or tubes, tucking body/truck; sucking; position changes	Examine using blanket swaddle or nest to support infant regulation by removing only a small part of the body at a time while keeping most of body contained during exam.

(continued)

Table 14.1. Neurobehavioral Organization and Facilitation *(Continued)*

System	Signs of Stress	Signs of Stability	Interventions
			Ask a parent or nurse to provide support during exams, tests, or procedures; swaddle or contain as needed to keep limbs close to body during care or exams and to provide boundaries for grasping or foot bracing.
			Position for sleep with hands to face or mouth.
			Provide pacifier intermittently when awake and at times other than exams, care, or procedures.
			Give older infants something to hold (maybe a finger or blanket).
			Encourage parent to support parenting skill; teach parents communication cues and behaviors; model appropriate responses to cues.

State	Rapid state transitions, unable to move to drowsy or sleep state when stressed, states are not clear to observers	Transitions smoothly from high arousal states to quiet alert or sleep state; focused attention on an object or person; maintains quiet alert state without stress or with some facilitation	Consistently avoid rapid disruption of state behavior (e.g., starting an exam without preparing the baby for the intrusion) by awakening slowly with soft speech or touch; use indirect lighting or shield eyes depending on PMA during exams or care.
			Assist return to sleep or quiet alert state after handling.
			Provide auditory and facial visual stimulation for quietly alert infants based on cues; premature infants may need to start with only one mode of stimulation initially, adding others based on cues.
			Swaddling or containment to facilitate state control or maintenance

Source: Modified from Als H. Toward a synactive theory of development: promise for the assessment and support of infant individuality. *Infant Ment Health J* 1982;3:229–243; Als H. A synactive model of neonatal behavioral organization: framework for the assessment of neurobehavioral development of the premature infant and his parents in the environment of the neonatal intensive care unit. *Phys Occup Ther Pediatr* 1986;6:3–55; Hunter JG. The neonatal intensive care unit. In: Case-Smith J, Allen AS, Pratt PN, eds. *Occupational Therapy for Children.* St. Louis, MO: Mosby; 2001:593; Carrier CT, Walden M. Wilson D. The high-risk newborn and family. In: Hockenberry MJ, ed. *Wong's Nursing Care of Infants and Children.* 7th ed. St. Louis, MO: Mosby; 2003.

as visceral changes such as gagging, hiccupping, vomiting, and stooling. Motoric signs of stress include facial grimacing, gaping mouth, twitching, hyperextension of limbs, finger splaying, back arching, flailing, and generalized hyper- or hypotonia. State alterations suggesting stress include rapid state transitions, diffuse sleep states, irritability, and lethargy. Changes in attention or interactional availability, exhibited by covering eyes/face, gaze aversion, frowning, and hyperalert or panicky facial presentation, represent signs of stress in preterm infants.

B. **Self-regulating behavior.** Preterm infants employ a number of self-consoling behaviors to cope with stress including hand or foot bracing; sucking; bringing hands to face; flexed positioning; cooing; and grasping of linens, tubing, or own body parts. Because painful procedures may overwhelm an infant's ability to self-console, support of the infant by parents or staff during these activities is needed.

III. GOALS OF DEVELOPMENTAL SUPPORT.

Developmental support necessitates attention by caregivers to observe cues (autonomic, motor, state) and respond to them. Infant cues provide clues to the type of intervention that may be most effective in decreasing stress and the subsequent physiologic cost. The individual caregiver must learn to recognize and appropriately respond when an infant communicates stress, pain, or the need for attention. A priority of IDSC is for infants to experience auditory, visual, and social input without disrupting autonomic, motor, or state function and integration. Once this objective is achieved, infants can begin to explore their world and relate to their parents during meaningful and reciprocal exchanges.

A. **Supporting autonomic system stability.** Because the autonomic and visceral systems cannot be impacted directly, interventions are used to assist an infant's return to a state that supports autonomic stability. Swaddling, hand-containment (facilitated tuck), and nesting with boundaries are supportive interventions that have been shown to be efficacious. Anticipatory planning for a quiet, calm environment, swaddling to reduce motor arousal, and letting the infant guide the pace of a feeding are strategies that will elicit less stress behaviors during feeding and may result in better feeding tolerance. Autonomic stability is especially important during handling not only to assist the infant with coping but also to allow the clinician to perform a physical exam or diagnostic test that reflects an infant's condition.

B. **Intervening through the motor system.** Support of the motor system is focused first on development and function and second on the prevention of acquired positioning deformities or functional limitations. Containment or "facilitated tuck" is useful for calming or support during care and/or procedures. Positioning aids may be needed when an infant cannot sustain a flexed, aligned posture with midline orientation that is also comfortable. Term infants who cannot maintain age-appropriate posture and/or movement due to neuromuscular disease, congenital anomalies, severity of illness, or medications can develop musculoskeletal problems or loss of skin integrity and also need positioning support. Movement is necessary for musculoskeletal growth and development. Thus, it is imperative that boundaries or swaddling provide containment without being restrictive.

C. **Creating environments that cultivate state organization.** Preterm infants have less ability to maintain a state and have more variable transition between states compared to term infants. Environmental modifications are made to promote quiet, focused attentional states and foster periods of well-defined, restful sleep with regular respirations and little movement. To promote the development of state organization, it is important to avoid activities that cause abrupt state transitions, such as rousing an infant from sleep by suddenly repositioning for an examination. Letting an infant know when a caregiver approaches to perform care at the bedside by using soft speech (infant's name), gentle touch, and containment while slowly repositioning can alleviate abrupt state disruption. Staff, parents, and others need to be consistent in their approach.

IV. **DEVELOPMENTALLY SUPPORTIVE ENVIRONMENT.** By providing a developmentally supportive NICU environment, neonatal caregivers can support neurologic and sensory development and potentially minimize later developmental issues in preterm and medically fragile infants. The acutely ill term infant also requires environmental modifications that reduce stress and promote sleep and recovery. Environments may be modified at the bedside to respond appropriately to an infant's ongoing requirements. Environments on a larger, more complex scale occur when NICUs are remodeled or newly designed. Health care professionals, architects, interior design consultants, health care facility regulators, and acoustic designers have revolutionized the NICU environment with continuously evolving standards of design based on research findings and clinical experience. When possible, anticipation of an infant's environmental needs prior to admission is ideal. The influence of the environment is of practical concern for short- and long-term development (e.g., both light and sound impact sleep).

A. **Sound.** Increased noise levels in the NICU are associated with physiologic stress and autonomic instability. Intense noise levels at 55 to 60 dBA and above disrupt sleep and may impact brain development occurring during both active/light sleep and quiet sleep. The development of sleep state organization may also be altered. The American Academy of Pediatrics (AAP) recommends that NICU sound levels not exceed an hourly equivalent sound level of 45 dB and hourly L_{10} (noise level exceeded for 10% of 1 hour) of 50 dB. Transient sounds should not exceed 65 dB. Infants cared for in incubators may be exposed to increased ambient noise from personnel tapping on the incubator walls or using the top of the incubator as a shelf. Music or recording devices placed within the incubator also increase ambient sound levels.

An IDSC program includes systematic efforts to manage environmental sound (e.g., low conversational tones, rounding away from the bedside, placing pagers on vibrate mode, care in opening and closing portholes). Baseline sound levels need to be measured occasionally during the year along with an evaluation of sources contributing to noise intensity or sudden loud sounds. Random monitoring of sound levels is helpful in sustaining noise abatement.

Limited information is available on the impact of sound frequencies on infants in the NICU. Early investigations have reported frequencies ranging from <500 Hz to 16,000 Hz or more over 50% of the time in the NICU. Inside the womb, the fetus is exposed to frequencies of <500 Hz until later in gestation when the womb thins closer to delivery. Around 33 weeks, fetuses can respond to high-frequency sounds; however, the effects of repeated exposure over time are unknown. The preterm infant may experience high-frequency, high-intensity sounds repeatedly throughout his or her hospital stay without the natural protection of mother's womb; this may influence the developing architecture and functional organization of cortical auditory connections. Because the effects of such exposure are unknown at this time, spectral analysis along with sound intensity require further study. As a precaution, both sound intensity and frequency should be monitored in the NICU and a plan developed to minimize the infant's exposure to potentially deleterious levels of sound.

The most natural source of sound for the infant is mother's voice. If a baby cannot distinguish the maternal voice from ambient noise, auditory development may be altered from the natural evolution that occurs in the womb.

B. **Light.** The relationship between ambient light and neurodevelopment is less clear. Reduced illumination is associated with increased autonomic stability in preterm infants and more frequent eye opening by both preterm and term infants. An additional developmental benefit of reducing environmental light is a concurrent reduction in environmental noise and less handling of infants. Early preterm infants may experience discomfort when exposed to intense light due to very thin eyelids that cannot block light and an immature pupillary reflex. Visual stimulation before 30 to 32 weeks' PMA is often accompanied by stress responses. Protection from light for the early preterm infant can be accomplished with thick, quilted covers that have dark material on the side facing the incubator. Lighting for staff needs to be at a level that allows safe and efficient functioning. During procedures, the infant's eyes should be protected from direct light using blanket tents or other methods that do not require tactile input. Eye covers should only be used when phototherapy is indicated. Reduction of light in the NICU does not appear to affect the incidence or progression of retinopathy of prematurity or alter visually evoked potentials measured in early childhood. These are relatively short-term outcomes; long-term effects of early, atypical lighting and visual stimulation are unknown.

The AAP Guidelines for Perinatal Care recommend adjustable ambient light levels from 10 to 600 lux (1 to 60 foot-candles) in infant areas. Procedure lighting that can be controlled or reduced as needed is recommended for each NICU bed. Procedure lights need to be focused so they do not alter the illumination of other infants.

The AAP also supports the recommendations of both the Illuminating Engineering Society and the 2012 Consensus Committee on NICU design. New or renovated NICUs typically provide ambient lighting of 10 to 20 lux. The light levels used in cycled lighting research for the nighttime cycle are within this range and can be used for light variation in the development of circadian rhythms. Cycled lighting may be beneficial for preterm infants, but the gestational age at which light intensity, day/night pattern, and light duration is safe and beneficial is not known. Preterm infants who have been exposed to cycled lighting at 30 weeks' gestational age and beyond have greater weight gain, earlier oral feeding, and more regulated patterns of rest/activity after discharge than control groups. However, atypical stimulation to one sensory system may adversely affect the function of another sensory system. Until more is understood about light exposure, a conservative approach is best.

C. **NICU design.** Single family rooms support the infant and family bond and create an environment that is readily adapted to meet an individual infant's requirements. Whether single family rooms are more beneficial than the traditional open-bay design is not certain. In one study, preterm infants cared for in single family rooms were found to have delayed cerebral maturation on magnetic resonance imaging (MRI) at term and significantly inferior language scores at 2 years of age compared to a peer cohort cared for in open bays. These results are thought to be related to sensory and social deprivation. On the other hand, another study noted that infants cared for in single family rooms experienced a lower infection rate, decreased stress, better weight gain, improved feeding tolerance, and better attention and tone. Regardless of design, thoughtful consideration of the needs of an individual infant must be considered to provide an environment that supports optimal outcomes.

V. DEVELOPMENTALLY SUPPORTIVE CARE PRACTICES. Developmental
support in the NICU requires collaboration and teamwork to integrate the developmental needs of infants within the context of medical treatment and nursing care. This entails a coordinated, primary team that includes the family and is designed to work in partnership around the infant's state of alertness, sleep cycles, communication cues, medical condition, and family presence. The goal is to maximize rest, minimize stress, and optimize healing and growth in a framework that supports family participation.

A. **Positioning.** The goals of positioning are to facilitate flexed and midline positioning of extremities, stabilize respiratory patterns, and lessen physiologic stress. Interventions include flexion, containment, midline alignment, and comfort. The use of "nesting materials" (e.g., soft blanket rolls, commercially available positioning devices) or swaddling is useful in minimizing the upper/lower extremity abduction, scapular retraction, and cervical hyperextension typical of preterm infants. More mature infants with congenital neuromuscular or skeletal disorders may also need positioning support.

Nesting needs to allow sufficient room for the infant to push against boundaries, to facilitate continuing development of the neuromotor and skeletal systems.

B. **Feeding.** Oral feeding is a complex task requiring physiologic maturation, coordination of suck–swallow–breathe mechanics, and development of oral motor skills. Breastfeeding is the preferred method, and breast milk is recommended for both preterm and term infants (see Chapter 22). The transition to oral feeding from tube feeding requires skilled assessment and judgment on the part of the caregiver. An infant who is successful in learning to nipple feed is less likely to develop feeding problems after discharge. It is important that the infant learns to feed properly and that family members are able to feed their infant. Progression to oral feeds is highly contingent on elements of IDSC and occurs predictably in several phases. Pre–non-nutritive suck (NNS) is characterized by weak suck and instability of motor, autonomic, and state regulation systems; NNS is characterized by more optimal suck patterns and should be encouraged during gavage feeds. Nutritive suck typically begins at approximately 33 weeks' PMA and progresses to full oral intake as autonomic stability and oral motor coordination improve. Strategies to promote successful progression through these phases include identifying and minimizing signs of physiologic stress; environmental modification to promote autonomic stability; feeding in a flexed, midline position; pacing techniques; and use of slow-flow nipples. Considerations for a feeding plan include the infant's opportunities to practice, environmental preparation to minimize stressors, and using the infant's feeding readiness cues to start feedings rather than strict adherence to a specific PMA, specific time intervals, and feeding duration. Infants fed using feeding readiness cues experience significantly fewer adverse events during feedings, reach full oral feeding sooner, are discharged earlier, gain the same amount of weight as controls, and demonstrate about three cues per feeding. In addition, experiential feeding, that is, feeding frequently during the day without regard for duration, also results in less time to full oral feeding. Leaving a gavage tube in place during initial feeding attempts or repeated insertions may cause discomfort and interfere with feeding progression or generate oral aversion and later feeding disorders. Research is needed to understand more about the risk factors for feeding behavior disorders associated with aversive or repeated noxious stimulation of the oropharynx and gastrointestinal tract.

C. Touch

1. **Hand containment or facilitated tuck** can be done by parents soon after admission. This technique reduces pain responses during painful and nonpainful events. Parents can be taught how to touch their infant in ways that are nurturing and won't create stress.

2. **Kangaroo care** sometimes referred to as skin-to-skin holding is a technique consistently associated with improved infant outcomes (i.e., fewer respiratory complications, improved weight gain, and temperature regulation) and maternal outcomes (i.e., improved maternal competence and longer breastfeeding duration). Mothers who use kangaroo holding produce a greater volume of breast milk than mothers who hold in the traditional way. Kangaroo care can be initiated as soon as infants are medically stable. Infants are held on their mother or father's chest wearing only a diaper and are covered with a blanket and hat as needed. A minimum of 1 hour is recommended for kangaroo holding. A NICU protocol for kangaroo holding ensures safety and minimizes an infant's stress response to handling/positioning. Kangaroo holding impacts several developing sensory systems including tactile (skin), olfactory, and vestibular (rise/fall of chest). Soft speech by the parent will be audible to their infant if ambient noise is minimized. The preterm infant's visual capacity is not challenged because eye-to-eye contact is not a necessary component for kangaroo care. Parents can be with their infant earlier in a way that is satisfying for them and supportive for their baby.

D. Team collaboration and consistency of care. Developmental care should be considered as part of routine care. The unpredictable nature of care in the NICU can be diminished by consistent caregivers who are familiar with an infant's clinical and behavioral baseline, provide care in a similar manner, respond quickly to cues, and provide relevant information to all members of the infant's team including the family to create an individualized plan of care. The developmental plan is complementary to the medical plan and uses developmental principles, techniques, and environmental modifications to reduce stressors that challenge an infant's physiologic stability through behavioral instability.

VI. PAIN AND STRESS. Pain assessment and management is a basic right of *all* patients. Evidence-based assessment and practice guidelines facilitate the use of pain management by physicians, nurses, and other practitioners. A streamlined approach using algorithms may enhance utilization at the bedside.

A. Pain. Effective nonpharmacologic interventions incorporate developmental principles such as swaddling, NNS, kangaroo holding, hand containment/facilitated tuck, breastfeeding, and administration of an oral sucrose solution (see Chapter 70). Nonpharmacologic measures are used as an adjunct to pharmacologic treatment of moderate-to-severe pain.

B. The AAP and the Canadian Pediatric Society advocate management of both pain and stress. High-stress situations need to be identified and modified to minimize the impact on the ill or preterm infant. Examples of potential high-stress conditions include delivery room care, transport to NICU, admission process, and diagnostic procedures that often produce pain or discomfort along with stress. During stressful events, developmental support based on infant cues guides the NICU team's care and needs to be ongoing with every episode of care.

VII. PARENT SUPPORT/EDUCATION. Effective IDSC is dependent on implementation of the principles of family-centered care during NICU stay as well as upon transition to home.

A. In the NICU. Preterm birth and NICU hospitalization negatively impact parent–infant interactions, which, in turn, is associated with long-term adverse developmental sequelae. Individual family-centered interactions (i.e., family-based developmental evaluations, support, and education) have been associated with reduced parent stress and more positive parent–infant interactions. Family-centered NICU policies include welcoming families 24 hours per day, promotion of family participation in infant care, creation of parent advisory boards, implementation of parent support groups, and comfortable rooming-in areas for parents.

B. Discharge teaching. Because brain growth and maturation may occur at a slower rate in the extrauterine environment, parents must understand that their baby may not behave as a term baby would when he or she has reached 40 weeks' PMA. Many parents report being ill-prepared for discharge from the NICU with respect to recognizing signs of illness, employing effective calming strategies, being aware of typical and delayed development, and using strategies to promote infant development. Teaching that begins well before discharge can help parents be better prepared to assume their role as the primary caregiver.

C. **Postdischarge family supports.** Parents report feeling frightened and alone following discharge of their preterm infant from the NICU, even when services are provided by a visiting nurse and early intervention specialists. Support groups for parents of preterm infants designed to provide long-term emotional and educational support are available in many communities. In addition, magazines, books, and web-based materials related to parenting preterm infants are available. A promising approach to facilitating seamless transition to community-based services includes referral to the federally mandated Early Intervention (EI) program before the infant's discharge and collaboration between NICU and EI professionals to create a developmentally supportive transition plan.

D. **Infant follow-up and EI programs.** The focus of a follow-up program is to prevent or minimize developmental delay through early identification of risk factors and referral to appropriate treatment programs. Close follow-up is paramount to maximizing developmental outcome. Every center that cares for medically fragile and preterm neonates needs to have a follow-up program available. Which group of infants to follow and the frequency of follow-up assessments are dependent on state and medical center resources.

Suggested Readings

Laadt VL, Woodward BJ, Papile LA. System of risk triage: a conceptual framework to guide referral and developmental intervention decisions in the NICU. *Infants Young Child* 2007;20(4):336–344.

Shepley MM. *Design for Pediatric and Neonatal Critical Care.* New York, NY: Routledge; 2014.

Spruill CT. Developmental support. In: Verklan T, Verklan MT, eds. *Core Curriculum for Neonatal Intensive Care Nursing.* 5th ed. Philadelphia, PA: WB Saunders; 2015:197–215.

Temperature Control
Kimberlee E. Chatson

KEY POINTS
- Immediate postnatal hypothermia is a worldwide issue with implications of significant morbidity and mortality.
- The preterm infant is especially vulnerable, and extra measures need to be taken to provide a neutral thermal environment.
- Induced hypothermia is a new modality that can reduce neuronal loss and subsequent brain injury after hypoxic-ischemic insult. Recognition and timely treatment of infants is needed to be effective.

I. **BACKGROUND.** Neonatal hypothermia after delivery is a worldwide issue, occurs in all climates, and if prolonged can cause harm and affect survival. Thermoregulation in adults is achieved by both metabolic and muscular activity (e.g., shivering). During pregnancy, maternal mechanisms maintain intrauterine temperature. After birth, newborns must adapt to their relatively cold environment by the metabolic production of heat because they are not able to generate an adequate shivering response. Brown fat is a source for thermogenesis in term newborns. It is highly vascularized and innervated by sympathetic neurons. When these infants face cold stress, norepinephrine levels increase and act in the brown fat tissue to stimulate lipolysis. Most of the free fatty acids (FFAs) are re-esterified or oxidized; both reactions produce heat. Factors that can increase risk for hypothermia include prematurity, intrauterine growth restriction, asphyxia, and certain congenital anomalies (e.g., abdominal wall defects, central nervous system [CNS] anomalies).

II. **TEMPERATURE MAINTENANCE**

A. **Premature infants** experience increased mechanisms of heat loss combined with decreased heat production capabilities. These special problems in temperature maintenance put them at a disadvantage. Compared with term infants, premature infants have

1. A higher ratio of skin surface area to weight

2. Highly permeable skin which leads to increased transepidermal water loss

3. Decreased subcutaneous fat with less insulative capacity

4. Less-developed stores of brown fat and decreased glycogen stores

5. Poor vasomotor control

6. Challenges with adequate caloric intake to provide nutrients for thermogenesis and growth

7. Limited oxygen delivery if pulmonary conditions coexist

B. Cold stress. In the setting of resuscitation, newborn infants can be subject to acute hypothermia and respond with a cycle of peripheral vasoconstriction, causing anaerobic metabolism, metabolic acidosis, and pulmonary vasoconstriction. Hypoxemia further compromises the infant's response to cold. Premature infants are at the highest risk for hypothermia and its sequelae (i.e., hypoglycemia, metabolic acidosis, increased oxygen consumption). After the immediate newborn period, the more common and chronic problem facing premature infants than actual hypothermia is caloric loss from unrecognized chronic cold stress, resulting in excess oxygen consumption and inability to gain weight. The use of low-reading thermometers (from 29.4°C/85.0°F) is recommended because temperature readings <34.4°C (94.0°F) can go undetected with routine thermometers.

C. Neonatal cold injury is a rare, extreme form of hypothermia that may be seen in low birth weight (LBW) infants and term infants with CNS disorders. Core temperature can fall below 32.2°C (90°F). It occurs more often in home deliveries, emergency deliveries, and settings where there is inadequate support regarding the thermal environment and practices needed to minimize heat loss. These infants may have a bright red color because of the failure of oxyhemoglobin to dissociate at low temperature. They may have central pallor or cyanosis. The skin may show edema and sclerema. Signs may include hypotension; bradycardia; slow, shallow, irregular respiration; poor sucking reflex; abdominal distention or vomiting; decreased activity; decreased response to stimulus; and decreased reflexes. Metabolic acidosis, hypoglycemia, hyperkalemia, azotemia, and oliguria can be present. Sometimes, there is generalized bleeding, including pulmonary hemorrhage. It is controversial whether warming should be rapid or slow. Setting the abdominal skin temperature to 1°C higher than the core temperature or setting it to 36.5°C on a radiant warmer will produce slow rewarming. In addition to rewarming, hypoglycemia should be corrected. The infant may benefit from a normal saline bolus (10 to 20 mL/kg), supplemental oxygen, and correction of metabolic acidosis. These infants should not be fed and should be carefully evaluated and treated for possible infection, bleeding, or injury.

D. Hyperthermia, defined as an elevated core body temperature, may be caused by a relatively hot environment, infection, dehydration, CNS dysfunction, or medications. Although the issue of infection is of clinical concern, awareness of environmental contributors such as phototherapy, incubators or warming table settings, or proximity to sunlight should be considered. If environmental temperature is the cause of hyperthermia, the trunk and extremities are the same temperature and the infant appears vasodilated. In contrast, infants with sepsis are often vasoconstricted and the extremities are cooler than the trunk.

E. Induced hypothermia. In recent years, there is experimental and clinical evidence that induction of controlled hypothermia can reduce neuronal loss and subsequent brain injury after a hypoxic-ischemic insult. It is a time-sensitive therapy and needs to be instituted within the first 6 hours after birth to be most effective. Passive cooling in the delivery room and during stabilization, followed by transfer to a center that performs the treatment, should be considered when there is a history of an acute perinatal event (nonreassuring fetal heart tracings, cord prolapse, placental abruption), pH ≤7.0/base deficit ≥16 on cord gas or gas obtained within 1 hour of life, 10-minute Apgar score ≤5, or assisted ventilation initiated at birth and continued for at least 10 minutes. Target temperature range is 32.5°C to 34.5°C. Core temperature (typically measured rectally at referring hospital and on transport) should be monitored every 15 minutes (see Chapter 55).

III. MECHANISMS OF HEAT LOSS

A. **Radiation.** Heat dissipates from the infant to a colder object in the environment.

B. **Convection.** Heat is lost from the skin to moving air. The amount lost depends on air speed and temperature.

C. **Evaporation.** Heat is lost through conversion of water to gas. The amount of loss depends primarily on air velocity and relative humidity. Wet infants in the delivery room are especially susceptible to evaporative heat loss.

D. **Conduction.** Heat is lost due to transfer of heat from the infant to the surface on which he or she lies.

IV. NEUTRAL THERMAL ENVIRONMENTS minimize heat loss. Thermoneutral conditions exist when heat production (measured by oxygen consumption) is minimal and core temperature is within the normal range (Table 15.1).

V. MANAGEMENT TO PREVENT HEAT LOSS

A. **Healthy term infant**

1. Standard thermal care guidelines include maintaining the delivery room temperature at 72°F (American Academy of Pediatrics [AAP])/25°C (World Health Organization [WHO]), immediately drying the infant (especially the head), removing wet blankets, and wrapping the newborn in prewarmed blankets. It is also important to prewarm contact surfaces and minimize drafts. A cap is useful in preventing significant heat loss through the scalp.

2. Examination in the delivery room should be performed with the infant under a radiant warmer. A skin probe with servocontrol to keep skin temperature at 36.5°C (97.7°F) should be used for prolonged examinations.

3. Skin-to-skin care during the first 1 to 2 hours of life offers a practical and effective approach to achieving a neutral thermal environment. This method has the added benefit of promoting early breastfeeding.

B. **Premature infant**

1. Standard thermal care guidelines should be followed.

2. Additional interventions immediately after birth can optimize thermoregulation.
   a. Barriers to prevent heat loss should be used in extremely premature infants. These infants should be placed in a polyethylene bag immediately

Table 15.1. Neutral Thermal Environmental Temperatures

Age and weight	Temperature*	
	At start (°C)	Range (°C)
0–6 hours		
Under 1,200 g	35.0	34.0–35.4
1,200–1,500 g	34.1	33.9–34.4
1,501–2,500 g	33.4	32.8–33.8
Over 2,500 g (and >36 weeks' gestation)	32.9	32.0–33.8
6–12 hours		
Under 1,200 g	35.0	34.0–35.4
1,200–1,500 g	34.0	33.5–34.4
1,501–2,500 g	33.1	32.2–33.8
Over 2,500 g (and >36 weeks' gestation)	32.8	31.4–33.8
12–24 hours		
Under 1,200 g	34.0	34.0–35.4
1,200–1,500 g	33.8	33.3–34.3
1,501–2,500 g	32.8	31.8–33.8
Over 2,500 g (and >36 weeks' gestation)	32.4	31.0–33.7
24–36 hours		
Under 1,200 g	34.0	34.0–35.0
1,200–1,500 g	33.6	33.1–34.2
1,501–2,500 g	32.6	31.6–33.6
Over 2,500 g (and >36 weeks' gestation)	32.1	30.7–33.5
36–48 hours		
Under 1,200 g	34.0	34.0–35.0
1,200–1,500 g	33.5	33.0–34.1
1,501–2,500 g	32.5	31.4–33.5
Over 2,500 g (and >36 weeks' gestation)	31.9	30.5–33.3
		(continued)

Table 15.1. *(Continued)*

Age and weight	Temperature*	
	At start (°C)	Range (°C)
48–72 hours		
Under 1,200 g	34.0	34.0–35.0
1,200–1,500 g	33.5	33.0–34.0
1,501–2,500 g	32.3	31.2–33.4
Over 2,500 g (and >36 weeks' gestation)	31.7	30.1–33.2
72–96 hours		
Under 1,200 g	34.0	34.0–35.0
1,200–1,500 g	33.5	33.0–34.0
1,501–2,500 g	32.2	31.1–33.2
Over 2,500 g (and >36 weeks' gestation)	31.3	29.8–32.8
4–12 days		
Under 1,500 g	33.5	33.0–34.0
1,501–2,500 g	32.1	31.0–33.2
Over 2,500 g (and >36 weeks' gestation)	—	—
4–5 days	31.0	29.5–32.6
5–6 days	30.9	29.4–32.3
6–8 days	30.6	29.0–32.2
8–10 days	30.3	29.0–31.8
10–12 days	30.1	29.0–31.4
12–14 days		
Under 1,500 g	33.5	32.0–34.0
1,501–2,500 g	32.1	31.0–33.2
Over 2,500 g (and >36 weeks' gestation)	29.8	29.0–30.8
2–3 weeks		
Under 1,500 g	33.1	32.2–34.0
1,501–2,500 g	31.7	30.5–33.0

(continued)

Table 15.1. Neutral Thermal Environmental Temperatures *(Continued)*

Age and weight	Temperature*	
	At start (°C)	Range (°C)
3–4 weeks		
Under 1,500 g	32.6	31.6–33.6
1,501–2,500 g	31.4	30.0–32.7
4–5 weeks		
Under 1,500 g	32.0	31.2–33.0
1,501–2,500 g	30.9	29.5–32.2
5–6 weeks		
Under 1,500 g	31.4	30.6–32.3
1,501–2,500 g	30.4	29.0–31.8

*Generally speaking, the smaller infants in each weight group will require a temperature in the higher portion of the temperature range. Within each time range, the younger infants require the higher temperatures.
Source: Fanaroff AA, Klaus MH. The physical environment. In: Fanaroff AA, Fanaroff JM, eds. *Klaus and Faranoff's Care of the High Risk Neonate*. 6th ed. Philadelphia, PA: Elsevier Saunders; 2013:132–150.

after birth; the wet body is placed in the bag from the neck down. Plastic wraps and plastic caps are also effective in infants born at <29 weeks.

b. A radiant warmer should be used during resuscitation and stabilization. A heated incubator should be used for transport.

c. External heat sources including skin-to-skin care (>28 weeks) and transwarmer mattresses have demonstrated a reduction in the risk of hypothermia.

3. In the neonatal intensive care unit (NICU), infants require a thermoneutral environment to minimize energy expenditure and optimize growth; skin mode or servocontrol can be set so that the incubator's internal thermostat responds to changes in the infant's skin temperature to ensure a normal temperature despite any environmental fluctuation. If a skin probe cannot be used due to the potential damage to skin in small premature infants, the incubator should be kept at an appropriate temperature on air mode (see Table 15.1).

4. Humidification of incubators has been shown to reduce evaporative heat loss and decrease insensible water loss, typically used for patients <1,200 g or 30 to 32 weeks' gestation for the first 10 to 14 days after birth. Risks and concerns for possible bacterial contamination have been addressed in current incubator designs which include heating devices that elevate the water temperature to a level that destroys most organisms. Notably, the water transforms into a gaseous vapor and not a mist, thus eliminating the airborne water droplet as a medium for infection.

5. Servocontrolled open warmer beds may be used for very sick infants when access is important. The use of a tent made of plastic wrap or barrier creams such as Aquaphor (or sunflower seed oil in resource-limited settings) prevent both convection heat loss and insensible water loss (see Chapter 23). Due to potential infectious risk, these creams and oils should be used sparingly and not for longer than 72 hours after birth.

6. Incubators are designed to decrease all four forms of heat loss, namely, evaporation, conduction, radiation, and convection. Double-walled incubators further decrease heat loss primarily due to radiation and, to a lesser degree, conduction.

7. Current technology includes hybrid devices such as the Versalet Incuwarmer (Hill-Rom Air-Shields, Batesville, IN) and the Giraffe OmniBed (Ohmeda Medical, Madison, WI). They offer the features of both a traditional radiant warmer bed and an incubator in a single device. This allows for the seamless conversion between modes, which minimizes thermal stress and allows for ready access to the infant for routine and emergency procedures.

8. Premature infants in relatively stable condition can be dressed in clothes and caps and covered with a blanket. This intervention offers a broader range of safe environmental temperatures. Heart rate and respiration should be continuously monitored because the clothing may limit observation.

VI. HAZARDS OF TEMPERATURE CONTROL METHODS

A. **Hyperthermia.** A servocontrolled warmer can generate excess heat, which can cause severe hyperthermia if the probe becomes detached from the infant's skin. Temperature alarms are subject to mechanical failure.

B. **Undetected infections.** Servocontrol of temperature may mask the hypothermia, hyperthermia, or temperature instability associated with infection. A record of both environmental and core temperatures, along with observation for other signs of sepsis, will help detect infections.

C. **Volume depletion.** Radiant warmers can cause increased insensible water loss. Body weight, urine output, and fluid balance should be closely monitored in infants cared for on radiant warmers.

Suggested Readings

Fanaroff AA, Klaus MH. The physical environment. In: Fanaroff AA, Fanaroff JM, eds. *Klaus and Fanaroff's Care of the High Risk Neonate*. 6th ed. Philadelphia, PA: Elsevier Saunders; 2013:132–150.

McCall EM, Alderdice F, Halliday HL, et al. Interventions to prevent hypothermia at birth in preterm and/or low birthweight infants. *Cochrane Database Syst Rev* 2008;(1):CD004210.

Papile LA, Baley JE, Benitz JE, et al. Hypothermia and neonatal encephalopathy. *Pediatrics* 2014;133:1146–1150.

Sherman TI, Greenspan JS, St. Clair N, et al. Optimizing the neonatal thermal environment. *Neonatal Netw* 2006;25(4):251–260.

16 Follow-up Care of Very Preterm and Very Low Birth Weight Infants

Jane E. Stewart, Frank Hernandez, and
Andrea F. Duncan

KEY POINTS

- Children born very preterm and very low birth weight are at high risk for neurodevelopmental deficits and respiratory, cardiovascular, and growth abnormalities.
- Children born preterm require long-term, specialized follow-up care to monitor for medical and neurodevelopmental problems to allow for early identification and intervention to optimize their long-term outcomes.
- Children born preterm have increased risk for learning disabilities, attentional problems requiring special educational services.
- Children born preterm have an increased risk of abnormal visual and auditory function and require additional early screening and follow-up evaluations in the first years of life.

I. **INTRODUCTION.** Of the over 4 million children born each year in this country, 2% (88,000) are born very preterm, which is defined as <32 weeks' gestational age (GA). Advances in obstetric and neonatal care have resulted in increased survival of these infants. The ramifications of this improvement are vast because these infants are at increased risk for long-term complication including neurodevelopmental sequelae, such as cognitive delay, cerebral palsy, fine and gross motor coordination problems, learning disabilities, visual and hearing problems, and medical problems, such as respiratory, cardiovascular, and growth issues. The more preterm an infant, the greater the risk of such difficulties. It is thus critical that these children have appropriate long-term follow-up care which includes provision of close monitoring of the most common problems of the preterm infant.

II. MEDICAL CARE ISSUES

A. **Respiratory issues** (see Chapter 34). Very preterm infants are at high risk for respiratory ailments, especially during the first year. Many present to primary care practitioners and specialists with chronic wheezing and recurrent respiratory tract infections. Children of the lowest gestations and birth weights suffer the greatest burden of respiratory illness. Very low birth weight (VLBW; birth weight <1,500 g) infants are 4 times more likely to be rehospitalized during the first year than are higher birth weight infants; up to 60% are rehospitalized at least once by the time they reach school age. The increased risk of hospitalization persists into early school age; 7% of VLBW children are hospitalized in a given year, compared with 2% of higher birth weight children. In a recent study of extremely premature infants, 57% of infants born between 23 and 25 weeks' gestation, and 49% of those born between 26 and 28 weeks' gestation required rehospitalization in the first 18 months of life. Admissions during the first year of life are most commonly for complications of respiratory infections among very preterm and VLBW infants.

Lung development continues during the postnatal period, and exposure to volutrauma and barotrauma along with hyperoxia may impede this process. This can damage lung tissue and decrease pulmonary blood flow. The resultant lung disease can extend into adulthood.

Approximately 23% of VLBW infants and 40% of extremely low birth weight (ELBW; birth weight <1,000 g) infants develop bronchopulmonary dysplasia (BPD) (defined as O_2 dependence beyond 28 days with the severity assessed at 36 weeks' postmenstrual age [PMA]). Very preterm infants with BPD are most likely to suffer respiratory ailments in the short and long term and should be monitored for related morbidities, including acute respiratory exacerbations, upper and lower respiratory infections, pulmonary hypertension, cor pulmonale, growth failure, and developmental delay. Infants with severe BPD may require treatment with tracheostomy and long-term ventilator support. More commonly, infants with significant BPD may be discharged home on some combination of supplemental oxygen, bronchodilator, steroid, and/or diuretic therapy. In the longer term, children with BPD may develop asthma-like symptoms in childhood which are not uniformly responsive to bronchodilators. In later life, survivors of BPD also lack catch-up growth in lung function and have an accelerate decline in lung function. It is important to note that children born preterm who do not develop BPD are also at increased risk for these respiratory illnesses.

1. **Home oxygen**. Some infants discharged home from the neonatal intensive care unit (NICU) on supplementary oxygen may be weaned off within the first few months following discharge, whereas others may remain on oxygen for 2 years or more. Infants with BPD who are discharged home on oxygen are rehospitalized at twice the rate during the first 2 years of life compared to those who were not.

2. **Respiratory syncytial virus (RSV)**. RSV is the most important cause of respiratory infection in premature infants, particularly in those with chronic lung disease. To minimize illness caused by RSV, VLBW infants should receive prophylactic treatment with palivizumab (Synagis) monoclonal antibody. The American Academy of Pediatrics (AAP) recommends treatment during RSV season for at least the first year of life for infants born ≤28 weeks' gestation and for at least the first 6 months of life for those born between 28 and 32 weeks' gestation. To prevent

illness caused by respiratory viruses, families should be counseled regarding good hand hygiene by all those in close contact with infants, avoidance of exposure to others with respiratory infections (especially young children during the winter season), and avoidance of passive cigarette smoke exposure. The influenza vaccine is also recommended for VLBW infants when they are older than 6 months; until then, care providers in close contact with the infant should strongly consider receiving the influenza vaccine.

3. **Air travel**. In general, air travel is not recommended for infants with BPD because of the increased risk of exposure to infection and because of the lowered cabin pressure resulting in lower oxygen content in the cabin air. If an infant's PaO_2 is ≤ 80 mm Hg, supplemental oxygen will be needed while flying.

B. **Immunizations.** VLBW infants should receive their routine pediatric immunizations according to the same schedule as term infants, with the exception of hepatitis B vaccine. Medically stable, thriving infants should receive the hepatitis B vaccine as early as 30 days of age regardless of GA or birth weight. If the baby is ready for discharge to home before 30 days of age, it can be given at the time of discharge to home. Although studies evaluating the long-term immune response to routine immunizations have shown antibody titers to be lower in preterm infants, most achieve titers in the therapeutic range.

C. **Growth.** VLBW infants have a high incidence of feeding and growth problems for multiple reasons. Infants with severe BPD have increased caloric needs for appropriate weight gain. Many of these infants also have abnormal or delayed oral motor development and have oral aversion because of negative oral stimulation during their early life. Growth should be followed carefully on standardized growth curves (the World Health Organization [WHO] International Growth Curves 2006) using the child's age corrected for prematurity for the first 2 years of life and then using the Centers for Disease Control and Prevention (CDC) standardized curves. Supplemental caloric density is commonly required to optimize growth. Specialized preterm infant formulas with increased protein, calcium, and phosphate (either added to human milk or used alone) should be considered for the first 6 to 12 months of life for infants who have borderline growth. ELBW infants may demonstrate growth that is close to or below the fifth percentile. However, if their growth runs parallel to the normal curve, they are usually demonstrating a healthy growth pattern. Infants whose growth curve plateaus or whose growth trajectory falls off warrant further evaluation to assess caloric intake. If growth failure persists, consultation with a gastroenterologist or endocrinologist to rule out gastrointestinal pathology such as severe gastroesophageal reflux disease or endocrinologic problems such as growth hormone deficiency should be considered. Monitoring for excessive weight gain is also recommended with adjustment of caloric density if weight has normalized to the 50th percentile or demonstrates a rapid acceleration over a short period of time. There is some evidence that links rapid weight gain of low birth weight (LBW) infants to excess accretion of adipose and subsequent risks of adult obesity and associated morbidities.

Gastrostomy tube placement may be necessary in a small subset of patients with severe feeding problems. Long-term feeding problems are frequent in this population of children, and they usually require specialized feeding and oral motor therapy to ultimately wean from gastrostomy tube feedings.

1. **Anemia.** VLBW infants are at risk for iron deficiency anemia and should receive supplemental iron for the first 12 to 15 months of life.

2. **Rickets.** VLBW infants who have had nutritional deficits in calcium, phosphorous, or vitamin D intake are at increased risk for rickets. Infants who are at highest risk are those treated with long-term parenteral nutrition, furosemide, and those with decreased vitamin D absorption due to fat malabsorption. Infants with rickets diagnosed in the NICU may need continued supplementation of calcium, phosphorous, and vitamin D during the first year of life. Supplemental vitamin D (400 IU/day) should also be provided to all infants discharged home on human milk or who are not taking 1 L of formula per day, which is enough to provide 400 IU/day.

D. **Sensory issues** that need special follow-up include vision and hearing.

1. **Ophthalmologic follow-up** (see Chapter 67). Infants with severe retinopathy of prematurity (ROP) are at increased risk for significant vision loss or blindness in the setting of retinal detachment. The risk of severe ROP is highest in the ELBW population in whom the incidence of blindness is 2% to 9%. Infants who have required treatment with laser therapy or bevacizumab (Avastin) warrant additional close monitoring to ensure that the infant's retina becomes fully vascularized without complications.

In addition to ROP, other ophthalmologic conditions seen in NICU graduates include the following:

a. **Refractive errors** are more frequent in premature than term infants. Myopia is the most common problem and may be severe. Hyperopia also occurs more commonly in premature infants. Vision is corrected with eyeglasses.

b. **Amblyopia** (reduced vision caused by lack of use of one eye during the critical age for visual development) is more frequent in premature infants usually related to strabismus, anisometropia, and bilateral high refractive error (bilateral ametropia). Amblyopia can become permanent if it is not treated before 6 to 10 years of age.

c. **Strabismus**, or misalignment of the eyes, is more common in premature infants, especially in those with a history of ROP, intracranial hemorrhage, or white matter injury; the most common form is esotropia (crossed eyes), although exotropia (also known as wall-eye) and hypertropia (vertical misalignment of the eyes so that one eye is higher than the other) also occur. Strabismus may be treated with eye patching, atropine drops, corrective lenses, or surgery depending on the cause.

d. **Anisometropia**, defined as a substantial difference in refractive error between the two eyes, occurs more often in premature than term infants. Because the eyes cannot accommodate (focus) separately, the eye with the higher refractive error can develop amblyopia. Treatment for anisometropia is vision correction with eye glasses.

In patients who have had severe ROP including those treated with laser therapy, there is an increased risk of cataracts, glaucoma, late retinal detachment, abnormal color vision development, and visual field deficits. Infants who have received intravitreal bevacizumab (Avastin) treatment are known to have delayed maturation of their retinal vessels. Potential long-term outcomes of this treatment are still unknown and are currently being studied.

All VLBW infants should have follow-up with an ophthalmologist who has experience with ophthalmologic problems related to prematurity. Close monitoring until the retinal vessels have reached maturity should occur in the first months of life. Subsequent assessments should occur by 8 to 12 months of age and then according to the ophthalmologist's recommendation, usually annually or again at 3 years of age at the latest.

2. **Hearing follow-up.** Hearing loss occurs in approximately 2% to 11% of VLBW infants. Prematurity increases the risk of both sensorineural and conductive hearing loss. All VLBW infants should be screened both in the neonatal period and again before 1 year of age (earlier if parental concerns are noted or if the infant has additional risk factors for hearing loss) (see Chapter 68). There is also evidence that VLBW infants are at increased risk for auditory dyssynchrony (also called auditory neuropathy) and central auditory processing problems.

E. **Dental problems.** VLBW infants have been noted to have an increased incidence of enamel hypoplasia and discoloration. Long-term oral intubation in the neonatal period may result in palate and alveolar ridge deformation affecting tooth development. Initiation of routine supplemental flouride at 6 months PMA is recommended, as is referral to a pediatric dentist in the first 12 months of life.

III. NEURODEVELOPMENTAL OUTCOMES.
Infants with intracranial hemorrhage, in particular parenchymal hemorrhage, or periventricular white matter injury are at increased risk for neuromotor and cognitive delay. Infants with white matter injury are also at increased risk for visuomotor problems, as well as visual field deficits. Among ELBW infants with neonatal complications including BPD, brain injury (defined on ultrasonographic imaging as intraparenchymal echodensity, periventricular leukomalacia, porencephalic cyst, "grade 3" intraventricular hemorrhage [IVH], "grade 4" intraparenchymal hemorrhage), and severe ROP (threshold or stage 4 or 5 ROP in one or both eyes), 88% had poor neurosensory outcomes at 18 months of age with either cerebral palsy, cognitive delay, severe hearing loss, or bilateral blindness. Infants with cerebellar hemorrhage are at increased risk for abnormal motor development as well as cognitive, behavioral, functional, and social developmental problems. Although less common, injury to the developing gray matter and basal ganglia, thalami, and brainstem are associated with an even higher rate of severe neurodevelopmental morbidity.

A. **Neuromotor problems.** The incidence of cerebral palsy is 7% to 12% in VLBW infants and 11% to 15% in ELBW infants. The most common type of cerebral palsy is spastic diplegia. This correlates with the anatomic location of the corticospinal tracts in the periventricular white matter. VLBW infants are also at risk for other types of abnormal motor development including motor coordination problems and later problems with motor planning.

1. Both transient and long-term motor problems in infants require assessment and treatment by physical therapists and occupational therapists. These services are usually provided in the home through local early intervention programs. Infants with sensorineural handicaps require coordination of appropriate clinical services and developmental programs. For older children, consultation with the schools and participation in an educational plan are important.

2. Early diagnosis and referral to a neurologist and orthopedic surgeon will prompt referral for appropriate early intervention services such as physical and occupational therapy. Some infants with cerebral palsy are candidates for treatment with orthotics or other adaptive equipment. Children with hemiparesis may be candidates for constraint therapy. Children with significant spasticity are candidates for treatment with botulinum-A toxin (Botox) injections. In the case of severe spasticity, treatment with baclofen (oral or through an intrathecal catheter with a subcutaneous pump) may be helpful. Older children are candidates for surgical procedures. Hippotherapy (horseback riding therapy) and aquatherapy are also beneficial for young patients with cerebral palsy.

B. **Cognitive impairment.** Risk of cognitive disability in preterm infants is associated with degree of prematurity, presence of cerebral injury on neuroimaging, low parental education, and socioeconomic status. Progress is typically assessed by use of some form of IQ or development quotient (DQ) on an established scale such as the Bayley Scales of Infant Development or the Mullen Scales of Early Learning. Additional instruments are available but their psychometric properties may not be as robust. Scales with excellent psychometric properties such as the Early Childhood Stanford-Binet Intelligence Scales (5th edition) can only be empirically used for those 24 months and older.

1. VLBW infants tend to have scores somewhat lower on such scales than term infants, but many still fall within the normal range. The percentage of infants with scores >2 standard deviations below the mean is between 5% and 20% for VLBW infants and between 14% and 40% for ELBW infants. Most studies reflect the status of children younger than age 2 years. Among older children, the percentage of children who are severely affected appears to be the same, but the percentage with school failure or school problems is as high as 50%, with rates of 20% even among children with average IQ scores. When children were tested at ages 8 to 11 years, learning disabilities particularly related to visual spatial and visual motor abilities, written output, and verbal functioning were more common in ELBW infants (without neurologic problems diagnosed) compared to term infants of similar sociodemographic status. There is also increasing evidence that VLBW schoolchildren have significant difficulties with simultaneous processing when compared to term children, thereby having an impact on visual motor integration and logical reasoning. More than 50% of ELBW infants require some type of special education assistance

compared to <15% of healthy term infants. Studies of teen and adult survivors born preterm are limited but reflect ongoing problems including lower rates of educational achievement, lower income, and higher level of unemployment. However, a report of ELBW infants assessed in the teenage years with measures of self-esteem noted that they do not differ from term controls. Likewise, studies assessing VLBW teen and young adults in their perception of their quality of life report positive values comparable to term controls. Further longitudinal follow-up of these children into early adulthood assessing quality of life measures in addition to the incidence of neurodevelopmental disability is essential.

2. Referral to **early intervention programs** at the time of discharge from the NICU allows early identification of children with delays and referral for therapy from educational specialists and speech therapists when appropriate. Children with severe language delays may also benefit from referral to special communication programs that use adaptive technology to enhance language and communication. Caretakers will traditionally require significant assistance not only in understanding the importance of specialized interventions but also in navigating the idiosyncrasies of available programs. Managed care pressures, the availability of specific specialists within programs, and the quality and frequency of each direct service to be delivered can vary significantly from program to program. Parents and caretakers may not be aware of these factors, and this in turn could affect the delivery of crucial services at a most important developmental critical period.

3. **Social and communication development** difficulties are also increasingly a concern in the population of preterm infants. Several recent studies have noted prematurity as a risk factor for autism and have noted that in prospective studies of preterm infants at the toddler age, they are more likely to screen positive for autism. Neuroimaging techniques, diagnostic instruments, and biologic markers geared to accurately assess these more serious potential consequences at the earliest possible age have been developed. Psychometric instruments such as the Autism Diagnostic Observation Schedule (ADOS) and early electroencephalographic signatures promise better sensitivity and specificity than previously available. These studies are ongoing, and the true positive rate for autism will be better understood with further follow-up research.

During school-aged years, these children and their parents report more social difficulties with their peers, with risk being directly associated with cognitive and behavioral development.

4. Another population to consider is the late preterm infant (34 to 37 weeks gestation). Although outcomes in general are good, recent studies looking at these infants when they reach school age reveal that they perform at a lower level on measures of total school readiness, reading, math, and expressive language scores compared with term control infants.

C. Emotional and behavioral health

1. **Sleep.** Preterm infants have a higher rate of sleep problems compared to those born at term. The cause is frequently multifactorial with medical and behavioral components. Smaller preterm infants may have the

lightest sleep related to their brain immaturity, and their potential exposure in the NICU to an environment with light and noise that is not conducive to appropriate sleep–wake cycle routines. Patience and predictability are important caveats to remember when caring for preterm infants. It is important to remind parents that their infant should sleep supine in a crib or bassinet per the AAP Guidelines for Infant Sleep Safety and SIDS Risk Reduction. Co-sleeping with parents and allowing infants to sleep in infant swings or car seats should be advised against. Formal, behaviorally based sleep cycle remediation efforts are not recommended until the child is at least 1 year old. Parents may benefit from books on sleep training or in more severe cases, referral to a sleep specialist.

2. **Behavior.** VLBW children are at increased risk for behavior problems related to hyperactivity and/or attention deficit. Recent research findings indicate that parenchymal lesions/ventricular enlargement during the neonatal period predict attentional difficulties without hyperactivity in these children, a finding that is important for developing interventions. The risk factors for behavioral problems also include stress within the family, maternal depression, financial difficulties, and smoking. Behavior problems can contribute to school difficulties. In relation to both school problems and other health issues, VLBW children are seen as less socially competent than normal birth weight (BW) children. Detection of behavioral problems is achieved most commonly using scales developed to elicit parental and teacher concerns. The youngest children for whom such standardized scales are available are 2 years old. Parents and educators may struggle to identify the source of a behavioral issue and will question whether normal developmental factors or the prematurity itself may be responsible for the maladaptive behavior. Management depends on the nature of the problem and the degree of functional disruption. Some problems may be managed with special educational programs; others may involve referral to appropriate behaviorally based psychotherapy services. Screening of NICU mothers for postpartum depression or posttraumatic stress disorder is also recommended; the incidence of depressive symptoms in mothers who have delivered a premature infant is higher and, when identified, provides an opportunity for intervention that will enhance both maternal and child health. Many pediatric hospitals have behavioral medicine specialists who focus not only on the baby's individual needs but also on the impact that a new preterm baby can have on each of the family members.

3. **Mental health.** VLBW children tend to experience internalizing problems, such as depression and anxiety when compared to their term gestation peers.

IV. DEVELOPMENTAL FOLLOW-UP PROGRAMS support optimization of health outcomes for NICU graduates and provide feedback information for improvement of medical care. Activities can include the following:

A. **Management of sequelae associated with prematurity.** As ever smaller infants survive, the risk of chronic sequelae increases.

B. **Consultative assessment and referral.** Regardless of specific morbidity at the time of discharge, NICU graduates require surveillance for the emergence of a variety of problems that may require referral to and coordination of multiple preventive and rehabilitative services.

C. **Monitoring outcomes.** Information on health problems and use of services by NICU graduates is integral to both the assessment of the effect of services and the counseling of parents regarding an individual child's future.

D. **Program structure**

1. The population requiring follow-up care differs with each NICU and the availability and quality of community resources. Most programs use as criteria some combination of birth weight and specific complications. The criteria must be explicit and well understood by all members of the NICU team, with mechanisms developed for identifying and referring appropriate children.

2. Visits depend on the infant's needs and community resources. Some programs recommend a first visit within a few weeks of discharge to assess the transition to home. If not dictated by acute problems, future visits are scheduled to assess progress in key activities. In the absence of acute care needs, we assess patients routinely at 6-month intervals.

3. Because the focus of follow-up care is enhancement of individual and family function, personnel must have a breadth of expertise, including (i) clinical skill in the management of sequelae of prematurity; (ii) the ability to perform neurologic and cognitive diagnostic assessment; (iii) familiarity with general pediatric problems presenting in premature infants; (iv) the ability to manage children with complex medical, motor, and cognitive problems; and (v) knowledge of the availability of and referral process to community programs. Families will require varying degrees of advice and guidance.

4. Methods for assessing an individual's progress depend on the need for direct assessment by health professionals and the quality of primary care and early intervention services. A variety of indirect approaches of assessing developmental progress including parental surveys exist that provide information identifying children who have delays or other developmental concerns and warrant further assessment and/or intervention. This strategy of initial assessment may be helpful when it is difficult for families to travel the distance back to the medical centers or to reduce program costs. Recommended staff team members and consultants include pediatrician (developmental specialist or neonatologist), neonatology fellows or pediatric residents (for training), pediatric neurologist, pulmonologist, physical therapist, psychologist, occupational therapist, dietician, speech and language specialist, and social worker.

5. **Family/parent function and support.** Having a premature infant is often an extremely stressful experience for the parents. Providing specialized care in assessment, supportive counseling, and resources to families caring for the VLBW infant is essential and includes particular attention to issues of postpartum affective conditions and anxiety following the potentially traumatic experience of having a critically

ill infant. Provision of specialized behavioral guidance and supportive counseling in addition to facilitating referrals to community providers for additional care should be provided by the team. Addressing the basic needs of families including health insurance issues, respite, advocating for services in the community, financial resources, and marital stress are also important.

Suggested Readings

Bhutta AT, Cleves MA, Casey PH, et al. Cognitive and behavioral outcomes of school-aged children who were born preterm: a meta-analysis. *JAMA* 2002;288(6):728–737. doi:10.1001/jama.288.6.728.

Delobel-Ayoub M, Arnaud C, White-Koning M, et al. Behavioral problems and cognitive performance at 5 years of age after very preterm birth: the EPIP-AGE study. *Pediatrics* 2009;123(6):1485–1492.

Glass H, Costarino AT, Stayer SA, et al. Outcomes for extremely premature infants. *Anesth Analg* 2015;120(6):1337–1351.

Greenough A. Long-term respiratory consequences of premature birth at less than 32 weeks of gestation. *Early Hum Dev* 2013;89:S25–S27.

Larroque B, Ancel PY, Marret S, et al. Neurodevelopmental disabilities and special care of 5-year-old children born before 33 weeks of gestation (the EPIPAGE study): a longitudinal cohort study. *Lancet* 2008;371:813–820.

Pike KC, Lucas JS. Respiratory consequences of late preterm birth. *Paediatr Respir Rev* 2015;16(3):182–188.

Wadhawan R, Oh W, Vohr BR, et al. Neurodevelopmental outcomes of triplets or higher-order extremely low birth weight infants. *Pediatrics* 2011;127: e654–e660.

Wilson-Costello D, Friedman H, Minich N, et al. Improved neurodevelopmental outcomes for extremely low birth weight infants in 2000–2002. *Pediatrics* 2007;119(1):37–45.

Wood NS, Costeloe K, Gibson AT, et al. The EPICure study: associations and antecedents of neurological and developmental disability at 30 months of age following extremely preterm birth. *Arch Dis Child Fetal Neonatal Ed* 2005;90:F134–F140.

Woodward LJ, Anderson PJ, Austin NC, et al. Neonatal MRI to predict neurodevelopmental outcomes in preterm infants. *N Engl J Med* 2006;355:685–694.

17 Neonatal Transport

Monica E. Kleinman

KEY POINTS

- Whenever possible, transport of the mother and fetus prior to delivery is preferable to a postnatal transport.
- Newborns transported by air are subject to specific physiologic stresses associated with altitude.
- The risk of interfacility transport can be reduced by the use of specially trained and equipped neonatal transport teams.

I. **INTRODUCTION.** Regionalization of perinatal services necessitates that newborns requiring intensive care or specialty treatment be transported between facilities. Most experts agree that whenever possible, it is preferable to safely and expeditiously transfer the mother to a center with the necessary resources prior to delivery of a high-risk newborn. Unfortunately, some infants requiring expert neonatal care are not identified prior to birth, and others deliver too quickly to permit maternal transfer. It is important that a system exists for timely referral, clear communication of information and recommendations, and access to specially trained personnel who can provide neonatal resuscitation and stabilization before and during transport.

II. INDICATIONS

A. Interhospital transport should be considered if the medical resources or personnel needed for specialized neonatal care are not available at the birth hospital. Because the birth of a high-risk infant cannot always be predicted, all facilities providing maternity services should ensure that personnel caring for infants at birth or in the immediate newborn period are proficient in basic neonatal resuscitation and stabilization.

B. Transfer to the regional tertiary neonatal center should be expedited following initial stabilization. Medical personnel from the referring center should contact their affiliated neonatal intensive care unit (NICU) transport service to arrange transfer and to discuss a management plan to optimize the patient's condition before the transport team's arrival.

C. **Criteria for neonatal transfer** depend on the capability of the referring hospital as defined by the American Academy of Pediatrics (AAP) policy statement on levels of neonatal care and as dictated by local and state public health regulations. The AAP defines neonatal levels of care as shown in Table 17.1.

Table 17.1. Levels of Neonatal Care

Level of Care	Services
Level 1 (including well newborn nurseries)	Neonatal resuscitation at delivery Postnatal care for stable term newborns Postnatal care for late preterm newborns who are physiologically stable Stabilization of the preterm or critically ill newborn prior to transfer to a higher level of care
Level 2 (special care nurseries)	Level 1 capabilities plus: Care for newborns born <32 weeks or >1,500 g with physiologic immaturity or transient conditions related to prematurity Ongoing care of infants recovering from critical conditions Time-limited provision of mechanical ventilation or continuous positive airway pressure Stabilization prior to transfer for any infant needing transfer to a higher level of care
Level 3 (neonatal intensive care units)	Level 2 capabilities plus: Provision of life support and comprehensive neonatal intensive care Subspecialty medical and surgical expert consultation Mechanical ventilation (all forms) Diagnostic imaging capabilities
Level 4 (regional neonatal intensive care units)	Level 3 capabilities plus: Specialized surgical capabilities for repair of congenital or acquired conditions Critical care transport services and outreach education

Source: American Academy of Pediatrics Committee on Fetus and Newborn. Levels of neonatal care. *Pediatrics* 2012;130:587–597, reprinted with permission.

All hospitals with level 1 or 2 neonatal care services should have agreements with regional perinatal centers outlining criteria for perinatal consultations and neonatal transfer. Conditions that typically require transfer to a center that provides neonatal intensive care include the following:

1. Prematurity (<32 weeks' gestation) and/or birth weight <1,500 g
2. Respiratory distress requiring continuous positive airway pressure (CPAP) or high concentrations of oxygen (FiO_2 >0.6).

3. Hypoxic respiratory failure requiring invasive mechanical ventilation

4. Persistent pulmonary hypertension

5. Congenital heart disease or cardiac arrhythmias

6. Congenital anomalies and/or inborn errors of metabolism

7. Hypoxic-ischemic encephalopathy

8. Seizures

9. Other conditions that may be indications for neonatology consultation and/or transfer

   a. Severe hyperbilirubinemia that may require exchange transfusion

   b. Infant of diabetic mother with hypoglycemia or other complications

   c. Severe intrauterine growth restriction

   d. Birth weight between 1,500 and 2,000 g and gestational age between 32 and 36 weeks

   e. Procedures or therapies unavailable at referring hospital (ECHO, surgery, extracorporeal membrane oxygenation [ECMO], etc.)

III. ORGANIZATION OF TRANSPORT SERVICES

A. The regional NICU transport team should have an appointed **medical director**. The transport team should follow practice guidelines detailed in easily accessible written protocols and procedures, which should be reviewed on a periodic basis. A medical control physician, who may be the attending neonatologist or fellow, should supervise each individual patient transport. The medical control physician should be readily available by telephone for consultation to assist in the management of the infant during transport.

B. **Transport teams.** Qualified transport teams should be composed of individuals with pediatric/neonatal critical care experience and training in the needs of infants and children during transport and who participate in the transport of such patients with sufficient frequency to maintain their expertise. Such teams typically consist of a combination of at least two or three trained personnel and can include one or more of the following: neonatal nurse practitioners, critical care nurses, respiratory therapists, paramedics, and physicians. Senior pediatric residents and subspecialty fellows can participate in transports for those services that include physician team members. The transport team's skills should be assessed periodically, and procedural and situational training should be part of routine ongoing education.

C. **Types of transport teams**

1. Unit-based transport teams consist of personnel (nurses, respiratory therapists, neonatal nurse practitioners, etc.) who are involved in routine patient care in the NICU and are deployed when a request for transport is received. If few infants are transported to the NICU, this type of staffing may be most cost-effective; however, each team member has little opportunity to gain experience or maintain skills specific to transport.

2. Dedicated transport teams are staffed separately from NICU personnel specifically for the purpose of transport of patients to and from the hospital. These personnel do not have patient assignments, although they

may assist NICU staff when they are not on transport. A large volume of transports is necessary to justify a dedicated transport team, which must consist of sufficient personnel for around the clock coverage. This arrangement allows dedicated personnel to maintain specialized skills for transport and facilitates rapid mobilization to transport requests.

D. **Modes of transport** include ambulance, rotor-wing (helicopter), and fixed-wing (airplane) aircraft. The type of vehicle(s) operated will depend on each program's individual needs, specifically the distance of transports anticipated, acuity of patients, and geographic terrain to be covered by the vehicle. Some hospitals own, maintain, and insure their own vehicles, whereas others contract with commercial vendors for vehicles that can accommodate a transport incubator and appropriate equipment. Although the type(s) of vehicle chosen for transport will vary depending on the individual program's needs, the vehicles chosen must be outfitted to conform to standards that ensure safety and efficiency of transport. Vehicles should comply with all local, state, and federal guidelines for air transport and/or ground ambulances. The vehicles should be large enough to allow the transport team to adequately assess and treat patients as needed *en route* to the referral hospital and should be equipped with appropriate electrical power supply, medical gases (with reserve capacity, in case of a breakdown), and communication systems. All equipment and stretchers should be properly secured, and transport team personnel should use appropriate passenger safety restraints.

Each mode of transport—ground, rotor-wing, and fixed-wing—has advantages and disadvantages. **Ground transport** is used most commonly among neonatal transport programs. Advantages include a larger workspace than air ambulances, ability to accommodate multiple team members and passengers, and the option to stop the vehicle to assess the patient or perform procedures. **Rotor-wing transport** has the advantage of a rapid response with hospital-to-hospital service for patients up to a distance of ~100 to 150 miles or less each way, although a rotor-wing service is more expensive to operate, has limitations with regard to weather and weight, and has inherently more safety considerations. **Fixed-wing transport** is advisable for transport of patients over greater distances (over ~150 miles each way), is moderately expensive to operate, and requires an airport to land and an ambulance at either end of the flight to transport the patient between the airport and the hospital. Fixed-wing aircraft have fewer restrictions for weather than do helicopters.

E. **Equipment.** The team should carry with them all equipment, medications, and other supplies that might be needed to stabilize an infant at a referring hospital. Teams should use checklists prior to departure to ensure that vital supplies and equipment are not forgotten. Packs especially designed for neonatal transport are commercially available. These packs or other containers should be stocked by members of the transport team, which ensures that they will know where to find required items promptly. The weight of the stocked packs should be documented for air transport (Tables 17.2 to 17.4).

F. **Legal issues.** The process of neonatal transport may raise legal issues, which vary among states. Transport teams should periodically review all routine procedures and documentation forms with their hospital legal counsel to

Table 17.2. Neonatal Transport Team Equipment

Transport incubator equipped with neonatal-capable ventilator and gas supply (oxygen and compressed air tanks), blender, and flow meter

Monitors for heart rate, invasive and noninvasive blood pressures, oxygen saturation, and temperature, with associated electrodes/probes/transducers/cuffs

Defibrillator with neonatal-appropriate energy settings and paddles/pads

Suction device and suction catheters

Feeding tubes, sump tubes (e.g., Replogle)

Oxygen tubing, masks, nasal cannulas, CPAP devices

Nitric oxide tank and delivery equipment

Infusion pumps

Gel-filled mattress

Glucometer or other point-of-care testing device

Airway equipment

Flow-inflating bag with manometer and oxygen tubing

Face masks (premature and term infant)

Oropharyngeal airways

Laryngoscopes with no. 00, 0, and 1 blades, with extra batteries/bulbs (if needed)

Endotracheal tubes sizes 2.5–4.0 mm

Magill forceps

Laryngeal mask airways

CO_2 detectors or waveform capnography

Instrument tray for chest tubes and umbilical vessel catheters

Chest tubes and connectors, Heimlich valves, closed suction/water seal system

Vascular access supplies, including intraosseous needles

Medication delivery supplies, including needles and syringes

Stethoscope

Gloves, masks, disposable gowns, eye protection

Source of electrical power, heat, and light

(continued)

Table 17.2. *(Continued)*

Adaptors to plug into both hospital and vehicle power
Clipboard with transport data forms, permission forms, progress notes, and booklet for parents
Medication guide for dosing and infusion preparation
CPAP, continuous positive airway pressure; CO_2, carbon dioxide.

ensure compliance with changing laws that govern the transport of infants and accompanying family members (if present). The team should have the ability to contact via telephone appropriate hospital legal counsel as needed.

G. **Quality assurance and performance improvement** activities should be performed routinely using established benchmarks whenever possible.

H. **Malpractice insurance coverage** is required for all team members. The tertiary hospital should decide whether transport is considered as an off-site or extended on-site activity because this can affect the necessary coverage.

I. **Ambulance regulations** vary from state to state and may conflict with transport team goals. For example, some states require that an ambulance stop at the scene of an unattended accident to render aid until a second ambulance arrives.

IV. REFERRING HOSPITAL RESPONSIBILITIES

A. **Identify the appropriate tertiary care facility for transfer.** If it is known before birth that the infant will need transfer to a tertiary care facility (e.g., an infant with congenital cyanotic heart disease), both the parents and the appropriate tertiary care facility can be prepared for the transfer. Prompt notification of the receiving hospital will allow timely deployment of the transport team and verify that the required services are available. Any risk posed by the patient for communicable diseases must be disclosed to the tertiary center at the time of the request for transfer.

B. **Documentation.** Staff at the referring hospital should complete the administrative forms required for transfer, which include parental consent. A transfer summary should document the care given to the infant at the referring hospital. Transport team documentation begins upon the team's arrival and should note all treatment rendered to the patient by either the referring hospital staff or the transport team.

V. TRANSPORT TEAM RESPONSIBILITIES

A. When receiving the initial request for transfer, the medical control physician should obtain a sufficiently detailed summary from the referring clinician to decide the appropriate team composition and equipment required, in consultation with the transport team.

Table 17.3. Medications Used during Neonatal Transport

Adenosine
Albumin 5%
Ampicillin
Atropine
Calcium chloride
Calcium gluconate
Dexamethasone
Dextrose 10% in water ($D_{10}W$)
Dextrose 5% in water (D_5W)
Dobutamine
Dopamine
Epinephrine (1:10,000; 0.1 mg/mL)
Erythromycin eye ointment
Fentanyl
Fosphenytoin
Furosemide
Gentamicin
Heparin
Lidocaine
Lorazepam
Midazolam
Morphine
Naloxone
Normal saline (0.9% NaCl)
Phenobarbital
Potassium chloride
Prostaglandin E_1 (requires refrigeration)
Rocuronium

(continued)

Table 17.3. *(Continued)*
Sodium bicarbonate 4.2% (0.5 mEq/mL)
Sterile water for injection
Surfactant (bovine surfactant products require refrigeration)
Vecuronium
Vitamin K_1

B. The medical control physician should discuss the patient's condition, anticipated problems, and potential therapies with the transport team members before their departure. This provides an opportunity for the team members to ask questions and to determine if there is any additional equipment or medications that might be needed.

C. Upon arrival at the referring NICU, transport team members should introduce themselves clearly and politely to the referring hospital staff and family members. Appropriate photo identification should be worn. The referring and/or primary physicians should be identified and their names documented.

D. Transfer of patient information (handoff) should be clear. Use of checklists for communication decreases the likelihood of important items being overlooked during handoff.

E. The team should work collegially with the referring hospital staff and be objective in their assessment and stabilization. The transfer of care from referring hospital staff to the transport team is a stepwise process that requires clear communication about roles and responsibilities. Any differences of opinion related to the care of the infant should be discussed with the medical control physician.

Table 17.4. Barometric Pressure and Partial Pressure of Oxygen with Increasing Altitude

	Sea Level	2,000	4,000	6,000	8,000	10,000
Barometric pressure (torr)	760	706	656	609	565	523
Partial pressure of FiO_2 0.21 (torr)	160	148	138	128	119	110

$$F_iO_2 \text{ required} = \frac{F_iO_2 \times BP_1}{BP_2}$$

F_iO_2, fraction of inspired oxygen patient is currently receiving; BP_1, barometric pressure prior to flight; BP_2, barometric pressure at altitude.

F. Parents should be given an opportunity to see the infant before the team leaves the referring hospital. While meeting with the family, the team should obtain consent for transfer and other anticipated procedures (including blood transfusion, if indicated), as well as review the team's policy regarding parents traveling with their newborn on transport.

G. Following completion of the transport, the team should call the referring hospital staff with pertinent follow-up of the patient's condition and how he or she tolerated the transport to the tertiary facility.

H. Transport teams should consider an active outreach education program for referring hospital staff that could include conferences, in-service presentations, and case reviews.

VI. MEDICAL MANAGEMENT BEFORE TRANSPORT

A. The medical control physician should support the medical management and stabilization of the neonate while the transport team is mobilizing and *en route*. The extent of pretransport diagnostic testing and treatment depends on the urgency of the patient's condition as well as the resources available at the referring hospital. In general, pretransport interventions should focus on respiratory, cardiac, neurologic, and metabolic stabilization.

B. **Pretransport management should include attention to the following:**

1. Establish and maintain a neutral thermal environment or allow for passive cooling if the infant meets criteria for therapeutic hypothermia.

2. Ensure airway patency and security and support oxygenation and ventilation.

3. Support hemodynamics and perfusion with fluids and/or vasoactive infusions.

4. Ensure adequate blood glucose concentration.

5. Obtain vascular access (PIV, UVC, UAC) as indicated.

6. Obtain appropriate cultures and give first doses of antibiotics, if indicated.

7. Obtain copies of obstetric and neonatal charts for the transport team, including copies of radiographic studies.

8. Prepare the parents for transport of their infant and, if possible, allow them time to visit with their infant.

VII. MEDICAL MANAGEMENT DURING RETURN TRANSPORT

A. **The mobile environment.** The period of time after leaving the referring hospital and arriving at the receiving hospital is the most vulnerable for the patient due to challenges with monitoring, assessment, and interventions in the mobile environment. Most modern monitors are built to withstand interference from road vibration and 60 cycle electrical signals. Direct observation of the patient may be challenging due to the use of the isolette, movement of the vehicle, and restraint use by the transport team members, so it is essential that monitoring devices are functioning and easily visible.

B. **Adverse events.** Dislodgment of lines and tubes can occur with movement of the ambulance or patient. Properly securing tubes and lines prior to transport is the most effective prevention strategy, and team members should carefully coordinate transfers into and out of the isolette so that someone is responsible for supporting the endotracheal tube. Travel in both the ground and air environments involves physiologic stressors that are different than in the hospital setting, and judicious use of sedation may be indicated to maintain the patient's comfort and safety and, in particular, avoid inadvertent extubation. In the event of an unexpected clinical deterioration, auscultation may be unreliable due to background noise, and capnography may be more reliable to assess endotracheal tube position. If the patient continues to deteriorate, it may be appropriate during ground transport to ask the driver to pull over so that the team can accurately assess breath sounds and perform necessary interventions. Ambulance sirens and flashing lights should be used only in rare circumstances because they increase the risk of causing accidents and have not been shown to save substantial time or reduce mortality.

C. **Communication.** The transport team should notify the medical control physician of any significant changes in the patient's condition during transport. On rare occasions, it may be appropriate to return to the referring hospital or divert to a closer hospital if the patient is not responding to interventions. Cellular phones are most commonly used to communicate during transport, but a back-up system (i.e., radio) should be available in the event there is no cellular phone service due to terrain or distance. If indicated, the medical control physician should notify subspecialty services that may need to be involved urgently in the care of the patient on arrival, such as cardiology or surgery.

VIII. ARRIVAL AT THE NEONATAL INTENSIVE CARE UNIT

A. The team should give the NICU caregivers a succinct and complete summary of the infant's clinical condition and copies of the referring hospital's medical record and radiographic studies. Use of a standardized handoff script will ensure relevant information is not inadvertently omitted.

B. A team member should telephone the parents to let them know that their infant has arrived safely.

C. Relevant documentation regarding the transport should be completed and a copy added to the patient's medical record, including contact information for the parents.

D. All transport medications should be immediately restocked, and all equipment checked and prepared for subsequent transports.

E. If an untoward incident occurred during transport, appropriate documentation should be completed, and the transport team's medical director should be notified to allow appropriate investigation and debriefing.

IX. SPECIFIC CONDITIONS AND MANAGEMENT

A. **Premature infants with respiratory distress syndrome** (RDS) who have not responded to early application of CPAP may benefit from exogenous surfactant administration. When a preterm infant requires intubation and mechanical ventilation, the transport team should consider administration of surfactant. Ideally, a chest x-ray should be obtained after intubation and prior to surfactant delivery to avoid administration of surfactant into one lung. The transport team should anticipate rapid changes in lung compliance and be prepared to wean ventilatory support during the first 30 minutes after surfactant delivery due to the risk of pneumothorax.

B. Hypoxic respiratory failure and pulmonary hypertension. Management should focus on ensuring optimal lung recruitment using ventilatory strategies and, in some cases, surfactant administration, while avoiding injurious ventilator settings and/or hyperventilation. If the infant has signs of severe pulmonary hypertension (e.g., tachycardia, pre- and postductal oxygen saturation difference, systemic hypotension), transport teams should be prepared to institute inhaled nitric oxide at the referring hospital and continue administration during transport. If inhaled nitric oxide has been started at the referring hospital, it is important to avoid interruption during transport due to the risk of rebound pulmonary hypertension.

C. Cardiac disease. Ideally, a cardiologist or cardiac intensive care specialist at the tertiary care facility should be available to make recommendations for care prior to and during transport of the infant. For infants with suspected ductal-dependent congenital heart disease, prostaglandin E_1 (PGE_1) may be initiated prior to transport. Apnea, fever, and hypotension are common side effects of PGE_1 and appear to be dose-dependent. In the past, endotracheal intubation was routinely recommended for neonates receiving PGE_1. More recently, many transport teams have adopted the approach of using low-dose PGE_1 for infants without significant respiratory distress or impaired perfusion. In such cases, it may not be necessary to secure the airway prior to transport, which may be beneficial to the balance of pulmonary and systemic blood flow in infants with single ventricle physiology.

D. Surgical conditions. Special consideration should be given to infants being transported by air (see section X.B) who may benefit from gastric decompression if there is suspicion of intestinal obstruction.

X. PHYSIOLOGIC CONSIDERATIONS OF AIR TRANSPORTS. Rotor-wing aircraft are not pressurized, so the interior pressure will vary with altitude. Fixed-wing aircraft are pressurized but typically operate at an equivalent altitude of 5,000 to 8,000 ft where barometric pressure is decreased.

A. Alveolar hypoxia (Dalton's law). As altitude increases, the barometric pressure and partial pressure of oxygen in the air decrease (see Table 17.4), leading to a decrease in alveolar oxygen tension. Even in aircraft with pressurized cabins, because the cabin pressure is usually maintained at a level equal to 5,000 to 8,000 ft above sea level, it may be necessary to increase the FiO_2 delivered to the infant to compensate. The FiO_2 required at altitude to approximate the same oxygen tension that the patient is receiving at sea level can be calculated by the formula in Table 17.4. If neonates with severe lung disease are transported by air, it may be necessary to request the pilot to pressurize the cabin closer to sea level to avoid severe hypoxemia. Ultimately, pulse oximetry and blood gas estimations should be used to guide adjustments in delivered FiO_2 to maintain adequate oxygen delivery.

B. Gas expansion (Boyle's law). As altitude increases and barometric pressure decreases, the volume of gases will increase. As a result, gases trapped in closed spaces will expand. This can result in a small pneumothorax or the normal gaseous distention of the gastrointestinal tract causing clinical deterioration in an infant that was stable at sea level. To prevent decompensation in flight, pneumothoraces should be drained and the stomach vented with a nasogastric tube before an air transport.

XI. SIMULATION IN TRANSPORT MEDICINE. Transport of critically ill infants involves high-stress situations where it is crucial for the team members to work well together to ensure patient and team member safety using clear communication and principles of crisis resource management. Simulation-based training allows teams to practice working together to enhance their interactions and efficiency in a safe environment.

Suggested Readings

American Academy of Pediatrics. *Guidelines for Air and Ground Transport of Neonatal and Pediatric Patients*. 4th ed. Elk Grove Village, IL: American Academy of Pediatrics; 2016.

Schwartz HP, Bigham MT, Schoettker PJ, et al. Quality metrics in neonatal and pediatric critical care transport: a national Delphi project. *Pediatr Crit Care Med* 2015;16:711–717.

18 Neonatal Intensive Care Unit Discharge Planning

Vincent C. Smith and Theresa M. Andrews

KEY POINTS

- Begin discharge planning shortly after admission and continue until families are prepared to bring their infants home.
- Follow the tenets of family-centered care involving the family as a member of the team as much as possible.
- Include a structured family education program that is tailored to a family's specific needs and circumstance with frequent evaluations of progress and the capacity for adjustment as necessary.

A successful transition from the neonatal intensive care unit (NICU) to home is critical in order to ensure a safe and confident transition home for newborns and their families. In keeping with the rest of newborn care, there is a progressive trend toward increased family centeredness and efficiency that requires careful and organized discharge planning. The optimal safe and successful discharge requires mutual participation between the family and the medical faculty and should begin at admission and follow the continuum of the infant's hospital stay. This chapter discusses the infant's discharge readiness as well as the discharge preparation for the family.

NICU **discharge readiness** is the attainment of technical skills and knowledge, emotional comfort, and confidence with infant care by the primary caregivers at the time of discharge. NICU **discharge preparation** is the process of facilitating discharge readiness to successfully make the transition from the NICU to home. Discharge readiness is the desired outcome, and discharge preparation is the process.

I. **INFANT'S DISCHARGE READINESS.** The American Academy of Pediatrics (AAP) recommends the transition to home occur when the infant achieves physiologic maturity and has completed all predischarge testing and treatment.

A. Healthy growing preterm infants are considered ready for discharge when they meet the following criteria:

1. Able to maintain temperature in an open environment

2. Able to take all feedings by bottle or breast without respiratory compromise

3. Demonstrates steady weight gain evidenced by a weight gain of 20 to 30 g/day

4. Free of apnea or bradycardia for 5 days (see Chapter 31)

5. Able to sleep with head of bed flat without compromising the infant's health and safety

B. Complete routine screening tests and immunizations according to AAP, local, and regional guidelines (Table 18.1).
For all infants

1. Newborn screening (see Chapter 8)

2. Hearing screening (see Chapter 68)

3. Immunizations administered according to AAP guidelines based on chronologic, not postmenstrual, age (http://www.cdc.gov/vaccines and see Chapter 7)

For preterm infants

4. Head ultrasound and ophthalmologic evaluation if indicated screening (see Chapter 67)

5. Car seat/bed use (see Table 18.1). Prior to discharge, each preterm infant requires a car seat or car bed evaluation as appropriate.

C. When planning discharge, it is important to consider the infant's relative fragility and the complexity of care needs. Infants with specialized needs require a complex, flexible, ongoing discharge care plan. Because medications, special formulas, and/or dietary supplements may be challenging for the parents to obtain, the need for these items should be identified early so they can be obtained as soon as possible to optimize discharge teaching opportunities. If an infant will require in-home respiratory support, make a referral to a durable medical equipment (DME) company. A respiratory therapist (RT) must assess the home to evaluate outlets in the infant's area, measure door openings, inquire about electrical panel location and capacity, and ensure a safe environment.

Table 18.1. Guidelines for Routine Screening, Testing, Treatment, and Follow-up at Neonatal Intensive Care Unit (NICU)
Newborn Screening
Criteria
▪ All infants admitted to the NICU
Initial
▪ Day 3 or discharge (D/C) date (whichever comes first)
(continued)

Table 18.1. Guidelines for Routine Screening, Testing, Treatment, and Follow-up at Neonatal Intensive Care Unit (NICU) *(Continued)*

Follow-up

- Day 14 or D/C date (whichever comes first)

- Day 30 or D/C date (whichever comes first)

- Continue monthly

- On D/C date if more than 7 days since prior screen

Head Ultrasound (see Chapter 54)

Criteria

- All infants with gestational age (GA) <32 weeks

Initial

- Days 7–10 (in the case of critically ill infants, when results of an earlier ultrasonography may alter clinical management, an ultrasonography should be performed at the discretion of the clinician)

Follow-up (minimum if no abnormalities noted)

- If no hemorrhage or germinal hemorrhage only
  Week 4 and at 40 weeks' postmenstrual age (or discharge if <40 weeks)

- If intraventricular (grade 2+) or intraparenchymal hemorrhage: Follow up at least weekly until stable (more frequently if unstable posthemorrhagic hydrocephalus). (Daily head circumference measurement should also be performed in the case of ventricular dilatation.)

Note: An ultrasound should be done at any GA at any time if thought to be clinically indicated.

Audiology Screening (see Chapter 68)

Criteria

- All infants being discharged home from NICU or who are at 34 weeks PMA or greater at the time of transfer to a level 2 nursery

Timing

- Examine at 34 weeks gestation or greater.

(continued)

Table 18.1. *(Continued)*

Car Seat and Car Bed Fit Assessment and Screening

Criteria

- All infants to be discharged home from NICU and born at <37 weeks or BW <2,500 g or with other conditions that may compromise respiratory status (e.g., chronic lung disease, airway anomalies, and tracheostomy).

Timing

- Fit assessment or screening prior to discharge home

Ophthalmologic Examination (see Chapter 67)

Criteria

- All infants with birth weight ≤1,500 g or GA <31 0/7 weeks

- Infants with a birth weight between 1,500 g and 2,000 g or GA 31 0/7–34 0/7 weeks with high-illness severity (e.g., those who have had severe respiratory distress syndrome, hypotension requiring pressor support, or surgery in the first several weeks of life) per the discretion of the attending neonatologist

Timing of Initial Exam

GA	Postmenstrual Age	Week after Birth
22*	29	7
23*	30	7
24	31	7
25	31	6
26	31	5
27	31	4
28	32	4
29	33	4
30	34	4
31+	—	4

*Guidelines have been adjusted slightly from the AAP recommendations per BCH Ophthalmology's discretion.

- If the infant is transferred to another nursery prior to 4 weeks of age, recommend exam at the receiving hospital.

- If the infant is discharged home prior to 4 weeks of age, examine prior to discharge.

(continued)

Table 18.1. Guidelines for Routine Screening, Testing, Treatment, and Follow-up at Neonatal Intensive Care Unit (NICU) *(Continued)*

Follow-up (Based on Most Recent Exam Findings)

■ Follow-up examinations should be recommended by the examining ophthalmologist on the basis of retinal findings classified according to the international classification. The following schedule is suggested:

Stage	Zone	Follow-up
Immature (no ROP)	I	≤1 week
Immature (no ROP)	posterior II	1–2 weeks
Immature (no ROP)	mid-anterior II	2 week
Immature (no ROP)	III	3 week
I	I	≤1 week
I	II	2 weeks
I	III	2–3 weeks
II	I	≤1 week
II	II	1–2 weeks
II	III	2–3 weeks
III	II	≤1 week
Regressing	I	1–2 weeks
Regressing	II	2 weeks
Regressing	III	2–3 weeks

■ Follow up after resolution of ROP depends on the severity of the active phase of ROP but should occur by age 1 year. The following findings warrant consideration of treatment:

Stage	Zone
I, II, or III with plus disease	I
III no plus disease	I
II or III with plus disease	II

*Guidelines have been adjusted slightly from the AAP recommendations per BCH Ophthalmology's Discretion

Hepatitis B Vaccination (see Chapter 48)

Criteria

■ All infants being discharged home from NICU

(continued)

Table 18.1. *(Continued)*

Initial

- If weight ≥2,000 g and stable: Vaccinate at birth or shortly thereafter.

- If weight ≥2,000 g and unstable: Defer vaccination until the infant's clinical condition has stabilized.

- If weight <2,000 g: Vaccinate at 30 days or discharge (whichever comes first).

Synagis RSV Prophylaxis

Criteria

- Synagis RSV prophylaxis should be considered from November through March for infants who meet any of the following criteria:

  □ GA at birth <29 0/7 weeks

  □ GA at birth 29 0/7–31 6/7 weeks with chronic lung disease defined as need for supplemental oxygen for at least 28 days after birth

  □ Certain types of hemodynamically significant congenital heart disease

  □ Pulmonary abnormality or neuromuscular disease that impairs ability to clear secretions from upper airways

  □ Profound immunocompromised condition

Timing

- Give first dose 48–72 hours before discharge.

Infant Follow-up Program (IFUP)—Offered at Many Hospitals That Have a Level 3 NICU

Criteria

- All infants with GA <32 weeks at birth

Timing

- Referral completed before discharge

- First appointment to be scheduled at 3 months post due date

Neonatal Neurology Program

Criteria

- All infants meeting one of the following conditions:

  □ Neurologic disorders (e.g., intracranial hemorrhage, neonatal seizures, and stroke)

(continued)

Table 18.1. Guidelines for Routine Screening, Testing, Treatment, and Follow-up at Neonatal Intensive Care Unit (NICU) *(Continued)*

☐ Neuromuscular disorders
☐ Recipient of therapeutic hypothermia for HIE
Timing
▪ Referral completed before discharge
Note: Infants with GA <32 weeks at birth should also be referred to IFUP
Early Intervention Program (EIP)
Criteria
▪ Infant meeting four or more of the following criteria:
☐ BW <1,200 g
☐ GA <32 weeks
☐ NICU admission >5 days
☐ Apgar <5 at 5 minutes
☐ Intrauterine growth restriction (IUGR) or small for gestational age (SGA) (refer to growth curves)
☐ Chronic feeding difficulties
☐ Suspected central nervous system abnormality
☐ Maternal age <17 years or 3 or more births at maternal age <20 years
☐ High school education <10 years
☐ Parental chronic illness or disability affecting caregiving
☐ Lack of family supports
☐ Inadequate food, shelter, and clothing
☐ Open or confirmed protective service investigation ("51-A")
☐ Substance abuse in the home
☐ Violence in the home
Timing
▪ Referral completed before discharge
PMA, postmenstrual age; BW, birth weight; AAP, American Academy of Pediatrics; BCH, Boston Children's Hospital; ROP, retinopathy of prematurity; RSV, respiratory syncytial virus.

II. PARENT'S DISCHARGE PREPARATION. The AAP recommends that there is an active program for parental involvement and preparation for care of the infant at home, arrangements for health care of the infant after discharge in a medical home by a physician or other health care professional who is experienced in the care of high-risk infants, and an organized program of tracking and surveillance to monitor growth and development.

Part 1: Discharge Teaching

A. Discharge teaching concepts

1. Identification of caregivers: Designate at least two individuals who will be familiar with the infant's care in the event that one is unavailable.

2. Family-centered care (FCC) is the concept that parents are an integral part of the care team who work in partnership with the medical providers on decision making and providing care for the infant. FCC may ameliorate the stressors that families experience due to the separation of family and infant, inability to experience a traditional parenting role, and the inclusion of multiple caregivers in daily care.

   a. The four central tenets of FCC are dignity and respect, information sharing, family participation in care, and collaboration with the family.

   b. FCC can shorten the length of stay, decrease the risk for readmission, enhance breastfeeding outcomes, boost families' confidence with infant care, and increase staff satisfaction.

   c. FCC should be incorporated in all aspects of discharge preparation for the families.

   d. Family presence/participation in medical rounds is an easy opportunity to help promote FCC and prepare families for the transition home.

   e. The early establishment of parents as partners and participants in their infants care helps a family cope with the stress and separation associated with NICU care and promotes an easier transition home.

3. **Discharge planning team includes the following:**

   a. Family

   b. Staff including some combination of the following: clinical nurses, physicians, mid-level providers (e.g., neonatal advance practice nurses and physician assistants), case managers, other providers (e.g., primary care pediatric provider or subspecialist) as appropriate

4. **Support of families with limited English proficiency**

   a. Families with limited English proficiency are at increased risk for not understanding discharge teaching and to have poor transitions home.

   b. Support for families with limited English proficiency should include the following:

      i. Use of appropriately trained interpreters for all discharge teaching

      ii. Verification of comprehension of discharge teaching and needed medical follow-up with interpreters

      iii. Provision of supplemental materials in the families' preferred language when possible

B. Discharge teaching structure

1. Discharge teaching should begin early and be distributed throughout the NICU hospitalization to prevent the family from being overwhelmed with a large volume of content near the end of the hospitalization.

2. The education program should be structured to include all the skills and knowledge they are expected to master, tailored to their specific circumstance. It should offer repetition and frequent opportunities to evaluate progress and the capacity for adjustment as necessary.

3. Checklist can be helpful to make sure educational content is consistent and provides the family with an idea of what they will be expected to master (Table 18.2). A nursing discharge planning worksheet will allow all staff providing family education to be aware of which topics already have and which ones need to be covered (see Table 18.3).

4. Skills demonstration

   a. Provide parents with adequate opportunities to practice skills initially under direct supervision and then with supervisory support as needed.

   b. Repetition and return demonstrations (i.e., teach-back technique) can be used to increase parental retention of the education content.

   c. Provide specific, practical information with examples that are meaningful to the family's everyday experiences.

   d. Supplement discharge teaching with other materials to reinforce the teaching and increasing retention of the material.

      i. Written information presented in a manner that is simple, clear, and devoid of medical jargon, with complex words and concepts defined in precise terms

      ii. Some families may have limited functional health literacy; therefore, pictographs, visual aids, multimedia, and recorded information are helpful to illustrate key concepts.

C. Discharge teaching content. Parents need instruction in all of the following:

1. Technical infant care skills

   a. Breast/bottle-feeding and mixing formula

   b. Bathing and dressing an infant

   c. Caring for the infant's skin, umbilical cord, and genitalia

   d. Placing the infant in a safe sleeping position and environment

   e. Administering and storing medications properly

   f. Using medical equipment as appropriate

   g. Cardiopulmonary resuscitation (CPR)

2. Normal and abnormal preterm infant behavior

   a. Typical preterm infant behaviors include breast- and bottle-feeding patterns commonly seen, normal bowel and bladder function, and usual infant sleep–wake cycles.

   b. Some typical preterm infant behaviors are normal but may seem abnormal to those not accustomed to preterm infants. Specifically, preterm infants frequently do not engage socially in the same way as term infants including being less active, alert, and responsive as well as more irritable and having more gaze aversion.

   c. Changes in behavior that may be signs of illness that require close monitoring: not hungry or eating less well than baseline, sleepier or less active than usual, more irritable or fussy than usual

   d. Physical signs that may be signs of illness that require close monitoring: changes from the infant's normal breathing pattern; cyanosis (blueness) of the lips or mouth; flushed, very pale, or mottled (spotted or blotched) skin; or lower muscle tone than usual

e. Abnormal signs and symptoms that should prompt a discussion with the medical home: vomiting and/or diarrhea, dry diapers for more than 12 hours, no stool for more than 4 days, black or bright red stool, a rectal temperature over 100° F, or an axillary (armpit) temperature over 99.6° F or below 97° F.

3. Home environment preparation
  a. Equipment and supplies to acquire in anticipation of discharge:
    i. Feeding-related supplies: breast pump, nipples/bottles, formula
    ii. Crib or bassinet (safety approved)
    iii. Diapers
    iv. Infant clothes
    v. Thermometer (axillary or forehead for common use and rectal to be used when directed by a medical provider)
    vi. Smoke and carbon monoxide detectors

4. Anticipatory guidance
  a. Provide a realistic idea of what their home life will be like during the immediate and more longer term period following discharge including:
    i. Anticipated and potential infant developmental or growth-related issues
    ii. Expected number and type of physician visits for routine infant health maintenance and illness
  b. Families must be taught how to cope with and soothe their crying infant and learn about shaken baby syndrome and the harm caused by shaking, slamming, hitting, or throwing the infant.
  c. Families may also be given anticipatory guidance related to potential parental mental health issues such as anxiety and depression that can arise in the period following discharge.

5. Special circumstances
  a. Infants going home on oxygen should notify local emergency care providers including community hospital emergency departments and local emergency medical technicians (EMTs) or first responders of the child's condition, medical needs, and possible problems. This will help optimize appropriate emergency response. Helping the family to prepare a succinct summary of the infant's medical conditions and current medications can be extremely useful. An electronic copy is preferable so that the information can be updated easily. Local utility companies such as telephone, electricity, fuel, and public works for snow removal should be notified in writing of the child's presence in the home so they will assign priority resumption of services if there is an interruption.
  b. Emergency management at home: management of a life-threatening emergency associated with equipment malfunction, instruction on emergency procedures (e.g., CPR), availability of community resources, a list of relevant individuals or organizations to call with questions and concerns
  c. Home care services are becoming more widely available; however, their ability to provide specialized pediatric or neonatal services is

variable. Consult the NICU case manager to assess the infants home care needs, review insurance, and make community referrals.

d. Home nursing care

  i. Nurses from visiting nurse associations provide home visits for reinforcement of teaching, health and psychosocial assessments, and short-term treatments or nursing care.

  ii. Private duty nursing or block nursing may be provided to infants who are discharged home with complex medical needs, such as with a tracheostomy. Case management should be consulted as soon as it is known that an infant with complex medical needs will be discharged to home. The case manager will make referrals to have an infant's care reviewed to determine the allotment of hours. This level of in-home care will require secondary insurance. In some circumstances, the hours may be approved but it is difficult to secure nurses with appropriate training and experience to fill those hours.

D. Family assessment. Family assessment is a key component of a successful discharge process. Families are able to build on their strengths if given the opportunity to participate in the care early and be an active participant in the discharge process. Early partnership with the family promotes confidence and decreases stress by enhancing the parents' feeling of control. The ability to provide adequate parent education is vital for the successful transition to home. With early planning, ongoing teaching, and attention to the family's needs and resources, the transition to home can be smooth, even in the most complex cases. The family assessment should address the following questions:

  1. Who will be the primary care giver(s) for the infant? How willingly is this responsibility assumed?

  2. What is the family structure? Do they have a support system? Does one need to be developed or strengthened?

  3. Are there language or learning barriers? If so, address them as soon as they are identified.

  4. How do they learn best? The nursing team should maximize the use of educational tools, written materials, visual props, and demonstrations.

  5. How do previous or present experiences with the infant's care affect the family's ability to oversee care after discharge?

  6. What are the actual and perceived complexities of the skills required to care for the infant?

  7. What are their coping habits and styles?

  8. Do the parents have any medical or psychological concerns that may have an impact on caretaking abilities?

  9. What are the cultural beliefs and how might this affect the care of the infant?

  10. What are the financial concerns? Will the family's income change? If so, what resources are available to compensate?

11. Are there issues related to the family's living conditions that will be challenging? Families can become overwhelmed by the volume of medical equipment that will be delivered to the home in the days before discharge. Have the parents describe the home nursery and other spaces for the infant/caregivers and supplies. Ask them to take pictures to evaluate layout options. Discuss supply storage recommendations such as plastic bins on wheels, baskets, etc.

Part 2: Transfer and/or Coordination of Care

A. The medical home

1. The AAP recommends that high-risk infants receive their primary care in a medical home with a primary care provider who has expertise in caring for patients who have required NICU care.

2. The medical home is usually staffed by a pediatrician, family practitioner, and/or nurse practitioner. Ongoing communication between NICU staff and the primary care provider begins long before discharge. This maintains continuity and facilitates appropriate medical care after discharge. A family should make a pediatrician appointment for 1 to 3 days after discharge, preferably not on the same day as a visiting nurse appointment, if applicable.

3. The communication between the NICU team and the primary care provider should, at a minimum, include a written discharge.

4. A phone call or in-person meeting between the NICU provider and pediatrician is appropriate for complex medical or social situations.

B. Discharge summary

1. A standardized format for the discharge summary improves clarity and helps to ensure that all the pertinent information is included and organized in a useful fashion. Define complex words and concepts with precise terms.

2. Discharge summary suggested content (Table 18.4)
  a. The pertinent maternal history
  b. Infant's birth history
  c. Infant's neonatal history
  d. NICU medical course synopsis
  e. Infant's discharge diagnoses
  f. Infant's condition at discharge
  g. Prognosis if guarded
  h. Home feeding plan
  i. Discharge medications, dosages, and intervals
  j. Medical equipment needs (e.g., oxygen, gastrostomy tube, etc.)
  k. Follow-up appointments that were either arranged prior to discharge or recommended but not yet arranged
  l. Newborn hearing screen results
  m. State newborn screenings dates and (if known) results
  n. Car seat challenge results if relevant
  o. Any immunizations administered
  p. Any pending test or lab results

      q. Referrals made to community service programs (e.g., community health nursing agencies, early intervention services)

C. Early intervention

    1. Early intervention programs are community-based and offer multidisciplinary services for children from birth to age 3 years.

    2. Children deemed at biologic, environmental, or emotional risk are eligible. Programs are partially federally funded and are offered at a reduced rate based on household income.

    3. They provide multidisciplinary services including physical therapy, occupational therapy, speech and feeding therapy, early childhood education, social services, and parental support groups.

    4. Services may be home-based or center-based. For further detailed criteria, see Table 18.1.

III. ALTERNATIVES TO HOME DISCHARGE.
Alternatives to home discharge may be temporary or permanent. Integrating the child into the home may be difficult because of medical needs or family situation. Decisions regarding alternative placement may be painful for the family and therefore require extra support. Alternatives vary widely from community to community.

A. Inpatient pediatric ward or level 2 nurseries may be options for the infant who is stable but needs a less intense level of hospital care before going home. Pediatric wards may have a place for parents to room in, and community hospitals may be closer to home. Both options can offer more opportunities for families to be together to participate in care and have more time to learn.

B. Pediatric rehabilitation hospitals can be used for the high-risk infant who requires ongoing but less acute hospital care.

C. Pediatric nursing homes provide extended care at a skilled level.

D. Medical foster care places the special needs infant in a home setting with specially trained caregivers. The ultimate goal is to place the infant back with the family.

E. Hospice care may be institutional or home-based. It focuses on maximizing the quality of life when cure is not expected.

Going Home from the NICU

Baby's name in hospital: _____   Baby's name after discharge: _____

	Please check off items as they occur.	Additional Information	Parent Initials
In NICU	Discharge planning meeting		
	Pediatrician chosen Dr. _____ # _____		
	Baby added to insurance policy		
	CPR class complete		
	Handouts received and/or discussed with nurse ☐ Safe travels (car seat safety) ☐ Safe sleep practices ☐ Shaken baby syndrome ☐ Carbon monoxide and smoke detectors ☐ Protecting babies from infection	☐ Temperature taking ☐ When to call the pediatrician ☐ Flu/pertussis vaccines for families/caregivers ☐ Suction bulb use ☐ Bathing techniques ☐ Tummy time and activities for 1st year	
Preparing for Home	Car seat brought to NICU and base installed in car		
	Supplies at home:		
	• Crib/bassinet (safety approved)		
	• Diapers, wipes, ointments		
	• Thermometer, suction bulb		
	• Feeding supplies	☐ Breast pump (if needed) ☐ Nipple/bottles ☐ Formula (if needed)	
	• Circumcision care education	☐ N/A	
	Hearing screen results received*	*If referral needed, add to specialists.	
	Written home feeding plan received		
	Recipe for breast milk/formula received		
	Car seat screen result received*	*If not passed, arrange for car bed.	
Going Home	Pediatrician visit date: __ / __ / __ Time: __ : __	Visiting nurse date: __ / __ / __	
	Early intervention arranged with _____		
	Specialists: _____ Name: _____ Date: __ / __ Time: __ : __ Name: _____ Date: __ / __ Time: __ : __		
	Med: _____ Dose/frequency: _____ Med: _____ Dose/frequency: _____ Med: _____ Dose/frequency: _____	☐ Medications/syringes obtained ☐ Medication teaching complete	
	Received immunization booklet (blue book)		
	Parents Completed Discharged Readiness Questionnaire		

Table 18.2. Sample family discharge checklist.

Nurse Discharge Planning Worksheet

Baby's name in hospital: _____ Medical record #: _____

Baby's name after discharge: _____

During discharge meeting	Date	Completed by (RN Initials)	Not Required	Family Declined	Comments
Discharge meeting held				☐	
Family given discharge packet					
Family obtained a car seat					
Family offered CPR class				☐	
Family received "shaken baby" brochure					
Pediatrician chosen					
No later than 1 week prior to anticipated discharge					
Early intervention (EI) arranged			☐	☐	
Visiting nurse (VNA) arranged Agency: _____ Phone: _____ Fax: _____ Anticipated visit date: __ / __ / __			☐	☐	
Infant data sent to infant follow-up program (IFUP)			☐	☐	
Ophthalmology follow-up Dr. _____ Date/time: _____ Phone: _____			☐	☐	
Other follow-up appointments Specialty: _____ Dr. _____ Date/time: _____ Phone: _____			☐		Other: ___
Specialty: _____ Dr. _____ Date/time: _____ Phone: _____			☐		
Specialty: _____ Dr. _____ Date/time _____ Phone: _____			☐		
Palivizumab (Respiratory syncytial virus [RSV] season only) Patient meets requirements? Yes ☐ No ☐					
Palivizumab parent information sheet given			☐	☐	
Palivizumab parent consent obtained			☐	☐	
Palivizumab injection given			☐	☐	
Hepatitis B vaccine Hepatitis B vaccine information statement given					

Table 18.3. Sample nurse discharge planning worksheet. (Courtesy of Dr. Vincent Smith, Beth Israel Deaconess Medical Center.)

			Not Required	Family Declined	
Hepatitis B vaccine consent obtained			☐	☐	
Hepatitis B vaccine given			☐	☐	

No later than 1 week prior to anticipated discharge	Date	Completed by (RN Initials)	Not Required	Family Declined	Comments
Discharge Teaching Feeding/nutrition reviewed				☐	
Bowel and bladder patterns reviewed				☐	
Bulb syringe use reviewed				☐	
Bathing, skin care, cord care reviewed				☐	
Temperature taking reviewed				☐	
Circumcision care			☐	☐	
Protection from infection reviewed				☐	
Feeding Infant transitioned to discharge feeding: (BM/formula: _____ kcal/oz: _____)			☐		
Family received written feeding plan			☐		
Family received milk/formula recipe			☐		
Appropriate WIC forms given to family			☐	☐	
Medication/Medical Equipment Family received discharge prescriptions			☐		
Medication administration teaching completed Med: _____ Dose/frequency: _____			☐		
Med: _____ Dose/frequency: _____					
Med: _____ Dose/frequency: _____					
Requires home equipment? Yes ☐ No ☐					
If equipment required; case management contacted					

Equipment (e.g., O$_2$ monitor)	**Company Contact Information**				Date Teaching Completed

No later than 1–2 days prior to anticipated discharge	Date	Completed by (RN Initials)	Not Required	Family Declined	Comments
Pediatrician appointment scheduled Dr. _____ Date/time: _____ Phone: _____					
Family given immunization book				☐	

Table 18.3. *(Continued)*

Family learned how to administer home medications			☐	☐	
Hearing screening complete Passed ☐ Referred L ☐ R ☐					
Car seat form complete			☐		
Discharge newborn screen sent					
Family attended CPR class				☐	
Family offered CPR refresher video				☐	
When to call your baby's doctor reviewed			☐	☐	
Car seat instruction reviewed			☐	☐	
Attending completed discharge summary					If not, reason:
Family received a copy of discharge summary					If not, reason:
Completed Nurse Discharge Readiness Questionnaire					

RNs, please provide quality improvement feedback/comments on this form and discharge process:

Table 18.3. *(Continued)*

Table 18.4. Sample Neonatal Intensive Care Unit (NICU) Discharge/Interim Summary Dictation Guideline/Discharge Summary Content

1. Name of attending
2. Service ("Neonatology")
3. Patient's name as it appears in the hospital records
4. Patient's medical record number
5. Date of birth
6. Sex of patient
7. Date of admission
8. Date of discharge
9. History
a. The patient's postdischarge name (*spell name*)
b. Reason for admission, birth weight, and gestational age
c. Maternal history including prenatal labs, pregnancy, labor, and birth history
10. Physical examination at discharge including weight, head circumference, and length with percentiles at birth and discharge
11. Summary of hospital course by systems (*concise*). Include pertinent lab results:
■ *Respiratory:* initial impression. Surfactant given? Maximum level of support. Days on ventilation, CPAP, supplemental oxygen. If apnea, report how patient was treated, when treatment ended, and condition resolved.
■ *Cardiovascular:* diagnoses/therapies in summary form. Echo/ECG results
■ *Fluids, electrolytes, nutrition:* Brief feeding history. Include most recent weight, length, and head circumference.
■ *GI:* maximum bilirubin and therapy used
■ *Hematology:* patient's blood type, brief transfusion summary, most recent Hct
■ *Infectious disease:* white blood counts, cultures, colonization if appropriate, antibiotic courses
■ *Neurology:* Describe findings on head imaging.
■ *Psychosocial:* relevant observations of family function and psychosocial needs
(continued)

Table 18.4. Sample Neonatal Intensive Care Unit (NICU) Discharge/Interim Summary Dictation Guideline/Discharge Summary Content *(Continued)*

- *Sensory*

    i. *Audiology:* "Hearing screening results." (*If didn't pass, indicate date/place of follow-up test. If not done, recommend test prior to discharge.*)

    ii. *Ophthalmology*

    - Indicate if infant did not meet criteria for eye exam.

    - Indicate if infant has not yet been examined but does require exam.

    - If ROP was ever detected, include maximum stage of ROP and date of that exam.

    - For all, include date and results of last exam.

    - If not mature, state plans for follow-up including date and time of scheduled appointment.

    - If mature, state time frame for routine follow-up.

12. Condition at discharge (e.g., "stable") including prognosis if guarded.

13. Discharge disposition (e.g., "home," "level 2," "level 3," "chronic care")

14. Name of primary pediatrician.   Phone #:   Fax #:

15. Care/recommendations

    a. Feeds at discharge including volume, caloric density, and frequency

    b. Medications including each medication's dose (concentration if volume), route, frequency

    c. Medical equipment and supply needs

    d. Car seat challenge *if indicated*

    e. State newborn screening status including dates and known results

    f. Immunizations received including dates

    g. Follow-up appointments scheduled/recommended

16. Discharge diagnoses list

CPAP, continuous positive airway pressure; Echo, echocardiogram; ECG, electrocardiogram; GI, gastrointestinal; Hct, hematocrit; ROP, retinopathy of prematurity.

Table 18.5. Additional Discharge Instruction Sheet

Community Resources

- **Poison Control Center**..(800) 222-1222
- **Parental Stress Line** ....(800) 632-8188
- **Battered Women's Hotline (24-hour)**...................................(800) 799-SAFE
- **Alcohol and Addictions Resource Center** ....(574) 234-6024
- **Alcohol and Drug Addiction Resource Center**....................(877) 322-6766
- **Mother of Twins Association** ....(248) 231-4480

Breastfeeding

- **La Leche League**..(877) 4-LaLeche

Guidelines for When Parents Should Call Their Infant's Doctor

Any sudden changes in infant's usual patterns of behavior:

- Increased sleepiness
- Increased irritability
- Poor feeding

Any of the following:

- Breathing difficulty
- Blueness around lips, mouth, or eyes
- Fever (by rectal temperature) over 100.0°F or (under the arm) over 99.6°F or low temperature (rectal) under 97.0°F
- Vomiting or diarrhea
- Dry diaper for >12 hours
- No bowel movement for >4 days
- Black or bright red color in stool

Suggested Readings

American Academy of Pediatrics Committee on Fetus and Newborn. Hospital discharge of the high-risk neonate. *Pediatrics* 2008;122(5):1119–1126.

Broedsgaard A, Wagner L. How to facilitate parents and their premature infant for the transition home. *Int Nurs Rev* 2005;52:196–203.

Bruder MB, Cole M. Critical elements of transition from NICU to home and follow-up. *Child Health Care* 1991;20:40–49.

Griffin JB, Pickler RH. Hospital-to-home transition of mothers of preterm infants. *MCN Am J Matern Child Nurs* 2011;36:252–257.

Griffin T. Family-centered care in the NICU. *J Perinat Neonatal Nurs* 2006;20: 98–102.

Maroney D. Evidence-based practice within discharge teaching of the premature infant 2005. http://www.premature-infant.com/evidencebased.pdf. Accessed December 15, 2011.

Moore KA, Coker K, DuBuisson AB, et al. Implementing potentially better practices for improving family-centered care in neonatal intensive care units: successes and challenges. *Pediatrics* 2003;111:e450–e460.

Smith VC, Dukhovny D, Zupancic JA, et al. Neonatal intensive care unit discharge preparedness: primary care implications. *Clin Pediatr (Phila)* 2012;51(5):454–461.

Smith VC, Hwang SS, Dukhovny D, et al. Neonatal intensive care unit discharge preparation, family readiness and infant outcomes: connecting the dots. *J Perinatol* 2013;33(6):415–421.

Smith VC, Young S, Pursley DM, et al. Are families prepared for discharge from the NICU? *J Perinatol* 2009;29:623–629.

Sneath N. Discharge teaching in the NICU: are parents prepared? An integrative review of parents' perceptions. *Neonatal Netw* 2009;28:237–246.

Weiss ME, Lokken L. Predictors and outcomes of postpartum mothers' perceptions of readiness for discharge after birth. *J Obstet Gynecol Neonatal Nurs* 2009;38:406–417.

19 Decision-Making and Ethical Dilemmas

Frank X. Placencia and Christy L. Cummings

KEY POINTS

- Parents are generally accorded the right to make decisions on behalf of their child, in their best interests, as surrogate decision makers (parental authority and responsibility).
- Shared decision making should involve the medical team and family and should incorporate the most current medical evidence along with parental values and perspectives.
- Parental authority may be challenged when parental medical decisions clearly oppose their child's best interests.
- Withholding and withdrawing life-sustaining interventions are morally equivalent and ethically acceptable in certain situations in the neonatal intensive care unit (NICU), although in practice, withdrawing may sometimes feel more difficult for families and staff.
- Ethics committee consultation may be an invaluable resource and should be sought in ethically challenging cases.

I. BACKGROUND. The practice of neonatology necessitates decision making in all aspects of care. Most neonatologists feel comfortable making routine clinical decisions regarding management of pulmonary or cardiac function, infection, nutrition, and neurodevelopment care. On the other hand, clinical situations with ethical implications are often more difficult for professionals and families. These include decisions regarding instituting, withholding, or withdrawing life-sustaining therapy in patients with irreversible or terminal conditions such as extreme immaturity, severe hypoxic-ischemic encephalopathy, certain congenital anomalies, or other conditions that are refractory to the best available treatments.

A. The **ethical principles** that must be considered in the decision-making process in the neonatal intensive unit (NICU) care include beneficence, non-maleficence, respect for autonomy, justice, and other principles and ethical frameworks associated with the physician–patient relationship, such as narrative ethics, feminist ethics, or care ethics.[1,2] Other principles that must be considered include the following:

1. Treatment decisions must be based on the infant's best interests, free from considerations of race, ethnicity, ability to pay, or other influences. The American Academy of Pediatrics (AAP), the judicial system, and

various bioethicists have all embraced some form of this standard, although their interpretations have differed.

2. The infant's parents generally serve as the legal and moral fiduciaries (or advocates) for their child. The relationship of parents to children is that of responsibility, not rights. Because infants are incapable of making decisions for themselves, the parents become their surrogate decision makers. Therefore, the parents are owed respect for autonomy in making decisions for their infants as long as their decisions do not conflict with the best interests of their child.

3. The physician serves as a fiduciary who acts in the best interest of the patient using the most current evidence-based medical information. In this role as infant advocate, the physician oversees the responses (decisions) of his or her patient's parents. It is the responsibility of the physician to involve the court system when he or she perceives that the infant's interests are inappropriately threatened by the parents' decision.

B. There is considerable debate on how to define the "best interests" of the infant. The most controversial issue is whether the primary focus should be the preservation of life (the vitalist approach) or the maintenance of a particular quality of life (the nonvitalist approach). This debate enters into difficult decisions more frequently as it becomes technically possible to sustain smaller and sicker infants. Staff and parents often struggle with identifying the medical and moral choices and with making decisions based on those choices. These choices, including the understanding of what defines a fulfilling or adequate quality of life, vary substantially among families and professionals.

C. Informed consent versus parental permission. The 1995 AAP Committee on Bioethics policy statement "Informed Consent, Parental Permission, and Assent in Pediatric Practice" embraced the concept of parental permission. Parental permission, such as informed consent, requires that parents be informed of the various treatment options, as well as their risks and benefits, and allows them to make decisions in cooperation with the physician. It differs from informed consent in that it is derived from the obligation shared by the parents and physicians to make decisions in the best interest of the infant, thereby enabling the physician to proceed with a treatment plan without parental permission (or even against parental wishes) if doing so is clearly in the best interests of the infant.

II. DEVELOPING A PROCESS FOR ETHICAL DECISION MAKING. An ethically sound, well-defined, and rigorous process for making decisions in ethically challenging cases is key to avoiding unwanted outcomes or intervention by a state agency or court. A NICU should define the decision-making process and identify the individuals (primary medical team, nursing staff, subspecialists, social services, ethicists, hospital legal counsel) that may need to participate in that process. Developing this process in advance allows for healthy discussions among NICU personnel that incorporate ethical knowledge and values at a time and place separate from a specific patient. Ideally, this preparation will ease the stress when an actual decision needs to be made.

A. **Develop an educational program to prepare NICU caregivers to** address difficult decisions regarding patient care. Focus on process (who, when, where) as well as on substance (how). Identifying areas of frequent consensus and disagreement within a NICU and outlining a general approach to those situations can provide helpful guidance. The educational program should be available for NICU staff and discussed during the orientation of new personnel. The hospital ethics committee can serve as an educational resource for personnel regarding how to approach ethical decision making.

B. **Identify common ethical situations** (e.g., extreme prematurity, multiple congenital anomalies, severe asphyxia) that might produce conflict and have a series of multidisciplinary discussions about these models as part of an educational program. These conversations should include a review of updated evidence and the common underlying ethical principles likely to be in conflict and illuminate common areas of agreement or disagreement. These discussions help develop a consensus on group values, promote a tolerance for individual differences, and establish trust and respect among professionals. The overall goal is to better prepare caregivers when actual situations arise, while recognizing that each situation will be unique.

C. **Define and support the role of the parents** who should be seen as the primary decision makers for their infant unless they have indicated otherwise. The parents' desired decision making should be explored with them in open and honest discussions. The ethical and legal presumption is that they will make decisions that are in the best interests of their child (best interests standard) and within the context of accepted legal and social boundaries. If the health care providers believe that the parental choice is not in the child's best interest, then they have an obligation as the infant advocate to override the parental decision. Although every effort must be made to align the views of the parents and medical team, in cases of continued disagreement regarding the treatment course most likely to serve the best interests of the infant, the hospital ethics committee, hospital legal counsel, and social services should be consulted and the court system may need to be involved. In this situation, the physician should continue to serve as the infant's advocate, while also maintaining open communication with the parents.

D. **Develop consensus among the primary clinical team** and consultants prior to meeting with the parents. Team meetings prior to family meetings provide the opportunity for caregivers to clarify the dilemmas and options that will be offered to the family and, hopefully, to reach a consensus regarding recommendations. It also allows the team to establish who will communicate with the family to help maintain consistency during the discussion of complicated medical and ethical issues.

In large practices, a diverse array of opinions is common. Establishing a forum in which the primary team may solicit the opinions of other staff members on the medical and ethical questions specific to the case serves multiple purposes: (i) identification of alternative treatment options, (ii) identification of staff members (physicians, nurses, etc.) comfortable with pursuing a course of action that current members may not be, and (iii) creation of consensus within the group on a specific course of action that can be presented to the hospital ethics committee if need be.

E. **Identify available resources.** Determine the roles of social service, chaplain, hospital attorney, and the hospital ethics committee. Individuals with a general knowledge of existing hospital policies on common situations such as "do not attempt resuscitation" orders or withdrawal of life support should be included in the multidisciplinary discussion above. One or two key resource people with additional expertise who are easily accessible should also be identified. These professionals should be familiar with hospital policies, the ethics codes of the hospital as well as those of national organizations such as the AAP or the American Medical Association, and applicable federal and state laws. These key resource people are often members of the hospital ethics committee who can be available without necessarily pursuing a formal ethics consult.

F. **Base decisions on the most accurate, up-to-date medical information.** Good ethics begins with good facts. Take the time to accumulate the relevant data. Consultation services are likely to provide valuable input. Be consistent in asking the same appropriate questions in each clinical setting. The answers to these questions may vary from case to case, but the questions regarding the ethical principles must always be asked. Be wary of setting certainty as a goal because it is almost never achievable in the NICU. Instead, a reasonable degree of medical certainty is often more achievable. As the weight of a decision's consequences increases, so does the rigor of the requirement for a reasonable degree of certainty and the importance of parental involvement in the decision-making process.

G. **People of good conscience can disagree.** Individual caregivers must feel free to remove themselves from patient care if their ethical sense conflicts with the decision of the primary team and parents. This conflict should be handled with the medical or nursing director of the NICU. Parents and caregivers must be able to appeal decisions to an individual such as the NICU medical director or to the hospital's ethics committee. No system will provide absolute certainty that the "right" decision will always be made. However, a system that is inclusive, systematic, and built on an approach that establishes a procedure for handling these difficult issues is most likely to produce acceptable decisions.

III. **EXTREMELY PREMATURE INFANTS.** Nearly all NICUs have struggled with decisions about infants born at the threshold of viability and the question of "how small is too small." The practice of resuscitating extremely preterm infants presents difficult medical and ethical challenges. Current technology allows some of these infants to survive but with a great risk of substantial neurodevelopmental impairment. Parents may ask that neonatologists pursue aggressive therapies despite poor prognoses. Neonatologists are concerned that instituting those therapies may not be the most appropriate course of action. The AAP statement on perinatal care at the threshold of viability stresses several key areas: (i) Parents must receive adequate and current information about potential infant survival and short- and long-term outcomes, (ii) physicians are obligated to be aware of the most current national and local survival data, and (iii) parental choice should be respected as much as possible with joint decision making by both the parents and the physicians as the standard. As more experience is gained with these very difficult situations, further debate and discussion are likely to lead to greater consensus in this area. Guidelines for resuscitation by gestational age or birth weight are intentionally vague because these are only a few of the factors involved in predicting outcome. In making these decisions and recommendations, clinicians should take into account the specifics of each pregnancy as well as the local outcomes data (see National Institute of Child Health and Human Development perinatal outcome calculator: http://www.nichd.nih.gov/about/org/cdbpm/pp/prog_epbo/epbo_case.cfm).

IV. **THE DECISION TO REDIRECT LIFE-SUSTAINING TREATMENT TO COMFORT MEASURES.** One of the most difficult issues is deciding when to withhold or withdraw life-sustaining therapies. Philosophies and approaches vary among caregivers and NICUs. The AAP statement on noninitiation or withdrawal of intensive care for high-risk newborns stresses several key areas: (i) Decisions about noninitiation or withdrawal of intensive care should be made by the health care team in collaboration with the parents, who must be well informed about the condition and prognosis of their infant; (ii) parents should be active participants in the decision-making process; (iii) compassionate comfort care should be provided to all infants, including those for whom intensive care is not provided; and (iv) it is appropriate to provide intensive care when it is thought to be of benefit to the infant and not when it is thought to be harmful, of no benefit, or futile.

One model to consider emphasizes an objective, interdisciplinary approach to determine the best course of action.

A. The goal of the process is to identify the action that is in the **baby's best interest**. The interests of others, including family and caregivers, are of less priority than are the baby's but should also be considered.

B. **Shared decision making should be guided by data.** Caregivers should explore every reasonable avenue to maximize collection of data relevant to the ethical question at hand. Information about alternative therapies and prognosis should be sought. The objective data are evaluated in the context of the primary team's meetings. Subspecialty consultations should be obtained when indicated and included in the primary team's deliberations. Often, these consultations may add extra input to assist in the questions that the primary team is trying to address. It is important that these consultants' input be reviewed with the primary team before discussing such findings with the parents.

C. **Shared decision making should be guided by parental values and goals.** As the decision to withhold or withdraw life-sustaining medical treatment becomes the focus, the team discusses the best data available, their implications, and their degree of certainty. The goal should be to build a **consensus** regarding the best plan of care for the baby and/or recommendations for the parents. Sometimes, there will be strong scientific support for a particular option. In other instances, the best course of action must be estimated. During this time, it is especially important to actively seek feedback from the parents regarding their thoughts, feelings, and understanding of the clinical situation. It should be emphasized that different caregivers reach the consensus at different rates and times. Supporting each participant through this process is important until all understand and accept the consensus and can then readily agree on a decision.

D. **The parents' role as surrogate decision makers should be respected.** This starts with communication that is completely transparent. The primary care team should meet regularly with the parents to discuss the baby's progress, current status, plan of care, and to summarize the team's medical and ethical discussions. Parental views are always considered; they are most likely to influence decisions when it remains unclear which option (e.g., continuing vs. discontinuing life-sustaining treatment) is in the child's best interest. Parents are not expected to evaluate clinical data in isolation. Even in instances of medical uncertainty, the primary team objectively assesses what is known, as well as what remains uncertain about the infant's condition and/or prognosis, in conjunction with parental values and wishes. The team should also provide the parents with their best assessment and recommendation. In the face of true medical uncertainty, parental wishes should be supported in deference to those of the primary medical team.

E. There is agreement among ethical and legal scholars that no ethical distinction exists between **withholding and withdrawing life-sustaining treatments**. Therefore, a therapeutic trial of life-sustaining treatment is acceptable, and parents and staff should not feel remorse in withdrawing those treatments if they no longer, or never did, improve the infant's condition and therefore serve his or her best interests. In practice, this may be more difficult emotionally and psychologically for families and even staff. However, not using the approach of starting and then stopping therapy that is nonbeneficial may result in one of two adverse outcomes: (i) Nonbeneficial, possibly even harmful, treatment may be continued longer than necessary and (ii) some infants who might benefit from treatment may be excluded if it is feared that treatment would needlessly prolong the lives of a greater number of infants whose condition would not respond. The president's Commission on Medical Ethics argues that withdrawal of life-sustaining treatment after having shown no efficacy, may be more justifiable than presuming futility and thus withholding treatment. This approach supports the concept of a "trial of intensive care" wherein the staff and family agree to start life-sustaining treatment and to discontinue it if it becomes clear that continued treatment is no longer in the infant's best interest.

The 1984 Amendment to the Child Abuse and Neglect Prevention and Treatment Act (CAPTA) defines treatment as NOT medically indicated if the infant is irreversibly comatose; if it would merely prolong dying, not be effective in ameliorating or correcting all of the life-threatening conditions; if it would be futile in terms of survival; or if it would be virtually futile in terms of survival and be inhumane. These conditions both protect the rights of children to treatment despite underlying conditions or potential disabilities and support the importance of quality of life determinations in the provision of care. Substantial conflict can arise if the caregivers and parents disagree about the goals of care. A NICU must be prepared for these circumstances.

F. The **hospital ethics committee** is helpful when the primary team is unable to reach consensus or disagrees with the parents' wishes when they are clearly harmful and/or opposed to the child's best interests. Consultation with the ethics committee helps encourage communication among all involved parties and improve collaborative decision making. They can often ease tensions between parents and caregivers, allowing for a resolution to the dilemma.

Suggested Readings

Amendments to Child Abuse Prevention and Treatment Act (CAPTA), 42 USC §5101 (1984).

American Academy of Pediatrics. Informed consent, parental permission, and assent in pediatric practice. *Pediatrics* 1995;95:314–317.

Batton DG. Clinical report—antenatal counseling regarding resuscitation at an extremely low gestational age. *Pediatrics* 2009;124:422–427.

Bell EF. Noninitiation or withdrawal of intensive care for high-risk newborns. *Pediatrics* 2007;119:401–403.

Goldworth A, Silverman W, Stevenson DK, et al. *Ethics and Perinatology.* New York, NY: Oxford University Press; 1995.

Mercurio MR. The ethics of newborn resuscitation. *Semin Perinatol* 2009;33(6): 354–363.

Mercurio MR. The role of a pediatric ethics committee in the newborn intensive care unit. *J Perinatol* 2011;31(1):1–9.

President's Commission for the Study of Ethical Problems in Medicine and Biomedical and Behavioral Research. *Deciding to Forego Life-Sustaining Treatment: A Report on the Ethical, Medical, and Legal Issues in Treatment Decisions.* Washington, DC: U.S. Government Publishing Office; 1983.

References

1. American College of Obstetrics and Gynecology. ACOG Committee Opinion No. 390, December 2007. Ethical decision making in obstetrics and gynecology. *Obstet Gynecol* 2007;110(6):1479–1487.

2. Cummings C, Mercurio M. Maternal–fetal conflicts. In: Diekema DS, Mercurio MR, Adam MB, eds. *Clinical Ethics in Pediatrics: A Case-Based Textbook.* Cambridge, United Kingdom: Cambridge University Press; 2011:51–56.

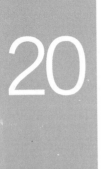

20 Management of Neonatal End-of-Life Care and Bereavement Follow-up

Caryn E. Douma and Patrick Jones

KEY POINTS

- Neonatal deaths are more common than in any other time in childhood; most follow a decision to withdraw life-sustaining treatment.
- High-quality end-of-life and bereavement care is the natural extension of a family-centered approach in the neonatal intensive care unit (NICU).
- Combining available guidelines with family preferences ensures sensitive and appropriate end-of-life and bereavement care.

I. INTRODUCTION. Providing compassionate, family-centered, end-of-life care in the neonatal intensive care unit (NICU) environment is challenging for caregivers. The care team must balance the medical needs of the infant with those of the parents and family. Parents are profoundly affected by the compassion and treatment they receive from health care providers during end-of-life care. Although the death of a baby is a devastating event, the knowledge and skill of the multidisciplinary team can greatly influence the ability of the parents to effectively cope with their loss.

Despite advances in neonatal care, more children die in the perinatal and neonatal period than in any other time in childhood. The majority of neonatal deaths in the United States are due to congenital malformations and disorders related to short gestation and low birth weight.

For many families, a lethal or life-limiting condition may be diagnosed early in the pregnancy; thus, the opportunity to begin the decision-making process occurs prior to admission to the NICU. Perinatal hospice is an alternative to termination of the pregnancy and provides a structured approach for the parents and the care team when developing a plan to create the best possible outcome for the baby and family.

II. FAMILY-CENTERED END-OF-LIFE CARE PRINCIPLES AND DOMAINS. The provision of quality end-of-life care is a process that allows for clear and consistent communication delivered by a compassionate multidisciplinary team within a framework of shared decision making. Providing physical and emotional support and follow-up care enables the parents to begin the healing process as they return home.

End-of-life domains comprise family-centered care in the intensive care unit. These domains provide guidance and process measures to assess and provide quality of care at the end of life.

A. Patient- and family-centered decision making

B. Communication among the multidisciplinary team members and between the team and the parents and families

C. Spiritual support of families

D. Emotional and practical support of families

E. Symptom management and comfort care

F. Continuity of care

G. Emotional and organizational support for health care workers

III. COORDINATION OF CARE

A. **Communication and collaboration.** Family support in the NICU relies heavily on communication between the family and the health care team and the relationship among the members of the care team. A collaborative care model that allows physicians, nurses, and other team members to work co-operatively and share decisions, while respecting each professional's unique contribution, promotes an environment where the best care can be delivered.

1. Care provided at the end of life is an extension of the relationship already in place between the care providers and the infant and family. Staff can facilitate this relationship in the following ways:

   a. Communicate with families through frequent meetings with the primary team.

   b. Include the obstetrical care team and other consultants when appropriate.

   c. Encourage sibling visitation and extended family support.

   d. Encourage incorporation of cultural and spiritual customs.

   e. Provide an environment that allows parents to develop a relationship with their infant, visiting and holding as often as medically appropriate.

2. Parents want to be given information in a clear, concise manner and value honesty and transparency.

3. Clear recommendations about the goals of care (life support vs. comfort care) from the health care team are appropriate and may relieve parents of the some of the burden of decision making in the end-of-life context.

4. Most neonatal deaths occur following a decision to remove life-sustaining treatment.

5. Prior to meeting with the family to discuss redirection of care from treatment to comfort, it is important for the multidisciplinary team to agree on goals of care and identify the needs of the patient and family.

6. Address conflicts within the team early in the process, utilizing available professional supports, such as ethical or spiritual consultants.

7. It is essential for the team to reach agreement prior to meeting with the family.

8. One spokesperson (usually the attending physician) is recommended to maintain continuity of communication.

B. Patient- and family-centered decision making

1. Most parents want to be involved in the decision to transition care from treatment to comfort, yet not all are able to participate or want to feel responsible for the final decision. They rely on the care team to interpret the information and deliver the choices in a compassionate, sensitive manner that incorporates their individual needs and desired level of involvement.

2. The parents need to feel supported regardless of the decision that is made.

3. The quality of the relationship and the communication style of the team members can influence the ability of the parents to understand the information presented and to reach consensus with the heath care team.

4. Shared decision making involves the support and participation of the entire team.

5. Meet with the family in a private, quiet area and allow ample time for the family to understand the information presented and the recommendations of the team.
a. Provide a medical translator if needed.
b. Refer to the baby by name.
c. Ask the parents how they feel and how they perceive the situation.
d. Once the decision has been made to redirect care away from supporting life to comfort measures, develop a specific plan with the family that involves a description of how life-sustaining support will be withdrawn and determine their desired level of participation.

C. Withdrawing life-sustaining treatment

1. Once a decision has been made to withdraw life-sustaining treatment and provide comfort care, the family should be provided an environment that is quiet, private, and will accommodate everyone the family wishes to include.

2. Staffing should be arranged so that one nurse and one physician will be readily available to the family at all times.

3. Allow parents ample time to create memories and become a family. Allow them to hold, photograph, bathe, and dress their infant before, during, or after withdrawing mechanical ventilation or other life support.

4. Discuss the entire process with parents, including endotracheal tube removal and pain control. Gently describe how the infant will look and measures that the staff will take to provide the infant with a comfortable, pain-free death. Let them know that death will not always occur immediately.

5. Arrange for baptism and spiritual support if desired; incorporate spiritual and cultural customs into the plan of care if desired.

6. The goal of comfort care is to provide a pain-free comfortable death. Anticipate medications that may be required, leaving intravenous access in place. Discontinue muscle relaxation before extubation. The goal of medication use should be to ensure that the infant is as comfortable as possible.

7. When the infant is extubated, discontinue all unnecessary intravenous catheters and equipment.

8. Allow parents to hold their infant for as long as they desire after withdrawing life support. The nurse and attending physician should be nearby to assist the family and assess heart rate and comfort of the infant.

9. When the family has a surviving multiple, it is important that the care team acknowledge the difficulty that this will present both at the time of death and during the grieving process.

10. Autopsy should be discussed before or after death at the discretion of the attending physician.

11. Create a memory box including crib cards, photographs, clothing, a lock of hair, footprints, handprints, and any other mementos accumulated during the infant's life. Keep them in a designated place if the family does not desire to see or keep them at the time of death. Parents often change their minds later and are grateful that these items have been retained.

12. Be sure that photographs of the infant have been taken. Parents of multiples will often want a photograph of their children together or a family picture. It is helpful for the NICU to have a digital camera and printer available. Now I Lay Me Down To Sleep (NILMDTS) is an organization that utilizes volunteer professional photographers and is available in many communities.

D. Emotional and organizational support for staff

1. A debriefing meeting for all members of the health care team after a baby's death provides an opportunity for those involved with the death to share their thoughts and emotions, if desired. Chaplains and social workers are often good resources for staff support and are usually considered a part of the care team.

2. Reviewing the events surrounding the death helps to identify what went well and opportunities for improvement.

3. Institutional support may include paid funeral leave, counseling, and remembrance ceremonies.

4. Recognizing and addressing staff response to grief in the workplace is a necessary part of providing end-of-life care.

5. Many institutions have developed formal programs to support staff working with dying patients. Programs often include support groups, counseling, writing workshops, and other interventions. Creating rituals around the time of death and providing time to reflect before returning to care for patients can be helpful.

IV. BEREAVEMENT FOLLOW-UP

A. **General principles.** Bereavement follow-up provides continuing support to families as they return home to continue the grieving process. Some families may not wish any contact with the team after they return home, and others may desire more frequent meetings or calls. Prior to leaving the hospital, it is important for a member of the team to review the follow-up support that will be provided. A bereavement packet with literature and a summary of hospital-specific programs is useful to provide the family with grief resources and contact information. Most programs include follow-up calls and cards within the first week and again between 4 and 6 weeks after the death of the infant. A follow-up meeting with the team allows the family the opportunity to review the events that surrounded the death, including the autopsy results if appropriate. In addition to providing support to the family, the meeting allows the team to assess the need for further support and provide referrals that might include support groups or counseling.

B. **Hospital care**

1. A designated team member or bereavement coordinator should review the program and bereavement materials with the parents or a family member. Often, a family support person is best able to absorb this information and communicate to the parents at the appropriate time.

2. Briefly describe the normal grieving process and what to expect in the following days and weeks.

3. Lactation support should be offered if appropriate and a plan made for lactation suppression and follow-up.

4. Provide assistance in making burial or cremation arrangements.

5. The family's obstetrician, pediatrician, and other community supports should be notified of the infant's death.

6. A representative from the primary team or appropriately trained designee should assume responsibility for coordinating bereavement follow-up. This person will be responsible for arranging and documenting the follow-up process.

7. Provide assistance to the family as they leave the hospital without their child. If possible, arrange for prepaid valet parking or an escort to the door.

C. **Follow-up after discharge**

1. Contact the family within the first week to provide an opportunity for questions and offer support. The designated follow-up coordinator usually takes responsibility for placing the call and documentation. Other members of the care team may wish to maintain contact if they developed a close relationship with the family. It is important to discuss specific follow-up details with the family prior to discharge home.

2. Parents appreciate receiving a sympathy card, signed by members of the primary team sent to their home within the first few weeks, and communication at selected intervals.

3. Schedule a follow-up meeting with the family approximately 4 to 6 weeks after the infant's death. Timing will depend on availability of autopsy results and parental preference. In some cases, the family will

not want to return to the hospital or continue contact. The coordinator will be sure this is documented and arrange for the family to be followed through a primary care provider or other community agency. Follow-up calls can still be made if the family consents.

4. Meetings should include a review of events surrounding the infant's death, results of the autopsy or other studies, and implications for future pregnancies.

5. Assessment should be made to determine the coping ability of the family as they continue with the grieving process and referrals made to appropriate professionals or agencies including bereavement support groups if needed.

6. Send a card and initiate a phone call around the 1-year anniversary of the infant's death. This can be a difficult time for the family. Many families develop their own rituals to celebrate the life of their child during this time. Contact from members of their care team is greatly appreciated.

7. Plan for future meetings if the family desires.

Suggested Readings

Balaguer A, Martín-Ancel A, Ortigoza-Escobar D, et al. The model of palliative care in the perinatal setting: a review of the literature. *BMC Pediatr* 2012;12:25. doi:10.1186/1471-2431-12-25.

Koopmans L, Wilson T, Cacciatore J, et al. Support for mothers, fathers and families after perinatal death. *Cochrane Database Syst Rev* 2013;(6):CD000452. doi:10.1002/14651858.CD000452.pub3.

Online Resources/Websites

British Association of Perinatal Medicine Working Group Report. Palliative care (supportive and end of life care): a framework for clinical practice in perinatal medicine. http://nebula.wsimg.com/c84cb7310f1d226b1072c40c0c77 54ac?AccessKeyId=BE16207C1CC3A18A9A3A&disposition=0&allow origin=1. Accessed August 1, 2015.

Gundersen Health System. Resolve through Sharing: bereavement services home. http://www.gundersenhealth.org/resolve-through-sharing. Accessed August 1, 2015.

Texas Pediatric Society. Palliative care toolkit. https://txpeds.org/palliative-care-toolkit. Accessed August 1, 2015.

21

Nutrition

Diane M. Anderson, Brenda B. Poindexter, and
Camilia R. Martin

KEY POINTS
- Human milk is the best nutrition for term and premature infants.
- Early nutrition influences childhood growth and neurodevelopment.
- Growth assessment is essential to ensure optimal nutrition.

Following birth, term infants rapidly adapt from a relatively constant intrauterine supply of nutrients to intermittent feedings of milk. Preterm infants, however, are at increased risk for nutritional compromise. These infants are born with limited nutrient accretion and reserves due to their premature delivery, immature metabolic pathways, and increased nutrient demands. In addition, medical and surgical conditions commonly associated with prematurity have the potential to alter nutrient requirements and complicate adequate nutrient delivery. As survival for these high-risk newborns continues to improve, current data suggest that early nutrition can improve both short- and long-term outcomes.

I. GROWTH

A. Fetal body composition changes throughout gestation, with accretion of most nutrients occurring primarily in the late second and throughout the third trimester. Term infants will normally have sufficient glycogen and fat stores to meet energy requirements during the relative starvation of the first days after birth. In contrast, preterm infants will rapidly deplete their limited nutrient reserves of glycogen and nitrogen, becoming both hypoglycemic and catabolic unless appropriate nutritional therapy is provided. In practice, it is generally assumed that the severity of nutrient insufficiency is inversely related to gestational age at birth and birth weight.

B. Postnatal growth varies from intrauterine growth in that it begins with a period of weight loss, primarily through the loss of extracellular fluid. The typical postnatal weight loss in the term infant is 5% to 10% of birth weight. Historically, in preterm infants, this postnatal weight loss can be as much as 15% of birth weight, with the nadir by 4 to 6 postnatal days and a regain to birth weight by 14 to 21 days. This postnatal weight loss pattern, however, can be attenuated in most preterm infants with optimized, early nutrition. Although currently, there is no widely accepted measure of neonatal growth that captures both the weight loss and subsequent gain characteristic of this period, in general, the goals in practice are to limit the degree and duration of initial weight loss in preterm infants and to facilitate regain of birth weight within 7 to 10 postnatal days.

C. After achieving birth weight, intrauterine growth and nutrient accretion rate data are used as reference standards for assessing growth and nutrient requirements for the growing preterm infant. Goals for weight gain are 15 to 20 g/kg/day for infants <2 kg and 20 to 30 g/day for larger infants. Approximately 1 cm/week in length and 1 cm/week in head circumference are used as a goal for growth in these parameters. Although these goals may not be initially attainable in some ill preterm infants, replicating growth of the fetus at the same gestational age remains an appropriate goal as recommended by the American Academy of Pediatrics (AAP). Efforts to minimize cumulative postnatal nutrient deficits begin in the first postnatal days and require a combined approach with parenteral and enteral nutrition.

D. Serial measurements of weight, head circumference, and length plotted on growth curves provide valuable information in the nutritional assessment of the preterm infant. Gender-specific growth charts are available based on intrauterine growth curves for weights, lengths, and head circumferences. The Revised Fenton growth charts[1] combine intrauterine growth with the World Health Organization (WHO) chart to construct a growth chart from 22 to 50 weeks' postmenstrual age (PMA). Preterm growth is taken from six countries, and the growth curve is smoothed from the preterm to the term WHO curve. The smoothing reflects the rapid growth demonstrated by preterm infants (Figs. 21.1A,B). The Olsen growth curves[2] are drawn from a large, contemporary, racially diverse U.S. sample (Figs. 21.2A–D). Infants can be plotted from 23 to 42 weeks' PMA on gender-specific weight, length, and head circumference curves. Postnatal growth curves and body mass index (BMI) curves are also available. Postnatal growth curves follow the same infants over time (i.e., longitudinal growth curves) and are available from a number of single-NICU studies and from the National Institute of Child Health and Human Development (NICHD) multicenter study (2000). These curves, however, show *actual*, not ideal growth. Intrauterine growth remains the gold standard for comparison.

E. When an infant is in full-term–corrected gestational age, the Centers for Disease Control and Prevention (CDC) recommends the WHO Child Growth Standards 2006 be used for monitoring of growth. Infants should be plotted by corrected age and followed for catch-up growth. The charts can be downloaded from http://www.cdc.gov/growthcharts/who_charts.htm.

II. NUTRIENT RECOMMENDATIONS

A. Sources for nutrient recommendations for preterm infants include the American Academy of Pediatrics, Committee on Nutrition (AAP-CON), the European Society for Paediatric Gastroenterology, Hepatology and Nutrition Committee on Nutrition (ESPGHAN-CON), and in the textbook *Nutritional Care of Preterm Infants: Scientific Basis and Practical Guidelines* (page 298) (Table 21.1). These recommendations are based on (i) intrauterine accretion rate data, (ii) the nutrient content of human milk, (iii) the assumed decreased nutrient stores and higher nutritional needs in preterm infants, and (iv) the available data on biochemical measures reflecting

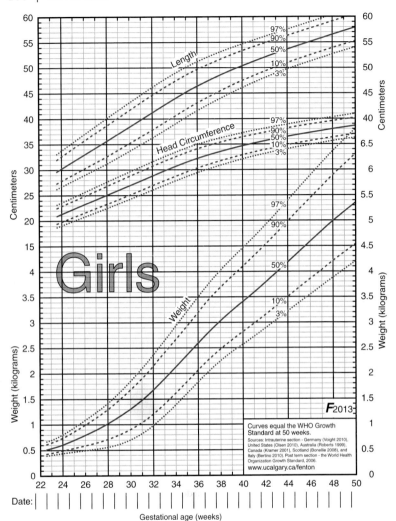

Figure 21.1. A: Fenton growth chart for girls. (From Fenton TR, Kim JH. A systematic review and meta-analysis to revise the Fenton growth chart for preterm infants. *BMC Pediatr* 2013; 13:59. http://www.ucalgary.ca/fenton. Accessed June 23, 2016.)

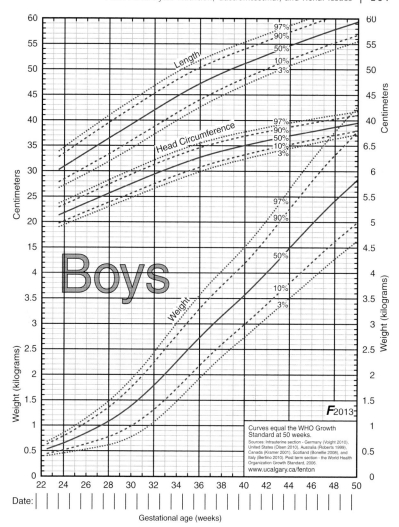

Figure 21.1. B: Fenton growth chart for boys. (From Fenton TR, Kim JH. A systematic review and meta-analysis to revise the Fenton growth chart for preterm infants. *BMC Pediatr* 2013; 13:59. http://www.ucalgary.ca/fenton. Accessed June 23, 2016.)

Intrauterine Growth Curves   Name _____

Record # _____

FEMALES

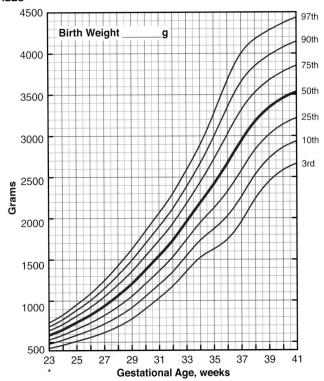

BIRTH SIZE ASSESSMENT

Date of birth: / / (wks GA)	Select one
Large-for-gestational age (LGA) >90th percentile	☐
Appropriate-for-gestational age (AGA) 10-90th percentile	☐
Small-for-gestational age (SGA) <10th percentile	☐

* 3rd and 97th percentiles on all curves for 23 weeks should be interpreted cautiously given the small sample size.

Figure 21.2. A: Olsen weight chart for girls. (Reproduced with permission from Olsen IE, Groveman S, Lawson ML, et al. New intrauterine growth curves based on United States data. *Pediatrics* 2010;125:e214–e224. http://www.nursing.upenn.edu/media/infantgrowthcurves/Documents/Olsen-NewIUGrowthCurves_2010permission.pdf. Accessed June 23, 2016. Copyright 2010 by the American Academy of Pediatrics. Data source: Pediatrix Medical Group.)

Page 2

Name _____

Record # _____

FEMALES

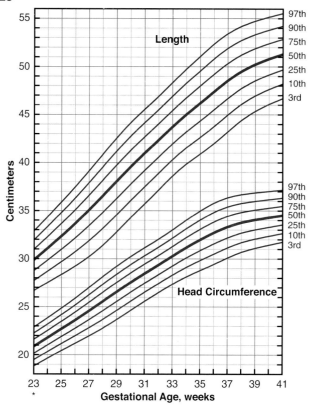

Date																
GA (wks)																
WT (g)																
L (cm)																
HC (cm)																

* 3rd and 97th percentiles on all curves for 23 weeks should be interpreted cautiously given the small sample size.

Figure 21.2. B: Olsen length and head circumference chart for girls. (Reproduced with permission from Olsen IE, Groveman S, Lawson ML, et al. New intrauterine growth curves based on United States data. *Pediatrics* 2010;125:e214–e224. http://www.nursing.upenn.edu/media/infantgrowthcurves/Documents/Olsen-NewIUGrowthCurves_2010permission.pdf. Accessed June 23, 2016. Copyright 2010 by the American Academy of Pediatrics. Data source: Pediatrix Medical Group.)

Intrauterine Growth Curves

Name _____

Record # _____

MALES

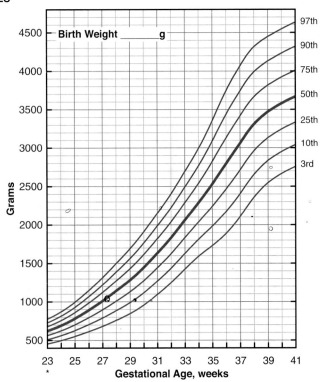

BIRTH SIZE ASSESSMENT:

Date of birth: / / (wks GA)	Select one
Large-for-gestational age (LGA) >90th percentile	☐
Appropriate-for-gestational age (AGA) 10-90th percentile	☐
Small-for-gestational age (SGA) <10th percentile	☐

* 3rd and 97th percentiles on all curves for 23 weeks should be interpreted cautiously given the small sample size.

Figure 21.2. C: Olsen weight chart for boys. (Reproduced with permission from Olsen IE, Groveman S, Lawson ML, et al. New intrauterine growth curves based on United States data. *Pediatrics* 2010;125:e214–e224. http://www.nursing.upenn.edu/media/infantgrowthcurves/Documents/Olsen-NewIUGrowthCurves_2010permission.pdf. Accessed June 23, 2016. Copyright 2010 by the American Academy of Pediatrics. Data source: Pediatrix Medical Group.)

Name _____

Record # _____

MALES

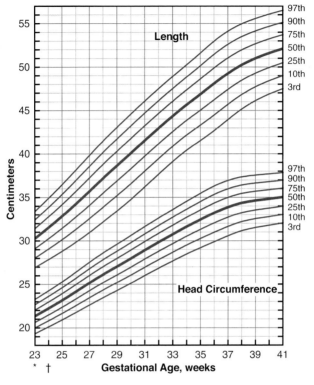

Date																		
GA (wks)																		
WT (g)																		
L (cm)																		
HC (cm)																		

* 3rd and 97th percentiles on all curves for 23 weeks should be interpreted cautiously given the small sample size.
† Male head circumference curve at 24 weeks all percentiles should be interpreted cautiously as the distribution of data is skewed left.

Figure 21.2. D: Olsen length and head circumference chart for boys. (Reproduced with permission from Olsen IE, Groveman S, Lawson ML, et al. New intrauterine growth curves based on United States data. *Pediatrics* 2010;125:e214–e224. http://www.nursing.upenn.edu/media/infantgrowthcurves/Documents/Olsen-NewIUGrowthCurves_2010permission.pdf. Accessed June 23, 2016. Copyright 2010 by the American Academy of Pediatrics. Data source: Pediatrix Medical Group.)

Table 21.1. Comparison of Enteral Intake Recommendations and Selected Feeding Regimens* for the Preterm Infant

Nutrient	Unit	Enteral Intake Recommendations for Preterm Infants†	Mature Human Milk‡	Mature Human Milk plus Four Vials Enfamil Liquid HMF/dL	Mature Human Milk plus Four Packets Similac HMF/dL	Mature Human Milk plus Prolact +6	Enfamil Premature High Protein 24 kcal/oz with Iron	Similac Special Care 24 High Protein with Iron	Gerber Good Start Premature 24 High Protein
Protein‡	g/kg/day	3.5–4.5	1.4	3.9	3.6	3.7	4.4	4.0	4.4
Carbohydrate	g/kg/day	10–14	12	11.4	13.8	12.6	13.1	12.1	11.8
Fat	g/kg/day	5–7	5.3	7.3	5.4	7.7	6.1	6.6	6.3
Docosahexaenoic acid	mg/kg/day	18–60					20.7	16.5	20
Arachidonic acid	mg/kg/day	18–45					42	26.4	40
Vitamin A	IU/kg/day	400–1,500	240	1,650	1,185	306	1,633	1,512	1,220
Vitamin D	IU/day	200–400**	2	236	176	60	363	181	220
Vitamin E	IU/kg/day	2.2–12	0.9	7.8	5.8	1.5	7.6	4.8	7.3
Vitamin K	µg/kg/day	4.4–28	0.4	7.4	12.3	0.6	10.9	14.5	9.8
Thiamine	µg/kg/day	140–300	30	255	265	30	242	302	244
Riboflavin	µg/kg/day	200–400	75	388	433	86	363	750	366
Vitamin B_6	µg/kg/day	50–300	30	200	275	30	181	302	244

Vitamin B$_{12}$	µg/kg/day	0.1–0.8	0.11	0.89	0.74	0.18	0.3	0.67	0.3
Niacin	mg/kg/day	1–5.5	0.6	5.1	5.4	0.53	4.8	6.0	4.9
Folate	µg/kg/day	25–100	16.5	52.5	48.8	23.7	48.4	44.8	54.9
Pantothenic acid	mg/kg/day	1.2–1.7	0.34	1.43	0.28	0.41	1.45	2.3	1.7
Biotin	µg/kg/day	3.6–6	1.1	5.1	19.9	0.7	4.8	45	6.1
Vitamin C	mg/kg/day	18–25	15	32	51	10.8	24.2	45	37
Choline	mg/kg/day	8–35					29	12	18.1
Inositol	mg/kg/day	4.4–81					53	48	43
Taurine	mg/kg/day	4.5–9					7.4		12
Carnitine	mg/kg/day	~2.9					2.9		3.2
Calcium	mg/kg/day	100–220	35	174	217.5	183	200	218	200
Phosphorus	mg/kg/day	60–140	20	95	121.9	96	109	121	104
Magnesium	mg/kg/day	7.9–15	5	9.7	15.6	11	10.9	14.5	12.2
Iron	mg/kg/day	2–4	0.09	2.3	0.6	0.29	2.2	2.2	2.2
Zinc	µg/kg/day	1,000–3,000	300	1,450	1,683	1,300	1,810	1,810	1,590
Manganese	µg/kg/day	0.7–7.5	0.5	13	11.8	25.8	7.6	14.5	8.5
Copper	µg/kg/day	120–230	45	113	292.8	137	145	302	183
Iodine	µg/kg/day	10–60	23	19		16	30	7	43

(continued)

Table 21.1. Comparison of Enteral Intake Recommendations and Selected Feeding Regimens* for the Preterm Infant _(Continued)_

Nutrient	Unit	Enteral Intake Recommendations for Preterm Infants†	Mature Human Milk‡	Mature Human Milk plus Four Vials Enfamil Liquid HMF/dL	Mature Human Milk plus Four Packets Similac HMF/dL	Mature Human Milk plus Prolact +6	Enfamil Premature High Protein 24 kcal/oz with Iron	Similac Special Care 24 High Protein with Iron	Gerber Good Start Premature 24 High Protein
Selenium	μg/kg/day	1.3–10	3	2	4	2	6	2	2
Sodium	mEq/kg/day	3–5	1.2	2.5	2.2	3.4	3.7	2.3	2
Potassium	mEq/kg/day	2–5	1.8	2.91	4.4	3.4	3.1	4	3.8
Chloride	mEq/kg/day	3–7	1.8	2.5	3.4	2.7	3.7	2.8	2.9

*Calculated intakes of human milk feedings and formulas are based on an intake of 150 mL/kg/day.
†The American Academy of Pediatrics[3] suggests the estimated requirements based on the fetal accretion rate of protein are 3.5 to 4 g/kg/day. The current recommendations from Koletzko et al.[4] and the European Society for Paediatric Gastroenterology, Hepatology and Nutrition Committee [5] are 3.5 to 4.5 g/kg/day to provide catch-up growth for extremely low birth weight infants.
‡Denotes mature milk post 2 weeks of lactation of mothers who deliver term infants.
**Aim for 400 IU/day.
HMF, human milk fortifier.

adequate intake. However, due to the limitations of the currently available data, the goals for nutrient intake for preterm infants are considered to be recommendations only.

B. **Fluid** (see Chapters 13 and 23). The initial step in nutritional support is to determine an infant's fluid requirement, which is dependent on gestational age, postnatal age, and environmental conditions. Generally, baseline fluid needs are inversely related to gestational age at birth and birth weight. During the first postnatal week, very low birth weight (VLBW) infants are known to experience increased water loss because of the immaturity of their skin, which has a higher water content and increased permeability, and the immaturity of their renal function with a decreased ability to concentrate urine. Environmental factors, such as radiant warmers, phototherapy, and incubators, also impact insensible losses and may affect fluid requirements. Conversely, restriction of fluid intake is often utilized for the prevention and/or treatment of patent ductus arteriosus, renal insufficiency, and bronchopulmonary dysplasia (BPD). Fluid requirements in the first few postnatal weeks are, therefore, continually reassessed, as the transition is made from fetal to neonatal life and at least daily afterward.

C. **Energy.** Estimates suggest that preterm infants in a thermoneutral environment require approximately 40 to 60 kcal/kg/day for maintenance of body weight, assuming adequate protein is provided. Additional calories are needed for growth, with the smallest neonates tending to demonstrate the greatest need, because their rate of growth is highest (Table 21.2). The three sources, AAP, ESPGHAN-CON, and Koletzko et al. recommend a range of 105 to 135 kcal/kg/day. Practice generally strives for energy intakes of 110

Table 21.2. Estimation of Energy Requirement of the Low Birth Weight Infant

	Average Estimation (kcal/kg/day)
Energy expended	40–60
Resting metabolic rate	40–50*
Activity	0–5*
Thermoregulation	0–5*
Synthesis	15†
Energy stored	20–30†
Energy excreted	15
Energy intake	90–120

*Energy for maintenance.
†Energy cost of growth.
Source: American Academy of Pediatrics, Committee on Nutrition. *Pediatric Nutrition Handbook*. 7th ed. Elk Grove Village, IL: American Academy of Pediatrics; 2014.

to 130 kcal/kg/day. Infants with severe and/or prolonged illness frequently require a range of 130 to 150 kcal/kg/day. Lesser intakes (85 to 100 kcal/kg/day) may sustain intrauterine growth rates, when parenteral nutrition (PN) is used.

III. PARENTERAL NUTRITION

A. Nutrient goals. The initial goal for PN is to provide adequate calories and amino acids to prevent negative energy and nitrogen balance. Goals thereafter include the promotion of appropriate weight gain and growth while awaiting the attainment of adequate enteral intake.

B. Indications for initiating parenteral nutrition. PN is started the first postnatal day for infants who are <1,500 g birth weight. For infants for whom significant enteral intake is not anticipated by 3 to 5 days of age or for those with cardiac disease requiring calcium supplementation, PN may also be considered.

C. Peripheral versus central parenteral nutrition

1. Parenteral solutions may be infused through a peripheral or central vein. Historically, the AAP has recommended that peripheral solutions maintain an osmolarity between 300 and 900 mOsm/L. Because of this limitation, peripheral solutions often cannot adequately support growth in extremely low birth weight (ELBW) infants. Central PN not only allows for the use of more hypertonic solutions but also incurs greater risks, particularly catheter-related sepsis. Umbilical venous catheters are commonly used for parenteral administration.

2. Central PN is considered to be warranted under the following conditions:
   a. Nutritional needs exceed the capabilities of peripheral PN.
   b. An extended period (e.g., >7 days) of inability to take enteral feedings, such as in infants with necrotizing enterocolitis (NEC) and in some postoperative infants
   c. Imminent lack of peripheral venous access

D. Carbohydrate. Dextrose (D-glucose) is the carbohydrate source in intravenous (IV) solutions (see Chapter 24).

1. The caloric value of dextrose is 3.4 kcal/g.

2. Because dextrose contributes to the osmolarity of a solution, it is generally recommended that the concentration administered through peripheral veins be limited to ≤12.5% dextrose. Higher concentrations of dextrose may be used for central venous infusions. Infants receiving extracorporeal membrane oxygenation (ECMO) therapy may require up to 40% dextrose due to fluid restriction. The use of ultrafiltration with ECMO allows for an increase in fluid administration and a decrease in dextrose to 22% to meet the infant's glucose needs.

3. Dextrose infusions are typically referred to in terms of the milligrams of glucose per kilogram per minute (mg/kg/minute) delivered, which expresses the total glucose load and accounts for infusion rate, dextrose concentration, and the patient's weight (Fig. 21.3).

Dextrose %	5	6	7	7.5	8	9	10	11	12	12.5	14	15	20
mL/kg/day													
10	0.3	0.4	0.5	0.5	0.6	0.6	0.7	0.8	0.8	0.9	1.0	1.0	1.4
20	0.7	0.8	1.0	1.0	1.1	1.3	1.4	1.5	1.7	1.7	1.9	2.1	2.8
30	1.0	1.3	1.5	1.6	1.7	1.9	2.1	2.3	2.5	2.6	2.9	3.1	4.2
40	1.4	1.7	1.9	2.1	2.2	2.5	2.8	3.1	3.3	3.5	3.9	4.2	5.6
50	1.7	2.1	2.4	2.6	2.8	3.1	3.5	3.8	4.2	4.3	4.9	5.2	6.9
60	2.1	2.5	2.9	3.1	3.3	3.8	4.2	4.6	5.0	5.2	5.8	6.3	8.3
70	2.4	2.9	3.4	3.6	3.9	4.4	4.9	5.3	5.8	6.1	6.8	7.3	9.7
80	2.8	3.3	3.9	4.2	4.4	5.0	5.6	6.1	6.7	6.9	7.8	8.3	11.1
90	3.1	3.8	4.4	4.7	5.0	5.6	6.3	6.9	7.5	7.8	8.8	9.4	12.5
100	3.5	4.2	4.9	5.2	5.6	6.3	6.9	7.6	8.3	8.7	9.7	10.4	13.9
110	3.8	4.6	5.3	5.7	6.1	6.9	7.6	8.4	9.2	9.5	10.7	11.5	15.3
120	4.2	5.0	5.8	6.3	6.7	7.5	8.3	9.2	10.0	10.4	11.7	12.5	16.7
130	4.5	5.4	6.3	6.8	7.2	8.1	9.0	9.9	10.8	11.3	12.6	13.5	18.1
140	4.9	5.8	6.8	7.3	7.8	8.8	9.7	10.7	11.7	12.2	13.6	14.6	19.4
150	5.2	6.3	7.3	7.8	8.3	9.4	10.4	11.5	12.5	13.0	14.6	15.6	20.8
160	5.6	6.7	7.8	8.3	8.9	10.0	11.1	12.2	13.3	13.9	15.6	16.7	22.2

Figure 21.3. Chart to quickly calculate glucose infusion rate in neonates. (From Chowning R, Adamkin DH. Table to quickly calculate glucose infusion rates in neonates. *J Peri* 2015;35:463.)

4. The initial glucose requirement for term infants is defined as the amount that is necessary to avoid hypoglycemia. In general, this may be achieved with initial infusion rates of approximately 4 to 6 mg/kg/minute.

5. Preterm infants usually require higher rates of glucose because they have a higher brain-to-body weight ratio and higher total energy needs. Initial infusion rates of 4 to 8 mg/kg/minute may be required to maintain euglycemia.

6. Initial rates may be advanced, as tolerated, by 1 to 2 mg/kg/minute daily to a goal of 11 to 12 mg/kg/minute. This may be accomplished by increasing dextrose concentration, by increasing infusion rate, or by a combination of both. Infusion rates above 11 to 12 mg/kg/minute may exceed the infant's oxidative capacity and are generally not recommended because this may cause the excess glucose to be converted to fat, particularly in the liver. This conversion may also increase oxygen consumption, energy expenditure, and CO_2 production.

7. The quantity of dextrose that an infant can tolerate will vary with gestational and postnatal age. Signs of glucose intolerance include hyperglycemia and secondary glucosuria with osmotic diuresis.

E. **Protein.** Crystalline amino acid solutions provide the nitrogen source in PN.

1. The caloric value of amino acids is 4 kcal/g.

2. Three pediatric amino acid formulations are commercially available in the United States: TrophAmine (B. Braun), Aminosyn-PF (Hospira), and Premasol (Baxter). In theory, these products are better adapted to

the needs of newborns than are standard adult formulations because they have been modified for improved tolerance and contain conditionally essential amino acids. However, the optimal amino acid composition for neonatal PN has not yet been defined. The addition of cysteine is recommended because this amino acid may be conditionally essential in premature infants.

3. It has been demonstrated that VLBW infants who do not receive amino acids in the first postnatal days catabolize body protein at a rate of at least 1 g/kg/day. Studies investigating the use of early amino acids have consistently shown a reversal of this catabolism without adverse metabolic consequences. Current recommendations support the infusion of amino acids at a dose of 2 to 3 g/kg/day beginning in the first 24 hours after birth.

4. Infants with a birth weight <1,500 g are provided with 2 to 3 g/kg/day shortly after birth. Infants >1,500 g are also initiated on 2 to 3 g/kg/day if indicated, depending on their size, clinical condition, and estimated time to achieve significant enteral volumes.

5. Protein infusion rates are increased to a target of 3.5 to 4 g/kg/day for premature infants and up to 3 g/kg/day for the term neonates.

F. **Lipid.** Currently, in the United States, soybean oil provides the fat source for IV fat emulsions.

1. The caloric value of 20% lipid emulsions is 2 kcal/mL (~10 kcal/g). The use of 20% emulsions is preferred over 10% because the higher ratio of phospholipids to triglyceride in the 10% emulsion interferes with plasma triglyceride clearance. Twenty percent emulsions also provide a more concentrated source of calories. For these reasons, only 20% lipid emulsions are used.

2. Current data suggest that preterm infants are at risk for essential fatty acid (EFA) deficiency within 72 hours after birth, if an exogenous fat source is not delivered. This deficiency state can be avoided by the administration of 0.5 to 1 g/kg/day of lipid emulsion.

3. The optimal initiation and advancement rates for lipid emulsions have not been well studied and have not been defined. The most recent recommendation synthesizing the available data to date reports that in infants <1,500 g at birth, 2 g/kg/day of lipids should be provided within the first 24 hours after birth. This rate should be advanced by the next day to a goal of 3 g/kg/day.

4. Decreased tolerance to IV lipids is frequently seen with infants <1,000 g birth weight, <27 weeks' gestation, are small for gestational age, suffer from intrauterine growth restriction, or have sepsis. IV lipids may need to be advanced more slowly for these infants. Monitoring of blood triglycerides (TGs) may be considered; however, the acceptable range of TG levels balancing safety and nutritional needs for preterm infants has not been determined.

5. Tolerance also correlates with hourly infusion rate. No benefit to a rest period has been identified. Therefore, lipid emulsions are infused over 24 hours for optimal clearance.

G. Electrolytes

1. Sodium and potassium concentrations are adjusted daily based on individual requirements (see Chapter 23). Maintenance requirements are estimated at approximately 2 to 4 mEq/kg.

2. Increasing the proportion of anions provided as acetate aids in the treatment of metabolic acidosis in VLBW infants.

H. Vitamins.
The current pediatric vitamin formulations (M.V.I. Pediatric, Hospira, Lake Forest, IL; INFUVITE Pediatric, Baxter, Deerfield, IL) do not maintain blood levels of all vitamins within an acceptable range for preterm infants. However, there are no products currently available that are specifically designed for preterm infants. Table 21.3 provides guidelines for the use of the available formulations for term and preterm infants. For infants <2,500 g, the AAP suggests a dose of 40% of the M.V.I. Pediatric (INFUVITE Pediatric) 5 mL vial/kg/day. For infants 2,500 g or greater, the AAP suggests the 5 mL M.V.I. Pediatric (INFUVITE Pediatric) per day. Vitamin A is the most difficult to provide in adequate amounts to the VLBW infant without providing excess amounts of the other vitamins because it is subject to losses through photodegradation and absorption to plastic tubing and solution-containing bags. B vitamins may also be affected by photodegradation. This is of particular concern with long-term PN use, and for this reason, consideration should be given to shielding the PN-containing plastic bags and tubing from light.

I. Minerals.
The amount of calcium and phosphorus that can be administered through IV is limited by the precipitation of calcium phosphate. Unfortunately, the variables that determine calcium and phosphate compatibility in PN are complex and what constitutes maximal safe concentrations is controversial. The aluminum content of these preparations should also be considered.

1. Calcium-to-phosphorus ratios of approximately 1.3:1 to 1.7:1 by weight (1:1 to 1.3:1 molar) are suggested. However, despite efforts to optimize mineral intake, preterm infants receiving prolonged PN remain at increased risk for metabolic bone disease (see Chapter 59).

2. Three-in-one PN solutions are not used (dextrose, amino acid, and lipid mixed in single bag) for the following reasons:

a. The pH of lipid emulsions is more basic and increases the pH of the total solution, which decreases the solubility of calcium and phosphorus and limits the amount of these minerals in the solution.

b. If the calcium and phosphorus in a three-in-one solution did precipitate, it would be difficult to detect because the solution is already cloudy.

c. Three-in-one solutions require either a larger micron filter or no filter, which may pose a greater sepsis risk.

J. Trace elements

1. Currently, 1.0 mL/kg of Peditrace (Fresenius Kabi) or 0.2 mL/dL of NeoTrace and 1.5 μg/dL of selenium are added, beginning in the first days of PN. However, when PN is supplementing enteral nutrition or limited to <2 weeks, only zinc may be needed.

2. As copper and manganese are excreted in bile, these trace elements are routinely reduced or omitted if impaired biliary excretion and/or

Table 21.3. Suggested Intakes of Parenteral Vitamins in Infants

Vitamins	Estimated Needs		(2 mL) of a 5 mL Single-Dose Vial M.V.I. Pediatric (Hospira), INFUVITE Pediatric (Baxter)
	Term Infants (≥2.5 kg) (dose/day)	Preterm Infants (≤2.5 kg)*	
Lipid soluble			
A (μg)†	700	280	280
D (IU)†	400	160	160
E (mg)†	7	2.8	2.8
K (μg)	200	80	80
Water soluble			
Thiamine (mg)	1.2	0.48	0.48
Riboflavin (mg)	1.4	0.56	0.56
Niacin (mg)	17	6.8	6.8
Pantothenate (mg)	5	2	2
Pyridoxine (mg)	1	0.4	0.4
Biotin (μg)	20	8	8
Vitamin B_{12} (μg)	1	0.4	0.4
Ascorbic acid (mg)	80	32	32
Folic acid (μg)	140	56	56

*Dose/kg of body weight per day for preterm infants, not to exceed daily dose for term (>2.5 kg) infants.
†700 μg retinol equivalent = 2,300 IU; 7 mg alpha-tocopherol = 7 IU; 10 μg vitamin D = 400 IU.

cholestatic liver disease is present. Trace minerals may be provided on Monday, Wednesday, and Friday to limit intakes of these nutrients. Zinc may be provided as a separate supplement on the remaining days.

3. Infants with ostomy outputs lose excessive zinc and copper. Additional supplementation may be indicated.

Table 21.4. Schedule for Nutrition Laboratory Monitoring

	Parenteral Nutrition	**Enteral Nutrition**
Electrolytes	Daily, till stable; then as clinically indicated	As clinically indicated (consider with use of diuretics, history of electrolyte abnormality, poor growth)
Triglycerides	Consider during initiation and/or advancement for extremely low gestational age or growth restricted infants receiving parenteral lipid nutrition.	Not indicated
Calcium, phosphorus, alkaline phosphatase	After 14 days of PN and as clinically indicated	Consider in low birth weight infants 2 and 4 weeks after achieving full enteral feedings and thereafter as clinically indicated.
Alanine aminotransferase (ALT) Direct bilirubin	After 14 days of PN and as clinically indicated	Not indicated

 K. Metabolic monitoring for infants receiving PN. Infants receiving PN are typically monitored according to the schedule indicated in Table 21.4.

 L. Potential complications associated with PN

  1. Cholestasis (see Chapter 26) may be seen and is more often transient than progressive. Experimentally, even short-term PN can reduce bile flow and bile salt formation.

   a. Risk factors include the following:

    i. Prematurity

    ii. Duration of PN administration

    iii. Duration of fasting (lack of enteral feeding also produces bile inspissation and cholestasis)

    iv. Infection

    v. Narcotic administration

   b. Recommended management:

    i. Attempt enteral feeding. Even minimal enteral feedings may stimulate bile secretion.

    ii. Avoid excess nutrition with PN.

    iii. Provision of a mixed fuel source may be helpful.

    iv. When conjugated bilirubin is >1.5 mg/dL, lipids may be decreased to 1 g/kg. If this change is made, the glucose infusion rate may need to be increased to 14 to 16 mg glucose/kg/minute to meet energy needs. However, recent investigations have not shown that low-dose lipids will prevent cholestasis in preterm neonates.

v. Research is ongoing regarding the use of lipid emulsions for the prevention and/or treatment of cholestasis (see Chapter 26). Omegaven made from fish oil and SMOF made from soy oil, medium-chain triglycerides (MCTs), olive oil, and fish oil are under investigation. They are available by approval of the U.S. Food and Drug Administration for compassionate use only in the United States.

2. **Metabolic bone disease** (see Chapter 59). The use of earlier enteral feedings and central PN, with higher calcium and phosphorus concentrations, has reduced the incidence of metabolic bone disease. However, this continues to be seen with the prolonged use of PN in place of enteral nutrition or the feeding of enteral formulations designed for the term infant.

3. **Metabolic abnormalities.** Azotemia, hyperammonemia, and hyperchloremic metabolic acidosis have become uncommon since introduction of the current crystalline amino acid solutions. These complications may occur, however, with amino acid intakes exceeding 4 g/kg/day.

4. **Metabolic abnormalities related to lipid emulsions**
   a. **Hyperlipidemia/hypertriglyceridemia.** The incidence tends to be inversely related to gestational age at birth and postnatal age. A short-term decrease in the lipid infusion rate usually is sufficient to normalize serum lipid levels. The AAP suggests serum triglyceride concentrations be maintained below 200 mg/dL.
   b. **Indirect hyperbilirubinemia.** Because free fatty acids can theoretically displace bilirubin from albumin-binding sites, the use of lipid emulsions during periods of neonatal hyperbilirubinemia has been questioned. Research, however, suggests that infusion of lipid, at rates up to 3 g/kg/day, is unlikely to displace bilirubin. However, during periods of extreme hyperbilirubinemia (e.g., requiring exchange transfusion), rates <3 g/kg/day are typically provided.
   c. **Sepsis** has been associated with decreased lipoprotein lipase activity and impaired triglyceride clearance. Therefore, during a sepsis episode, it may be necessary to temporarily reduce and/or limit the lipid infusion to avoid hypertriglyceridemia.
   d. Due to the concern about toxic products of lipid peroxidation, protecting lipid emulsions from both ambient and phototherapy lights may also be considered.

M. **Other additives**

1. **Carnitine** facilitates the transport of long-chain fatty acids into the mitochondria for oxidation. However, this nutrient is not routinely added to PN solutions. Preterm infants who receive prolonged, unsupplemented PN are at risk for carnitine deficiency due to their limited reserves and inadequate rates of carnitine synthesis. Infants who are able to tolerate enteral nutrition receive a source of carnitine via human

milk and/or carnitine-containing infant formula. However, for infants requiring prolonged (e.g., >2 to 4 weeks) PN, a parenteral source of carnitine may be provided 10 mg/kg/day until enteral nutrition can be established.

2. **Cysteine** is not a component of current crystalline amino acid solutions because it is unstable over time and will form a precipitate. Cysteine is ordinarily synthesized from methionine and provides a substrate for taurine. However, this may be considered an essential amino acid for preterm infants due to low activity of the enzyme hepatic cystathionase, which converts methionine to cysteine. Supplementation with L-cysteine hydrochloride lowers the pH of the PN solution and may necessitate the use of additional acetate to prevent acidosis. However, the lower pH also enhances the solubility of calcium and phosphorus and allows for improved mineral intake. Cysteine is routinely supplemented in PN at a rate of approximately 30 to 40 mg/g protein.

3. **Glutamine** is an important fuel for intestinal epithelial cells and lymphocytes; however, due to its instability, it is presently not a component of crystalline amino acids solutions. Studies to date have not proven its addition to PN as helpful for the neonate.

4. **Insulin** is not routinely added to PN. Its use must be weighed against the risk of wide swings in blood glucose levels as well as the concerns surrounding the overall effects of the increased uptake of glucose. When hyperglycemia is severe or persistent, an insulin infusion may be useful (see Chapter 24).

5. **Vitamin A** is important for normal growth and differentiation of epithelial tissue, particularly the development and maintenance of pulmonary epithelial tissue. ELBW infants are known to have low vitamin A stores at birth, minimal enteral intake for the first several weeks after birth, reduced enteral absorption of vitamin A, and unreliable parenteral delivery. Studies have suggested that vitamin A supplementation can reduce the risk of BPD. At present, infants weighing <1,000 g at birth are supplemented with 5,000 IU vitamin A intramuscularly three times per week for the first 4 postnatal weeks, beginning in the first 72 hours (see Chapter 34).

IV. ENTERAL NUTRITION

A. **Early enteral feeding**

1. The structural and functional integrity of the gastrointestinal (GI) tract is dependent on the provision of enteral nutrition. Withholding enteral feeding after birth places the infant at risk for all the complications associated with luminal starvation, including mucosal thinning, flattening of the villi, and bacterial translocation. **Minimal enteral nutrition** (also referred to as "gut priming" or "trophic feedings") may be described as the nonnutritive use of very small volumes of human milk or formula, for the intended purpose of preservation of gut maturation rather than nutrient delivery. Definitive conclusions cannot be drawn as to what constitutes the optimal volume for minimal enteral nutrition.

2. **Benefits associated with minimal enteral nutrition include the following:**

   a. Improved levels of gut hormones

   b. Less feeding intolerance

   c. Earlier progression to full enteral feedings

   d. Improved weight gain

   e. Improved calcium and phosphorus retention

   f. Fewer days on PN

3. **The following are guidelines for the use of gut priming in preterm infants:**

   a. Begin as soon after birth as possible, ideally by postnatal days 1 to 2. A standardized feeding protocol will help to accomplish this goal.

   b. Use full-strength colostrum/preterm maternal milk or pasteurized donor human milk (PDHM). In instances where the supply of maternal milk is insufficient for 100% gut priming volume, and PDHM has been declined or is unavailable, full-strength 20 kcal/oz preterm formula may be used. Gut priming may be administered as a fixed dose (i.e., 0.5 mL every 4 hours for infants, 800 g at birth). Alternatively, a low volume per kilogram may be delivered (i.e., 10 to 20 mL/kg/day divided into eight aliquots for infants <1,250 g birth weight).

   c. Gut priming is not used in infants with severe hemodynamic instability, suspected or confirmed NEC, evidence of ileus, or clinical signs of intestinal pathology. Infants who are undergoing medical treatment for patent ductus arteriosus may receive gut priming, pending the discretion of the care team.

   d. Controlled trials of gut priming with umbilical arterial catheters (UACs) in place have not shown an increased incidence of NEC. Therefore, the presence of a UAC is not considered to be a contraindication to minimal enteral nutrition. However, the clinical condition accompanying the prolonged use of a UAC may serve as a contraindication.

B. Preterm infants

1. **Fortified human milk.** Human milk provides the gold standard for feeding term infants, and fortified human milk will meet the needs of premature infants. The use of human milk offers many nutritional and nonnutritional advantages for the premature infant. Feeding tolerance is improved, and the incidence of sepsis and NEC is decreased. Earlier discharge is facilitated by better feeding tolerance and less illness. The use of fortified human milk is considered to be the preferred feeding for preterm infants.

   a. Preterm human milk contains higher amounts of protein, sodium, chloride, and magnesium than term milk. However, the levels of these nutrients remain below preterm recommendations, the differences only persist for approximately the first 21 days of lactation, and composition is known to vary.

   b. For these reasons, human milk for preterm infants is routinely supplemented with human milk fortifier (HMF). The use of HMF is recommended for infants <1,500 g birth weight and may also be considered for infants with birth weights up to 1,800 to 2,000 g and <34 weeks' gestation. Powdered and liquid, bovine milk–based HMF as well as liquid donor human milk–based HMF are available. The U.S. Food and Drug Administration[6] recommends that powdered preparations not be used in premature infants given the risk of bacterial contamination. The addition of bovine milk–based HMF to human milk (see Table 21.1) increases energy, protein, vitamin, and mineral contents to levels more appropriate for preterm infants. Iron supplementation is indicated for the low iron bovine milk–based HMF. The donor human milk–based fortifier increases energy, protein, and mineral intake. However, as vitamin content of the feeding is not appreciably increased with the use of this product, a multivitamin and iron supplement is typically administered daily.

c. HMF is added at 2 to 4 kcal/oz prior to the infant reaching 100 mL/kg/day. Studies are ongoing to determine the optimal timing for introducing HMF.

d. When 100% maternal milk is unavailable, PDHM may be offered to infants who are considered to be at highest risk for feeding intolerance and NEC. Most typically, this includes VLBW newborns and/or those born at <32 weeks' gestation. Donor milk may also be used to supplement a new mother's supply for older or larger infants. Depending on the hospital's guidelines, assent or consent is obtained from the parent or guardian prior to administering PDHM. Maternal milk is preferentially fed, as available, with PDHM being used, as needed, to reach goal volumes. PDHM is typically offered until 100% maternal milk is achieved or an established endpoint have been reached. These endpoints may be full-volume feedings for a certain period of time (i.e., full feedings for 48 hours) or until a goal weight or PMA has been reached (i.e., 34 weeks' PMA and infant weight of >1,500 to 1,800 g). Once the established endpoint is achieved, the infant is slowly transitioned off PDHM by gradually adding in formula feedings. This process usually occurs over several days.

e. When human milk is fed through continuous infusion, incomplete delivery of nutrients may occur, in particular, the nonhomogenized fat and nutrients in the HMF may cling to the tubing. Small, frequent bolus feedings may result in improved nutrient delivery and absorption compared with continuous feedings.

f. Protocols for the collection and storage of human milk are outlined in Chapter 22.

2. **Preterm formulas** (see Tables 21.1 and 21.5) are designed to meet the nutritional and physiologic needs of preterm infants and have some common features:

a. Whey-predominant, taurine-supplemented protein source, which is better tolerated and produces a more normal plasma amino acid profile than casein-predominant protein

b. Carbohydrate mixtures of 40% to 50% lactose and 50% to 60% glucose polymers to compensate for preterm infants' relative lactase deficiency

c. Fat mixtures containing approximately 40% to 50% MCTs, to compensate for limited pancreatic lipase secretion and small bile acid pools, as well as 50% to 60% long-chain TGs to provide a source of EFAs

Table 21.5. Nutrient Composition of Human Milk and Select Infant Formula

	kcal/ 30 mL	Protein (g/dL)	Fat (g/dL)	DHA (mg/dL)	ARA (mg/dL)	Carbohydrate* (g/dL)	Electrolytes (mEq/dL) Na K Cl	Minerals (mg/dL) Ca P Fe†	Vitamins (IU/dL) A D E	Folic Acid (µg/dL)	Osmolality (mOsmol/ kg H$_2$O)	PRSL (mOsmol/L)
Mature Human Milk (composition varies)	20	0.9	3.5			8	0.8 1.2 1.2	23 13 0.03	160 1 0.6	16.5	295	88
Formula (manufacturer‡)												
Preterm Formulas												
Enfamil Premature (Mead Johnson)	20	2.2	3.4	11.5	23	7.3	2.0 1.7 2.1	112 61 1.22	910 200 4.3	27	260	201
Enfamil Premature (Mead Johnson)	24	2.7	4.1	13.8	28	8.8	2.5 2.1 2.5	134 73 1.46	1,100 240 5.1	32	320	239
Enfamil Premature High Protein (Mead Johnson)	24	2.9	4.1	13.8	28	8.5	2.5 2.1 2.5	134 73 1.46	1,100 240 5.1	32	300	260
Enfamil Premature (Mead Johnson)	30	3.3	5.1	17.2	34	10.9	3.1 2.5 3.1	167 91 1.83	1,370 300 6.4	41	320	302
Gerber Good Start Premature (Nestlé)	20	2.0	3.5	11.2	22.4	7.1	1.6 2.1 1.6	111 57 1.2	676 122 4.1	30	229	187
Gerber Good Start Premature (Nestlé)	24	2.4	4.2	13.4	26.9	8.5	2.0 2.5 2.0	133 69 1.5	812 146 4.9	37	275	225

Gerber Good Start Premature High Protein (Nestlé)	24	2.9	4.2	13.4	26.9	7.9	2.0	2.5	2.0	133	69	1.5	812	146	4.9	37	299	254
Gerber Good Start Premature (Nestlé)	30	3.0	5.3	17.0	33.9	10.7	2.4	3.1	2.5	166	86	1.8	1,015	183	6.1	46	341	277
Similac Special Care (Abbott)	20	2.0	3.7	9.3	14.8	7.0	1.3	2.2	1.6	122	68	1.2	845	101	2.7	25	235	188
Similac Special Care (Abbott)	24	2.4	4.4	11.0	17.6	8.4	1.6	2.7	1.9	146	73	1.5	1,014	122	3.3	30	280	225
Similac Special Care High Protein (Abbott)	24	2.7	4.4	11.0	17.6	8.1	1.5	2.7	1.9	146	73	1.5	1,014	122	3.3	30	280	240
Similac Special Care (Abbott)	30	3.0	6.7	14.1	22.1	7.8	1.9	3.4	2.3	183	101	1.8	1,268	152	4.1	38	325	282
Nutrient-Enriched Postdischarge Formulas																	
Enfamil EnfaCare (Mead Johnson)	22	2.1	3.9	12.6	25	7.7	1.2	2.0	1.7	89	49	1.3	330	56	3.0	19	Liquid 230 Powder 310	182
Similac NeoSure (Abbott)	22	2.1	4.1	10.3	16.4	7.5	1.1	2.7	1.6	78	46	1.3	260	52	2.6	19	250	187
Standard Cow's Milk-Based Formula																	
Enfamil (Mead Johnson)	20	1.4	3.6	11.5	23	7.6	0.8	1.9	1.2	53	29	1.2	200	41	1.4	11	300	124

(continued)

Table 21.5. Nutrient Composition of Human Milk and Select Infant Formula (Continued)

	kcal/ 30 mL	Protein (g/dL)	Fat (g/dL)	DHA (mg/dL)	ARA (mg/dL)	Carbohydrate* (g/dL)	Electrolytes (mEq/dL) Na K Cl	Minerals (mg/dL) Ca P Fe†	Vitamins (IU/dL) A D E	Folic Acid (µg/dL)	Osmolality (mOsmol/ kg H₂O)	PRSL (mOsmol/L)
Gerber Good Start Gentle (Nestlé)	20	1.5	3.4	10.9	10.9	7.8	0.8 1.9 1.3	45 26 1.0	203 51 1.4	10	250	133
Similac Advance (Abbott)	20	1.4	3.6			7.6	0.7 1.8 1.2	53 28 1.2	203 51 1.0	10	310	127
Similac Advance (Abbott)	19	1.3	3.5			7.2	0.7 1.8 1.2	53 28 1.2	192 48 1.0	10	310	120
Specialized Formulas												
Similac Alimentum (Abbott)	20	1.9	3.7	5.6	14.8	6.9	1.3 2.0 1.6	71 51 1.2	202 41 2.0	10	320	253
EleCare (Abbott)	20	2.1	3.3	5.0	13.2	7.3	1.4 2.7 1.2	79 57 1.2	186 41 1.4	20	350	279
Nutramigen (Liquids) (Mead Johnson)	20	1.9	3.6			7.0	1.4 1.9 1.7	64 35 1.2	203 34 1.4	11	320	169

Product																		
Pregestimil (Mead Johnson)	20	1.9	3.8	11.5	23	6.9	1.4	1.9	1.7	64	35	1.2	240	34	2.7	11	320	167
Pregestimil (Mead Johnson)	24	2.3	4.5	13.6	27	8.2	1.6	2.3	2.0	76	42	1.5	282	40	3.2	13	340	200
PurAmino DHA & ARA (Mead Johnson)	20	1.9	3.6	11.5	23	7.2	1.4	1.9	1.7	64	35	1.2	200	34	1.4	11	350	169
Neocate (Nutricia)	20	1.9	3.5	12.3	12.3	7.3	1.2	1.9	1.5	79	56	1.0	190	50	1.0	9	340	168
Alfamino (Nestlé)	20	1.9	3.4	10.9	10.9	7.4	1.1	1.8	1.6	80	53	1.2	214	38	1.5	10	330	154
Enfaport (Mead Johnson)	20	2.4	3.7	11.4	22.8	6.8	0.9	2.0	1.7	64	35	1.2	240	34	2.7	11	250	290
Similac PM 60/40 (Abbott)	20	1.5	3.8			6.9	0.7	1.4	1.1	38	19	0.5	202	41	1.0	10	280	124

*See text for types of carbohydrates used in formulas.

†In instances where high- and low-iron formulations are available, the iron-fortified value appears.

‡Additional product information and nutrient composition data may be found at the following websites: http://www.meadjohnson.com, http://www.abbott.com, http://www.nutricia-na.com, http://www.medical.gerber.com.

DHA, docosahexaenoic acid; ARA, arachidonic acid; Na, sodium; K, potassium; Cl, chloride; Ca, calcium; P, phosphorus; Fe, iron.

    d. Higher concentrations of protein, vitamins, minerals, and electrolytes to meet the increased needs associated with rapid growth and limited fluid tolerance.

   3. Feeding advancement. When attempting to determine how best to advance a preterm infant to full enteral nutrition, there is very limited data to support any one method as optimal. The following guidelines reflect current practice:

    a. Use full-strength human milk or 24 kcal/oz preterm formula and advance feeding volume according to the guidelines in Table 21.6 for any infant being fed by tube feedings.

    b. As previously discussed, for human milk–fed infants, the caloric density may be advanced by 2 to 4 kcal/oz with liquid bovine or human milk–based HMF before the infant reaches 100 mL/kg/day. Volume, at the new caloric density, is typically maintained for approximately 24 hours before the advancement schedule is resumed.

    c. As enteral volumes are increased, the rate of any IV fluid is calculated to achieve total fluid goals. Nutrient intake from parenteral and enteral feedings is calculated to prevent nutrient overload such as protein.

C. Term infants

   1. Human milk is considered the preferred feeding choice for term infants.

Table 21.6. Tube Feeding Guidelines

Birth Weight (g)	Initial Rate (mL/kg/day)	Volume Increase (mL/kg every 12 hours)
<1,000	10	10
1,001–1,250	10–20	10
1,251–1,500	20–30	10–15
1,501–1,800	30	15
1,801–2,500	30–40	15–20

The initial volume should be administered for at least 24 hours prior to advancement. The guidelines should be individualized based on the infant's clinical status/history of present illness. Once feeding volume has reached approximately 80 mL/kg/day, infants weighing <1,250 g should be considered for feeding intervals of every 2 hours or every 3 hours, as opposed to every 4 hours. Once feeding volume has reached approximately 100 mL/kg per day, consider advancing to 22 kcal/oz or 24 kcal/oz for all infants weighing <1,500 g. Consider advancing feeding volume more rapidly than the above guidelines once tolerance of >100 mL/kg/day is established but do not exceed increments of 15 mL/kg every 12 hours in most infants weighing <1,500 g. The recommended volume goal for feedings is 140 to 160 mL/kg/day. These guidelines do not apply to infants capable of *ad libitum* feedings.

2. Term formulas. The Infant Formula Act provides specific guidelines for the composition of infant formulas so that term infant formulas approximate human milk in general composition. Table 10.5 describes the composition of commonly available formulas, many of which are derived from modified cow's milk.

D. **Specialized formulas** have been designed for a variety of congenital and neonatal disorders, including milk protein allergy, malabsorption syndromes, and several inborn errors of metabolism. Indications for the most commonly used of these specialized formulas are briefly reviewed in Table 21.7, whereas composition is outlined in Table 21.5. However, it is important to note that **these formulas were not designed to meet the special nutritional needs of preterm infants**. Preterm infants who are fed these formulas require close nutritional assessment and monitoring for potential protein, mineral, and multivitamin supplementation.

E. **Caloric/energy-enhanced feedings.** Many ill term and preterm infants require increased energy/nutrient intakes in order to achieve optimal rates of growth.

   1. Preterm infants. Many different strategies are currently utilized to maximize energy content to achieve recommended postnatal growth. Practice should be individualized to the infant, and the general goal is to maximize all macronutrients. Principles to guide increasing caloric/energy content of enteral feedings include the following:

   a. HMF

   i. Bovine milk–based HMF can provide 2 to 4 additional kcal/oz.

   ii. For infants receiving a **liquid donor human milk–based HMF**, the fortifiers are designed to make 24 to 30 kcal/oz milk. The energy and protein content of the milk will be increased with the higher caloric fortifier, and the mineral content will stay constant. In addition, a donor human milk cream supplement is available to increase energy intake when protein needs have been met by the donor human milk–based HMF.

   b. Protein supplementation, with an extensively hydrolyzed protein modular, may be considered for VLBW infants in order to increase the protein content to approximately 4.5 g/kg/day, as needed.

   c. Maximize total daily volume delivered as tolerated.

   d. If additional calories/energy are needed after the earlier measures have been taken, high-calorie (30 kcal/oz) liquid preterm formula can be added to the feedings.

   e. The use of vegetable oils and powdered products should be avoided, if possible.

   f. Formula-fed, fluid-restricted preterm infants may be switched to a 26 to 30 kcal/oz premature infant formula once they are tolerating appropriate volumes of 24 kcal/oz feedings.

   2. Term infants

   a. Human milk–fed term infants requiring caloric enhancement may utilize infant formula powder, MCT or corn oil, and/or SolCarb (maltodextrin), added in increments of 2 to 3 kcal/oz (typically not to exceed a maximum caloric density of 30 kcal/oz). As with preterm infants,

Table 21.7. Indications for Use of Infant Formulas

Clinical Condition	Suggested Type of Infant Formula	Rationale
Allergy to cow's milk protein or soy protein	Extensively hydrolyzed protein or free amino acids	Impaired digestion/ utilization of intact protein
Bronchopulmonary dysplasia	High-energy, nutrient-dense	Increased energy requirement, fluid restriction
Biliary atresia	Semi-elemental, containing reduced LCT (~45%), with supplemented MCT (~55%)	Impaired intraluminal digestion and absorption of long-chain fats
Chylothorax (persistent)	Significantly reduced LCT (~15%), with supplemented MCT (~84%)	Decreased lymphatic absorption of fats
Congestive heart failure	High-energy formula	Lower fluid and sodium intake; increased energy requirement
Cystic fibrosis	Semi-elemental formula, containing reduced LCT (~45%), with supplemented MCT (~55%) or standard formula with pancreatic enzyme supplementation	Impaired intraluminal digestion and absorption of long-chain fats
Galactosemia	Soy protein–based formula	Lactose-free
Gastroesophageal reflux	Standard formula, Enfamil AR	Consider small, frequent feedings.
Hepatic insufficiency	Semi-elemental formula, containing reduced LCT (~45%), with supplemented MCT (~55%)	Impaired intraluminal digestion and absorption of long-chain fats
Lactose intolerance	Low lactose formula	Impaired digestion or utilization of lactose
Lymphatic anomalies	Significantly reduced LCT (~15%), with supplemented MCT (~84%)	Impaired absorption of long-chain fats

(continued)

Table 21.7. *(Continued)*		
Clinical Condition	**Suggested Type of Infant Formula**	**Rationale**
Necrotizing enterocolitis	Preterm formula or semi-elemental formula, if indicated	Impaired digestion
Renal insufficiency	Standard formula	
	Similac PM 60/40	Low phosphate content, low renal solute load
LCT, long-chain triglyceride; MCT, medium-chain triglyceride.		

adjustments should be made gradually with feeding tolerance assessed after each change. Hindmilk may also be used.

b. For term infants receiving standard formula, the formula density may be increased as needed by concentration or with formula concentrate diluted to a more calorically dense feeding and/or modulars. The overall nutrient composition of these feedings should be considered.

3. Supplements are further described in Table 21.8.

4. Growth patterns of infants receiving these supplements are monitored closely, and the nutritional care plan is adjusted accordingly.

Table 21.8. Oral Dietary Supplements Available for Use in Infants			
Nutrient	**Product**	**Source**	**Energy Content**
Fat	MCT oil (Novartis)	Medium-chain triglycerides	8.3 kcal/g 7.7 kcal/mL
	Microlipid (Novartis)	Long-chain triglycerides	4.5 kcal/mL
	Corn oil	Long-chain triglycerides	8.6 kcal/g 8 kcal/mL
Carbohydrate	SolCarb (Solace) (for term infants only)	Maltodextrin	3.8 kcal/g 8 kcal/tsp (powder)
Protein	Abbott liquid protein	Extensively hydrolyzed casein protein	3.6 kcal/g 4 kcal/6 mL

F. **Feeding method.** These should be individualized based on gestational age, clinical condition, and feeding tolerance.

1. **Nasogastric/orogastric feedings.** Nasogastric tube feedings are utilized more frequently because orogastric tubes tend to be more difficult to secure.

   a. **Candidates**
      i. Infants <34 weeks' gestation, as most do not yet have the ability to coordinate suck-swallow-breathe patterns
      ii. Infants with impaired suck/swallow coordination due to conditions such as encephalopathy, hypotonia, and maxillofacial abnormalities.

   b. **Bolus versus continuous.** Studies may be found in support of either method and, in practice, both are utilized. Feedings are usually initiated as bolus, divided every 3 to 4 hours. If difficulties with feeding tolerance occur, the amount of time over which a feeding is given may be lengthened by delivery via a syringe pump for 30 to 120 minutes.

2. **Transpyloric feedings**

   a. **Candidates.** There are only a few indications for transpyloric feedings.
      i. Infants intolerant to nasogastric/orogastric feedings
      ii. Infants at increased risk for aspiration
      iii. Severe gastric retention or regurgitation
      iv. Anatomic abnormalities of the GI tract such as microgastria

   b. **Other considerations**
      i. Transpyloric feedings should be delivered continuously because the small intestine does not have the same capacity for expansion as does the stomach.
      ii. There is an increased risk of fat malabsorption, because lingual and gastric lipase secretions are bypassed.
      iii. These tubes are routinely placed under guided fluoroscopy.

3. **Transition to breast/bottle-feedings** is a gradual process.
      i. Nonnutritive attempts at the breast should be encouraged before 33 to 34 weeks, if tolerated. Early, nonnutritive sucking facilitates milk production and increases the likelihood the infant is still breastfeeding at the time of hospital discharge.
      ii. Infants who are approximately 33 to 34 weeks' gestation, who have coordinated suck-swallow-breathe patterns and respiratory rates <60 breaths per minute, are appropriate candidates for introducing breast/bottle-feedings.
      iii. If able, nutritive oral feeding attempts at the breast should precede oral feeding attempts with the bottle.

4. **Gastrostomy feedings**
   a. **Candidates**
      i. Infants with neurologic impairment and/or those who are unable to take sufficient volumes through breast/bottle-feeding to maintain adequate growth/hydration status.

G. **Iron.** The AAP recommends that growing preterm infants receive a source of iron, provided at 2 to 4 mg/kg/day, after 2 weeks of age. The AAP further suggests that preterm infants on iron-fortified preterm formula do not need additional iron. However, the current recommendations[4] recommend 2 to 3 mg/kg/day for VLBW infants. It has been suggested that >2 mg/kg/day may be needed, when adjusted for noncompensated phlebotomy losses and the number of days during which the infant does not receive iron due to feeding intolerance or illness. Iron supplementation is recommended until the infant is 12 months of age. Iron-fortified formulas and iron-fortified HMF provide approximately 2.2 mg/kg/day when delivered at a rate of 150 mL/kg/day. Low iron formulas are not recommended for use.

H. Vitamin E is an important antioxidant that acts to prevent fatty acid peroxidation in the cell membrane. The recommendation for preterm infants is 2.2 to 12 IU vitamin E/kg/day. Preterm infants are not initiated on iron supplements until they are tolerating full enteral volumes of 24 kcal/oz feedings, which provides vitamin E at the low to midrange of the recommendations.

I. Other immunonutrients

1. Glutamine and **arginine** are important sources of fuel and substrates for distal protective compounds (e.g., glutathione and nitric oxide, respectively). However, evidence-based replacement strategies for these elements are lacking. Thus, as with parenteral glutamine supplementation, there are presently no recommendations for enteral glutamine and/or arginine supplementation in preterm infants.

2. Specific immunonutrients have been shown to be involved with lung development and the protection from lung injury. Providing immunonutrients to premature infants may aid in the prevention and treatment of BPD. Selected immunonutrients include **vitamin A, vitamin D, inositol,** and **long-chain polyunsaturated fatty acids (LCPUFAs)**, such as docosahexaenoic acid and arachidonic acid.
a. The use of intramuscular (IM) administration vitamin A with premature infants has been linked to a reduction in BPD, but the use is not universal. There is a lack of consensus on the ease to implement the vitamin A protocol and the concern with the use of IM injections.
b. Animal and limited human research suggests improved lung growth and development with the use of other immunonutrients such as vitamin D, inositol, and LCPUFA. More research in timing, dosing, and delivery is indicated with these immunonutrients before clinical use can occur for the preterm infant.

V. SPECIAL CONSIDERATIONS

A. Gastroesophageal reflux (GER). Episodes of GER, as monitored by esophageal pH probes, are common in both preterm and full-term infants. The majority of infants, however, do not exhibit clinical compromise from GER.

1. Introduction of enteral feedings. Emesis can be associated during the introduction and advancement of enteral feedings in preterm infants. These episodes are most commonly related to intestinal dysmotility secondary to prematurity and will respond to modifications of the feeding regimen.
a. Temporary reductions in the feeding volume, lengthening the duration of the feeding (sometimes to the point of using continuous feeding),

removal of nutritional additives, and temporary cessation of enteral feedings are all possible strategies depending on the clinical course of the infant. Continuous human milk feedings can lead to milk fat adherence to the feeding tube and decreased infant growth. When the infant has demonstrated feeding tolerance, the feedings can be switched back to bolus feedings. Transitioning to bolus feedings by decreasing the pump time in a gradual fashion may be helpful.

b. Rarely, specialized formulas are used when all other feeding modifications have been tried without improvement. In general, these formulas should only be used for short periods of time with close nutritional monitoring.

c. Infants who have repeated episodes of symptomatic emesis that prevent achievement of full-volume enteral feedings may require evaluation for anatomic problems such as malrotation or Hirschsprung disease. In general, radiographic studies are not undertaken unless feeding problems have persisted for 2 or more weeks or unless bilious emesis occurs (see Chapter 62).

2. **Established feedings.** Preterm infants on full-volume enteral feedings may have occasional episodes of emesis. If these episodes do not compromise the respiratory status or growth of the infant, no intervention is required other than continued close monitoring of the infant. If symptomatic emesis is associated with respiratory compromise, repeated apnea, or growth restriction, therapeutic maneuvers are indicated.

   a. Positioning. Reposition the infant to elevate the head and upper body, in either a prone or right side down position.

   b. Feeding intervals. Shortening the interval between feedings to give a smaller volume during each feeding may sometimes improve signs of GER. Infants fed by gavage may have the duration of the feeding increased.

3. **Apnea.** Studies using pH probes and esophageal manometry have not shown an association between GER and apnea episodes. Treatment with promotility agents should not be used.

B. **NEC** (see Chapter 27). Nutritional support of the patient with NEC focuses around providing complete PN during the acute phase of the disease, followed by gradual introduction of enteral nutrition after the patient has stabilized and the gut has been allowed to heal.

   1. **PN.** For at least 5 to 14 days after the initial diagnosis of NEC, the patient is kept nothing by mouth (NPO) and receives total PN. The goals for PN were delineated previously in section III.

   2. **Initiation of feedings.** If the patient is clinically stable after a minimum of 5 to 14 days of bowel rest, feedings are generally introduced at approximately 10 to 20 mL/kg/day, preferably with maternal milk or PDHM, although a standard formula appropriate for the gestational age of the patient may also be used (i.e., preterm formula for the typical neonatal intensive care unit [NICU] infant). More specialized formulas containing elemental proteins are rarely indicated.

   3. **Feeding advancement.** If low-volume feedings (10 to 20 mL/kg/day) are tolerated for 24 to 48 hours, gradual advancement is continued at

approximately 10 mL/kg every 12 to 24 hours for the next 2 to 3 days. If this advancement is tolerated, further advancement proceeds according to the guidelines in Table 21.6. Supplemental PN is continued until enteral feedings are providing approximately 100 to 120 mL/kg/day volume.

   4. Feeding intolerance. Signs of feeding intolerance include emesis, abdominal distension, and increased numbers of apnea episodes. Reduction of feeding volume or cessation of feeding is usually indicated. If these clinical signs prevent attainment of full-volume enteral feedings despite several attempts to advance feedings, radiographic contrast studies may be indicated to rule out intestinal strictures. Gastric residuals alone in absence of other physical signs and symptoms of feeding intolerance are not helpful.

   5. Enterostomies. If one or more enterostomies are created as a result of surgical therapy for NEC, it may be difficult to achieve full nutritional intake by enteral feedings. Depending on the length and function of the upper intestinal tract, increasing feeding volume or nutritional density may result in problems with malabsorption, dumping syndrome, and poor growth.

   a. Refeeding. Output from the proximal intestinal enterostomy can be refed into the distal portion(s) of the intestine through the mucous fistula(s). This may improve the absorption of both fluid and nutrients.

   b. PN support. If growth targets cannot be achieved using enteral feedings, continued use of supplemental PN may be indicated depending on the patient's overall status and liver function. Enteral feedings should be continued at the highest rate and nutritional density tolerated, and supplemental PN should be given to achieve the nutritional goals and growth outcomes as previously outlined.

C. **BPD.** Preterm infants who have BPD have increased caloric requirements due to their increased metabolic expenditure and, at the same time, have a lower tolerance for excess fluid intake (see Chapter 34).

   1. Fluid restriction. Total fluid intake is typically restricted from the usual 150 mL/kg/day to 140 mL/kg/day or less depending on severity of lung disease. In cases of severe chronic lung disease (CLD), further restriction to 130 mL/kg/day may be required. Careful monitoring is required when fluid restrictions are implemented to ensure adequate caloric and micronutrient intake. Growth parameters must also be monitored so that continued growth is not compromised.

   2. Caloric density. Infants with CLD may require up to 30 kcal/oz feedings in order to achieve the desired growth targets. Infants with severe BPD should be carefully monitored for proportional growth.

VI. NUTRITIONAL CONSIDERATIONS IN DISCHARGE PLANNING. Recent
data describing postnatal growth in the United States suggest that a significant number of VLBW and ELBW infants continue to have catch-up growth requirements at the time of discharge from the hospital. However,

there is a paucity of data regarding what to feed the preterm infant after discharge.

A. **Human milk.** The use of human milk and efforts to transition to full breastfeeding in former preterm infants who continue to require enhanced caloric density feedings poses a unique challenge. Individualized care plans are indicated in order to support the transition to full breastfeeding while continuing to allow for optimal rates of growth. Usually, this is accomplished by a combination of a specified number of nursing sessions per day, supplemented by two to three feedings of nutrient-enriched postdischarge formula. This method allows the infant to nurse and receive nutrient-dense feedings. Another approach is to continue use of HMF postdischarge. The use of ready-to-feed postdischarge formula will help avoid the exposure to infant formula powder. Infant formula powder is not sterile and does present the risk of *Cronobacter* spp. contamination for the immunocompromised infant. Growth rate data obtained in the hospital is typically forwarded to infant follow-up clinics and the private pediatrician for VLBW and ELBW infants.

B. **Formula choices**

1. **Nutrient-enriched postdischarge formulas.** A meta-analysis of randomized controlled trials concluded that postdischarge formulas have limited benefits for growth and development up to 18 months after term compared with standard infant formulas. In some of the trials, infants on standard formula increased their volume of intake, therefore mostly compensating for any additional nutrients from the postdischarge formulas. The ESPGHAN suggested that preterm infants who demonstrate subnormal weight for age at discharge should be fed with fortified human milk or special formula fortified with high contents of protein, minerals and trace elements as well as LCPUFAs until at least 40 weeks' PMA but possibly for another 3 months thereafter. In practice, preterm infants are considered to be appropriate candidates for the use of these formulas, either as an additive to human milk or as a sole formula choice, once they are >2,000 g and 35 weeks' corrected age. However, the length of time after discharge these formulas should be continued remains unclear.

2. **Term formulas** may also be utilized; however, careful monitoring of growth after discharge should continue.

C. **Vitamin and iron supplementation**

1. The AAP recommends 400 IU vitamin D per day for all infants. Unless they are consuming at least 1,000 mL/day of vitamin D–fortified formula, they will not meet this goal.

2. Preterm infants who are >2,000 g and 35 weeks' corrected gestational age, and human milk–fed, are supplemented daily with 1 mL pediatric multivitamin (MVI) without iron, and with ferrous sulfate drops administered separately. Often, MVI with iron will be given at discharge to infants who weigh >2,000 g to facilitate supplementation adherence by parents. This supplement provides 10 mg iron/mL, and the infant will quickly grow into a goal of 2 to 4 mg iron/kg/day.

3. Preterm infants who are >2,000 g and 35 weeks' corrected gestational age, and fed a combination of human milk and formula, are supplemented with 1 mL vitamin D drops to provide 400 IU per day. Ferrous sulfate drops are administered separately, as needed. The upper limit of vitamin D intake for infants is 1,000 IU per day. The infant would need to consume >1 quart of formula with the 400 IU per day supplement to reach >1,000 IU per day of vitamin D.

4. Preterm infants who are >2,000 g and 35 weeks' corrected gestational age, and formula-fed, are supplemented with 0.5 mL (400 IU/mL) vitamin D drops to provide a 200 IU vitamin D per day supplement + 200 IU per day from the formula. Ferrous sulfate drops are administered separately, if needed.

5. Term infants, who are exclusively human milk–fed, are supplemented daily with 1 mL (400 IU/mL) vitamin D drops, once feedings have been established. Iron supplementation is not indicated until 4 months of age. Earlier iron supplementation of 1 mg/kg is indicated for term infants who have received numerous blood drawings. Low birth weight infants should receive 2 mg/kg of iron.

6. Term infants, who are fed iron-fortified infant formula do not require vitamin D or iron supplements. In a few weeks, their formula volume intakes should provide goal intake of 400 IU per day of vitamin D.

References

1. Fenton TR, Kim JH. A systematic review and meta-analysis to revise the Fenton growth chart for preterm infants. *BMC Pediatr* 2013;13:59. http://www.ucalgary.ca/fenton. Accessed June 23, 2016.

2. Olsen IE, Groveman SA, Lawson ML, et al. New intrauterine growth curves based on United States data. *Pediatrics* 2010;125:e214–e224. http://www.nursing.upenn.edu/media/infantgrowthcurves/Documents/Olsen-NewIUGrowthCurves_2010permission.pdf. Accessed June 23, 2016.

3. American Academy of Pediatrics, Committee on Nutrition. *Pediatric Nutrition Handbook*. 7th ed. Elk Grove Village, IL: American Academy of Pediatrics; 2014.

4. Koletzko B, Poindexter B, Uauy R, eds. *Nutritional Care of Preterm Infants: Scientific Basis and Practical Guidelines*. Basel, Switzerland: Karger; 2014.

5. Agostoni C, Buonocore G, Carnielli VP, et al. Enteral nutrient supply for preterm infants: commentary from the European Society of Paediatric Gastroenterology, Hepatology and Nutrition Committee on Nutrition. *J Pediatr Gastroenterol Nutr* 2010;50:85–91.

6. U.S. Food and Drug Administration, Center for Food Safety and Applied Nutrition. Health professionals letter on Enterobacter sakazakii infections associated with use of powdered (day) infant formulas in neonatal intensive care units. http://www.fda.gov/Food/RecallsOutbreaksEmergencies/SafetyAlertsAdvisories/ucm111299.htm. Published April 2002. Accessed June 23, 2016.

Suggested Readings

Centers for Disease Control and Prevention. Birth to 24 months: boys head circumference-for-age and weight-for-length percentiles. http://www.cdc.gov/

growthcharts/data/who/GrChrt_Boys_24HdCirc-L4W_rev90910.pdf. Accessed June 23, 2016.

Centers for Disease Control and Prevention. Birth to 24 months: boys length-for-age and weight-for-age percentiles. http://www.cdc.gov/growthcharts/data/who/GrChrt_Boys_24LW_9210.pdf. Accessed June 23, 2016.

Centers for Disease Control and Prevention. Birth to 24 months: girls head circumference-for-age and weight-for-length percentiles. http://www.cdc.gov/growthcharts/data/who/GrChrt_Girls_24HdCirc-L4W_9210.pdf. Accessed June 23, 2016.

Centers for Disease Control and Prevention. Birth to 24 months: girls length-for-age and weight-for-age percentiles. http://www.cdc.gov/growthcharts/data/who/GrChrt_Girls_24LW_9210.pdf. Accessed June 23, 2016.

Grummer-Strawn LM, Reinold C, Krebs NF. Use of World Health Organization and CDC growth charts for children aged 0–59 months in the United States. *MMWR Recomm Rep* 2010;59(RR-9):1–15. http://www.cdc.gov/mmwr/pdf/rr/rr5909. Accessed June 23, 2016.

Breastfeeding and Maternal Medications

Nancy Hurst and Karen M. Puopolo

KEY POINTS

- Breastfeeding is beneficial for mother, baby, and society.
- Hospital policies should include strategies to promote nonseparation of mothers and babies and exclusive breastfeeding.
- All breastfeeding infants should be seen by their primary health provider at 3 to 5 days of age to ensure adequacy of milk intake.

I. **RATIONALE FOR BREASTFEEDING.** Breastfeeding enhances maternal involvement, interaction, and bonding; provides species-specific nutrients to support normal infant growth; provides nonnutrient growth factors, immune factors, hormones, and other bioactive components that can act as biologic signals; and can decrease the incidence and severity of infectious diseases, enhance neurodevelopment, decrease the incidence of childhood obesity and some chronic illnesses, and decrease the incidence and severity of atopic disease. Breastfeeding is beneficial for the mother's health because it increases maternal metabolism; has maternal contraceptive effects with exclusive, frequent breast-feeding; is associated with decreased incidence of maternal premenopausal breast cancer and osteoporosis; and imparts community benefits by decreasing health care costs and economic savings related to commercial infant formula expenses.

II. **RECOMMENDATIONS ON BREASTFEEDING FOR HEALTHY TERM INFANTS INCLUDE THE FOLLOWING GENERAL PRINCIPLES**

A. Promote hospital policies that support exclusive breastfeeding and nonsepa-ration of mother and infant during hospital stay, beginning with immediate skin-to-skin contact after birth.

B. Encourage frequent feeding (8 to 12 feeds per 24 hours) in response to early infant cues.

C. When direct breastfeeding is not possible, instruct mother to hand express and/or pump to promote milk production.

D. Supplements to breast milk (i.e., water or formula) should not be given un-less medically indicated.

E. Breastfeeding should be well established (about 2 weeks postbirth) before pacifiers are used.

F. Complementary foods should be introduced around 6 months with continued breastfeeding up to and beyond the first year.

G. Oral vitamin D drops (400 IU daily) should be given to the infant beginning within the first few days of age.

H. Supplemental fluoride should not be provided during the first 6 months of age.

III. MANAGEMENT AND SUPPORT ARE NEEDED FOR SUCCESSFUL BREASTFEEDING

A. **Prenatal period.** During pregnancy, all mothers should receive the following:

1. Information on the benefits of breastfeeding for mothers and infants

2. General information on the importance of exclusive breastfeeding during the maternity hospital stay in order to lay the foundation for adequate milk production

B. **Early postpartum period.** Prior to hospital discharge, all mothers should receive the following:

1. Breastfeeding assessment by a maternal–child nurse or lactation specialist

2. General breastfeeding information about the following:
   a. Basic positioning of infant to allow correct infant attachment at the breast
   b. Minimum anticipated feeding frequency (8 times/24-hour period)
   c. Expected physiologically appropriate small colostrum intakes (about 15 to 20 mL in first 24 hours)
   d. Infant signs of hunger and adequacy of milk intake
   e. Common breast conditions experienced during early breastfeeding and basic management strategies
   f. Postdischarge referral sources for breastfeeding support

C. All breastfeeding infants should be seen by a pediatrician or other health care provider within 1 to 3 days after discharge from the birth hospital to ensure appropriate milk intake, assessed by weight change from birth weight and urine and stool output. By 3 to 5 days of age, the infant should have yellow, seedy stools (~3/day) and no more meconium stools and at least six wet diapers per day. A validated nomogram for assessing newborn weight loss can be accessed at http://www.newbornweight.org/.

1. At 3 to 5 days postdelivery, the mother should experience some breast fullness and notice some dripping of milk from opposite breast during breastfeeding, demonstrate ability to latch infant to breast, understand infant signs of hunger and satiety, understand expectations and treatment of minor breast/nipple conditions.

2. Expect a return to birth weight by 12 to 14 days of age and a continued rate of growth of at least ½ oz/day during the first month.

3. If infant growth is inadequate, after ruling out any underlying health conditions in the infant, breastfeeding assessment should include adequacy of infant attachment to the breast, presence or absence of signs of

normal lactogenesis (i.e., breast fullness, leaking), and maternal history of conditions (i.e., endocrine, breast surgery) that may affect lactation.

a. The ability of infant to transfer milk at breast can be measured by weighing the infant before and after feeding using the following guidelines:

    i. Weighing the diapered infant before and immediately after the feeding (without changing the diaper)

    ii. 1 g infant weight gain equals 1 mL milk intake

4. If milk transfer is inadequate, supplementation (preferably with expressed breast milk) may be indicated.

5. Instructing the mother to express her milk with a mechanical breast pump following or in place of a feeding will allow additional breast stimulation to increase milk production.

IV. MANAGEMENT OF BREASTFEEDING PROBLEMS

A. Sore, tender nipples. Most mothers will experience some degree of nipple soreness most likely a result of hormonal changes and increased friction caused by the infant's sucking action. A common description of this soreness includes an intense onset at the initial latch-on with a rapid subsiding of discomfort as milk flow increases. Nipple tenderness should diminish during the first few weeks until no discomfort is experienced during breastfeeding. Purified lanolin and/or expressed breast milk applied sparingly to the nipples following feedings may hasten this process.

B. Traumatized, painful nipples (may include bleeding, blisters, cracks). Nipple discomfort associated with breastfeeding that does not follow the scenario described previously requires immediate attention to determine cause and develop appropriate treatment modalities. Possible causes include ineffective, poor latch-on to breast; improper infant sucking technique; removing infant from breast without first breaking suction; and underlying nipple condition or infection (i.e., eczema, bacterial, fungal infection). Management includes (i) assessment of infant positioning and latch-on with correction of improper techniques. Ensure that mother can duplicate positioning technique and experiences relief with adjusted latch-on. (ii) Diagnose any underlying nipple condition and prescribe appropriate treatment. (iii) In cases of severely traumatized nipples, temporary cessation of breastfeeding may be indicated to allow for healing. It is important to instruct the mother to maintain lactation with mechanical/hand expression until direct breastfeeding is resumed.

C. Engorgement is a severe form of increased breast fullness that usually presents on day 3 to 5 postpartum signaling the onset of copious milk production. Engorgement may be caused by inadequate and/or infrequent breast stimulation resulting in swollen, hard breasts that are warm to the touch. The infant may have difficulty latching on to the breast until the engorgement is resolved. Treatment includes (i) application of warm, moist heat to the breast alternating with cold compresses to relieve edema of the breast tissue, (ii) gentle hand expression of milk to soften areola to facilitate infant attachment to the breast, (iii) gentle massage of the breast during feeding and/or milk expression, and (iv) mild analgesic (acetaminophen) or anti-inflammatory (naproxen) for pain relief and/or reduction of inflammation.

D. Plugged ducts usually present as a palpable lump or area of the breast that does not soften during a feeding or pumping session. It may be the result of an ill-fitting bra, tight, constricting clothing, or a missed or delayed feeding/pumping. Treatment includes (i) frequent feedings/pumpings beginning with the affected breast, (ii) application of moist heat and breast massage before and during feeding, and (iii) positioning infant during feeding to locate the chin toward the affected area to allow for maximum application of suction pressure to facilitate breast emptying.

E. Mastitis is an inflammatory and/or infectious breast condition—usually affecting only one breast. Signs and symptoms include rapid onset of fatigue, body aches, headache, fever, and tender, reddened breast area. Treatment includes (i) continued breastfeeding on affected and unaffected breasts, (ii) frequent and efficient milk removal—using an electric breast pump when necessary (it is not necessary to discard expressed breast milk), (iii) appropriate antibiotics for a sufficient period (10 to 14 days), and (iv) comfort measures to relieve breast discomfort and general malaise (i.e., analgesics, moist heat/massage to breast).

V. SPECIAL SITUATIONS.
Certain conditions in the infant, mother, or both may indicate specific strategies that require a delay and/or modification of the normal breastfeeding relationship. Whenever breastfeeding is delayed or suspended for a period of time, frequent breast emptying with an electric breast pump is recommended to ensure maintenance of lactation.

A. Infant conditions

1. **Hyperbilirubinemia** is not a contraindication to breastfeeding. Special attention should be given to ensuring infant is breastfeeding effectively in order to enhance gut motility and facilitate bilirubin excretion. In **rare** instances of severe hyperbilirubinemia, breastfeeding may be interrupted temporarily for a short period of time.

2. **Congenital anomalies** may require special management.
   a. Craniofacial anomalies (i.e., cleft lip/palate, Pierre Robin) present challenges to the infant's ability to latch effectively to the breast. Modified positioning and special devices (i.e., obturator, nipple shield) may be utilized to achieve an effective latch.
   b. Cardiac or respiratory conditions may require fluid restriction and special attention to pacing of feeds to minimize fatigue during feeding.
   c. Restrictive lingual frenulum (ankyloglossia/tongue tie) may interfere with the infant's ability to effectively breastfeed. The inability of the infant to extend the tongue over the lower gum line and lift the tongue to compress the underlying breast tissue may compromise effective milk transfer. Frenulotomy is often the treatment of choice.

3. **Premature infants** receive profound benefits from breastfeeding and the receipt of mother's own milk. Mothers should be encouraged to express their milk (see breast milk collection and storage in the subsequent text)—even if they do not plan on direct breastfeeding—in order to provide their infant with the special nutritional and nonnutritional human milk components.

Although mother's own milk imparts the greatest benefit to pre-term and high-risk infants, pasteurized donor breast milk may be an alternative when mother's own milk is not available. When considering donor milk feeding, the product should be obtained from milk banks that adhere to the guidelines established by the Human Milk Banking Association of North America (HMBANA). These guidelines ensure safe handling and maintain the maximum amount of active human milk components. We obtain parental assent prior to using donor milk.

a. Special attention should be given to late preterm and near-term infants (35 to 37 weeks' gestation) who are often discharged from the hospital before they are breastfeeding effectively. Management considerations include (i) mechanical milk expression concurrent with breastfeeding until the infant is breastfeeding effectively, (ii) systematic assessment (and documentation) of breastfeeding by a trainer observer, and (iii) weighing the infant before and after breastfeeding to evaluate adequacy of milk intake and determine need for supplementation.

b. For premature infants <35 weeks, mothers should be encouraged to practice early and frequent skin-to-skin holding and suckling at the breast to facilitate early nipple stimulation to enhance milk volume and enable infant oral feeding assessment.

B. **Maternal conditions**

1. **Endocrine diseases** have the potential to affect lactation and milk production.

   a. Women with diabetes should be encouraged to breastfeed, and many find an improvement in their glucose metabolism during lactation. Early, close monitoring to ensure the establishment of lactation and adequacy of infant growth are recommended due to a well-documented delay (1 to 2 days) in the secretory phase of lactogenesis.

   b. Thyroid disease does not preclude breastfeeding, although without proper treatment of the underlying thyroid condition, poor milk production (hypothyroidism) or maternal loss of weight, agitation, and heart palpitations (hyperthyroidism) may negatively affect lactation. With proper pharmacologic treatment, the ability to lactate does not appear to be effected.

   c. Gestational ovarian theca lutein cysts and retained placental fragments are conditions that prevent the secretory phase of lactogenesis.

2. Women with a **history of breast or chest surgery** should be able to breastfeed successfully. Prenatal assessment should include documenting the type of procedure (i.e., augmentation, reduction mammoplasty) and surgical approach (i.e., submammary, periareolar, free nipple transplantation) utilized in order to evaluate the level of follow-up indicated in the early postpartum period to monitor the progress of breastfeeding and adequacy of milk production and infant growth.

VI. CARE AND HANDLING OF EXPRESSED BREAST MILK.
When possible, direct breastfeeding provides the greatest benefit for mother and infant, especially in terms of provision of specific human milk components and maternal–infant interaction. However, when direct breastfeeding is not possible, expressed

breast milk should be encouraged with special attention to milk expression and storage techniques. Mothers separated from their infants immediately following delivery due to infant prematurity or illness must initiate lactation by mechanical milk expression. Milk expression and storage techniques can affect the composition and bacterial content of mother's own milk. Guidelines for milk collection and storage vary depending upon the condition of the infant: healthy term infant (Centers for Disease Control and Prevention [CDC]) or hospitalized preterm infant (HMBANA and American Diabetes Association [ADA]).

A. **Breast milk expression and collection.** Recommendations for initiation and maintenance of mechanical milk expression for pump-dependent mothers of hospitalized infants include (i) breast stimulation with a hospital-grade electric breast pump combined with hand expression/breast massage initiated within the first few hours following delivery, (ii) frequent pumping/hand expression (8 to 12 times daily) during the first 2 weeks following birth theoretically stimulates mammary alveolar growth and maximizes potential milk yield, (iii) pumping 10 to 15 minutes per session during the first few days until the onset of increased milk flow at which time pumping time per session can be modified to continue 1 to 2 minutes beyond a steady milk flow, and (iv) a target daily milk volume of 800 to 1,000 mL at the end of the second week following delivery is optimal.

B. **Guidelines for breast milk collection** include (i) instructing the mother to wash hands prior to each milk expression; (ii) all milk collection equipment coming in contact with the breast and breast milk should be thoroughly cleaned prior to and following each use; (iii) sterilizing milk collection equipment once a day (HMBANA); (iv) collecting milk in sterile glass or hard plastic containers—plastic bags are not recommended for milk storage for preterm infants; and (v) label each milk container with infant's identifying information, date, and time of milk expression.

C. **Guidelines for breast milk storage** include (based on HMBANA/ADA recommendations for the hospitalized preterm infant with CDC recommendations for healthy term infants included in parenthesis) (i) use fresh, unrefrigerated milk within 4 hours of milk expression (CDC: 6 to 8 hours); (ii) refrigerate milk immediately following expression when the infant will be fed within 96 hours (CDC: 5 days); (iii) freeze milk when infant is not being fed or the mother is unable to deliver the milk to the hospital within 24 hours of expression; (iv) in the event that frozen milk partially thaws, either complete thawing process and feed the milk or refreeze. Milk may be stored in a freezer compartment WITHIN a refrigerator compartment for 2 weeks, in a freezer compartment SEPARATE FROM the refrigerator compartment for 3 to 6 months, or a chest or upright deep freezer for up 6 to 12 months. Milk stored in these conditions for longer periods may be safe but will be of lower nutritional quality due to lipid degradation.

VII. CONTRAINDICATIONS AND CONDITIONS *NOT* CONTRAINDICATED TO BREASTFEEDING. There are a few contraindications to breastfeeding or expressed breast milk feeding. Maternal health conditions should be evaluated and appropriate treatments prescribed in order to support continued breastfeeding and/or minimal interruption of feeding when possible. Most maternal medications

enter breast milk to some degree; however, with few exceptions, the concentrations of most are relatively low and the dose delivered to the infant often subclinical.

A. Contraindications to breastfeeding

1. An infant with **galactosemia** will be unable to breastfeed or receive breast milk.

2. A mother with **active untreated tuberculosis** will be isolated from her newborn for initial treatment. She can express her milk to initiate and maintain her milk volume during this period, and once it is deemed safe for her to have contact with her infant, she can begin breastfeeding.

3. The CDC recommends that **women who test positive for HIV in the United States** should not breastfeed.

4. Some maternal medications are contraindicated during breastfeeding. Clinicians should maintain reliable resources for information on the transfer of drugs into human milk (see section VIII).

B. Conditions that are **not** contraindications to breastfeeding

1. Mothers who are hepatitis B surface antigen–positive. Infants should receive hepatitis B immune globulin and hepatitis B vaccine to eliminate risk of transmission.

2. Although hepatitis C virus has been found in breast milk, transmission through breastfeeding has not been shown (see Chapter 48).

3. In full-term infants, the benefits of breastfeeding appear to outweigh the risk of transmission from cytomegalovirus (CMV)-positive mothers. The extremely preterm infant is at increased risk for perinatal CMV acquisition. Although freezing or pasteurizing mother's own milk may reduce the risk of transmission, there is no evidence that such approaches will benefit very low birth weight infant (VLBW) infants.

4. Mothers who are febrile

5. Mothers exposed to low-level environmental chemical agents

6. Although tobacco smoking is not contraindicated, mothers should be advised to avoid smoking in the home and make every effort to stop smoking while breastfeeding.

7. Alcohol use should be avoided because it is concentrated in milk and it can inhibit short-term milk production. Although an occasional, small alcoholic drink is acceptable, breastfeeding should be avoided for 2 hours after the drink.

VIII. MATERNAL MEDICATIONS AND BREASTFEEDING. Questions commonly arise regarding the safety of maternal medication use during breastfeeding. A combination of the biologic and chemical properties of the drug and the physiology of the mother and infant determine the safety of any individual medication. Consideration is given to the amount of drug that is found in breast milk, the half-life of the drug in the infant, and the biologic effect of the drug on the infant.

A. Drug properties that affect entry into breast milk. Molecular size, pH, pKa, lipid solubility, and protein-binding properties of the drug all affect the **milk-to-plasma (M/P) concentration ratio**, which is defined as the relative concentration of the protein-free fraction of the drug in milk and maternal plasma. Small molecular size, slightly alkaline pH, nonionization, high lipid solubility, and lack of binding to serum proteins all favor entry of a drug into breast milk. The half-life of the medication and frequency of drug administration are also important; the longer the cumulative time the drug is present in the maternal circulation, the greater the opportunity for it to appear in breast milk.

B. **Maternal factors.** The total maternal dose and mode of administration (intravenous vs. oral) as well as maternal illness (particularly renal or liver impairment) can affect the persistence of the drug in the maternal circulation. Medications taken in the first few days postpartum are more likely to enter breast milk as the mammary alveolar epithelium does not fully mature until the end of the first postpartum week.

C. **Infant factors.** The maturity of the infant is the primary factor determining the persistence of a drug in the infant's system. Preterm infants and term infants in the first month after birth metabolize drugs more slowly because of renal and hepatic immaturity. The total dose of drug that the infant is exposed to is determined by the volume of milk ingested (per kilogram of body weight) as well as the frequency of feeding (or frequency of milk expression in the case of preterm infants).

IX. DETERMINATION OF DRUG SAFETY DURING BREASTFEEDING. A

number of available resources evaluate the risk of individual medications to the breastfed infant. Ideally, direct measurements of the entry of a drug into breast milk and the level and persistence of the drug in the breastfed infant, as well as experience with exposure of infants to the drug, are all used to make a judgment regarding drug safety. This type of information is available for relatively few medications. In the absence of specific data, a judgment is made on the basis of both the known pharmacologic properties of the drug and the known or predicted effects of the drug on the developing infant. Clinicians providing advice to the nursing mother about the safety of a particular medication should be aware of the following points.

A. **Resources may differ in their judgment of a particular drug.** Information about some medications (especially newer ones) is in flux, and safety judgments may change over a relatively short period of time. Different resources approach the question of medication use in breastfeeding with different perspectives. For example, drug manufacturers generally do not make a definitive statement about the safety of drugs in breastfeeding. Resources specifically designed to address breastfeeding will take the available data and make a judgment about relative safety of the drug.

B. **The safety of a drug in pregnancy may not be the same as the safety of the drug during breastfeeding.** Occasionally, a medication that is contraindicated in pregnancy (e.g., warfarin or ibuprofen) is safe to use while breastfeeding.

C. **Definitive data are not available for most medications or for specific clinical situations.** There is a need for individualized clinical judgment in many cases, taking into account the available information, the need of the mother for the medication, the combination of different medications taken, and the risk to the infant of both exposure to the drug and of exposure to breast milk substitutes. Consultation with the **Breastfeeding and Human Lactation Study Center** at the University of Rochester can aid the clinician in making specific clinical judgments.

D. The U.S. Food and Drug Administration (FDA) published in 2014 the **Content and Format of Labeling for Human Prescription Drug and Biological Products; Requirements for Pregnancy and Lactation Labeling**, referred to as the **"Pregnancy and Lactation Labeling Rule"** (PLLR or final rule). "The PLLR requires changes to the content and format for information presented in prescription drug labeling in the Physician Labeling Rule (PLR) format to assist health care providers in assessing benefit versus risk and in subsequent counseling of pregnant women and nursing mothers who need to take medication, thus allowing them to make informed and educated decisions for themselves and their children. The PLLR removes pregnancy letter categories—A, B, C, D, and X. The PLLR also requires the label to be updated when information becomes outdated" (http://www .fda.gov/Drugs/DevelopmentApprovalProcess/DevelopmentResources/ Labeling/ucm093307.htm).

X. RESOURCES

A. **LactMed is the drugs and lactation database, maintained by the U.S. National Library of Medicine's Toxicology Data Network (TOXNET).** It is found at http://toxnet.nlm.nih.gov/cgi-bin/sis/htmlgen?LACT. This database includes information on the expected transfer of substances in breast milk, anticipated absorption of substances by the infant, data on maternal and infant blood levels, and possible adverse effects in the nursing infant. Suggested therapeutic alternatives are listed where appropriate. This resource does not offer a specific rating system but provides summary guidance based on available data (or lack of data). All data are derived from the scientific literature and fully referenced; links to PubMed are provided for cited literature.

B. **American Academy of Pediatrics, "The Transfer of Drugs and Therapeutics into Human Breast Milk: An Update on Selected Topics,"** *Pediatrics* **2013.** The American Academy of Pediatrics no longer publishes safety ratings of medications, referring medical professionals to the LactMed web-based resource. This clinical report specifically addresses breastfeeding and the use of antidepressant medications, prescription pain medications, alcohol and drugs of abuse, medications used to treat substance dependence, substances used as galactogogues, common herbal supplements, vaccines, and radioactive substances used in diagnostic imaging.

C. **Hale T.** *Medications and Mother's Milk*, **16th ed.** Amarillo, TX: Hale Publishing; 2014. This book is a comprehensive listing of hundreds of prescription and over-the-counter medications, radiopharmaceuticals, contrast agents, contraceptives, vitamins, herbal remedies, and vaccines, with primary references cited for most. The author provides a "Lactation Risk

Category" rating for each entry as follows: **L1**: safest; **L2**: safer; **L3**: moderately safe; **L4**: possibly hazardous; and **L5**: contraindicated. Many drugs fall into the **L3 category**, which is defined as follows: "There are no controlled studies in breastfeeding women; however, the risk of untoward effects to a breastfed infant is possible, or controlled studies show only minimal, nonthreatening adverse effects. Drugs should be given only if the potential benefit justifies the potential risk to the infant."

D. **Briggs GG, Freeman RK, eds.** *Drugs in Pregnancy and Lactation: A Reference Guide to Fetal and Neonatal Risk*, **10th ed.** Philadelphia, PA: Wolters Kluwer Health; 2015. This book lists primary references and reviews data for medications with respect to the risk to the developing fetus and the risk in breastfeeding. For drug use in pregnancy, the book provides a recommendation from 17 potential categories based on available human and animal reproduction data. For drug use in lactation, the book provides a recommendation from seven potential categories based on available human and pharmacologic data.

E. **Lawrence RA, Lawrence RM.** *Breastfeeding: A Guide for the Medical Profession*, **8th ed.** Philadelphia, PA: Elsevier; 2015. This book includes an extended discussion of the pharmacology of drug entry into breast milk. An appendix contains medications listed by category (analgesics, antibiotics, etc.) and provides available safety ratings as well as extensive pharmacokinetic data for each drug, including values for the M/P ratio and maximum amount (milligram per milliliter) of drug found in breast milk.

F. **The Breastfeeding and Human Lactation Study Center.** The Study Center maintains a drug data bank that is regularly updated. Health professionals may call (585) 275-0088 to speak with staff members regarding the safety of a particular drug in breastfeeding. The Study Center will only take calls from health care professionals (not parents). The Study Center is part of the Division of Neonatology, Golisano Children's Hospital at the University of Rochester Medical Center.

G. **InfantRisk Center—http://www.infantrisk.com.** This center is staffed by knowledgeable personnel providing up-to-date evidence-based information on the use of medications during pregnancy and breastfeeding. They can be contacted at (806) 352-2519 Monday to Friday 8 am to 5 pm CST or online at the address above.

Suggested Readings

American Dietetic Association. Infant Feedings: Guidelines for Preparation of Formula and Breast milk in Health Care Facilities; 2011. http://www.neogenii.com/wp-content/themes/enfold/pdfs/ADA.pdf

Hale T. *Medications and Mother's Milk*. 16th ed. Amarillo, TX: Pharmasoft Medical; 2014.

Hurst NM, Meier PP. Breastfeeding the preterm infant. In: Riordan J, Wambach K, eds. *Breastfeeding and Human Lactation*. 4th ed. Boston, MA: Jones & Bartlett; 2010:425–470.

Jones F. *Best Practice for Expressing, Storing and Handling Human Milk in Hospitals, Homes, and Child Care Settings*. 3rd ed. Fort Worth, TX: Human Milk Banking Association of North America; 2011.

Lawrence RA. *Breastfeeding: A Guide for the Medical Profession*. 7th ed. Maryland Heights, MO: Elsevier-Mosby; 2010.

Philipp BL. ABM Clinical Protocol #7: model breastfeeding policy (Revision 2010). *Breastfeed Med* 2010;5(4):173–177.

Sachs HC; and the Committee on Drugs. The transfer of drugs and therapeutics into human breast milk: an update on selected topics. *Pediatrics* 2013;132: e796–e809. **http://pediatrics.aappublications.org/content/pediatrics/132/3/e796.full.pdf**

Section on Breastfeeding. Breastfeeding and the use of human milk. *Pediatrics* 2012;129(3):e827–e841.

Online Resources

Academy of Breastfeeding Medicine. **http://www.bfmed.org/**. Accessed June 21, 2016.

Baby Friendly Hospital Initiative in the United States. **http://www.babyfriendlyusa.org/**. Accessed June 21, 2016.

Centers for Disease Control and Prevention. **http://www.cdc.gov/breastfeeding/**. Accessed June 21, 2016.

Human Milk Banking Association of North America. **http://www.hmbana.org/**. Accessed June 21, 2016.

InfantRisk Center. **http://www.infantrisk.com**. Accessed June 21, 2016.

International Lactation Consultants Association. **http://www.ilca.org/**. Accessed June 21, 2016.

LactMed database. **http://toxnet.nlm.nih.gov/cgi-bin/sis/htmlgen?LACT**. Accessed June 21, 2016.

La Leche League International. **http://www.lalecheleague.org/**. Accessed June 21, 2016.

United States Breastfeeding Committee. **http://www.usbreastfeeding.org/**. Accessed June 21, 2016.

Weight loss nomograms. **http://www.newbornweight.org/** Accessed June 21, 2016.

Wellstart International. **http://www.wellstart.org/**. Accessed June 21, 2016.

23

Fluid and Electrolyte Management

Elizabeth G. Doherty

KEY POINTS

- Transition from fetal to neonatal life is associated with significant changes in water and electrolyte homeostatic control.
- Sources of water loss in the neonate include kidneys, skin, and lungs.
- Preterm infants are most vulnerable to fluid and electrolyte imbalance.
- Assessment and management of fluid requirement is an essential component of newborn care.

Careful fluid and electrolyte management in term and preterm infants is an essential component of neonatal care. Developmental changes in body composition in conjunction with functional changes in skin, renal, and neuroendocrine systems account for the fluid balance challenges faced by neonatologists on a daily basis. Fluid management requires the understanding of several physiologic principles.

I. DISTRIBUTION OF BODY WATER

A. **General principles.** Transition from fetal to newborn life is associated with major changes in water and electrolyte homeostatic control. Before birth, the fetus has constant supply of water and electrolytes from the mother across the placenta. After birth, the newborn assumes responsibility for its own fluid and electrolyte homeostasis. The body composition of the fetus changes during gestation with a smaller proportion of body weight being composed of water as gestation progresses.

B. **Definitions**

1. Total body water (TBW) = intracellular fluid (ICF) + extracellular fluid (ECF) (Fig. 23.1)

2. ECF is composed of intravascular and interstitial fluid.

3. Insensible water loss (IWL) = fluid intake − urine output + weight change

C. **Perinatal changes in TBW.** A proportion of diuresis in both term and preterm infants during the first days of life should be regarded as physiologic. This diuresis results in a weight loss of 5% to 10% in term infants and up to 15% in

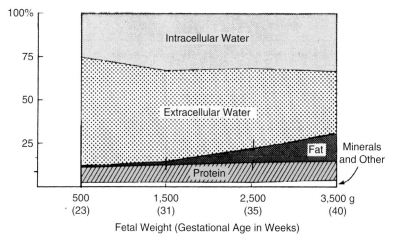

Figure 23.1. Body composition in relation to fetal weight and gestational age. (From Dweck HS. Feeding the prematurely born infant. Fluids, calories, and methods of feeding during the period of extrauterine growth retardation. *Clin Perinatol* 1975;2:183. Data from Widdowson EM. Growth and composition of the fetus and newborn. In: Assali NS, ed. *Biology of Gestation*. Vol. 2. New York, NY: Academic Press; 1968.)

preterm infants. At lower gestational ages, ECF accounts for a greater proportion of birth weight (see Fig. 23.1). Therefore, very low birth weight (VLBW) infants must lose a greater percentage of birth weight to maintain ECF proportions equivalent to those of term infants. Larger weight loss is possibly beneficial to the preterm infant, as administration of excessive fluid and sodium (Na) may increase risk of chronic lung disease (CLD) and patent ductus arteriosus (PDA).

D. Sources of water loss

1. **Renal losses.** Renal function matures with increasing gestational age (GA). Immature Na and water homeostasis is common in the preterm infant. Contributing factors leading to varying urinary water and electrolyte losses include the following:

   a. Decreased glomerular filtration rate (GFR)

   b. Reduced proximal and distal tubule Na reabsorption

   c. Decreased capacity to concentrate or dilute urine

   d. Decreased bicarbonate, potassium (K), and hydrogen ion secretion

2. **Extra renal losses.** In VLBW infants, IWL can exceed 150 mL/kg/day owing to increased environmental and body temperatures, skin breakdown, radiant warmers, phototherapy, and extreme prematurity (Table 23.1). Respiratory water loss increases with decreasing GA and with increasing respiratory rate; in intubated infants, inadequate humidification of the inspired gas may lead to increased IWL. Other fluid losses that should be replaced if amount is deemed significant include stool (diarrhea or ostomy drainage), cerebrospinal fluid (from ventriculotomy or serial lumbar punctures), and nasogastric tube or thoracostomy tube drainage.

Table 23.1. Insensible Water Loss (IWL)

Birth Weight (g)	IWL (mL/kg/day)
750–1,000	82
1,001–1,250	56
1,251–1,500	46
>1,501	26

Values represent mean IWL for infants in incubators during the first week of life. IWL is increased by phototherapy (up to 40%), radiant warmers (up to 50%), and fever. IWL is decreased by the use of humidified gas with respirators and heat shields in incubators. *Source*: Bell et al. 1980, Fanaroff et al., 1972, and Okken et al., 1979.

Incubators for newborn infants are being designed to improve maintenance of warmth and humidity and may lead to decreased IWL (e.g., the Giraffe Isolette).

II. ASSESSMENT OF FLUID AND ELECTROLYTE STATUS

A. History

1. **Maternal.** The newborn's fluid and electrolyte status partially reflects maternal hydration status and drug administration. Excessive use of oxytocin, diuretics, or hyponatremic intravenous (IV) fluid can lead to maternal and fetal hyponatremia. Antenatal steroids may increase skin maturation, subsequently decreasing IWL and the risk of hyperkalemia.

2. **Fetal/perinatal.** The presence of oligohydramnios may be associated with congenital renal dysfunction, including renal agenesis, polycystic kidney disease, or posterior urethral valves. Severe *in utero* hypoxemia or birth asphyxia may lead to acute tubular necrosis.

B. Physical examination

1. **Change in body weight.** Acute changes in an infant's weight generally reflect a change in TBW. The compartment affected will depend on the gestational age and clinical course of the infant. For example, long-term use of paralytic agents and peritonitis may lead to increased interstitial fluid volume and increased body weight but decreased intravascular volume. Therefore, weight should be measured at least daily.

2. **Skin and mucosal manifestations.** Altered skin turgor, sunken anterior fontanelle, and dry mucous membranes are not sensitive indicators of fluid or electrolyte balance.

3. **Cardiovascular.** Tachycardia can result from ECF excess (e.g., heart failure) or hypovolemia. Capillary refill time can be delayed with reduced cardiac output or peripheral vasoconstriction, and hepatomegaly can occur with increased ECF volume. Blood pressure changes occur late in the sequence of responses to reduced cardiac output.

C. Laboratory studies

1. **Serum electrolytes and plasma osmolarity** reflect the composition and tonicity of the ECF. Frequent monitoring, every 4 to 6 hours, should be done in the extremely low birth weight (ELBW) infants during the first few days of life owing to high IWL.

2. **Fluid balance** with input and output measurements should be monitored. Normal urine output is 1 to 3 mL/kg/hour. With ECF depletion (dehydration), urine output may fall to <1 mL/kg/hour. However, in neonates with immature renal function, urine output may not decrease despite ECF volume depletion.

3. **Urine electrolytes and specific gravity (SG)** can reflect renal capacity to concentrate or dilute urine and reabsorb or excrete Na. Increases in SG can occur when the infant is receiving decreased fluids, has decreased urine output, or is spilling glucose. Neither urine electrolytes nor SG is very helpful when infant is on diuretics.

4. **Fractional excretion of Na (FENa)** reflects the balance between glomerular filtration and tubular reabsorption of Na.

   FENa = (urine Na × plasma creatinine) / (plasma Na × urine creatinine) × 100

   a. Level of <1% indicates prerenal factors reducing renal blood flow.
   b. Level of 2.5% occurs with acute renal failure (ARF).
   c. Level of >2.5% is frequently seen in infants of <32 weeks' gestation.

5. **Blood urea nitrogen (BUN) and serum creatinine (Cr)** values provide indirect information about ECF volume and GFR. Values in the early postnatal period reflect placental clearance.

6. **Arterial pH, carbon dioxide tension (PCO_2), and Na bicarbonate** determinations can provide indirect evidence of intravascular volume depletion because poor tissue perfusion leads to high anion gap metabolic acidosis (lactic acidosis).

III. MANAGEMENT OF FLUIDS AND ELECTROLYTES. The goal of early management is to allow initial ECF loss over the first 5 to 6 days as reflected by weight loss, while maintaining normal tonicity and intravascular volume as reflected by blood pressure, heart rate, urine output, serum electrolyte levels, and pH. Subsequent fluid management should maintain water and electrolyte balance, including requirements for body growth.

A. The term infant. Body weight decreases by 3% to 5% over the first 5 to 6 days. Subsequently, fluids should be adjusted so that changes in body weight are consistent with caloric intake. Clinical status should be monitored for maldistribution of water (e.g., edema). Na supplementation is not usually required in the first 24 hours unless ECF expansion is necessary. Small for gestational age term infants may require early Na supplementation to maintain adequate ECF volume.

B. The premature infant. Allow a 5% to 15% weight loss over the first 5 to 6 days. Table 23.2 summarizes initial fluid therapy. Then, adjust fluids to maintain stable weight until an anabolic state is achieved and growth occurs. Frequently assess response to fluid and electrolyte therapy during the

Table 23.2. Initial Fluid Therapy*

Birth Weight (kg)	Dextrose (g/100 mL)	Fluid Rate (mL/kg/day)		
		<24 hour	24–48 hour	>48 hour
<1	5–10	100–150†	120–150	140–190
1–1.5	10	80–100	100–120	120–160
>1.5	10	60–80	80–120	120–160

*Infants in humidified incubators. Infants under radiant warmers usually require higher initial fluid rates.
†Very low birth weight (VLBW) infants frequently require even higher initial rates of fluid administration and frequent reassessment of serum electrolytes, urine output, and body weight.

first 2 days of life. **Physical examination and urine output and SG and serum electrolyte determinations may be required initially as frequently as every 6 to 8 hours in infants <1,000 g** (see section VIII.A).

Water loss through skin and urine may exceed 200 mL/kg/day, which can represent up to **one-third of TBW**. IV Na supplementation is not required for the first 24 hours unless ECF volume loss exceeds 5% of body weight per day (see Chapter 13). If ECF volume expansion is necessary, **normal saline (NS) is preferred over 5% albumin solutions** in order to reduce risk of CLD.

IV. APPROACH TO DISORDERS OF NA AND WATER BALANCE. Abnormalities can be grouped into disorders of **tonicity** or **ECF volume**. The conceptual approach to disorders of tonicity (e.g., hyponatremia) depends on whether the newborn exhibits normal ECF (euvolemia), ECF depletion (dehydration), or ECF excess (edema).

A. **Isonatremic disorders**

1. **Dehydration**

a. **Predisposing factors** frequently involve equivalent losses of Na and water (through thoracostomy, nasogastric, or ventriculostomy drainage) or third-space losses that accompany peritonitis, gastroschisis, or omphalocele. Renal Na and water losses in the VLBW infant can lead to hypovolemia despite normal body tonicity.

b. **Diagnosis.** Dehydration is usually manifested by weight loss, decreased urine output, and increased urine SG. However, infants of <32 weeks' gestation may not demonstrate oliguria in response to hypovolemia. Poor skin turgor, tachycardia, hypotension, metabolic acidosis, and increasing BUN may coexist. A low FENa (<1%) is usually only seen in infants of >32 weeks' gestational age (see section II.C.4).

c. **Therapy. Administer Na and water** to first correct deficits and then adjust to equal maintenance needs plus ongoing losses. Acute isonatremic dehydration may require IV infusion of 10 mL/kg of NS if acute weight loss is >10% of body weight with signs of poor cardiac output.

2. Edema

a. Predisposing factors include excessive isotonic fluid administration, heart failure, sepsis, and neuromuscular paralysis.

b. Diagnosis. Clinical signs include periorbital and extremity edema, increased weight, and hepatomegaly.

c. Therapy includes **Na restriction** (to decrease total-body Na) and water restriction (depending on electrolyte response).

B. Hyponatremic disorders (see Table 23.3). Consider **factitious hyponatremia** due to hyperlipidemia or **hypoosmolar hyponatremia** due to osmotic agents. True hypoosmolar hyponatremia can then be evaluated.

1. Hyponatremia due to ECF volume depletion

a. Predisposing factors include diuretic use, osmotic diuresis (glycosuria), VLBW with renal water and Na wasting, adrenal or renal tubular salt-losing disorders, gastrointestinal losses (vomiting, diarrhea), and third-space losses of ECF (skin sloughing, early necrotizing enterocolitis [NEC]).

b. Diagnosis. Decreased weight, poor skin turgor, tachycardia, rising BUN, and metabolic acidosis are frequently observed. If renal function is mature, the newborn may develop decreased urine output, increased urine SG, and a low FENa.

c. Therapy. If possible, reduce ongoing Na loss. Administer Na and water to replace deficits and then adjust to match maintenance needs plus ongoing losses.

2. Hyponatremia with normal ECF volume

a. Predisposing factors include excess fluid administration and the syndrome of inappropriate antidiuretic hormone (SIADH) secretion. Factors that cause SIADH include pain, opiate administration, intraventricular hemorrhage (IVH), asphyxia, meningitis, pneumothorax, and positive-pressure ventilation.

b. Diagnosis of SIADH. Weight gain usually occurs without edema. Excessive fluid administration without SIADH results in low urine SG and high urine output. In contrast, SIADH leads to **decreased urine output** and **increased urine osmolarity**. Urinary Na excretion in infants with SIADH varies widely and reflects Na intake. The diagnosis of SIADH presumes no volume-related stimulus to antidiuretic hormone (ADH) release, such as reduced cardiac output or abnormal renal, adrenal, or thyroid function.

c. Therapy. Water restriction is therapeutic unless (i) serum Na concentration is less than approximately 120 mEq/L or (ii) neurologic signs such as obtundation or seizure activity develop. In these instances, **furosemide** 1 mg/kg IV q6h can be initiated while replacing urinary Na excretion with **hypertonic NaCl (3%) (1 to 3 mL/kg initial dose).** This strategy leads to loss of free water with no net change in total-body Na. Fluid restriction alone can be utilized once serum Na concentration is >120 mEq/L and neurologic signs abate.

3. Hyponatremia due to ECF volume excess

a. Predisposing factors include sepsis with decreased cardiac output, late NEC, heart failure, abnormal lymphatic drainage, and neuromuscular paralysis.

Table 23.3. Hyponatremic Disorders

Clinical Diagnosis	Etiology	Therapy
Factitious hyponatremia	Hyperlipidemia	
Hypertonic hyponatremia	Mannitol	
	Hyperglycemia	
ECF volume normal	Syndrome of inappropriate antidiuretic hormone (SIADH)	Restrict water intake
	Pain	
	Opiates	
	Excess intravenous fluids	
ECF volume deficit	Diuretics	Increase Na intake
	Late-onset hyponatremia of prematurity	
	Congenital adrenal hyperplasia	
	Severe glomerulotubular imbalance (immaturity)	
	Renal tubular acidosis	
	Gastrointestinal losses	
	Necrotizing enterocolitis (third-space loss)	
ECF volume excess	Heart failure	Restrict water intake
	Neuromuscular blockade (e.g., pancuronium)	
	Sepsis	
ECF, extracellular fluid.		

b. Diagnosis. Weight increase with edema is observed. Decreasing urine output, increasing BUN and urine SG, and a low FENa are often present in infants with mature renal function.

c. Therapy. Treat the underlying disorder and **restrict water** to alleviate hypotonicity. Na restriction and improving cardiac output may be beneficial.

C. Hypernatremic disorders

1. **Hypernatremia with normal or deficient ECF volume**

   a. Predisposing factors include increased renal and IWL in VLBW infants. Skin sloughing can accelerate water loss. ADH deficiency secondary to IVH can occasionally exacerbate renal water loss.

   b. Diagnosis. Weight loss, tachycardia and hypotension, metabolic acidosis, decreasing urine output, and increasing urine SG may occur. Urine may be dilute if the newborn exhibits central or nephrogenic diabetes insipidus.

   c. Therapy. Increase **free water administration** to reduce serum Na no faster than 1 mEq/kg/hour. If signs of ECF depletion or excess develop, adjust Na intake. **Hypernatremia does not necessarily imply excess total-body Na**. For example, **in the VLBW infant, hypernatremia in the first 24 hours of life is almost always due to free water deficits** (see section VIII.A.1).

2. **Hypernatremia with ECF volume excess**

   a. Predisposing factors include excessive isotonic or hypertonic fluid administration, especially in the face of reduced cardiac output.

   b. Diagnosis. Weight gain associated with edema is observed. The infant may exhibit normal heart rate, blood pressure, and urine output and SG, but an elevated FENa.

   c. Therapy. Restrict Na administration.

V. OLIGURIA exists if urine flow is <1 mL/kg/hour. Although delayed micturition in a healthy infant is not of concern until 24 hours after birth, urine output in a critically ill infant should be assessed by 8 to 12 hours of life, using urethral catheterization if indicated. Diminished urine output may reflect abnormal prerenal, renal parenchymal, or postrenal factors (Table 23.4). The most common causes of neonatal ARF are asphyxia, sepsis, and severe respiratory illness. It is important to exclude other potentially treatable etiologies (see Chapter 28). In VLBW infants, oliguria may be normal in the first 24 hours of life (see section VIII.A.1).

A. **History and physical examination.** Screen the maternal and infant history for maternal diabetes (renal vein thrombosis), birth asphyxia (acute tubular necrosis), and oligohydramnios (Potter syndrome). Force of the infant's urinary stream (posterior urethral valves), rate and nature of fluid administration and urine output, and nephrotoxic drug use (aminoglycosides, indomethacin, furosemide) should be evaluated. **Physical examination** should determine blood pressure and ECF volume status; evidence of cardiac disease, abdominal masses, or ascites; and the presence of any congenital anomalies associated with renal abnormalities (e.g., Potter syndrome, epispadias).

B. **Diagnosis**

1. **Initial laboratory examination** should include urinalysis, BUN, Cr, and FENa determinations. These aid in diagnosis and provide baseline values for further management.

2. **Fluid challenge**, consisting of a total of 20 mL/kg of NS, is administered as two infusions at 10 mL/kg/hour if no suspicion of structural heart

Table 23.4. Etiologies of Oliguria

Prerenal	Renal Parenchymal	Postrenal
Decreased inotropy	Acute tubular necrosis	Posterior urethral valves
	Ischemia (hypoxia, hypovolemia)	
Decreased preload	Disseminated intravascular coagulation	
	Renal artery or vein thrombosis	Neuropathic bladder
Increased peripheral resistance	Nephrotoxin	
	Congenital malformation	Prune belly syndrome
	Polycystic disease	
	Agenesis	
	Dysplasia	Uric acid nephropathy

disease or heart failure exists. Decreased cardiac output not responsive to ECF expansion may require the institution of inotropic/chronotropic pressor agents. Dopamine at a dose of 1 to 5 μg/kg/minute may increase renal blood flow and a dose of 2 to 15 μg/kg/minute may increase total cardiac output. These effects may augment GFR and urine output (see Chapter 40).

3. **If no response to fluid challenge occurs**, one may induce diuresis with **furosemide** 2 mg/kg IV.

4. Patients who are unresponsive to increased cardiac output and diuresis should be evaluated with an **abdominal ultrasonography** to define renal, urethral, and bladder anatomy. IV pyelography, renal scanning, angiography, or cystourethrography may be required (see Chapter 28).

C. **Management. Prerenal** oliguria should respond to increased cardiac output. **Postrenal** obstruction requires urologic consultation, with possible urinary diversion and surgical correction. If parenchymal **ARF** is suspected, minimize excessive ECF expansion and electrolyte abnormalities. If possible, eliminate reversible causes of declining GFR, such as nephrotoxic drug use.

1. **Monitor** daily weight, input and output, and BUN, Cr, and serum electrolytes.

2. **Fluid restriction.** Replace insensible fluid loss plus urine output. **Withhold K supplementation** unless hypokalemia develops. Replace urinary Na losses unless edema develops.

3. **Adjust dosage and frequency of drugs** eliminated by renal excretion. Monitor serum drug concentrations to guide drug-dosing intervals.

4. **Peritoneal or hemodialysis** may be indicated in patients whose GFR progressively declines causing complications related to ECF volume or electrolyte abnormalities (see Chapter 28).

VI. METABOLIC ACID–BASE DISORDERS

A. **Normal acid–base physiology.** Metabolic acidosis results from excessive loss of buffer or from an increase of volatile or nonvolatile acid in the extracellular space. Normal sources of acid production include the metabolism of amino acids containing sulfur and phosphate as well as hydrogen ion released from bone mineralization. Intravascular buffers include bicarbonate, phosphate, and intracellular hemoglobin. Maintenance of normal pH depends on excretion of volatile acid (e.g., carbonic acid) from the lungs, skeletal exchange of cations for hydrogen, and renal regeneration and reclamation of bicarbonate. Kidneys contribute to maintenance of acid–base balance by reabsorbing the filtered load of bicarbonate, secreting hydrogen ions as titratable acidity (e.g., H_2PO_4), and excreting ammonium ions.

B. **Metabolic acidosis** (see Chapter 60)

1. **Anion gap.** Metabolic acidosis can result from accumulation of acid or loss of buffering equivalents. Anion gap determination will suggest mechanism. Na, Cl, and bicarbonate are the primary ions of the extracellular space and exist in approximately electroneutral balance. The **anion gap**, calculated as the difference between the Na concentration and sum of the Cl and bicarbonate concentrations, reflects the unaccounted-for anion composition of the ECF. An increased anion gap indicates an accumulation of organic acid, whereas a normal anion gap indicates a loss of buffer equivalents. Normal values for the neonatal anion gap are 5 to 15 mEq/L and vary directly with serum albumin concentration.

2. **Metabolic acidosis associated with an increased anion gap (>15 mEq/L).** Disorders (Table 23.5) include renal failure, inborn errors of metabolism, lactic acidosis, late metabolic acidosis, and toxin exposure. Lactic acidosis results from diminished tissue perfusion and resultant anaerobic metabolism in infants with asphyxia or severe cardiorespiratory disease. Late metabolic acidosis typically occurs during the second or third week of life in premature infants who ingest high casein-containing formulas. Metabolism of sulfur-containing amino acids in casein and increased hydrogen ion release due to the rapid mineralization of bone cause an increased acid load. Subsequently, inadequate hydrogen ion excretion by the premature kidney results in acidosis.

3. **Metabolic acidosis associated with a normal anion gap (<15 mEq/L)** results from buffer loss through the renal or gastrointestinal systems (see Table 23.5). Premature infants <32 weeks' gestation frequently manifest a proximal or distal renal tubular acidosis (RTA). Urine pH persistently >7 in an infant with metabolic acidosis suggests a distal

Table 23.5. Metabolic Acidosis

Increased Anion Gap (>15 mEq/L)	Normal Anion Gap (<15 mEq/L)
Acute renal failure	Renal bicarbonate loss
Inborn errors of metabolism	Renal tubular acidosis
Lactic acidosis	Acetazolamide
Late metabolic acidosis	Renal dysplasia
Toxins (e.g., benzyl alcohol)	Gastrointestinal bicarbonate loss
	Diarrhea
	Cholestyramine
	Small-bowel drainage
	Dilutional acidosis
	Hyperalimentation acidosis

RTA. Urinary pH <5 documents normal distal tubule hydrogen ion secretion, but proximal tubular bicarbonate resorption could still be inadequate (proximal RTA). IV Na bicarbonate infusion in infants with proximal RTA will result in a urinary pH >7 before attaining a normal serum bicarbonate concentration (22 to 24 mEq/L).

    4. **Therapy.** Whenever possible, **treat the underlying cause**. Lactic acidosis due to low cardiac output or due to decreased peripheral oxygen delivery should be treated with specific measures. The use of a low-casein formula may alleviate late metabolic acidosis. Treat normal anion gap metabolic acidosis by decreasing the rate of bicarbonate loss (e.g., decreased small-bowel drainage) or providing buffer equivalents. **IV Na bicarbonate or Na acetate** (which is compatible with Ca salts) is most commonly used to treat arterial pH <7.25. Oral buffer supplements can include citric acid (Bicitra) or Na citrate (1 to 3 mEq/kg/day). Estimate bicarbonate deficit from the following formula:

$$\text{Deficit} = 0.4 \times \text{body weight} \times (\text{desired bicarbonate} - \text{actual bicarbonate})$$

    The premature infant's acid–base status can change rapidly, and frequent monitoring is warranted. The infant's ability to tolerate an increased Na load and to metabolize acetate is an important variable that influences acid–base status during treatment.

   C. **Metabolic alkalosis.** The etiology of metabolic alkalosis can be clarified by determining urinary Cl concentration. Alkalosis accompanied by ECF depletion is associated with decreased urinary Cl, whereas states of mineralocorticoid excess are usually associated with increased urinary Cl (Table 23.6). Treat the underlying disorder.

Table 23.6. Metabolic Alkalosis

Low Urinary Cl (<10 mEq/L)	High Urinary Cl (>20 mEq/L)
Diuretic therapy (late)	Bartter syndrome with mineralocorticoid excess
Acute correction of chronically compensated respiratory acidosis	Alkali administration
Nasogastric suction	Massive blood product transfusion
Vomiting	Diuretic therapy (early)
Secretory diarrhea	Hypokalemia
Cl, chloride.	

VII. DISORDERS OF K BALANCE. K is the fundamental intracellular cation. Serum K concentrations do not necessarily reflect total-body K because extracellular and intracellular K distribution also depends on the pH of body compartments. **An increase of 0.1 pH unit in serum results in approximately 0.6 mEq/L fall in serum K concentration due to an intracellular shift of K ions**. Total-body K is regulated by balancing K intake (normally 1 to 2 mEq/kg/day) and excretion through urine and the gastrointestinal tract.

A. **Hypokalemia** can lead to arrhythmias, ileus, renal concentrating defects, and obtundation in the newborn.

   1. **Predisposing factors** include nasogastric or ileostomy drainage, chronic diuretic use, and renal tubular defects.

   2. **Diagnosis.** Obtain serum and urine electrolytes, pH, and an electrocardiogram (ECG) to detect possible conduction defects (prolonged QT interval and U waves).

   3. **Therapy.** Reduce renal or gastrointestinal losses of K. Gradually increase intake of K as needed.

B. **Hyperkalemia.** The normal serum K level in a nonhemolyzed blood specimen at normal pH is 3.5 to 5.5 mEq/L; symptomatic hyperkalemia may begin at a serum K level >6 mEq/L.

   1. **Predisposing factors.** Hyperkalemia can occur unexpectedly in any patient but should be **anticipated** and **screened** for in the following scenarios:

     a. Increased K release secondary to tissue destruction, trauma, cephalhematoma, hypothermia, bleeding, intravascular or extravascular hemolysis, asphyxia/ischemia, and IVH

     b. Decreased K clearance due to renal failure, oliguria, hyponatremia, and congenital adrenal hyperplasia

     c. Miscellaneous associations including dehydration, birth weight <1,500 g (see section VIII.A.2), blood transfusion, inadvertent excess (KCl) administration, CLD with KCl supplementation, and exchange transfusion.

d. Up to 50% of VLBW infants born before 25 weeks' gestation manifest serum K levels >6 mEq/L in the first 48 hours of life (see section VIII.A.2). **The most common cause of sudden unexpected hyperkalemia in the neonatal intensive care unit (NICU) is medication error**.

2. **Diagnosis.** Obtain serum and urine electrolytes, serum pH, and Ca concentrations. The hyperkalemic infant may be asymptomatic or may present with a spectrum of signs including bradyarrhythmias or tachyarrhythmias, cardiovascular instability, or collapse. The ECG findings progress with increasing serum K from peaked T waves (increased rate of repolarization), flattened P waves and increasing PR interval (suppression of atrial conductivity), to QRS widening and slurring (conduction delay in ventricular conduction tissue as well as in the myocardium itself), and finally, supraventricular/ventricular tachycardia, bradycardia, or ventricular fibrillation. The ECG findings may be the first indication of hyperkalemia (see Chapter 41).

   Once hyperkalemia is diagnosed, remove all sources of exogenous K (change all IV solutions and analyze for K content, check all feedings for K content), rehydrate the patient if necessary, and eliminate arrhythmia-promoting factors. The pharmacologic therapy of neonatal hyperkalemia consists of three components:

   a. Goal 1: stabilization of conducting tissues. This can be accomplished by Na or Ca ion administration. **Ca gluconate (10%) given carefully at 1 to 2 mL/kg IV (over 0.5 to 1 hour)** may be the most useful in the NICU. Treatment with hypertonic NaCl solution is not done routinely. However, if the patient is both hyperkalemic and hyponatremic, NS infusion may be beneficial. Use of antiarrhythmic agents such as lidocaine and bretylium should be considered for refractory ventricular tachycardia (see Chapter 41).

   b. Goal 2: dilution and intracellular shifting of K. Increased serum K in the setting of dehydration should respond to fluid resuscitation. Alkalemia will promote intracellular K-for-hydrogen-ion exchange. **Na bicarbonate 1 to 2 mEq/kg/hour IV** may be used, although the resultant pH change may not be sufficient to markedly shift K ions. Na treatment as described in goal 1 may be effective. **In order to reduce risk of IVH, avoid rapid Na bicarbonate administration, especially in infants born before 34 weeks' gestation and younger than 3 days**. Respiratory alkalosis may be produced in an intubated infant by hyperventilation, although the risk of hypocarbia-diminishing cerebral perfusion may make this option more suited to emergency situations. Theoretically, every 0.1 pH unit increase leads to a decrease of 0.6 mEq/L in serum K.

   Insulin enhances intracellular K uptake by direct stimulation of the membrane-bound Na–K ATPase. Insulin infusion with concomitant glucose administration to maintain normal blood glucose concentration is relatively safe as long as serum or blood glucose levels are frequently monitored. **This therapy may begin with a bolus of insulin and glucose (0.05 unit/kg of human regular insulin with 2 mL/kg of dextrose 10% in water [$D_{10}W$]) followed by continuous infusion of $D_{10}W$ at 2 to 4 mL/kg/hour and human regular insulin (10 units/100 mL) at 1 mL/kg/hour**. To minimize the effect of binding to IV tubing, insulin diluted in $D_{10}W$ may be flushed through the tubing. Adjustments in infusion rate of either glucose or insulin in response to hyperglycemia or hypoglycemia may be simplified if the two solutions are prepared individually (see Chapter 24).

β2-Adrenergic stimulation enhances K uptake, probably through stimulation of the Na–K ATPase. The immaturity of the β-receptor response in preterm infants may contribute to nonoliguric hyperkalemia in these patients (see section VIII.A.2). To date, β stimulation is not primary therapy for hyperkalemia in the pediatric population. However, if cardiac dysfunction and hypotension are present, use of dopamine or other adrenergic agents could, through β-2 stimulation, lower serum K.

c. Goal 3: enhanced K excretion. Diuretic therapy (e.g., **furosemide 1 mg/kg IV**) may increase K excretion by increasing flow and Na delivery to the distal tubules. In the clinical setting of inadequate urine output and reversible renal disease (e.g., indomethacin-induced oliguria), **peritoneal dialysis** and **double volume exchange transfusion** are potentially lifesaving options. Peritoneal dialysis can be successful in infants weighing <1,000 g and should be considered if the patient's clinical status and etiology of hyperkalemia suggest a reasonable chance for good long-term outcome. **Use fresh whole blood (<24 hours old) or deglycerolized red blood cells reconstituted with fresh frozen plasma for double volume exchange transfusion**. Aged, banked blood may have K levels as high as 10 to 12 mEq/L; aged, washed packed red blood cells will have low K levels (see Chapter 42).

Enhanced K excretion using cation exchange resins such as Na or Ca polystyrene sulfonate has been studied primarily in adults. The resins can be administered orally per gavage (PG) or rectally. A study involving uremic and control rats demonstrated that Na polystyrene sulfonate (Kayexalate) administered by rectum with sorbitol was toxic to the colon, but rectal administration after suspension in distilled water produced only mild mucosal erythema in 10% of animals. Another possible complication of resins is bowel obstruction secondary to bezoar or plug formation.

The reported experience with resin use in neonates covers those born at 25 to 40 weeks' gestation. **PG administration of Kayexalate is not recommended in preterm infants because they are prone to hypomotility and are at risk for NEC. Rectal administration of Kayexalate (1 g/kg at 0.5 g/mL of NS) with a minimum retention time of 30 minutes should be effective in lowering serum K levels by approximately 1 mEq/L. The enema should be inserted 1 to 3 cm using a thin silastic feeding tube.** Published evidence supports the efficacy of this treatment in infants. Kayexalate prepared in water or NS (eliminating sorbitol as a solubilizing agent) and delivered rectally should be a therapeutic agent with an acceptable risk–benefit ratio.

The clinical condition, ECG, and actual serum K level all affect the choice of therapy for hyperkalemia. Figure 23.2 contains guidelines for treatment of hyperkalemia.

VIII. COMMON CLINICAL SITUATIONS

A. VLBW infant

1. **VLBW infants undergo three phases of fluid and electrolyte homeostasis:** prediuretic (first day of life), diuretic (second to third day of life), and

Remove All Sources of Exogenous Potassium

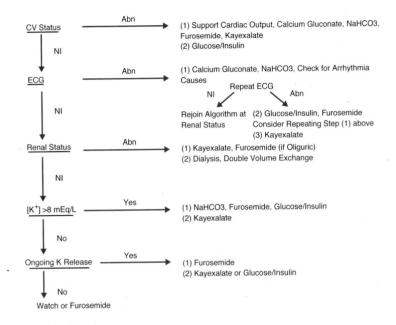

Figure 23.2. Treatment of hyperkalemia. CV, cardiovascular; Nl, normal; Abn, abnormal; ECG, electrocardiogram; IV, intravenous; $D_{10}W$, dextrose in 10% water; GI, gastrointestinal. For a given algorithm outcome, proceed by administering the entire set of treatments labeled (1). If unsuccessful in lowering $[K^+]$ or improving clinical condition, proceed to the next set of treatments, for example, (2) and then (3).

postdiuretic (fourth to fifth day of life). Marked diuresis can occur during the diuretic phase leading to **hypernatremia** and the need for frequent serum electrolyte determinations (q6–8h) and increased rates of parenteral fluid administration. Increased free water loss through skin and dopamine-associated natriuresis (due to increased GFR) can further complicate management. Hypernatremia often occurs despite a total-body Na deficit. Lack of a brisk diuretic phase has been associated with increased CLD incidence.

In addition, **impaired glucose tolerance** can lead to hyperglycemia, requiring reduced rates of parenteral glucose infusion (see Chapter 24). This combination frequently leads to administration of reduced dextrose concentrations (<5%) in parenteral solutions. Avoid the infusion of parenteral solutions containing <200 mOsmol/L (i.e., D_3W), to minimize local osmotic hemolysis and thereby reduce renal K load.

2. **VLBW infants often develop a nonoliguric hyperkalemia** in the first few days of life. This is caused by a relatively low GFR combined with an intracellular to extracellular K shift due to decreased Na–K ATPase activity. Postnatal glucocorticoid use may further inhibit Na–K ATPase activity. Insulin infusion to treat hyperkalemia may be necessary but elevates the risk of iatrogenic hypoglycemia. Treatment with Kayexalate (see section VII.B.2.c) can occasionally be beneficial in infants born before 32 weeks' gestation despite the obligate Na load and potential irritation of bowel mucosa by rectal administration. Na restriction can reduce the risk of CLD.

3. **Late-onset hyponatremia of prematurity** often occurs 6 to 8 weeks postnatally in the growing premature infant. Failure of the immature renal tubules to reabsorb filtered Na in a rapidly growing infant often causes this condition. Other contributing factors include the low Na content in breast milk and diuretic therapy for CLD. Infants at risk should be monitored with periodic electrolytes measurements and if affected, treated with simple Na supplementation (start with 2 mEq/kg/day).

B. **Severe CLD** (see Chapter 34). CLD requiring **diuretic** therapy often leads to **hypokalemic, hypochloremic metabolic alkalosis**. Affected infants frequently have a chronic respiratory acidosis with partial metabolic compensation. Subsequently, vigorous diuresis can lead to total-body K and ECF volume depletion, causing a superimposed metabolic alkalosis. If the alkalosis is severe, alkalemia (pH >7.45) can supervene and result in central hypoventilation. If possible, gradually reduce urinary Na and K loss by reducing the diuretic dose and/or increase K intake by administration of KCl (starting at 1 mEq/kg/day). Rarely, administration of ammonium chloride (0.5 mEq/kg) is required to treat the metabolic alkalosis. Long-term use of loop diuretics such as furosemide promotes excessive urinary Ca losses and nephrocalcinosis. Urinary Ca losses may be reduced through concomitant thiazide diuretic therapy (see Chapter 34).

Suggested Readings

Baumgart S. What's new from this millennium in fluids and electrolyte management for the VLBW and ELBW prematures. *J Neonatal-Perinatal Med* 2009;2:1–9.

Bell EF, Gray JC, Weinstein MR, et al. The effects of thermal environment on heat balance and insensible water loss in low-birth-weight infants. *J Pediatr* 1980;96:452–459.

Bhatia J. Fluid and electrolyte management in the very low birth weight neonate. *J Perinatol* 2006;26:S19–S21.

Lorenz JM, Kleinman LI, Ahmed G, et al. Phases of fluid and electrolyte homeostasis in the extremely low birth weight infant. *Pediatrics* 1995;96(3, pt 1): 484–489.

24 Hypoglycemia and Hyperglycemia

Heather H. Burris

KEY POINTS

- Hypoglycemia is common in the newborn period but remains controversial due to the difficulty in defining hypoglycemia.
- The American Academy of Pediatrics recommends screening asymptomatic at-risk infants (preterm, small for gestational age [SGA], large for gestational age [LGA], and infants of diabetic mothers [IDMs]) and treating hypoglycemia once it is recognized.
- The Pediatric Endocrine Society states that by 48 to 72 hours of life, *plasma* glucose levels should be similar to that of older children and adults (>60 mg/dL).
- *Plasma* glucose is the gold standard, and whole blood glucoses (often measured at bedside) may be approximately 15% lower than plasma levels.
- Hyperglycemia is very rarely seen in the newborn nursery but frequently occurs in very low birth weight (VLBW) infants in the neonatal intensive care unit (NICU).

Hypoglycemia is one of the most common metabolic problems seen in both the newborn nursery and neonatal intensive care unit (NICU). Confirming a diagnosis of clinically significant hypoglycemia requires interpretation of blood glucose values within the clinical context. The definition of hypoglycemia as well as its clinical significance and management remain controversial. Blood glucose levels in the first hours of life are typically lower than normal values of older children or adults. In healthy infants, blood glucose levels can often be maintained in the appropriate range by initiating feeding soon after birth. Most cases of neonatal hypoglycemia are transient, respond readily to treatment, and are associated with an excellent prognosis. Persistent hypoglycemia is more likely to be associated with abnormal endocrine conditions, including hyperinsulinemia, as well as possible neurologic sequelae, but it is not possible to validly quantify the effects of neonatal hypoglycemia on subsequent neurodevelopment.

Hyperglycemia is very rarely seen in the newborn nursery but frequently occurs in very low birth weight (VLBW) infants in the NICU.

I. **HYPOGLYCEMIA.** Glucose provides approximately 60% to 70% of fetal energy needs. Almost all fetal glucose derives from the maternal circulation by the process of transplacental-facilitated diffusion that maintains fetal glucose levels at approximately two-thirds of maternal levels. The severing of the umbilical cord at birth abruptly interrupts the source of glucose. Subsequently, the newborn must rapidly respond by glycogenolysis of hepatic stores, inducing gluconeogenesis, and utilizing exogenous nutrients from feeding to maintain adequate glucose levels. During this normal transition, newborn glucose levels fall to a low point in the first 1 to 2 hours of life (to as low as 30 mg/dL) and then increase to >45 mg/dL, stabilizing at mean levels of 65 to 70 mg/dL by 3 to 4 hours of age.

A. Incidence. The incidence of hypoglycemia varies by population and definition used. Furthermore, blood glucose levels change markedly within the first hours of life, and it is necessary to know the infant's exact age in order to interpret the glucose level and diagnose hypoglycemia. However, a recent prospective New Zealand study of infants at risk for hypoglycemia (defined as a blood glucose <2.6 mOsm [<46.8 mg/dL]) demonstrated that 47% of large for gestational age (LGA) infants, 52% of small for gestational age (SGA) infants, 48% of infants of diabetic mothers (IDMs), and 54% of late preterm infants were found to be hypoglycemic.

B. Definition. In 2011, the American Academy of Pediatrics (AAP) published a clinical report by David Adamkin and the Committee on Fetus and Newborn focused on postnatal glucose homeostasis in late-preterm and term infants. The report provides a practical guideline for screening and management of neonatal hypoglycemia. In the absence of consensus in the literature of exact definitions of hypoglycemia (glucose values or duration), the report guides clinicians to develop hypoglycemia screening protocols to avoid prolonged hypoglycemia in symptomatic infants and asymptomatic at-risk newborns. The Pediatric Endocrine Society also released hypoglycemia guidelines in 2015 which specify that infants >48 hours of age should have higher glucose levels and be evaluated for hypoglycemia with higher thresholds (<60 mg/dL) specifically of *plasma* glucose which is approximately 15% higher than whole blood glucose. The thresholds for treating hypoglycemia depend on the presence of symptoms, the age of the infant in hours, and the persistence of hypoglycemia.

In the AAP report, the authors recommend measuring **blood glucose levels** and treatment for the following:

1. **Symptomatic** infants with blood glucose <40 mg/dL with intravenous (IV) glucose (for symptoms, see section I.D.1)

2. **Asymptomatic** infants at risk for hypoglycemia defined as late preterm (34 to 36 6/7 weeks of gestation), term SGA, IDM, or LGA
   a. First 4 hours of life

   i. Initial screen <25 mg/dL (should be done within first hours after birth), infant should be fed and rechecked, and if the next level, 1 hour later, is <25 mg/dL, treatment with IV glucose should be administered.

   ii. If the second check is 25 to 40 mg/dL, feeding may be considered as an alternative to IV glucose.

   b. Four to 24 hours of life

   i. Glucose <35 mg/dL, infants should be fed and glucose rechecked in 1 hour.

   ii. If glucose continues to be <35 mg/dL, IV glucose should be administered.

    iii. If recheck after initial feeding is 35 to 45 mg/dL, feeding may be attempted.

    iv. Recommendation is to target glucose >45 mg/dL.

c. According to the Pediatric Endocrine Society, by **48 to 72 hours** of life, glucose control should be similar to that of older children and adults. *Plasma* glucose levels should be >60 mg/dL. Bedside reagent strips will be within ±10 to 15 mg/dL and less accurate in the hypoglycemic range. Furthermore, typically bedside whole blood glucose measurements are ~15% lower than plasma levels.

C. Etiology

1. **Hyperinsulinemic** hypoglycemia causes persistent, recurrent hypoglycemia in newborns, and it may be associated with an increased risk of brain injury because it not only decreases serum glucose levels but also prevents the brain from utilizing secondary fuel sources by suppressing fatty acid release and ketone body synthesis. Some cases of hyperinsulinemic hypoglycemia are transient and resolve over the course of several days, whereas others require more aggressive and prolonged treatment.

    a. The most common example of hyperinsulinism is the **IDM** (see Chapter 62). Additionally, LGA infants are at risk for hyperinsulinism. Although women are screened for gestational diabetes during pregnancy, some women either have mild glucose intolerance that is subthreshold for diagnosis or develop late-onset glucose intolerance, and their infants are sometimes LGA and hypoglycemic.

    b. Congenital genetic. Hyperinsulinism is seen in mutations of genes encoding the pancreatic beta cell adenosine triphosphate (ATP)-sensitive potassium channel, such as ABCC8 and KCNJ11 which encode for SUR1 and Kir6.2. Elevated insulin levels are also associated with loss of function mutations in HNF4A gene. Additional mutations continue to be identified.

    c. Secondary to other conditions

        i. Birth asphyxia

        ii. Syndromes such as Beckwith-Wiedemann syndrome (macrosomia, mild microcephaly, omphalocele, macroglossia, hypoglycemia, and visceromegaly)

        iii. Congenital disorders of glycosylation and other metabolic conditions

        iv. Erythroblastosis (hyperplastic islets of Langerhans) (see Chapter 26)

        v. Maternal tocolytic therapy with beta-sympathomimetic agents (terbutaline)

        vi. Malpositioned umbilical artery catheter used to infuse glucose in high concentration into the celiac and superior mesenteric arteries T11–T12, stimulating insulin release from the pancreas

        vii. Abrupt cessation of high glucose infusion

        viii. After exchange transfusion with blood containing high glucose concentration

        ix. Insulin-producing tumors (nesidioblastosis, islet cell adenoma, or islet cell dysmaturity)

2. **Decreased production/stores**

    a. Prematurity (Among 193 late preterm infants in a prospective New Zealand study, 54% were hypoglycemic.)

b. Intrauterine growth restriction (**IUGR**) or **SGA**. Among 152 SGA infants in New Zealand study, 52% were hypoglycemic.

c. Inadequate caloric intake

d. Delayed onset of feeding

3. **Increased utilization and/or decreased production.** Any infant with one of the following conditions should be evaluated for hypoglycemia; parenteral glucose may be necessary for the management of these infants.

a. Perinatal stress

    i. Sepsis

    ii. Shock

    iii. Asphyxia

    iv. Hypothermia (increased utilization)

    v. Respiratory distress

    vi. Postresuscitation

b. After exchange transfusion with heparinized blood that has a low glucose level in the absence of a glucose infusion; reactive hypoglycemia after exchange with relatively hyperglycemic citrate-phosphate-dextrose (CPD) blood

c. Defects in carbohydrate metabolism (see Chapter 60)

    i. Glycogen storage disease

    ii. Fructose intolerance

    iii. Galactosemia

d. Endocrine deficiency

    i. Adrenal insufficiency

    ii. Hypothalamic deficiency

    iii. Congenital hypopituitarism

    iv. Glucagon deficiency

    v. Epinephrine deficiency

e. Defects in amino acid metabolism (see Chapter 60)

    i. Maple syrup urine disease

    ii. Propionic acidemia

    iii. Methylmalonic acidemia

    iv. Tyrosinemia

    v. Glutaric acidemia type II

    vi. Ethylmalonic adipic aciduria

f. Polycythemia. Hypoglycemia may be due to higher glucose utilization by the increased mass of red blood cells. Additionally, decreased amount of serum per drop of blood may cause a reading consistent with hypoglycemia on whole blood measurements but may yield a normal glucose level on laboratory analysis of serum (see Chapter 46).

g. Maternal or infant therapy with **beta-blockers** (e.g., labetalol or propranolol). Possible mechanisms include the following:

    i. Prevention of sympathetic stimulation of glycogenolysis

    ii. Prevention of recovery from insulin-induced decreases in free fatty acids and glycerol

    iii. Inhibition of epinephrine-induced increases in free fatty acids and lactate after exercise

D. Diagnosis

1. **Symptoms** that have been attributed to hypoglycemia are nonspecific.
   a. Irritability
   b. Tremors
   c. Jitteriness
   d. Exaggerated Moro reflex
   e. High-pitched cry
   f. Seizures
   g. Lethargy
   h. Hypotonia
   i. Cyanosis
   j. Apnea
   k. Poor feeding
   l. Many infants have no symptoms.

2. **Screening.** Serial blood glucose levels should be routinely measured in infants who have risk factors for hypoglycemia and in infants who have symptoms that could be due to hypoglycemia (see section I.B).

3. **Reagent strips with reflectance meter.** Although in widespread use as a screening tool, reagent strips are of unproven reliability in documenting hypoglycemia in neonates.
   a. Reagent strips measure whole blood glucose, which is 15% lower than plasma levels.
   b. Reagent strips are subject to false-positive and false-negative results as a screen for hypoglycemia, even when used with a reflectance meter.
   c. A valid confirmatory laboratory glucose determination is required before one can diagnose hypoglycemia; however, if the sample awaits analysis in the laboratory, the glucose level can be falsely low (see section I.D.4.a)
   d. If a reagent strip reveals a concentration <45 mg/dL, treatment should not be delayed while one is awaiting confirmation of hypoglycemia by laboratory analysis. If an infant has either symptom that could be due to hypoglycemia and/or a low glucose level as measured by a reagent strip, treatment should be initiated immediately after the confirmatory blood sample is obtained.
   e. New point of care devices are available to allow for the accurate and rapid determination of glucose levels on small volume samples, but we do not yet use them for routine screening.

4. **Laboratory diagnosis**
   a. The laboratory sample must be obtained and analyzed promptly to avoid the measurement being falsely lowered by glycolysis. The glucose level can fall up to 6 mg/dL per hour in a blood sample that awaits analysis.

5. **Subcutaneous continuous glucose monitors** have been shown to be accurate but have primarily been used in research settings.

6. **Additional evaluation** for persistent hypoglycemia. Most hypoglycemia will resolve in 2 to 3 days. A requirement of more than 8 to 10 mg of glucose per kilogram per minute suggests increased utilization due to hyperinsulinism. This condition is usually transient, but if it persists, endocrine evaluation may be necessary to specifically evaluate for hyperinsulinism or other rare causes of hypoglycemia as listed in section I.D.1.

Many evaluations are not productive because they are done too early in the course of a transient hypoglycemic state or the samples to determine hormone levels are drawn when the glucose level is normal.

a. Critical lab sample. Diagnosing hyperinsulinemia requires measuring an insulin level that is inappropriately high for a simultaneous serum glucose. Evaluation requires drawing blood for insulin, cortisol, and amino acids at a time when the glucose level is <40 mg/dL. The typical critical lab sample includes the following:

    i. Glucose

    ii. Insulin

    iii. Cortisol. Cortisol levels can be used to screen for the integrity of the hypothalamic-pituitary-adrenal axis.

    iv. Beta-hydroxybutyrate and free fatty acid levels. Measurement of plasma beta-hydroxybutyrate and free fatty acid levels can be useful because decreased levels of these substances can indicate excessive insulin action even if insulin levels are not significantly elevated.

b. If the insulin level is normal for the blood glucose level, consider additional testing as indicated below to evaluate for other causes of persistent hypoglycemia such as defects in carbohydrate metabolism (see section I.C.3.c), endocrine deficiency (see section I.C.3.d), and defects in amino acid metabolism (see section I.C.3.e).

    i. Growth hormone

    ii. Adrenocorticotropic hormone (ACTH)

    iii. Thyroxine (T4) and thyroid-stimulating hormone (TSH)

    iv. Glucagon

    v. Plasma amino acids

    vi. Urine ketones

    vii. Urine-reducing substance

    viii. Urine amino acids

    ix. Urine organic acids

    x. Genetic testing for various mutations such as SUR1 and KiR6.2.

7. Differential diagnosis. The symptoms mentioned in section I.D.1 can be due to many other causes with or without associated hypoglycemia. If symptoms persist after the glucose concentration is in the normal range, other etiologies should be considered. Some of these are as follows:

a. Sepsis

b. Central nervous system (CNS) disease

c. Toxic exposure

d. Metabolic abnormalities

    i. Hypocalcemia

    ii. Hyponatremia or hypernatremia

    iii. Hypomagnesemia

    iv. Pyridoxine deficiency

e. Adrenal insufficiency

f. Heart failure

g. Renal failure

h. Liver failure

E. **Management.** Anticipation and prevention, when possible, are key to the management of infants at risk for hypoglycemia (see section I.B.2).

1. **Feeding.** Some asymptomatic infants with early glucose levels in the 30s (mg/dL) will respond to feeding (breast milk or formula). A follow-up blood glucose should be measured 1 hour after the start of the feeding. If the glucose level does not rise, IV glucose infusions are required. Feeding of glucose water is not recommended. The early introduction of milk feeding is preferable and will often result in raising glucose levels to normal, maintaining normal stable levels, and avoiding problems with rebound hypoglycemia. We sometimes find it useful to add calories to feedings in infants who feed well but have marginal glucose levels when weaning off of IV fluids.

2. **Breastfeeding.** Breastfed infants have lower glucose levels but higher ketone body levels than those who are formula fed. The use of alternate fuels may be an adaptive mechanism during the first days of life as the maternal milk supply and the infant's feeding ability both increase. Early breastfeeding enhances gluconeogenesis and increases the production of gluconeogenic precursors. Some infants will have difficulty in adapting to breastfeeding, and symptomatic hypoglycemia has been reported to develop in breastfed infants after hospital discharge. Late preterm infants will sometimes have a delay in achieving adequate oral feeding volumes and should have glucose levels measured. It is important to document that breastfed infants are latching on and appear to be sucking milk, but there is no need to routinely monitor glucose levels in healthy full-term breastfed infants who do not have additional risk factors and are asymptomatic. Although data are emerging about the potential benefits of hand expression of colostrum for IDM for storage prior to delivery, this practice remains controversial and not yet standard of care.

3. **Dextrose gel.** In 2013, the Sugar Babies study demonstrated that use of 40% dextrose gel administration to treat mild hypoglycemia in infants at risk for hypoglycemia decreased NICU admissions for hypoglycemia and led to lower formula feeding rates at 2 weeks of life. Some units are incorporating dextrose gel into their hypoglycemia protocols.

4. **IV therapy**
   a. Indications
      i. Inability to tolerate oral feeding
      ii. Persistent symptoms of hypoglycemia after feeding
      iii. Oral feedings do not maintain normal glucose levels.
      iv. Severe hypoglycemia (see section I.B.2)
   b. Urgent treatment
      i. 200 mg/kg of glucose over 1 minute; to be followed by continuing therapy below
         This initial treatment is equivalent to 2 mL/kg of dextrose 10% in water ($D_{10}W$) infused intravenously.
   c. Continuing therapy
      i. Infusion of glucose at a rate of 6 to 8 mg of glucose per kilogram per minute (see Fig. 24.1).

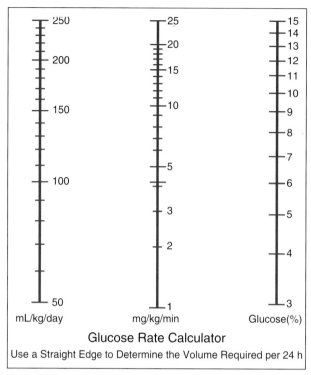

Figure 24.1. Interconversion of glucose infusion units. (From Klaus MH, Faranoff AA, eds. *Care of the High-risk Neonate.* 2nd ed. Philadelphia, PA: WB Saunders; 1979:430.)

ii. Glucose infusion rate (GIR) may be calculated using the following formula:

$$\text{GIR in mg/kg/minute} = \frac{(\text{dextrose \% concentration} \times \text{mL/kg/day})}{144}$$

For example, in an infant receiving $D_{10}W$ at 80 mL/kg/day, the GIR would be $\frac{(10 \times 80)}{144} = 5.6$ mg/kg/minute.

Another way to calculate the GIR can be easily remembered (as it rhymes):

$$\frac{(D \times \text{rate})}{(6 \times \text{weight})}$$

This is equivalent to (dextrose % concentration × mL/hour on the pump) / (6 × weight [kg])

For example, for a 4-kg infant receiving 13.3 mL/hour (80 mL/kg/day) of $D_{10}W$, the GIR would be

$$\frac{(10 \times 13.33)}{(6 \times 4)} = 5.6 \text{ mg/kg/minute}$$

Many hospitals now have computerized provider order entry systems that automatically calculate the GIR.

Additionally, Figure 24.1 helps visualize the GIR depending on total fluid goal and dextrose concentration.

iii. Recheck glucose level 20 to 30 minutes after IV bolus and then hourly until stable, to determine if additional therapy is needed.

iv. Additional bolus infusions of 2 mL/kg of $D_{10}W$ may be needed.

v. If glucose is stable and in acceptable range, feedings may be continued and the glucose infusion tapered as permitted by glucose measurements prior to feeding.

vi. For most infants, IV $D_{10}W$ at daily maintenance rates will provide adequate glucose. The required concentration of dextrose in the IV fluids will depend on the daily water requirement. It is suggested that calculation of both glucose intake (i.e., milligrams of glucose per kilogram per minute) and water requirements be done each day or more frequently if glucose levels are unstable. For example, on the first day the fluid requirement is generally about 80 mL/kg/day or 0.055 mL/kg/minute; therefore, $D_{10}W$ provides about 5.6 mg of glucose/kg/minute, and $D_{15}W$ at 80 mL/kg/day provides 8.25 mg of glucose per kilogram per minute.

vii. Some infants with hyperinsulinism and infants with IUGR will require 12 to 15 mg of dextrose per kilogram per minute (often as $D_{15}W$ or $D_{20}W$).

viii. The concentration of glucose and the rate of infusion are increased as necessary to maintain a normal blood glucose level. A central venous catheter may be necessary to give adequate glucose ($D_{15}W$ to $D_{20}W$) in an acceptable fluid volume. After glucose levels have been stable in the normal range, it is appropriate to taper the GIR and concentration while monitoring glucose levels before feeding. IV fluids should be weaned slowly while feedings are advanced.

5. Historically, providers have administered **hydrocortisone**, 10 mg/kg/day intravenously in two divided doses, if it is difficult to maintain glucose values in the normal range despite 12 to 15 mg of glucose per kilogram per minute. Hydrocortisone reduces peripheral glucose utilization, increases gluconeogenesis, and increases the effects of glucagon. The hydrocortisone will usually result in stable and adequate glucose levels, and it can then be rapidly tapered over the course of a few days. Before administering hydrocortisone, providers might consider drawing a cortisol level. We do not use hydrocortisone routinely for hypoglycemia.

6. **Diazoxide** (8 to15 mg/kg/day in divided doses every 8 to 12 hours) may be given orally for infants who are persistently hyperinsulinemic. This drug inhibits insulin release by acting as a specific ATP-sensitive

potassium channel agonist in normal pancreatic beta cells and decreases insulin release. It can take up to 5 days for a positive effect to be seen. Side effects include fluid retention, and coadministration with a diuretic such as hydrochlorothiazide may be considered.

7. **Octreotide** (5 to 20 μg/kg/day subcutaneously or intravenously divided every 6 to 8 hours). A long-acting somatostatin analog that inhibits insulin secretion. It can be used when diazoxide does not successfully control the glucose level. Tachyphylaxis can develop.

8. **Glucagon** (0.2 mg/kg intramuscularly, subcutaneous (SC), or IV, maximum 1.0 mg) is rarely used. It may be given to hypoglycemic infants with good glycogen stores, but it is only a temporizing measure to mobilize glucose for 2 to 3 hours in an emergency until IV glucose can be given. The glucose level will often fall after the effects of glucagon have worn off, and it remains important to obtain IV access to adequately treat these infants. For IDMs, the dose is 0.3 mg/kg (maximum dose is 1.0 mg) (see Chapter 62).

9. If medical treatment does not control the blood glucose level, consider a 18F-fluoro-L-DOPA positron emission tomography (PET) scan to identify focal lesions in the pancreas and consider surgical treatment by subtotal **pancreatectomy**. Referral to a subspecialty center with experience in these procedures should be considered if a genetic defect of glucose control is suspected or confirmed.

F. **Long-term follow-up and evaluation**

1. Infants with hypoglycemia have been reported to exhibit a typical pattern of CNS injury particularly in the parietooccipital cortex and subcortical white matter. However, it is often difficult clinically to separate isolated hypoglycemia from hypoxic-ischemic encephalopathy plus hypoglycemia. Some clinicians believe it is useful to obtain a magnetic resonance imaging **(MRI) scan** on infants with symptomatic hypoglycemia, but this is not yet standard of care. Close follow-up of neurodevelopmental status is warranted.

II. **HYPERGLYCEMIA** is usually defined as a whole blood glucose level higher than 125 mg/dL or plasma glucose values higher than 145 mg/dL. This problem is not only commonly encountered in low birth weight preterm infants receiving parenteral glucose but is also seen in other sick infants. There are usually not any specific symptoms associated with neonatal hyperglycemia, but the major clinical problems associated with hyperglycemia are hyperosmolarity and osmotic diuresis. Osmolarity of more than 300 mOsm/L usually leads to osmotic diuresis (each 18 mg/dL rise in blood glucose concentration increases serum osmolarity 1 mOsm/L). Subsequent dehydration may occur rapidly in small preterm infants with large insensible fluid losses.

The hyperosmolar state, an increase of 25 to 40 mOsm or a glucose level of more than 450 to 720 mg/dL, can cause water to move from the intracellular compartment to the extracellular compartment. The resultant contraction of the intracellular volume of the brain may be a cause of intracranial hemorrhage.

Although rarely seen in the first months of life, diabetes mellitus can present with severe clinical symptoms including polyuria, dehydration, and ketoacidosis that require prompt treatment. The genetic basis of neonatal diabetes is beginning to be understood and has implications for its treatment (see following discussion).

A. Etiology

1. **Iatrogenic.** Exogenous parenteral glucose administration of more than 4 to 5 mg/kg/minute of glucose in preterm infants weighing <1,000 g may be associated with hyperglycemia.

2. **Drugs.** The most common association is with glucocorticoids. Other drugs associated with hyperglycemia are caffeine, theophylline, phenytoin, and diazoxide.

3. **Extremely low birth weight infants** (<1,000 g), possibly due to variable insulin response, to persistent endogenous hepatic glucose production despite significant elevations in plasma insulin, or to insulin resistance that may in part be due to immature glycogenolysis enzyme systems. Extremely low birth weight infants sometimes must be administered fluids in excess of 200 mL/kg/day, and a minimum glucose concentration of dextrose 5% must be used to avoid infusing a hypotonic solution. When this amount of fluid is administered, the infant is presented with a large glucose load. Modifications to the physical environment (i.e., humidified incubators, see Chapters 15 and 23) that decrease free water loss help limit the amount of IV fluid needed to treat these infants.

4. **Lipid infusion.** Free fatty acids are associated with increased glucose levels.

5. **Sepsis**, possibly due to depressed insulin release, cytokines, or endotoxin, resulting in decreased glucose utilization. Stress hormones such as cortisol and catecholamines are elevated in sepsis. In an infant who has normal glucose levels and then becomes hyperglycemic without an excess glucose load, sepsis should be the prime consideration.
   a. **"Stressed"** preterm infants requiring mechanical ventilation or other painful procedures, from persistent endogenous glucose production due to catecholamines and other "stress hormones." Insulin levels are usually appropriate for the glucose level.

6. **Hypoxia**, possibly due to increased glucose production in the absence of a change in peripheral utilization.

7. **Surgical procedures**. Hyperglycemia in this setting is possibly due to the secretion of epinephrine, glucocorticoids, and glucagon as well as excess administration of glucose-containing IV fluids.

8. **Neonatal diabetes mellitus**. In this rare disorder, infants present with significant hyperglycemia that requires insulin treatment in the first months of life. They characteristically are SGA term infants, without gender predilection, and a third have a family history of diabetes mellitus. They present with marked glycosuria, hyperglycemia (240 to 2,300 mg/dL), polyuria, severe dehydration, acidosis, mild or absent ketonuria, reduced subcutaneous fat, and failure to thrive. Insulin values are either absolutely or relatively low for the corresponding blood glucose elevation. Approximately half of the infants have a transient need for insulin treatment and are at risk for recurrence of diabetes in the second or third decade. Many of the patients with permanent diabetes have

mutations involving regulation of the ATP-sensitive potassium channels of the pancreatic beta cells. Activating mutations of either the KCNJ11 gene that encodes the Kir6.2 subunit or the ABCC8 gene that encodes the sulfonylurea receptor (SUR1) have been implicated in the cause of neonatal diabetes. Repeated plasma insulin values are necessary to distinguish transient from permanent diabetes mellitus. Molecular genetic diagnosis can help distinguish the infants with transient diabetes from those with permanent diabetes, and it can also be important for determining which infants are likely to respond to treatment with sulfonylureas.

9. Diabetes due to **pancreatic lesions** such as pancreatic aplasia or hypoplastic or absent pancreatic beta cells is usually seen in SGA infants who may have other congenital defects. They usually present soon after birth, and survival has been rare.

10. Transient hyperglycemia associated with ingestion of **hyperosmolar formula**. Clinical presentation may mimic transient neonatal diabetes with glycosuria, hyperglycemia, and dehydration. A history of inappropriate formula dilution is key. Treatment consists of rehydration, discontinuation of the hyperosmolar formula, and appropriate instructions for mixing concentrated or powder formula.

11. **Hepatic glucose production** can persist despite normal or elevated glucose levels.

12. **Immature development of glucose transport proteins**, such as GLUT-4

B. **Treatment.** The primary goal is prevention and early detection of hyperglycemia by carefully adjusting GIRs and frequent monitoring of blood glucose levels and urine for glycosuria. If present, evaluation and possible intervention are indicated.

1. Measure glucose levels in preterm infants or infants with abnormal symptoms.

2. Extremely low birth weight preterm infants ($<$1,000 g) should start with a GIR of at least 4 to 6 mg/kg/minute. Glucose levels and fluid balance need to be followed closely to provide data for adjusting the concentration and/or the rate of glucose infusion. Hypotonic fluids (dextrose solutions with concentrations under 5%) should be avoided.
   a. As appropriate, decrease the GIR and closely follow the blood glucose levels.

3. Begin parenteral nutrition as soon as possible in low birth weight infants. Some amino acids promote insulin secretion.
   a. Feed if condition allows. Feeding can promote the secretion of hormones that promote insulin secretion.
   b. Many small infants will initially be unable to tolerate a certain glucose load (e.g., 6 mg/kg/minute) but will eventually develop tolerance if they are presented with just enough glucose to keep their glucose level high yet not enough to cause glycosuria.

4. **Exogenous insulin** therapy has been used when glucose values exceed 250 mg/dL despite efforts to lower the amount of glucose delivered or when prolonged restriction of parenterally administered glucose would substantially decrease the required total caloric intake. Neonates may be extremely

sensitive to the effects of insulin. It is desirable to decrease the glucose level gradually to avoid rapid fluid shifts. Very small doses of insulin are used, and the actual amount delivered may be difficult to determine because some of the insulin is adsorbed on the plastic surfaces of the IV tubing. Unlike in adult intensive care units (ICUs) where insulin and tight glucose control has been shown to increase survival, the routine use of insulin is not recommended in the NICU. The 2011 Cochrane Report on routine strategies to prevent hyperglycemia among VLBWs reported that prophylactic insulin use was associated with higher risk of death by 28 days and no improvements in long-term outcomes among survivors. We use insulin on a limited basis when even low GIRs ($\sim$4 mg/kg/minute) are ineffective at reducing blood glucose levels below approximately 250 mg/dL.

a. Insulin infusion

   i. The standard dilution is 15 units regular human insulin (0.15 mL) added to 29.85 mL normal saline for a concentration of 0.5 units/mL.

   ii. Prior to starting the infusion, purge the IV tubing with a minimum of 2 times the volume of the connecting tubing using the insulin-containing solution to saturate the plastic binding sites.

   iii. Bolus insulin infusion

     a) Dose 0.05 to 0.1 units/kg every 4 to 6 hours as needed (PRN)

     b) Infuse over 15 minutes via syringe pump

     c) Monitor glucose every 30 minutes to 1 hour

     d) If glucose remains >200 mg/dL after three doses, consider continuous infusion of insulin.

   iv. Continuous insulin infusion

     a) Rate of infusion is 0.05 to 0.2 units/kg/hour (usual starting dose is 0.05 units/kg/hour).

$$\text{Flow rate (mL/hour)} = \frac{(\text{dose [units/kg/hour]} \times \text{weight [kg]})}{\text{concentration (units/mL)}}$$

For example:
Ordered dose is 0.05 units/kg/hour, and infant weighs 600 g (0.6 kg).
0.05 units/kg/hour $\times$ 0.6 kg = 0.03 units/hour
Concentration is 0.5 units/mL.

$$\text{Infusion rate is: } \frac{0.03 \text{ units/hour}}{0.5 \text{ mL}} = (0.06 \text{ mL/hour})$$

     b) Check glucose levels every 30 minutes until stable to adjust the infusion rate.

     c) If glucose remains >180 mg/dL, titrate in increments of 0.01 unit/kg/hour.

     d) If hypoglycemia occurs, discontinue insulin infusion and administer IV bolus of $D_{10}W$ at 2 mL/kg $\times$ 1 dose.

     e) Monitor potassium level.

     f) Monitor for rebound hyperglycemia.

b. Subcutaneous insulin lispro

   i. This is rarely used except in neonatal diabetes. A typical dose is 0.03 unit/kg PRN for glucose >200 mg/dL.

ii. Do not administer more frequently than every 3 hours to avoid hypoglycemia.

iii. Rotate administration sites.

iv. Monitor glucose level frequently.

v. Monitor electrolytes including potassium level every 6 hours initially.

vi. Insulin lispro has a rapid onset of action (15 to 30 minutes) and peak effect is 30 minutes to 2½ hours.

c. Oral sulfonylureas have been used in the long term management of infants with Kir6.2 and SUR1 defects.

Suggested Readings

Adamkin DH; and the Committee on Fetus and Newborn. Postnatal glucose homeostasis in late-preterm and term infants. *Pediatrics* 2011;127(3): 575–579. doi:10.1542/peds.2010-3851.

Beardsall K, Vanhaesebrouck S, Ogilvy-Stuart AL, et al. Early insulin therapy in very-low-birth-weight infants. *N Engl J Med* 2008;359(18):1873–1884. doi:10.1056/NEJMoa0803725.

Harris DL, Weston PJ, Harding JE. Incidence of neonatal hypoglycemia in babies identified as at risk. *J Pediatr* 2012;161(5):787–91. doi:10.1016/j .jpeds.2012.05.022.

Harris DL, Weston PJ, Signal M, et al. Dextrose gel for neonatal hypoglycaemia (the Sugar Babies Study): a randomised, double-blind, placebo-controlled trial. *Lancet* 2013;382(9910):2077–2083. doi:10.1016/S0140-6736(13)61645-1.

Thornton PS, Stanley CA, De Leon DD, et al. Recommendations from the Pediatric Endocrine Society for Evaluation and Management of Persistent Hypogly-cemia in Neonates, Infants, and Children. *J Pediatr* 2015;167(2):238–245. doi:10.1016/j.jpeds.2015.03.057.

25 Abnormalities of Serum Calcium and Magnesium

Steven A. Abrams

KEY POINTS

- Hypocalcemia is common in preterm infants but is more likely to occur at a higher ionized calcium level and present as seizures in full-term or near-term infants.
- Intravenous treatment of hypocalcemia must be done cautiously with continuous cardiac monitoring in neonates.
- Hypomagnesemia is commonly seen with hypocalcemia and should be treated.
- Hypercalcemia is also common especially in extremely small preterm infants and requires adjustment of calcium intake when severe in the first days of life.

I. HYPOCALCEMIA

A. General principles

1. **Definition.** Neonatal hypocalcemia is defined as a total serum calcium concentration of <7 mg/dL or an ionized calcium concentration of <4 mg/dL (1 mmol/L). In very low birth weight (VLBW) infants, ionized calcium values of 0.8 to 1 mmol/L are common and not usually associated with clinical symptoms. In larger infants, and in infants of >32 weeks' gestation, symptoms may more readily occur with an ionized calcium concentration of <1 mmol/L.

2. **Pathophysiology**

   a. Calcium ions (Ca^{2+}) in cellular and extracellular fluid (ECF) are essential for many biochemical processes. Significant aberrations of serum calcium concentrations are frequently observed in the neonatal period.

      i. **Hormonal regulation of calcium homeostasis.** Regulation of serum and ECF-ionized calcium concentration within a narrow range is critical for blood coagulation, neuromuscular excitability, cell membrane integrity and function, and cellular enzymatic and secretory activity. The principal calciotropic or calcium-regulating hormones are parathyroid hormone (PTH) and 1,25-dihydroxyvitamin D, (1,25(OH)$_2$D, also referred to as *calcitriol*).

    ii. When the ECF-ionized calcium level declines, parathyroid cells secrete PTH. PTH mobilizes calcium from bone, increases calcium resorption in the renal tubule, and stimulates renal production of 1,25(OH)$_2$D. PTH secretion causes the serum calcium level to rise and the serum phosphorus level to either be maintained or fall.

    iii. Vitamin D is synthesized from provitamin D in the skin after exposure to sunlight and is also ingested in the diet. Vitamin D is transported to the liver, where it is converted to 25(OH)D (the major storage form of the hormone). This is transported to the kidney, where it is converted to the biologically active hormone 1,25(OH)$_2$D (calcitriol). Calcitriol increases intestinal calcium and phosphate absorption and mobilizes calcium and phosphate from bone.

3. Etiology

    a. Prematurity. Preterm infants are capable of mounting a PTH response to hypocalcemia, but target organ responsiveness to PTH may be diminished.

    b. Infants of diabetic mothers (IDMs) have a 25% to 50% incidence of hypocalcemia if maternal control is poor. Hypercalcitoninemia, hypoparathyroidism, abnormal vitamin D metabolism, and hyperphosphatemia have all been implicated, but the etiology remains uncertain.

    c. Severe neonatal birth depression is frequently associated with hypocalcemia, hypomagnesemia, and hyperphosphatemia. Decreased calcium intake and increased endogenous phosphate load are likely causes.

    d. Congenital. Parathyroids may be absent in DiGeorge sequence (hypoplasia or absence of the third and fourth branchial pouch structures) as an isolated defect in the development of the parathyroid glands or as part of the Kenny-Caffey syndrome.

    e. Pseudohypoparathyroidism. Maternal hyperparathyroidism

    f. Magnesium deficiency (including inborn error of intestinal magnesium transport) impairs PTH secretion.

    g. Vitamin D deficiency (frequency in newborn period is uncertain)

    h. Alkalosis and bicarbonate therapy

    i. Rapid infusion of citrate-buffered blood (exchange transfusion) chelates ionized calcium.

    j. Shock or sepsis

    k. Phototherapy may be associated with hypocalcemia by decreasing melatonin secretion and increasing uptake of calcium into the bone.

    l. For late-onset hypocalcemia, high phosphate intakes lead to excess phosphorus and decreased serum calcium.

B. Diagnosis

1. Clinical presentation

    a. Hypocalcemia increases both cellular permeability to sodium ions and cell membrane excitability. The signs are usually nonspecific: apnea, seizures, jitteriness, increased extensor tone, clonus, hyperreflexia, and stridor (laryngospasm).

b. Early-onset hypocalcemia in preterm newborns is often asymptomatic but may show apnea, seizures, or abnormalities of cardiac function although identifying these as primarily due to the calcium level is often difficult.

c. Late-onset syndromes, in contrast, frequently presents as hypocalcemic seizures. Often, they must be differentiated from other causes of newborn seizures, including "fifth-day" fits.

2. **History**

   a. For late-onset presentation, mothers may report partial breastfeeding but rarely, if ever, exclusive breastfeeding. Abnormal movements and lethargy may precede obvious seizure activity. Rarely, use of goat's milk or whole milk of cow may be reported. Symptoms are usually described beginning from the third to fifth days of life.

   b. Hispanic background as a risk factor has been described but is unproven.

   c. Overfeeding may also be identified in the history although this can be difficult to ascertain.

3. **Physical examination**

   a. General physical findings associated with seizure disorder in the newborn may be present in some cases. Usually, there are no apparent physical findings.

4. **Laboratory studies**

   a. There are three definable fractions of calcium in serum: (i) ionized calcium (~50% of serum total calcium); (ii) calcium bound to serum proteins, principally albumin (~40%); and (iii) calcium complexed to serum anions, mostly phosphates, citrate, and sulfates (~10%). Ionized calcium is the only biologically available form of calcium.

   b. Assessment of calcium status using ionized calcium is preferred, especially in the first week of life. Correction nomograms, used to convert total calcium into ionized calcium, are not reliable in the newborn period.

   c. Calcium concentration reported as milligrams per deciliter can be converted to molar units by dividing by 4 (e.g., 10 mg/dL converts to 2.5 mmol/L).

   d. Postnatal changes in serum calcium concentrations. At birth, the umbilical serum calcium level is elevated (10 to 11 mg/dL). In healthy term babies, calcium concentrations decline for the first 24 to 48 hours; the nadir is usually 7.5 to 8.5 mg/dL. Thereafter, calcium concentrations progressively rise to the mean values observed in older children and adults.

   e. Although an association with vitamin D deficiency is uncommon, an assessment of both maternal and neonatal serum 25-hydroxyvitamin D level may be warranted. Values <10 to 12 ng/dL are suggestive of severe deficiency that may be associated with clinical symptoms in some, but probably not most, infants.

   f. Hypomagnesemia is often seen in association with late-onset hypocalcemia.

5. **Monitoring**

   a. Suggested schedule for monitoring calcium levels in infants such as VLBW, IDM, and birth depression who are at risk for developing hypocalcemia:

   i. Ionized calcium: at 12, 24, and 48 hours of life
   ii. Total serum phosphorus and total serum magnesium for infants with hypocalcemia

iii. Other lab tests, including serum concentrations of PTH, 25(OH)D, and 1,25(OH)$_2$D are not usually needed unless neonatal hypocalcemia does not readily resolve with calcium therapy. It is extremely rare that 1,25(OH)$_2$D is ever measured in neonates.

iv. A prolonged electrocardiographic QTc interval is a traditional indicator that is typically not clinically useful in the newborn period.

6. Imaging

a. Absence of a thymic shadow on a chest radiograph and the presence of conotruncal cardiac abnormalities may suggest a diagnosis of 22q11 syndrome, also known as *CATCH22* or *DiGeorge sequence*. Genetic consultation and evaluation may be of value if this is suspected.

C. Treatment

1. Medications

a. Therapy with calcium is usually adequate for most cases. In some cases (see the following text), concurrent therapy with magnesium is indicated.

b. Rapid intravenous infusion of calcium can cause a sudden elevation of serum calcium level, leading to bradycardia or other dysrhythmias. Intravenous calcium should be given for treatment of hypocalcemic crisis (e.g., seizures) with careful cardiovascular monitoring.

c. Infusion by means of the umbilical vein may result in hepatic necrosis if the catheter is lodged in a branch of the portal vein.

d. Rapid infusion by means of the umbilical artery can cause arterial spasms and, at least experimentally, intestinal necrosis and thus is not indicated.

e. Intravenous calcium solutions are incompatible with sodium bicarbonate because calcium carbonate will precipitate.

f. Extravasation of calcium solutions into subcutaneous tissues can cause severe necrosis and subcutaneous calcifications.

g. Calcium preparations. Calcium gluconate 10% solution is preferred for intravenous use. Calcium glubionate syrup (Neo-Calglucon) is a convenient oral preparation. However, the high sugar content and osmolality may cause gastrointestinal irritation or diarrhea.

i. If the ionized calcium level drops to 1 mmol/L or less (>1,500 g) or 0.8 mmol/L or less (<1,500 g), a continuous intravenous calcium infusion may be commenced. For infants with early hypocalcemia, this may be done using total parenteral nutrition (TPN). For use without other TPN components, a dose of 40 to 50 mg/kg/day of elemental calcium is typical.

ii. It may be desirable to prevent the onset of hypocalcemia for newborns who exhibit cardiovascular compromise (e.g., severe respiratory distress syndrome, asphyxia, septic shock, and persistent pulmonary hypertension of the newborn). Use a continuous calcium infusion, preferably by means of a central catheter, to maintain an ionized calcium 1.0 to 1.4 mmol/L (<1,500 g) or 1.2 to 1.5 mmol/L (>1,500 g).

    iii. Emergency calcium therapy (for active seizures or profound cardiac failure thought to be associated with severe hypocalcemia) consists of 100 to 200 mg/kg of 10% calcium gluconate (9 to 18 mg of elemental calcium per kilogram) by intravenous infusion over 10 to 15 minutes.

h. Monitor heart rate and rhythm and the infusion site throughout the infusion.

i. Repeat the dose in 10 to 20 minutes if there is no clinical response.

j. Following the initial dose(s), maintenance calcium should be given through continuous intravenous infusion.

k. Hypocalcemia associated with hyperphosphatemia presenting after day of life (DOL) 3

    i. The goal of initial therapy is to reduce renal phosphate load while increasing calcium intake. Reduce phosphate intake by feeding the infant human milk or a low-phosphorus formula (Similac PM 60/40 is most widely used but other relatively low mineral formulas, including Nestle Good Start, may be used).

    ii. Avoid the use of preterm formulas, lactose-free or other special formulas, or transitional formulas. These have high levels of phosphorus or may be more limited in calcium bioavailability.

    iii. Increase the oral calcium intake using supplements (e.g., 20 to 40 mg/kg/day of elemental calcium added to Similac PM 60/40). Phosphate binders are generally not necessary and may not be safe for use, especially in premature infants.

    iv. Gradually wean calcium supplements over 2 to 4 weeks. Monitor serum calcium and phosphorus levels one to two times weekly.

    v. The use of vitamin D or active vitamin D (1,25 dihydroxyvitamin D) in this circumstance is not usually necessary. If a serum 25-hydroxyvitamin D level is obtained and is <15 to 18 ng/mL, then 1,000 IU of vitamin D should be given daily and the value rechecked in 14 to 21 days. Rarely should higher doses of vitamin D be given to neonates.

l. Rare defects in vitamin D metabolism are treated with vitamin D analogs, for example, dihydrotachysterol (Hytakerol) and calcitriol (Rocaltrol). The rapid onset of action and short half-life of these drugs lessen the risk of rebound hypercalcemia.

II. HYPERCALCEMIA

A. General principles

1. Definition

a. Neonatal hypercalcemia (serum total calcium level >11 mg/dL, serum ionized calcium level >1.45 mmol/L) may be asymptomatic and discovered incidentally during routine screening. Alternatively, the presentation of severe hypercalcemia (>16 mg/dL or ionized calcium >1.8 mmol/L) can require immediate medical intervention. Very mild hypercalcemia (serum calcium 11 to 12 mg/dL) is common and does not require any intervention at all.

2. Etiology

a. Imbalance in intake or use of calcium

b. Clinical adjustment of TPN by completely removing the phosphorus (due to, e.g., concern about excess sodium or potassium intake) can rapidly lead to hypercalcemia, especially in VLBW infants. This commonly leads to ionized calcium values from 1.45 to 1.6 mmol/L.

c. Extreme prematurity. Moderate to extreme hypercalcemia is not uncommon in infants <750 g birth weight on usual TPN mineral intakes. Values up to 2.2 mmol/L of ionized calcium occur. This is likely due to inability to utilize calcium in these infants and may or may not be associated with a high serum phosphorus.

d. Hyperparathyroidism

   i. Congenital hyperparathyroidism associated with maternal hypoparathyroidism usually resolves over several weeks.

   ii. Neonatal severe primary hyperparathyroidism (NSPHP). The parathyroids are refractory to regulation by calcium, producing marked hypercalcemia (frequently 15 to 30 mg/dL).

   iii. Self-limited secondary hyperparathyroidism associated with neonatal renal tubular acidosis

e. Hyperthyroidism. Thyroid hormone stimulates bone resorption and bone turnover.

f. Hypophosphatasia, an autosomal recessive bone dysplasia, produces severe bone demineralization and fractures.

g. Increased intestinal absorption of calcium

h. Hypervitaminosis D may result from excessive vitamin D ingestion by the mother (during pregnancy) or the neonate. Because vitamin D is extensively stored in fat, intoxication may persist for weeks to months (see Chapter 21).

i. Decreased renal calcium clearance

j. Familial hypocalciuric hypercalcemia, a clinically benign autosomal dominant disorder, can present in the neonatal period. The gene mutation is on chromosome 3q21–24.

k. Idiopathic neonatal/infantile hypercalcemia occurs in the constellation of Williams syndrome (hypercalcemia, supravalvular aortic stenosis or other cardiac anomalies, "elfin" facies, psychomotor retardation) and in a familial pattern lacking the Williams phenotype. Increased calcium absorption has been demonstrated; increased vitamin D sensitivity and impaired calcitonin secretion are proposed as possible mechanisms.

l. Subcutaneous fat necrosis is a sequela of trauma or asphyxia. Only the more generalized necrosis seen in asphyxia is associated with significant hypercalcemia. Granulomatous (macrophage) inflammation of the necrotic lesions may be a source of unregulated $1,25(OH)_2D_3$ synthesis.

m. Acute renal failure usually during the diuretic or recovery phase

B. Diagnosis

1. Clinical presentation

a. Hyperparathyroidism—includes hypotonia, encephalopathy, poor feeding, vomiting, constipation, polyuria, hepatosplenomegaly, anemia, and extraskeletal calcifications, including nephrocalcinosis

b. Milder hypercalcemia may present as feeding difficulties or poor linear growth.

2. History

a. Maternal/family history of hypercalcemia or hypocalcemia, parathyroid disorders, and nephrocalcinosis

b. Family history of hypercalcemia or familial hypocalciuric hypercalcemia

c. Manipulations of TPN

3. Physical examination

a. Small for dates (hyperparathyroidism, Williams syndrome)

b. Craniotabes, fractures (hyperparathyroidism), or characteristic bone dysplasia (hypophosphatasia)

c. Elfin facies (Williams syndrome)

d. Cardiac murmur (supravalvular aortic stenosis and peripheral pulmonic stenosis associated with Williams syndrome)

e. Indurated, bluish-red lesions (subcutaneous fat necrosis)

f. Evidence of hyperthyroidism

4. Laboratory evaluation

a. The clinical history, serum and urine mineral levels of phosphorus, and the urinary calcium:creatinine ratio ($[U_{Ca}/U_{Cr}]$) should suggest a likely diagnosis.

    i. A very elevated serum calcium level (>16 mg/dL) usually indicates primary hyperparathyroidism or, in VLBW infants, phosphate depletion or the inability to utilize calcium for bone formation.

    ii. Low serum phosphorus level indicates phosphate depletion, hyperparathyroidism, or familial hypocalciuric hypercalcemia.

    iii. Very low U_{Ca}/U_{Cr} suggests familial hypocalciuric hypercalcemia.

b. Specific serum hormone levels (PTH, 25(OH)D) may confirm the diagnostic impression in cases where obvious manipulations of diet/TPN are not apparent. Measurement of 1,25 dihydroxyvitamin D is rarely indicated unless hypercalcemia persists in infants $>1,000$ g with no other apparent etiology.

c. A very low level of serum alkaline phosphatase activity suggests hypophosphatasia (confirmed by increased urinary phosphoethanolamine level).

d. Radiography of hand/wrist may suggest hyperparathyroidism (demineralization, subperiosteal resorption) or hypervitaminosis D (submetaphyseal rarefaction).

C. Treatment

1. Emergency medical treatment (symptomatic or calcium >16 mg/dL, ionized Ca >1.8 mmol/L)

a. Volume expansion with isotonic saline solution. Hydration and sodium promote urinary calcium excretion. If cardiac function is normal, infuse normal saline solution (10 to 20 mL/kg) over 15 to 30 minutes.

b. Furosemide (1 mg/kg intravenously) induces calciuria.

2. Inorganic phosphate may lower serum calcium levels in hypophosphatemic patients by inhibiting bone resorption and promoting bone mineral accretion.

a. Glucocorticoids are effective in hypervitaminosis A and D and subcutaneous fat necrosis by inhibiting both bone resorption and intestinal calcium absorption; they are ineffective in hyperparathyroidism.

b. Low-calcium, low-vitamin D diets are an effective adjunctive therapy for subcutaneous fat necrosis and Williams syndrome.

c. Calcitonin is a potent inhibitor of bone resorption. The antihypercalcemic effect is transient but may be prolonged if glucocorticoids are used concomitantly. There is little reported experience in neonates.

d. Parathyroidectomy with autologous reimplantation may be indicated for severe persistent neonatal hyperparathyroidism.

III. DISORDERS OF MAGNESIUM: HYPO- AND HYPERMAGNESEMIA

A. Etiology

1. Hypermagnesemia is usually due to an exogenous magnesium load exceeding renal excretion capacity.

   a. Magnesium sulfate therapy for maternal preeclampsia or preterm labor

   b. Administration of magnesium-containing antacids to the newborn

   c. Excessive magnesium in parenteral nutrition

   d. Hypomagnesemia is uncommon but is often seen with late-onset hypocalcemia.

B. Diagnosis

1. Elevated serum magnesium level (>3 mg/dL) suggests hypermagnesemia although symptoms are uncommon with serum values <4 to 5 mg/dL. Low serum magnesium level of <1.6 mg/dL suggests hypomagnesemia.

2. Severe hypermagnesemic symptoms are unusual in neonates with serum magnesium level <6 mg/dL. The common curariform effects include apnea, respiratory depression, lethargy, hypotonia, hyporeflexia, poor suck, decreased intestinal motility, and delayed passage of meconium.

3. Hypomagnesemia is usually seen along with hypocalcemia in the newborn. Hypomagnesemic symptoms can also include apnea and poor motor tone.

4. Hypomagnesemia may be seen with therapeutic cooling in the newborn.

C. Treatment

1. Hypocalcemic seizures with concurrent hypomagnesemia should include treatment for the hypomagnesemia.

   a. The preferred preparation for treatment is magnesium sulfate. The 50% solution contains 500 mg or 4 mEq/mL

   b. Correct severe hypomagnesemia (<1.6 mg/dL) with 50 mg/kg of magnesium sulfate intravenously given over 1 to 2 hours. When administering intravenously, infuse slowly and monitor heart rate. The dose may be repeated after 12 hours. Obtain serum magnesium levels before each dose.

2. Often, the only intervention necessary for hypermagnesemia is removal of the source of exogenous magnesium.

3. Exchange transfusion, peritoneal dialysis, and hemodialysis are not used in the newborn period.

4. For hypermagnesemic babies, begin feedings only after suck and intestinal motility are established. Rarely, respiratory support may be needed.

Suggested Readings

Abrams SA. Committee on Nutrition. Calcium and vitamin D requirements of enterally fed preterm infants. *Pediatrics* 2013;131(5):e1675–e1683.

Abrams SA, Tiosano D. Disorders of calcium, phosphorus, and magnesium metabolism in the neonate. In: Martin RJ, Fanaroff AA, Walsh MC, eds. *Fanaroff and Martin's Neonatal Perinatal Medicine*. 10th ed. Philadelphia, PA: Elsevier Saunders; 2015;1460–1489.

Tsang RC. Calcium, phosphorus, and magnesium metabolism. In: Polin RA, Fox WW, eds. *Fetal and Neonatal Physiology*. 2nd ed. Philadelphia, PA: WB Saunders; 1992;2308–2329.

Neonatal Hyperbilirubinemia

Ann R. Stark and Vinod K. Bhutani

KEY POINTS

- Visual inspection is **not** a reliable measure of bilirubin level.
- Jaundice identified prior to age 24 hours is a medical emergency and may result from excessive bilirubin production.
- Bilirubin measurement and identification of risk factors before discharge of healthy term and late preterm infants predicts need for phototherapy and guides timing of follow-up.
- Evaluation of cholestasis in infants with jaundice at 2 weeks of age ensures prompt therapy of treatable disorders.

I. **BACKGROUND.** Almost all newborn infants have a serum or plasma total bilirubin (TB) level >1 mg/dL in contrast to normal adults in whom the normal TB level is <1 mg/dL. Approximately 85% of all term newborns and most preterm infants develop clinical jaundice. Also, 6.1% of well term newborns have a peak TB level >12.9 mg/dL. A TB level >15 mg/dL is found in 3% of normal term infants.

II. **BILIRUBIN METABOLISM.** The TB level results from the balance of bilirubin production and excretion.

A. **Bilirubin production.** Bilirubin is derived from the breakdown of heme-containing proteins in the reticuloendothelial system. A normal newborn produces 6 to 10 mg of bilirubin/kg/day, greater than the adult production of 3 to 4 mg/kg/day.

1. **Red blood cell (RBC) hemoglobin** is the major heme-containing protein. Hemoglobin released from senescent RBCs in the reticuloendothelial system or from ineffective erythropoiesis accounts for 80% to 90% of bilirubin production. One gram of hemoglobin produces 34 mg of bilirubin. Breakdown of other heme-containing proteins such as cytochromes and catalase contributes the remaining 10% to 20% of bilirubin.

2. **Bilirubin metabolism.** The microsomal enzyme heme oxygenase located in the liver, spleen, and nucleated cells oxidizes the heme ring from heme-containing proteins to **biliverdin** and **carbon monoxide (CO)**

(excreted from the lung); the **iron** that is released is reused. The enzyme **biliverdin reductase** reduces biliverdin to bilirubin. Because heme breakdown yields equimolar amounts of CO and biliverdin, bilirubin production can be indirectly assessed by measuring CO production.

B. Bilirubin clearance and excretion

1. **Transport.** Bilirubin is nonpolar, insoluble in water, and is transported to liver cells bound to serum **albumin**. Bilirubin bound to albumin does not usually enter the central nervous system (CNS) and is thought to be nontoxic. Displacement of bilirubin from albumin by acidosis, drugs, such as ceftriaxone, or by free fatty acids (FFAs) at high molar ratios of FFA:albumin may increase bilirubin toxicity.

2. **Hepatic uptake.** Nonpolar, fat-soluble bilirubin (dissociated from albumin) crosses the hepatocyte plasma membrane and is bound mainly to cytoplasmic **ligandin** (Y protein) for transport to the smooth endoplasmic reticulum.

3. **Conjugation.** In hepatocytes, the enzyme **uridine diphosphoglucuronate glucuronosyltransferase (UGT1A1)** catalyzes the conjugation of bilirubin with glucuronic acid, resulting in mostly bilirubin diglucuronides and some monoglucuronides that are more water-soluble than unconjugated bilirubin. Both forms of conjugated bilirubin are excreted into the bile canaliculi against a concentration gradient.

   Inherited deficiencies and polymorphisms of the conjugating enzyme gene can cause severe hyperbilirubinemia in newborns. **Polymorphisms in the UGT1A gene due to differences in the number of thymine-adenine repeats in the promotor gene** diminish the expression of the UGT1A1 enzyme and result in increased TB levels (Gilbert syndrome). Differences in these polymorphisms in individuals of different ancestry contribute to the racial variation in conjugating ability and neonatal hyperbilirubinemia among Caucasian, Asian, and African populations. In addition, a mutation in the UGT1A1 gene that is common in East Asians contributes to an increased risk of severe neonatal hyperbilirubinemia in that population.

4. **Excretion.** Conjugated bilirubin is secreted into the bile and then excreted into the gastrointestinal (GI) tract where it is eliminated in the stool. Conjugated bilirubin is not reabsorbed from the bowel unless it is deconjugated by the intestinal enzyme **β-glucuronidase**, present in the neonatal intestinal mucosa. Resorption of bilirubin from the GI tract and delivery back to the liver for reconjugation is called the **enterohepatic circulation**. Intestinal bacteria, present in adults but to a limited extent in newborns, can prevent enterohepatic circulation of bilirubin by reducing conjugated bilirubin to **urobilin**, which is not a substrate for β-glucuronidase.

5. **Fetal bilirubin metabolism.** Most unconjugated bilirubin formed by the fetus is cleared by the placenta into the maternal circulation. Formation of conjugated bilirubin is limited in the fetus because of decreased fetal hepatic blood flow, decreased hepatic ligandin, and decreased UGT1A1 activity. The small amount of conjugated bilirubin excreted into the fetal gut is usually hydrolyzed by β-glucuronidase and resorbed.

Bilirubin is normally found in amniotic fluid by 12 weeks' gestation and is usually absent by 37 weeks' gestation. Increased amniotic fluid bilirubin is found in hemolytic disease of the newborn and in fetal intestinal obstruction below the bile ducts.

III. NONPATHOLOGIC HYPERBILIRUBINEMIA. The serum TB level of most newborn infants rises to >2 mg/dL in the first week after birth. This level usually rises in full-term infants to a peak of 6 to 8 mg/dL by 3 to 5 days of age and then falls. A rise to 12 mg/dL is in the physiologic range. In preterm infants, the peak may be 10 to 12 mg/dL on the fifth day after birth, and can rise further in the absence of treatment without any specific abnormality of bilirubin metabolism, and may not be benign based on the infant's gestational age. Levels <2 mg/dL may not be seen until 1 month of age in both full-term and preterm infants. This nonpathologic jaundice is attributed to the following mechanisms:

A. **Increased bilirubin production due to the following:**

1. Increased RBC volume per kilogram and decreased RBC survival (90 days vs. 120 days) in infants compared to adults

2. Increased ineffective erythropoiesis and increased turnover of nonhemoglobin heme proteins

B. **Defective uptake** of bilirubin from plasma caused by decreased ligandin and binding of ligandin by other anions

C. **Decreased clearance** due to decreased UGT1A1 activity. In term infants at 7 days of age, UGT activity is approximately 1% that of adults and does not reach adult levels until at least 3 months of age.

D. **Decreased hepatic excretion** of bilirubin. Increased enterohepatic circulation caused by high levels of intestinal β-glucuronidase, preponderance of bilirubin monoglucuronide rather than diglucuronide, decreased intestinal bacteria, and decreased gut motility with poor evacuation of bilirubin-laden meconium

IV. HYPERBILIRUBINEMIA is defined as a TB >95th percentile on the hour-specific Bhutani nomogram (Fig. 26.1).

A. The following situations suggest severe hyperbilirubinemia and require evaluation:

1. Onset of jaundice before 24 hours of age

2. An elevation of TB that requires phototherapy (Fig. 26.2)

3. Rate of rise in total serum bilirubin (TSB) or transcutaneous bilirubin (TcB) level of >0.2 mg/dL/hour

4. Associated signs of illness such as vomiting, lethargy, poor feeding, excessive weight loss, apnea, tachypnea, or temperature instability

5. Jaundice persisting after 14 days in a term infant

B. **Causes of hyperbilirubinemia**

1. **Increased bilirubin production.** Hemolytic disease is the most common cause of hyperbilirubinemia (see Chapter 45). This includes

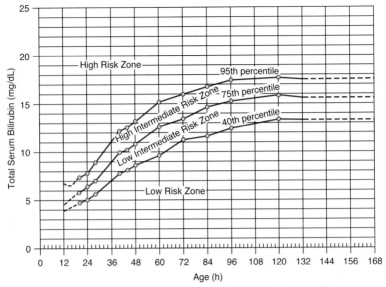

Risk designation of term and near-term well newborns based on their hour-specific serum bilirubin values. The high-risk zone is designated by the 95th percentile track. The intermediate-risk zone is subdivided to upper- and lower-risk zones by the 75th percentile track. The low-risk zone has been electively and statistically defined by the 40th percentile track. (Dotted extensions are based on <300 TSB values/epoch). This study is based on heel stick venous bilirubins.

Figure 26.1. Hour-specific bilirubin nomogram. Predictive ability of a predischarge hour-specific serum bilirubin for subsequent significant hyperbilirubinemia in healthy term and near-term newborns. (Reprinted with permission from Bhutani VK, Johnson L, Sivieri EM. Predictive ability of predischarge hour-specific serum bilirubin for subsequent significant hyperbilirubinemia in healthy term and near-term newborns. *Pediatrics* 1999;103:6–14.)

RBC disorders such as isoimmunization (e.g., Rh ABO and minor blood group incompatibility), erythrocyte biochemical abnormalities such as glucose-6-phosphate dehydrogenase or pyruvate kinase deficiencies, or abnormal erythrocyte morphology such as hereditary spherocytosis (HS). Other causes of increased RBC breakdown are sepsis, sequestered blood due to bruising or cephalohematoma, and polycythemia.

2. **Decreased bilirubin clearance**
   a. Mutations in the gene that encodes UGT1A1 decrease bilirubin conjugation, reducing hepatic clearance and increasing serum TB levels.
   b. Crigler-Najjar syndrome due to either absent UGT activity (type I) or reduced UGT activity (type II) results in severe hyperbilirubinemia.
   c. Gilbert syndrome results from a mutation in the promoter region of the UGT1A1 gene, reducing production of UGT, and is the most common inherited disorder of bilirubin glucuronidation. Although the

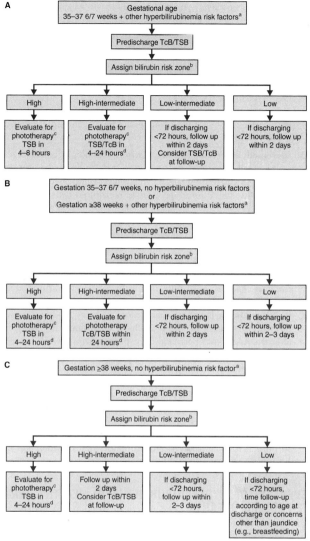

- Provide lactation evolution and support for all breastfeeding mothers.
- Recommendation for timing of repeat TSB measurement depends on age at measurement and how far the TSB level is above the 95th percentile (Fig 26.1). Higher and earlier initial TSB levels require an earlier repeat TSB measurement.
- Perform standard clinical evaluation at all follow-up visits.
- For evaluation of Jaundice, see 2004 AAP guideline.
- [a] Table 26.1. [b] Fig 26.1. [c] Fig 26.3. [d] In hospital or as outpatient. [e] Follow-up recommendations can be modified according to level of risk for hyperbilirubinemia; depending on the circumstances in infants at low risk, later follow-up can be considered.

Figure 26.2. Algorithm providing recommendations for management and follow-up according to predischarge bilirubin measurements, gestation, and risk factors for subsequent hyperbilirubinemia. (From Maisels MJ, Bhutani VK, Bogen D, et al. Hyperbilirubinemia in the newborn infant ≥35 weeks' gestation: an update with clarifications. *Pediatrics* 2009;124:1193–1198.)

Gilbert genotype alone is not associated with increased hyperbilirubinemia, severe hyperbilirubinemia can result when an affected newborn also has increased bilirubin production or increased enterohepatic circulation.

d. Polymorphisms of the organic anion transporter protein OATP-2 may lead to severe hyperbilirubinemia, especially when combined with a UGT1A1 mutation.

e. Decreased clearance may occur in infants of diabetic mothers and with congenital hypothyroidism, galactosemia, and other inherited metabolic disorders.

3. **Increased enterohepatic circulation.** Pathologic conditions leading to increased enterohepatic circulation include decreased enteral intake, including breastfeeding failure; breast milk jaundice; or impaired intestinal motility due to intestinal atresias, meconium ileus, or Hirschsprung disease.

a. Breastfeeding failure jaundice. Infants who are breastfed have higher bilirubin levels on day 3 of age compared to formula-fed infants. Breastfeeding failure jaundice typically occurs with lactation failure during the first postnatal week that leads to insufficient intake, with weight loss and sometimes hypernatremia. Hyperbilirubinemia is attributed mainly to the decreased intake of milk that leads to slower bilirubin elimination and increased enterohepatic circulation.

b. "Breast milk jaundice" (condition that may be due to genetic predisposition) **occurs in about 2.4% of all infants.** Typically, it begins after the first 3 to 5 postnatal days, peaks within 2 weeks of age, and if breastfeeding is continued, gradually returns to normal levels over 3 to 12 weeks. If breastfeeding is stopped, the bilirubin level may fall rapidly in 48 hours. If nursing is then resumed, the bilirubin may rise by 2 to 4 mg/dL but usually will not reach the previous high level. Affected infants have good weight gain, normal liver function test (LFT) results, and no evidence of hemolysis. The mechanism of breast milk jaundice is thought to be either associated with Gilbert disease or perhaps a factor in human milk, possibly β-glucuronidase, that deconjugates intestinal bilirubin and promotes its absorption.

V. PREVENTION OF HYPERBILIRUBINEMIA IN HEALTHY TERM AND LATE-PRETERM INFANTS.
The American Academy of Pediatrics (AAP) practice guideline for the treatment of unconjugated hyperbilirubinemia in healthy newborn infants at 35 weeks' gestation and greater is based on three general principles to reduce the occurrence of severe hyperbilirubinemia while also reducing unintended harm: universal systematic assessment before discharge, close follow-up, and prompt intervention when indicated.

A. Risk assessment is performed prior to discharge of otherwise healthy infants ≥35 weeks' gestation to predict the development of severe hyperbilirubinemia that requires treatment. This is accomplished with a measurement of serum/plasma or TcB. Visual inspection is **not** a reliable measure of bilirubin level.

1. A **screening TB** collected by heelstick sampling at the time of the metabolic screen is plotted on an hour-specific bilirubin nomogram (Fig. 26.1) and combined with clinical risk factors (see section V.B),

especially lower gestational age, helps to identify infants at increased risk for developing hyperbilirubinemia and that require close follow-up.

2. **TcB** measurement is sometimes used to avoid blood sampling, and TcB hour-specific nomograms are available. However, TcB measurements are not reliable in certain circumstances such as during or after phototherapy, after sunlight exposure, or at TB levels ≥15 mg/dL. TcB can overestimate TB in darkly pigmented infants and underestimate TB in light-skinned infants. As a result, if TcB is used to screen infants, TB should be measured if TcB is ≥75th percentile on the TB nomogram for phototherapy, ≥95th percentile on the TcB nomogram, if the TcB is ≥13 mg/dL on follow-up after discharge, or if therapy is being considered.

3. **End-tidal carbon monoxide (ETCO)**, corrected to ambient CO_2, does not improve the sensitivity or specificity of predicting severe hyperbilirubinemia over TB alone. However, it identifies infants with increased bilirubin production due to hemolytic conditions who need closer monitoring and earlier intervention.

B. **Major risk factors** for development of severe hyperbilirubinemia include the following:

1. Predischarge TB in a high-risk zone (>95th percentile for age in hours according to the Bhutani nomogram) or high intermediate risk zone (Fig. 26.1).

2. Jaundice within the first 24 hours after birth

3. Immune or other hemolytic disease

4. Gestational age 35 to 36 weeks

5. Previous sibling with jaundice

6. Cephalohematoma or significant bruising

7. East Asian race

C. **Follow-up.** Because the peak bilirubin level typically occurs at 72 to 96 hours, after healthy newborns are discharged from their birth hospital, follow-up is essential. Infants discharged before 72 hours should be seen within the next 2 days. Infants at lower gestational ages or who have other risk factors should be seen earlier (see Fig. 26.2). Suggested management and follow-up are guided by predischarge bilirubin level and risk factors including gestational age. Parents should receive written and verbal instructions about the need for follow-up.

VI. EVALUATION OF INFANT WITH HYPERBILIRUBINEMIA

A. **History**

1. **Family history**

a. A family history of jaundice, anemia, splenectomy, or early gallbladder disease suggests hereditary hemolytic anemia (e.g., spherocytosis, glucose-6-phosphate dehydrogenase [G6PD] deficiency).

b. A family history of liver disease may suggest galactosemia, α1-antitrypsin deficiency, tyrosinosis, hypermethioninemia, Gilbert disease, Crigler-Najjar syndrome types I and II, or cystic fibrosis.

    c. Ethnic or geographic origin associated with hyperbilirubinemia (East Asian, Greek, and American Indian)

    d. A sibling with jaundice or anemia may suggest blood group incompatibility or breast milk jaundice.

2. Pregnancy history

    a. Illness during pregnancy may suggest congenital viral or toxoplasmosis infection.

    b. Infants of diabetic mothers are more likely to develop hyperbilirubinemia (see Chapter 2).

    c. Maternal drugs may interfere with bilirubin binding to albumin, making bilirubin toxic at relatively low levels (sulfonamides) or may trigger hemolysis in a G6PD-deficient infant (sulfonamides, nitrofurantoin, antimalarials).

3. Labor and delivery history

    a. Birth trauma may be associated with extravascular bleeding and hemolysis.

    b. Oxytocin use may be associated with neonatal hyperbilirubinemia, although this is controversial.

    c. Infants with hypoxic-ischemic insult may have elevated bilirubin levels; causes include inability of the liver to process bilirubin and intracranial hemorrhage.

    d. Delayed cord clamping may be associated with neonatal polycythemia and increased bilirubin load.

4. Infant history

    a. Delayed or infrequent stooling may be caused by poor caloric intake or intestinal obstruction and lead to increased enterohepatic circulation of bilirubin.

    b. Poor caloric intake may decrease bilirubin uptake by the liver.

    c. Vomiting can be due to sepsis, pyloric stenosis, or galactosemia.

B. Physical examination. Jaundice results from deposition of bilirubin in the skin and subcutaneous tissues. Blanching the skin with finger pressure makes it easier to observe jaundice. However, **visual inspection is not a reliable indicator of serum TB level or the detection of rapidly rising levels, especially in infants with dark skin.** Jaundice typically progresses in a cephalocaudal direction, starting in the face. The highest bilirubin levels are typically associated with jaundice below the knees and in the hands, although there is substantial overlap of bilirubin levels associated with jaundice progression. Jaundiced infants should have a bilirubin measurement and be examined for the following contributing factors:

1. **Lower gestational age**

2. **Small for gestational age (SGA)** may be associated with polycythemia and intrauterine infections.

3. **Microcephaly may be** associated with congenital infections.

4. **Extravascular blood** bruising, cephalohematoma, or other enclosed hemorrhage

5. **Pallor** associated with hemolytic anemia or extravascular blood loss

6. **Petechiae** may suggest congenital infection, sepsis, or erythroblastosis.

7. **Hepatosplenomegaly** may be associated with hemolytic anemia, congenital infection, or liver disease.

8. **Omphalitis** or other sign of infection

9. **Chorioretinitis** associated with congenital infection

10. Evidence of **hypothyroidism** (see Chapter 61)

C. **Additional laboratory tests** should be performed when serum TB is ≥95th percentile for age in hours or at or near the threshold for initiation of phototherapy.

1. **The mother's blood type, Rh, and antibody screen** should have been done during pregnancy and the antibody screen repeated at delivery.

2. **The infant's blood type, Rh, and direct Coombs test** to assess for iso-immune hemolytic disease. Infants of Rh-negative women should have a blood type, Rh, and Coombs test performed at birth. Routine blood typing and Coombs testing of infants born to O Rh-positive mothers to determine risk for ABO incompatibility is unnecessary. Such testing is indicated in infants with clinically significant hyperbilirubinemia and can be considered in those in whom follow-up is difficult or whose increased skin pigmentation may limit recognition of jaundice. Blood typing and Coombs testing should be considered for infants who are discharged early, especially if the mother is type O.

3. **Peripheral smear for RBC morphology and reticulocyte count** to detect causes of Coombs-negative hemolytic disease (e.g., spherocytosis). HS occurs in about 1 per 2,000 births and may be missed if family history alone is used for screening, as many cases are *de novo*, and HS may be autosomal recessive in infants of Japanese ancestry. In one report, a mean corpuscular hemoglobin concentration (MCHC) of ≥36.0 g/dL has 82% sensitivity and 98% specificity for diagnosing HS.

4. **Hematocrit** or hemoglobin measurement will identify polycythemia or suggest blood loss from occult hemorrhage.

5. Identification of specific **antibody on the infant's RBCs** (if result of direct Coombs test is positive)

6. **Direct or conjugated bilirubin** should be measured when bilirubin levels are at or above the 95th percentile or when the phototherapy threshold is approaching. Direct bilirubin should also be measured when jaundice persists beyond the first 2 weeks of age or with signs of cholestasis (light-colored stools and bilirubin in urine). If direct bilirubin is elevated, obtain urinalysis and urine culture, check state newborn screen for hypothyroidism and galactosemia, and check urine for reducing substances (see section IX, cholestatic jaundice).

7. With prolonged jaundice, tests for liver disease, congenital infections, sepsis, metabolic defects, or hypothyroidism are indicated.

8. **G6PD measurement** may be helpful, especially in infants of African, East Asian, Mediterranean, or Middle Eastern descent or if the TB is ≥18 mg/dL. The incidence of G6PD deficiency among African Americans males is 11% to 13%, comprising the most affected subpopulation in the United States.

VII. MANAGEMENT OF UNCONJUGATED HYPERBILIRUBINEMIA.

Management of hyperbilirubinemia is directed at prevention of severe hyperbilirubinemia, defined as TB >25 g/dL in term and late preterm infants, and presumably lower in preterm infants. **Initiation of therapy** is directed by the hour-specific TB value, modified by the presence of any risk factors that increase the risk of brain damage because they interfere with binding of bilirubin to albumin, increase permeability of the blood–brain barrier, or make brain cells more susceptible to damage by bilirubin (Fig. 26.3). These neurotoxicity risk factors include isoimmune hemolytic disease, G6PD deficiency, asphyxia, lethargy, temperature instability, sepsis, acidosis, or albumin <3 g/dL (if measured) (Table 26.1). Lower gestational age increases risk of toxicity. Intervention in preterm infants is guided by gestational and postmenstrual age (Table 26.2). **Phototherapy** is the initial intervention used to treat and prevent severe hyperbilirubinemia in asymptomatic infants and should be provided to infants with signs of acute bilirubin encephalopathy (ABE) while preparations are made for exchange transfusion. TB typically begins to decline within a few hours of treatment initiation. The rate of decline is increased by increased irradiance, more exposed surface area, and a higher initial TB value.

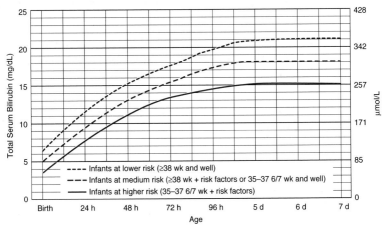

- Use total bilirubin. Do not subtract direct reacting or conjugated bilirubin.
- Risk factors = isoimmune hemolytic disease, G6PD deficiency, asphyxia, significant lethargy, temperature instability, sepsis, acidosis, or albumin <3.0 g/dL (if measured).
- For well infants 35–37 6/7 wk, can adjust TSB levels for intervention around the medium risk line. It is an option to intervene at lower TSB levels for infants closer to 35 wk and at higher TSB levels for those closer to 37 6/7 wk.
- It is an option to provide conventional phototherapy in hospital or at home at TSB levels 2–3 mg/dL (35–50 mmol/L) below those shown, but home phototherapy should not be used in any infant with risk factors.

Figure 26.3. Guidelines for phototherapy in hospitalized infants of 35 or more weeks' gestation. TSB, total serum bilirubin. Management of hyperbilirubinemia in the newborn infant 35 or more weeks of gestation. (Reprinted with permission from the American Academy of Pediatrics Subcommittee on Hyperbilirubinemia. Management of hyperbilirubinemia in the newborn infant 35 or more weeks of gestation. *Pediatrics* 2004;114:297–316.)

Table 26.1. Risk Factors for Hyperbilirubinemia Neurotoxicity

| Isoimmune hemolytic disease |
| G6PD deficiency |
| Asphyxia |
| Sepsis |
| Acidosis |
| Albumin <3.0 mg/dL |

G6PD, glucose-6-phosphate dehydrogenase.
Source: From Maisels MJ, Bhutani VK, Bogen D, et al. Hyperbilirubinemia in the newborn infant ≥35 weeks' gestation: an update with clarifications. *Pediatrics* 2009;124:1193–1198.

A. Mechanisms of bilirubin reduction by phototherapy
  1. The main mechanism is **structural isomerization** by light that irreversibly converts bilirubin to lumirubin, a more soluble substance that can be excreted into bile and urine without conjugation.
  2. **Photoisomerization** rapidly converts about 15% of the 4Z, 15Z bilirubin isomer to the less toxic 4Z, 15E form. Although the less toxic isomer

Table 26.2. Suggested Use of Phototherapy and Exchange Transfusion in Preterm Infants <35 Weeks Gestational Age

Gestational Age (week)	Phototherapy: Initiate Phototherapy Total Serum Bilirubin (mg/dL)	Exchange Transfusion: Total Serum Bilirubin (mg/dL)
<28 0/7	5–6	11–14
28 0/7–29 6/7	6–8	12–14
30 0/7–31 6/7	8–10	13–16
32 0/7–33 6/7	10–12	15–18
34 0/7–34 6/7	12–14	17–19

Source: Maisels MJ, Watchko JF, Bhutani VK, et al. An approach to the management of hyperbilirubinemia in the preterm infant less than 35 weeks of gestation. *J Perinatol* 2012;32:660–664.

can be excreted into bile without conjugation, the process is reversible and clearance is slow. Standard laboratory tests do not distinguish between the isomers, so TB levels may not change although may be less toxic.

3. Photo-oxidation is a slow process that converts bilirubin to small polar products that are excreted in the urine and is the least important mechanism of bilirubin elimination.

B. **Characteristics of devices.** Although multiple devices are available for phototherapy, according to an AAP Technical Report, the most effective are characterized by the following:

  1. Light emission in the blue-green spectrum (460 to 490 nm), which includes the region (460 nm) where bilirubin most strongly absorbs light

  2. Irradiance of at least 30 $\mu W/cm^2/nm$

  3. Illumination of maximal body surface area

  4. Shown to decrease TB during first 4 to 6 hours of exposure

C. **Light sources**

  1. Blue light-emitting diodes (LEDs) provide optimal high-intensity light in the absorption spectrum of bilirubin and are available as either overhead or underneath (mattress or fiberoptic pad) devices.

  2. Fluorescent special blue light F20T12/BB and TL52 tubes lower TB most effectively because they deliver light in the blue-green spectrum, providing maximal absorption and good skin penetration.

  3. Halogen white lights are placed at the recommended distance from the infant because they are hot and can cause thermal injury.

  4. Fiberoptic blankets or pads can be placed directly under the infant, generate little heat, and provide higher irradiance than fluorescent lights. Due to their small size, they rarely cover enough surface area to be effective when used alone in term infants and thus are typically used together with overhead lights.

D. **Phototherapy administration**

  1. Exposure during phototherapy should be as extensive as possible, minimizing the area covered by a diaper.

  2. An opaque mask should shield the eyes, avoiding occlusion of the nose.

  3. Fluorescent lights should be used with the infant in an open crib, bassinet, or warmer because the top of an incubator would prevent the lights from being close enough to the infant.

E. **Sunlight exposure.** Although sunlight exposure effectively lowers TB level, safety concerns, including exposure to ultraviolet light, potential sunburn, and thermal effects, preclude use of sunlight as a reliable therapeutic tool. In low-resource settings, use of appropriate filters and thermal monitoring may allow use of sunlight for phototherapy.

F. **Monitoring**

  1. **TB level** is measured to monitor the response to therapy. The frequency of measurement depends on the initial TB value and the baby's age at initiation. When phototherapy is started during the birth hospitalization

for a rising TB, TB is measured 4 to 6 hours after initiation and then repeated in 8 to 12 hours if TB has declined. For babies readmitted after birth hospitalization with a TB value that exceeds the 95th percentile for age in hours, TB is measured 2 to 3 hours after phototherapy is begun to ensure that TB is decreasing. TB is measured 18 to 24 hours after discontinuation of phototherapy.

G. Adverse effects. Phototherapy is generally considered safe. Temperature is monitored to avoid temperature instability. Monitoring of urine output and weight allows early detection of increased insensible water loss that may lead to dehydration. Occurrence of loose stools or an erythematous rash, if present, is typically transient.

  1. **"Bronze baby" syndrome**, a dark bronze discoloration of the skin thought to be related to impaired excretion of photoproducts of bile pigment, may occur with phototherapy in infants with direct hyperbilirubinemia (cholestatic jaundice) and usually resolves gradually within a few weeks after phototherapy is discontinued. The etiology is unknown, and whether the bronze pigments cause neurotoxicity is uncertain.

  2. Due to risk of retinal degeneration seen in animals after 24 hours of fluorescent phototherapy exposure and for reasons of infant comfort, eyes are covered in all newborns undergoing phototherapy.

H. Adequate hydration and urine output should be maintained to promote urinary excretion of lumirubin. Oral feedings by breast or bottle should continue during phototherapy unless TB is approaching the exchange transfusion level; in that case, phototherapy should not be interrupted by feeding until TB has fallen below 20 mg/dL. Breastfed infants with inadequate intake or excessive weight loss should be supplemented with expressed breast milk or formula. Breastfeeding, if interrupted, should resume as soon as possible.

I. Pharmacologic therapy. Intravenous immunoglobulin (IVIG) has been used in infants with hemolytic disease caused by Rh or ABO incompatibility when TB continues to rise in infants receiving intensive phototherapy or is within 2 or 3 mg/dL of the threshold recommended for exchange transfusion. The mechanism is unknown, but IVIG may act by occupying the Fc receptors on macrophages, decreasing removal of antibody-coated red cells from the circulation. Although data on efficacy of reducing the need for exchange transfusion are conflicting, current data suggest that the balance of risks and benefits of the two interventions favors IVIG administration to prevent exchange transfusion. We administer 0.5 to 1 g/kg IVIG over 2 hours and repeat the dose in 12 hours if needed.

J. Exchange transfusion is used to remove bilirubin when intensive phototherapy fails to prevent a rise in bilirubin to potentially toxic levels or in infants with neurologic signs suggestive of bilirubin toxicity (Fig. 26.4). Exchange transfusion is the most effective method for rapid removal of bilirubin. In cases of isoimmune hemolytic disease, exchange transfusion also removes antibody and sensitized RBCs which are replaced with donor RBCs lacking the sensitizing antigen.

  1. Immediately after a double volume exchange transfusion (about 160 to 180 mL/kg), TB values are typically half the value prior to the procedure. Thirty to 60 minutes, extravascular bilirubin rapidly equilibrates

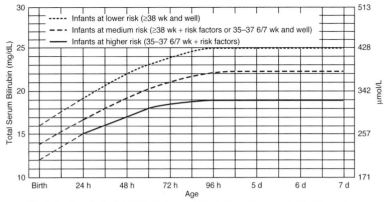

- The dashed lines for the first 24 h indicate uncertainty due to a wide range of clinical circumstances and a range of responses to phototherapy.
- Immediate exchange transfusion is recommended if infant shows signs of acute bilirubin encephalopathy (hypertonia, arching, retrocollis, opisthotonos, fever, high pitched cry) or if TSB is ≥5 mg/dL (85 μmol/L) above these lines.
- Risk factors–isoimmune hemolytic disease, G6PD deficiency, asphyxia, significant lethargy, temperature instability, sepsis, acidosis.
- Use total bilirubin. Do not subtract direct reacting or conjugated bilirubin.
- If infant is well and 35–37 6/7 wk (medium risk) can individualize TSB levels for exchange based on actual gestational age.

Figure 26.4. Guidelines for exchange transfusion in hospitalized infants of 35 or more weeks' gestation. TSB, total serum bilirubin; G6PD, glucose-6-phosphate dehydrogenase. (Reprinted with permission from the American Academy of Pediatrics Subcommittee on Hyperbilirubinemia. Management of hyperbilirubinemia in the newborn infant 35 or more weeks of gestation. *Pediatrics* 2004;114:297–316.)

with the reduced vascular level, so that TB levels return to approximately two-thirds of preexchange levels. This procedure replaces approximately 85% of the circulating RBCs.

2. We use fresh type O Rh-negative irradiated packed RBCs that are resuspended in AB plasma and cross-matched against maternal plasma and cells. The unit is reconstituted to a hematocrit of 50% to 55%. In isoimmune non-ABO hemolytic disease, the blood should not contain the sensitizing antigen. The volume ordered should be twice the infant's estimated blood volume (2 times 80 to 90 mL/kg plus additional volume to account for tubing losses [~30 mL]). A blood warmer is used to maintain temperature at 37°C.

3. Exchange transfusion is usually performed through an umbilical venous catheter using a push–pull technique in which aliquots of the patient's blood are removed and replaced with the donor blood. Individual aliquots should be approximately 10% or less of the infant's blood volume, with a maximum volume of 20 mL for a term baby who weighs more than 3 kg and smaller volumes in babies with physiologic instability. Alternatively, in a very small or unstable baby, blood can be steadily withdrawn from an umbilical artery catheter at a rate of 2 to 4 mL/kg/

minute while an equivalent volume is slowly infused at the same rate through a venous catheter (an isovolumic procedure).

4. Albumin infused 1 to 2 hours prior to the exchange transfusion promotes removal of more bilirubin because more extravascular bilirubin is drawn into the circulation.

5. Intensive phototherapy should be resumed after the transfusion, and TB should be monitored at 2, 4, and 6 hours after the transfusion and then at least every 12 to 24 hours until TB declines sufficiently to discontinue phototherapy. Increasing TB or recurrent neurologic signs are followed to assess need for repeat exchange transfusion.

6. Infants should be monitored for complications that are related to the procedure and use of blood products. Common complications include thrombocytopenia and coagulation abnormalities; hypoglycemia, hyperkalemia, and hypocalcemia; and acid–base abnormalities. Less frequent complications include necrotizing enterocolitis (see Chapter 27), portal vein thrombosis, cardiac arrhythmias, and infection.

7. Home phototherapy is effective, cheaper than hospital phototherapy, and easy to implement with the use of fiberoptic blankets but may not have the same irradiance or surface area exposure as hospital phototherapy. The AAP recommends the use of home phototherapy only for infants with bilirubin levels in the "phototherapy optional" range (see Fig. 26.3).

VIII. BILIRUBIN TOXICITY

A. Brain injury by bilirubin. Unconjugated bilirubin that is not bound to albumin is a potential toxin that can enter the brain and cause apoptosis and/or necrosis. FFAs and certain drugs (e.g., ceftriaxone) may displace bilirubin from albumin and promote entry into the brain. If the blood–brain barrier is disrupted by factors including hyperosmolarity, asphyxia, and hypercarbia, bilirubin can also enter the brain bound to albumin. Acidosis affects bilirubin solubility and promotes its deposition into brain tissue. The blood–brain barrier may be more vulnerable in preterm than in term infants.

B. Bilirubin deposited in the brain can result in bilirubin-induced neurologic dysfunction (BIND). Severe hyperbilirubinemia (TB >25 mg/dL) is associated with increased risk of BIND in term or late preterm infants; the level of risk in preterm infants is uncertain but presumed to be lower. The brain regions typically affected by bilirubin toxicity include the basal ganglia, cerebellum, white matter, and the brainstem nuclei for oculomotor and auditory function.

C. Neurologic manifestations of bilirubin toxicity reflect the areas of the brain that are most often affected and can be reversible or permanent.

1. ABE is the clinical manifestation of bilirubin toxicity seen in the neonatal period. The clinical presentation consists of three phases:
a. Early phase. Signs are subtle and may include lethargy, hypotonia, high-pitched cry, and poor suck.
b. Intermediate phase progresses in the absence of intervention for hyperbilirubinemia and is characterized by hypertonia of extensor muscles (rigidity, opisthotonus, and retrocollis), oculogyric crisis, irritability,

fever, and seizures. Some infants die in this phase. All infants who survive this phase are likely to develop chronic bilirubin encephalopathy (clinical diagnosis of kernicterus).

c. Advanced phase. Signs include pronounced opisthotonus and retrocollis, cry that can be weak or shrill, apnea, seizures, and coma. Affected infants die from intractable seizures or respiratory failure.

2. **Kernicterus** refers to the chronic and permanent sequelae of bilirubin toxicity that develop during the first year of age. Most infants who develop kernicterus have had signs of ABE in the neonatal period although some have a history of high TB level with few or no signs of ABE. The signs of kernicterus are as follows:

   a. Choreoathetoid cerebral palsy with neuromotor impairments

   b. Sensorineural hearing loss (auditory neuropathy), characterized by abnormal brainstem auditory evoked response with normal otoacoustic emission testing

   c. Limitation of upward gaze

   d. Dental enamel dysplasia

IX. CHOLESTASIS, OR CONJUGATED HYPERBILIRUBINEMIA, is due to failure to excrete bile. This may be caused by defects in intrahepatic bile production, defects in transmembrane transport of bile, or mechanical obstruction to flow. Conjugated hyperbilirubinemia is defined by a direct or conjugated bilirubin level >1 mL/dL or >15% of the TB level. It may be associated with hepatomegaly, splenomegaly, pale stools, and dark urine. An infant with jaundice at 2 weeks of age should be evaluated for cholestasis by measuring total and direct bilirubin level. Rapid diagnosis is important so that therapy for treatable disorders can be started promptly.

A. **Many disorders cause neonatal cholestasis**; a complete list is beyond the scope of this chapter.

1. **Obstructive bile duct disorders.** Biliary atresia is a frequent cause and must be identified promptly so that intervention (hepatoportoenterostomy) can be performed before 2 months of age. This condition may be associated with situs inversus, polysplenia or asplenia, and cardiac anomalies. Another cause is Alagille syndrome, which is characterized by unusual facial appearance, ocular abnormality (posterior embryotoxon), cardiac abnormalities (pulmonic stenosis), and vertebral anomalies (butterfly vertebrae). Choledochal duct cysts are an uncommon but surgically treatable cause of cholestasis.

2. **Infectious causes** include sepsis and urinary tract infections as well as infections caused by numerous viral, bacterial, and other organisms.

3. **Metabolic disorders** include α1-antitrypsin deficiency, cystic fibrosis, galactosemia, tyrosinemia, galactosemia, storage diseases (Gaucher, Niemann-Pick), Zellweger syndrome, mitochondrial disorders, and congenital disorders of glycosylation.

4. **Immunologic disorders** include gestational alloimmune liver disease (formerly neonatal hemochromatosis) and neonatal lupus erythematosus.

5. **Endocrine disorders** include hypothyroidism and panhypopituitarism.

6. Toxic disorders. A frequent cause of cholestasis in the neonatal intensive care unit (NICU) occurs in infants unable to take enteral feeding who have prolonged courses of total parenteral nutrition (PN) including lipid. This condition typically resolves with introduction of enteral feedings.

7. Isoimmune hemolysis. Conjugated hyperbilirubinemia occurs in a small proportion of infants with excessive hemolysis such as ABO/Rh incompatibility and may persist for 2 weeks.

B. Diagnosis

1. History and findings on physical examination may support a specific diagnosis. Acholic stools suggest obstruction.

2. Laboratory studies to evaluate liver function should include total and direct or conjugated bilirubin, serum alanine aminotransferase (ALT), aspartate aminotransferase (AST), gamma-glutamyl transpeptidase (GGT), alkaline phosphatase, and coagulation studies. Specific laboratory studies should be performed based on findings from the history and physical examination. These include tests for infections and metabolic, genetic, or endocrine disorders.

3. Abdominal ultrasonography may suggest biliary atresia by failure to visualize the gall bladder or presence of the triangular cord sign. Choledochal duct cyst, gallstones, or vascular malformations may be identified.

4. Hepatobiliary scintigraphy with technetium-labeled iminodiacetic acid analogs may distinguish biliary atresia from other causes of cholestasis such as neonatal hepatitis. Bilirubin concentration measured in a duodenal aspirate and compared to serum concentration is an alternative to scintigraphy to assess bile excretion.

5. Percutaneous liver biopsy is recommended to evaluate cholestatic jaundice in a guideline of the North American Society for Pediatric Gastroenterology, Hepatology and Nutrition.

6. If studies support a diagnosis of biliary atresia, intraoperative cholangiography is performed. If biliary obstruction is demonstrated, a hepato-portoenterostomy (Kasai procedure) is performed.

C. Management of PN-associated cholestasis. Most cholestasis in the NICU is due to inability to tolerate enteral feeding and prolonged exposure to PN.

1. Enteral feedings, even at minimal volumes of 10 mL/kg/day, are initiated as soon as possible. If enteral feedings can be established, infants with persistent cholestasis and abnormal LFTs are supplemented with fat-soluble vitamin supplements (ADEK). If cholestasis persists as enteral feedings are increased, we consider use of ursodiol.

2. In infants unable to take enteral feedings and who continue on PN, LFTs are checked weekly. Copper and manganese, trace metals that are excreted in bile, are reduced or eliminated. We discontinue intralipid administration and substitute parenteral fish oil (Omegaven 10% fish oil emulsion, 1 g/kg/day—Fresenius Kabi, Homburg, Germany) on an investigational protocol in infants with PN-associated liver disease (http://www.fda.gov/Drugs/DevelopmentApprovalProcess/HowDrugs areDevelopedandApproved/ApprovalApplications/InvestigationalNew DrugINDApplication/ucm368740.htm).

Suggested Readings

American Academy of Pediatrics Subcommittee on Hyperbilirubinemia. Practice parameter: management of hyperbilirubinemia in the newborn infant 35 or more weeks of gestation. *Pediatrics* 2004;114:297–316.

Bhutani VK; and the American Academy of Pediatrics Committee on Fetus and Newborn. Phototherapy to prevent severe neonatal hyperbilirubinemia in the newborn infant 35 or more weeks of gestation. *Pediatrics* 2011;128(4):e1046–1052.

Götze T, Blessing H, Grillhösl C, et al. Neonatal cholestasis—differential diagnoses, current diagnostic procedures, and treatment. *Front Pediatr* 2015;3:43.

Maisels MJ, Bhutani VK, Bogen D, et al. Hyperbilirubinemia in the newborn infant ≥35 weeks' gestation: an update with clarifications. *Pediatrics* 2009;124: 1193–1198.

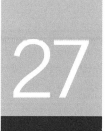

27 Necrotizing Enterocolitis

Jörn-Hendrik Weitkamp, Muralidhar H. Premkumar, and Camilia R. Martin

KEY POINTS

- Necrotizing enterocolitis (NEC) remains the most common and most devastating surgical emergency in the neonatal intensive care unit (NICU).
- The etiology is multifactorial and different for preterm and term infants. Immature intestinal function, formula feeding, bacterial dysbiosis, and a hyperinflammatory host response are key factors in typical NEC of the preterm infant.
- The diagnosis is made by combination of clinical and radiographical signs and can be confirmed by histopathology.
- Treatment includes gastric decompression, bowel rest, and broad-spectrum antimicrobial therapy. Transfer to a surgical center may be indicated.
- Current best evidence for NEC prevention exists for antenatal steroid use, standardized enteral feeding guidelines, exclusive use of human milk, avoidance of acid blockade, and minimization of empiric antibiotic exposure.
- The standard use of probiotics remains controversial due to the lack of U.S. Food and Drug Administration (FDA)-approved, pharmaceutical grade products and no clear benefit in recent, large clinical trials.

I. **BACKGROUND.** Necrotizing enterocolitis (NEC) is the most common and most serious gastrointestinal (GI) emergency of the neonate. Its pathogenesis is complex and multifactorial, and the etiology remains unclear. In spite of the advances in neonatology over the last few decades, the mortality and morbidity secondary to NEC remains high. Current clinical practice is directed mainly toward prompt, early diagnosis and institution of proper intensive care management.

A. **Definition.** NEC is an acute inflammatory injury of the distal small and often proximal large intestine. Surgical pathology reveals segmental coagulative necrosis of the mucosa with focal hemorrhage as evidence for ischemia. Other features include intramural gas (pneumatosis) and sloughing of mucosa, submucosa, and muscularis mucosa, which is in contrast to the preserved mucosal integrity in spontaneous intestinal perforation. Universally accepted risk factors include prematurity, bacterial dysbiosis, and formula feeding.

B. **Epidemiology.** Despite decades of research, NEC remains the most common serious surgical disorder among infants in a neonatal intensive care unit (NICU) and is a significant cause of neonatal morbidity and mortality.

1. The **incidence** of NEC varies from center to center and from year to year within centers. There are endemic and epidemic occurrences. An estimated 0.3 to 2.4 cases occur in every 1,000 live births. In most centers, NEC occurs between 1% and 5% of all NICU admissions and 5% to 10% of very low birth weight (VLBW) infants. Mortality ranges from 20% to 40% but can approach 100% in case of NEC totalis. Overall, NEC is responsible for 12% of deaths in extreme premature infants <27 weeks of gestational age.

2. At least 30% of NEC cases result in surgical resection of affected tissue. However, the timing for surgical intervention and the type of surgery remain controversial. Severe NEC that requires surgical intervention increases the average length of stay by 43 days and is associated with increased morbidity (e.g., short bowel syndrome) and mortality.

3. **Prematurity** is the single greatest risk factor. Decreasing gestational age is associated with an increased risk of NEC. The postnatal age at onset is inversely related to birth weight and gestational age, with a mean age at onset of 12 days. The mean postmenstrual age of infants with NEC is between 30 and 32 weeks.

4. Approximately 10% of infants with NEC are **term**. Risk factors for this population include congenital heart disease with presumed decreased intestinal perfusion (e.g., hypoplastic left heart syndrome, coarctation of the aorta), polycythemia, intrauterine cocaine exposure, and intestinal anomalies such as gastroschisis. The colon appears to be the most commonly affected site.

5. NEC pathogenesis is **multifactorial**. Additional risk factors for the disease include histologic plus clinical chorioamnionitis, IUGR, maternal smoking, polycythemia, and other—less well supported—maternal or neonatal conditions. Antenatal steroids improve the maturity of the GI tract and have been shown to reduce the incidence of NEC.

6. Recently, prolonged empiric antimicrobial use has been associated with increased NEC occurrence and matches other studies that documented decreased microbial diversity and overgrowth of potential pathogenic bacteria (dysbiosis) prior to clinical presentation of NEC.

7. Although bacteria are clearly involved in the pathogenesis of the disease, no single infectious organisms have been isolated except in relative rare outbreak situations. NEC should be differentiated from infectious (viral) or allergic (milk intolerance) colitis.

8. Transfusion-associated NEC (TANEC) has been described in numerous reports and although blood transfusions were independent risk factors in several retrospective studies, a causal relationship has not yet been confirmed in larger prospective trials.

9. A rare, more benign form of NEC has been described: *pneumatosis coli*. Neonates without the typical risk factors for NEC present with grossly

bloody stools, minimal or absent abdominal and systemic signs, and isolated colonic pneumatosis without small bowel involvement.

10. Almost all infants with NEC have received enteral feedings prior to disease onset. Formula feeding increases the risk of NEC (relative risk is 2.8). However, up to 6% of infants <1,250 g birth weight still develop the disease despite receiving exclusively breast milk.

C. **Pathogenesis**

1. The pathogenesis of NEC remains a conundrum. NEC is a multifactorial disease resulting from complex interactions between immaturity, mucosal injury, and bacterial imbalances. Because these factors affect most preterm infants, infants who develop NEC must also exhibit an especially harmful inflammatory response to intestinal antigens.

2. Genetic polymorphisms have been described in patients at higher risk for severe NEC such as in genes encoding toll-like receptor (TLR) 4 or interleukin 18 (IL-18) signaling. Polymorphism in the secretor gene fucosyltransferase (FUT) 2 encoding low secretor status have been associated with earlier and more severe disease.

3. Intestinal immaturity plays an important role in the pathogenesis of NEC: increased permeability of the intestinal epithelium, decreased motility, a thinner mucus layer, low or absent levels of secretory IgA, and lack of regulatory adaptation of the intestinal mucosal immune system.

4. Experiments in germ-free animals and TLR4 knockout mice strongly suggest that bacterial antigen is critical for the initiation of intestinal inflammation and NEC development. Previous studies have been hampered by the inability of conventional microbial culture techniques to thoroughly characterize the human GI microbiota because 80% of bacteria colonizing humans are not detected by culture methods. Sequencing the 16S small subunit bacterial ribosomal RNA (16S rRNA) gene or the entire bacterial genome discovered reduction in microbial community diversity with a shift toward increased abundance of potentially pathogenic subgroups. Although not representative for the vast majority of sporadic NEC cases, the literature contains numerous reports of NEC "outbreaks" with detection of various specific bacteria or viruses.

5. An excessive and inappropriate intestinal inflammatory response appears to be the key inciting event that leads to NEC. Although specific antigenic triggers may vary, failure to downregulate the innate immune receptor TLR4 on intestinal epithelial cells and lower ratios of FOXP3$^+$ T regulatory cells in the mucosa are examples that can explain why the poorly adapted premature intestine is prone to inflammatory injury. Prenatal factors (e.g., corticosteroids vs. chorioamnionitis) may influence the "inflammatory set-up" of the preterm gut at birth.

6. Evidence supports a critical role for inflammatory mediators. **Platelet activating factor (PAF), bacterial** endotoxin, lipopolysaccharide (LPS), tumor necrosis factor (TNF), proinflammatory interleukins, and nitric oxide are some of the inflammatory mediators that have been studied in the pathophysiology of NEC. Both animal studies and samples from human infants demonstrate the association of elevated levels of PAF

in infants with NEC compared with those without. In animal models, exogenous administration of PAF mimics NEC-like injury and PAF antagonists limit such injury. Various other inflammatory mediators such as cyclooxygenase (COX-2), reactive oxygen species, tumor necrosis factor alpha (TNF-α), and IL-18 have been implicated in NEC pathogenesis mostly in animal models.

These data also point to the multifactorial etiology of the disease and underline the fact that not one but several strategies are necessary for the prevention of NEC.

7. Several retrospective studies have suggested a temporal association of packed red blood cell (PRBC) transfusions with the onset of NEC, but this link remains to be confirmed by prospective matched case-control studies. Hypothesized mechanisms include T cell activation, immune-mediated hemolysis, and splanchnic vasoconstriction associated with the transfusion. However, it remains unclear if blood transfusions play a causal role for NEC or are just indicators of impending or ongoing disease.

8. A large number of other factors such as low Apgar scores, timing and volumes of feeding, umbilical catheterization, hypoxic-ischemic insults, presence of a patent ductus arteriosus (PDA), or treatment with indomethacin or vasopressors have not been uniformly confirmed as independent pathophysiologic contributors.

II. DIAGNOSIS.
Early diagnosis of NEC may be an important factor in determining outcome. This is accomplished by a high index of suspicion and careful clinical observation for nonspecific signs in infants at risk.

A. **Clinical characteristics.** There is a broad spectrum of disease manifestations. The clinical features of NEC can be divided into systemic and abdominal signs. Most infants have a combination of both, although abdominal signs usually predominate.

1. **Systemic signs.** Respiratory distress, apnea and/or bradycardia, lethargy, temperature instability, irritability, poor feeding, hypotension (shock), decreased peripheral perfusion, acidosis, oliguria, bleeding diathesis

2. **Abdominal (enteric) signs.** Abdominal distension or tenderness, gastric aspirates (feeding residuals), vomiting (of bile, blood, or both), ileus (decreased or absent bowel sounds), hematochezia (grossly bloody stools), abdominal wall erythema or induration, persistent localized abdominal mass, or ascites

3. The **course of the disease** varies among infants. Most frequently, it will appear (i) as a fulminant, rapidly progressive presentation of signs consistent with intestinal necrosis and sepsis or (ii) as a slow, paroxysmal presentation of abdominal distension, ileus, and possible infection. The latter course will vary with the rapidity of therapeutic intervention and require consistent monitoring and anticipatory evaluation (see section III).

B. **Laboratory features.** The diagnosis is suspected from clinical presentation but must be confirmed by diagnostic radiographs, surgery, or autopsy.

No laboratory tests are specific for NEC; nevertheless, some tests are valuable in confirming diagnostic impressions.

1. **Imaging studies.** The abdominal **radiograph** will often reveal an abnormal gas pattern consistent with ileus. Both anteroposterior (AP) and cross-table lateral or left lateral decubitus views should be included. These films may reveal bowel wall edema, a fixed-position loop on serial studies, the appearance of a mass, pneumatosis intestinalis (the radiologic hallmark used to confirm the diagnosis), gasless abdomen indicating ascites, portal or hepatic venous air, pneumobilia, or pneumoperitoneum with the appearance of gas under the diaphragm. Of note, extremely low birth weight (ELBW) infants often present with abdominal distension and ileus because intramural gas or pneumoperitoneum become more commonly presenting features after 30 weeks' postmenstrual age. Spontaneous intestinal perforation (SIP) may present with pneumoperitoneum without other clinical signs.

   Abdominal **ultrasound** can be a more sensitive method to detect intramural air and portal venous gas in experienced hands. Doppler studies can confirm bowel necrosis by absent blood flow. These techniques are particularly helpful to confirm radiographic appearance of pneumatosis intestinalis in well-appearing infants with feeding intolerance.

2. **Blood and serum studies.** Thrombocytopenia, persistent metabolic acidosis, and severe refractory hyponatremia constitute the most common triad of signs and help to confirm the diagnosis. Serial measurements of C-reactive protein (CRP) may also be helpful in the diagnosis and assessment of response to therapy of severe NEC. Blood cultures are positive in ~40% of cases.

3. **Analysis of stool** for blood has been used to detect infants with NEC based on changes in intestinal integrity. Although grossly bloody stools may be an indication of NEC, routine testing of stool for occult blood has no value for NEC diagnosis. Approximately 60% of infants will have Hemoccult-positive stools at any given time during hospitalization without any evidence for NEC.

C. **Bell staging criteria** with the Walsh and Kleigman modification allow for uniformity of diagnosis across centers. Bell staging is not a continuum; babies may present with advanced NEC without earlier signs or symptoms.

1. **Stage I** (suspect) includes clinical signs and symptoms, including abdominal signs and nondiagnostic radiographs.

2. **Stage II** (definite) includes clinical and laboratory signs and pneumatosis intestinalis and/or portal venous gas on radiographs.
   a. Mildly ill
   b. Moderately ill with systemic toxicity

3. **Stage III** (advanced) includes more severe clinical signs and laboratory abnormalities, pneumatosis intestinalis, and/or portal venous gas on radiographs.
   a. Critically ill (e.g., disseminated intravascular coagulation [DIC], shock) and impending intestinal perforation
   b. Critically ill as in section II.C.3.a but with pneumoperitoneum

D. **Differential diagnosis**

1. **Pneumonia and sepsis** are common and frequently associated with intestinal ileus. The abdominal distension, discoloration, and tenderness characteristic of NEC should be absent, however, in infants with ileus not due to NEC.

2. **Surgical abdominal catastrophes** include malrotation with obstruction (complete or intermittent), malrotation with midgut volvulus, intussusception, ulcer, gastric perforation, and mesenteric vessel thrombosis. The clinical presentation of these disorders may overlap with that of NEC. Occasionally, the diagnosis is made only at the time of exploratory laparotomy.

3. **SIP** is a distinct clinical entity occurring in approximately 2% of ELBW infants. It often presents as a gasless abdomen or as an asymptomatic pneumoperitoneum, although other clinical and laboratory abnormalities may be present. SIP tends to occur at an earlier postnatal age than NEC, has significantly lower morbidity and mortality, and is not associated with feeding. The risk of SIP is increased with early postnatal glucocorticoid exposure and indomethacin treatment for PDA. Concurrent treatment with glucocorticoids and indomethacin increases the risk of SIP.

4. **Infectious enterocolitis** is rare in this population but must be considered if diarrhea is present. Etiologies can be viral (e.g., cytomegalovirus [CMV] colitis) or bacterial (e.g., *Campylobacter* sp.). These infants typically lack any other systemic or enteric signs of NEC.

5. Severe forms of **inherited metabolic disease** (e.g., galactosemia with *Escherichia coli* sepsis) may lead to profound acidosis, shock, and vomiting and may initially overlap with some signs of NEC.

6. Severe **allergic colitis** can present with abdominal distension and bloody stools. Usually, these infants are well appearing and have normal abdominal radiographs and laboratory studies.

7. **Feeding intolerance** is a common but ill-defined problem in premature infants. Despite adequate GI function *in utero*, some premature infants will have periods of gastric residuals and abdominal distension associated with advancing feedings. The differentiation of this problem from NEC can be difficult. Cautious evaluation by withholding enteral feedings and administering parenteral nutrition (PN) and antibiotics for 48 to 72 hours may be indicated until this benign disorder can be distinguished from NEC. Serial monitoring of CRP, platelet counts, and kidney-ureter-bladder x-rays (KUBs) can sometimes help distinguish feeding intolerance from NEC.

E. **Additional diagnostic considerations**

1. Because the early abdominal signs may be nonspecific, at present, **a high index of suspicion** is the most reliable approach to early diagnosis. The goal has been to prevent the initiation of a cascade that results in tissue injury, necrosis, and inflammatory sequelae characteristic of NEC. Several biomarkers such as inflammatory cytokines, intestinal or liver fatty acid binding protein (I-FABP or L-FABP), heart rate characteristics,

protcomics, microbiome changes, and machine learning algorithms have been studied with this endpoint in mind, but none have been clinically established to date. Although traditionally persistent or worsening abnormalities in WBCs, platelet counts, CRPs, and/or lactate levels have been used to indicate a relative indication for surgical intervention, newer biomarkers and algorithms may help with risk stratification to identify infants with high likelihood for surgical disease more precisely and earlier.

2. **Radiographic findings** can often be subtle and confusing. For example, intestinal perforation in ELBW infants can present as ileus or gasless abdomen, and conversely, pneumoperitoneum does not necessarily indicate abdominal perforation from NEC. Serial review of the radiographs with a pediatric radiologist is indicated to assist in interpretation and to plan for further appropriate studies, which may increasingly include abdominal ultrasound with Doppler.

III. MANAGEMENT

A. **Immediate medical management** (Table 27.1). Treatment should begin promptly when a diagnosis of NEC is suspected. Therapy is based on intensive care measures and the anticipation of potential problems.

1. **Respiratory function.** Rapid assessment of ventilatory status (physical examination, arterial blood gases) should be made, and supplemental oxygen and mechanical ventilatory support should be provided as needed.

2. **Cardiovascular function.** Assessment of circulatory status (physical examination, blood pressure) should be made, and circulatory support provided as needed. Volume in the form of normal saline, fresh frozen plasma, or packed red cells (dose 10 mL/kg) may be used if circulatory volume is compromised. Pharmacologic support may be necessary to ensure adequate blood pressure and tissue perfusion. Impending circulatory collapse will often be reflected by poor perfusion and oxygenation, although arterial blood pressure may be maintained. Intra-arterial blood pressure monitoring is often necessary. Further monitoring of central venous pressure (CVP) may become necessary if additional pharmacologic support of the circulation or failing myocardium is needed (see Chapter 40).

3. **Metabolic function.** Metabolic acidosis will generally respond to volume expansion. The use of sodium bicarbonate is controversial and should be reserved for severe metabolic acidosis with concerns for cardiac dysfunction (dose 1 to 2 mEq/kg). The blood pH and lactate level should be monitored; in addition, serum electrolyte levels, blood glucose, and cardiac and liver function should be measured.

4. **Nutrition.** All GI feedings are discontinued, and the bowel is decompressed by suctioning through a naso- or orogastric tube. Length of withholding enteral nutrition varies between 5 and 14 days for medical NEC and 10 to 14 days for surgical disease. Guidance from randomized controlled trials is not available, but one study suggested safe refeeding once CRP levels have normalized. PN is given through

Table 27.1. Management of Necrotizing Enterocolitis

Bell Staging Criteria	Diagnosis	Management (Usual Attention to Respiratory, Cardiovascular, and Hematologic Resuscitation Presumed)
Stage I (suspected)	Clinical signs Nondiagnostic radiograph	NPO with IV fluids Gastric decompression CBC, C-reactive protein, electrolytes Blood culture Ampicillin and gentamicin × 48 hours KUB q8–12h × 48 hours Abdominal ultrasound with Doppler
Stage II (definite)	Clinical signs Pneumatosis intestinalis and/or portal venous gas on radiograph	NPO with parenteral nutrition Gastric decompression CBC, C-reactive protein, electrolytes KUB (AP and lateral) q6–8h × 24–48 hours and then PRN Abdominal ultrasound with Doppler CBC, C-reactive protein, electrolytes Blood culture Ampicillin, gentamicin, and metronidazole × 10–14 days Surgical consultation
Stage III (advanced)	Clinical signs	NPO with parenteral nutrition
	Critically ill	Nasogastric drainage
	Pneumatosis intestinalis or pneumoperitoneum on radiograph	Gastric decompression CBC, C-reactive protein, electrolytes KUB (AP and lateral) q6–8h × 24–48 hours and then PRN Abdominal ultrasound with Doppler Ampicillin, gentamicin, and metronidazole Surgical consultation

NPO, nothing by mouth; IV, intravenous; CBC, complete blood count; KUB, kidney, urethra, bladder x-ray; AP, anteroposterior; PRN, as needed.

peripheral or central access as soon as possible, with the aim of providing 90 to 110 cal/kg/day once amino acid solutions and intralipid are both tolerated. A central venous catheter is almost always necessary to provide adequate calories in the VLBW infant. We wait to place a central catheter for this purpose until the blood cultures are negative, during which time adaptation to peripheral PN can take place (see Chapter 21).

5. **Infectious disease.** Blood and sometimes urine cultures are obtained and sent for culture and sensitivities. Traditional culture and 16S rRNA gene sequencing from blood and peritoneal fluid of patients with NEC have identified a vast variety of aerobic and anaerobic gram-positive and gram-negative bacteria including *Klebsiella pneumoniae, E. coli, Pseudomonas* sp., *Clostridium* sp., *Bacteroides* sp., and *Staphylococcus* sp. Therefore, typical combination therapy is indicated such as ampicillin, gentamicin, and metronidazole. Alternatively, treatments include clindamycin, piperacillin-tazobactam, or meropenem, sometimes in combination with vancomycin. *Candida* spp. are early colonizers of the premature intestine and can be identified in preterm infants with NEC especially in case of intestinal perforation and lack of antifungal prophylaxis. Safety and efficacy of a particular antibiotic regimen has not been established in infants with NEC, and therefore none of these drugs or combinations are U.S. Food and Drug Administration (FDA)-labeled for this population.

   With changing antibiotic sensitivities, providers must be aware of the predominant local NICU flora, the organisms associated with NEC, and their resistance patterns and adjust antibiotic coverage accordingly. Antibiotic therapy is adjusted on the basis of culture results, but only 10% to 40% of blood cultures will be positive, necessitating continued broad-spectrum coverage in most cases. In infants requiring surgery, peritoneal fluid cultures may also help target appropriate antibiotic treatment. Treatment is generally maintained for 10 to 14 days in cases of definite NEC (≥Bell II). There is no evidence to support the use of enteral antibiotics.

6. **Hematologic aspects.** Analysis of the complete blood count and differential is mostly helpful to detect clinically significant anemia and/or thrombocytopenia. PRBCs are often transfused to maintain the hematocrit above 35%. The prothrombin time, partial thromboplastin time, fibrinogen, and platelet count should be evaluated for evidence of DIC. Fresh frozen plasma is often used to treat coagulation problems.

7. **Renal function.** Oliguria often accompanies the initial hypotension and hypoperfusion of NEC; measurement of urine output is indicated. In addition, serum blood urea nitrogen (BUN), creatinine, and serum electrolyte levels should be monitored. Impending renal failure from acute tubular necrosis, coagulative necrosis, or vascular accident must be anticipated, and fluid therapy adjusted accordingly (see Chapter 28).

8. **Neurologic function.** Evaluation of the infant's condition may be difficult given the degree of illness, but one must be alert to the problems of associated meningitis and intraventricular hemorrhage (IVH). Seizures are rare but may occur secondary to either meningitis, IVH, or from the metabolic perturbations associated with NEC. These complications must be anticipated and promptly recognized and treated.

9. **GI function.** Physical examination and serial (every 6 to 8 hours during the first 2 to 3 days) radiographs are used to assess ongoing GI damage. Unless perforation occurs or full-thickness necrosis precipitates severe

peritonitis, management remains medical. The evaluation for surgical intervention, however, is controversial and complex (see section III.B).

10. **Family support.** Any family of an infant in the NICU may be overwhelmed by the crisis. Infants with NEC present a particular challenge because the disease often causes sudden deterioration for "no apparent reason." Furthermore, the impending possibility of surgical intervention and the high mortality and uncertain prognosis make this situation most difficult for parents. Careful anticipatory sharing of information supports a trusting alliance with the family.

B. **Surgical intervention**

1. **Prompt early consultation** should be obtained with a pediatric surgeon. This will allow the surgeon to become familiar with the infant and will provide an additional evaluation by another skilled individual. If a pediatric surgeon is not available and advancement to more severe disease is likely, the infant should be transferred to a high-level center with pediatric surgery service.

2. **GI perforation** is probably the only absolute indication for surgical intervention. Unfortunately, there is no reliable or absolute indicator of imminent perforation; therefore, frequent monitoring is necessary. Perforation occurs in 20% to 30% of patients, usually 12 to 48 hours after the onset of NEC, although it can occur later. In some cases, the absence of pneumoperitoneum on the abdominal radiograph can delay the diagnosis, and paracentesis may aid in establishing the diagnosis. In general, an infant with increasing abdominal distension, an abdominal mass, a worsening clinical picture despite medical management, or a persistent fixed loop on serial radiographs may have a perforation and may require operative intervention.

3. **Full-thickness necrosis of the GI tract** may require surgical intervention, although this diagnosis is difficult to establish in the absence of perforation. In most cases, the infant with bowel necrosis will have signs of peritonitis, such as ascites, abdominal mass, abdominal wall erythema, induration, persistent thrombocytopenia, progressive shock from third-space losses, or refractory metabolic acidosis. Paracentesis may help to identify these patients before perforation occurs.

4. The specific type of **surgical treatment** varies by center and extent of disease. It includes peritoneal drainage, laparotomy with diverting ostomy alone, laparotomy with intestinal resection and primary anastomosis, "clip and drop," or stoma creation, with or without second-look procedure. To date, no randomized controlled trial has demonstrated a clear benefit for one procedure over another. In very unstable infants, surgery in the NICU rather than transfer to the operating room is a commonly used option, especially in single-room NICUs. Mortality in these cases is high, likely due to the critical status of patients already before surgery. The goal is to excise complete necrotic bowel while preserving as much bowel length as possible. If large areas are resected, the length and position of the remaining bowel are noted because this will affect the long-term outcome. In case of "NEC totalis" (bowel necrosis from duodenum to rectum), mortality is almost certain and resection is typically not attempted.

5. In ELBW infants (<1,000 g) and extremely unstable infants, **peritoneal drainage** under local anesthesia may be a management option. In many cases, this temporizes laparotomy until the infant is more stable, and in some cases, no further operative procedure is required. Prospective studies have found no difference in mortality between laparotomy and peritoneal drainage for surgical NEC. However, approximately half of patients with peritoneal drainage eventually receive laparotomy (35% to 74%), potentially limiting the validity of the intention-to-treat analyses. The cost burden of peritoneal drainage followed by laparotomy is large compared to laparotomy alone, and given the absence of survival benefit and reported worse long-term neurodevelopmental outcome after peritoneal drainage, its utility is questionable.

C. Long-term management. Once the infant has been stabilized and effectively treated, feedings can be reintroduced. This process typically starts after 7 to 14 days of treatment by stopping gastric decompression. If infants can tolerate their own secretions, feedings are begun very slowly while parenteral alimentation is gradually tapered. No conclusive data are available on the best method or type of feeding, but breast milk may be tolerated best and is preferred. The occurrence of strictures may complicate feeding plans. The incidence of recurrent NEC is 4% and appears to be independent of type of management. Recurrent disease should be treated as before and will generally respond similarly. If surgical intervention was required and an ileostomy or colostomy has been created, intestinal reanastomosis can be electively undertaken after an adequate period of healing. If an infant tolerates enteral feedings, reanastomosis may be performed after a period of growth at home. However, earlier surgical intervention may be indicated in infants who cannot be advanced to full volume or strength feedings because of malabsorption and intestinal dumping. Before reanastomosis, a contrast study of the distal bowel is frequently obtained to establish the presence of a stricture that can be resected at the time of ostomy closure.

IV. PROGNOSIS. Few detailed and accurate studies are available on prognosis. In uncomplicated cases of NEC, the long-term prognosis may be comparable with that of other low birth weight infants; however, those with stage IIB and stage III NEC have a higher incidence of mortality (of over 50%), growth delay (delay in growth of head circumference is of most concern), and poor neurodevelopmental outcome. NEC requiring surgical intervention may have more serious sequelae, including mortality secondary to infection, respiratory failure, PN-associated hepatic disease, rickets, and significant developmental delay.

A. Sequelae of NEC can be directly related to the disease process or to the long-term NICU management often necessary to treat it. GI sequelae include strictures, enteric fistulas, short bowel syndrome, malabsorption and chronic diarrhea, dumping syndromes related to loss of terminal ileum and ileocecal valve, fluid and electrolyte losses with rapid dehydration, and hepatitis or cholestasis related to long-term PN. Strictures occur in 25% to 35% of patients with or without surgery and are most common in the large bowel. However, not all strictures are clinically significant and may not preclude advancement to full feeding volumes. Short bowel syndrome occurs in approximately 10% to 20% following surgical treatment. Metabolic sequelae include failure to thrive, metabolic bone disease, and problems related to central nervous system (CNS) function in the VLBW infant. NEC is a significant predictor of lasting neurodevelopmental morbidity independent of other factors. Survivors of NEC have significantly impaired motor and cognitive outcomes with on average 11 IQ points lower intelligence than matched control children. Although the outcomes for many prematurity-related illnesses have improved over the past decades, mortality and morbidity rates for NEC have remained constant.

B. **Prevention of NEC is the ultimate goal.** Unfortunately, this can best be accomplished only by preventing premature birth. If prematurity cannot be avoided, several preventive strategies may be of benefit.

1. **Induction of GI maturation.** The incidence of NEC is significantly reduced after prenatal steroid therapy.

2. **Exclusive feeding of human milk–based diet.** Premature infants who are fed exclusively with expressed human milk are at decreased risk for developing NEC. Mothers should be strongly encouraged to provide expressed milk for their premature babies when able. **Donor breast milk reduces the risk of NEC compared to formula.** Formula-fed infants had greater increases in weight, length, and head circumference in several studies, but no difference was found on growth rates or neurodevelopmental outcome after discharge. Future trials should compare growth, development, and adverse outcomes in infants who receive formula milk versus nutrient-fortified donor breast milk given as a supplement to maternal expressed breast milk or as sole diet.

3. **Optimization of enteral feedings** (see Chapter 21). Because of the lack of adequately sized randomized trials in ELBWs, currently there is not enough evidence to support either early versus delayed feedings or an optimum rate of advancement of feedings. However, from the available evidence, it is clear that adoption and strict adherence to a particular standardized feeding regimen reduces the risk of NEC; therefore, individual NICUs should agree on a feeding regimen and monitor adherence.

4. **Enterally fed probiotics** are a promising new approach to the prevention of NEC. Probiotics fed to preterm infants may help to normalize intestinal microflora colonization. A recent meta-analysis has shown reduced incidence of NEC by over 50% in infants fed probiotics (e.g., *Lactobacillus GG, Bifidobacterium breve, Saccharomyces boulardii, Lactobacillus acidophilus*) compared with controls. However, the studies included in the meta-analysis were quite disparate in the type of probiotics and in their use. More recently, neither the large Probiotics in Preterm babies Study (PiPS) trial in the United Kingdom nor the ProPrems trial in Australia (together over 2,500 babies) demonstrated any reduction in death, sepsis, or NEC in infants *below 28 weeks'* gestational age. In addition, fatal infectious complications have been reported in association with unregulated use of live probiotic supplementation. Until further evidence is available to help determine the most effective probiotic(s), their optimum dosage, and long- and short-term safety, the routine use of probiotics in the prevention and treatment of NEC cannot be universally recommended.

5. A number of nutritional **supplements** (e.g., polyunsaturated fatty acids [PUFA], L-arginine); **growth factors** such as transforming growth factor beta (TGF-β) and heparin-binding epidermal growth factor (HB-EGF); **immune modulators** such as immunoglobulins, trefoil factors, lactoperoxidase, superoxide dismutase, platelet-activating factor (PAF) acetylhydrolase, alkaline phosphatase, and inhibitors of TLR4 and others have been explored in animal models and even clinical trials but are not ready yet for routine clinical use. One currently explored promising agent is oral bovine or human lactoferrin. **Lactoferrin** is a glycoprotein with broad-spectrum antimicrobial activity found in colostrum and milk. Current evidence suggests that oral lactoferrin with or without probiotics decreases late-onset sepsis and NEC in preterm infants without adverse events. However, these data need to be confirmed after completion of ongoing trials for dosing optimization and type of lactoferrin. Long-term outcomes of lactoferrin use are unknown. Other mostly experimental therapy options include TLR4 inhibitors and HB-EGF. Currently, best evidence for **NEC prevention** strategies exists for prenatal steroids, standardized enteral feeding guidelines, exclusive use of human milk, avoidance of acid blockade, and minimization of empiric antibiotic exposure.

Suggested Readings

Coggins S, Wynn J, Weitkamp JH. Infectious causes for necrotizing enterocolitis. *Clin Perinatol* 2015;42(1):133–154.

Cotten CM, Taylor S, Stoll B, et al; for NICHD Neonatal Research Network. Prolonged duration of initial empirical antibiotic treatment is associated with increased rates of necrotizing enterocolitis and death for extremely low birth weight infants. *Pediatrics* 2009;123(1):58–66.

Neu J, Walker WA. Necrotizing enterocolitis. *N Engl J Med* 2011;364(3):255–264.

Patole S, de Klerk N. Impact of standardised feeding regimens on incidence of neonatal necrotising enterocolitis: a systematic review and meta-analysis of observational studies. *Arch Dis Child Fetal Neonatal Ed* 2005;90(2): F147–F151.

Sharma R, Hudak ML. A clinical perspective of necrotizing enterocolitis: past, present, and future. *Clin Perinatol* 2013;40(1):27–51.

28 Neonatal Kidney Conditions

Joshua A. Samuels, Haendel Muñoz, and
Rita D. Swinford

KEY POINTS

- Glomerular filtration rate (GFR) at birth is lower in the most premature infants and rises after birth dependent on the degree of prematurity.
- In term babies, GFR rises quickly, doubling by 2 weeks of age and reaching adult levels by 1 year of age.
- Management of infants who develop acute kidney injury should focus on treating the underlying etiology, avoiding further injury, and addressing consequences of decreased renal function.
- Congenital anomalies of the kidney and urinary tract may become apparent with prenatal ultrasound, discovered at birth, or present later in life.

Kidney problems in the neonate may be the result of specific inherited, developmental abnormalities or the result of acquired events either in the prenatal or in the postnatal period. For this reason, evaluation includes a detailed review of the history (family history, gestational history, and the neonatal events) as well as a review of the presenting clinical features and relevant laboratory/radiologic findings. An understanding of the developmental processes and the differences in renal physiology in the neonatal period compared to that at later ages is necessary for evaluation.

I. RENAL EMBRYOGENESIS AND FUNCTIONAL DEVELOPMENT

A. Embryogenesis

The development of the human kidney is a self-regulating process in which kidney function directs multiple interdependent cellular processes of the developing nephrons and tubules. Nephrogenesis requires a fine balance of numerous factors that can be disturbed by various genetic and/or epigenetic prenatal events including nutritional deficiencies, toxic insults, hypertension, pharmacology, prematurity, and low birth weight resulting in low nephron number at birth.

The mature human kidney is the final product of three embryonic organs: the pronephros, the mesonephros, and the metanephros. The transient pronephros, the first structure containing rudimentary tubules, disappears at the end of the fourth week of gestation. Despite its transient nature, the pronephros is required for normal kidney development. The mesonephros follows and develops concomitantly and contains well-developed nephrons comprising vascularized glomeruli connected to proximal and distal tubules draining into a mesonephric duct. Ultimately, the mesonephros fuses with the cloaca, contributes to the formation of the urinary bladder and in the male, the genital system. The metanephros is the final developmental stage and can be identified around the fifth or sixth week of gestation. The metanephros has two components: the ureteric bud (UB) and the metanephric mesenchyme. The UB is the origin of the metanephros, originating from the Wolffian mesonephric duct.

The UB is a branching epithelial tube of programmed intermediate mesenchymal cells whose inductive signals stimulate development of epithelial precursors. It induces mesenchymal cells to migrate closer to each other in preparation for their conversion into epithelial cells. With each division of the UB, a new layer of nephrons is induced from stem cells; as development proceeds, the metanephros is located at progressively higher levels, reaching the lumbar position by 8 weeks of gestation.

The developmental history of the nephron and collecting system differ: Whereas the nephron arises from mesenchymal cells undergoing mesenchymal–epithelial transitions, the tubules form from reiterated UB branching.

The beginning of the UB from the Wolffian duct begins at the 28th day of gestation, branching in a highly reproducible manner with a nephron induced at each of its tips. These branches eventually form the collecting system (ducts, renal pelvis, ureter, and bladder trigone). Multiple gene regulatory networks have been reported to act either as inducers (e.g., c-Ret, GDNF, ETv4, ETv5, SOX8, SOX9, Wnt11, Angiotensin II, PAX2, AT2R) or inhibitors (e.g., FoxC1, FoxC2, BMP4, Slit2). The GDNF/c-Ret/Wnt1 pathway, for example, is considered a major positive regulator of UB development, playing multiple crucial roles in cell movements and growth. In its absence, kidneys display severe branching abnormalities, lack of UB leading to renal hypoplasia, renal agenesis, abnormal ureter–bladder connections, etc.

Most nephrons in human kidneys are endowed by 36 weeks of gestation; nephron number varies from 300,000 to 1,800,000 (average 900,000) nephrons per kidney. Nephrons cannot regenerate; therefore, nephron endowment has profound implications for future chronic kidney disease (CKD) development. Four stages of nephron development have been defined: stage I, where the renal vesicle appears; stage II, transformation of renal vesicle to a comma-shaped body; stage III, capillary loop stage; and stage IV, maturing nephron stage including proximal tubules, the loop of Henle, distal tubules, and development of the juxtaglomerular complex and part of the afferent arterioles. During this stage, the renal interstitium differentiates into the various components of cortex, medulla, etc. Disruption of any part of this sequence leads to reduced nephron numbers. Once the nephron number has been determined, postnatal factors (such as acute kidney injury or chronic illness) can only further decrease the nephron population.

Gene-targeting experiments have greatly improved our understanding of kidney and urinary tract morphogenesis, but our understanding is incomplete with respect to the complete contribution of genetic expression regulating the ups and downs of UB and epithelial cell interactions, as well as the metanephric mesenchyme and in stromal cells during renal development. This complex picture demonstrates that mutations or altered epigenetic modulation of genes expressed during nephrogenesis compromises ureteric elongation and branching and therefore the process of mesenchymal–epithelial transition. The consequence of even subtle changes in the reciprocal and complex interactions between these cell types has severe consequences on the ultimate development of the human kidney.

B. Functional Development

At birth, the kidneys replace the placenta as the major homeostatic organs, maintaining fluid and electrolyte balance and removing harmful waste products. This transition occurs with increases in renal blood flow (RBF), glomerular filtration rate (GFR), and tubular functions. Because of this postnatal transition, the level of renal function relates more closely to the postnatal age than to the gestational age at birth.

1. **RBF** remains low during fetal development, accounting for only 2% to 3% of cardiac output. At birth, RBF rapidly increases to 15% to 18% of cardiac output because of (i) a decrease in renal vascular resistance, which is proportionally greater in the kidney compared to other organs, (ii) an increase in systemic blood pressure, and (iii) increase in inner to outer cortical blood flow.

2. **Glomerular filtration** begins soon after the first nephrons are formed and GFR increases in parallel with body and kidney growth ($\sim$1 mL/minute/kg of body weight). Once all the glomeruli are formed by 34 weeks' gestation, the GFR continues to increase until birth because of decreases in renal vascular resistance. GFR is less well autoregulated in the neonate than in older children. It is controlled by maintenance of glomerular capillary pressure by the greater vasoconstrictive effect of angiotensin II at the efferent than afferent arteriole where the effect is attenuated by concurrent prostaglandin-induced vasodilatation.

   GFR at birth is lower in the most premature infants and rises after birth dependent on the degree of prematurity. In term babies, GFR rises quickly, doubling by 2 weeks of age and reaching adult levels by 1 year of age. Similar values are reached by premature infants, although over a longer time interval (see Table 28.5).

3. **Tubular function**
   a. Sodium (Na^+) handling. The ability of the kidneys to reabsorb Na^+ is developed by 24 weeks' gestation, although tubular resorption of Na^+ is low until after 34 weeks' gestation. This is important when evaluating a preterm infant for prerenal azotemia because they will be unable to reabsorb sodium maximally and thus will have elevated fractional excretion of sodium (FENa; see Table 28.1). Very premature infants cannot conserve Na^+ even when Na^+ balance is negative. Hence, premature infants below 34 weeks' gestation often develop hyponatremia when receiving formula or breast milk even in the absence of kidney injury or damage. Na^+ supplementation is warranted. After 34 weeks' gestation, Na^+ reabsorption becomes more efficient so that 99% of filtered Na^+ can be reabsorbed, resulting in an FENa of $<$1% if challenged with renal hypoperfusion (prerenal state). Full-term neonates can retain Na^+ when in negative Na^+ balance but, like premature infants, are also limited in their ability to excrete a Na^+ load because of their low GFR.

Table 28.1. Commonly Used Equations and Formulas

$\text{CrCl (mL/min/1.73 m}^2) = K \times \text{Length (cm)}/P_{Cr}$

$\text{CrCl (mL/min/1.73 m}^2) = U_{Cr} \times U_{vol} \times 1.73/P_{Cr} \times \text{BSA}$

$\text{FENa} = 100 \times (U_{Na}{+} \times P_{Cr})/(P_{Na}{+} \times U_{Cr})$

$\text{TRP} = 100 \times [1 - (U_P \times P_{Cr})/(P_P \times U_{Cr})]$

$\text{Calculated } P_{osm} \geq 2 \times \text{plasma } [Na^+] + [\text{glucose}]/18 + \text{BUN}/2.8$

$\text{Plasma anion gap} = [Na^+] - [Cl^-] - [HCO_3{}^-]$

K, 0.34 in premature infants <34 weeks and 0.41 in infants from 35 weeks to term; CrCl, creatinine clearance; U_{Cr}, urinary creatinine; U_{vol}, urinary volume per minute; P_{Cr}, plasma creatinine; BSA, body surface area; FENa, fractional excretion of sodium; U_{Na}, urinary sodium; P_{Na}, plasma sodium; TRP, tubular reabsorption of phosphorus; U_P, urinary phosphorus; P_P, plasma phosphous; P_{osm}, plasma osmolarity; BUN, blood urea nitrogen.

b. Water handling. The newborn infant has a limited ability to concentrate urine due to limited urea concentration within the renal interstitium (because of low protein intake and anabolic growth). The resulting decreased osmolality of the interstitium leads to a decreased concentrating ability and thus a diminished capacity to reabsorb water by the neonatal kidney. The maximal urine concentration (osmolality) is only 500 mOsm/L in premature infants and 800 mOsm/L in term infants. Although this is of little consequence in infants receiving appropriate amounts of water with hypotonic feeding, it can become clinically relevant in infants receiving higher osmotic loads. In contrast, both premature and full-term infants can dilute their urine normally with a minimal urine osmolality of 35 to 50 mOsm/L. Their low GFR, however, limits their ability to handle water loads.

c. Potassium (K^+) handling. The limited ability of premature infants to excrete large K^+ loads is related to decreased distal tubular K^+ secretion, a result of decreased aldosterone sensitivity, low $Na^+-K^+-ATPase$ activity, and their low GFR. Premature infants often have slightly higher serum K^+ levels than older infants and children. If there is a question of renal potassium handling and possible abnormal hyperkalemia, potassium should be accurately measured using a central blood draw (as opposed to a heel stick).

d. Acid and bicarbonate handling are limited by a low serum bicarbonate threshold in the proximal tubule (14 to 16 mEq/L in premature infants, 18 to 21 mEq/L in full-term infants) which improves as maturation of $Na^+-K^+-ATPase$ and Na^+-H transporter occurs. Essentially, premature infants are born with a mild proximal RTA that improves with maturation. In addition to proximal tubular handling of bicarbonate, the production of ammonia in the distal tubule and proximal tubular glutamine synthesis are decreased. The lower rate of phosphate excretion limits the generation of titratable acid, further limiting infants ability to eliminate an acid load. Very low birth weight infants can develop mild metabolic acidosis during the second to fourth week after birth that may require administration of additional sodium bicarbonate.

e. Calcium and phosphorous handling in the neonate is characterized by a pattern of increased phosphate retention associated with growth. Serum phosphorus levels are higher in newborns than in older children and adults. The intake and filtered load of phosphate, parathyroid hormone (PTH), and growth factors modulate renal phosphate transport. The higher phosphate level and higher rate of phosphate reabsorption are not explained by the low GFR or to tubular unresponsiveness to extrarenal factors (PTH, vitamin D). More likely, there is a developmental mechanism that favors renal conservation of phosphate in part due to growth hormone effects, as well as a growth-related Na^+-dependent phosphate transporter, so that a positive phosphate balance for growth is maintained. Tubular reabsorption of phosphate (TRP) is also altered by gestational age, increasing from 85% at 28 weeks to 93% at 34 weeks and 98% by 40 weeks.

Calcium levels in the fetus and cord blood are higher than those in the neonate. Calcium levels fall in the first 24 hours, but low levels of PTH persist. This relative hypoparathyroidism in the first few days after birth may be the result of this physiologic response to hypercalcemia in the normal fetus. Although total plasma Ca^+ values <8 mg/dL in premature infants are common, they are usually asymptomatic because the ionized calcium level is usually normal. Factors that favor this normal ionized Ca^+ fraction include lower serum albumin and the relative metabolic acidosis in the neonate.

Urinary calcium excretion is lower in premature infants and correlates with gestational age. At term, urinary calcium excretion rises and persists until approximately 96 months of age. The urine calcium excretion in premature infants varies directly with Na^+ intake, urinary Na^+ excretion, and inversely with plasma Ca^{2+}. Neonatal stress and therapies such as aggressive fluid use or furosemide administration increase Ca^{2+} excretion, aggravating the tendency to hypocalcemia or nephrocalcinosis.

4. Fetal urine contribution to amniotic fluid volume is minimal in the first half of gestation (10 mL/hour) but increases significantly to an average of 50 mL/hour and is a necessary contribution to pulmonary development. Oligohydramnios or polyhydramnios may reflect dysfunction of the developing kidney and warrants a more thorough evaluation of the fetal kidneys.

II. CLINICAL ASSESSMENT OF KIDNEY FUNCTION. Assessment of kidney function is based on the patient's history, physical examination, and appropriate laboratory and radiologic tests.

A. History

1. **Prenatal history** includes any maternal illness, drug use, or exposure to known and potential teratogens.

   a. Maternal use of angiotensin-converting enzyme (ACE) inhibitors, angiotensin receptor blockers, or indomethacin decreases glomerular capillary pressure and GFR and has been associated with neonatal kidney failure.

b. Oligohydramnios may indicate a decrease in fetal urine production. It may be associated with kidney agenesis, dysplasia, polycystic kidney disease, or severe obstruction of the urinary tract system. It most often is a sign of poor fetal perfusion due to placental insufficiency as seen in preeclampsia or maternal vascular disease (see Chapters 2 and 4).

Conversely, polyhydramnios is seen in pregnancies complicated by maternal diabetes (see Chapter 2) and in fetal anomalies such as esophageal atresia (see Chapter 64) or anencephaly (see Chapter 57). It also may be a result of renal tubular dysfunction with inability to fully concentrate urine.

c. Elevated serum/amniotic fluid alpha-fetoprotein and enlarged placenta are associated with congenital nephrotic syndrome.

2. **Family history.** The risk of renal disease is increased if there is a family history of urinary tract anomalies, polycystic kidney disease, consanguinity, or inherited renal tubular disorders. Familial diseases (congenital nephrotic syndrome, autosomal recessive polycystic disease of kidney [ARPKD], hydronephrosis, or dysplasia) may be recognized *in utero* or remain asymptomatic until later life.

3. **Delivery history.** Fetal distress, perinatal asphyxia, sepsis, and volume loss may lead to ischemic or anoxic injury. Although often multiorgan, the neonatal kidneys are at particular risk for ischemic injury due to their low GFR and relative hypoxia at baseline.

4. **Micturition.** Seventeen percent of newborns void in the delivery room, approximately 90% void by 24 hours, and 99% void by 48 hours. The rate of urine formation ranges from 0.5 to 5.0 mL/kg/hour at all gestational ages. The most common cause of delayed or decreased urine production is improper recording of initial void or inadequate perfusion of the kidneys. Delay in micturition may also be due to intrinsic kidney abnormalities or obstruction of the urinary tract.

B. **Physical examination.** Careful examination will detect abdominal masses in 0.8% of neonates. Most of these masses are either renal in origin or related to the genitourinary (GU) system. It is important to consider in the differential diagnosis whether the mass is unilateral or bilateral (Table 28.2). Edema may be present in infants with congenital nephrotic syndrome (due to low oncotic pressure) or from fluid overload if input exceeds output. Tubular defects and use of diuretics can cause salt and water losses which can lead to dehydration.

Many congenital syndromes may affect the kidneys; thus, a thorough evaluation is necessary in those presenting with congenital renal anomalies. Findings associated with congenital kidney anomalies include low-set ears, ambiguous genitalia, anal atresia, abdominal wall defect, vertebral anomalies, aniridia, meningomyelocele, tethered cord, pneumothorax, pulmonary hypoplasia, hemihypertrophy, persistent urachus, hypospadias, and cryptorchidism among others (Table 28.3). Spontaneous pneumothorax may occur in those who have pulmonary hypoplasia associated with renal abnormalities.

Table 28.2. Abdominal Masses in the Neonate

Type of Mass	Total Percentage
Renal	55
Hydronephrosis	
Ureteropelvic junction obstruction	
Multicystic dysplastic kidney	
Polycystic kidney disease	
Mesoblastic nephroma	
Renal ectopia	
Renal vein thrombosis	
Nephroblastomatosis	
Wilms tumor	
Genital	15
Hydrometrocolpos	
Ovarian cyst	
Gastrointestinal	20

Source: From Pinto E, Guignard JP. Renal masses in the neonate. *Biol Neonate* 1995;68:175–184.

    C. **Laboratory evaluation.** Kidney function tests must be interpreted in relation to gestational and postnatal age (see Tables 28.4 and 28.5).

        1. Urinalysis reflects the developmental stages of renal physiology.

            a. Specific gravity. Full-term infants have a limited concentrating ability with a maximum specific gravity of 1.021 to 1.025.

            b. Protein excretion varies with gestational age. Urinary protein excretion is higher in premature infants and decreases progressively with postnatal age (see Table 28.4). In normal full-term infants, protein excretion is minimal after the second week of life.

            c. Glycosuria is commonly present in premature infants of <34 weeks' gestation. The tubular resorption of glucose is <93% in infants born before 34 weeks' gestation compared with 99% in infants born after 34 weeks' gestation. Glucose excretion rates are highest in infants born before 28 weeks' gestation.

            d. Hematuria is abnormal and rare in the term newborn. It is more frequent in the premature infants and may indicate intrinsic kidney damage or result from a bleeding or clotting abnormality (see section III.G).

Table 28.3. Congenital Syndromes with Renal Components

Dysmorphic Disorders, Sequences, and Associations	General Features	Renal Abnormalities
Oligohydramnios sequence (Potter syndrome)	Altered facies, pulmonary hypoplasia, abnormal limb and head position	Renal agenesis, severe bilateral obstruction, severe bilateral dysplasia, autosomal recessive polycystic kidney disease
VATER and VACTERL syndrome	Vertebral anomalies, anal atresia, tracheoesophageal fistula, radial dysplasia, cardiac and limb defects	Renal agenesis, renal dysplasia, renal ectopia
MURCS association and Rokitansky sequence	Failure of paramesonephric ducts, vaginal and uterus hypoplasia/atresia, cervicothoracic somite dysplasia	Renal hypoplasia/agenesis, renal ectopia, double ureters
Prune belly	Hypoplasia of abdominal muscle, cryptorchidism	Megaureters, hydronephrosis, dysplastic kidneys, atonic bladder
Spina bifida	Meningomyelocele	Neurogenic bladder, vesicoureteral reflux, hydronephrosis, double ureter, horseshoe kidney
Caudal dysplasia sequence (caudal regression syndrome)	Sacral (and lumbar) hypoplasia, disruption of the distal spinal cord	Neurogenic bladder, vesicoureteral reflux, hydronephrosis, renal agenesis
Anal atresia (high imperforate anus)	Rectovaginal, rectovesical, or rectourethral fistula tethered to the spinal cord	Renal agenesis, renal dysplasia
Hemihypertrophy	Hemihypertrophy	Wilms tumor, hypospadias
Aniridia	Aniridia, cryptorchidism	Wilms tumor
Drash syndrome	Ambiguous genitalia	Mesangial sclerosis, Wilms tumor
Small deformed or low-set ears		Renal agenesis/dysplasia

(continued)

Table 28.3. Congenital Syndromes with Renal Components (Continued)

Dysmorphic Disorders, Sequences, and Associations	General Features	Renal Abnormalities
Autosomal Recessive		
Cerebrohepatorenal syndrome (Zellweger syndrome)	Hepatomegaly, glaucoma, brain anomalies, chondrodystrophy	Cortical renal cysts
Jeune syndrome (asphyxiating thoracic dystrophy)	Small thoracic cage, short ribs, abnormal costochondral junctions, pulmonary hypoplasia	Cystic tubular dysplasia, glomerulosclerosis, hydronephrosis, horseshoe kidneys
Meckel-Gruber syndrome (dysencephalia splanchnocystica)	Encephalocele, microcephaly, polydactyly, cryptorchidism, cardiac anomalies, liver disease	Polycystic/dysplastic kidneys
Johanson-Blizzard syndrome	Hypoplastic alae nasi, hypothyroidism, deafness, imperforate anus, cryptorchidism	Hydronephrosis, caliectasis
Schinzel-Giedion syndrome	Short limbs, abnormal facies, bone abnormalities, hypospadias	Hydronephrosis, megaureter
Short rib–polydactyly syndrome	Short horizontal ribs, pulmonary hypoplasia, polysyndactyly, bone and cardiac defects, ambiguous genitalia	Glomerular and tubular cysts
Bardet-Biedl syndrome	Obesity, retinal pigmentation, polydactyly	Interstitial nephritis
Autosomal Dominant		
Tuberous sclerosis	Fibrous-angiomatous lesions, hypopigmented macules, intracranial calcifications, seizures, bone lesions	Polycystic kidneys, renal angiomyolipoma
Melnick-Fraser syndrome (branchio-oto-renal [BOR] syndrome)	Preauricular pits, branchial clefts, deafness	Renal dysplasia, duplicated ureters

(continued)

Table 28.3. *(Continued)*

Dysmorphic Disorders, Sequences, and Associations	General Features	Renal Abnormalities
Nail-patella syndrome (hereditary osteo-onychodysplasia)	Hypoplastic nails, hypoplastic or absent patella, other bone anomalies	Proteinuria, nephrotic syndrome
Townes syndrome	Thumb, auricular, and anal anomalies	Various renal abnormalities
X-Linked		
Oculocerebrorenal syndrome (Lowe syndrome)	Cataracts, rickets, mental retardation	Fanconi syndrome
Oral–facial–digital (OFD) syndrome type I	Oral clefts, hypoplastic alae nasi, digital asymmetry (X-linked, lethal in men)	Renal microcysts
Trisomy 21 (Down syndrome)	Abnormal facies, brachycephaly, congenital heart disease	Cystic dysplastic kidney and other renal abnormalities
X0 syndrome (Turner syndrome)	Small stature, congenital heart disease, amenorrhea	Horseshoe kidney, duplications and malrotations of the urinary collecting system
Trisomy 13 (Patau syndrome)	Abnormal facies, cleft lip and palate, congenital heart disease	Cystic dysplastic kidneys and other renal anomalies
Trisomy 18 (Edwards syndrome)	Abnormal facies, abnormal ears, overlapping digits, congenital heart disease	Cystic dysplastic kidneys, horseshoe kidney, or duplication
XXY, XXX syndrome (Triploidy syndrome)	Abnormal facies, cardiac defects, hypospadias and cryptorchidism in men, syndactyly	Various renal abnormalities
Partial trisomy 10q	Abnormal facies, microcephaly, limb and cardiac abnormalities	Various renal abnormalities

Table 28.4. Normal Urinary and Renal Values in Term and Preterm Infants

	Preterm Infants <34 Weeks	Term Infants at Birth	Term Infants 2 Weeks	Term Infants 8 Weeks
GFR (mL/minute/1.73 m^2)	13–58	15–60	63–80	
Bicarbonate threshold (mEq/L)	14–18	21	21.5	
TRP (%)	>85	>95		
Protein excretion (mg/m^2/24 hours) (mean ± 1 SD)	60 ± 96	31 ± 44		
Maximal concentration ability (mOsmol/L)	500	800	900	1,200
Maximal diluting ability (mOsmol/L)	25–30	25–30	25–30	25–30
Specific gravity	1.002–1.015	1.002–1.020	1.002–1.025	1.002–1.030
Dipstick				
pH	5.0–8.0	4.5–8.0	4.5–8.0	4.5–8.0
Proteins	Neg to ++	Neg to +	Neg	Neg
Glucose	Neg to ++	Neg	Neg	Neg
Blood	Neg	Neg	Neg	Neg
Leukocytes	Neg	Neg	Neg	Neg

GFR, glomerular filtration rate; TRP, tubular reabsorption of phosphate; SD, standard deviation; Neg, negative.

e. The urinary sediment examination will usually demonstrate multiple epithelial cells (thought to be urethral mucosal cells) for the first 24 to 48 hours. In infants with asphyxia, an increase in epithelial cells and transient microscopic hematuria with leukocytes is common. Further investigation is necessary if these sediment findings persist. Hyaline and fine granular casts are common in dehydration or hypotension. Uric acid crystals are common in dehydration states and concentrated urine samples. They may be seen as pink or reddish brown diaper staining (particularly with the newer absorptive diapers).

2. **Method of collection**

   a. Suprapubic aspiration is the most reliable method to obtain an uncontaminated sample collection for urine culture. Ultrasound guidance will improve chance of success.

   b. Bladder catheterization is used if an infant has failed to pass urine by 36 to 48 hours and is not apparently hypovolemic (see section III.B), if precise determination of urine volume is needed, or to optimize urine drainage if functional or anatomic obstruction is suspected.

   c. Bag collections are adequate for most studies such as determinations of specific gravity, pH, electrolytes, protein, glucose, and sediment but should never be used for urine culture. Bagged samples are not appropriate when urinary tract infection (UTI) is suspected. Bladder catheterization can cause trauma of the urethral mucosa; therefore, bag collection is the preferred method if hematuria is suspected.

   d. Diaper urine specimens are reliable for estimation of pH and qualitative determination of the presence of glucose, protein, and blood.

3. **Evaluation of renal function**

   a. Serum creatinine at birth reflects maternal kidney function. In healthy term infants, serum creatinine levels fall from 0.8 mg/dL at birth to 0.5 mg/dL at 5 to 7 days and reach a stable level of 0.3 to 0.4 mg/dL by 9 days. Premature infants' serum creatinine may rise transiently for the first few days and then will reduce slowly over weeks to months depending on the level of prematurity. The rate of decrease in serum creatinine in the first few weeks is slower in younger gestational age infants with lower GFR (Table 28.5).

   b. Blood urea nitrogen (BUN) is another potential indicator of kidney function. However, BUN can be elevated as a result of increased production of urea nitrogen in hypercatabolic states or increased protein intake, sequestered blood, tissue breakdown, or from hemoconcentration.

Table 28.5. Normal Serum Creatinine Values in Term and Preterm Infants (Mean ± SD)

Age (Day)	<28 Weeks	28–32 Weeks	32–37 Weeks	>37 Weeks
3	1.05 ± 0.27	0.88 ± 0.25	0.78 ± 0.22	0.75 ± 0.2
7	0.95 ± 0.36	0.94 ± 0.37	0.77 ± 0.48	0.56 ± 0.4
14	0.81 ± 0.26	0.78 ± 0.36	0.62 ± 0.4	0.43 ± 0.25
28	0.66 ± 0.28	0.59 ± 0.38	0.40 ± 0.28	0.34 ± 0.2

Source: From Rudd PT, Hughes EA, Placzek MM, et al. Reference ranges for plasma creatinine during the first month of life. *Arch Dis Child* 1983;58:212–215; van den Anker JN, de Groot R, Broerse HM, et al. Assessment of glomerular filtration rate in preterm infants by serum creatinine: comparison with inulin clearance. *Pediatrics* 1995;96:1156–1158.

Table 28.6. Inulin Clearance Glomerular Filtration Rate in Healthy Premature Infants

Age	mL/minute/1.73 m^2
1–3 days	14.0 ± 5
1–7 days	18.7 ± 5.5
4–8 days	44.3 ± 9.3
3–13 days	47.8 ± 10.7
1.5–4 months	67.4 ± 16.6
8 years	103 ± 12

    c. GFR can be measured directly by clearance studies of either exogenous substances (inulin, chromium ethylenediaminetetraacetic acid [Cr-EDTA], sodium iothalamate) or endogenous substances such as creatinine or cystatin C (Table 28.6). Practical considerations such as frequent blood sampling, urine collection, or infusion of an exogenous substance limit their use and are used only for research purposes. GFR is most often estimated from serum creatinine and body length (see Table 28.1), although the equation must be used with caution because it is strictly an estimate with significant predictive variability in determining true GFR. Newer estimates using cystatin C, although only experimental now, are likely to come to clinical use soon.

    d. Measurement of serum and urine electrolytes is used to guide fluid and electrolyte management and in assessing kidney tubular function. One must consider serum values and clinical context in order to interpret urine electrolyte measurements.

  D. Radiologic studies

    1. Ultrasonography is the initial imaging study to delineate kidney parenchymal architecture. This is a noninvasive, low-cost study that can be done at the bedside, especially useful in unstable infants. It can easily confirm the presence of gross renal abnormalities seen in a previous antenatal ultrasound, such as hydronephrosis or dysplastic kidney disease. As a general rule, the length of the kidneys in millimeters is approximately the gestational age in weeks. Normative data is presented on Figure 28.1. Larger kidneys may suggest the presence of hydronephrosis, polycystic kidney disease (PKD), multicystic dysplastic kidney disease (MCDK), or rarely, congenital nephrotic syndrome or renal tumors. Smaller kidneys may suggest dysplasia or hypoplasia. The kidney cortex has echogenicity similar to that of the liver or spleen in the neonate, in contrast to the hypoechoic renal cortex seen in adults and older children. Hyperechogenic kidneys can be seen in PKD, cystic dysplasia, glomerulocystic disease, or kidney injury. In addition, the medullary pyramids in the neonate are much more hypoechoic than the cortex and hence

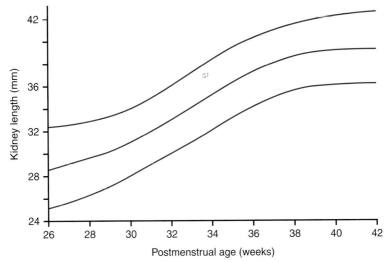

Figure 28.1. Kidney length for postmenstrual age. Smoothed cross-sectional growth charts showing the mean (± 2 SD) for postmenstrual age 26–42 weeks. (From de Vries L, Levene MI. Measurement of renal size in preterm and term infants by real-time ultrasound. *Arch Dis Child* 1983;58[2]:145–147.)

are more prominent in appearance. Color Doppler flow techniques have significant intraoperator variability but can visualize and measure RBF and renal artery resistive index (RI). Preterm infants tend to have higher RI compared to term infants; higher RI can suggest renal parenchymal disease and urinary tract obstruction.

2. **Voiding cystourethrography (VCUG)**, with fluoroscopy, is an excellent method to determine vesicoureteral reflux (VUR), bladder anatomy, and define lower tract anatomy such as in posterior urethral valves (PUV). Radionuclide cystography is often used to evaluate VUR because of its lower radiation dose. However, VCUG produces better static imaging for anatomical defects and is preferred for the initial evaluation of obstructive uropathy. Most radiologists perform VCUGs without sedation, the use of which has been associated with false-positive results.

3. **Radionuclide scintography** is useful in demonstrating the position and relative function of the kidneys in infants who have sufficient GFR. Isotopes such as technetium-99m-diethylenetriaminepentacetic acid (DTPA) or mercaptoacetyltriglycine (MAG3) are handled by glomerular filtration and can be used to assess RBF and kidney function. In conjunction with intravenously administered furosemide, it can help differentiate obstructive from nonobstructive hydronephrosis. Isotopes that bind to the renal tubules, such as technetium-99m-dimercaptosuccinic acid (DMSA), produce static images of the renal cortex. This may be helpful for assessing acute pyelonephritis and renal scarring from renal artery emboli or renal vascular disorders and to

quantify the amount of renal cortex in patients with renal dysplasia and hypoplasia. Most of these nuclear techniques rely on renal filtration and are thus of questionable use in very preterm infants.

III. COMMON CLINICAL KIDNEY PROBLEMS IN NEONATES

A. **Conditions diagnosed by prenatal ultrasonography.** Routine maternal ultrasonographic screening detects an incidence of fetal GU abnormalities of 0.3% to 0.5%.

1. **Hydronephrosis** is the most common abnormal finding, reported in >80% of the cases with a kidney abnormality. Approximately 75% of these are confirmed postnatally.

   a. Initial management of a newborn with prenatally identified hydronephrosis depends on the clinical condition of the patient and the suspected nature of the lesion.

   b. Unilateral hydronephrosis is more common and is not associated with systemic or pulmonary complications if the contralateral kidney is normal. Postnatal ultrasonographic confirmation may be carried out electively at approximately 2 to 4 weeks of life, depending on severity. Earlier ultrasonographic examination might miss abnormalities because hydronephrosis may not be detected because of physiologic dehydration. It is important to repeat the study if done in the first few days after birth.

   c. Bilateral hydronephrosis is more worrisome, especially if oligohydramnios or pulmonary disease is present. In the male infant, postnatal evaluation (ultrasonography and VCUG) should be performed within the first day to determine the etiology (PUV, ureteropelvic junction [UPJ] obstruction, ureterovesical junction [UVJ] obstruction, prune belly syndrome, or VUR). With postbladder obstruction such as PUV, ultrasonography will often demonstrate a trabeculated and thickened bladder wall. Concomitant tortuous ureters are an ominous finding for overall kidney function and development.

   d. Antibiotic prophylaxis is recommended until VCUG rules out VUR. Nitrofurantoin (1 to 2 mg/kg/day) or trimethoprim-sulfamethoxazole (2 mg of trimethoprim plus 10 mg of sulfamethoxazole per kilogram) are used for UTI prophylaxis in older infants. In infants with postgestational age <48 weeks, nitrofurantoin can cause hemolytic anemia and sulfa displaces bilirubin from albumin and kernicterus can develop. Due to these reasons, amoxicillin (10 mg/kg/day) is the initial drug of choice in infants under a postgestational age of 48 weeks (see section III.H).

   e. In the presence of VUR, long-term prophylactic antibiotics have been shown in one trial to reduce the number of symptomatic UTIs. Despite the improvement in clinical infections, there was no difference in the rate of renal scarring between children given prophylaxis or not. This finding might indicate the underlying renal dysplasia is often present during renal development even when early prophylaxis is initiated.

2. **Multicystic dysplastic kidney (MCDK)** is being diagnosed more by routine prenatal ultrasonography, especially those with unilateral involvement. An MCDK is one in which no functional parenchyma is present and a lobulated "ball of grapes"–like structure is present. Infants with

unilateral MCDK are usually asymptomatic, and by definition, the affected kidney has no renal function as demonstrated by DMSA renal scan. There is general agreement that surgical removal is indicated only rarely in cases with infection or with respiratory compromise secondary to abdominal compression by the abnormal kidney. Although surgical removal had been suggested to decrease the potential of renal cell carcinoma, there is no evidence that surgical removal of asymptomatic MCDK improves long-term outcomes. In asymptomatic patients, medical observation is the current practice and surgical removal is reserved only if symptoms develop. Although the affected kidney may initially grow (due to cyst growth) during infancy, the affected kidney usually involutes and is often no longer visible on imaging by age 5 years.

3. Renal abnormalities may be associated with other congenital anomalies including neural tube defects, congenital heart lesions, intestinal obstructive lesions, abdominal wall defects, central nervous system (CNS) or spinal abnormalities, and urologic abnormalities of the lower urinary tract.

B. Acute kidney injury (AKI), previously termed acute renal failure, is defined as an abrupt decrease in glomerular filtration, with or without underlying structural abnormalities. The condition often presents with diminished urinary output and/or elevation of serum creatinine (Table 28.7) and other electrolyte abnormalities. AKI correlates with mortality as in older pediatric and adult patients. AKI may be secondary to prerenal azotemia, intrinsic (tubular, glomerular, or interstitial disease), or postrenal disorders (obstructive) (Table 28.8).

1. Prerenal azotemia occurs when the kidney becomes underperfused. The most common causes of prerenal azotemia are loss of effective blood volume, relative loss of intravascular volume from increased capillary leak, poor cardiac output, medications, or intra-abdominal compartment syndrome. These conditions can lead to intrinsic renal tubular damage if not corrected expeditiously.

Table 28.7. Acute Kidney Injury Criteria in Neonates

Stage	Serum Creatinine Criteria	Urinary Output Criteria
1	SCr increase of ≥0.3 mg/dL or SCr increase to 150%–199% of baseline	UOP >0.5 mL/kg/hour and ≤1 mL/kg/hour
2	SCr increase to 200%–299% of baseline	UOP >0.1 mL/kg/hour and ≤0.5 mL/kg/hour
3	SCr increase to ≥300% of baseline or SCr ≥2.5 mg/dL or receipt of dialysis	UOP ≤0.1 mL/kg/hour

Baseline serum creatinine (SCr) will be defined as the lowest previous SCr value.
UOP, urine output.

Table 28.8. Causes of Acute Kidney Injury in the Neonatal Period

1. Prerenal

   a. Reduced effective circulatory volume

      i. Hemorrhage dehydration

      ii. Sepsis

      iii. Necrotizing enterocolitis

      iv. Congenital heart disease

      v. Hypoalbuminemia

   b. Increased renal vascular resistance

      i. Polycythemia

      ii. Indomethacin

      iii. Adrenergic drugs (e.g., tolazoline)

   c. Hypoxia/asphyxia

2. Intrinsic or renal parenchymal

   a. Sustained hypoperfusion leading to acute tubular necrosis

   b. Congenital anomalies

      i. Agenesis

      ii. Hypoplasia/dysplasia

      iii. Polycystic kidney disease

   c. Thromboembolic disease

      i. Bilateral renal vein thrombosis

      ii. Bilateral renal arterial thrombosis

   d. Nephrotoxins

      i. Aminoglycosides

      ii. Radiographic contrast media

      iii. Maternal use of ACE inhibitors or indomethacin

3. Obstructive

   a. Urethral obstruction

      i. Posterior urethral valves

      ii. Stricture

(continued)

Table 28.8. *(Continued)*

b. Ureterocele
c. Ureteropelvic/ureterovesical obstruction
d. Extrinsic tumors
e. Neurogenic bladder
f. Megacystis or megaureter syndrome
ACE, angiotensin-converting enzyme.

2. **Intrinsic AKI** implies direct damage to the glomeruli, interstitium, or tubules. In neonates, tubular injury is most commonly caused by prolonged or severe ischemia, nephrotoxins, or sepsis. Glomerular and primary interstitial injury is very rare in neonates.

3. **Postrenal AKI** results from obstruction to urinary flow in both kidneys. In boys, the most common lesion is PUV; however, acquired obstruction (from masses, stones, or fungal balls) can also occur. Renal function may be abnormal even after correction of the obstruction.

   Evaluation to determine the underlying etiology of rising creatinine or decreased urine output is critical to AKI management.

4. Evaluate history for oligohydramnios, perinatal asphyxia, bleeding disorders, polycythemia, thrombocytosis, thrombocytopenia, sepsis, or maternal drug use. Evaluate for the presence of nephrotoxic medication. Aminoglycoside drugs such as gentamicin for sepsis rule out, nonsteroidal anti-inflammatory drugs (NSAIDs) such as ibuprofen or indomethacin for patent ductus arteriosus (PDA) closure, and ACE inhibitors such as captopril or enalapril commonly used in infants with congenital heart defects can cause AKI.

5. Place an indwelling urinary catheter for accurate output measurement.

6. Evaluate for signs and symptoms of intravascular depletion (tachycardia, sunken fontanelle, poor skin turgor, dry mucous membranes).

7. If edema is present, evaluation to determine whether intravascular volume is depleted (e.g., in hypoalbuminemia) or elevated is helpful in determining the etiology and plan of action.

8. A fluid challenge with normal saline 10 to 20 mL/kg over 30 minutes can not only replete intravascular volume but also help to determine if intravascular depletion is present. Evaluation for cardiac failure is imperative prior to aggressive fluid resuscitation for renal failure.

9. Renal ultrasonogram should be performed to rule out bladder obstruction and to assess for congenital anomalies of the kidney and urinary tract.

10. Laboratory evaluation can help determine the underlying etiology. Table 28.9 lists laboratory tests that are helpful in differentiating

Table 28.9. Renal Failure Indices in the Oliguric Neonate

Indices	Prerenal Failure	Intrinsic Renal Failure
Urine sodium (mEq/L)	10–50	30–90
Urine/plasma creatinine	29.2 ± 1.6	9.7 ± 3.6
FENa*	0.9 ± 0.6	4.3 ± 2.2

*Fractional excretion of sodium (FENa) defined in Chapter 9.
Source: Modified from Mathew OP, Jones AS, James E, et al. Neonatal renal failure: usefulness of diagnostic indices. *Pediatrics* 1980;65:57.

prerenal azotemia from intrinsic and obstructive causes. Test samples should be obtained before fluid challenge if possible.

Management of those who develop AKI should focus on treating the underlying etiology, avoiding further injury, and addressing consequences of decreased renal function.

11. As mentioned, response to fluid challenge not only provides information about the underlying cause of AKI but also serves as the beginning of the management plan. Close evaluation of the cause of the intravascular volume depletion should be sought and appropriate fluid management should be given. Intravenous albumin should be considered for those with low serum albumin (1 g/kg of 5% albumin).

12. Avoidance of nephrotoxic medications to prevent further insult and dose adjustment of concurrent medications based on estimated renal function are critical to early recovery. Remember that rising creatinine is a late (and slow) manifestation of diminished GFR. Avoidance of further injury to damaged kidneys might prevent further complications.

13. Furosemide may be given to correct fluid overload but has not been shown to prevent or diminish AKI. Adequate urine output does not signify adequate or recovered GFR. If patient has response to diuresis, careful monitoring of electrolytes and fluid status should be followed; hypokalemia, metabolic alkalosis, or hypovolemia can result after several days of treatment in ongoing AKI. Low-dose or "renal dose" (2 µg/kg/day) dopamine has *not* been shown to prevent AKI, although it may also increase urine output.

14. If blood pressure is low in relation to vascular congestion and/or abdominal pressures, consider increasing blood pressure with inotropes to increase glomerular filtration (see Chapter 40).

15. **Management of complications**
    a. Discontinue or minimize potassium (K+) intake. Low-K+ formula such as Similac PM 60/40 or K+-free IV solution are used. Treatment of hyperkalemia (K+ >6 mEq/L) is as follows:
    i. Calcium is given as 1 to 2 mL/kg of calcium gluconate 10% over 2 to 4 minutes for cardioprotection. The electrocardiogram (ECG) is monitored.

ii. **Sodium bicarbonate will shift K into the cells and can temporarily lower serum K^+**. The 1 mEq/kg given intravenously over 5 to 10 minutes will decrease serum potassium by 1 mEq/L.

iii. **Glucose and insulin will also shift K^+ into cells to temporarily lower serum K^+ levels.** Begin with a bolus of regular human insulin (0.05 units/kg) and dextrose 10% in water (2 mL/kg) followed by a continuous infusion of dextrose 10% in water at 2 to 4 mL/kg/hour and human regular insulin (10 units per 100 mL) at 1 mL/kg/hour. Monitor blood glucose level frequently. Maintain a ratio of 1 or 2 units of insulin to 4 g glucose.

iv. **Furosemide** can be given for kaliuresis as well as natriuresis. A trial of 1 mg/kg intermittently is given. Avoid volume depletion due to overdiuresis.

v. **Sodium polystyrene sulfonate (Kayexalate)** is administered rectally in a dose of 1.0 to 1.5 g/kg (dissolved in normal saline at 0.5 g/mL saline) or orally in a dose of 1.0 g/kg (dissolved in dextrose 10% in water) as needed to decrease serum K levels. The enema tube, a thin silastic feeding tube, is inserted 1 to 3 cm. If possible, we avoid using Kayexalate in low birth weight infants due to the risk of bowel perforation. Kayexalate 1 g/kg removes approximately 1 mEq/L of potassium. Kayexalate is active in the colon, so rectal doses lower potassium quicker than oral doses.

vi. **Dialysis** is considered when hyperkalemia cannot be controlled with the above medical therapy. Although hemodialysis (HD) is the most rapid way to remove K^+, peritoneal dialysis (PD) or continuous venovenous hemoperfusion (CVVH) can be used (see section III.B.15.i in the following text).

b. **Fluid management** is based on the patient's fluid status and determination of ongoing losses. Unless dehydration or polyuric states are present, volume should be limited to replacement of insensible losses and urine output (see Chapter 23). The inability to adequately prescribe nutrition due to fluid restriction and/or significant fluid overload is indication for dialysis.

c. Sodium (Na^+) is restricted and Na^+ concentration is monitored, accounting for fluid balance. Hyponatremia is usually secondary to excess free water and the inability of the injured kidneys to appropriately reabsorb filter Na^+. Close monitoring of electrolytes, especially sodium, is needed during diuretic therapy or with dialysis.

d. Phosphorus is restricted in AKI by using a low-phosphorus formula (e.g., Similac PM 60/40). Oral calcium carbonate can be used as a phosphate-binding agent.

e. Calcium supplementation is given if ionized calcium is decreased or the patient is symptomatic. In infants with CKD, 1,25-dihydroxyvitamin D or its analog is given to maximize intestinal Ca^{2+} absorption and prevent renal osteodystrophy (see Chapter 25).

f. Metabolic acidosis is usually mild unless there is (i) significant tubular dysfunction with decreased ability to reabsorb bicarbonate or (ii) increased lactate production due to decreased perfusion due to heart failure or volume loss from hemorrhage (see section III.B). Use sodium bicarbonate or sodium citrate to correct severe metabolic acidosis.

g. Nutrition is critical to the growing newborn. Infants who can take oral feeding are given a low-phosphate and low-potassium formula with a low renal solute load (e.g., Similac PM 60/40). Caloric density can be progressively increased to a maximum of 50 kcal/oz with glucose polymers (Polycose) and oil. Adequate protein for neonates with otherwise normal renal function should be provided unless they are on continuous HD or PD. Because these therapies can cause protein losses of 1.0 to 1.5 g/kg/day, additional protein supplementation is necessary.

h. Hypertension (see section III.D).

i. Dialysis is indicated when conservative management has been unsuccessful in correcting severe fluid overload, hyperkalemia, acidosis, and uremia. Inadequate nutrition because of severe fluid restriction in the anuric infant is a relative indication for dialysis. Because the technical aspects and the supportive care are specialized and demanding, this procedure must be performed in centers where the staff has experience with acute dialysis in infants and neonates. When using either HD or CVVH, the smaller blood volume of neonates results in a relatively large extracorporeal circuit volume. A blood prime is required for each treatment, and the infant may experience temperature instability and rapid fluid shifts. PD must be performed manually with individual exchanges due to the small volumes initially used. Despite recent advances in dialysis devices and more broadly based expertise, dialysis-dependent AKI in a neonate is still a disease with high morbidity and mortality.

C. Congenital anomalies of the kidney and urinary tract (CAKUT) may become apparent with prenatal ultrasound, discovered at birth, or present later in life.

Common lesions are hydronephrosis, dysplastic kidneys (with or without cysts), MCDK, and obstruction of the urinary system either at the level of the UPJ, UVJ, or by valves at the urethra (UPJ). Besides CAKUT anomalies, ARPKD which is associated with liver fibrosis is another cause of renal failure in neonates. Autosomal dominant polycystic kidney disease (ADPKD) is more common in the general population but does not generally present until later in life. Differential diagnosis includes other renal masses (see Table 28.2). The severity of renal impairment in these diseases varies from extreme oligohydramnios and *in utero* compromise to late presentation in adulthood. Ultimately, the prognosis depends on the severity of the anomaly, whether the contralateral kidney is viable, and on extrarenal organ dysfunction. In the newborn course, the degree of pulmonary hypoplasia will dictate the likelihood of viability of the infant. Long term, CAKUT remains the most common cause of CKD and end-stage renal disease (ESRD) in childhood.

D. Blood pressure in the newborn is much lower than in older children and adults. Specific values are related to weight and gestational age. Blood pressure rises with postnatal age, 1 to 2 mm Hg/day during the first week and 1 mm Hg/week during the next 6 weeks in both the preterm and full-term infant (Fig. 28.2).

1. Normative values of blood pressure are shown for full-term infants and premature infants in Tables 28.10 to 28.12. All normative values for blood pressure are based on pressures measured in the arm of calm infants. Leg pressures are often higher than arm pressures, as are measurements taken during crying or distress.

A

Measurements in Boys Birth to 12 Months

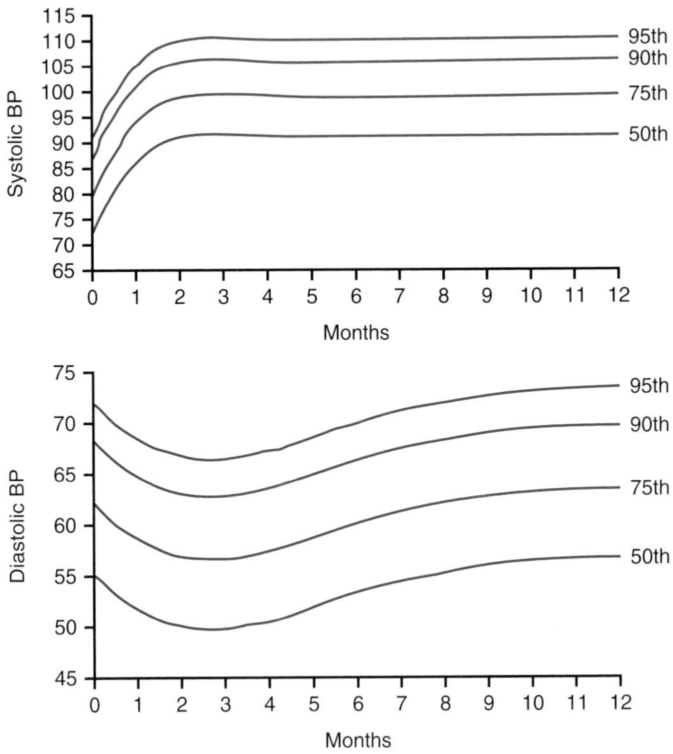

Both Percentile													
Systolic BP	87	101	106	106	106	106	106	106	106	106	106	106	106
Diastolic BP	58	58	63	63	63	65	66	67	68	68	69	69	69
Height cm	51	59	63	66	68	70	72	73	74	76	77	78	83
Weight kg	4	4	5	5	6	7	8	9	9	10	10	11	11

Figure 28.2. Age-specific percentiles for blood pressure (BP). (From Task Force on Blood Pressure Control in Children. *Report of the Second Task Force on Blood Pressure Control in Children—1987.* Bethesda, MD: National Heart, Lung and Blood Institute, National Institutes of Health; 1987.)

2. **Hypertension** is defined as persistent blood pressure >2 standard deviations above the mean. The clinical signs and symptoms, which are all nonspecific and may even be absent, include cardiorespiratory abnormalities such as tachypnea, cardiomegaly, or heart failure; neurologic findings such as irritability, lethargy, or seizure; failure to thrive; or gastrointestinal (GI) difficulties. All infants in the neonatal intensive care unit (NICU) should have their blood pressures measured, preferably in

B

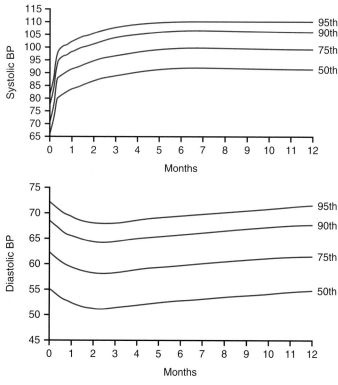

Measurements in Girls Birth to 12 Months

Both Percentile													
Systolic BP	76	88	101	104	105	106	106	106	106	106	106	106	106
Diastolic BP	48	55	64	64	65	65	66	66	66	67	67	67	67
Height cm	54	56	56	58	61	63	66	68	70	72	74	76	77
Weight kg	4	4	4	5	5	6	7	8	9	9	10	10	11

Figure 28.2. *(Continued)*

the arm when calm. Persistently elevated blood pressures should lead to a more thorough evaluation of etiology.

3. Neonatal hypertension has many causes (Table 28.13). The three most common causes of hypertension in newborns are secondary to umbilical artery thrombi, bronchopulmonary dysplasia, and coarctation of the aorta. Evaluation includes history and physical examination, a review of fluid status, medications, history of umbilical or arterial line placement, and four extremity blood pressure measurements. Renin-mediated hypertension and fluid overload may both contribute to renal causes of hypertension. Urinalysis, renal function studies, serum electrolyte levels,

Table 28.10. Normal Longitudinal Blood Pressure in Full-term Infants (mm Hg)

	Boys		Girls	
Age	Systolic	Diastolic	Systolic	Diastolic
First day	67 ± 7	37 ± 7	68 ± 8	38 ± 7
Fourth day	76 ± 8	44 ± 9	75 ± 8	45 ± 8
1 month	84 ± 10	46 ± 9	82 ± 9	46 ± 10
3 months	92 ± 11	55 ± 10	89 ± 11	54 ± 10
6 months	96 ± 9	58 ± 10	92 ± 10	56 ± 10

Source: From Gemeilli M, Managanaro R, Mamì C, et al. Longitudinal study of blood pressure during the 1st year of life. *Eur J Pediatr* 1990;149:318.

and renal ultrasonographic examination should also be obtained. Color Doppler flow studies may detect aortic or renal vascular thrombosis, although this test is not reliable in neonates and carries the possibility of both false positives and false negatives. A DMSA renal scan may detect segmental renal arterial infarctions. Plasma renin levels are difficult to interpret in neonates. Echocardiogram is indicated if coarctation is suspected and can determine if left ventricular hypertrophy has occurred from sustained hypertension.

Table 28.11. Systolic and Diastolic Blood Pressure Ranges in Infants of 500 to 2,000 g Birth Weight at 3 to 6 Hours of Life

Birth Weight (g)	Systolic (mm Hg)	Diastolic (mm Hg)
501–750	50–62	26–36
751–1,000	48–59	23–36
1,001–1,250	49–61	26–35
1,251–1,500	46–56	23–33
1,501–1,750	46–58	23–33
1,751–2,000	48–61	24–35

Source: From Hegyi T, Carbone MT, Anwar M, et al. Blood pressure ranges in premature infants. I. The first hours of life. *J Pediatr* 1994;124:627–633.

Table 28.12. Estimated Blood Pressure Values after 2 Weeks of Age in Infants from 26 to 44 Weeks Postconceptional Age

Postconceptual Age	50th Percentile	95th Percentile	99th Percentile
44 weeks			
SBP	88	105	110
DBP	50	68	73
MAP	63	80	85
42 weeks			
SBP	85	98	102
DBP	50	65	70
MAP	62	76	81
40 weeks			
SBP	80	95	100
DBP	50	65	70
MAP	60	75	80
38 weeks			
SBP	77	92	97
DBP	50	65	70
MAP	59	74	79
36 weeks			
SBP	72	87	92
DBP	50	65	70
MAP	59	72	77
34 weeks			
SBP	70	85	90
DBP	40	55	60
MAP	50	65	70

(continued)

Table 28.12. *(Continued)*

Postconceptual Age	50th Percentile	95th Percentile	99th Percentile
32 weeks			
SBP	68	83	88
DBP	40	55	60
MAP	49	64	69
30 weeks			
SBP	65	80	85
DBP	40	55	60
MAP	48	63	68
28 weeks			
SBP	60	75	80
DBP	38	50	54
MAP	45	58	63
26 weeks			
SBP	55	72	77
DBP	30	50	56
MAP	38	57	63

SBP, systolic blood pressure; DBP, diastolic blood pressure; MAP, mean arterial pressure.
Source: From Dionne JM, Abitbol CL, Flynn JT. Hypertension in infancy: diagnosis, management and outcome. *Pediatr Nephrol* 2012;27:17–32.

4. Management is directed at correcting the underlying cause whenever possible. Antihypertensive therapy (Table 28.14) is administered for sustained hypertension that is not related to volume overload or concomitant medications. Hydralazine is most commonly used acutely or as a PRN medication. Amlodipine or lisinopril are often used for persistent hypertension. Regardless of the need for antihypertensive medications, most neonatally acquired hypertension resolves within a few years. Because of their early course, NICU graduates are at increased risk for developing hypertension during adolescence, especially those who require treatment with antihypertensive medications.

E. Renal vascular thrombosis

1. **Renal artery thrombosis (RAT)** is often related to the use of indwelling umbilical artery catheters which can obstruct or emit an embolus into

Table 28.13. Causes of Hypertension in the Neonate

1. Vascular

    a. Renal artery thrombosis

    b. Renal vein thrombosis

    c. Coarctation of the aorta

    d. Renal artery stenosis

    e. Idiopathic arterial calcification

2. Renal

    a. Obstructive uropathy

    b. Polycystic kidney disease

    c. Acute kidney injury

    d. Chronic kidney disease

    e. Renal tumor

    f. Wilms tumor

    g. Glomerulonephritis

    h. Pyelonephritis

3. Endocrine

    a. Congenital adrenal hypoplasia

    b. Primary hyperaldosteronism

    c. Hyperthyroidism

4. Neurologic

    a. Increased intracranial pressure

    b. Cushing disease

    c. Neural crest tumor

    d. Cerebral angioma

    e. Drug withdrawal

5. Pulmonary

    a. Bronchopulmonary dysplasia

(continued)

Table 28.13. *(Continued)*
6. Drugs
a. Corticosteroids
b. Caffeine
c. Theophylline
d. Adrenergic agents
e. Phenylephrine
7. Other
a. Fluid/electrolyte overload
b. Abdominal surgery
c. Associated with extracorporeal membrane oxygenation (ECMO)

the renal artery. Other rare causes include congenital hypercoagulable states and severe hypotension. Although the management is controversial, potential options include surgical thrombectomy, thrombolytic agents, and conservative medical care including antihypertensive therapy. The surgical renal salvage rate is no better than medical management. As with other etiologies of neonatal hypertension, patients with unilateral RAT who receive conservative medical treatment are usually normotensive by 2 years of age, no longer requiring antihypertensive medications, and have normal creatinine clearance, although some have unilateral renal atrophy with compensatory contralateral hypertrophy. There have been reports of long-term complications with hypertension and/or proteinuria and progression to renal failure in adolescence (see Chapter 44).

2. **Renal vein thrombosis (RVT)** has the predisposing conditions of hyperosmolarity, polycythemia, hypovolemia, and hypercoagulable states and is therefore often associated with infant of diabetic mothers, or use of umbilical venous catheters. Cases of intrauterine renal venous thrombosis have been described and present with calcification of the clot in the inferior vena cava (IVC). The classic clinical findings include gross hematuria often with clots, enlarged kidneys, hypertension, and thrombocytopenia. Other symptoms are nonspecific and include vomiting, shock, lower extremity edema, and abdominal distention. The diagnosis of RVT is confirmed by ultrasonography, which typically shows an enlarged kidney with diffuse homogenous hyperechogenicity; Doppler flow studies may detect thrombi in the IVC or renal vein leading to absent renal flow. The differential diagnosis includes renal masses or hemolytic uremic syndrome.

    The management of RVT is also controversial. Initial therapy should focus on the maintenance of circulation, fluid, and electrolyte

Table 28.14. Antihypertensive Agents for the Newborn (See Appendix A for Specific Dosing Recommendations)

	Dose	Comment
Diuretics		
Furosemide	0.5–1.0 mg/kg/dose IV, IM, PO	May cause hyponatremia, hypokalemia, hypercalciuria
Chlorothiazide	20–40 mg/kg/day PO; divided q12h	
Hydrochlorothiazide	2–3mg/kg/day; usually divided BID	
Vasodilators		
Hydralazine	0.25–1.0 mg/kg/dose; q6–8h	May cause tachycardia
Calcium Channel Blockers		
Amlodipine	0.1–0.4 mg/kg/dose PO; q12–24h	Slower onset of action, less likely to cause sudden hypotension
Nifedipine	0.2 mg/kg/dose SL, PO	Limited in neonates; may cause tachycardia
Nicardipine	Titrated, starting dose 0.5 μg/kg/minute IV continuous infusion. Up to 2 μg/kg/minute reported	Requires IV infusion
Isradipine	0.05–0.15 mg/kg/dose given q6–8h	May cause sudden hypotension
β-Receptor Antagonist		
Propranolol	0.5–1.0 mg/kg/dose PO; q6–8h	May cause bronchospasm
α- or β-Receptor Antagonist		
Labetalol	0.5–1.0 mg/kg/dose IV; q4–6h	Limited use in neonates
ACE Inhibitor		
Lisinopril	0.07–0.6 mg/kg/day PO; q24h	May cause oliguria hyperkalemia renal failure
Captopril	<3 months: 0.01–0.5 mg/kg/dose PO; q8h >3 months: 0.15–0.3 mg/kg/dose PO; q8h	
Enalapril	0.1–0.6 mg/kg/dose IV; 8–24 hours	

IV, intravenous; IM, intramuscular; PO, by mouth, BID, twice daily; SL, sublingual; ACE, angiotensin-converting enzyme.

balance while examining for underlying predisposing clinical conditions. Assessment of the coagulation status includes platelet count, prothrombin time (PT), partial thromboplastin time (PTT), fibrinogen, and fibrin split products and, if suggested by maternal history, lupus antiphospholipid antibodies.

No consensus exists on the use of heparin. If there is unilateral involvement without evidence of disseminated intravascular coagulation (DIC), conservative management is warranted. If there is bilateral involvement and evidence of DIC, more aggressive therapy is indicated because the infant is at risk for complete loss of kidney function. Heparin therapy should be initiated with an initial bolus of 50 to 100 units/kg followed by continuous infusion at 25 to 50 units/kg to maintain PTT of 1.5 times normal. Antithrombin III (AT III) activity should be reassessed before heparin therapy is instituted as AT III is required for the anticoagulant action of heparin. Recently, low molecular weight heparin has been used both as initial treatment for thrombosis and as prophylactic therapy after recannulization of the occluded vessel. In the treatment of patients with thrombosis, dosages of 200 to 300 anti-Fxa U/kg are reported to reach a therapeutic level of 0.5 to 1.0 anti-Fxa U/mL. Reported dosages range from 45 to 100 anti-Fxa units/kg to reach prophylactic levels of 0.2 to 0.4 anti-Fxa U/mL.

Thrombolytic therapy with streptokinase and urokinase has been used in both RAT and RVT, with variable success but are no longer commercially available. There is limited experience with the use of thromboplastin activator (TPA). This is used in low dose (0.02 to 0.03 mg/kg) if there is evidence of bleeding and titrated to PTT value of 1.5 times normal. Plasma infusion may be necessary to provide thromboplastin activation. Protamine and e-caproic acid should be present at the bedside because significant bleeding can occur. Surgical intervention should be considered if there has been an indwelling umbilical vein catheter, the thrombosis is bilateral, and involves the main renal veins leading to renal failure. This type of thrombosis is likely to have started in the IVC rather than intrarenal and hence is more likely amenable to surgical attention (see Chapter 44).

F. **Proteinuria** in small quantities during the first weeks of life is frequently found. After the first week, persistent proteinuria >250 mg/m^2/day should be investigated (see Table 28.4).

   1. In general, **mild proteinuria** reflects a vascular or tubular injury to the kidney or the inability of the immature tubules to reabsorb protein. Administration of large amounts of colloid can exceed the reabsorptive capacity of the neonatal renal tubules and may result in mild proteinuria.

   2. **Massive proteinuria** (>1.5 g/m^2/day), hypoalbuminemia with serum albumin levels <2.5 g/dL, and edema are all components of congenital nephrotic syndrome. Prenatal clues to the diagnosis include elevated maternal/amniotic alpha-fetoprotein levels and enlarged placenta. Children with severe forms of congenital nephrotic syndrome require daily intravenous albumin and Lasix for fluid removal, high caloric diets, replacement of thyroid, iron and vitamins due to excess losses of binding proteins, and ultimately, require bilateral nephrectomies and

renal transplantation. They are at high risk for infections and thrombosis due to immunoglobin losses and loss of anticoagulant proteins.

3. No specific treatment is required for mild proteinuria. Treat the underlying disease and monitor the proteinuria until resolved.

4. Glomerular disease is rare and usually associated with congenital nephrotic syndrome if presentation is in the nursery.

G. **Hematuria** is defined as >5 red blood cells (RBCs) per high-power field. It is uncommon in newborns and should always be investigated.

1. Hematuria has many causes (Table 28.15) including hemorrhagic disease of the newborn if vitamin K supplementation has not been given. The differential diagnosis for hematuria includes urate staining of the diaper, myoglobinuria, or hemoglobinuria. A negative dipstick with benign sediment suggests urates, whereas a positive dipstick with negative

Table 28.15. Etiology of Hematuria in the Newborn
1. Acute tubular necrosis
2. Cortical necrosis
3. Vascular disease
a. Renal vein thrombosis
b. Renal artery thrombosis
4. Bleeding and clotting disorders
a. Disseminated intravascular coagulation
b. Severe thrombocytopenia
c. Clotting factors deficiency
5. Urologic anomalies
6. Glomerular disease
7. Tumors
a. Wilms tumor
b. Neuroblastoma
c. Angiomas
8. Nephrocalcinosis
9. Trauma
a. Suprapubic bladder aspiration
b. Urethral catheterization

sediment for RBCs indicates the presence of globin pigments. Vaginal bleeding ("pseudomenses") in girls or a severe diaper rash is also a possible cause of blood in the diaper or positive dipstick for heme.

2. Evaluation of neonatal hematuria depends on the clinical situation. Depending on the clinical situation, one may consider performing the following tests: urinalysis with examination of the sediment, urine culture, ultrasonography of the upper and lower urinary tract, evaluation of renal function (serum creatinine and BUN), and coagulation studies.

H. Urinary tract infection

1. Infections of the urinary tract in newborns can present with a spectrum of findings: from asymptomatic bacteriuria to pyelonephritis and/or sepsis. A urine culture should be obtained from every infant with fever, poor weight gain, poor feeding, unexplained prolonged jaundice, or any clinical signs of sepsis. A UTI is uncommon in the first 48 hours of life.

2. The diagnosis is confirmed by positive urine culture obtained by suprapubic bladder aspiration or a catheterized specimen with a colony count exceeding 1,000 colonies per millimeter. A blood culture should also be obtained prior to antibiotic administration, even from asymptomatic infants with UTI. Although most newborns with UTIs have leukocytes in the urine, an infection can be present in the absence of leukocyturia.

3. *Escherichia coli* accounts for approximately 75% of the infections. The remainders are caused by other gram-negative bacilli (*Klebsiella*, *Enterobacter*, *Proteus*) and by gram-positive cocci (enterococci, *Staphylococcus epidermidis*, *Staphylococcus aureus*).

4. Evaluation of the urinary tract by ultrasonography is required to rule out hydronephrosis, obstructive uropathy, severe vesicoureteral reflux, or neurogenic bladder with inability to empty the bladder. Adequate drainage or relief of obstruction is necessary for antibiotic control of the infection. Although controversial in older children, a VCUG is needed in neonates following a UTI to define lower tract abnormalities and to detect reflux. VUR occurs in 40% of neonates with UTIs and predominates slightly in boys. Inadequate therapy, particularly in the presence of urologic abnormalities, could lead to renal scarring with potential development of hypertension and loss of renal function.

5. The initial treatment is antibiotics, usually a combination of ampicillin and gentamicin, given parenterally. The final choice of antibiotic is based on the sensitivity of the cultured organism. Treatment is continued for 10 to 14 days, and amoxicillin prophylaxis (10 mg/kg/day) is administered until a VCUG is performed. If VUR is present, prophylactic treatment should be continued. For later onset infections (>7 days) in hospitalized infants, some experts would suggest using vancomycin rather than ampicillin to cover the possibility of hospital-acquired organisms until definitive culture results are available.

6. The decision for circumcision is based primarily on cultural or ethnic background. Data on risk of UTIs, penile cancer, and protection from sexually transmitted diseases in circumcised and uncircumcised men are insufficient to recommend routine circumcisions. Medical indications for

circumcision include urinary retention due to adhesions of the foreskin or to tight phimosis. Circumcision should be avoided in cases of hypospadias, ambiguous genitalia, and bleeding disorders (see Chapter 9).

I. **Tubular disorders**

1. **Fanconi syndrome** is a group of disorders with generalized dysfunction of the proximal tubule resulting in excessive urinary losses of amino acids, glucose, phosphate, and bicarbonate. The glomerular function is usually normal.

   a. **Clinical and laboratory findings** include the following:

      i. Hypophosphatemia due to the excessive urinary loss of phosphate. In these patients, the TRP is abnormally low. Rickets and osteoporosis are secondary to hypophosphatemia and can appear in the neonatal period.

      ii. Metabolic acidosis is secondary to bicarbonate wasting (proximal renal tubular acidosis [RTA]).

      iii. Aminoaciduria and glycosuria do not result in significant clinical signs or symptoms.

      iv. These infants are often polyuric and therefore at risk for dehydration.

      v. Hypokalemia, due to increased excretion by the distal tubule to compensate for the increased sodium reabsorption, is also frequent and sometimes profound.

   b. **Etiology.** The primary form of Fanconi syndrome is rare in the neonatal period and is a diagnosis of exclusion. Although familial cases (mainly autosomal dominant) have been reported, it is generally sporadic. Most secondary forms of the syndrome in the neonatal period are related to inborn errors of metabolism, including cystinosis, hereditary tyrosinemia, hereditary fructose intolerance, galactosemia, glycogenosis, Lowe syndrome (oculocerebrorenal syndrome), and mitochondrial disorders. Cases associated with heavy metal toxicity have also been described.

2. **RTA** is defined as metabolic acidosis resulting from the inability of the kidney to excrete hydrogen ions or to reabsorb bicarbonate. Poor growth may result from RTA.

   a. **Distal RTA (type I)** is caused by a defect in the secretion of hydrogen ions by the distal tubule. The urine cannot be acidified below 6 pH. It is frequently associated with hypercalciuria. Nephrocalcinosis (NC) is common later in life. In the neonatal period, distal RTA may be primary, due to a genetic defect, or secondary to several disorders.

   b. **Proximal RTA (type II)** is a defect in the proximal tubule with reduced bicarbonate reabsorption leading to bicarbonate wasting. Serum bicarbonate concentration falls until the abnormally low threshold for bicarbonate reabsorption is reached in the proximal tubule (generally <16 mEq/L). Once this threshold has been reached, no significant amount of bicarbonate reaches the distal tubule, and the urine can be acidified at that level. Proximal RTA can occur as an isolated defect or in association with Fanconi syndrome (see section III.I.1).

   c. **Hyperkalemic RTA (type IV; remember, there is no type III)** is a result of a combined impaired ability of the distal tubule to excrete hydrogen ions and potassium. In the neonatal period, this disorder is seen in infants with aldosterone deficiency, adrenogenital syndrome, reduced tubular responsiveness to aldosterone, or associated obstructive uropathies such as in older patients.

d. The treatment of RTA is based on correction of the acidosis with alkaline therapy. Bicitra or sodium bicarbonate, 2 to 3 mEq/kg/day in divided doses, is usually sufficient to treat type I and type IV RTA. The treatment of proximal RTA requires larger doses, sometimes as high as 10 mEq/kg/day bicarbonate. In secondary forms of RTA, the treatment of the primary cause often results in the resolution of the RTA.

J. Nephrocalcinosis is detected by ultrasound examinations.

1. Nephrocalcinosis (NC) is generally associated with a hypercalciuric state. Drugs that are associated with NC and increased urinary calcium excretion include loop diuretics such as furosemide, methylxanthines, glucocorticoids, and vitamin D in pharmacologic doses. In addition, hyperoxaluria, often associated with parenteral nutrition, and hyperphosphaturia facilitate the deposition of calcium crystals in the kidney.

2. Kidney stones and NC secondary to primary hyperoxaluria/oxalosis, RTA, or UTIs are rare in newborns, although these conditions might present within a few months of birth.

3. Few follow-up studies of NC in premature infants are available. In general, kidney function is not significantly impaired, and 75% of cases resolve spontaneously often within the first year of life as demonstrated by ultrasonography. Resolution may take up to 5 to 7 years, however, and significant tubular dysfunction at 1 to 2 years of age has been reported.

4. It is unclear whether NC requires a specific treatment. If possible, drugs such as furosemide that cause hypercalciuria should be discontinued. Change to or addition of thiazide diuretics and supplemental magnesium in patients with bronchopulmonary dysplasia with a need for long-term diuretic therapy may be helpful. Monitoring of urinary calcium excretion (urine calcium:creatinine ratio) helps in determining response to therapy.

K. Cystic disease of the kidney may result from abnormalities in development, such as multicystic dysplasia, or from genetically induced diseases. The principal differential diagnosis of bilateral cystic kidney disease in the newborn includes **ARPKD**, **ADPKD**, and glomerulocystic kidney disease.

1. In ARPKD, the genetic defect has been mapped to chromosome 6p21, which encodes a novel protein product named fibrocystin or polyductin. In infants with ARPKD, the kidneys appear markedly enlarged and hyperechogenic by ultrasonography, with a typical "snowstorm" appearance with concurrent liver fibrosis and/or dilated bile ducts. In contrast, macroscopic cysts are usually detected in cases of ADPKD and glomerulocystic disease and the liver is spared. The clinical findings of ARPKD are variable and include bilateral smooth enlarged kidneys, varying degrees of renal insufficiency, which usually progresses to renal failure over time, and severe renin-mediated hypertension. Infants with more severe involvement may have oligohydramnios with pulmonary hypoplasia and Potter syndrome, but those patients who survive the neonatal period can be carried to renal transplantation in later childhood or adolescence.

ARPKD is always associated with liver involvement, which may progress to liver failure requiring transplantation in adolescence.

2. In ADPKD, an abnormal gene PKD1 has been identified and located on the short arm of chromosome 16, and a second gene PKD2 located on the long arm of chromosome 4. These two genes account for most of the ADPKD patients. Clinical manifestations include bilateral renal masses that are usually less symmetrical than in ARPKD. Because of its dominant genetics, ADPKD is much more common than ARPKD, even in neonates.

3. Other hereditary syndromes that can manifest as renal cystic disease include tuberous sclerosis; von Hippel-Lindau disease; Jeune asphyxiating thoracic dysplasia; oral-facial-digital syndrome type 1; brachymesomelia-renal syndrome; and trisomy 9, 13, and 18.

L. Kidney tumors are rare in the neonatal period. These include mesoblastic nephroma and nephroblastomatosis. The differential diagnosis includes other causes of renal masses (see Table 28.2).

Suggested Readings

Bailie MD. Renal function and disease. *Clin Perinatol* 1992;19(1):91–92.

Bateman DA, Thomas W, Parravicini E, et al. Serum creatinine concentration in very-low-birth-weight infants from birth to 34-36 wk postmenstrual age. *Pediatr Res* 2015;77:696–702.

Blowey DL, Duda PJ, Stokes P, et al. Incidence and treatment of hypertension in the neonatal intensive care unit. *J Am Soc Hypertens* 2011;5:478–483.

Chiara A, Chirico G, Barbarini M, et al. Ultrasonic evaluation of kidney length in term and preterm infants. *Eur J Pediatr* 1989;149(2):94–95.

Coulthard MG, Vernon B. Managing acute renal failure in very low birthweight infants. *Arch Dis Child Fetal Neonatal Ed* 1995;73:F187–F192.

de Vries L, Levene MI. Measurement of renal size in preterm and term infants by real-time ultrasound. *Arch Dis Child* 1983;58(2):145–147.

Dionne JM, Abitbol CL, Flynn JT. Hypertension in infancy: diagnosis, management and outcome. *Pediatr Nephrol* 2012;27:17–32.

dos Santos AC Jr, de Miranda DM, Simões e Silva AC. Congenital anomalies of the kidney and urinary tract: an embryogenic review. *Birth Defects Res C Embryo Today* 2014;102:374–381.

Giapros V, Tsoni C, Challa A, et al. Renal function and kidney length in preterm infants with nephrocalcinosis: a longitudinal study. *Pediatr Nephrol* 2011; 26:1873–1880.

Guignard JP, Drukker A. Clinical neonatal nephrology. In: Barratt TM, Avner ED, Harmon WE, eds. *Pediatric Nephrology*. Philadelphia, PA: Lippincott Williams & Wilkins; 1999.

Moghal NE, Embleton ND. Management of acute renal failure in the newborn. *Semin Fetal Neonatal Med* 2006;11:207–213.

Vieux R, Hascoet JM, Merdariu D, et al. Glomerular filtration rate reference values in very preterm infants. *Pediatrics* 2010;125:e1186–e1192.

29 Mechanical Ventilation

Eric C. Eichenwald

KEY POINTS

- Use of noninvasive respiratory support often avoids the need for mechanical ventilation in preterm infants with respiratory distress.
- Volume-targeted, patient-triggered ventilators reduce the risk of bronchopulmonary dysplasia in preterm infants.
- Ventilatory support strategy should target the pathophysiology of the pulmonary condition causing respiratory failure.

I. **GENERAL PRINCIPLES.** Mechanical ventilation is an invasive life support procedure with many effects on the cardiopulmonary system. The goal is to optimize both gas exchange and clinical status at minimum fractional concentration of inspired oxygen (FiO_2) and ventilator pressures/tidal volume (V_T). The ventilator strategy employed to accomplish this goal depends, in part, on the infant's disease process. In addition, recent advances in technology have brought more options for ventilatory therapy of newborns.

II. **TYPES OF VENTILATORY SUPPORT**

A. Continuous positive airway pressure

1. **Continuous positive airway pressure (CPAP) is usually administered by means of a ventilator, stand-alone CPAP delivery system, or "bubble" CPAP systems.** Any system used to deliver CPAP should allow continuous monitoring of the delivered pressure and be equipped with safety alarms to indicate when the pressure is above or below the desired level. Alternatively, CPAP may be delivered by a simplified system providing blended oxygen flowing past the infant's airway, with the end of the tubing submerged in 0.25% acetic acid in sterile water solution to the desired depth to generate pressure ("bubble CPAP"). Stand-alone variable flow CPAP devices, in which expiratory resistance is decreased via a "fluidic flip" of flow at the nosepiece during expiration, are also available.

2. **General characteristics.** A continuous flow of heated, humidified gas is circulated past the infant's airway, typically at a set pressure of 3 to 8 cm H_2O, maintaining an elevated end-expiratory lung volume while the infant breathes spontaneously. The air–oxygen mixture and airway pressure can be adjusted. Variable flow CPAP systems may decrease the work of breathing and improve lung recruitment in infants on CPAP

but have not been shown to be clearly superior to conventional means of delivery. CPAP is usually delivered by means of nasal prongs, nasopharyngeal tube, or nasal mask. Endotracheal CPAP should not be used because the high resistance of the endotracheal tube increases the work of breathing, especially in small infants. Positive-pressure hoods and continuous-mask CPAP are not recommended.

3. Advantages

a. CPAP is less invasive than mechanical ventilation and causes less lung injury.

b. When used early in infants with respiratory distress syndrome (RDS), CPAP can help prevent alveolar and airway collapse and thereby reduce the need for mechanical ventilation.

c. Use of immediate CPAP in the delivery room for spontaneously breathing immature infants ≥ 24 weeks' gestation decreases the need for mechanical ventilation and administration of surfactant. Although individual trials comparing initial CPAP and mechanical ventilation and early surfactant treatment show similar rates of bronchopulmonary dysplasia (BPD), meta-analyses of the prospective randomized trials of early CPAP show that initial CPAP use is associated with a decreased risk of death or BPD.

d. CPAP decreases the frequency of obstructive and mixed apneic spells in some infants.

4. Disadvantages

a. CPAP is not effective in patients with frequent apnea or inadequate respiratory drive.

b. CPAP provides inadequate respiratory support in the face of severely abnormal pulmonary compliance and resistance.

c. Maintaining nasal or nasopharyngeal CPAP in large, active infants may be technically difficult.

d. Infants on CPAP frequently swallow air, leading to gastric distension and elevation of the diaphragm, necessitating decompression by a gastric tube.

5. Indications (see section III.A)

B. High flow nasal cannula

1. Many units have switched to use of high flow nasal cannula (HFNC) as an alternative to conventional CPAP devices. HFNC allows delivery of distending pressure to the infant's airway with a simpler patient interface.

2. **General characteristics.** HFNC usually refers to the delivery of blended, heated, and humidified oxygen at flows >1 L/minute via small binasal prongs. Two commercial devices for delivery of HFNC are available for use in newborns.

3. Advantages

a. Reported advantages to HFNC include ease of use, a simpler patient interface, and a lower incidence of nasal breakdown compared with conventional CPAP.

b. Randomized trials to date comparing HFNC to CPAP as postextubation support in extremely preterm infants are limited but suggest that HFNC may be an acceptable alternative to CPAP in many infants.

Data suggest that the failure of HFNC may be higher than conventional CPAP in infants <26 weeks' gestation.

4. Disadvantages

a. Potential disadvantages include more variable distending pressure delivery (both low and high) and a tendency for a longer duration of respiratory support compared with CPAP.

C. Pressure-limited, time-cycled, continuous flow ventilators have historically been used in newborns with respiratory failure but have been replaced in most U.S. neonatal intensive care units (NICUs) by patient-triggered, volume-targeted ventilators (see the following text).

1. General characteristics of pressure-limited ventilation. A continuous flow of heated and humidified gas is circulated past the infant's airway; the gas is a mixture of air, blended with oxygen to maintain the desired oxygen saturation level. Peak inspiratory pressure (PI or PIP), positive end-expiratory pressure (PEEP), and respiratory timing (rate and duration of inspiration and expiration) are selected.

2. Advantages

a. The continuous flow of fresh gas allows the infant to make spontaneous respiratory efforts between ventilator breaths (intermittent mandatory ventilation [IMV]).

b. Good control is maintained over respiratory pressures.

c. Inspiratory and expiratory time can be independently controlled.

d. The system is relatively simple and inexpensive.

3. Disadvantages

a. VT is poorly controlled.

b. The system does not respond to changes in respiratory system compliance.

c. Spontaneously breathing infants, who breathe out of phase with too many IMV breaths ("bucking" or "fighting" the ventilator), may receive inadequate ventilation and are at increased risk for air leak.

D. Synchronized and patient-triggered (assist/control or pressure support) ventilators are adaptations of conventional pressure-limited ventilators used for newborns.

1. General characteristics. These ventilators combine the features of pressure-limited, time-cycled, continuous flow ventilators with an airway pressure, airflow, or respiratory movement sensor. By measuring inspiratory flow or movement, these ventilators deliver intermittent positive-pressure breaths at a fixed rate, in synchrony with the baby's inspiratory efforts ("synchronized IMV," or synchronized intermittent mandatory ventilation [SIMV]). During apnea, SIMV ventilators continue to deliver the set IMV rate. In patient-triggered ventilation, a positive pressure breath is delivered with every inspiratory effort. As a result, the ventilator delivers more frequent positive pressure breaths, usually allowing a decrease in the inspiratory pressure (PIP) needed for adequate gas exchange. During apnea, the ventilator in patient-triggered mode delivers an operator-selected IMV ("control") rate. In some ventilators, synchronized IMV breaths can be supplemented by pressure-supported breaths in the spontaneously breathing infant. Ventilators equipped with a flow sensor can also be used to monitor delivered VT continuously by integration of the flow signal. Two types of patient-triggered ventilation are commonly available to the following:

a. In assist/control (A/C) ventilation, the ventilator delivers a breath with each inspiratory effort. The clinician sets the inspiratory time and peak inflation pressure or target VT. The clinician also sets a minimum mandatory ventilator rate to maintain adequate minute ventilation should the spontaneous respiratory rate fall below the minimum selected rate.

b. Pressure support ventilation (PSV) is similar to A/C mode in that each spontaneous patient breath results in a ventilator support breath. However, each breath is terminated when inspiratory gas flow falls to a predetermined proportion of peak flow (usually 15% to 20%). As a result, the patient determines the rate and pattern of breathing (inspiratory time or inspiratory:expiratory ratio). PSV counteracts the resistance imposed by the endotracheal tube and ventilator circuit by providing additional inspiratory flow that is limited to a preset pressure selected by the clinician. A higher inspiratory flow rate (shorter inspiratory rise time or slope) shortens the time to reach maximal airway pressure, which decreases the work of breathing.

2. **Advantages**

   a. Synchronizing the delivery of positive pressure breaths with the infant's inspiratory effort reduces the phenomenon of breathing out of phase with IMV breaths ("fighting" the ventilator). This may decrease the need for sedative medications and aid in weaning mechanically ventilated infants.

   b. Pronounced asynchrony with ventilator breaths, during conventional IMV, has been associated with the development of air leak and intraventricular hemorrhage. Whether the use of SIMV or A/C ventilation reduces these complications is not known.

3. **Disadvantages**

   a. Under certain conditions, the ventilators may inappropriately trigger a breath because of signal artifacts or fail to trigger because of problems with the sensor.

   b. Limited data are available comparing patient-triggered ventilation to other modes of ventilation in newborns. PSV may not be appropriate for small premature infants with irregular respiratory patterns and frequent apnea because of the potential for significant variability in ventilation. However, some data suggest that use of patient-triggered modes of ventilation in premature infants may decrease markers of lung inflammation and facilitate earlier extubation, when used as the initial mode of mechanical ventilator support.

4. **Indications.** SIMV can be used when a conventional pressure-limited ventilator is indicated. If available, it is the preferable mode of ventilator therapy in infants who are breathing spontaneously while on IMV. The indications for A/C and PSV have not been established, although many NICUs use these modes because of perceived advantages of using lower peak inspired pressure and smaller VTs.

E. **Volume-targeted ventilators.** Advances in technology for measuring delivered VTs have made these ventilators first-line therapy for newborns with respiratory failure. Only volume-targeted ventilators specifically designed for newborns should be used. Volume-targeted ventilators are always patient-triggered.

1. **General characteristics.** Volume-targeted ventilators are similar to pressure-limited ventilators except that the operator selects the VT delivered rather than the PIP. "Volume guarantee" is a mode of pressure-limited SIMV, in which the ventilator targets an operator-chosen VT (usually 4 to 6 mL/kg) during mechanically delivered breaths. Volume guarantee allows rapid response of the ventilator pressures to changing lung compliance and may be particularly useful in infants with RDS who receive surfactant therapy. Pressure-regulated volume control (PRVC) is a modified pressure-targeted ventilatory mode, in which inspiratory pressure is sequentially adjusted to deliver a target inspiratory volume with the lowest possible pressures.

2. **Advantages.** The pressure automatically varies with respiratory system compliance to deliver the selected VT, therefore minimizing variability in minute ventilation and avoiding wide swings in VT frequently seen with pressure-limited ventilators. Recent data suggest that volume-targeted ventilation reduces the risk of death or BPD in extremely low birth weight infants, presumably by reduction of the risk of volutrauma.

3. **Disadvantages**
   a. The system can be complicated and requires more skill to operate.
   b. Because VTs in infants are small, some of the VTs selected are lost in the ventilator circuit or from air leaks around uncuffed endotracheal tubes. Some ventilators compensate for these losses by targeting expired rather than inspired VTs or by accounting for dead space in the circuit.

4. **Indications.** Volume-targeted ventilators are particularly useful if lung compliance is rapidly changing, as in infants receiving surfactant therapy.

F. **High-frequency ventilation** (HFV) is an important adjunct to conventional mechanical ventilation in newborns. Three types of high-frequency ventilators are approved for use in newborns in the United States: a high-frequency oscillator (HFO), a high-frequency flow interrupter (HFFI), and a high-frequency jet (HFJ) ventilator.

1. **General characteristics.** Available high-frequency ventilators are similar despite considerable differences in design. All are capable of delivering extremely rapid rates (300 to 1,500 breaths per minute, 5 to 25 Hz; 1 Hz = 60 breaths per minute), with VTs equal to or smaller than anatomic dead space. These ventilators apply continuous distending pressure to maintain an elevated lung volume; small VTs are superimposed at a rapid rate. HFJ ventilators are paired with a conventional pressure-limited device, which is used to deliver intermittent "sigh" breaths to help prevent atelectasis. Sigh breaths are not used with HFO ventilation. Expiration is passive (i.e., dependent

on chest wall and lung recoil) with HFFI and HFJ machines, whereas expiration is active with HFO. The mechanisms of gas exchange are incompletely understood.

2. Advantages

   a. HFV can achieve adequate ventilation while avoiding the large swings in lung volume required by conventional ventilators and associated with lung injury. Because of this, HFV may be useful in pulmonary air leak syndromes (pulmonary interstitial emphysema [PIE], pneumothorax) or in infants failing conventional mechanical ventilation.

   b. HFV allows the use of a high mean airway pressure (MAP) for alveolar recruitment and resultant improvement in ventilation–perfusion ($\dot{V}/\dot{Q}$) matching. This may be advantageous in infants with severe respiratory failure, requiring high MAP to maintain adequate oxygenation on a conventional mechanical ventilator.

3. Disadvantages. Despite theoretical advantages of HFV, no significant benefit of this method has been demonstrated in routine clinical use over more conventional ventilators. Only one rigorously controlled study found a small reduction in BPD in infants at high risk treated with HFO ventilation as the primary mode of ventilation. This experience is likely not generally applicable, however, because other studies have shown no difference. These ventilators are more complex and expensive, and there is less long-term clinical experience. The initial studies with HFO suggested an increased risk of significant intraventricular hemorrhage, although this complication has not been observed in recent clinical trials. Studies comparing the different types of high-frequency ventilators are unavailable; therefore, the relative advantages or disadvantages of HFO, HFFI, and HFJ, if any, are not characterized.

4. Indications. HFV is primarily used as a rescue therapy for infants failing conventional ventilation. Both HFJ and HFO ventilators have been shown to be superior to conventional ventilation in infants with air leak syndromes, especially PIE. Because of the potential for complications and equivalence to conventional ventilation in the incidence of BPD, we do not use HFV as the primary mode of ventilatory support in infants.

G. Noninvasive mechanical ventilation. Neonatal nasal intermittent positive pressure ventilation (NIPPV) provides noninvasive respiratory support to preterm infants who otherwise would require endotracheal intubation and ventilation. It is a supplement to CPAP. NIPPV superimposes inflations set to a peak pressure delivered through nasal prongs or mask. Some devices attempt to synchronize inflations with the infant's spontaneous inspirations. It remains unclear if NIPPV is superior to conventional CPAP or prevents the need for mechanical ventilation.

1. NIPPV has been used for the following clinical settings:

   a. Apnea of prematurity

   b. Following extubation, NIPPV compared with nasal CPAP has been reported shown to reduce extubation failure in infants who required intubation and ventilation.

   c. Primary mode of ventilation in preterm infants with RDS

III. INDICATIONS FOR RESPIRATORY SUPPORT

A. **Indications** for CPAP in the preterm infant with RDS include the following:

1. Recently delivered preterm infant with minimal respiratory distress and low supplemental oxygen requirement (to prevent atelectasis)

2. Respiratory distress and requirement of FiO_2 above 0.30 by hood

3. FiO_2 above 0.40 by hood

4. Initial stabilization in the delivery room for spontaneously breathing, extremely preterm infants (25 to 28 weeks' gestation)

5. Initial management of premature infants with moderate respiratory distress

6. Clinically significant retractions and/or distress after recent extubation

7. In general, infants with RDS who require FiO_2 above 0.35 to 0.40 on CPAP should be intubated, ventilated, and given surfactant replacement therapy. In some NICUs, intubation for surfactant therapy in infants with RDS is followed by immediate extubation to CPAP. We generally use mechanical ventilation for all infants who are given surfactant.

8. After extubation to facilitate maintenance of lung volume

9. HFNC is likely equivalent to CPAP in postextubation stabilization; it remains unclear if it is as effective in stabilization of infants with more severe respiratory distress or in infants <26 weeks' gestation.

B. **Relative indications for mechanical ventilation** in any infant include the following:

1. Frequent intermittent apnea unresponsive to methylxanthine therapy

2. Early treatment when use of mechanical ventilation is anticipated because of deteriorating gas exchange.

3. Relieving "increased work of breathing" in an infant with signs of moderate-to-severe respiratory distress

4. Administration of surfactant therapy in infants with RDS

C. **Absolute indications for mechanical ventilation**

1. Prolonged apnea

2. PaO_2 below 50 mm Hg, or FiO_2 above 0.80. This indication may not apply to the infant with cyanotic congenital heart disease.

3. $PaCO_2$ above 60 to 65 mm Hg with persistent acidemia

4. General anesthesia

IV. HOW VENTILATOR CHANGES AFFECT BLOOD GASES

A. **Oxygenation** (see Table 29.1)

1. **FiO_2.** The goal is to maintain adequate tissue oxygen delivery. Generally, this can be accomplished by achieving a PaO_2 of 50 to 70 mm Hg and results in a hemoglobin saturation of 88% to 95% (see Fig. 29.1). Increasing inspired oxygen is the simplest and most direct means of improving oxygenation. In premature infants, the risk of retinopathy

Table 29.1. Ventilator Manipulations to Increase Oxygenation

Parameter	Advantage	Disadvantage
↑ FiO_2	Minimizes barotrauma	Fails to affect $\dot{V}/\dot{Q}$ matching
	Easily administered	Direct toxicity, especially >0.6
↑ PIP or V_T	Improves $\dot{V}/\dot{Q}$	Lung injury: air leak, BPD
↑ PEEP	Maintains FRC/prevents collapse	Shifts to stiffer part of compliance curve
	Splints obstructed airways	May impede venous return
		Increases expiratory work and CO_2
		Increases dead space
↑ T_I	Increases MAP	Results in slower rates; may need to increase PIP
	"Critical opening time"	Lower minute ventilation for given PIP–PEEP combination
↑ Flow	Square wave—maximizes MAP	Greater shear force, more lung injury
		Greater resistance at greater flows
↑ Rate	Increases MAP while using lower PIP	Inadvertent PEEP with high rates or long time constant

Increase in any setting (except FiO_2) results in higher mean airway pressure.
↑, increase; FiO_2, fractional concentration of inspired oxygen; $\dot{V}/\dot{Q}$, ventilation–perfusion ratio; PIP, peak inspiratory pressure; V_T, tidal volume; BPD, bronchopulmonary dysplasia; PEEP, positive end-expiratory pressure; FRC, functional residual capacity; T_I, inspiratory time; MAP, mean airway pressure.

and pulmonary oxygen toxicity argue for minimizing PaO_2 and closely monitoring oxygen saturations. For infants with other conditions, the optimum PaO_2 may be higher. Direct pulmonary oxygen toxicity begins to occur at FiO_2 values >0.60 to 0.70.

2. MAP

a. MAP is the average area under the curve of the pressure waveform. Most ventilators now display MAP or can be equipped with a device to do so; it may also be calculated using the following equation: MAP = [(PIP – PEEP) (T_I) / T_I + T_E] + PEEP. MAP is increased by increases in

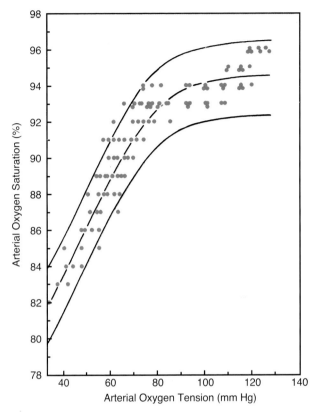

Figure 29.1. Comparison of paired measurements of oxygen saturation by pulse oximetry and of oxygen tension by indwelling umbilical artery oxygen electrode. The lines represent ±2 standard deviations. (Modified from Wasunna A, Whitelaw AG. Pulse oximetry in preterm infants. *Arch Dis Child* 1987;62[9]:957.)

PEEP, PIP, Ti, and rate; all these changes lead to higher PaO_2, but each has different effects on $PaCO_2$. For a given rise in MAP, increasing PEEP gives the greatest improvement in PaO_2.

b. Optimum MAP results from a balance between optimizing PaO_2, minimizing direct oxygen toxicity, minimizing barotrauma and volutrauma, achieving adequate ventilation, and minimizing adverse cardiovascular effects. Ventilator-induced lung injury is probably most closely related to peak-to-peak swings in lung volume, although changes in airway pressure are also implicated.

c. MAP as low as 5 cm H_2O may be sufficient in infants with normal lungs, whereas 15 cm H_2O or more may be necessary in severe RDS. Excessive MAP may impede venous return and adversely affect cardiac output.

Table 29.2. Ventilator Manipulations to Increase Ventilation and Decrease PaCO$_2$

Parameter	Advantage	Disadvantage
↑ Rate	Easy to titrate	Maintains same dead space/V$_T$
	Minimizes lung injury	
		May lead to inadvertent PEEP
↑ PIP or V$_T$	Better bulk flow (improved dead space/V$_T$)	More barotrauma
		Shifts to stiffer compliance curve
↓ PEEP	Increases V$_T$	Decreases MAP
	Decreases dead space	Decreases oxygenation; may result in alveolar collapse
	Shifts to steeper part of compliance curve	Decreases splinting of obstructed/closed airways
↑ Flow	Permits shorter T$_I$, longer T$_E$	More barotrauma
↑ T$_E$	Allows longer time for passive expiration in face of prolonged time constant	Shortens T$_I$
		Decreases MAP
		Decreases oxygenation

PaCO$_2$, partial pressure of carbon dioxide, arterial; ↑, increase; V$_T$, tidal volume; PEEP, positive end-expiratory pressure; PIP, peak inspiratory pressure; ↓, decrease; MAP, mean airway pressure; T$_I$, inspiratory time; T$_E$, expiratory time.

3. Ventilation (see Table 29.2)

a. CO$_2$ elimination depends on minute ventilation. Because minute ventilation is the product of respiratory rate and V$_T$, increases in ventilator rate will lower PaCO$_2$. Increases in V$_T$ can be achieved by increasing the PIP on pressure-cycled ventilators or by increasing targeted volume on volume-limited or volume guarantee machines. Because V$_T$ is a function of the difference between PIP and PEEP, a reduction in PEEP also improves ventilation. At very low V$_T$s, the volume of dead space becomes important and may lead to CO$_2$ retention.

b. Optimal PaCO$_2$ varies according to disease state. For very immature infants or infants with air leak, a PaCO$_2$ of 50 to 60 mm Hg may be tolerated to minimize ventilator-induced lung injury, provided pH can be maintained >7.20 to 7.25.

V. DISEASE STATES

A. **Effects of diseases.** Respiratory failure can result from numerous illnesses through a variety of pathophysiologic mechanisms. Optimal ventilatory strategy must take into account the pathophysiology, expected time course, and particular vulnerabilities of the patient.

B. **Pulmonary mechanics influence the ventilator strategy selected.**

1. **Compliance is the stiffness** or distensibility of the lung and chest wall; that is, the change in volume (ΔV) produced by a change in pressure (ΔP), or $\Delta V/\Delta P$. It is decreased with surfactant deficiency, excess lung water, and lung fibrosis. It is also decreased when the lungs are hyperexpanded.

2. **Resistance is the impediment** to airflow due to friction between gas and airways (airway resistance) and between tissues of the lungs and chest wall (viscous tissue resistance); that is, the change in pressure (cm H_2O) divided by the change in flow (L/second). Almost half of airway resistance is in the upper airways, including the endotracheal tube when in use. Resistance is high in diseases characterized by airway obstruction, such as meconium aspiration and BPD. Resistance can change rapidly if, for example, secretions partially occlude the endotracheal tube.

3. **Time constant** is the product of compliance (mL/cm H_2O) and resistance (cm H_2O/mL/second). This is a measure of the time it takes to equilibrate pressure between the proximal airway and the alveoli. Expiratory time constants are somewhat longer than inspiratory ones. When time constants are long, as in meconium aspiration, care must be taken to set ventilator inspiratory times and rates that permit adequate inspiration to deliver the required V_T and adequate expiration to avoid inadvertent PEEP.

4. **Functional residual capacity (FRC)** is a measure of the volume of the lungs at end expiration. FRC is decreased in diseases that permit alveolar collapse, particularly surfactant deficiency.

5. **$\dot{V}/\dot{Q}$ matching.** Diseases that reduce alveolar surface area (through atelectasis, inflammatory exudates, or obstruction) permit intrapulmonary shunting of desaturated blood. The opposite occurs in persistent pulmonary hypertension when extrapulmonary shunting diverts blood flow away from the ventilated lung. Both mechanisms result in systemic recirculation of desaturated blood.

6. **Work of breathing** is especially important in the smallest infants and those with chronic lung disease whose high airway resistance, decreased lung compliance, compliant chest wall, and weak musculature may overwhelm their metabolic energy requirements and impede growth.

C. **Specific disease states.** Several of the more common neonatal disease processes are described in the subsequent text and are presented in Table 29.3, along with the optimal ventilatory strategies. Before initiating ventilatory

Table 29.3. Neonatal Pulmonary Physiology by Disease State

Disease	Compliance mL/cm H$_2$O	Resistance cm H$_2$O/mL/s	Time Constant (s)	FRC (mL/kg)	$\dot{V}/\dot{Q}$ Matching	Work
Normal term	4–6	20–40	0.25	30	—	—
RDS	↓↓	—	↓↓	↓	↓/↓↓	↑
Meconium aspiration	—/↓	↑↑	↑	↑/↑↑	↓↓	↑
BPD	↑/↓	↑↑	↑	↑↑	↓↓/↓	↑↑
Air leak	↓↓	—/↑	—/↑	↑↑	↓/↓↓-	↑↑
VLBW apnea	↓	—	↓↓	—/↓	↓/—	—/↑

FRC, functional residual capacity; $\dot{V}/\dot{Q}$, ventilation–perfusion ratio; —, little or no change; RDS, respiratory distress syndrome; ↓, decrease; /, either/or; ↑, increase; BPD, bronchopulmonary dysplasia; VLBW, very low birth weight.

support, clinicians must evaluate for mechanical causes of distress, including pneumothorax or airway obstruction.

1. **RDS** (see Chapter 33)
    a. **Pathophysiology.** RDS is caused by surfactant deficiency, which results in a severe decrease in compliance (stiff lung). This causes diffuse alveolar collapse with $\dot{V}/\dot{Q}$ mismatching and increased work of breathing.
    b. **Surfactant replacement.** Early initiation of CPAP, usually starting in the delivery room, may avoid the need for mechanical ventilation and surfactant therapy in many infants, even at very early gestational ages. Alternatively, some recommend intubation and initiation of mechanical ventilation early in the course of RDS in order to provide surfactant therapy promptly. Surfactant therapy modifies the distinctive time course of escalation, plateau, and weaning in classic RDS. Ventilatory strategy should anticipate the increased risk of pneumothorax because compliance increases and time constants lengthen, especially with the rapid improvement that can be seen after surfactant administration. In all approaches, a PaCO$_2$ value higher than the physiologic value is acceptable to minimize ventilator-induced lung injury.
    c. **Ventilator strategy**
        i. **CPAP.** In mild to moderately affected infants who may not require intubation and surfactant administration, CPAP is used very early in the disease course to prevent further atelectasis. CPAP is initiated at 5 to 6 cm H$_2$O and increased to a maximum of 7 to 8 cm H$_2$O. The risk of pneumothorax may be

increased at higher levels of CPAP pressure. CPAP is titrated by clinical assessment of retractions and respiratory rate and by observation of O_2 saturation. NIPPV may be an alternative approach to CPAP in this setting. Additionally, in infants with more severe RDS, consideration may be given to intubation for surfactant administration with prompt extubation followed by CPAP (INSURE technique).

ii. **Mechanical ventilation** is used when $\dot{V}/\dot{Q}$ mismatching is so severe that increased FiO_2 and CPAP are inadequate to maintain gas exchange, or in infants who tire from the increased work of breathing. Data suggest that a ventilator strategy that avoids large changes in VT may reduce ventilator-induced lung injury; hence, volume-targeted ventilation, as described earlier, is the preferred mode in infants with RDS. The objective of all strategies of assisted ventilation in the infant with RDS should be to provide the lowest level of ventilatory support possible to support adequate oxygenation and ventilation while attempting to reduce acute and chronic lung injury secondary to barotrauma/volutrauma and oxygen toxicity. Our preferred approach is to maintain the appropriate MAP with a TI initially set at 0.3 second and rate of approximately 20 to 40 breaths per minute. Rarely, a longer TI is required to provide adequate oxygenation.

iii. **VT** is usually initially set at 4 to 6 mL/kg and adjusted for adequate minute ventilation. If pressure-limited ventilation is used, PIP is initially estimated by visible chest excursion and is usually 20 to 25 cm H_2O.

iv. **PEEP.** PEEP is usually set at 4 to 6 cm H_2O. Higher PEEP may interfere with cardiac output.

v. **Flow.** Flow rates of 7 to 12 L/minute are needed to provide a relatively square pressure waveform. Higher flows may be required at very high PIP (>35 cm H_2O).

vi. **Rates** are generally set initially at 20 to 40 breaths per minute and adjusted according to blood gas results.

vii. **Weaning.** When the patient improves, FiO_2 and PIP or VT are weaned first, alternating with rate, in response to assessment of chest excursion, oxygen saturation, and blood gas results. In volume-targeted ventilation, the PIP will decrease automatically in response to improved compliance; weaning may be accomplished by decreasing the targeted level of VT. In patient-triggered modes, the back-up rate of the ventilator is usually not changed, and progressive decreases in PIP are used to wean the ventilator. Extubation is usually successful when ventilator rates are <20 to 25 breaths per minute, or PIP is below 16 to 18 cm H_2O to deliver the desired VT. Prior to extubation, caffeine citrate therapy should be started to facilitate spontaneous breathing. Prophylactic caffeine increases the success rate of extubation in very low birth weight infants.

viii. **Advantages and disadvantages.** This ventilatory strategy maximizes alveolar recruitment but with a potential for greater lung injury secondary to higher PIP and volutrauma secondary to higher VT.

ix. HFV may be initiated if conventional ventilation fails to maintain adequate gas exchange at acceptable settings. HFV should be used only by clinicians familiar with its use. We consider the use of HFV when the MAP required for adequate gas exchange exceeds 10 to 11 cm H_2O in small infants, and 12 cm H_2O in larger infants, or if air leak occurs. Strategies differ depending on whether HFJ, HFO, or HFFI is used. We prefer HFO ventilation over other available HFV because of its ease of use and applicability in a wide range of pulmonary diseases and infant weights.

a) **HFJ ventilation.** HFJ requires a special adapter for a standard endotracheal tube to allow connection to the jet port of the ventilator.

1) **PIP and PEEP.** Peak pressures on the jet ventilator are initially set approximately 20% lower than on those being used with conventional ventilation and adjusted to provide adequate chest vibration assessed clinically and by blood gas determinations. PIP, PEEP, and FiO_2 are adjusted as needed to maintain oxygenation. CO_2 elimination is dependent on the pressure difference (PIP – PEEP). Because of the lower peak pressures required to ventilate, PEEP may be increased to 8 to 10 cm H_2O if needed to improve oxygenation.

2) **Rate.** The frequency is usually set at 420 breaths per minute, with an inspiratory jet valve on-time of 0.02 second.

3) **Conventional ventilator settings.** Once the HFJ is properly adjusted, the conventional ventilator rate is decreased to 2 to 10 breaths per minute to help maintain alveolar recruitment, with PIP set at 2 to 3 cm H_2O lower than the jet PIP. In air leak syndromes, it may be advantageous to provide no sigh breaths from the conventional ventilator as long as the PEEP is set high enough to maintain lung volume.

4) **Weaning** from HFJ ventilation is accomplished by decreasing the jet PIP in response to blood gas determinations and the FiO_2. PEEP is weaned as tolerated if pressures higher than 4 to 5 cm H_2O are used. Frequency and jet valve on-time are generally not adjusted.

5) **Similar strategies** outlined for the HFJ apply in use of the HFFI.

b) **HFO ventilation.** With HFO, operator-selected parameters include MAP, frequency, and piston amplitude.

1) **MAP.** In RDS, the initial MAP selected is usually 2 to 5 cm H_2O higher than that being used on the conventional ventilator to enhance alveolar recruitment. MAP used with HFO is titrated to O_2 requirement and to provide adequate lung expansion on chest x-ray. Care must

be exercised to avoid lung hyperinflation, which might adversely affect oxygen delivery by reducing cardiac output.

2) **Frequency is usually set at 10 to 15 Hz.** Inspiratory time is set at 33%.

3) **Amplitude.** Changes in piston amplitude primarily affect ventilation. It is set to provide adequate chest vibration, assessed clinically and by blood gas determinations.

4) **Flow rates** of 8 to 15 L/minute are usually adequate.

5) **Weaning.** In general, FiO_2 is weaned first, followed by MAP in decrements of 1 to 2 cm H_2O once the FiO_2 falls below 0.6. Piston amplitude is adjusted by frequent assessment of chest vibration and blood gas determinations. Frequency is usually not adjusted unless adequate oxygenation or ventilation cannot otherwise be achieved. In contrast to conventional mechanical ventilation, decreasing the frequency of breaths in HFO ventilation will improve ventilation because of effects on delivered VT. In both HFJ and HFO, we usually wean to extubation after transfer back to conventional ventilation, although infants can be extubated directly from HFV.

2. **Meconium aspiration syndrome (MAS)** (see Chapter 35)

   a. Pathophysiology. MAS results from aspiration of meconium-stained amniotic fluid. The severity of the syndrome is related to the associated asphyxial insult and the amount of fluid aspirated. The aspirated meconium causes acute airway obstruction, markedly increased airway resistance, scattered atelectasis with V̇/Q̇ mismatching, and hyperexpansion due to obstructive ball-valve effects. The obstructive phase is followed by an inflammatory phase 12 to 24 hours later, which results in further alveolar involvement. Aspiration of other fluids (such as blood or amniotic fluid) has similar but milder effects.

   b. Ventilator strategy. Because of the ball-valve effects, the application of positive pressure may result in pneumothorax or other air leak, so initiating mechanical ventilation requires careful consideration of the risks and benefits. Low levels of PEEP (4 to 5 cm H_2O) are helpful in splinting open partially obstructed airways and equalizing V̇/Q̇ matching. Higher levels may lead to hyperinflation. If airway resistance is high and compliance is normal, a slow-rate, moderate-pressure/volume strategy is needed. If pneumonitis is more prominent, more rapid rates can be used. Sedation or muscle relaxation may be used to minimize the risks of air leak in severe MAS because of the high transpulmonary pressures these large infants can generate when "fighting" the ventilator and the ball-valve hyperexpansion caused by their disease. Use of patient-triggered ventilation may be helpful in some infants and avoid the need for muscle relaxation. Weaning may be rapid if the illness is primarily related to airway obstruction or prolonged if complicated by lung injury and severe inflammation. Due to secondary surfactant inactivation, the use of surfactant therapy may improve lung compliance and oxygenation and should be considered in more severe cases of MAS.

HFV has also been successfully used in infants with MAS who are failing conventional ventilation or who have air leak. The strategies are similar to those described in the preceding text. During HFO, slower frequencies (8 to 10 Hz) may be useful to improve oxygenation and ventilation in severe cases.

3. **BPD** (see Chapter 34)

   a. Pathophysiology. BPD results from injury to the alveoli and airways. Bleb formation may lead to poor recoil. Fibrosis and excess lung water may cause stiffer compliance. Airways may be narrowed and fibrotic or hyperreactive. The upper airways may be overdistended and conduct airflow poorly. BPD is marked by shifting focal atelectasis, hyperinflation with $\dot{V}/\dot{Q}$ mismatch, chronic and acute increases in airway resistance, and a significant increase in the work of breathing.

   b. Ventilator strategy. The optimal strategy is to wean infants off the ventilator as soon as possible to prevent further mechanical injury and oxygen toxicity. If this is not feasible, ventilator settings should be minimized to permit tissue repair and long-term growth. Rates less than about 20 breaths per minute should generally be avoided to prevent increased work of breathing, but longer T_I (0.4 to 0.5 second) may be used to maintain FRC. Some centers use SIMV in combination with PSV in severe cases to improve work of breathing and ventilation. Higher PIPs are sometimes required (20 to 30 cm H_2O) because of the stiff lungs, although the high resistance prevents transfer of most of this to the alveoli. Oxygenation should be maintained (saturations of 90% to 92%), but higher $PaCO_2$ values can be permitted (55 to 65 mm Hg), provided the pH is acceptable. Acute decompensations can result from bronchospasm and interstitial fluid accumulation. These must be treated with adjustment of PIP, bronchodilators, and diuretics. Acute BPD "spells" in which oxygenation and airway resistance worsen rapidly are usually due to larger airway collapse and may be treated successfully with higher PEEP (7 to 8 cm H_2O). Frequent rapid desaturations secondary to acute decreases in FRC with crying or infant movement respond to changes in FiO_2 but may also be partially ameliorated by using higher PEEP. Weaning is a slow and difficult process, decreasing rate by 1 to 2 breaths per minute or 1 cm H_2O decrements in PIP every day when tolerated. Fortunately, with improved medical and ventilatory care of these infants, it is rare for infants with BPD to require tracheostomy for chronic ventilation.

4. **Air leak** (see Chapter 38)

   a. Pathophysiology. Pneumothorax and PIE are the two most common air leak syndromes. Pneumothorax results when air ruptures into the pleural space. In PIE, the interstitial air substantially reduces tissue compliance as well as recoil. In addition, peribronchial and perivascular air may compress the airways and vascular supply, causing "air block."

   b. Ventilator strategy. Because air is driven into the interstitium throughout the ventilatory cycle, the primary goal is to reduce MAP through any of its components (PIP or V_T, T_I, or PEEP) and to rely on increased FiO_2 to provide oxygenation. This strategy holds for all air leak syndromes. If dropping the MAP is not tolerated, other techniques may be tried. Because the time constants for interstitial air are much longer than those for the alveoli, we sometimes use very rapid conventional rates (up to 60 breaths per minute), which may preferentially ventilate the alveoli.

HFV is an important alternative therapy for severe air leak and, if available, may be the ventilatory treatment of choice. HFV strategies for air leak differ from those used in diffuse alveolar disease. As described for conventional ventilation, the ventilatory goal in air leak syndromes is to decrease MAP, relying on FiO_2 to provide oxygenation. With HFJ and HFFI, PEEP is maintained at lower levels (4 to 6 cm H_2O), and few to no-sigh breaths are provided. With HFO, the MAP initially used is the same as that being used on the conventional ventilator and the frequency set at 15 Hz. While weaning, MAP is decreased progressively, tolerating higher FiO_2 in the attempt to limit the MAP exposure.

5. Apnea (see Chapter 31)

a. Pathophysiology. Occasionally, apnea is severe enough to warrant ventilator support, even in the absence of pulmonary disease. This may result from apnea of prematurity, or during or following general anesthesia.

b. Ventilator strategy. For infants completely dependent on the ventilator, the goal should be to provide "physiologic" ventilation using moderate PEEP (3 to 4 cm H_2O), low gas flow, and normal rates (30 to 40 breaths per minute), with PIP or V_T adjusted to prevent hyperventilation (10 to 18 cm H_2O). Prolonged T_I is unnecessary. For infants requiring a ventilator because of intermittent but prolonged apnea, low rates (12 to 15 breaths per minute) may be sufficient.

VI. ADJUNCTS TO MECHANICAL VENTILATION

A. Sedation (see chart on intubation sedation guidelines and Chapters 69 and 70) can be used when agitation or distress is associated with excessive lability of oxygenation and hypoxemia. Although this problem is more common in the neonate receiving long-term ventilation, acutely ill newborns may occasionally benefit from sedation. Morphine (0.05 to 0.1 mg/kg) or fentanyl (1 to 3 µg/kg) can be used but may cause neurologic depression. Prolonged use may lead to dependence. Lorazepam (0.05 to 0.1 mg/kg/dose given every 4 to 6 hours) or midazolam (0.05 to 0.1 mg/kg/dose given every 2 to 4 hours) has been used in more mature infants and in more chronic situations. In preterm infants, nonpharmacologic methods, such as limiting environmental light and noise and providing behavioral supports, may help decrease agitation and limit the need for sedative medications. As discussed, synchronized IMV or patient-triggered ventilation may also help diminish agitation and ventilatory lability.

B. Muscle relaxation with pancuronium bromide (0.1 mg/kg/dose, repeated as needed) or vecuronium (0.1 mg/kg/dose) is rarely used but may be indicated in some infants who continue to breathe out of phase with the ventilator after attempts at finding appropriate settings and sedation have failed; the need for muscle relaxation is reduced in patient-triggered ventilation as babies will breathe "in sync" with the delivered ventilator breaths.

Although unequivocal data are not available, gas exchange may be improved in some infants following muscle relaxation. Prolonged muscle relaxation leads to fluid retention and may result in deterioration in compliance. Sedation is routinely administered to infants receiving muscle relaxants.

C. **Blood gas monitoring** (see Chapter 30). All infants receiving mechanical ventilation require continuous monitoring of oxygen saturation and intermittent blood gas measurements.

VII. COMPLICATIONS AND SEQUELAE.
As a complex and invasive technology, mechanical ventilation can result in numerous adverse outcomes, both iatrogenic and unavoidable.

A. **Lung injury and oxygen toxicity**

1. **BPD** is related to increased airway pressure and changes in lung volume, although oxygen toxicity, anatomic and physiologic immaturity, and individual susceptibility also contribute.

2. **Air leak** is directly related to increased airway pressure. Risk is increased at MAPs in excess of 14 cm H_2O.

B. **Mechanical**

1. Obstruction of endotracheal tubes may result in hypoxemia and respiratory acidosis.

2. Equipment malfunction, particularly disconnection, is not uncommon and requires functioning alarm systems and vigilance.

C. **Complications of invasive monitoring**

1. Peripheral arterial occlusion with infarction (see Chapter 44)

2. Aortic thrombosis from umbilical arterial catheters, occasionally leading to renal impairment and hypertension

3. Emboli from flushed catheters, particularly to the lower extremities, the splanchnic bed, or even the brain

D. **Anatomic**

1. Subglottic stenosis from prolonged intubation; risk increases with multiple reintubations

2. Acquired tracheobronchomalacia from prolonged mechanical intubation

3. Palatal grooves from prolonged orotracheal intubation

4. Vocal cord damage

Suggested Reading

Goldsmith J, Karotkin E. *Assisted Ventilation of the Neonate.* 5th ed. Philadelphia, PA: Saunders-Elsevier; 2010.

Blood Gas and Pulmonary Function Monitoring

Lawrence M. Rhein

KEY POINTS

- Assessment of oxygenation and ventilation is critical to assess respiratory function.
- Pulse oximetry is the primary tool for noninvasive oxygen monitoring in newborns.
- A neonatal intensive care unit (NICU) policy is essential to guide target saturation values and alarm limits in infants treated with supplemental oxygen.

I. **GENERAL PRINCIPLES.** Both invasive and noninvasive techniques are used to monitor respiratory health in the clinical setting. Although both methods have limitations, monitoring of oxygenation and ventilation is critical to assess respiratory function. Invasive techniques, including blood gas monitoring, allow (i) assessment of pulmonary gas exchange; (ii) determination of hemoglobin oxygen saturation and arterial oxygen content; and (iii) evaluation, although limited, of adequacy of tissue oxygen delivery. Noninvasive techniques may be less specific but allow easier determination of serial measurements and identification of trends.

II. **OXYGEN USE AND MONITORING.** Causes of hypoxemia include hypoventilation, mismatch of ventilation and perfusion, diffusion impairment, and shunt. Supplemental oxygen is most effective for diffusion abnormalities but ineffective to treat hypoventilation. In emergency situations, sufficient oxygen to abolish cyanosis should be administered. Oxygen monitoring with pulse oximetry should be initiated as soon as possible, and the concentration of oxygen should be adjusted to maintain saturation values within a targeted range. An oxygen blender and pulse oximeter should be used whenever supplemental oxygen is administered. Monitoring of oxygen use is necessary to reduce both hypoxic injury to tissues and to minimize oxidative injury to the lungs or the immature retina of the preterm infant.

   A. **Arterial blood gas (ABG) measurements.** Arterial PO_2 (PaO_2) and PCO_2 ($PaCO_2$) are direct indicators of efficiency of pulmonary gas exchange in infants with acute lung disease. PaO_2 measured under steady state conditions from an indwelling catheter is the "gold standard" for oxygen monitoring.

1. **Usual values.** Most sources consider 50 to 80 mm Hg to be an acceptable target range for newborn PaO_2. Preterm infants who require respiratory support may exhibit wide swings in PaO_2 values. In such circumstances, a single blood gas value may not accurately reflect the overall trend of oxygenation.

2. **Sampling.** To minimize sampling and dilutional artifacts, ABG samples should be collected in dry heparin syringes that are commercially available for this purpose. Most blood gas analyzers allow determination of blood gas values as well as other whole blood parameters on 0.2- to 0.3-mL samples. Samples should be analyzed within 15 minutes or preserved on ice if sent to a remote laboratory site. Blood gas sampling by percutaneous puncture is used when the need for measurement is infrequent or an indwelling catheter is not available. However, the discomfort of the puncture may result in agitation and a fall in PaO_2 so that the value obtained underestimates the true steady state value.

B. **Noninvasive oxygen monitoring** provides real-time trend data that is particularly useful in infants exhibiting frequent swings in PaO_2 and oxygen saturation. Noninvasive devices also may reduce the frequency of blood gas sampling in more stable patients.

1. **Pulse oximetry** is the primary tool for noninvasive oxygen monitoring in newborns. Pulse oximeters provide continuous measurement of hemoglobin oxygen saturation (SpO_2) with a high level of accuracy ($\pm3\%$) when compared to control values measured by co-oximetry, at least down to the range of 70%.

   a. **General characteristics.** Oximeters depend on different absorption characteristics of oxygenated versus reduced hemoglobin for various wavelengths of light. Differences in transmission of two (usually red and near infrared [IR]) or more wavelengths through tissues with pulsatile blood flow are measured. Using the measured values, the proportion of oxygenated and reduced hemoglobin is calculated and displayed as percent saturation. Modern pulse oximeters can efficiently discriminate artifactual values from valid measurements. Sensitivity of detection of hypoxemia by pulse oximeters is dependent on the averaging time of the oximeters; shorter averaging times detect hypoxemia more sensitively compared to longer averaging times.

   b. **Disadvantages.** Pulse oximetry does not measure the PaO_2 and thus is insensitive in detecting hyperoxemia. Due to the shape of the oxyhemoglobin dissociation curve, if SpO_2 is >95%, PaO_2 is unpredictable. Under such conditions, PaO_2 may be >100 mm Hg. Patient movement and the low amplitude pulse wave of small preterm infants may introduce artifacts that result in false episodes of desaturation, although software modifications have reduced this problem. Other potential sources of artifact include inappropriate sensor placement, presence of high-intensity light (some phototherapy devices), fetal hemoglobin values >50%, and presence of carboxyhemoglobin or methemoglobin.

c. Targeted saturation values. The optimal range of oxygen saturation, especially for preterm infants, remains unknown. One systematic review and meta-analysis of several well-designed multicenter randomized controlled trials concluded that targeting oxygen saturations to 85% to 89% is associated with an increased risk of mortality and necrotizing enterocolitis but a lower risk of retinopathy of prematurity. However, more recent meta-analyses suggest that too much uncertainty exists to make a clear recommendation. In older studies that targeted oxygen saturation values in preterm infants after the immediate newborn period (supplemental therapeutic oxygen for prethreshold retinopathy of prematurity [STOP-ROP,] benefits of oxygen saturation targeting [BOOST]), SpO_2 values >95% in preterm infants receiving supplemental oxygen was associated with increased need for prolonged supplemental oxygen. Determination of an optimal target saturation in preterm infants may be elusive because some babies may be more vulnerable to oxidative injury and others to hypoxia. These vulnerabilities may affect end organs (e.g., the eye, the brain, and the gut) differently and may vary over time with organ maturation.

Because the optimal oxygen target is not certain, a neonatal intensive care unit (NICU) policy is essential. One approach is as follows: For infants who require supplemental oxygen, we maintain SpO_2 in the 88% to 92% range for infants <29 weeks' gestation or 1,250 g (monitor alarm limits 85% to 93%) until 36 weeks' postmenstrual age, when the upper target changes to >93%. For infants 29 weeks' gestation or more, or when infants reach 29 weeks' postmenstrual age, we maintain SpO_2 88% to 95% (monitor alarm limits 85% to 97%). If these targets are maintained, arterial PO_2 will rarely exceed 90 mm Hg. Other NICUs may target a slightly higher SpO_2 range and a wider set of alarm limits.

2. **Transcutaneous oxygen monitoring** ($PtcO_2$) can be useful in management of acute cardiopulmonary disease during the first 2 postnatal weeks or if arterial catheterization is not possible. However, this technique has been largely supplanted in the NICU by pulse oximetry.

III. ASSESSMENT OF PULMONARY VENTILATION. Alveolar ventilation is assessed by direct or noninvasive measurement of PCO_2. Low values should be avoided because lung injury has been associated with excessive volume distension of the immature lung. A strategy of "permissive hypercapnia" in mechanically ventilated infants generally tolerates PCO_2 values in the range of 50 to 65 mm Hg.

A. **Blood gas determination.** As is the case with oxygen monitoring, a $PaCO_2$ value obtained at steady state from an indwelling arterial catheter provides the most accurate indicator of alveolar ventilation. Lack of a catheter, however, limits the availability of this sampling for many patients, especially infants with chronic pulmonary insufficiency. Blood obtained by percutaneous arterial puncture is an alternative but may not reflect steady state values because of artifacts introduced by pain and agitation.

1. **Venous blood** from a central catheter may be useful in certain circumstances. If alveolar ventilation and circulatory function are normal,

venous PCO_2 usually exceeds arterial values by 5 to 6 mm Hg. However, if significant hypoventilation or circulatory dysfunction is present, this relationship is unpredictable.

2. Capillary blood gases. PCO_2 and pH values obtained from properly collected capillary blood samples can closely reflect arterial values. The extremity must be warmed and a free-flowing blood sample collected under strictly anaerobic conditions without squeezing the extremity. In smaller premature infants, these conditions may be difficult to achieve.

B. Noninvasive carbon dioxide monitoring. Measurement of $PaCO_2$ by ABG sampling and analysis is the gold standard for assessing ventilation. Unfortunately, $PaCO_2$ can be a dynamic and rapidly changing value not accurately reflected in a single invasive measurement. To overcome these limitations, noninvasive monitors can be used to provide a continuous estimate of $PaCO_2$. The two most available noninvasive monitoring methods are transcutaneous monitoring and capnography.

1. Transcutaneous CO_2 monitoring ($PtcCO_2$) estimates the $PaCO_2$ through electrochemical measurements of CO_2 gas diffusing through body tissue and skin. A sensor at the skin surface measures the pH of an electrolyte solution that is separated from the skin by a permeable membrane. The sensor is warmed to approximately 42° to 43°C to induce a local hyperemia, resulting in vasodilation of the dermal capillary bed below the sensor, increasing arterial blood flow. This vasodilation also facilitates diffusion of CO_2. $PtcCO_2$ is often slightly higher than the corresponding measured $PaCO_2$ value. This is likely due to two main factors. First, the elevated temperature alters the solubility of CO_2. Second, the hyperemia increases the metabolism of the skin cells, which contributes to CO_2 levels. The $PtcCO_2$ may therefore require a corrective algorithm to more closely align monitor values with the $PaCO_2$.

a. Transcutaneous monitoring is generally considered safe; however, tissue injury may occur at the measuring site, including blisters, burns, and skin tears. Because the technology involves hyperemia where the probe is applied, continuous monitoring is generally avoided because skin-related complications primarily occur when the $PtcCO_2$ is in place for long periods of time. Patients with poor skin integrity or adhesive allergy are not good candidates for $PtcCO_2$.

b. Some clinical situations may lead to an increased discrepancy between the $PtcCO_2$ and $PaCO_2$. These include improper probe placement or application, factors associated with increased distance from probe to capillaries (such as body wall edema or thickness of the patient's skin or subcutaneous tissue), poor perfusion of the site of probe placement, or hyperoxemia ($PaO_2 > 100$ torr).

c. Transcutaneous carbon dioxide tension exceeds that of arterial blood by a mean of 4 mm Hg in the normal range, but this gradient may more than double in the presence of hypercapnia. The need for a high level of user attention and expertise has limited the use of this technique.

2. Capnography refers to the noninvasive measurement of the partial pressure of carbon dioxide in exhaled breaths, expressed as the CO_2 concentration over time. The relationship of CO_2 concentration to time can be represented graphically as a waveform or capnogram, or can be used to determine the maximum CO_2 concentration at the end of each tidal breath, or end-tidal CO_2 (EtCO_2). Capnography has been widely used in the United States since the 1980s; its many clinical uses include assessment of disease severity or response to therapy or the confirmation of proper endotracheal tube placement.

a. Capnography uses IR radiation and absorption to detect CO_2. Molecules of CO_2 absorb IR radiation at a specific wavelength (4.26 µm). CO_2 monitors use lightweight IR sensors to emit IR light through adapter windows to a photodetector that is sensitive to the IR band of CO_2. The IR radiation absorption is highly correlated with the CO_2 concentration present.

b. Capnography devices are categorized based on their location for sampling and therefore also on the types of patients for whom they are effective.

 i. Mainstream devices measure CO_2 directly from the airway, with the sensor located on the airway adapter at the hub of the endotracheal tube, between the breathing circuit and the endotracheal tube. The signals detected are amplified and transmitted via cable to a monitor where the partial pressure of the CO_2 is calculated and displayed. Mainstream sensors are heated to slightly above body temperature to prevent condensation of water vapor because this can cause falsely high CO_2 readings. Potential disadvantages of mainstream capnography include relative fragility of adapters, increased mechanical dead space, additional weight on the airway, and use limited to intubated patients.

 ii. Sidestream devices measure CO_2 via nasal or nasal–oral cannula by aspirating a small sample from the exhaled breath through cannula tubing to a sensor located inside the CO_2 monitor. This allows monitoring of nonintubated patients because sampling of the expiratory gases can be obtained from the nasal cavity. Gases can even be sampled from the nasal cavity during the administration of oxygen using nasal cannula. Sidestream systems used in infants usually use low flow rates of approximately 50 mL/minute. These devices may require additional safeguards, including a gas scavenging system to collect anesthetic gases in the sample if present, and a water trap to collect condensation from humidified sample gas or patient secretions. Disadvantages of sidestream capnography include variation in humidity and temperature between the sampling and measurement sites, pressure drops through the tubing that may affect CO_2 measurement, and a delay of up to several seconds to display the measurement.

 iii. Several factors limit the utility of EtCO_2 measurements in newborns.

  a) Mechanical ventilation typically uses relatively rapid rates compared to adult strategies, and most ventilator circuits deliver a continuous fresh flow of gas throughout the respiratory cycle. This limits the ability to obtain a true end-expiratory plateau.

b) Arterial–alveolar CO_2 gradients are elevated in babies with serious parenchymal lung disease because of maldistribution of ventilation (mean 6 to 10 mm Hg). As a result, end-tidal measurements may significantly underestimate arterial PCO_2 values. However, in babies with more uniform distribution of ventilation, end-tidal measurements may be useful to monitor trends.

c. Confirming endotracheal intubation placement. The Neonatal Resuscitation Program recommends use of an exhaled CO_2 detector (colorimetric device or capnograph) to confirm correct tube placement during endotracheal intubation.

d. Monitoring during anesthesia. The Standards for Basic Anesthetic Monitoring of the American Society of Anesthesiology specifies the use of continuous $EtCO_2$ monitoring of all patients, including newborns, during general anesthesia with endotracheal tube or laryngeal mask airway.

IV. PULMONARY GRAPHICS MONITORING.

Several devices are marketed for bedside pulmonary function testing in infants and young children. In addition, most newer generation ventilators graphically display various measured or calculated parameters. Despite the added cost and increasing availability of these modalities, evidence of beneficial effect on neonatal outcomes is lacking. Several techniques have been advocated in limited studies.

A. Tidal volume measurements may be used to assist in manual adjustment of ventilator settings. Alternatively, such measurements may be used for software-automated ventilator adjustments designed to maintain a defined range of delivered tidal volume (volume guarantee) or consistent tidal volume delivery using minimal peak airway pressure (pressure-limited volume control). However, technical issues may limit efficacy of these modalities. Measured tidal volume varies markedly in devices from different manufacturers. These discrepancies result from differences in measurement sites, variations in tubing system compliance, and use of different strategies to compensate for endotracheal tube leaks. In addition, some software algorithms average adjustments in tidal volume over several breaths. Although newer ventilator modes may improve consistency of delivered tidal volume, a substantial proportion of values remain outside the target range. Despite these shortcomings, tidal volume measurements using the same device consistently over time may provide clinically useful information during chronic mechanical ventilation and may be helpful with weaning following surfactant treatment when lung compliance changes rapidly.

B. Flow volume loops. Positive end-expiratory pressure (PEEP) is an important tool in management of infants with congenital or acquired bronchomalacia, a common complication of severe bronchopulmonary dysplasia (BPD). In limited case studies, real-time flow volume loop tracings have been used to guide determination of optimal PEEP to oppose airway collapse. However, indices that quantitate the flow-volume relationship have not been validated in young infants. Because of rapid breathing, onset of inspiration often occurs before end-expiratory closure of the loop is achieved. As a result, "normal" tracings are difficult to obtain and clinical application of this technique in small infants is limited.

Suggested Readings

Manja V, Lakshminrusimha S, Cook DJ. Oxygen saturation target range for extremely preterm infants: a systematic review and meta-analysis. *JAMA Pediatr* 2015;169(4):332–340.

Pretto JJ, Roebuck T, Beckert L, et al. Clinical use of pulse oximetry: official guidelines from the Thoracic Society of Australia and New Zealand. *Respirology* 2014;19:38–46.

Reiterer F, Sivieri E, Abbasi S. Evaluation of bedside pulmonary function in the neonate: from the past to the future. *Pediatr Pulmonol* 2015;50(10):1039–1050.

Apnea

Ann R. Stark

KEY POINTS

- Apnea spells typically resolve by 36 to 37 weeks' postmenstrual age (PMA) in infants born at 28 weeks of gestation or more but may persist to or beyond 40 weeks' PMA in more preterm infants.
- Caffeine is a safe and effective treatment for apnea.
- Evidence does not support treatment of gastroesophageal reflux to reduce apnea frequency.
- Prior to discharge, a 5- to 7-day period after discontinuation of caffeine therapy without recorded apnea events predicts a low likelihood of recurrent symptomatic apnea.

I. BACKGROUND

A. Definition. Apnea is defined as the cessation of airflow. Apnea is pathologic (an apneic spell) when absent airflow is prolonged (usually 20 seconds or more) or accompanied by bradycardia (heart rate <100 beats per minute) or hypoxemia that is detected clinically (cyanosis) or by oxygen saturation monitoring. Bradycardia and desaturation are usually present after 20 seconds of apnea, although they typically occur more rapidly in the small premature infant. As the spell continues, pallor and hypotonia are seen, and infants may be unresponsive to tactile stimulation. The level or duration of bradycardia or desaturation that may increase the risk of neurodevelopmental impairment is not known.

B. Classification of apnea is based on whether absent airflow is accompanied by continued inspiratory efforts and upper airway obstruction. Most spells in preterm infants are mixed.

1. Central apnea occurs when inspiratory efforts are absent.

2. Obstructive apnea occurs when inspiratory efforts persist in the presence of airway obstruction, usually at the pharyngeal level.

3. Mixed apnea occurs when airway obstruction with inspiratory efforts precedes or follows central apnea.

C. Incidence. Apneic spells occur frequently in premature infants. The incidence of apnea increases with decreasing gestational age. Essentially, all infants <28 weeks' gestational age have apnea. As many as 25% of all premature infants who weigh <1,800 g (~34 weeks' gestational age) have at least one apneic episode.

1. **Onset.** Apneic spells generally begin at 1 or 2 days after birth; if they do not occur during the first 7 days, they are unlikely to occur later.

2. **Duration.** Apneic spells persist for variable periods postnatally and usually cease by 36 to 37 weeks' postmenstrual age (PMA) in infants born at 28 weeks' gestation or more. In infants born before 28 weeks' gestation, however, spells often persist beyond term PMA. After resolution of apnea, preterm infants may also have intermittent hypoxemic events that are not clinically apparent or detected by routine monitoring. Furthermore, in a study in which infants were monitored at home, significant apnea and/or bradycardia were recorded up to 43 weeks' PMA in 20% of preterm infants who were free of spells for at least 5 days before discharge and in 33% of those who had spells observed during that period (Collaborative Home Infant Monitoring Evaluation [CHIME] study). The clinical significance of these events is uncertain.

3. **Term infants.** Apneic spells occurring in infants at or near term are always abnormal and are nearly always associated with serious, identifiable causes, such as birth asphyxia, intracranial hemorrhage, seizures, or depression from medication. Failure to breathe at birth in the absence of drug depression or asphyxia is generally caused by irreversible structural abnormalities of the central nervous system.

II. **PATHOGENESIS.** Several mechanisms have been proposed to explain apnea in premature infants, although those responsible for this disorder are unknown. Many clinical conditions have also been associated with apneic spells, and some may be causative.

A. **Developmental immaturity of central respiratory drive** is a likely contributing factor because apneic spells occur more frequently in immature infants.

1. The occurrence of apnea may correlate with brainstem neural function. The frequency of apnea decreases over a period in which brainstem conduction time of the auditory-evoked response shortens as gestational age increases.

2. Breathing in infants is strongly influenced by sleep state. Active or rapid eye movement (REM) sleep is marked by irregularity of tidal volume and respiratory frequency. REM sleep predominates in preterm infants, and apneic spells occur more frequently in this state than in quiet sleep.

B. **Chemoreceptor response**

1. In preterm infants, hypoxia results in transient hyperventilation, followed by hypoventilation and sometimes apnea, in contrast to the response in adults. In addition, hypoxia makes the premature infant less responsive to increased levels of carbon dioxide. This suggests that immaturity of peripheral chemoreceptors may be involved in the pathogenesis of apnea. Although most infants do not appear to be hypoxemic before the onset of apnea, hypoxemia might play a role in prolonging the spell.

2. The ventilatory response to increased carbon dioxide is decreased in preterm infants with apnea compared with a matched group without

apnea and is also decreased compared to term infants or adults. This suggests the possible contribution of immature central chemoreceptors to the pathogenesis of apnea.

C. **Reflexes.** Active reflexes invoked by stimulation of the posterior pharynx, lung inflation, fluid in the larynx, or chest wall distortion can precipitate apnea in infants. These reflexes may be involved in the apnea that is sometimes associated, for example, with vigorous use of suction catheters in the pharynx or with fluid in the upper airway during feeding.

D. **Respiratory muscles.** Ineffective ventilation may result from impaired coordination of the inspiratory muscles (diaphragm and intercostal muscles) and the muscles of the upper airway (larynx and pharynx).

1. Airway obstruction contributes to mixed and obstructive apneic spells. The site of this obstruction is usually the upper pharynx, which is vulnerable because of poor muscle tone, especially in REM sleep. Passive neck flexion, pressure on the lower rim of a face mask, and submental pressure (all encountered during nursery procedures) can obstruct the airway in infants and lead to apnea, especially in a small premature infant. Spontaneously occurring airway obstruction is seen more frequently when preterm infants assume a position of neck flexion.

2. Nasal obstruction can lead to apnea, especially in preterm infants who usually do not switch to oral breathing after nasal occlusion.

E. Gastroesophageal reflux is common in preterm infants. However, no association has been demonstrated between apnea of prematurity and gastroesophageal reflux.

F. Many inhibitory neurotransmitters are thought to play a role in the pathogenesis of apnea.

III. MONITORING AND EVALUATION

A. All infants <35 weeks' gestational age should be monitored for apneic spells for at least the first week after birth because of the risk of apneic spells in this group. Monitoring should continue until no significant apneic episode has been detected for at least 5 days. Because impedance apnea monitors may not distinguish respiratory efforts during airway obstruction from normal breaths, heart rate should be monitored in addition to, or instead of, respiration. Pulse oximetry should be monitored to detect episodes of desaturation. Even with careful monitoring, some prolonged spells of apnea and bradycardia may not be recognized.

When a monitor alarm sounds, one should remember to respond to the infant, not the monitor, checking for bradycardia, cyanosis, and airway obstruction.

Most apneic spells in preterm infants respond to tactile stimulation. Infants who fail to respond to stimulation should be ventilated during the spell with bag and mask, generally starting with a fractional concentration of inspired oxygen (FiO_2) equal to the FiO_2 used before the spell to avoid marked elevations in arterial oxygen tension.

After the first apneic spell, the infant should be evaluated for a possible underlying cause (Table 31.1); if a cause is identified, specific treatment

Table 31.1. Evaluation of an Infant with Apnea		
Potential Cause	**Associated History or Signs**	**Evaluation**
Infection	Feeding intolerance, lethargy, temperature instability	Complete blood count, cultures, if appropriate
Impaired oxygenation	Desaturation, tachypnea, respiratory distress	Continuous oxygen saturation monitoring, arterial blood gas measurement, chest x-ray examination
Metabolic disorders	Jitteriness, poor feeding, lethargy, CNS depression, irritability	Glucose, calcium, electrolytes
Drugs	CNS depression, hypotonia, maternal history	Magnesium; screen for toxic substances in urine
Temperature instability	Lethargy	Monitor temperature of patient and environment.
Intracranial pathology	Abnormal neurologic examination, seizures	Cranial ultrasonographic examination
CNS, central nervous system.		

can then be initiated. One should be particularly alert to the possibility of a precipitating cause in infants who are >34 weeks' gestational age. Evaluation should include a history and physical examination and may include arterial blood gas measurement; complete blood count; and measurement of blood glucose, calcium, and electrolyte levels.

B. Although sudden infant death syndrome (SIDS) occurs more frequently in preterm infants, a history of apnea of prematurity does not increase this risk.

IV. TREATMENT

A. General measures

1. **Specific therapy** should be directed at an underlying cause, if one is identified.

2. The optimal range of oxygen saturation for preterm infants is not certain. However, supplemental oxygen should be provided if needed to maintain values in the targeted range (see Chapter 30).

3. **Care should be taken** to avoid reflexes that may trigger apnea. Suctioning of the pharynx should be done carefully, and tolerance of oral feedings when appropriate should be closely monitored.

4. **Positions of extreme flexion** or extension of the neck should be avoided to reduce the likelihood of airway obstruction. Prone positioning stabilizes the chest wall and may reduce apnea.

B. **Caffeine. Treatment with caffeine, a methylxanthine**, markedly reduces the number of apneic spells and the need for mechanical ventilation. The primary mechanism by which methylxanthines may decrease apnea is antagonism of adenosine, a neurotransmitter that can cause respiratory depression by blocking both its inhibitory A_1 receptor and its excitatory A_{2A} receptors. Respiratory effects include increased carbon dioxide sensitivity, decreased hypoxic depression of breathing, and decreased periodic breathing.

In the Caffeine for Apnea of Prematurity (CAP) study, survival without neurodevelopmental disability at 18 to 21 months of age, the primary outcome, was improved in infants 500 to 1,250 g birth weight treated early with caffeine compared to placebo. Caffeine treatment also reduced the rate of bronchopulmonary dysplasia. We therefore begin caffeine citrate treatment in all infants <1,250 g birth weight soon after birth and continue until it is deemed no longer necessary to treat apnea. In preterm infants >1,250 g birth weight who require mechanical ventilation, we begin caffeine treatment prior to extubation. In other infants with apnea of prematurity, we begin caffeine to treat frequent and/or severe apnea.

1. We use a loading dose of 20 mg/kg of caffeine citrate (10 mg/kg caffeine base) orally or intravenously >30 minutes, followed by maintenance doses of 5 to 10 mg/kg in one daily dose beginning 24 hours after the loading dose.

a. If apnea continues at the lower range of maintenance doses, we give an additional dose of 10 mg/kg caffeine citrate and increase the maintenance dose by 20%.

b. Caffeine serum levels of 5 to 20 μg/mL are considered therapeutic. We do not routinely measure serum drug concentration because of the wide therapeutic index and the lack of an established dose–response relationship.

c. Caffeine is generally discontinued at 33 to 34 weeks' PMA if no apneic spells have occurred for 5 to 7 days. As noted previously, apnea in infants born at <28 weeks' gestation frequently persists beyond this PMA, and caffeine is continued until the spells resolve. The effect of caffeine likely remains for approximately 1 week after it has been discontinued. We continue monitoring until no apnea has been detected for at least 5 days after that period.

2. Additional long-term benefits or risks of caffeine therapy are uncertain. In the CAP trial, weight gain was less during the first 3 weeks after randomization in infants treated with caffeine but not at 4 and 6 weeks, and head circumference was similar in the two groups during the 6-week observation period. Mean percentiles for growth parameters were similar at 18 to 21 months corrected age.

3. Most reports of side effects of methylxanthines in newborns are based on experience with theophylline. Caffeine appears to be less toxic than theophylline and is well tolerated.

C. **Nasal continuous positive airway pressure** (CPAP) at moderate levels (4 to 6 cm H_2O) can reduce the number of mixed and obstructive apneic spells. By helping to maintain a higher end-expiratory volume, CPAP may limit the depth and duration of desaturation that occurs during central apnea spells. Humidified high-flow nasal cannula can be used to provide increased end-expiratory volume, although its effect on reduction of apnea frequency has not been specifically evaluated. Nasal intermittent positive pressure ventilation (NIPPV) may reduce extubation failure due to apnea following mechanical ventilation (see Chapter 29).

D. **Whether blood transfusion reduces the frequency of apneic spells** in some infants remains controversial because results of studies are conflicting. We consider a transfusion of packed red blood cells (PRBCs) if the hematocrit is <25% to 30% and the infant has episodes of apnea and bradycardia that are frequent or severe while continuing treatment with caffeine (see Chapter 45).

E. Gastroesophageal reflex (GER) frequently occurs in preterm infants who are having apnea, although these events are rarely temporally related. Pharmacologic treatment of GER with agents that increase motility or decrease gastric acidity have not been shown to reduce apnea frequency. Because increased late onset sepsis and necrotizing enterocolitis have been associated with use of agents that decrease gastric acidity, we limit the use of these medications.

F. **Mechanical ventilation** may be required if the other interventions are unsuccessful.

V. DISCHARGE CONSIDERATIONS

A. We typically require that preterm infants have no apnea spells recorded for 5 to 7 days prior to discharge, although this may be extended for extremely low gestation infants or those with severe events. Because of the long half-life of caffeine (50 to 100 hours) and even longer effects in some infants, we typically start this "countdown" period several days to 1 week after caffeine is stopped. Feeding-associated events are generally not included, although severe events during feeding may suggest lack of discharge readiness. However, a monitored apnea-free period does not preclude later apnea, as shown by the CHIME study (see section I.C.2 earlier), and apnea may take longer to resolve in infants born at lower gestational ages.

B. Intercurrent viral illness, anesthesia, and ophthalmologic examinations may precipitate recurrent apnea in preterm infants. These infants should be monitored closely at least until 44 weeks' PMA. Immunizations (primarily 2 months and rarely 4 months) may also exacerbate apnea in very preterm infants who remain in the neonatal intensive care unit.

Suggested Reading

Eichenwald EC; and the Committee on Fetus and Newborn. Apnea of prematurity. *Pediatrics* 2016;137(1):1–7.

32

Transient Tachypnea of the Newborn

Mary Lucia P. Gregory

KEY POINTS

- Transient tachypnea of the newborn (TTN) is benign and self-limited.
- Management is supportive with oxygen or continuous positive airway pressure (CPAP), and symptoms resolve in 12 to 72 hours.
- Clinicians should exclude other respiratory, infectious, cardiac, or neurologic etiologies.

I. **DEFINITION.** Transient tachypnea of the newborn (TTN), first described by Avery and coworkers in 1966, results from delayed clearance of fetal lung fluid. As the name implies, it is usually a benign, self-limited process. It generally affects infants born at late preterm or term gestation. The disorder is characterized by tachypnea with signs of mild respiratory distress including retractions and cyanosis; decreased oxygen saturation is usually alleviated by supplemental oxygen with FiO_2 <0.04.

II. **PATHOPHYSIOLOGY.** To accommodate the transition to breathing air at birth, the lungs must switch from a secretory mode that provides the fetal lung fluid required for normal lung growth and development *in utero*, to an absorptive mode. This transition is thought to be facilitated by changes in the maternal–fetal hormonal milieu, including a surge in glucocorticoids and catecholamines, associated with physiologic events near the end of pregnancy and during spontaneous labor. Amiloride-sensitive sodium channels expressed in the apical membrane of the alveolar epithelium play an important role in lung fluid clearance. Adrenergic stimulation and other changes near birth lead to passive transport of sodium through the epithelial sodium channels, followed by transport into the interstitium via basolateral Na^+/K^+-ATPase, and passive movement of chloride and water through paracellular and intracellular pathways. Interstitial lung fluid pools in perivascular cuffs of tissue and in the interlobar fissures and is then cleared into pulmonary capillaries and lung lymphatics. Disruption or delay in clearance of fetal lung fluid results in the transient pulmonary edema that characterizes TTN. Compression of the compliant airways by fluid accumulated in the interstitium can lead to airway obstruction, air trapping, and ventilation–perfusion mismatch. Functional residual capacity may be reduced due to obstruction, whereas thoracic gas volume may increase secondary to air trapping. Because infants usually recover, a precise pathologic definition is lacking.

III. EPIDEMIOLOGY. The incidence of TTN is 0.3% to 0.6% of term deliveries and 1% of preterm deliveries. Risk factors for TTN include cesarean delivery with or without labor, precipitous birth, and preterm birth. These conditions are thought to result in delayed or abnormal fetal lung fluid clearance due to the absence of the hormonal changes that accompany spontaneous labor. The presence of labor and the gestational age at delivery impact the risk of respiratory complications for infants delivered by elective cesarean section; onset of labor and term gestation provide some degree of protection. Delivery at lower gestational ages, including late preterm birth, increases the risk of TTN. Diagnosis at earlier gestations is complicated by the presence of comorbidities such as respiratory distress syndrome (RDS). Other risk factors include male gender and family history of asthma (especially mother). The mechanism underlying the gender- and asthma-associated risks is unclear but may be related to altered sensitivity to catecholamines that play a role in lung fluid clearance. Genetic polymorphisms in β-adrenergic receptors in alveolar type II cells have been associated with TTN and may influence lung fluid clearance by regulating epithelial sodium channel expression as well as explain the correlation between TTN and wheezing in the first years of life. Macrosomia, maternal diabetes, and multiple gestations also increase the risk of TTN. The associations between TTN and other obstetric factors such as excessive maternal sedation, prolonged labor, and volume of maternal intravenous fluids have been less consistent. Several small trials suggest that antenatal corticosteroids prior to cesarean section at 37 to 38 weeks may also decrease risk.

IV. CLINICAL PRESENTATION. Affected term or late preterm infants usually present within the first 6 hours after birth with tachypnea; respiratory rates are typically 60 to 120 breaths per minute. The tachypnea may be associated with mild to moderate respiratory distress with retractions, grunting, nasal flaring, and/or mild cyanosis that usually responds to supplemental oxygen at <0.40 FiO_2. Respiratory failure and need for mechanical ventilation are rare. Infants may have an increased anteroposterior diameter of the chest (barrel-shaped) due to hyperinflation, which may also push down the liver and spleen, making them palpable. Auscultation usually reveals good air entry, and crackles may or may not be appreciated. Signs of TTN usually persist for 12 to 24 hours in cases of mild disease but can last up to 72 hours in more severe cases.

V. DIFFERENTIAL DIAGNOSIS. The diagnosis of TTN requires the exclusion of other potential etiologies for mild to moderate respiratory distress presenting in the first 6 hours of age. The differential diagnosis includes pneumonia/sepsis, RDS, pulmonary hypertension, meconium aspiration, cyanotic congenital heart disease, congenital malformations (e.g., congenital diaphragmatic hernia, congenital pulmonary airway malformation), central nervous system injury (subarachnoid hemorrhage, hypoxic-ischemic encephalopathy) causing central hyperventilation, pneumothorax, polycythemia, and metabolic acidosis.

VI. EVALUATION

    A. History and physical examination. A careful history identifies elements such as prematurity, infectious risk factors, meconium, or perinatal depression that may aid in directing the evaluation. Similarly, findings on physical examination such as cardiac or neurologic abnormalities may lead to a more targeted investigation.

B. **Radiographic evaluation.** The chest radiograph of an infant with TTN is consistent with retained fetal lung fluid, with characteristic prominent perihilar streaking (sunburst pattern) due to engorgement of periarterial lymphatics that participate in the clearance of alveolar fluid. Coarse, fluffy densities may reflect alveolar edema. Hyperaeration with widening of intercostal spaces, mild cardiomegaly, widened and fluid-filled interlobar fissure, and mild pleural effusions may also be observed. The radiographic findings in TTN usually improve by 12 to 18 hours and resolve by 48 to 72 hours. This rapid resolution helps distinguish the process from pneumonia and meconium aspiration. The chest radiograph can also be used to exclude other diagnoses such as pneumothorax, RDS, and congenital malformations. Lung ultrasound can differentiate TTN from RDS with good specificity but is not in common clinical use. Of note, the presence of increased pulmonary vascularity in the absence of cardiomegaly may represent total anomalous pulmonary venous return.

C. **Laboratory evaluation.** A complete blood count (CBC) and appropriate cultures can provide information concerning possible pneumonia or sepsis. If risk factors or laboratory data suggest infection, or if respiratory distress does not improve, broad-spectrum antibiotics should be initiated. An arterial blood gas may be used to determine the extent of hypoxemia and adequacy of ventilation. Infants with TTN may have mild hypoxemia and mild respiratory acidosis that typically resolves over 24 hours. With persistent or severe hypoxemia, a cardiac evaluation should be considered. Respiratory alkalosis may reflect central hyperventilation due to CNS pathology or metabolic disorder.

VII. **TREATMENT.** Treatment is mainly supportive with provision of supplemental oxygen as needed. More severe cases may respond to continuous positive airway pressure (CPAP) to improve lung recruitment. Infants often undergo an evaluation for infection and are treated with antibiotics for 48 hours until blood cultures are negative, although evidence is increasing that empiric antibiotic exposure may not be necessary if the infant is closely observed and there are no historical risk factors for infection. If tachypnea persists and is associated with increased work of breathing, gavage feedings or intravenous fluids may be needed. Relatively restricted fluid intake has been shown to decrease duration of respiratory support in severe cases of TTN. Strategies aimed to facilitate lung fluid absorption have not shown clinical efficacy. Oral furosemide has not been shown to decrease the duration of tachypnea or length of hospitalization. In a trial based on the hypothesis that infants with TTN have relatively low levels of catecholamines that facilitate fetal lung fluid absorption, treatment with racemic epinephrine did not change the rate of resolution of tachypnea compared to placebo.

VIII. **COMPLICATIONS.** Although TTN is a self-limited process, supportive therapy may be accompanied by complications. CPAP is associated with increased risk of air leak. Delayed initiation of oral feeds may interfere with parental bonding and establishment of breastfeeding and may prolong hospitalization.

IX. PROGNOSIS. By definition, TTN is a self-limited process with no risk of recurrence, and the prognosis is excellent. Generally, there are no significant long-term residual effects. However, observational studies suggest a possible link between TTN and reactive airway disease in childhood.

Suggested Reading

Stroustrup A, Trasande L, Holzman IR. Randomized controlled trial of restrictive fluid management in transient tachypnea of the newborn. *J Pediatr* 2012; 160(1):38–43.e1.

33 Respiratory Distress Syndrome

Susan Guttentag

KEY POINTS

- Respiratory distress syndrome (RDS), a disease affecting preterm infants, is caused by insufficient pulmonary surfactant.
- Antenatal corticosteroids given to a pregnant woman in anticipation of preterm birth prevents RDS.
- Treatment entails establishment and maintenance of functional residual capacity by application of continuous positive airway pressure and surfactant administration.

I. INTRODUCTION. Respiratory distress syndrome (RDS), formerly known as hyaline membrane disease (HMD), describes a disease typical of preterm infants that is caused by insufficient pulmonary surfactant in alveoli. Pulmonary surfactant is a complex mixture of phospholipids, neutral lipids, and surfactant-specific proteins that is synthesized, packaged, and secreted from alveolar type II cells of the lung. In the alveolar spaces and small respiratory bronchioles that have poor structural support, surfactant sits at the air-liquid interface over the residual and protective liquid layer overlying the epithelium and disrupts the surface tension generated by the lung liquid. This surface tension is forceful enough to promote alveolar collapse at low lung volumes and to oppose reinflation of atelectatic airspaces. Absent or insufficient surfactant due to developmental immaturity of alveolar type II cells or spontaneous or inherited mutations of surfactant-related genes, or inactivation of surfactant due to inflammation, chemical modification, or lung injury, result in high surface tension and atelectasis. Preterm infants are particularly prone to RDS because alveolar type II cells do not develop until early in the third trimester, and their number and capacity to produce surfactant increase throughout the third trimester. Advances in preventive and rescue treatment strategies, including antenatal glucocorticoids, exogenous surfactant, and continuous positive airway pressure (CPAP), have greatly reduced the impact of RDS on neonatal morbidity and mortality, but RDS remains a particularly vexing problem for extremely low birth weight (ELBW) infants.

II. DIAGNOSIS

A. Risk factors

1. **Lung maturity**, which is distinct from structural lung development, is the most significant risk factor for RDS. By 24 weeks of gestation,

structural lung development has advanced sufficiently to provide gas exchange across lung epithelial and endothelial cells and provide a surface area sufficient to meet the oxygen consumption needs of the ELBW infant. However, the fetal lung at that gestation has insufficient numbers of alveolar type II cells to generate enough surfactant to avoid RDS. In contrast, the fetal lung at 36 weeks of gestation generally has sufficient surfactant stores and large numbers of alveolar type II cells to avoid RDS. In between, the preparedness for air breathing of the fetal lung depends on the extent of lung maturation, which is influenced by multiple genetic and environmental factors.

2. **Factors that affect lung maturation**

a. Fetal sex. Male infants are at higher risk for RDS due to the presence of circulating weak fetal androgens that inhibit the production of surfactant phospholipids.

b. Race. Infants of African ancestry are at lower risk for developing RDS, due in part to the increased presence of protective genetic polymorphisms.

c. Maternal diabetes. Poorly controlled maternal diabetes, in the absence of microvascular disease, is associated with RDS due to enhanced production of fetal insulin which inhibits the production of proteins important for surfactant function.

d. Mutations in surfactant-related proteins, specifically surfactant protein B and ABCA3, result in severe RDS typically in term infants from either dysfunctional surfactant or severely limited production, respectively. Infants with these mutations die without lung transplantation. Some mutations in ABCA3 and mutations of surfactant protein C are associated with progressive interstitial lung disease, often diagnosed beyond the neonatal period.

e. Labor, due to the production of endogenous maternal glucocorticoids, may enhance lung maturation, but inflammation often associated with preterm labor (w) can downregulate the production of many surfactant components.

B. **Antenatal testing**

1. Because gestational age is a strong predictor of RDS risk, invasive testing (amniocentesis) to confirm lung maturity in amniotic fluid samples is reserved for instances in which surfactant deficiency in addition to other fetal conditions would significantly impact morbidity and mortality. These conditions include fetal anomalies such as congenital diaphragmatic hernia and congenital heart disease where more precise timing of delivery of a near-term infant is desirable. Although the risk of adverse outcomes is low with amniocentesis in the third trimester, the widespread use of antenatal glucocorticoids has made the risk unnecessary for the majority of fetuses facing preterm delivery.

2. If lung maturity testing is indicated, the most readily available tests assess the lecithin (disaturated phosphatidylcholine) component of surfactant. Lecithin is the most abundant surfactant phospholipid, and its production is developmentally regulated. However, it is also present

in cell membranes, necessitating correction for the presence of contaminants like blood.

a. The **lecithin/sphingomyelin (L/S) ratio** corrects for the presence of a neutral lipid in low abundance in surfactant, whereas the **TDx-FLM II** corrects for the presence of albumin in the amniotic fluid sample. In both cases, samples contaminated significantly by blood or meconium can be difficult to interpret. RDS risk is low when the L/S ratio is >2, but notable exceptions to this include maternal diabetes, erythroblastosis fetalis, and intrapartum asphyxia. The TDx-FLM II has established gestational age–specific cutoffs but in general is predictive of low RDS risk at >55 mg lecithin per gram albumin.

b. The presence of **lamellar bodies** in amniotic fluid samples is a rapid and inexpensive test that may be useful in resource-poor settings. Lamellar bodies are the organelles in alveolar type II cells that receive, concentrate, and store surfactant constituents for regulated secretion. Upon exocytosis at the plasma membrane, surfactant is extruded into the alveolar space and the constituents must unravel and disperse to form a monolayer at the air-liquid interface. Unwound phospholipid can be discriminated by light microscopy or fluorescence-activated cell sorting (FACS), and $>50,000$ lamellar bodies per microliter of amniotic fluid has been correlated with lung maturity. Alternatively, the optical density of the amniotic fluid sample can be used as a proxy for the presence of lamellar bodies in amniotic fluid.

C. **Diagnosis.** RDS should be suspected in a preterm infant, typically <34 weeks' gestation, with signs of respiratory distress that develop soon after birth. These include tachypnea, retractions, flaring of the nasal alae, grunting, and cyanosis. Blood gas measurement will demonstrate hypoxemia and hypercarbia.

1. Infants with RDS who are spontaneously breathing may overcome surfactant deficiency by using a set of physiologic maneuvers to establish functional residual capacity (FRC) and optimize gas exchange. These result in characteristic signs/symptoms of RDS (see section II.C).

a. Tachypnea. Inadequate FRC leads to inadequate tidal volumes. To maintain minute ventilation (the product of tidal volume × respiratory rate), infants with RDS increase respiratory rate.

b. Retractions. To maximize negative inspiratory pressure and thus lung inflation, affected infants use accessory muscles of breathing to supplement diaphragmatic contractions. The high negative inspiratory pressure draws in the highly compliant chest wall resulting in suprasternal, intercostal, and subcostal retractions.

c. Flaring of the alae nasi. To maximize air entry into the lungs in babies who are obligate nose breathers, flaring of the alae nasi reduces the resistance to air flow through the upper airways.

d. Grunting. Grunting is active exhalation against a partially closed glottis and results in a pressure gradient at the level of the vocal cords that provides expiratory distending pressure to stabilize patent but surfactant-poor alveoli.

D. Radiographic evidence. RDS is a homogeneous lung disease due to the developmental deficiency of surfactant throughout the lung parenchyma.

Typical radiographic findings include low lung volumes, homogeneous microatelectasis that has the appearance of ground glass, and air bronchograms highlighted by the surrounding microatelectasis.

1. **Differential diagnosis**

    a. Transient tachypnea of the newborn (see Chapter 32). Excess fetal lung fluid can mimic RDS and can complicate RDS. Signs are indistinguishable from RDS, but TTN often resolves rapidly over the first several hours after birth. Radiographic findings are consistent with retained fetal lung fluid, with characteristic prominent perihilar streaking (sunburst pattern) due to engorgement of periarterial lymphatics that participate in the clearance of alveolar fluid and often fluid retained in the lateral fissure of the right lung.

    b. Pneumonia, especially due to group B *Streptococcus*. Proinflammatory cytokines elaborated in the course of an infection can inactivate surfactant constituents and downregulate surfactant production. Signs and radiographic findings of group B *Streptococcus* (GBS) sepsis/pneumonia are indistinguishable from RDS; therefore, obtaining blood cultures and initiating antibiotics should be considered.

    c. Genetic disorders of the surfactant system. Although more common in term and near-term infants, the presentation and radiographic findings are identical to RDS. Respiratory signs may be evident at birth or may develop over hours in a vigorous term infant able to initially spontaneously recruit FRC. However, the infant shows little to no response to the administration of artificial surfactant. Genetic mutations in surfactant protein B and ABCA3 can result in an RDS picture in the immediate newborn period.

    d. Disordered lung development. Like genetic disorders of the surfactant system, these rare disorders typically present in term and near-term infants with severe respiratory failure at birth and do not show sustained improvement with surfactant therapy. This category includes alveolar capillary dysplasia with malalignment of the pulmonary veins, congenital alveolar dysplasia, and brain-heart-lung disease due to mutations in Nkx2.1/TTF1.

III. **PREVENTION.** The basis for prevention of RDS is the observation that maternal hormones, specifically glucocorticoids, enhance surfactant maturation. Numerous trials have shown that administration of antenatal corticosteroids (ANC) in anticipation of preterm birth is effective in preventing RDS. ANC modifies surfactant readiness as well as lung structure, including thinning of alveolar walls. The target population is pregnant women at 24 to 34 weeks of gestation with PTL, although emerging evidence suggests some benefit as low as 23 weeks of gestation. A complete course of ANC is considered to be EITHER betamethasone at 12 mg intramuscular (IM) q24h × 2 doses OR dexamethasone 6 mg IM q12h × 4 doses. Meta-analyses have not demonstrated clearly superiority of one drug over the other. No contraindications exist to treatment, including rapidly progressive labor, and animal studies have demonstrated effects on lung structure even after incomplete dosing. However, benefits of prior treatment on lung maturity may diminish if PTL stops and pregnancy continues more than a week after ANC use. A second course can be beneficial under such circumstances, but continued redosing has been associated with poor neurodevelopmental outcomes due to deleterious effects of glucocorticoids on brain development.

IV. MANAGEMENT. The key principles of treatment of RDS are to establish and maintain FRC. The most important role of pulmonary surfactant in the alveoli and distal respiratory bronchioles is to maintain a low surface tension that permits these delicate airways to remain patent at low lung volumes. These airspaces are protected by secretion of a liquid layer over the surface of the lung epithelium. The surface tension exerted by this lung liquid is sufficient to promote atelectasis in the distal lung and oppose reexpansion of atelectatic airspaces. The polar head groups of surfactant phospholipids interact with water molecules to break the hydrogen bonding that mediates surface tension. Therefore, inadequate or dysfunctional surfactant in infants with RDS leads to an inappropriately high alveolar surface tension, resulting in difficulties recruiting atelectatic alveoli and in progressive atelectasis of recruited airspaces.

A. **CPAP** has its physiologic basis in the grunting that infants with RDS do to maintain FRC. Application of CPAP via nasal prongs, nasal mask, or face mask enables spontaneously breathing infants to gradually recruit atelectatic airspaces while maintaining alveolar patency at end expiration despite the absence of surfactant. Meta-analyses of CPAP trials from the 1970s to 1980s demonstrated the effectiveness of CPAP in more mature babies with RDS, and more recent trials showed that this strategy could be applied to even the least mature preterm infants without increasing the incidence of bronchopulmonary dysplasia (BPD).

1. Practical guidelines

a. **Pressure device.** Options for application include bubble CPAP, variable flow devices, and mechanical ventilators. Bubble CPAP devices also provides a gentle oscillation of positive pressure that may assist in recruitment and CO_2 elimination in addition to supporting alveoli. Whichever device is used, flows of approximately 5 to 10 L/minute are needed to prevent rebreathing and hypercarbia.

b. The development of humidification devices enabling the administration of high flow oxygen via nasal cannulas has led to their uses a strategy to provide end-expiratory pressure with a patient interface that may be less traumatic than nasal prongs. A single study utilizing an esophageal balloon to measure intrathoracic pressures during high flow rates suggested that the delivered CPAP in cm H_2O pressure approximated the liter flow rate in L/minute. One trial that compared nasal CPAP to heated, humidified high-flow nasal cannula (HHHFNC) in infants with an average gestational age of 33 weeks (1/3 between 28 and 32 weeks) either following mechanical ventilation or CPAP (87%) or as initial therapy (13%) found no difference in the primary outcome of failure requiring intubation within 72 hours of study entry. However, the limited evidence available suggests that HHHFNC should be used with caution, especially as initial therapy in ELBW infants.

c. **Patient interface.** A variety of nasal prongs and nasal masks can be used to provide an occlusive interface for CPAP delivery. The need for occlusion may lead to pressure necrosis of the nasal septum that can be severe enough to require surgical intervention. This can often be alleviated by alternating interfaces during routine nursing care. Daily rounds should include a discussion of the interface and status of the nasal septum.

d. Initiation of CPAP. Initiate nasal CPAP at 5 to 6 cm H_2O pressure and adjust based on chest radiograph (goal inflation 8 to 9 rib expansion) and oxygen requirement. Optimal FRC should be associated with a gradual reduction in FiO_2 to 0.21 in the uninjured lung with pure surfactant deficiency as well as normalization of respiratory rate. Monitoring of blood gases in the acute phase of recruitment may be necessary, but once adequate ventilation is achieved and recruitment has been established, noninvasive monitoring is usually sufficient to guide therapy.

e. Weaning strategies. Because successful application of CPAP is defined by achieving and maintaining a normal FRC, weaning of support should initially focus on reduction of supplemental oxygen until oxygen requirements are at least <30%, preferably <25%. For the preterm infant >32 weeks of gestation, discontinuation of CPAP can generally be considered at CPAP 4 to 5 and <25% oxygen. For infants born at <32 weeks of gestation, poor chest wall compliance alone can lead to progressive atelectasis, and longer term use of low CPAP may be advantageous, even when oxygen supplementation is no longer needed. Atelectasis can occur with gradual weaning and discontinuation of CPAP due to insufficient endogenous surfactant stores and/or poor chest wall compliance and may take several hours to develop. Signs of unsuccessful CPAP weaning include increases in oxygen requirement and respiratory rates, as well as retractions.

f. Contraindications. Few contraindications exist to using CPAP. The most important is apnea because the success of this therapy depends on the infant supplying the minute ventilation for normal CO_2 elimination. A trial of CPAP is contraindicated in infants with frank apnea in the delivery room. However, spontaneously breathing infants with respiratory distress or those at high risk for developing RDS (<30 weeks of gestation) may benefit from a trial of CPAP combined with early initiation of caffeine therapy to minimize apnea. Air leak is a relative contraindication to CPAP because air leak may worsen in the face of continuous positive pressure.

g. Complications

i. Overdistention. Rapid changes in lung compliance as atelectatic regions are recruited and supported, especially after administration of surfactant, can lead to overdistention of airspaces. In turn, this can result in (i) inadequate tidal volumes leading to hypercarbia; (ii) tamponade of the alveolar capillary bed, with ventilation–perfusion ($\dot{V}/\dot{Q}$) mismatch leading to hypercarbia and hypoxemia; and (iii) poor venous return sufficient to reduce cardiac output.

ii. Air leak. Although overdistention alone may lead to air leak, more often, air leak is due to large changes in airway pressures at the level of the respiratory bronchiole where airways lose their supporting structure, leading to disruption of the airway wall.

This may occur in the context of an infant struggling to breathe or crying against CPAP.

    iii. Underdistention. Failure to establish FRC will result in persistent need for oxygen supplementation and persistent atelectrauma of poorly supported airspaces. This is often due to difficulty with the patient-device interface (see section IV.A.1.c earlier) and/or an open mouth that presents a path for release of distending pressure. Repositioning patients in a side-lying or prone position to prop the jaw closed, or use of soft chin straps, can be useful.

    iv. Nasal septum trauma (see section IV.A.1.c earlier)

B. Restore alveolar surfactant. The majority of RDS encountered in the neonatal intensive care unit (NICU) is due to developmental deficiency of surfactant due to premature delivery of an infant with immature lungs. The widespread use of maternal antenatal glucocorticoids has reduced the incidence and severity of RDS, but the risk remains high when precipitous delivery or other circumstances preclude glucocorticoid administration. Fortunately, surfactant maturation continues postnatally and is often accelerated by the stress of preterm delivery and intensive care. For infants with RDS, exogenous surfactant therapy can acutely supplement insufficient endogenous stores and participate in the natural recycling of alveolar surfactant to enhance production by alveolar type II cells. The combination of antenatal glucocorticoid exposure and postnatal surfactant administration is more effective in reducing the morbidity and mortality of RDS than either intervention alone. Treatment of RDS in preterm infants is currently the only U.S. Food and Drug Administration (FDA)-approved indication for the use of exogenous surfactant.

    1. Practical considerations

        a. Prophylaxis versus treatment. Evidence demonstrates an advantage to early treatment of infants before the onset of signs as compared to waiting to establish a diagnosis of RDS. However, universal prophylaxis would lead to many infants being intubated to receive surfactant who either might not develop RDS or who could be successfully managed with CPAP until their own surfactant production was sufficient. Therefore, surfactant should be considered in preterm infants with signs of RDS in the immediate perinatal period after a failed trial of CPAP or in infants for whom CPAP is contraindicated, i.e., apnea, air leak.

        b. Surfactant preparation. Available surfactants include a variety of animal-derived products that are enriched through the addition of phospholipids but preserve the content of the hydrophobic surfactant proteins B and C that contribute to surfactant function (see Table 33.1).

        c. Dosing and dosing interval. Surfactant is administered to achieve a phospholipid dose that is at least 100 mg/kg (see Table 33.1). The standard dosing interval is every 12 hours for a maximum of three doses. However, in the absence of a therapeutic response or if the initial response is waning, the next dose can occur as soon as 6 hours later, rather than waiting to complete the 12-hour dosing interval.

        d. Administration. Surfactant is typically given to infants with RDS through an endotracheal tube (ETT) that either remains in place for mechanical ventilation or is inserted for surfactant dosing in an infant

Table 33.1. Dosing Information, Source, and Phospholipid and Protein Concentration for Beractant (Survanta), Calfactant (Infasurf), and Poractant Alfa (Curosurf)

Trade Name	Active Ingredient	Source	Dosing	Phospholipid Concentration	Protein Concentration
Survanta	Beractant	Bovine lung extract	▪ 4 mL/kg (100 mg/kg phospholipid) divided into four-quarter doses through endotracheal tube. Prophylaxis: Give within 15 minutes of birth in infants at risk for surfactant deficiency. Rescue therapy: Give when diagnosis of surfactant deficiency is made. ▪ Can use up to four doses, given no more frequently than every 6 hours	25 mg/mL	<1 mg/mL (SP-B and SP-C; does not contain SP-A)
Infasurf	Calfactant	Calf lung lavage fluid	▪ 3 mL/kg (105 mg/kg phospholipid) through endotracheal tube for prophylaxis or rescue therapy ▪ Can use up to three doses, given 12 hours apart	35 mg/mL	0.7 mg/mL (SP-B and SP-C; does not contain SP-A)
Curosurf	Poractant alfa	Porcine lung extract	▪ Initial dose: 2.5 mL/kg through endotracheal tube (200 mg/kg phospholipid) ▪ Can use up to two subsequent doses of 1.25 mL/kg administered 12 hours apart (maximum volume 5 mL/kg)	76 mg/mL	1 mg/mL (SP-B and SP-C; does not contain SP-A)

Sources: Survanta package insert. Columbus, OH: Abbott Nutrition; Infasurf package insert. Amherst, NY: ONY Inc; Curosurf package insert. Parma, Italy: Chiesi Farmaceutici S.p.A.

on CPAP and removed following the procedure. The ETT should be secured after intubation to avoid malpositioning of the tube during dosing. A chest radiograph is not necessary prior to dosing if equal breath sounds can be confirmed by auscultation. To minimize reflux up the ETT, administration via a sterile feeding tube inserted into the ETT with the tip is at or above the end of the ETT is preferable. Alternatively, the dose can be given via closed in-line suction devices to enable continuous mechanical ventilation. Providing the dose in 2 to 4 aliquots and allowing for recovery on mechanical ventilation between aliquots can help to minimize obstruction of the ETT or large airways by the viscous surfactant preparation. Positional maneuvers that were initially recommended to assist in surfactant distribution are not necessary due to the large volume relative to surface area and rapid distribution of surfactant and should be avoided because they could result in ETT malposition or extubation. Early experience with minimally invasive surfactant therapy (MIST), administered by insertion of a small bore catheter or a gastric tube into the trachea, indicates feasibility; further studies are needed to ensure safety and efficacy. Aerosolization devices for surfactant administration are currently in clinical trials.

 e. Complications

  i. Airway obstruction. Hypoxemia, bradycardia, and apnea may occur acutely during surfactant administration due to obstruction of large airways until surfactant distributes fully. Divided dose administration and recovery on mechanical ventilation minimize these transient events.

  ii. Air leak. More serious complications may result from a rapid increase in lung compliance that occurs as surfactant lowers surface tension, fostering alveolar recruitment. Infants receiving pressure-limited mechanical ventilation may develop pneumothorax as delivered tidal volumes increase (see Chapter 38). This may be avoided by converting to volume-limited mechanical ventilation (see section IV.C.1.b in the following text).

  iii. Hemorrhagic pulmonary edema. As compliance improves, pulmonary vascular resistance drops and can result in altered Starling forces that contribute to hemorrhagic pulmonary edema, commonly referred to as pulmonary hemorrhage, especially in the presence of a patent ductus arteriosus that can exacerbate the process with pulmonary overcirculation (see Chapter 37).

C. Ensure appropriate CO_2 elimination. Although poor oxygenation is most often the dominant feature of RDS, atelectasis also reduces the gas exchange surface area for CO_2, and additional strategies are needed to manage hypercarbia.

 1. Practical considerations

  a. Caffeine therapy. Successful use of nasal CPAP to treat RDS depends on adequate spontaneous breathing which is facilitated by early use of caffeine (see Chapter 31).

  b. Mechanical ventilation (see Chapter 29). Optimal ventilator strategy for infants with RDS includes the application of sufficient positive end-expiratory pressure (PEEP) to allow maintenance of FRC, applying the same guidelines for the use of end expiratory pressure with CPAP. For infants who fail CPAP, we generally start at the same level of PEEP as provided by nasal CPAP because delivery of end-expiratory pressure via an ETT is more effective than noninvasive application. As discussed earlier, optimization of FRC should result in need for decreased concentration of supplemental oxygen to maintain appropriate oxygen saturation. As with CPAP, complications include overdistention, volutrauma, and air leak.

We typically use volume-limited, time-cycled ventilation in infants with RDS, especially during the period of surfactant administration. In this ventilator mode, setting delivered tidal volume at 4 to 6 mL/kg results in automatic weaning of peak inspiratory pressures as lung compliance drops in response to surfactant treatment, thus avoiding volutrauma and air leak.

In infants with a large leak around the ETT due to either severe RDS with very low lung compliance or a tube relatively small compared to the airway size, pressure-limited, time-cycled ventilation may be needed. In this case, we closely monitor for sometimes dramatic changes in lung compliance and reduce peak inspiratory pressures to avoid delivering supraphysiologic tidal volumes, volutrauma, and air leak.

D. Outcomes. In the presurfactant era, RDS in late preterm infants typically resolved at 2 to 4 days of age, often preceded by spontaneous diuresis. With the widespread use of antenatal glucocorticoids, early use of nasal continuous positive airway pressure (NCPAP), and availability of exogenous surfactant, the time course of RDS has become more difficult to define. In addition, the frequent association of preterm birth with chorioamnionitis or latent inflammation may affect the time to resolution. RDS in infants born at $\geq$32 weeks' gestational age and without other complications typically resolves fully with no long-term pulmonary sequelae. Infants <32 weeks' gestational age are at risk for BPD; risk increases with decreasing gestational age (see Chapter 34).

Suggested Readings

Hillman N, Jobe AH. Noninvasive strategies for management of respiratory problems in neonates. *NeoReviews* 2013;14:e227–e236. doi:10.1542/neo.14-5-e227.

Jobe A. Surfactant for respiratory distress syndrome. *NeoReviews* 2014;15:e236–e245. doi:10.1542/neo.15-6-e236.

34 Bronchopulmonary Dysplasia/Chronic Lung Disease

Richard B. Parad and John Benjamin

KEY POINTS

- Bronchopulmonary dysplasia (BPD) affects 30% to 50% of extremely low birth weight infants.
- Arrested lung development and reduced gas exchange surface area are hallmarks of "new" BPD.
- Contributing factors include inflammation and lung injury from oxygen toxicity and mechanical ventilation induced barotrauma.
- Glucocorticoids, diuretics, and bronchodilators are often used for treatment of characteristic respiratory symptoms in BPD, although evidence-based strategies are lacking.

I. **DEFINITION.** A 2001 National Institutes of Health (NIH) consensus conference proposed definitions for bronchopulmonary dysplasia (BPD) (also known by the more general term *chronic lung disease* [CLD] of prematurity)

   A. For infants born at <32 weeks' gestation who received supplemental oxygen for their first 28 days, the NIH defined BPD at 36 weeks' postmenstrual age (PMA) as

      1. Mild: no supplemental O_2 requirement

      2. Moderate: supplemental O_2 requirement <30%

      3. Severe: supplemental O_2 requirement ≥30% and/or continuous positive airway pressure (CPAP) or ventilator support

   B. For infants born at ≥32 weeks, the NIH defined BPD as supplemental O_2 requirement for the first 28 days with severity level based on O_2 requirement at 56 days.

   C. **Physiologic definition of BPD.** The need for supplemental oxygen is based on oxygen saturation (SpO_2) during a room air challenge performed at 36 weeks' PMA (or 56 days for infants >32 weeks' PMA) or before hospital discharge. Persistent SpO_2 <90% is the cutoff below which supplemental O_2 should be considered.

D. Operationally, many clinicians simply define BPD as requirement for oxygen supplementation at 36 weeks' PMA. Lung parenchyma usually appears abnormal on chest radiographs. This definition can also apply to term infants who require chronic ventilatory support following meconium aspiration syndrome, pneumonia, and certain cardiac and gastrointestinal (GI) anomalies. BPD is associated with the development of chronic respiratory morbidity (CRM).

II. EPIDEMIOLOGY. Approximately 10,000 to 15,000 new cases of BPD occur in the United States each year. The incidence of BPD increases with decreasing gestational age at birth. Infants <28 weeks' gestation or <1,000 g birth weight are most susceptible, with incidence rates of 35% to 50%. Differences in populations (race/ethnicity/socioeconomic status), clinical practices, and definitions account for wide variation in the rate reported among centers. The relative risk is decreased in African Americans and females. Of infants with BPD, 44% develop CRM (defined as a requirement for pulmonary medications at 18 months corrected age). Of similar preterm infants who do not require O_2 at 36 weeks' PMA, 29% also develop CRM.

III. ETIOLOGY AND PATHOGENESIS

A. Etiology. A number of factors have been associated with BPD, some of which may be causal.

1. Immature lung substrate. The lung is most susceptible before alveolar septation begins. Injury at this stage may lead to an arrest of alveolarization and simplified lung structures that are the hallmark of new BPD.

2. Volutrauma and lung injury from mechanical ventilation or bag-and-mask ventilation

3. Oxygen toxicity. Insufficient production of the antioxidant enzymes superoxide dismutase, catalase, glutathione peroxidase, and/or deficiency of free radical sinks such as vitamin E, glutathione, and ceruloplasmin may predispose the lung to O_2 toxicity. Similarly, inadequate antiprotease protection may predispose the lung to injury from the unchecked proteases released by recruited inflammatory cells.

4. Genetic factors may contribute to BPD risk, but the mechanism is uncertain.

5. Excessive early intravenous fluid administration, perhaps by contributing to pulmonary edema

6. Persistent left-to-right shunt through the patent ductus arteriosus (PDA). Although prophylactic PDA ligation or administration of indomethacin or ibuprofen does not prevent BPD, persistent left-to-right shunt and late PDA closure appear to be associated with increased BPD risk. However, surgical PDA closure is also associated with increased BPD risk.

7. Intrauterine or perinatal infection, with cytokine release, may contribute to the etiology of BPD or modify its course. *Ureaplasma urealyticum*

has been associated with BPD in premature infants, although whether this relationship is causal is uncertain. Intrauterine *Chlamydia trachomatis* and other viral infections have also been implicated.

8. Intrauterine growth restriction has been linked to later development of BPD, although whether this is a causal mechanism for disease or just an association is uncertain.

9. Increased inositol clearance may lead to diminished plasma inositol levels and decreased surfactant synthesis or impaired surfactant metabolism.

10. An increase in vasopressin and a decrease in atrial natriuretic peptide release may alter pulmonary and systemic fluid balance in the setting of obstructive lung disease.

B. **Pathogenesis**

1. **Acute lung injury** is caused by the combination of O_2 toxicity, barotrauma, and volutrauma from mechanical ventilation. Cellular and interstitial injury results in the release of proinflammatory cytokines (interleukin 1β [IL-1β], IL-6, IL-8, tumor necrosis factor alpha [TNF-α]) that cause secondary changes in alveolar permeability and recruit inflammatory cells into interstitial and alveolar spaces; further injury from proteases, oxidants, and additional chemokines, and chemoattractants cause ongoing inflammatory cell recruitment and leakage of water and protein. Airway and vascular tone may be altered. Sloughed cells and accumulated secretions not cleared adequately by the damaged mucociliary transport system cause inhomogeneous peripheral airway obstruction that leads to alternating areas of collapse and hyperinflation and proximal airway dilation. Inflammation may also alter critical molecular pathways required for lung development leading to impaired alveolarization and emphysematous changes in the lung. In the original report by Northway in 1967 of the "old" BPD affecting infants with mean gestational age of 33 weeks and birth weight of 2,000 g, pathology of nonsurvivors showed predominantly small airway injury, fibrosis, and emphysema. In contrast, in the postsurfactant therapy era, "new" BPD affects mostly extremely preterm infants and the most significant pathologic finding in nonsurvivors is decreased alveolarization.

2. In the **chronic** phase of lung injury, the interstitium may be altered by fibrosis and cellular hyperplasia that results from excessive release of growth factors and cytokines, leading to dysregulated repair. Interstitial fluid clearance is disrupted, resulting in pulmonary fluid retention. Airways develop increased muscularization and hyperreactivity. The physiologic effects are decreased lung compliance, increased airway resistance, and impaired gas exchange with resulting ventilation–perfusion mismatching and air trapping.

3. **Histopathology.** Arrest of alveolarization and dilated simplified terminal airspaces are characteristic histologic features of "new" BPD seen at lower gestational ages. The resultant emphysematous changes and impairment in alveolar development leads to diminished surface area for gas exchange. In severe cases, pathology may reflect that seen in "old" BPD with detectable changes observed within the first few days

after birth. In these cases, necrotizing bronchiolitis, obstruction of small airway lumens by debris and edema, and areas of peribronchial and interstitial fibrosis are present. Changes in both large airways (glandular hyperplasia) and small airways (smooth muscle hyperplasia) likely form the histologic basis for reactive airway disease. Pulmonary vascular changes associated with pulmonary hypertension (PH) may be seen.

IV. CLINICAL PRESENTATION

A. Physical examination typically reveals tachypnea, retractions, and rales on auscultation.

B. Arterial blood gas (ABG) analysis shows hypoxemia and hypercarbia with eventual metabolic compensation for the respiratory acidosis.

C. The **chest radiograph** appearance changes as the disease progresses. With "new" BPD, the initial appearance is often diffuse haziness, increased density, and normal-to-low lung volumes. In more severe disease, chronic changes may include inhomogeneous regions of opacification and hyperlucency with superimposed hyperinflation.

D. Cardiac evaluation. Nonpulmonary causes of respiratory failure should be excluded. Electrocardiogram (ECG) can show persistent or progressive right ventricular hypertrophy if *cor pulmonale* develops. Left ventricular hypertrophy may develop with systemic hypertension. Two-dimensional echocardiography may be useful in excluding left-to-right shunts (see Chapter 41) and PH. Biventricular failure is unusual when good oxygenation is maintained, and the development of PH is avoided.

E. Infant pulmonary function testing (iPFT). Increased respiratory system resistance (Rrs) and decreased dynamic compliance (Crs) are hallmarks of BPD. In the first year after birth, iPFTs reveal decreased forced expiratory flow rate, increased functional residual capacity (FRC), increased residual volume (RV), and increased RV/total lung capacity ratio and bronchodilator responsiveness, with an overall pattern of mild-to-moderate airflow obstruction, air trapping, and increased airway reactivity. Although such testing is feasible, it is not typically used in clinical practice.

V. INPATIENT TREATMENT. The goals of treatment during the neonatal intensive care unit (NICU) course are to prevent or minimize further lung injury (barotrauma and volutrauma, O_2 toxicity, inflammation), maximize nutrition, and diminish O_2 consumption.

A. Pharmacologic prevention

1. Vitamin A (5,000 IU intramuscular [IM], three times weekly for the first 28 days of age) reduced the incidence of chronic lung disease (CLD) in extremely low birth weight (ELBW) infants by 10%. Although some centers routinely treat ELBW infants with vitamin A using this protocol, the impact on long-term outcomes is uncertain.

2. Caffeine citrate (20 mg/kg loading dose and 5 mg/kg daily maintenance) started during the first 10 days after birth in infants 500 to 1,250 g birth weight reduced the rate of BPD from 47% to 36% and improved the rate of survival without neurodevelopmental disability at 18 to 21 months corrected age.

3. **Investigational therapies without proven efficacy**

a. Inhaled nitric oxide (iNO). In animal models of BPD, iNO may act to relax airway and pulmonary vascular tone and diminish lung inflammation. Several multicenter clinical trials assessed the potential efficacy of iNO in attenuating or preventing BPD using different treatment regimens. One trial found that BPD was reduced in infants >1,000 g although not for the overall group; another found overall benefit that was limited to those treated at 7 to 14 days. Because benefit is unclear and both safety and long-term impact have not been established, an NIH consensus panel recommended that use of iNO to prevent or treat BPD is not supported by available evidence.

b. In <27-week gestation infants, intratracheal **recombinant human Cu/Zn superoxide dismutase** administered intratracheally every 48 hours while intubated resulted in an approximately 50% reduction in use of asthma medications, emergency room visits, and hospitalizations in the first year of life. **Recombinant human club cell protein 10**, a natural innate anti-inflammatory protein abundant in the lung, is undergoing evaluation for intratracheal administration for prophylaxis against CRM.

c. Whether azithromycin may decrease the risk of developing BPD in infants with documented *Ureaplasma* colonization or infection is under investigation.

B. **Mechanical ventilation**

1. **Acute phase.** Volume targeted compared to pressure limited ventilation appears to reduce the incidence of the combined outcome of BPD or death and of BPD, as well as air leak. We initially target 3 to 5 mL/kg/breath while providing adequate gas exchange (see Chapter 29). It is possible that use of patient-controlled ventilator modalities such as patient-triggered breaths and pressure-supported spontaneous breaths may lower BPD risk. Early use of nasal CPAP may avoid the need for intubation and surfactant therapy, although this has not clearly reduced the risk of BPD and some studies suggest increased rates of pneumothorax. Nasal intermittent positive pressure ventilation (NIPPV) does not appear to be any more effective than standard nasal CPAP in avoiding need for intubation and surfactant therapy.

In most circumstances, we avoid hyperventilation and target arterial carbon dioxide tension (PaCO$_2$) at ≥55 mm Hg, with pH ≥7.25, and target SpO$_2$ at 90% to 95% and arterial oxygen tension (PaO$_2$) 55 to 80 mm Hg. Although routine use of high-frequency oscillatory ventilation (HFOV) does not prevent BPD, follow-up at 11 to 14 years of age of infants enrolled in a large trial found better lung function in those treated with HFOV compared to conventional ventilation. We sometimes use heated, humidified high-flow nasal cannula (HHHFNC) for postextubation care in preterm infants >28 weeks' gestation. HHHFNC therapy may decrease the risk of extubation failure with the additional benefit of inducing less nasal trauma than CPAP. The impact of HHHFNC use on BPD risk has not been evaluated.

2. **Chronic phase.** Baseline ventilator settings are maintained with an aim to keep $PaCO_2$ <70 mm Hg with a compensated respiratory acidosis. Although an effort to transition to CPAP or HHHFNC as soon as possible is encouraged, subsequent support is not aggressively weaned until a pattern of steady weight gain is established.

C. **Supplemental oxygen** is supplied to maintain the PaO_2 >55 mm Hg. The Surfactant, Positive Pressure, and Oxygenation Randomized Trial (SUPPORT) of low (85% to 89%) versus high (91% to 95%) SpO_2 targets in infants <28 weeks' gestation revealed a higher mortality rate and no reduction in BPD rate (physiologic definition) in the low SpO_2 group, although severe ROP was less frequent in survivors. One approach for infants who receive supplemental oxygen is to target SpO_2 at 92% to 95% with alarm limits at 84% to 96%. Another is to adjust the target saturations according to gestational age or PMA (Table 34.1). Oximeter alarm limits may be set 0% to 2% outside the appropriate target range.

When end-expiratory pressure is no longer needed and FiO_2 is <0.3, we supply O_2 by nasal cannula (NC). We use a flow meter that is accurate at low rates and gradually decrease the flow of 100% O_2 while maintaining the appropriate SpO_2. Alternatively, flow can be decreased to the lowest marking on the flow meter as tolerated, and then O_2 concentration can be decreased. Estimates of the actual concentration of O_2 delivered to the lungs by NC at different flows of 100% O_2 have been generated by hypopharyngeal measurements (see Fig. 34.1). Once the infant remains stable on a low flow rate, we attempt a trial of withdrawal of NC support with close monitoring of O_2 saturation to determine if continued O_2 supplementation is required. In general, SpO_2 should remain >90% during sleep, feedings, and active periods before supplemental O_2 is discontinued. An "oxygen challenge test" can be performed at 36 weeks' PMA to confirm whether an infant requires supplemental oxygen to maintain SpO_2 >90% and thus meets the physiologic definition of BPD.

D. **Surfactant replacement therapy** decreases the combined outcome of O_2 requirement or death at 28 days of age, although it has made little or no impact on the overall incidence of BPD. Meta-analyses suggest that the incidence is decreased in larger premature infants but is higher in smaller premature infants who would have died without surfactant therapy (see Chapter 33). Late surfactant exhaustion may contribute to the development

Table 34.1. Postmenstrual Age Target Oxygen Saturations

Gestational Age	Target SpO$_2$ on O$_2$	Target SpO$_2$ off O$_2$
<32 weeks	90%–95%	90%–100%
32–36 weeks	92%–97%	92%–100%
>36 weeks	94%–98%	94%–100%

SpO$_2$, oxygen saturation; O$_2$, supplemental oxygen.

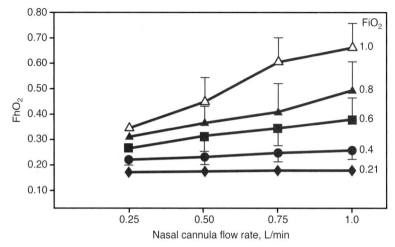

Figure 34.1. Approximate conversion from nasal cannula flow at different FiO_2 to hypopharyngeal FiO_2 (FhO_2). FiO_2, fraction of inspired O_2. (From Vain NE, Prudent LM, Stevens DP, et al. Regulation of oxygen concentration delivered to infants via nasal cannulas. *Am J Dis Child* 1989;143[12]:1458–1460. With permission.)

of BPD; although the TOLSURF trial of late surfactant dosing in ventilated preterm infants receiving iNO did not improve survival without BPD.

E. **PDA.** We consider treatment of a hemodynamically significant PDA in infants who have respiratory decompensation or cannot be weaned from mechanical ventilation (see Chapter 41).

F. **Fluid management.** Initial fluid intake is limited to the minimum required. Initially, we provide intake adequate to maintain urine output at least 1 mL/kg/hour and serum sodium concentration of 140 to 145 mEq/L. In the chronic phase, we may limit fluids to as low as 130 mL/kg/day with monitoring for adequate urine output and attention to higher caloric density nutrients to provide sufficient calories for growth. We regularly recalculate fluid intake for weight gain, once it is above birth weight. Later, when respiratory status is stable, fluid restriction is gradually relaxed.

G. **Medications.** When an infant remains ventilator-dependent on restricted fluid intake in the absence of PDA or intercurrent infection, we consider trying additional pharmacologic strategies.

1. **Diuretics** are used to treat pulmonary fluid retention. Diuretics indirectly attenuate signs of respiratory distress and result in decreased Rrs and increased Crs; gas exchange is variably affected. An acute clinical response may be seen within 1 hour, although maximal effect may not be achieved until 1 week of therapy. The clinical improvement is likely due to decreased lung water content, with decreased interstitial and peribronchial fluid resulting in less resistance and better compliance. The mechanisms of action may be due to either diuresis or nondiuretic

effects. Diuretics have not been shown to improve long-term clinical measures such as duration of ventilator dependence, hospital length of stay, or the incidence of BPD.

a. Furosemide is used initially at a dose of 1.0 mg/kg intravenously (or 2 mg/kg po/pg) daily. We give furosemide at the time of blood transfusions if these have been associated with increased pulmonary fluid and respiratory distress. Immature infants are at increased risk for toxicity from larger or more frequent doses because of the prolonged drug half-life. Side effects include hypercalciuria, nephrocalcinosis, ototoxicity, electrolyte imbalance, and nephrolithiasis.

b. Chlorothiazide. If a trial of furosemide given on three consecutive days suggests clinical improvement, we prefer treatment with chlorothiazide (20 to 40 mg/kg/day orally, divided BID) or hydrochlorothiazide (2 to 4 mg/kg/day orally, divided BID) to avoid furosemide toxicities. Thiazide diuretics decrease calcium excretion and, if used in combination with furosemide, may minimize calcium loss and reverse nephrocalcinosis due to furosemide. The combination may allow for the use of a lower furosemide dose, although we prefer to use a thiazide diuretic alone.

2. Bronchodilators. Acute obstructive episodes or chronically increased resistance may be related to increased airway tone or bronchospasm and may respond to bronchodilator therapy. In general, bronchodilators are most commonly used in older infants who remain ventilator-dependent; however, airway reactivity has been reported as early as 2 to 3 weeks of age in some infants.

a. Administration of nebulized β-adrenergic agonists (BAAs) like albuterol results in decreased Rrs and increased Crs and can be administered by metered-dose inhaler (MDI) with a spacer devise placed in line with the ventilator near the endotracheal tube.

b. MDI (1 puff) or nebulized (25 mg/kg/dose) ipratropium bromide, a muscarinic agent, increases Crs and decreases Rrs. Combination MDI containing both BAAs and muscarinic agents may provide a synergistic effect, but this has not been studied in preterm infants.

3. Caffeine citrate. The methylxanthine caffeine has airway dilation effects in asthmatics similar to aminophylline. This response has not been studied in the setting of BPD; however, infants with known airway reactivity who are weaning off caffeine should be observed for possible respiratory deterioration.

4. Postnatal corticosteroids. In early trials, treatment with glucocorticoids (usually dexamethasone) in infants who remained ventilator-dependent for 2 to 3 weeks resulted in increased Crs, decreased Rrs, and diminished O_2 requirement, and facilitated earlier extubation. However, glucocorticoid treatment does not appear to have a substantial impact on long-term pulmonary outcomes, such as duration of supplemental O_2 requirement, length of hospital stay, or mortality. Subsequent trials of earlier treatment, recurrent pulses, and lower doses have had inconsistent results as either a prophylactic or attenuating agent. Randomized trials of inhaled glucocorticoids also did not demonstrate improved pulmonary outcome. In addition to short-term side effects, including hypertension, hyperglycemia, and spontaneous GI perforation, long-term follow-up of infants treated with postnatal corticosteroids, primarily dexamethasone, has raised concerns about impaired neurodevelopment and growth. Because of this potential harm and lack of well-established long-term benefit, routine use of dexamethasone is discouraged and treatment reserved only for infants with progressive respiratory failure that is refractory to all other therapies. If treatment with dexamethasone is undertaken, we discuss the potential neurodevelopmental harm with parents before use.

Recent data suggest that hydrocortisone use may not be associated with the same neurodevelopmental concerns described with dexamethasone. One approach to **BPD prevention** is to estimate the risk of developing BPD using the National Institute of Child Health and Human Development (NICHD) Neonatal Research Network Neonatal BPD Outcome Estimator (https://neonatal.rti.org/index.cfm?fuseaction=BPDCalculator.start). If the risk of developing BPD is estimated at 2 weeks of age as ≥60%, a preventive course of hydrocortisone may be considered as follows: 1.25 mg/kg/dose IV/PO q6h × 7 days, then q8h × 5 days, then q12h × 5 days, then q24h × 5 days. A shorter hydrocortisone course is currently under evaluation in an NICHD multicenter trial.

a. Common acute complications of glucocorticoids include glucose intolerance, systemic hypertension, and transient catabolic state. Total neutrophil counts, band counts, and platelet counts increase during steroid treatment. Hypertrophic cardiomyopathy has been reported but is transient and does not appear to affect cardiac function. Intestinal perforation and gastric ulcerations can occur with early postnatal use, especially in combination with indomethacin, and resulted in termination of trials of dexamethasone and hydrocortisone. Adrenal suppression is transient.

b. Postextubation airway edema, with stridorous obstruction (see section VI.A) leading to respiratory failure, may be attenuated with three doses dexamethasone, 0.25 mg/kg/dose every 12 hours starting 8 to 12 hours before a planned extubation. Edema also may be acutely diminished with nebulized racemic epinephrine.

5. **Medications for pain control.** Pain management and sedation are used for physical or autonomic signs of pain or discomfort. These responses may interfere with the ability to ventilate and oxygenate. Oral sucrose, morphine sulfate or fentanyl, and short-acting benzodiazepines (in term infants) may be used (see Chapter 70).

6. **Electrolyte supplements.** Hyponatremia, hypokalemia, and hypochloremia with secondary hypercarbia are common side effects of chronic diuretic therapy that are corrected by lowering the diuretic dose or adding NaCl and KCl supplements. Adequate sodium intake should be provided. We provide NaCl supplement when serum sodium level falls to or below 130 mEq/L. Although hypochloremia may occur with compensated respiratory acidosis, low serum chloride concentration from diuretic-induced loss and inadequate intake can cause metabolic alkalosis and $PaCO_2$ elevation. Hypochloremia may also contribute

to poor growth. Chloride deficit should be corrected with KCl. Electrolytes should be monitored at regular intervals until equilibrium is reached (see Chapter 23).

H. Monitoring (see Chapter 30)

1. **ABG** analysis is used to monitor gas exchange and confirm correlation of noninvasive monitoring values.

2. We use **continuous pulse oximetry** for long-term monitoring of infants with BPD. The long-term goal is to keep the PaO_2 $\geq$55 mm Hg and avoid hyperoxemia.

3. **Capillary blood gas** (CBG) values are useful to monitor pH and PCO_2. Because pH and PCO_2 on CBGs sometimes vary from central values, we may compare them with ABG values if we have clinical concerns. If CBG and ABG values are similar, we monitor stable ventilator-dependent infants with pulse oximetry and one or two CBG analyses per day initially then less often if clinical condition remains unchanged. Less frequent CBG measurements are obtained for patients receiving supplemental oxygen with CPAP, HHHFNC, or by low-flow NC.

4. **Transcutaneous PCO_2 monitors** have undergone recent technical improvements so that they require less frequent calibration and operate at lower temperatures (minimizing skin injury). They may be useful to monitor PCO_2 trends, which allow more real-time ventilator adjustment to both minimize barotrauma and respond earlier to decompensations.

5. **Pulmonary function testing** is used in some centers to document functional responses to trials of bronchodilators and diuretics.

I. Nutrition (see Chapter 21)

1. **Metabolic rate** and energy expenditure are elevated in BPD although caloric intake may be poor. Providing more calories by the administration of lipids instead of carbohydrates lowers the respiratory quotient, thereby diminishing CO_2 production. To optimize growth, we try to minimize wasteful energy expenditure and maximize caloric and protein intake. Prolonged parenteral nutrition may be required. As enteral feeding is started, we feed by orogastric or nasogastric tube and advance oral feeding gradually to avoid tiring the infant. We increase the caloric density from 24 to 30 cal/oz human milk or formula, as required, to maintain daily growth of at least 10 to 15 mg/kg.

2. **Vitamin, trace element, and other dietary supplementation.** Vitamin E and antioxidant enzymes diminish oxidant toxicity, although vitamin E supplementation does not prevent BPD. Vitamin A may promote epithelial repair and minimize fibrosis. Selenium, zinc, and copper are trace elements vital to antioxidant enzyme function, and inadequate intake may interfere with protection.

J. Blood transfusions. We generally maintain hematocrit approximately 30% to 35% (hemoglobin 8 to 10 g/dL) as long as supplemental O_2 or ventilator support is needed. Fluid-sensitive patients may benefit from furosemide given immediately following the transfusion. Improved O_2 delivery may allow better reserves for growth in the infant with increased metabolic demands.

K. **Behavioral factors.** Attention to behavioral and environmental factors through individualized developmental care plans may minimize BPD risk and severity (see Chapter 14).

VI. ASSOCIATED COMPLICATIONS

A. Upper airway obstruction. Trauma to the nasal septum, larynx, trachea, or bronchi is common after prolonged or repeated intubation and suctioning. Abnormalities include laryngotracheobronchomalacia, granulomas, vocal cord paresis, edema, ulceration with pseudomembranes, subglottic stenosis, and congenital structural anomalies. Stridor may develop when postextubation edema is superimposed on underlying stenosis. Abnormalities are not excluded by the absence of stridor and may be asymptomatic, becoming symptomatic at the time of a viral upper respiratory tract infection. We consult otolaryngology specialists to perform flexible fiberoptic bronchoscopy to evaluate stridor, hoarseness, persistent wheezing, recurrent obstruction, or repeated extubation failures.

B. **Pulmonary Hypertension (PH)** is a major complication of BPD that is associated with a 2-year mortality rate of 38% to 43% after diagnosis. The development of PH in infants with BPD may involve both reversible and fixed components. Chronic hypoxemia leads to hypoxic vasoconstriction, PH, and eventual right ventricular hypertrophy and failure. Decrease in cross-sectional perfusion area and abnormal muscularization of more peripheral vessels have been documented. Left ventricular function also can be affected.

1. Supplemental O_2 is used to maintain SaO_2 between 92% and 95% or higher in infants with mature retinas. We obtain an echocardiogram by 36 to 37 weeks' PMA in infants with BPD who still require assisted ventilation or an inspired O_2 concentration of $>30\%$ to maintain adequate O_2 saturation, or have a PCO_2 of ≥ 60 mm Hg. In the more severely affected infants, we may begin monitoring as early as 32 weeks' PMA. These studies can exclude structural heart disease, assess left ventricular function, and estimate pulmonary vascular resistance and right ventricular function. Further studies are needed to determine if earlier screening echocardiograms in the first month of life can identify the development of PH in infants with BPD.

2. iNO is a useful therapy in the setting of acute PH and may improve oxygenation in infants with established BPD, although efficacy of iNO in long-term treatment of PH associated with BPD has not been determined. Sildenafil, a phosphodiesterase-5 inhibitor, may also improve oxygenation in patients with PH associated with BPD. Sildenafil offers the benefits of oral dosing and a long half-life, making administration at scheduled intervals of time possible. Because sildenafil has not been well evaluated in infants <1 year of age, it should be used with caution. Other pulmonary vasodilators, including calcium channel blockers such as nifedipine and endothelin receptor antagonists such as bosentan, remain investigational in infants with BPD. We monitor the response to therapy with serial echocardiograms to follow pulmonary vascular pressures and right ventricular function. Patients with persistent PH in

spite of treatment may need further evaluation by cardiac catheterization to delineate their pulmonary vascular anatomy and disease severity.

C. Systemic hypertension, sometimes with left ventricular hypertrophy, may develop in infants with BPD receiving prolonged O$_2$ therapy and should be treated (see Chapter 28).

D. Systemic-to-pulmonary shunting. Left-to-right shunt through collateral vessels (e.g., bronchial arteries) can occur in BPD. Risk factors include chest tube placement, thoracic surgery, and pleural inflammation. When left-to-right shunt is suspected and echocardiography fails to show intracardiac or PDA shunting, angiography may demonstrate collaterals. In this setting, occlusion of large vessels has been associated with clinical improvement.

E. Metabolic imbalance secondary to diuretics (see section V.G.1 and 6)

F. Infection. Because these chronically ill infants are at increased risk, episodes of pulmonary and systemic decompensation should be evaluated for infection. Monitoring tracheal aspirates with Gram stain may help distinguish endotracheal tube colonization from tracheobronchitis or pneumonia (presence of organisms and neutrophils). Viral and fungal infections should also be considered when fever or pneumonia develops. In infants with unresponsive clinical courses, we may assess tracheal aspirates for presence of *Ureaplasma* sp. and *Mycoplasma hominis* and treat if these organisms are identified.

G. Central nervous system (CNS) dysfunction. A neurologic syndrome presenting with extrapyramidal signs has been described in infants with CLD.

H. Hearing loss. Ototoxic drugs (furosemide, gentamicin) and ischemic or hypoxemic CNS injury increase the risk of sensorineural hearing loss. Screening with auditory brainstem responses should be performed at discharge (see Chapter 68).

I. Retinopathy of prematurity (ROP; see Chapter 67). ELBW infants with BPD are at high risk for developing ROP. Use of phenylephrine-containing eyedrops before eye examinations can cause an increase in airway resistance in some infants with BPD.

J. Nephrocalcinosis is frequently documented on ultrasonographic examination and has been linked to the use of furosemide and possibly steroids. Hematuria and passage of stones may occur. Most infants are asymptomatic, with eventual spontaneous resolution, but renal function should be followed (see Chapter 28).

K. Osteopenia may result from prematurity, inadequate calcium and phosphorus retention, and prolonged immobilization. Calcium loss due to furosemide and corticosteroids may also contribute. Supplementation with vitamin D, calcium, and phosphorus should be optimized (see Chapters 21 and 59).

L. Gastroesophageal reflux (GER). We try to document and treat GER in older infants when reflux or aspiration may contribute to pulmonary decompensation, apnea, or feeding intolerance with poor growth. Because trials have not shown acid neutralization and propulsive agents to be effective, we attempt management with optimized positioning, avoid excessive feeding volumes, and thicken feeds if needed. If decompensations associated with feeding may be related to swallow discoordination and microaspiration, we obtain fluoroscopic evaluations of swallowing while feeding contrast-laced human milk or formula to document aspiration. If aspiration is present, we sometimes test modification of feed viscosity. If nectar-thick feedings do not eliminate aspiration, we temporarily halt oral feeding and revert to nasogastric feeding until we confirm that aspiration with feeding has resolved. In severe cases, a gastrostomy tube and possible fundoplication may help avoid aspiration until swallow coordination has adequately matured.

M. Inguinal hernia. The incidence of inguinal hernia is increased by the presence of the patent processus vaginalis in very low birth weight (VLBW) infants, particularly boys, with BPD. If the hernia is reducible, surgical correction should be delayed until respiratory status is improved. Spinal, rather than general, anesthesia avoids reintubation and postoperative apnea.

N. Early growth failure may result from inadequate intake and excessive energy expenditure and may persist after clinical resolution of pulmonary disease. Premature withdrawal of supplemental O_2 may contribute to slowing of growth.

VII. **DISCHARGE PLANNING.** The timing of discharge depends on the availability of home care support systems and parental readiness (see Chapter 18).

A. Weight gain and oxygen therapy. Supplemental O_2 should be weaned when the SpO_2 is consistently maintained >92%, no significant periods of desaturations occur during feedings and/or sleep, good weight gain has been established, and respiratory status is stable. We prefer to delay discharge until O_2 has been discontinued. However, if long-term O_2 supplementation seems likely in an infant who is stable, growing, and has capable caretakers, we offer the option of home O_2 therapy.

B. Teaching. The involvement of parents in caregiving is vital to the smooth transition from hospital to home care. Parents should be taught cardiopulmonary resuscitation and early signs of decompensation. Teaching about equipment use, medication administration, and nutritional guidelines should begin when discharge planning is initiated.

C. Baseline values of vital signs, daily weight gain, discharge weight and head circumference, blood gases, SpO_2, hematocrit, electrolytes, and the baseline appearance of the chest radiograph and ECG are documented at discharge. Echocardiograms are obtained in more severely affected infants. This information is useful to evaluate subsequent changes in clinical status. Follow-up eye examination and hearing screening should be scheduled as needed.

D. Subspecialist and multidisciplinary management. Prior to discharge, we arrange for a baseline evaluation and interaction with the parents by the pulmonologist, cardiologist, and other subspecialists who will follow the infant as an outpatient.

VIII. **OUTPATIENT THERAPY**

A. Supplemental oxygen can be delivered by tanks or an O_2 concentrator. Portable tanks allow mobility. Weaning is based on periodic assessment of SpO_2.

B. Medications. We monitor electrolytes periodically in infants receiving diuretics. When the infant is stable, we allow him or her to outgrow the diuretic dose by 50% before discontinuing the drug. If bronchodilators have been used, they are tapered when respiratory status is stable in room air. Nebulized medications are tapered last. Discontinued medications should remain available for early use when symptoms recur.

C. Immunizations. In addition to standard immunizations, infants with BPD should receive pneumococcal and influenza vaccines and palivizumab (Synagis) (see Chapter 16).

D. Nutrition. Weight gain is a sensitive indicator of well-being and should be closely monitored. Infants often require caloric supplementation to maintain good growth after discharge. At discharge, we supplement calories in a transitional formula or, optimally, breast milk.

E. Passive smoke exposure. Because smoking in the home increases respiratory tract illness in children, parents of infants with BPD should be discouraged from smoking and should minimize the child's exposure to smoke-containing environments.

IX. OUTCOME

A. Mortality in severe BPD is estimated at 10% to 20% during the first year of life. The risk increases with duration of O_2 exposure and level of ventilatory support. Death is frequently caused by infection. The risk of sudden, unexpected death may be increased, but the cause is unclear.

B. Long-term morbidity

1. **Pulmonary.** Tachypnea, retractions, dyspnea, cough, and wheezing can be seen for months to years in seriously affected children. Reactive airway disease occurs more frequently, and infants with BPD are at increased risk for bronchiolitis and pneumonia. The rehospitalization rate for respiratory illness during the first 2 years of life in infants with BPD is approximately twice that of matched-control infants. Although complete clinical recovery can occur, underlying pulmonary function, gas exchange, and radiographic abnormalities may persist beyond adolescence. Persistent parenchymal and airway abnormalities are detectable on high resolution computed tomography (CT) scans of children and adults with a previous history of BPD. In addition, respiratory symptoms such as wheezing and lung functional abnormalities are also seen with higher frequency in these individuals. CRM measures at 6 and 12 months corrected age are being evaluated as potential outcomes to assess in studies of early therapeutic interventions aimed at preventing or attenuating BPD.

2. **Neurodevelopmental delay/neurologic deficits.** BPD is not an independent predictor of adverse neurologic outcome. However, infants with severe BPD may also have poor neurodevelopmental outcomes; respiratory and neural injury may be due to a common antecedent such as oxidative stress. Children with BPD have higher rates of motor, cognitive, educational, and behavioral impairments.

3. **Growth failure.** The degree of long-term growth delay is inversely proportional to birth weight and probably is influenced by the severity and
duration of CLD. Weight is most affected, and head circumference is
least affected. Delayed growth (<2 standard deviations below the mean)
persists for weight in approximately 20% and length or head circumference in approximately 10% at 20 months corrected age.

Suggested Readings

Islam JY, Keller RL, Aschner JL, et al. Understanding the short- and long-term
respiratory outcomes of prematurity and bronchopulmonary dysplasia. *Am
J Respir Crit Care Med* 2015;192(2):134–156.

Jain D, Bancalari E. Bronchopulmonary dysplasia: clinical perspective. *Birth Defects
Res A Clin Mol Teratol* 2014;100(3):134–144.

Jensen EA, Schmidt B. Epidemiology of bronchopulmonary dysplasia. *Birth Defects
Res A Clin Mol Teratol* 2014;100(3):145–157.

McEvoy CT, Jain L, Schmidt B, et al. Bronchopulmonary dysplasia: NHLBI workshop on the primary prevention of chronic lung diseases. *Ann Am Thorac
Soc* 2014;11(suppl 3):S146–153.

Meconium Aspiration
Erin J. Plosa

I. BACKGROUND

A. Cause. Acute or chronic hypoxia and/or infection can result in the passage of meconium *in utero*. In this setting, gasping by the fetus or newly born infant can cause aspiration of amniotic fluid contaminated by meconium. Meconium aspiration before or during birth can obstruct airways, interfere with gas exchange, and cause severe respiratory distress (Fig. 35.1).

B. Incidence. Meconium-stained amniotic fluid (MSAF) complicates approximately 10% to 15% of deliveries. The incidence of MSAF in preterm infants is very low. Most babies with MSAF are 37 weeks or older, and many meconium-stained infants are postmature and small for gestational age. Approximately 3% to 4% of neonates born through MSAF develop meconium aspiration syndrome (MAS), and approximately 30% to 50% of these infants require continuous positive airway pressure (CPAP) or mechanical ventilation.

II. PATHOPHYSIOLOGY.
Meconium is a sterile, thick, black-green odorless material that results from the accumulation of debris in the fetal intestine starting in the third month of gestation. The components of meconium include water (72% to 80%), desquamated cells from the intestine and skin, gastrointestinal mucin, lanugo hair, fatty material from the vernix caseosa, amniotic fluid, intestinal secretions, blood group–specific glycoproteins, bile, and enzymes including phospholipase A_2.

A. Passage of meconium *in utero*. MSAF occurs more commonly in term or postterm pregnancies and rarely prior to 34 weeks' gestation. MSAF may result from a postterm fetus with rising motilin levels and normal gastrointestinal function, vagal stimulation produced by cord or head compression, or *in utero* fetal stress. Amniotic fluid that is thinly stained is described

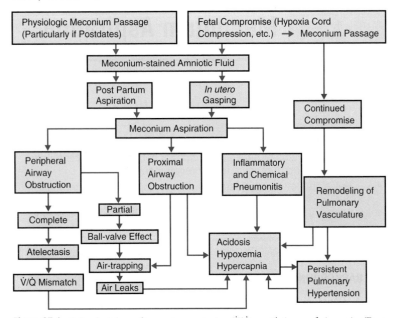

Figure 35.1. Pathophysiology of meconium aspiration. V̇/Q̇, ventilation–perfusion ratio. (From Wiswell T, Bent RC. Meconium staining and the meconium aspiration syndrome: unresolved issues. *Pediatr Clin North Am* 1993;40:955–981. Used with permission.)

as *watery*. Moderately stained fluid is opaque without particles, and fluid with thick meconium with particles is sometimes called *pea soup*.

B. Aspiration of meconium. In the presence of fetal stress, gasping by the fetus can result in aspiration of meconium before, during, or immediately following delivery. Severe MAS appears to be caused by pathologic intra-uterine processes, primarily chronic hypoxia, acidosis, and infection.

C. Effects of meconium aspiration. When aspirated into the lung, meconium may stimulate the release of cytokines and vasoactive substances that result in cardiovascular and inflammatory responses in the fetus and newborn. Meconium itself, or the resultant chemical pneumonitis, mechanically ob-structs the small airways, causes atelectasis, and a "ball-valve" effect with resultant air trapping and possible air leak. Aspirated meconium leads to vasospasm, hypertrophy of the pulmonary arterial musculature, and pul-monary hypertension that lead to extrapulmonary right-to-left shunting through the ductus arteriosus or the foramen ovale, resulting in worsened ventilation–perfusion (V̇/Q̇) mismatch and severe arterial hypoxemia. Approximately one-third of infants with MAS develop persistent pulmo-nary hypertension of the newborn (PPHN), which contributes to the mor-tality associated with this syndrome (see Chapter 36). Aspirated meconium also inhibits surfactant function. Several studies suggest that the enzymatic and sterol components of meconium disrupt the surfactant phospholipids and limit the ability for surfactant to lower surface tension.

D. Severity. MAS is considered mild in infants requiring <40% oxygen for <48 hours and moderate in infants requiring >40% oxygen for >48 hours without air leak. MAS is considered severe in infants who require assisted ventilation for >48 hours and is often associated with PPHN.

E. Sequelae. *In utero* passage of meconium in term infants has been associated with an increased risk of perinatal and neonatal mortality, severe acidemia, need for cesarean delivery, need for intensive care and oxygen administration, and adverse neurologic outcome. Preterm infants who pass meconium before delivery have similar adverse effects as well as an increased incidence of severe intraventricular hemorrhage, cystic periventricular leukomalacia, and cerebral palsy.

III. PREVENTION OF MECONIUM ASPIRATION SYNDROME

A. Prevention of passage of meconium *in utero.* Mothers at risk for uteroplacental insufficiency and thus MSAF include those with preeclampsia or increased blood pressure, chronic respiratory or cardiovascular disease, poor intrauterine fetal growth, postterm pregnancy, and heavy smokers. These women should be carefully monitored during pregnancy.

B. Amnioinfusion. The use of amnioinfusion in women whose labor is complicated by MSAF does not reduce neonatal morbidity related to meconium aspiration, although the technique effectively treats repetitive variable fetal heart rate decelerations by relieving umbilical cord compression in labor. A large randomized trial of amnioinfusion for women with thick meconium-stained fluid with or without variable fetal heart rate decelerations showed no reduction of the risk of moderate or severe MAS, perinatal death, or cesarean delivery. However, the study did not have adequate power to determine definitively if amnioinfusion may benefit the group with variable decelerations.

C. Timing and mode of delivery. In pregnancies that continue past the due date, induction as early as 41 weeks may help prevent MAS by avoiding passage of meconium. Delivery mode does not appear to significantly impact the risk of aspiration.

IV. MANAGEMENT OF INFANTS DELIVERED THROUGH MECONIUM-STAINED FLUID. Oropharyngeal and nasopharyngeal suctioning on the perineum and routine tracheal intubation and aspiration of meconium in vigorous infants are not effective in preventing MAS. Although intubation and endotracheal suctioning for meconium in nonvigorous infants was previously recommended, evidence to support this intervention in improving respiratory and neurodevelopmental outcomes is insufficient, and this procedure is no longer recommended. According to 2015 Neonatal Resuscitation Guidelines, emphasis should be placed on appropriate interventions to support ventilation and oxygenation as needed, which may include intubation and suction if the airway is obstructed (see Chapter 4).

If an infant does not improve with intubation and positive pressure ventilation, the trachea may be obstructed by thick secretions, including meconium. The trachea should be suctioned using a suction catheter inserted through the endotracheal tube or directly suctioned through the tube using a meconium aspirator attached to a suction source. The level of suction should be a pressure of 80 to 100 mm Hg.

V. MANAGEMENT OF MECONIUM ASPIRATION SYNDROME

A. Observation. Infants born through MSAF are at risk for meconium aspiration pneumonia and should be observed closely for respiratory distress.

1. A chest radiograph may help determine those infants who are most likely to develop respiratory distress, although a significant number of asymptomatic infants will have an abnormal-appearing chest film. The classic roentgenographic findings are diffuse, asymmetric patchy infiltrates, areas of consolidation, often worse on the right, and hyperinflation.

2. Monitoring of oxygen saturation during this period aids assessment of the severity of the infant's condition and avoids hypoxemia.

B. Care for neonate with meconium aspiration syndrome

1. The infant should be maintained in a neutral thermal environment, and tactile stimulation should be minimized.

2. Blood glucose and calcium levels should be assessed and corrected if necessary. Severely depressed infants may have severe metabolic acidosis that may need to be corrected.

3. Infants may also require specific therapy for hypotension and poor cardiac output, including cardiotonic medications such as dopamine.

4. Circulatory support with normal saline or packed red blood cells should be provided in patients with marginal oxygenation. In infants with substantial oxygen and ventilator requirements, we usually maintain a hemoglobin concentration above 15 g (hematocrit above 40%).

5. Renal function should be continuously monitored (see Chapter 28).

6. We avoid chest physiotherapy because of the potential adverse effect of exacerbating PPHN.

7. Airway and oral suctioning may be required to facilitate airway clearance, but potential benefits must be balanced against the risk of hypoxic episodes and subsequent worsening of PPHN.

C. Oxygen therapy. Management of hypoxemia should be accomplished by increasing the inspired oxygen concentration and by monitoring blood gases and pH. An indwelling arterial catheter is usually required for blood sampling. It is crucial to provide sufficient oxygen because repeated hypoxic insults may result in ongoing pulmonary vasoconstriction and contribute to the development of PPHN.

D. Assisted ventilation

1. **CPAP.** If FiO_2 requirements exceed 0.40, a trial of CPAP may be considered. CPAP is often helpful, and the appropriate pressures must be

individualized for each infant. However, CPAP may sometimes aggravate air trapping and should be instituted with caution if hyperinflation is apparent clinically or radiographically.

2. Mechanical ventilation. Infants with severe disease may have substantial gas exchange abnormalities. Mechanical ventilation is indicated for excessive carbon dioxide retention ($PaCO_2$ >60 mm Hg) or for persistent hypoxemia (PaO_2 <50 mm Hg).

a. In these infants, higher inspiratory pressures (approximately 30 to 35 cm H_2O) and larger tidal volumes are more often required than in infants with respiratory distress syndrome; the positive end-expiratory pressure (PEEP) selected (usually 4 to 6 cm H_2O) should depend on the individual's response. Adequate expiratory time should be permitted to prevent air trapping behind partly obstructed airways.

b. Useful starting points are an inspiratory time of 0.4 to 0.5 seconds at a rate of 20 to 25 breaths per minute. Some infants may respond better to conventional ventilation at more rapid rates with inspiratory times as short as 0.2 seconds.

c. High-frequency ventilation with jet or oscillatory ventilators may be effective in infants with severe MAS who fail to improve with conventional ventilation, and in those who develop air-leak syndromes. There are no prospective, randomized controlled trials comparing the efficacy of the various ventilator modes in MAS.

3. Extracorporeal membrane oxygenation (ECMO) may be required for infants with refractory respiratory failure.

E. Medications

1. Antibiotics. Differentiating between bacterial pneumonia and meconium aspiration by clinical course and chest x-ray findings may be difficult. Although few infants with MAS have documented infections, the use of broad-spectrum antibiotics (e.g., ampicillin and gentamicin) is usually indicated in infants when an infiltrate is seen on chest radiograph. Blood cultures should be obtained to identify bacterial disease, if present, and to determine length of antibiotic course.

2. Surfactant. Endogenous surfactant activity may be inhibited by meconium and is a secondary cause of surfactant deficiency. Surfactant replacement in MAS improves oxygenation, reduces the need for ECMO, and is recommended by the Committee on Fetus and Newborn of the American Academy of Pediatrics. A 2013 Cochrane review of four human studies of bronchoalveolar lavage for MAS demonstrated promising benefit for lavage with diluted surfactant but recommends additional studies to determine dosing and long-term outcomes.

3. Corticosteroids. We do not routinely recommend the use of corticosteroids in MAS. This approach has been proposed to reduce meconium-induced inflammation and to minimize prostaglandin-mediated pulmonary vasoconstriction. Several small randomized controlled trials demonstrated modest improvements in oxygenation and decreased length of NICU stay. However, these studies did not show a difference in mortality and did not address differences in neurodevelopmental outcomes.

4. Sedatives. The use of sedation and muscle relaxation may be warranted in infants who require mechanical ventilation (see Chapter 36).

5. Antioxidants. The use of antioxidants, in particular *N*-acetylcysteine, to mitigate reactive oxygen species (ROS)-induced lung injury in MAS has been recently investigated in animal models. Human studies are needed to define the efficacy and potential adverse effects in infants with MAS.

F. **Complications**

1. **Air leak.** Pneumothorax or pneumomediastinum occurs in approximately 15% to 33% of patients with MAS. Air leaks occur more frequently with mechanical ventilation, especially in the setting of air trapping. A high index of suspicion for air leak is necessary. Equipment should be available to evacuate a pneumothorax promptly (see Chapter 38).

2. **PPHN** is associated with MAS in approximately one-third of cases and contributes to the mortality associated with this syndrome (see Chapter 36). Depending on the extent of hypoxemia, echocardiography should be performed to ascertain the degree to which the right-to-left shunting is contributing to the infant's overall hypoxemia and to exclude congenital heart disease as the etiology. In severely ill infants with MAS and PPHN, inhaled nitric oxide (iNO) reduces the need for ECMO.

3. **Pulmonary sequelae.** Approximately 5% of survivors require supplemental oxygen at 1 month, and a substantial proportion may have abnormal pulmonary function, including increased functional residual capacity, airway reactivity, and higher incidence of pneumonia.

Suggested Readings

El Shahed AI, Dargaville PA, Ohlsson A, et al. Surfactant for meconium aspiration syndrome in term and late preterm infants. *Cochrane Database Syst Rev* 2014;(12):CD002054.

Hahn S, Choi HJ, Soll R, et al. Lung lavage for meconium aspiration syndrome in newborn infants. *Cochrane Database Syst Rev* 2013;(4):CD003486.

Swarnam K, Soraisham AS, Sivanandan S. Advances in the management of meconium aspiration syndrome. *Int J Pediatr* 2012;2012:359571.

36

Persistent Pulmonary Hypertension of the Newborn

Linda J. Van Marter and Christopher C. McPherson

KEY POINTS

- Higher pulmonary than systemic vascular resistance leads to right-to-left shunting and hypoxemia.
- An echocardiogram is an essential component of evaluation.
- Inhaled nitric oxide is a targeted evidence-based therapy.
- Selective vasopressor use avoids worsening pulmonary vascular resistance.

I. **DEFINITION.** Persistent pulmonary hypertension of the newborn (PPHN) reflects disruption of the normal perinatal fetal to neonatal circulatory transition. The disorder is characterized by sustained elevation in pulmonary vascular resistance (PVR) rather than the decrease in PVR that normally occurs at birth. Survivors of PPHN are at risk for adverse sequelae including chronic pulmonary disease and neurodevelopmental disabilities. Contemporary neonatal intensive care, including ventilator management, treatment with inhaled nitric oxide (iNO), and extracorporeal membrane oxygenation (ECMO), collectively have improved survival among infants with PPHN.

A. **Perinatal circulatory transition.** The normal perinatal circulatory transition is characterized by a rapid fall in PVR accompanying the first breath and a marked increase in systemic vascular resistance (SVR) associated with clamping of the umbilical cord. Circulating biochemical mediators released in response to increased arterial oxygen content and pH and lowered $PaCO_2$ cause constriction of the ductus arteriosus and vasorelaxation of the pulmonary circulation. These physiologic events raise SVR relative to PVR, cause functional closure of the foramen ovale, and signal the normal perinatal transition in pulmonary and systemic circulations. PPHN physiology mimics the fetal circulation in which PVR exceeds SVR and right-to-left hemodynamic shunting occurs through the foramen ovale and/or ductus arteriosus. Because of the similarity to the cardiovascular physiology of fetal life, PPHN also has been called "persistent fetal circulation." Before birth, this circulatory configuration results in systemic delivery of oxygenated blood from the placental circulation; in postnatal life, it causes diminished pulmonary perfusion and systemic hypoxemia.

II. **EPIDEMIOLOGIC ASSOCIATIONS.** PPHN occurs at a rate of 1 to 2 per 1,000 live births and is most common among full-term and postterm infants. Perinatal risk factors reported in association with PPHN include meconium-stained amniotic fluid and maternal conditions such as fever, anemia, and pulmonary disease. Case-control studies of risk factors for PPHN suggest associations between PPHN and a number of antenatal and perinatal factors, including maternal diabetes mellitus, urinary tract infection during pregnancy, selective serotonin reuptake inhibitor (SSRI) consumption during pregnancy, and cesarean section delivery. Male infants and those of black or Hispanic race are also at increased risk for PPHN. Although mechanisms of antenatal pathogenesis remain uncertain, there are a number of additional perinatal and neonatal conditions that have well-established links with PPHN.

A. Severe fetal hypoxemia ("asphyxia") is the most common associated diagnosis. Some speculate that prolonged fetal stress and hypoxemia lead to remodeling and abnormal muscularization of pulmonary arterioles. Acute birth asphyxia also causes release of vasoconstricting humoral factors and suppression of pulmonary vasodilators, thus contributing to pulmonary vasospasm.

B. Pulmonary parenchymal diseases, including surfactant deficiency, pneumonia, and aspiration syndromes, such as meconium aspiration, also are associated with increased risk of PPHN. In most such cases, the pulmonary hypertension is reversible, suggesting a vasospastic contribution; however, concomitant pulmonary vascular remodeling cannot be excluded. The risk of pulmonary hypertension appears to be greater when the fetus is of more advanced gestational age, suggesting that the stage of pulmonary vascular development might play a role in susceptibility to PPHN.

C. Abnormalities of pulmonary development contribute structurally to PPHN, either by pruning of the vascular tree, as occurs in congenital diaphragmatic hernia, Potter syndrome, and other forms of pulmonary parenchymal hypoplasia, or malalignment of pulmonary veins and arteries, as is seen in alveolar capillary dysplasia.

D. Myocardial dysfunction, myocarditis, intrauterine constriction of the ductus arteriosus, and several forms of congenital heart disease, including left- and right-sided obstructive lesions, can lead to pulmonary hypertension.

E. Pneumonia and/or sepsis of bacterial or viral origin can initiate PPHN. Underlying pathophysiologic mechanisms that contribute to pulmonary hypertension in this clinical setting include suppression of endogenous nitric oxide (NO) production, endotoxin-mediated myocardial depression, and pulmonary vasoconstriction associated with release of thromboxanes.

F. Although familial recurrence of PPHN is uncommon, genetic predisposition might play a role in PPHN risk. Infants with PPHN have low plasma levels of arginine and NO metabolites and also exhibit diminished endothelial nitric oxide synthase (eNOS) expression. Polymorphisms associated in case reports of PPHN involve several genes, including ABCA3, TMEM70 (mitochondrial), CRHR1, ACE, and SPINK5 (Netherton syndrome). Furthermore, PPHN associated with alveolar capillary dysplasia has been linked with mutation of FOXF1.

III. PATHOLOGY AND PATHOPHYSIOLOGY

A. **Pulmonary vascular remodeling** is pathognomonic of idiopathic PPHN and has been reported among a series of infants with fatal PPHN. Abnormal muscularization of the normally nonmuscular intra-acinar arteries, with increased medial thickness of the larger muscular arteries, results in a decreased cross-sectional area of the pulmonary vascular bed and elevated PVR. Mechanisms leading to the vascular remodeling of PPHN are under investigation. One possible stimulus to pulmonary vascular remodeling is fetal hypoxemia. Humoral growth factors released by hypoxia-damaged endothelial cells promote vasoconstriction and overgrowth of the pulmonary vascular muscular media. Laboratory and limited clinical data suggest that vascular changes might also occur following fetal exposure to nonsteroidal anti-inflammatory agents that cause constriction of the fetal ductus arteriosus and associated fetal pulmonary overcirculation.

B. **Pulmonary hypoplasia** affects both alveolar and pulmonary arteriolar development. It may be seen as an isolated anomaly or with congenital diaphragmatic hernia, oligohydramnios syndrome, renal agenesis (i.e., Potter syndrome), or remodeling or vasoconstriction of impaired fetal breathing.

C. **Reversible pulmonary vasospasm** is the likely pathophysiologic mechanism among infants with nonfatal PPHN. The underlying disease process, the associated conditions, and the developmental stage of the host each appear to modulate the pathophysiologic response. Hypoxia induces profound pulmonary vasoconstriction, and this response is exaggerated by acidemia. Neural and humoral vasoactive substances each might contribute to the pathogenesis of PPHN, the response to hypoxemia, or both. These include factors associated with platelet activation and production of arachidonic acid metabolites. Suppression of endogenous NO, prostacyclin, or bradykinin production and release of thromboxanes (A_2 and its metabolite, B_2), and leukotrienes (C_4 and D_4), appear to mediate the increased PVR seen with sepsis and hypoxemia.

D. **Myocardial dysfunction with elevated pulmonary vascular resistance**

1. **Right ventricular (RV) dysfunction** can be caused by intrauterine constriction of the ductus arteriosus, which results in altered fetal hemodynamics, postnatal pulmonary hypertension, RV failure, and an atrial right-to-left shunt. Furthermore, RV failure resulting in altered diastolic compliance causes right-to-left atrial shunting, even in the absence of elevated PVR.

2. **Left ventricular (LV) dysfunction** causes pulmonary venous hypertension and secondary pulmonary arterial hypertension, often to suprasystemic levels, contributing to right-to-left hemodynamic shunting through the ductus arteriosus. Treating this form of pulmonary hypertension requires an approach that improves LV function rather than simply lowering PVR.

E. **Mechanical factors** that influence PVR include cardiac output and blood viscosity. Low cardiac output recruits fewer pulmonary arteriolar channels and raises PVR by this mechanism as well as by its primary effect of lowering mixed venous oxygen content. Hyperviscosity, associated with polycythemia, reduces pulmonary microvasculature perfusion.

IV. DIAGNOSIS. PPHN should be routinely considered in evaluating the cyanotic newborn.

A. Among cases of suspected PPHN, the most common **alternative diagnoses** are congenital heart disease, sepsis, and severe pulmonary parenchymal disease.

B. The infant with PPHN appears distressed and has a **physical examination** that is most remarkable for evidence of cyanosis. In some infants, the extent of cyanosis might be appreciably different between regions perfused by pre- and postductal vasculature. The cardiac examination is notable for a prominent precordial impulse, a single or narrowly split and accentuated second heart sound, and sometimes, a systolic murmur consistent with tricuspid regurgitation.

C. A **gradient of 10% or more in oxygenation saturation** between simultaneous preductal (right upper extremity) and postductal (lower extremity) arterial blood gas (ABG) values or transcutaneous oxygen saturation (SaO_2) measurements documents the presence of a ductus arteriosus right-to-left hemodynamic shunt and, in the absence of structural heart disease, suggests PPHN. Because a subset of infants with PPHN has closure of the ductus arteriosus and their hemodynamic shunting occurs only at the foramen ovale, the absence of differential cyanosis or SaO_2 does not exclude PPHN.

D. The **chest radiograph** usually appears normal or shows associated pulmonary parenchymal disease. The cardiothymic silhouette is normal, and pulmonary blood flow is normal or diminished.

E. The **electrocardiogram (ECG)** most commonly shows RV predominance that is within the range considered normal for age. Less commonly, the ECG might reveal signs of myocardial ischemia or infarction.

F. An **echocardiographic study** should be performed in all infants with suspected PPHN to document hemodynamic shunting, evaluate ventricular function, and exclude congenital heart disease. Color Doppler examination is useful to assess the presence of intracardiac or ductal hemodynamic shunting. Additional echocardiographic markers, such as tricuspid valve regurgitation or a ventricular septum that is flattened or bowed to the left, suggest pulmonary hypertension. Pulmonary artery pressure can be estimated using continuous-wave Doppler sampling of the velocity of the tricuspid regurgitation jet, if present.

G. **Other diagnostic considerations.** A number of disorders, some of which are associated with secondary pulmonary hypertension, may be misdiagnosed as PPHN. Therefore, an important aspect of the evaluation of the infant with presumed PPHN is to rule out competing conditions, including the following:

1. Structural cardiovascular abnormalities associated with right-to-left ductal or atrial shunting include the following:
   a. Obstruction to pulmonary venous return: infradiaphragmatic total anomalous pulmonary venous return, hypoplastic left heart, cor triatriatum, congenital mitral stenosis
   b. Myopathic LV disease: endocardial fibroelastosis, Pompe disease
   c. Obstruction to LV outflow: critical aortic stenosis, supravalvar aortic stenosis, interrupted aortic arch, coarctation of the aorta

d. Obligatory left-to-right shunt: endocardial cushion defect, arteriovenous malformation, hemitruncus, coronary arteriovenous fistula
e. Miscellaneous disorders: Ebstein anomaly, transposition of the great arteries

2. Primary LV or RV dysfunction associated with right-to-left hemodynamic shunting. LV dysfunction, due to ischemia or obstruction caused by myopathic LV disease or obstruction to LV outflow, might present with a right-to-left ductus arteriosus shunt. RV dysfunction may be associated with right-to-left atrial shunting as a result of decreased diastolic compliance and elevated end-diastolic pressure. These diagnoses must be differentiated from idiopathic PPHN caused by pulmonary vascular remodeling or vasoconstriction.

H. Signs favoring cyanotic congenital cardiac disease over PPHN include cardiomegaly, grade 3+ murmur, weak pulses, active precordium, pulse differential between upper and lower extremities, pulmonary edema, and persistent pre- and postductal arterial oxygen tension (PaO_2) ≤ 40 mm Hg.

V. MANAGEMENT.

The infant with PPHN constitutes a medical emergency in which immediate appropriate intervention is critical to reverse hypoxemia, improve pulmonary and systemic perfusion, and preserve end-organ function. Adequate respiratory support providing normoxemia and neutral to slightly alkalotic acid–base balance facilitates the normal perinatal circulatory transition. Once stability is achieved, cardiorespiratory support should be tapered conservatively with careful attention to the infant's tolerance of each step in reducing support.

A. Supplemental oxygen. Hypoxia is a powerful pulmonary vasoconstrictor. Therefore, in the infant with suspected or documented PPHN, pre- and postductal SaO_2 should be continuously monitored. The use of supplemental oxygen to achieve normoxia is the most important therapy used to reduce abnormally elevated PVR. In the presence of hypoxemia, sufficient supplemental oxygen should be administered to any late preterm, near-term, or full-term newborn to maintain adequate oxygenation and minimize end-organ underperfusion and lactic acidemia. Laboratory data suggest that excessive oxygen exposure releases free radicals that worsen pulmonary hypertension; therefore, debate exists regarding the optimal set-point for SaO_2 among babies with PPHN. Currently, we aim to maintain postductal SaO_2 >93% to ensure adequate tissue oxygenation and avoid hypoxia-induced pulmonary vasoconstriction and <98% to modulate exposure to high inspired oxygen concentration (FiO_2) that might contribute to complications attributable to oxygen free radicals. Arterial access is indicated for blood gas and blood pressure monitoring.

B. Intubation and mechanical ventilation. Mechanical respiratory support is instituted when hypoxemia persists despite maximal administration of supplemental oxygen and/or respiratory failure is demonstrated by marked hypercapnia and acidemia. Specific approaches to respiratory support and mechanical ventilation vary among medical centers. Our approach maintains physiologic PaO_2 and $PaCO_2$ values but avoids hyperoxia and hyperventilation. Because infants with PPHN demonstrate marked lability, a conservative approach to tapering support is indicated until stability is achieved for 12 to 24 hours. Suggested target goals are SaO_2 94% to 97%, $PaCO_2$ 40 to 50 mm Hg, and pH 7.30 to 7.40.

1. Both the nature of the underlying pulmonary parenchymal abnormality, if any, and the infant's clinical lability or stability are important factors to consider when choosing a specific respiratory management strategy.

   a. In the absence of pulmonary alveolar disease, high intrathoracic pressure impedes cardiac output and elevates PVR. The optimal strategy for this group of infants involves mechanical ventilation with rapid, low-pressure, and short inspiratory time in an effort to minimize elevated intrathoracic pressure and modulate effects of ventilation on pulmonary venous return and cardiac output.

   b. When PPHN complicates parenchymal pulmonary disease, ventilator strategies should optimize treatment of the infant's primary pulmonary disease. High-frequency oscillatory ventilation (HFOV) has proven to be more effective than conventional mechanical ventilation in delivering iNO to infants whose PPHN is complicated by significant pulmonary parenchymal disease. High-frequency jet ventilation (HFJV) is especially useful for meconium aspiration pneumonitis and air leak.

   c. Surfactant has been shown to be a useful adjunctive therapy in cases of primary or secondary (e.g., meconium induced) surfactant deficiency.

C. **iNO.** NO is a naturally occurring substance produced by endothelial cells. Whether produced by pulmonary endothelium or delivered through the ventilator circuit, NO diffuses into smooth muscle cells, increases intracellular cyclic guanosine monophosphate (cGMP), relaxes the vascular smooth muscle, and causes pulmonary vasodilation. In the circulation, NO is bound by hemoglobin and biologically inactivated and, therefore, when delivered by inhalation, it causes little or no systemic vasodilation or hypotension. iNO administered by conventional or high-frequency ventilation in doses of 1 to 20 parts per million (ppm) causes pulmonary but not systemic vasodilation and, thus, selectively decreases PVR. In a systematic review conducted by the Cochrane Collaboration, iNO was deemed useful in reducing the need for ECMO among term infants with severe respiratory failure. A potential complication of iNO treatment is rebound hypoxemia that occurs when iNO is discontinued abruptly. For this reason, iNO should be tapered very gradually and not discontinued until adequate oxygenation can be maintained at an iNO dose of 1 ppm with an oxygen concentration of <50% to 60%. Methemoglobinemia is another potential toxicity of iNO treatment that is rare at doses of 20 ppm and below. At our center, we check methemoglobin (metHb) level at 24 hours of therapy and then subsequently as clinically indicated. Because not all infants with PPHN respond to iNO and some may deteriorate rapidly, we recommend treatment of critically ill infants with PPHN at a center in which both iNO and ECMO are readily accessible.

1. The usual starting dose of iNO is 20 ppm, and it is delivered via the ventilator circuit. As the baby improves and FiO_2 is <50% to 60%, iNO is tapered gradually at intervals no more frequent than every 4 hours: 20 to 15, 15 to 10, 10 to 5, 5 to 2, 2 to 1, and then off. The infant's

oxygen saturation in response to each step down is observed before further weaning and/or discontinuing the medication.

2. iNO is most effective when administered after adequate alveolar recruitment. This can be accomplished among infants with PPHN with diffuse pulmonary disease by the concomitant use of HFOV and/or surfactant treatment.

D. ECMO. In the absence of pulmonary hypoplasia, ECMO is lifesaving therapy for approximately 75% to 85% of infants with PPHN who fail conventional management and/or iNO treatment (see ECMO; Chapter 39). Among term or near-term infants meeting ECMO criteria (alveolar-arterial oxygen difference [AaDo$_2$] >600 or oxygenation index [OI] >30 on two ABGs ≥30 minutes apart), both iNO and HFOV appear to reduce the need for ECMO treatment. Therefore, when the infant's clinical status permits, a brief trial of HFOV and/or iNO is generally instituted before commencing ECMO.

E. Sedation and analgesia. Because catecholamine release activates pulmonary α-adrenergic receptors, thereby potentially raising PVR, an opioid analgesic that minimizes pain, such as fentanyl (1 to 4 μg/kg/hour infusion), is a useful adjunct therapy. Morphine sulfate (0.05 to 0.1 mg/kg/hour infusion) is an alternative analgesic that is best used when the infant is not hypotensive. Midazolam (0.06 mg/kg/hour infusion) may also be useful to provide adjunctive sedation in the absence of systemic hypotension. Infants with PPHN rarely require neuromuscular blockade to synchronize the infant's breathing with mechanical ventilation.

F. Hemodynamic support (see Chapter 40). Optimal cardiac output is necessary to maximize tissue oxygenation and mixed venous oxygen content. A limitation of current neonatal practice is the deficit of universally available technologies to assess cardiac output and end-organ perfusion. Although noninvasive means of assessing cardiac output are under development, at present, these are not widely available. In the absence of direct measures of cardiac output, hemodynamic support of infants with PPHN generally is guided by the systemic blood pressure needed to override the elevated PVR and reduce or eliminate the right-to-left hemodynamic shunt. End-organ perfusion is assessed indirectly via acid–base balance (i.e., presence or absence of lactic acidosis). Because many infants with PPHN experience PVR that is at or near-normal systemic blood pressure, we usually set initial treatment goals of gradually raising systemic blood pressure to levels of 50 to 70 mm Hg (systolic) and 45 to 55 mm Hg (mean) and assessing the hemodynamic shunt at each interval increase. As the infant improves and PVR falls, he or she will tolerate lower blood pressures without exhibiting a hemodynamic shunt; thus, ongoing reassessment of hemodynamic status and related revision of the treatment plan are essential components of the management of the infant with PPHN.

1. Volume expansion. Intravascular volume support can be an important adjunctive therapy for infants with PPHN accompanied by pathophysiologic conditions associated with intravascular volume depletion (e.g., hemorrhage, hydrops, capillary leak) or decreased SVR (e.g., septic shock). Normal saline (0.9% NS 10 mL/kg over 20 to 30 minutes) is used most often; in the case of hemorrhage or excessive capillary leak, packed red blood cells are used in addition when anemia is present. In treating infants with evidence of marked capillary leak, we avoid the use of 5% albumin because it also leaks from capillaries and worsens interstitial edema.

2. **Pharmacologic treatment** (Table 36.1). Evidence to guide specific vasopressor and/or inotrope therapy is limited to case reports and series. In the clinical setting of PPHN, inotropic agents, such as dobutamine or milrinone, and vasopressors, such as dopamine, epinephrine, and/or vasopressin, might be useful.

a. Dobutamine, a synthetic catecholamine, has been traditionally utilized for cardiac dysfunction in the setting of PPHN. However, high doses (5 to 10 µg/kg/minute) are associated with tachycardia and increased myocardial oxygen consumption, leading to the investigation of other inotropic agents.

b. Milrinone, a selective phosphodiesterase-3 inhibitor, has both inotropic and vasodilatory properties. Milrinone (0.33 to 1 µg/kg/minute) may be combined with iNO to augment pulmonary vasodilation as well as independently increase RV systolic performance. Systemic vasodilation is the most common dose-limiting adverse effect.

c. Vasopressor therapy in infants with PPHN has traditionally been composed of dopamine and epinephrine. Although these nonselective vasopressors may increase SVR, they have not been shown to improve pulmonary blood flow.

d. Norepinephrine (0.05 to 1 µg/kg/minute) is a potent adrenergic agent that stimulates both α1- and α2-adrenergic receptors, and, as a result, is expected to raise SVR disproportionately to PVR. There are limited data on the use of norepinephrine in neonates. In a single case series, norepinephrine treatment of infants with PPHN was associated with improved oxygenation. Responses to adrenergic stimulation can be highly variable and appear to be influenced by a multiplicity of factors, including disease state and developmental stage. We have rarely used norepinephrine in treating infants in our neonatal intensive care unit (NICU) and, at this time, cannot recommend it as a treatment for PPHN.

e. Any agent with α-adrenergic effects (epinephrine, norepinephrine, dopamine) ≥5 µg/kg/minute has the potential to increase PVR, and infants with PPHN should be evaluated closely for this potential complication and the therapy modified if associated with clinical deterioration.

f. Arginine vasopressin (AVP), a V1 receptor agonist, selectively vasodilates coronary, cerebral, pulmonary, and renal vascular beds while causing vasoconstriction in other systemic vascular beds. One case series suggests that low-dose AVP (0.1 mU/kg/minute to 1.2 mU/kg/minute) might be a potential adjunctive therapy in infants with PPHN refracting to iNO treatment, improving blood pressure, urine output, and OI.

G. **Correction of metabolic abnormalities.** Biochemical abnormalities might contribute to right-to-left shunting by impairing cardiac function. Correction of hypoglycemia and hypocalcemia is important in treating infants with PPHN in order to provide adequate substrates for myocardial function and appropriate responses to inotropic agents (see Chapters 40 and 41).

Table 36.1. Cardiovascular Effects of Vasopressors and Inotropes

| | Dose | Physiologic Goal | | Potential Adverse Cardiovascular Effects |
		Receptors Stimulated	Primary Indication	
Increase cardiac output				
Dobutamine	5–20 µg/kg/minute	β1, β2, α1	Cardiac dysfunction requiring rapid resolution	Tachycardia (++) Systemic vasodilation
Increase cardiac output and decrease pulmonary vascular resistance				
Milrinone	0.33–1 µg/kg/minute	PDE3 inhibition	Cardiac dysfunction Pulmonary hypertension	Systemic hypotension
Increase both cardiac output and systemic vascular resistance				
Dopamine*	0.5–2 µg/kg/minute	Dopaminergic	Poor urine output	Tachycardia (++) Pulmonary vasoconstriction
	2–6 µg/kg/minute	β1, dopaminergic	Cardiac dysfunction	
	>6 µg/kg/minute	α1, β1, dopaminergic	Hypotension	

(continued)

Table 36.1. Cardiovascular Effects of Vasopressors and Inotropes *(Continued)*

	Dose	Physiologic Goal		Potential Adverse Cardiovascular Effects
		Receptors Stimulated	Primary Indication	
Epinephrine*	0.05–0.1 μg/kg/minute	β1, β2	Cardiac dysfunction	Tachycardia (+++) Lactic acidosis Hyperglycemia
	0.1–0.5 μg/kg/minute	α1, α2, β1, β2	Hypotension refractory to dopamine	
Increase systemic vascular resistance				
Vasopressin	0.1–1.2 mU/kg/minute	V1, V2	Hypotension	Hyponatremia

*Dose ranges based on limited evidence and vary between patients.

H. Correction of polycythemia. Hyperviscosity, associated with polycythemia, increases PVR and is associated with release of vasoactive substances through platelet activation. Partial exchange transfusion to reduce the hematocrit to 50% to 55% should be considered in the infant with PPHN whose central hematocrit exceeds 65% (see Chapter 46).

I. Additional pharmacologic agents. Pharmacologic therapy is directed at the simultaneous goals of optimizing cardiac output, enhancing systemic blood pressure, and reducing PVR. Consideration of associated and differential diagnoses and the known or hypothetical pathogenesis of the right-to-left hemodynamic shunt might prove helpful in selecting the best agent or combination of agents for a particular infant.

    1. Sildenafil, a phosphodiesterase-5 inhibitor that increases endogenous NO by inhibiting its metabolism, offers promise for the treatment of PPHN. Small randomized controlled trials performed in circumstances in which iNO and high-frequency ventilation were not available have demonstrated the utility of oral therapy (1 to 2 mg/kg/dose every 6 hours). In an open-label dose-escalation study, oxygenation improved among infants treated with intravenous (IV) sildenafil therapy (0.4 mg/kg over 3 hours followed by 1.6 mg/kg/day), most of whom were receiving iNO. Systemic hypotension was observed in some infants treated with IV sildenafil. Because no randomized controlled trials have been reported to assess potential risks and benefits of IV sildenafil treatment of PPHN, this medication cannot be recommended for routine use in treating PPHN.

    2. Data also are insufficient to support the use of other proposed medical therapies for PPHN, including adenosine, bosentan, magnesium sulfate, calcium channel blockers, inhaled prostacyclin, inhaled ethyl nitrite, and inhaled or IV tolazoline.

VI. POSTNEONATAL OUTCOMES AMONG INFANTS WITH PPHN. The combined availability of iNO and ECMO led to reductions in PPHN-associated mortality from 25% to 50% to 10% to 15%. Survivors of PPHN remain at risk for medical and neurodevelopmental sequelae. Infants who develop PPHN are at approximately 20% risk of rehospitalization within 1 year of discharge and have a 20% to 46% risk of audiologic, neurodevelopmental, or cognitive impairments. We recommend close neurodevelopmental infant follow-up.

Suggested Readings

Giesinger RE, McNamara PJ. Hemodynamic instability in the critically ill neonate: an approach to cardiovascular support based on disease pathophysiology. *Semin Perinatol* 2016;40:174–188.

Jain A, McNamara PJ. Persistent pulmonary hypertension of the newborn: advances in diagnosis and treatment. *Semin Fetal Neonatal Med* 2015;20(4):262–271. doi:10.1016/j.siny.2015.03.001.

Lakshminrusimha S, Mathew B, Leach CL. Pharmacologic strategies in neonatal pulmonary hypertension other than nitric oxide. *Semin Perinatol* 2016;40:160–173.

Mohamed A, Nasef N, Shah V, et al. Vasopressin as a rescue therapy for refractory pulmonary hypertension in neonates: case series. *Pediatr Crit Care Med* 2014;15(2):148–154. doi:10.1097/PCC.0b013e31829f5fce.

37 Pulmonary Hemorrhage

Erin J. Plosa

KEY POINTS

- Pulmonary hemorrhage occurs in 3% to 5% of infants with severe respiratory distress syndrome (RDS).
- Symptomatic patent ductus arteriosus is an important risk factor.
- Treatment is largely supportive.

I. **DEFINITION.** Pulmonary hemorrhage is defined on **pathologic** examination as the presence of erythrocytes in the alveoli and/or lung interstitium. In infants who survive longer than 24 hours, interstitial hemorrhage predominates. Confluent hemorrhage involving at least two lobes of the lung is termed *massive* pulmonary hemorrhage. Although less agreement exists about the **clinical** definition, pulmonary hemorrhage is typically defined as the presence of hemorrhagic fluid in the trachea accompanied by respiratory decompensation that requires increased respiratory support or intubation within 60 minutes of the appearance of fluid.

II. **PATHOPHYSIOLOGY.** The precise mechanisms underlying pulmonary hemorrhage remain uncertain. Pulmonary hemorrhage likely results from heterogeneous conditions that converge in a common physiologic pathway.

   A. Based on studies of lung effluent demonstrating relatively low erythrocyte concentration compared to whole blood, pulmonary hemorrhage is thought to result from hemorrhagic pulmonary edema rather than direct bleeding into the lung.

   B. Acute left ventricular failure, caused by hypoxia and other conditions, may lead to increased pulmonary capillary pressure and injury to the capillary endothelium. This may result in increased transudation and leak into the interstitium and ultimately, pulmonary airspace.

   C. Factors that alter the integrity of the epithelial–endothelial barrier in the alveolus or that change the filtration pressure across these membranes may predispose infants to pulmonary hemorrhage.

   D. Disorders of coagulation may worsen pulmonary hemorrhage but are not thought to initiate the condition.

III. **EPIDEMIOLOGY.** Pulmonary hemorrhage complicates the course of 3% to 5% of preterm infants ventilated for respiratory distress syndrome (RDS).

Approximately 80% of pulmonary hemorrhages in preterm infants occur within 72 hours of birth. In autopsy studies, pulmonary hemorrhage is much more prevalent.

IV. PREDISPOSING FACTORS. Pulmonary hemorrhage has been linked to many predisposing factors and conditions, including RDS, intrauterine growth restriction, intrauterine and intrapartum asphyxia, infection, congenital heart disease, oxygen toxicity, maternal blood aspiration, severe hypothermia, diffuse pulmonary emboli, and urea cycle defects accompanied by hyperammonemia. Risk factors include conditions predisposing the infant to increased left ventricular filling pressures, increased pulmonary blood flow, compromised pulmonary venous drainage, or poor cardiac contractility. The following factors have been linked to pulmonary hemorrhage:

A. **Patent ductus arteriosus (PDA).** The presence of a PDA is a significant risk factor for pulmonary hemorrhage. Increased pulmonary blood flow and compromised ventricular function accompany decreasing pulmonary vascular resistance, leading to pulmonary microvascular injury and hemorrhagic pulmonary edema. In a cohort study of infants born at $<$29 weeks' gestation, early screening echocardiograms for PDA was associated with increased pharmacologic treatment for PDA and decreased rates of pulmonary hemorrhage and in-hospital mortality.

B. **Exogenous surfactant.** Pulmonary hemorrhage may complicate surfactant therapy, likely related to changes in lung compliance, increased left-to-right shunting across a PDA, and increased pulmonary blood flow. However, the overall benefits of surfactant treatment outweigh the risks.

C. **Sepsis.** Overwhelming sepsis appears to increase the risk of pulmonary hemorrhage, likely the result of increased pulmonary capillary permeability, and potentially exacerbated by the associated thrombocytopenia and coagulopathy.

V. CLINICAL PRESENTATION. The clinical diagnosis of pulmonary hemorrhage is made when sudden cardiorespiratory decompensation occurs in the setting of hemorrhagic fluid in the upper respiratory tract. Only a small percentage of pulmonary hemorrhages observed at autopsy are evident clinically. This is most likely due to the difficulty in diagnosing hemorrhage confined to the interstitial space without spread to the airways. In the absence of hemorrhagic secretions, respiratory deterioration is usually attributed to other causes.

VI. EVALUATION

A. **History and physical examination.** A thorough history may help identify predisposing factors such as risks for infection or the presence of a PDA. On physical examination, infants with pulmonary hemorrhage have pink or red frothy fluid in the airway and signs of respiratory decompensation. In the absence of respiratory deterioration, isolated bleeding may result from erosion or ulceration in the upper airway and not represent pulmonary hemorrhage.

B. **Radiographic evaluation.** The clinical diagnosis of pulmonary hemorrhage may be facilitated by the radiographic changes that accompany it. Nonspecific changes on chest radiograph include diffuse fluffy infiltrates or opacification of one or both lungs with air bronchograms.

C. **Laboratory studies.** The laboratory evaluation reflects the cardiopulmonary compromise with associated metabolic or mixed acidosis, a drop in hematocrit, and sometimes evidence of coagulopathy.

VII. **TREATMENT.** Because the underlying pathogenesis remains unclear, treatment remains supportive. The general approach involves clearing the airways of hemorrhagic fluid and restoring adequate ventilation.

A. **Provide positive end-expiratory pressure (PEEP).** The use of elevated PEEP of 6 to 8 cm of H_2O helps to decrease the efflux of interstitial fluid into the alveolar space.

B. **Restore hemodynamic stability.** Correct hemodynamic instability with volume resuscitation, including packed red blood cell replacement, and consider the addition of vasoactive medications as needed.

C. **Correct acidosis.** Restore both adequate ventilation and blood pressure to improve acidosis.

D. **Consider echocardiogram.** An echocardiographic evaluation may assist in the evaluation of ventricular function, need for vasoactive medications, and the possible contribution of a PDA. Consider pharmacologic or surgical closure of the PDA if hemodynamically significant.

E. **Identify other predisposing factors.** Additional potential contributing factors such as sepsis and coagulopathy must be addressed.

F. **Strategy for ventilation.** It is uncertain whether using high-frequency ventilation to provide high mean airway pressure while limiting tidal volume excursions is more effective than conventional ventilation to minimize further interstitial and alveolar fluid accumulation.

G. Limit aggressive airway suctioning.

H. **Role of surfactant therapy.** Surfactant therapy after pulmonary hemorrhage has been considered for continued treatment of primary surfactant deficiency in RDS or for treatment of secondary surfactant deficiency resulting from hemorrhagic airway edema. Following pulmonary hemorrhage, hemoglobin, plasma proteins, and cell membrane lipids present in the airspace may inactivate surfactant. Exogenous surfactant replacement may reverse the inhibition, as demonstrated in the setting of meconium aspiration. Case reports and case series suggest that surfactant may reduce mortality and morbidity from pulmonary hemorrhage. However, a 2012 Cochrane Review failed to identify any randomized controlled trials that address surfactant to treat pulmonary hemorrhage and suggests more studies are needed to recommend a change in clinical practice. Treatment should be decided on a case-by-case basis.

VIII. **PROGNOSIS.** The prognosis is difficult to establish in part due to the difficulty in establishing a clinical diagnosis for this condition. Pulmonary hemorrhage was thought to be uniformly fatal before mechanical ventilation, although this was based on pathologic diagnosis and therefore excluded infants with milder hemorrhages who survived. In a secondary analysis of the trial of indomethacin prophylaxis in preterm infants, prophylactic indomethacin reduced the rate of early serious pulmonary hemorrhage. The risks of death or survival with neurosensory impairment at 18 months of age were increased in infants with serious pulmonary hemorrhage.

Suggested Readings

Alfaleh K, Smyth J, Roberts R, et al. Prevention and 18-month outcomes of serious pulmonary hemorrhage in extremely low birth weight infants: results from the trial of indomethacin prophylaxis in preterms. *Pediatrics* 2008;121:e233–e238.

Aziz A, Ohlsson A. Surfactant for pulmonary haemorrhage in neonates. *Cochrane Database Syst Rev* 2012;(7):CD005254.

Rozé J, Cambonie G, Marchand-Martin L, et al. Association between early screening for patent ductus arteriosus and in-hospital mortality among extremely preterm infants. *JAMA* 2015;313(24):2441–2448.

Pulmonary Air Leak
Melinda Markham

KEY POINTS

- Pneumothorax in neonates is most commonly associated with underlying lung disease requiring mechanical ventilation.
- Signs of pneumothorax can be variable, and consideration of the diagnosis should be given for any infant with significant deterioration in respiratory or cardiovascular status.
- Chest tube or pigtail placement is often required for infants with pneumothorax on positive pressure ventilation.
- Spontaneous pneumothoraces in term infants may be managed conservatively if the infant remains clinically stable.

I. BACKGROUND

A. **Risk factors.** The primary risk factors for air leak are mechanical ventilation and lung disorders. Risk factors common in premature infants include respiratory distress syndrome (RDS), sepsis, and pneumonia. Surfactant therapy for RDS has markedly decreased the incidence of pneumothorax. Risk factors common in term infants are aspiration of meconium, blood, or amniotic fluid; pneumonia; and congenital malformations.

B. **Pathogenesis.** Air leak syndromes arise via a common mechanism. Transpulmonary pressures that exceed the tensile strength of the noncartilagenous terminal airways and alveolar saccules can damage the respiratory epithelium. Loss of epithelial integrity permits air to enter the interstitium, causing **pulmonary interstitial emphysema (PIE)**. Persistent elevation in transpulmonary pressure facilitates the dissection of air toward the visceral pleura and/or the hilum via the peribronchial and perivascular spaces. In rare circumstances, air can enter the pulmonary veins and result in **air embolism**. Rupture of the pleural surface allows the adventitial air to decompress into the pleural space, causing **pneumothorax**. Following a path of least resistance, air can dissect from the hilum and into the mediastinum, resulting in **pneumomediastinum**, or into the pericardium, resulting in **pneumopericardium**. Air in the mediastinum can decompress into the pleural space, the fascial planes of the neck and skin (**subcutaneous emphysema**), or the retroperitoneum. In turn, retroperitoneal air can rupture into the peritoneum (**pneumoperitoneum**) or dissect into the scrotum or labial folds.

1. **Elevations in transpulmonary pressure.** The infant's first breath may cause a negative inspiratory pressure up to 100 cm H_2O. Uneven

ventilation due to atelectasis, surfactant deficiency, pulmonary hemorrhage, or retained fetal lung fluid can increase transpulmonary pressure. In turn, this leads to alveolar overdistention and rupture. Similarly, aspiration of blood, amniotic fluid, or meconium can facilitate alveolar overdistention by a ball-valve mechanism.

2. **In the presence of pulmonary disease, positive pressure ventilation increases the risk of air leak.** The high airway pressure required to achieve adequate oxygenation and ventilation in infants with poor pulmonary compliance (e.g., pulmonary hypoplasia, RDS, inflammation, pulmonary edema) further increases this risk. Excessive transpulmonary pressures can occur when ventilator pressures are not decreased as pulmonary compliance improves. This situation sometimes occurs in infants with RDS after surfactant treatment when compliance increases rapidly. Mechanically ventilated preterm infants who make expiratory efforts against ventilator breaths are also at increased risk for pneumothorax.

3. **Direct trauma to the airways can also cause air leak.** Laryngoscopes, endotracheal tubes, suction catheters, and malpositioned feeding tubes can damage the lining of the airways and provide a portal for air entry.

II. TYPES OF AIR LEAKS

A. **Pneumothorax.** Spontaneous pneumothorax occurs in 0.07% of otherwise healthy-appearing neonates. One in 10 of these infants is symptomatic. The high inspiratory pressures and uneven ventilation that occur in the initial stages of lung inflation may contribute to this phenomenon. Pneumothorax is more common in newborns treated with mechanical ventilation for underlying pulmonary disease.

    Clinical signs of pneumothorax range from insidious changes in vital signs to the complete cardiovascular collapse that often accompanies a tension pneumothorax. As intrathoracic pressure rises, there is decreased lung volume, mediastinal shift, compression of the large intrathoracic veins, and increased pulmonary vascular resistance. The net effect is an increase in central venous pressure, a decrease in preload, and, ultimately, diminished cardiac output. A pneumothorax must be considered in mechanically ventilated infants who develop unexplained alterations in hemodynamics, pulmonary compliance, or oxygenation and ventilation.

1. **Diagnosis**
   a. **Physical examination**
      i. Signs of respiratory distress include tachypnea, grunting, flaring, and retractions.
      ii. Cyanosis
      iii. Chest asymmetry with expansion of the affected side
      iv. Shift in the point of maximum cardiac impulse
      v. Diminished or distant breath sounds on the affected side
      vi. Alterations in vital signs. With smaller collections of extrapulmonary air, compensatory increases may occur in heart rate and blood pressure. As the amount of air in the pleural space increases, central venous pressure rises, and severe hypotension, bradycardia, apnea, hypoxia, and hypercapnia may occur.

b. Arterial blood gases. Changes in arterial blood gas measurements are nonspecific but sometimes reflect a decreased PO_2 and increased PCO_2. The pH may be low as PCO_2 rises or with metabolic acidosis due to poor cardiac output with tension pneumothorax.

c. Chest radiograph. Anteroposterior (AP) views may show a hyperlucent hemithorax, a separation of the visceral from the parietal pleura, flattening of the diaphragm, and mediastinal shift. Smaller collections of intrapleural air can be detected beneath the anterior chest wall by obtaining a cross-table lateral view; however, an AP view is needed to identify the affected side. The lateral decubitus view, with the side of suspected pneumothorax up, may be helpful in detecting a small pneumothorax and may help differentiate skin folds, congenital lobar emphysema, congenital pulmonary airway (cystic adenomatoid) malformations, and surface blebs that occasionally give the appearance of intrapleural air.

d. Transillumination. A high-intensity fiberoptic light source may demonstrate a pneumothorax. This technique is less sensitive in infants with chest wall edema or severe PIE, in extremely small infants with thin chest walls, or in full-term infants with thick chest walls or dark skin.

e. Needle aspiration. In a rapidly deteriorating clinical situation, thoracentesis may confirm the diagnosis and be therapeutic (see section II.A.2.b).

2. **Treatment.** Note that prior to any procedure, a "time out" or "hold point" should be done with the nurse to confirm the correct patient, diagnosis, and laterality (side affected).

a. Conservative therapy. Close observation may be adequate for infants who are asymptomatic. The extrapulmonary air will usually resolve in 24 to 48 hours. Oxygen should only be administered if the baby develops hypoxemia. No evidence supports the use of 100% oxygen to hasten the resolution of pneumothorax. Furthermore, unnecessary oxygen exposure can lead to free radical injury.

b. Needle aspiration. Thoracentesis with a "butterfly" needle or intravenous (IV) catheter with an inner needle can be used to treat a symptomatic pneumothorax. Needle aspiration may be curative in infants not receiving mechanical ventilation and is frequently a temporizing measure in mechanically ventilated infants. In infants with severe hemodynamic compromise, thoracentesis may be a life-saving procedure.

    i. Attach a 23G or 25G butterfly needle or 22G or 24G IV catheter to a 10- to 20-mL syringe fitted with a three-way stopcock.

    ii. Identify the second intercostal space (ICS) in the midclavicular line, and prepare the overlying skin with an antibacterial solution.

    iii. Insert the needle firmly into the ICS in perpendicular fashion and pass it just above the top of the third rib. This will minimize the chance of lacerating an intercostal artery because these vessels are located on the inferior surface of the ribs. As the needle is inserted, have an assistant apply continuous suction with the syringe. A rapid flow of air into the syringe occurs when the needle enters the pleural space. Once the pleural space has been entered, stop advancing the needle. This will reduce the risk of puncturing the lung while the remaining air is evacuated. When the flow of air stops, the needle should be removed and pressure held over the site to minimize blood loss.

iv. A continuous air leak can be aspirated while a chest tube is being inserted (see section II.A.2.c). The "butterfly" needle can be left in place, and if an IV catheter is used, the needle can be removed and the plastic catheter left in place for further aspiration. A short piece of IV extension tubing, for example, a "T" connector, attached to the IV catheter hub will allow flexibility during repeated aspirations. It is important to remember that if the infant is spontaneously breathing, a needle left in place can serve as a conduit for air entry into the pleural space with negative pressure generated during inspiration. To prevent this, the butterfly tubing should be clamped or the stopcock left in the "off" position. This is less of a concern for babies who are on positive pressure ventilation.

c. Chest tube drainage. Chest tube drainage is generally needed to evacuate pneumothoraces that develop in infants receiving positive pressure ventilation. Frequently, these air leaks are continuous and will result in severe hemodynamic compromise if left untreated.

i. Insertion of a chest tube

a) Select a chest tube of the appropriate size; French size 10 (smaller) and 12 (larger) catheters are adequate for most infants.

b) Prepare the chest area with an antiseptic solution. The subcutaneous tissues overlying the fourth to sixth rib at the midaxillary line can be infiltrated with a 1% lidocaine solution for analgesia. Alternatively, we often give narcotic for pain management because local analgesia may obscure landmarks needed to guide the procedure.

c) In the midaxillary line in the sixth ICS, parallel to the rib, make a small incision (0.5 to 1.0 cm) through the skin. Avoid incision of breast tissue by locating the position of the nipple and surrounding tissue. An alternative site is in the anterior-superior portion of the chest wall; however, there is a risk of injury to the internal mammary artery and other regional vessels with this approach.

d) With a small curved hemostat, dissect the subcutaneous tissue overlying the rib. Make a subcutaneous track to the fourth ICS. Care should be taken to avoid the nipple area, the pectoralis muscle, and the axillary artery.

e) Enter the pleural space in the fourth ICS at the intersection of the nipple line and the anterior axillary line with the closed hemostat. Guide the tip over the top of the rib to avoid trauma to the intercostal artery. Push the hemostat through the intercostal muscles and parietal pleura. Listen for a rush of air to indicate pleural penetration, and a "pop" may be felt. Spread the tips to widen the opening and leave the hemostat in place. A trochar in the center of the chest tube can be used, but it increases the risk of lung or vascular injury, so it is not recommended.

f) Grasp the end of the chest tube with the tips of the mosquito hemostat. The chest tube and the hemostat should be in a parallel orientation. Direct the chest tube through the skin incision, into the pleural opening, and between the opened tips. After the pleural space has been entered, direct the chest tube anteriorly and cephalad by rotating the curved points of the hemostat. Release the hemostat and advance the chest tube a few centimeters. Be certain that the side ports of the chest tube are in the pleural space. Direct the chest tube to the location of the pleural air. The anterior pleural space is generally most effective for infants in the supine position.

g) Palpate the chest wall around the entry site to confirm that the chest tube is not in the subcutaneous tissues.

h) Attach the chest tube to a Heimlich valve (for transport) or an underwater drainage system such as a Pleur-evac®. Apply negative pressure (10 to 20 cm H_2O) to the underwater drainage system.

i) Using 3-0 or 4-0 silk, close the skin incision with a purse-string suture around the tube or a single interrupted suture on either side of the tube. Secure the chest tube by wrapping and then tying the skin suture tails around the tube.

j) Cover the insertion site with petrolatum gauze and a small, clear, plastic, adhesive surgical dressing. Avoid extensive taping or large dressings because they interfere with chest examination and may delay the discovery of a displaced chest tube.

k) AP and lateral chest radiographs are obtained to confirm tube position and ascertain drainage of the pleural air.

l) Radiographs may reveal that a chest tube is ineffective in evacuating extrapulmonary air. The most common cause of failure is tube placement in the posterior pleural space or the subcutaneous tissue. Other causes for ineffective drainage are tubes that perforate the lung, diaphragm, or mediastinum. Extrapulmonary air not in the pleural space, such as a pneumomediastinum or a subpleural pulmonary pseudocyst, will not be drained by a chest tube. Complications of chest tube insertion include hemorrhage, lung perforation, cardiac tamponade, and phrenic nerve injury.

ii. Insertion of a pigtail catheter

a) Pigtail catheters may be a less traumatic and faster way to relieve a pneumothorax and may be preferred to chest tube placement in premature infants.

b) Pigtail catheters 8 or 10 French gauge are inserted using a modified Seldinger technique. After locating and sterilizing the insertion site, an 18G needle or an 18G IV catheter is inserted into the pleural space. The guide wire is advanced through the catheter. The needle or the IV catheter is removed, keeping the guide wire in place, and a dilator is advanced over the wire. The pigtail catheter is then inserted in the pleural space over the guide wire. The catheter is advanced until the curve of the catheter is inside the chest.

d. Removal of a chest tube. When the infant's lung disease has improved and the chest tube has not drained air for 24 to 48 hours, discontinue suction and leave the tube under water seal. If radiographic examination shows no reaccumulation of extrapulmonary air in the next 12 to 24 hours, the chest tube should be removed. A narcotic is given for pain control prior to the chest tube removal. To reduce the chance of introducing air into the pleural space, cover the chest wound with a small occlusive dressing while removing the tube. Remove the chest tube during expiration in spontaneously breathing infants and during inspiration in mechanically ventilated infants. A manual mechanical breath for ventilated infants can ensure removing the chest tube during the inspiratory phase.

e. Persistent pneumothorax refractory to routine measures. High-frequency ventilation (HFV) can be used to minimize tidal volume and improve air leaks in mechanically ventilated infants. In patients with severe air leaks, oxygen supplementation is often increased so that mean airway pressure can be minimized. Interventional radiology may be needed to place catheters under ultrasound or fluoroscopic guidance to drain air collections that are inaccessible by standard techniques.

3. Complications

a. Profound ventilatory and circulatory compromise can occur and, if untreated, result in death.

b. Intraventricular hemorrhage may result, possibly secondary to a combination of fluctuating cerebrovascular pressures, impaired venous return, hypercapnia, hypoxia, and acidosis.

c. Inappropriate antidiuretic hormone secretion may occur.

B. PIE. PIE occurs most often in mechanically ventilated, extremely preterm infants with RDS or sepsis. Interstitial air can be localized or can spread to involve significant portions of one or both lungs. Interstitial air can dissect toward the hilum and the pleural surface via the adventitial connective tissue surrounding the lymphatics and pulmonary vessels. This can compromise lymphatic drainage and pulmonary blood flow. PIE alters pulmonary mechanics by decreasing compliance, increasing residual volume and dead space, and enhancing ventilation–perfusion mismatch. Rupture of interstitial air into the pleural space and mediastinum can result in pneumothorax and pneumomediastinum, respectively.

1. Diagnosis

a. PIE frequently develops in the first 48 hours after birth.

b. PIE may be accompanied by hypotension, bradycardia, hypercarbia, hypoxia, and acidosis.

c. PIE has two radiographic patterns: cyst-like and linear. Linear lucencies radiate from the lung hilum. Occasionally, large cyst-like blebs give the appearance of a pneumothorax.

2. Treatment

a. If possible, attempt to decrease mean airway pressure by lowering peak inspiratory pressure, positive end-expiratory pressure (PEEP), and inspiratory time. HFV can be utilized in infants with PIE to avoid large tidal volumes.

b. Unilateral PIE may improve if the infant is positioned with the affected lung dependent.

c. Endotracheal suctioning and manual positive pressure ventilation should be minimized.

d. Severe localized PIE that has failed to improve with conservative management may require collapse of the affected lung by selective bronchial intubation or occlusion or, rarely, surgical resection.

3. Complications. PIE may precede more severe complications such as pneumothorax, pneumopericardium, or an air embolism.

C. Pneumomediastinum. Mediastinal air can develop when pulmonary interstitial air dissects into the mediastinum or when direct trauma occurs to the airways or the posterior pharynx.

1. Diagnosis

a. Physical examination. Heart sounds may be distant.

b. Chest radiograph. Air collections are central and usually elevate or surround the thymus. This results in the characteristic "spinnaker sail" sign. A pneumomediastinum is best seen on a lateral view.

2. Treatment

a. Pneumomediastinum is of little clinical importance, and specific drainage procedures are usually unnecessary.

b. Rarely, cardiorespiratory compromise may develop if the air is under tension and does not decompress into the pleural space, the retroperitoneum, or the soft tissues of the neck. This situation may require mediastinotomy drainage. If the infant is mechanically ventilated, reduce mean airway pressure, if possible.

3. Complications. Pneumomediastinum may be associated with other air leaks.

D. Pneumopericardium. Pneumopericardium is the least common form of air leak in newborns but is a common cause of cardiac tamponade. Asymptomatic pneumopericardium is occasionally detected as an incidental finding on a chest radiograph. Most cases occur in preterm infants with RDS treated with mechanical ventilation, preceded by PIE and pneumomediastinum. The mortality rate for critically ill infants who develop pneumopericardium is high.

1. Diagnosis. Pneumopericardium should be considered in mechanically ventilated newborn infants who develop acute or subacute hemodynamic compromise.

a. Physical examination. Although infants may initially have tachycardia and decreased pulse pressure, hypotension, bradycardia, and cyanosis may ensue rapidly. Auscultation reveals muffled or distant heart sounds. A pericardial knock (Hamman sign) or a characteristic mill wheel–like murmur (bruit de moulin) may be present.

b. Chest radiograph. AP views show air surrounding the heart. Air under the inferior surface of the heart is diagnostic.

c. Transillumination. A high-intensity fiberoptic light source may illuminate the substernal region. Flickering of the light with the heart rate may help differentiate pneumopericardium from pneumomediastinum or a medial pneumothorax.

d. Electrocardiogram (ECG). Decreased voltages, manifest by a shrinking QRS complex, are consistent with pneumopericardium.

2. **Treatment.** Pediatric cardiology, if available, should be consulted when the diagnosis is made.

a. Conservative management. Asymptomatic infants not receiving positive pressure ventilation can be managed expectantly. Vital signs are closely monitored (especially changes in pulse pressure). Frequent chest radiographs are obtained until the pneumopericardium resolves.

b. Needle aspiration. Cardiac tamponade is a life-threatening event that requires immediate pericardiocentesis.

    i. Prepare the subxiphoid area with antiseptic solution.

    ii. Attach a 20G to 22G IV catheter with an inner needle to a short piece of IV extension tubing that, in turn, is connected to a three-way stopcock and a 20-mL syringe.

    iii. In the subxiphoid space, insert the catheter at a 30- to 45-degree angle and toward the infant's left shoulder.

    iv. Have an assistant aspirate with the syringe as the catheter is advanced.

    v. Once air is aspirated, stop advancing the catheter.

    vi. Slide the plastic catheter over the needle and into the pericardial space.

    vii. Remove the needle, reattach the IV tubing to the hub of the plastic catheter, evacuate the remaining air, and withdraw the catheter.

    viii. If air leak persists, prepare for pericardial tube placement.

    ix. If blood is aspirated, immediately withdraw the catheter to avoid lacerating the ventricular wall.

    x. The complications of pericardiocentesis include hemopericardium and laceration of the right ventricle or left anterior descending coronary artery.

c. Continuous pericardial drainage. Pneumopericardium often progresses to cardiac tamponade and may recur. A pericardial tube may be needed for continuous drainage.

3. **Complications.** Ventilated infants who have a pneumopericardium drained by needle aspiration frequently (80%) have a recurrence. Recurrent pneumopericardium can occur days after apparent resolution of the initial event.

E. **Other types of air leaks**

1. **Pneumoperitoneum.** Intraperitoneal air may result from extrapulmonary air that decompresses into the abdominal cavity. Usually, the pneumoperitoneum is of little clinical importance, but it must be differentiated from intraperitoneal air resulting from a perforated viscus. Rarely, pneumoperitoneum can impair diaphragmatic excursion and compromise ventilation. In these cases, continuous drainage may be necessary.

2. **Subcutaneous emphysema.** Subcutaneous air can be detected by palpation of crepitus in the face, neck, or supraclavicular region. Large collections of air in the neck, although usually of no clinical significance, can partially occlude or obstruct the compressible, cartilaginous trachea of the premature infant.

3. **Systemic air embolism.** An air embolism is a rare but usually fatal complication of pulmonary air leak. Air may enter the vasculature either by disruption of the pulmonary venous system or by inadvertent injection through an intravascular catheter. The presence of air bubbles in blood withdrawn from an umbilical artery catheter can be diagnostic.

Suggested Readings

Cates LA. Pigtail catheters used in the treatment of pneumothoraces in the neonate. *Adv Neonatal Care* 2009;9:7–16.

Clark SD, Saker F, Schneeberger MT, et al. Administration of 100% oxygen does not hasten resolution of symptomatic spontaneous pneumothorax in neonates. *J Perinatol* 2014;34:528–531.

Extracorporeal Membrane Oxygenation
Gerhard K. Wolf and John H. Arnold

KEY POINTS

- Indications for neonatal extracorporeal membrane oxygenation (ECMO) are severe respiratory failure and circulatory or cardiac failure that are considered reversible.
- Venovenous ECMO supports oxygenation and ventilation only; venoarterial ECMO supports gas exchange and circulation.
- Common ECMO complications include mechanical problems with the circuit, intracranial hemorrhage, other bleeding, and renal failure.

I. **BACKGROUND.** Extracorporeal membrane oxygenation (ECMO) is the application of a modified cardiopulmonary bypass for neonates in cardiac or respiratory failure not responding to conventional measures or treatments.

ECMO has been offered to 35,000 neonates worldwide to date (Tables 39.1 and 39.2). The use of ECMO for neonatal respiratory failure began to decline in the late 1990s due to improved strategies of lung protective ventilation and has been more constant since 2000. Approximately 40 centers in the United States offer neonatal ECMO.

II. INDICATIONS AND CONTRAINDICATIONS

A. **Respiratory failure.** The indications for neonatal ECMO are (i) reversible respiratory failure and (ii) a predicted mortality with conventional therapy great enough to warrant the risks of ECMO. ECMO is also considered in patients with life-threatening air leaks not manageable with optimal ventilatory support and chest drainage.

1. **Oxygenation index (OI)** is a measure of the severity of respiratory failure and is calculated as follows: $OI = $ mean airway pressure (MAP) $\times$ $FiO_2/PaO_2 \times 100$. It is essential to document OIs from serial blood gases over time because the OI may vary. ECMO indications vary among different centers. Commonly used criteria include two OIs of >40 within 1 hour, one OI of 60 on high-frequency ventilation, or one OI of 40 combined with cardiovascular instability. For infants hospitalized where ECMO is not available, an OI of 20 should prompt early outreach to an ECMO center for potential transfer because prolonged ventilation at high ventilator settings may worsen ventilator-induced

Table 39.1. Overall Outcomes for Neonatal Extracorporeal membrane oxygenation (ECMO) Worldwide by Indication, Extracorporeal Life Support Organization (ELSO) 2015

Neonatal	Total Patients	Survived ECLS	Survival to Discharge or Transfer
Respiratory	28,217	23,791 (84%)	20,978 (74%)
Cardiac	6,046	3,750 (62%)	2,497 (41%)
ECMO-CPR	1,188	766 (64%)	489 (41%)

Total Patients refers to all neonatal ECMO therapies reported in the ELSO registry. ECMO-CPR refers to neonatal patients placed emergently on ECMO during cardiopulmonary resuscitation. ECLS, extracorporeal life support; CPR, cardiopulmonary resuscitation.
Source: Published by the Extracorporeal Life Support Organization. *Extracorporeal Life Support Organization: ECMO and ECLS*. Ann Arbor, MI: Extracorporeal Life Support Organization; 2015.

lung injury and worsen the overall outcome. On a practical level, once ventilator support is maximally escalated, transport to an ECMO center may become impossible.

2. Total anomalous pulmonary venous return (TAPVR) may mimic neonatal respiratory distress syndrome (RDS), resulting from lung

Table 39.2. Neonatal Respiratory Runs by Diagnosis, Extracorporeal Life Support Organization (ELSO) 2015

Neonatal Categories	Total Runs	Percentage Survived
MAS	8,815	94
CDH	7,419	51
PPHN/PFC	4,915	77
Sepsis	2,873	73
RDS	1,553	84
Pneumonia	381	58
Air leak syndrome	133	74
Other	2,591	61

MAS, meconium aspiration syndrome; CDH, congenital diaphragmatic hernia; PPHN, persistent pulmonary hypertension of the newborn; PFC, persistent fetal circulation; RDS, respiratory distress syndrome.

congestion in the setting of inadequate drainage of the pulmonary veins in the left atrium. In any neonate with respiratory failure, hypoxia, and bilateral opacities on chest radiograph, TAPVR should be excluded prior to initiating ECMO support. Once venoarterial ECMO support is initiated, pulmonary blood flow is reduced and the diagnosis of TAPVR may be difficult to make using echocardiography alone; these patients may require cardiac catheterization on ECMO to demonstrate presence or absence of pulmonary veins entering the left atrium.

B. **Cardiac failure.** ECMO provides biventricular support for neonates with cardiac failure. General indications are low cardiac output (CO) syndrome despite maximal hemodynamic support or cardiac arrest with a potentially reversible underlying condition. ECMO for congenital heart defects can be offered as a bridge to definitive treatment until the newborn's condition has stabilized. Other cardiac indications are failure to wean from cardiopulmonary bypass, cardiomyopathy, and pulmonary hypertension.

C. **Rapid-response ECMO (ECMO-cardiopulmonary resuscitation [E-CPR]).** In the setting of a witnessed cardiorespiratory arrest, ECMO can be offered in centers with a rapid response team. Response times from the arrest to cannulation are ideally 15 to 30 minutes. A readily "clear-primed circuit" (an ECMO circuit primed with normal saline rather than with blood products) and an ECMO team must be available 24 hours per day in order to offer E-CPR. Effective cardiopulmonary resuscitation (CPR) before cannulation is essential for a favorable outcome during rapid-response ECMO.

D. *Ex utero* **intrapartum treatment (EXIT) to ECMO procedure.** The vessels are cannulated during a cesarean section while the newborn remains on placental support. Indications include severe congenital diaphragmatic hernia (CDH), lung tumors, and airway obstructing lesions such as large neck masses and mediastinal tumors.

E. **Contraindications.** ECMO should only be offered for reversible conditions. Contraindications are considered to be lethal chromosomal disorder (including trisomies 13 and 18 but not 21), irreversible brain damage, and grade 3 or greater intraventricular hemorrhage (IVH) or intraparenchymal hemorrhage. Relative contraindications include weight <1,500 g due to cannula size limitations (except for thoracic cannulations), gestational age <34 weeks due to increased risk of IVH, severe coagulopathy, progressive chronic lung disease, and continuous CPR for more than an hour before ECMO support.

III. PHYSIOLOGY

A. **Flow.** Venous drainage is passive from the patient to the ECMO circuit if nonocclusive roller pumps are used and active if centrifugal pumps are used. The cessation of venous drainage (due to cannula malposition, intravascular hypovolemia, cardiac tamponade, and pneumothorax) causes slowing of the pump speed because negative pressure could introduce air into the circuit. Flow is determined by venous return and the ECMO pump.

B. **Venoarterial (VA) ECMO.** VA ECMO supports the cardiac and the respiratory system and is indicated for primary cardiac failure or respiratory failure combined with secondary cardiac failure. In VA ECMO, the blood is drained from a single vein (internal jugular vein, femoral vein) and returned into the arterial system (internal carotid artery). Venovenous-arterial ECMO indicates drainage from two different veins and return to the arterial side. The patient's total CO is the sum of the native CO and the pump flow generated by the circuit: $CO_{total} = CO_{native} + CO_{circuit}$.

C. **Venovenous (VV) ECMO.** VV ECMO supports only the respiratory system and is indicated for isolated respiratory failure. VV ECMO refers to drainage from a single vein, VVV ECMO to drainage from two different veins. VV ECMO can also be considered in respiratory failure with hemodynamic instability, when hypotension and cardiovascular instability are thought to be caused by hypoxemia alone, because VV ECMO usually leads to rapid reversal of hypoxia and acidosis. VV ECMO spares accessing the carotid artery. Venovenous dual lumen (VVDL) refers to ECMO using specially designed double-lumen cannulas, providing drainage as well as return through different lumens of the same cannula. Some of the blood is immediately recirculated into the ECMO circuit. The rest of the oxygenated blood goes to the right side of the heart, into the pulmonary vascular bed, into the left side of the heart, and into the systemic circulation. As a requirement for VV ECMO, the internal jugular vein has to be large enough for a 14 French double-lumen cannula. Converting to VA ECMO is considered in the presence of additional hypotension, cardiac failure, or metabolic acidosis. Technical difficulties related to large recirculation in the venous cannula can also lead to the need to convert to VA ECMO. In our institution, the carotid artery is routinely identified at the time of VV cannulation. For conversion to VA ECMO, the venous cannula is left in place and an additional arterial cannula is inserted into the internal carotid artery.

D. **Oxygen delivery.** Oxygen delivery is the product of CO and arterial oxygen content. During ECMO, many factors contribute to oxygen delivery. Arterial oxygen content is determined by the gas exchange in the membrane oxygenator and the gas exchange from the neonate's lung. CO is only altered during VA ECMO and is determined by the ECMO flow and the infant's native CO.

E. **Carbon dioxide (CO_2) removal.** CO_2 removal is achieved by the membrane of the ECMO circuit and the patient's lung. The amount of CO_2 removed is dependent on the $PaCO_2$ of blood circulating through the membrane, the surface area of the membrane, and the gas flow through the membrane lung ("sweep gas flow"). As physiologic pulmonary function and tidal volume improve, the $PaCO_2$ decreases further and ECMO settings have to be adjusted. CO_2 removal is extremely efficient during ECMO, to the point that additional CO_2 has to be added into the circuit in order to prevent hypocarbia and respiratory alkalosis.

F. **Cerebral perfusion.** Cerebral perfusion during shock is rapidly restored after initiation of VA ECMO. In contrast, cerebral venous drainage and arterial perfusion to the brain are impaired by large bore cannulas during ECMO. Collateral circulation to the brain during VA ECMO in neonates is maintained through the circle of Willis. The carotid artery is frequently ligated after decannulation from ECMO, although reconstruction of the carotid artery has been successfully performed. Impairments to arterial reconstructions are an intimal flap, arterial thrombosis, infections, or excessive tension on attempt of reconstruction. Reconstructing the carotid artery may not have an impact on neurologic outcome, and arterial vascular stenosis postrepair may be a significant problem.

G. **Renal perfusion.** During VA ECMO, the arterial pulse-pressure wave may become dampened because the roller pump contributes significantly to the patient's CO. Animal models have suggested that renal perfusion is not different during VA as compared to VV ECMO. Unclamping the bridge during VA ECMO directs flow away from the patient and may be associated with a decrease in blood pressure and renal perfusion.

IV. MANAGEMENT

A. **Pre-ECMO.** In preparation for cannulation, the following should be available: central venous access to the patient, postductal arterial catheter, cross-matched blood in the blood bank, complete blood count, coagulation profile, head ultrasonographic examination. An echocardiogram should be done before ECMO in order to rule out structural cardiac abnormalities. During VA ECMO, it may be difficult to quantify pulmonary hypertension or identify certain congenital lesions such as total anomalous venous return because the right atrium is decompressed and blood flow through the lung is decreased. Platelets should be transfused for a platelet count <100,000/mL.

B. **Membrane.** The appropriate membrane for a neonate is a 0.8 m^2 or 1.5 m^2 silicone membrane oxygenator. The resulting total volume of a neonatal ECMO circuit is 600 mL.

C. **Saline priming.** Patients who are placed on ECMO emergently can be started on a saline-primed circuit. Instead of blood products, the circuit is primed with normal saline. In centers with rapid-response ECMO, a saline-primed, sterile circuit is always available, minimizing the time to initiate ECMO therapy. The neonate's own blood volume is initially diluted with the normal saline from the ECMO circuit. This causes a drop in hematocrit and a transient decrease in oxygen-carrying capacity. The hematocrit is later restored by using ultrafiltration and transfusing packed red blood cells (PRBCs).

D. **Blood priming.** Patients who are placed on ECMO nonemergently are started on a blood-primed circuit. Orders for the initial prime of a neonatal circuit are as follows: 500 mL of PRBC (cytomegalovirus [CMV] negative, <7 days old), 200 mL of fresh frozen plasma (FFP), 2 units of cryoprecipitate, and 2 units of platelets (not concentrated). Heparin and Tris-hydroxymethyl-aminomethane (THAM, also "Tris") buffer and calcium gluconate are added to the circuit. Once the circuit is fully primed with blood, the following laboratory measurements (with target ranges in parenthesis) are obtained from the ECMO circuit prior to connecting the patient: pH (7.35 to 7.45), PCO_2 (35 to 45 mm Hg), PO_2 (>300 mm Hg), HCO_3 (22 to 24 mEq/L), Na^+ (>125 mEq/L), K^+ (<8 mEq/L), ionized Ca^{++} (>0.8 mEq/L). This blood sample should be clearly marked indicating that the results are from the ECMO circuit prior to connection with the patient. Hyperkalemia of the circuit is treated with calcium and bicarbonate.

E. **Cannulation.** The ECMO cannulation is performed by cardiac or pediatric surgeons at the bedside, in the cardiac catheterization laboratory, or in the operating room. A surgical cutdown approach is preferred over transcutaneous cannulation. The infant is anesthetized and paralyzed with fentanyl, midazolam, and pancuronium. Heparin 30 units/kg is administered 3 minutes before cannulation. The following cannula sizes can be used: 8 to 14 French for the venous side, 8 to 10 French for the arterial side, or a 12 to 16 French VV double-lumen cannula. The vein is cannulated first. The catheter is introduced approximately 6.5 cm to the right atrium and sutured in place. In VA ECMO, the artery is cannulated in a similar manner. In full-term newborns, the arterial cannula is introduced 3.5 cm into the aortic arch. Once the patient is on ECMO, 2 units of platelets and 2 units of cryoprecipitate are administered. On initiation of ECMO, vasopressors can be rapidly weaned. The neonate may become markedly hypertensive on initiation of ECMO therapy. As hypertension in the setting of pre-ECMO acidosis and anticoagulation during ECMO is a significant risk factor for intracranial hemorrhage, any significant hypertension must be anticipated and treated without delay. Hydralazine 0.1 to 0.4 mg/kg/dose can be administered to treat hypertension.

F. **ECMO therapy.** ECMO pump flow rate is generally 100 to 120 mL/kg/minute in newborns. Sweep gas flow rate is 1.0 to 2.5 L/minute for a 0.8 m^2 and 1.0 to 4.5 L/minute for 1.5 m^2 membrane. A safety check is conducted every 4 hours. This safety check includes searching for blood clots and circuit inspection for leaks. Normothermia is maintained and temperature is regulated by adjustments in the heat exchanger water temperature. We use the following schedule for laboratory studies: (i) activated clotting time hourly; (ii) lactate levels twice daily; (iii) complete blood count, platelets, whole blood electrolytes, ionized calcium, and creatinine twice daily; (iv) antithrombin III (AT III) twice daily and prior to FFP administration and 3 hours post-FFP administration; and (v) liver function tests, alkaline phosphatase, lactate dehydrogenase (LDH), bilirubin, albumin, prealbumin, and total protein every week.

G. **Blood gas monitoring.** Arterial blood gas targets are PaO$_2$ >60 mm Hg and PaCO$_2$ 40 to 45 mm Hg. If PaO$_2$ is <60 mm Hg, the sweep gas to the ECMO membrane can be increased. If the fraction of delivered oxygen (FDO$_2$) is already maximized at 1.0, increasing the ECMO pump flow rate or increasing the patient's hematocrit may be helpful to increase oxygen delivery. On VV ECMO, it may be necessary to increase the ventilator settings to assist with oxygenation and ventilation.

H. **Anticoagulation.** Heparin is used in all patients to prevent clot formation. Antifactor Xa levels are used to monitor heparin infusion and avoid hemorrhagic complications. Anti-Xa levels are kept between 0.35 and 0.7. Heparin infusion is increased if anti-Xa values drop below 0.35 and decreased if anti-Xa values exceed 0.7. AT III levels may decrease over time during ECMO, and decreased AT III levels may result in heparin resistance and clotting of the ECMO circuit. If AT III levels drop below 60%, anti-Xa levels and heparin dosage should be optimized first, followed by replacement of AT III. If heparin-induced thrombocytopenia (HIT) is confirmed, argatroban, a synthetic direct thrombin inhibitor, can be used as an alternative anticoagulant during ECMO.

I. **Blood products.** Prothrombin time (PT) is maintained at <17 seconds. If PT is above 17 seconds, FFP at a dose of 20 mL/kg is administered.

Fibrinogen levels are kept above 100 mg/dL; for levels below 100 mg/dL, 1 to 2 units per 10 kg cryoprecipitate is administered. Platelet count is maintained above 100,000 using platelet transfusion. The hematocrit is kept above 35% to facilitate oxygen delivery.

J. ε-Aminocaproic acid (Amicar) lowers the incidence of hemorrhagic complications associated with ECMO, including intracranial and postoperative hemorrhage. Negative effects are increased clot formation in the circuit. Patients who are considered to be at high risk for bleeding complications are given Amicar. They include infants who (i) are <37 weeks' gestational age, (ii) have sepsis, (iii) have prolonged hypoxia or acidosis (pH 7.1) before ECMO, or (iv) have grade 1 or 2 IVH. A loading dose of Amicar (100 mg/kg) is given followed by a 30 mg/kg/hour infusion. After 72 hours of Amicar, the patient is assessed for further risks of bleeding complications. If these risks still exist, Amicar is continued and the circuit is changed at 120 hours. Otherwise, the Amicar infusion is discontinued. A surgical consult should be obtained in the setting of postoperative hemorrhage or bleeding from surgical sites. Factor VII at 90 μg/kg can be used in the setting of severe bleeding.

K. Antibiotics. We routinely administer broad-spectrum antibiotics to lower the risk of infection while on ECMO therapy. Infections during ECMO occur in about 5% of all ECMO runs.

L. Analgesia and sedation. Patients are sedated with an opioid/benzodiazepine combination. We typically use morphine 0.05 mg/kg/hour and lorazepam 0.05 to 0.1 mg/kg/dose every 4 to 6 hours. Fentanyl can be used during ECMO cannulation but should not be used during ECMO. Fentanyl is absorbed in large quantities by the ECMO membrane, leading to suboptimal analgesia.

M. Fluids and nutrition. Nutrition is administered through the parenteral route. Gastric feeding during ECMO is avoided because it may increase the risk of necrotizing enterocolitis. Lipid administration should not exceed 1 g/kg/day to prevent lipid accumulation and embolism in the circuit. Lipids should be administered directly to the patient and not to the circuit. Dextrose and amino acid solution (parenteral nutrition) can be administered through the circuit.

N. Ultrafiltration. An ultrafilter is placed in line with the ECMO circuit. The goal is to normalize fluid balance in patients who have excessive positive fluid balance. Indications are urine output of <0.5 mL/kg/hour, positive fluid balance >500 mL per 24 hours, and failed diuretic therapy.

O. Head imaging. Head ultrasonographic examinations are performed before ECMO, if possible, and serially during the ECMO run. Electroencephalograms are performed when seizure activity is suspected. An MRI of the brain is considered after the ECMO run is completed.

P. Ventilator strategy. The goal of the ventilator strategy on VA ECMO is to let the lung "rest," yet not to allow total lung collapse. Typical settings are peak inspiratory pressure (PIP) = 25 cm H_2O, positive end-expiratory pressure (PEEP) = 5 cm H_2O, rate = 10, inspiratory time 1 second, and FiO_2 = 0.4. With a patient on VA ECMO for pneumothorax and air leak, apneic oxygenation with $FiO_2 = 1$ should be considered starting at continuous positive airway pressure (CPAP) settings of 12 cm H_2O and decreasing until no further air leaks are present. On VV ECMO, ventilator settings may have to be adjusted to achieve adequate gas exchange because the patient's own lungs contribute to oxygenation and ventilation to a greater degree as compared to VA ECMO.

Endotracheal suctioning is performed every 4 hours. During ECMO, lung function is assessed as follows: (i) as lung function improves, CO_2 removal increases and oxygenation by the lung improves, resulting in better gas exchange. Sweep gases can be adjusted accordingly; (ii) chest radiographs show gradual resolution of pulmonary edema; (iii) as pulmonary edema resolves, lung mechanics improve and expired tidal volumes increase.

Q. **Conditioning and cycling.** "Conditioning" means challenging the patient by reducing the ECMO support to evaluate the gas exchange accomplished by the lungs. Sweep gas flow is reduced; FiO_2 is increased to 1 and the respiratory rate is increased to 25 breaths per minute; the flow of the ECMO pump is weaned to 100 mL/minute in 50-mL increments; and serial arterial blood gases are obtained. If the postductal saturation falls below 95%, the ECMO settings are resumed. "Cycling" means transiently removing the patient from the ECMO circuit. In VA ECMO, the venous and arterial cannulas are clamped, the bridge is opened, and the ECMO blood flow "cycles" from the arterial to the venous side through the bridge, without perfusing the patient. In VV ECMO, the sweep gas flow is interrupted ("capped"), whereas the circuit continues to flow.

R. **Decannulation.** When the patient's lung disease has improved enough to tolerate moderate ventilator settings, we consider decannulation. Our criteria for decannulation are as follows: PIP = 30 cm H_2O; PEEP = 5 cm H_2O; rate = 25 breaths per minute; $FiO_2 = 0.35$; PaO_2 over 60 mm Hg; $PaCO_2 = 40$ to 50 mm Hg; and pH <7.5. When these criteria are used, patients rarely require recannulation. At the time of decannulation from VA ECMO, we attempt to reconstruct the common carotid artery. The jugular vein is routinely ligated. Two units of concentrated platelets are given following decannulation.

Discontinuation of ECMO support is also considered in the following situations: when the disease process becomes irreversible, failure to wean successfully, neurologic events (devastating neurologic examination, significant intracranial hemorrhage), or multiorgan system failure.

V. SPECIAL SITUATIONS DURING EXTRACORPOREAL MEMBRANE OXYGENATION SUPPORT

A. **ECMO-circuit change.** A change of the entire ECMO circuit is considered (i) if premembrane pressures exceed 350 mm Hg with no change in postmembrane pressure, or if the circuit is extensively thrombosed by visual inspection of the tubing; (ii) if CO_2 removal is impaired despite maximum sweep gas flow rate and the circuit is extensively clotted; (iii) if there is a gas-to-blood leak and the circuit is extensively clotted; and (iv) if there is extensive platelet consumption. A new ECMO circuit may help to correct a persistent coagulopathy or platelet consumption. If a circuit needs to be changed, a new circuit is primed, the patient is cycled off ECMO, the old circuit is cut away, and the new circuit is connected, with care being taken to keep air out of the system and to maintain strict sterile barriers.

B. Lung biopsy. Irreversible causes of respiratory failure such as alveolar capillary dysplasia (ACD) or other forms of pulmonary hypoplasia are usually not known prior to ECMO support. If pulmonary function does not improve after a prolonged period (usually 1 to 2 weeks of ECMO support), a lung biopsy can be performed through a thoracotomy. Lung biopsy during ECMO and anticoagulation carries a significant risk of hemorrhage and should be performed by an experienced pediatric surgical team.

C. Left-sided heart failure and left atrial decompression. If left ventricular contractility is severely impaired, arterial blood will not be ejected through the left ventricular outflow tract, leading to an increase in both left ventricular end-diastolic pressure and left atrial pressures. This may lead to significant pulmonary edema from left atrial hypertension and to intravascular and intracardiac thrombosis secondary to stasis. In this circumstance, the left atrium may have to be decompressed ("vented") into the venous side of the ECMO circuit. This can either be achieved by creating an atrial septostomy in the cardiac catheterization lab or, if the patient is already cannulated through the open chest, by inserting a cannula directly into the left atrium.

VI. COMPLICATIONS

A. Mechanical. Common mechanical problems include clots in the circuit (most common in oxygenator, bladder, and bridge), cannula problems, oxygenator failure, and air in the circuit. Rupture of tubing is a rare but potentially significant problem. Poor venous return to the circuit causes the pump to shut down in order to avoid air entrainment. Causes for poor venous return from the patient to the ECMO circuit include hypovolemia, pneumothorax, or tamponade physiology. Mechanical reasons for poor venous return related to the ECMO circuit are poor catheter position, small venous catheter diameter, excessive catheter length, kinked tubing, and insufficient hydrostatic column length (height of patient above pump head). Initially, fluids are administered while other reasons for poor return are ruled out.

B. Cardiovascular. Hemodynamic instability during ECMO may be a result of hypovolemia, vasodilation during septic inflammatory response, arrhythmias, and pulmonary embolism. Volume overload, especially in the setting of capillary leak, may worsen chest wall compliance and further compromise gas exchange. Both hypo- and hypertension can occur during neonatal ECMO. In the extracorporeal life support (ECLS) registry, 22.3% of newborns on ECMO received inotropic support and 12% received vasodilators for hypertension.

C. Neurologic. Sequelae resulting in neurologic damage often originate from acidosis and hypoxia before commencement of ECMO. According to data through 2015 from the ECLS registry, intracranial hemorrhage occurred in

7.4% and infarction of the central nervous system (CNS) in 7% of neonates during ECMO therapy. Small intracranial hemorrhages are managed by optimizing clotting factors and using Amicar. Larger intracranial hemorrhages may force discontinuation of ECMO. Clinical seizures occurred in 8.9% of neonates on ECMO.

   D. Renal. Renal failure may warrant dialysis, whereas fluid overload may require hemofiltration during the ECMO run. Hemofiltration is common and was used in 15.6% of all neonatal ECMO runs (ECLS registry data).

VII. OUTCOME

   A. Survival. The ECLS database has reported the outcomes of ECMO therapies worldwide since 1985. A total of 28,271 ECMO runs (84% survival) for neonatal respiratory support were reported for neonatal respiratory disorders through July 2015 (see Table 39.1). For the most recently recorded year, the most common indication for ECMO therapy was CDH, followed by persistent pulmonary hypertension of the newborn (PPHN), meconium aspiration syndrome (MAS), sepsis, and neonatal RDS. Survival rates for these conditions are shown in Table 39.2. Mortality at 7 years of age after completion of the UK Collaborative ECMO trial was 33% in the ECMO group and 59% in the conventional group (Table 39.3).

Table 39.3. United Kingdom Neonatal ECMO Trial; Overall Status by 7 Years of Age

Overall Status by 7 Years of Age	ECMO ($n = 93$) (%)	Conventional ($n = 92$) (%)
Deaths	31 (33)	54 (59)
Lost to follow-up	6 (6)	4 (4)
Children with		
Severe disability	3 (3)	0
Moderate disability	9 (10)	6 (7)
Mild disability	13 (14)	11 (12)
Children with		
Impairment only	21 (23)	15 (16)
No abnormal signs or disability	10 (11)	2 (2)
Assessed survivors with no disability	31/56 (55)	17/34 (50)

ECMO, extracorporeal membrane oxygenation.
Source: Follow-up after completion of the McNally H, Bennett CC, Elbourne D, et al. United Kingdom collaborative randomized trial of neonatal extracorporeal membrane oxygenation: follow-up to age 7 years. *Pediatrics* 2006;117(5):e845–e854.

B. Neurodevelopment. Neurologic follow-up was assessed 7 years after completion of the UK Collaborative ECMO trial (see Table 39.3). Both the ECMO and conventional therapy groups had developmental problems and impaired neurologic outcome, but the ECMO group performed better in each task. Both groups had progressive sensorineural hearing loss and notable difficulties with learning and processing. Cognitive skills were not different, with cognitive level within the normal range for 76% of the children in each group. Among the survivors, 55% in the ECMO group and 50% in the conventional group were without disabilities. This study suggests that the underlying disease is the major influence on morbidity and that the beneficial effect of ECMO is still present after 7 years.

Suggested Readings

Extracorporeal Life Support Organization. Guidelines for neonatal respiratory failure. https://www.elso.org/Portals/0/IGD/Archive/FileManager/8588d1a580cusersshyerdocumentselsoguidelinesforneonatalrespiratoryfailure13.pdf. Accessed June 1, 2016.

McNally H, Bennett CC, Elbourne D, et al. United Kingdom collaborative randomized trial of neonatal extracorporeal membrane oxygenation: follow-up to age 7 years. *Pediatrics* 2006;117(5):e845–e854.

Short BL, Williams L, eds. *ECMO Specialist Training Manual*. 3rd ed. Ann Arbor, MI: Extracorporeal Life Support Organization; 2010.

Van Meurs K, Lally KP, Peek G, et al, eds. *ECMO: Extracorporeal Cardiopulmonary Support in Critical Care*. 3rd ed. Ann Arbor, MI: Extracorporeal Life Support Organization; 2005.

40 Shock

Amir M. Khan

KEY POINTS

- Shock remains an important cause of neonatal mortality and morbidity.
- Shock in neonates may be due to lower vascular tone (distributive shock), inadequate blood volume (hypovolemic shock), decreased cardiac function (cardiogenic shock), restricted blood flow (obstructive shock), and inadequate oxygen delivery (dissociative shock).
- Treatment for shock involves addressing the underlying etiology and managing its cardiovascular and systemic effects. Fluids, inotropes, vasopressors, and hydrocortisone replacement are used to treat shock in the neonate.

I. **DEFINITION.** Shock is defined as acute circulatory dysfunction resulting in insufficient oxygen and nutrient delivery to the tissues relative to their metabolic demand, leading to cellular dysfunction that may lead to lactic acidosis and if left uncorrected cause cell death. Shock remains an important cause of neonatal mortality and morbidity. Its prognosis depends on the duration and severity of shock and the resultant extent of vital organ damage. Shock can lead to long-term morbidity including severe neurologic compromise because of cerebral ischemia and reperfusion injury. Therefore, recognizing shock promptly and initiating therapy to address the cause of shock and maintaining hemodynamic stability is essential. In the extremely premature newborn, the lowest acceptable blood pressures (BPs) that may be associated with end organ damage are not well established; therefore, its treatment remains controversial.

II. **ETIOLOGY.** Shock in neonates may be due to lower vascular tone (distributive shock), inadequate blood volume (hypovolemic shock), decreased cardiac function (cardiogenic shock), restricted blood flow (obstructive shock), and inadequate oxygen delivery (dissociative shock). Distributive shock, with or without myocardial dysfunction, is the most frequent cause of hypotension underlying shock, especially in preterm infants.

A. **Distributive shock.** Changes in vascular tone in neonates can result in decreased flow to tissues due to the following:

1. Impaired vasoregulation from increased or dysregulated endothelial nitric oxide (NO) production in the perinatal transitional period, particularly in the preterm neonate

2. Neurologic injury such as in patients with severe hypoxic-ischemic injury which may affect neurovascular pathways

3. Sepsis-related release of proinflammatory cascades that lead to vasodilation

4. Anaphylactic shock is more common in children and rarely affects neonates.

B. Hypovolemic shock. The following conditions can reduce circulating blood volume:

1. Placental hemorrhage, as in abruptio placentae or placenta previa

2. Fetal-to-maternal hemorrhage

3. Twin-to-twin transfusion

4. Intracranial hemorrhage

5. Massive pulmonary hemorrhage (often associated with patent ductus arteriosus [PDA])

6. Blood loss due to disseminated intravascular coagulation (DIC) or other severe coagulopathies

7. Plasma leak into the extravascular compartment, as seen with low oncotic pressure states or capillary leak syndrome (e.g., sepsis)

8. Dehydration due to excessive insensible water loss or inappropriate diuresis as commonly observed in extremely low birth weight (ELBW) infants

C. Cardiogenic shock due to myocardial dysfunction. Decreased cardiac output either due to poor myocardial function or diverted flow through accessory channels results in cardiogenic shock. Some common causes of neonatal cardiogenic shock include the following:

1. Large PDA in a premature infant diverting left ventricular output to pulmonary circulation when uncompensated by an increase in left ventricular output

2. Intrapartum asphyxia leading to myocardial depression

3. Bacterial or viral myocarditis. Congenital viral infections such as enterovirus are more likely to cause severe myocarditis.

4. Fetal or neonatal arrhythmias compromising cardiac output

5. Large arteriovenous malformations (AVM) such as an intracranial AVM that divert a considerable amount of cardiac output away from the systemic circulation

6. Metabolic abnormalities (e.g., hypoglycemia), or cardiomyopathy seen in infants of diabetic mothers

D. Obstructive shock. Restricted venous inflow or arterial outflow will rapidly decrease cardiac output and lead to profound shock. Types of obstructions to blood flow include the following:

1. Venous obstructions
   a. Cardiac anomalies including total anomalous pulmonary venous return, cor triatriatum, tricuspid atresia, mitral atresia
   b. Acquired inflow obstructions can occur from intravascular air or thrombotic embolus.
   c. Increased intrathoracic pressure caused by high airway pressures, pneumothorax, pneumomediastinum, or pneumopericardium

2. Arterial obstructions

a. Cardiac anomalies including pulmonary stenosis or atresia, aortic stenosis or atresia

b. Vascular anomalies such as coarctation of the aorta or interrupted aortic arch

c. Hypertrophic subaortic stenosis due to ventricular hypertrophy seen in infants of diabetic mothers with compromised left ventricular outflow

III. DIAGNOSIS. At the onset of shock, normal compensatory mechanisms may be able to maintain adequate BP by diverting blood away from the skin, muscles, and other nonessential organs. This compensation allows BP to remain within the normal range and maintain perfusion to vital organs and is aptly named "compensated shock." During compensated shock, clinical findings may be subtle and include increased systemic vascular resistance (SVR) presenting as decreased peripheral perfusion (cold, pale skin with delayed capillary refill), tachycardia to maintain cardiac output, weak peripheral pulses and narrow pulse pressure (raised diastolic BP), ileus (decreased splanchnic circulation), and oliguria (decreased renal perfusion). If the clinical condition that results in shock remains unabated or if the underlying etiology is severe (e.g., sudden tension pneumothorax), compensatory mechanisms are usually insufficient to maintain BP and systemic hypotension ensues. "Uncompensated shock" refers to the phase of shock when the patient develops hypotension, and its clinical presentation will reflect decreased perfusion to vital organs. Lack of perfusion to the brain may cause changes in consciousness and lethargy. Lack of coronary perfusion increases the risk of cardiac arrest. In preterm infants, the associated decrease in brain blood flow and oxygen supply during hypotension predisposes to intraventricular/cerebral hemorrhages and periventricular leukomalacia with long-term neurodevelopmental abnormalities. In addition, in ELBW infants, the vasculature of the cerebral cortex may respond to transient myocardial dysfunction/shock with vasoconstriction rather than vasodilatation, further diminishing cerebral perfusion and increasing the risk of neurologic injury.

The physiologic response to increased SVR is altered in septic shock with the release of inflammatory mediators causing vasodilation and increased capillary permeability. In such cases, hypotension and wide pulse pressure is an early indicator of shock.

IV. INVESTIGATIONS. Monitoring vital signs and indicators of organ dysfunction may be helpful in diagnosing and monitoring shock, but the initiation of treatment as described in the following text should not be delayed during the investigation for laboratory indicators of shock. Uncompensated shock results in inadequate oxygen delivery to the tissues so that cellular metabolism becomes predominantly anaerobic, producing lactic and pyruvic acid. Hence, metabolic acidosis often indicates inadequate circulation. Periodic serum lactate measurements may help predict outcome, and serial measurements may be helpful in assessing response to medical interventions.

Other investigations should focus on identifying the underlying etiology of shock based on clinical findings. Such evaluation may include an echocardiogram to assess cardiovascular anatomy and function, appropriate laboratory studies to evaluate the presence of infection, anemia, dehydration, etc.

In addition to defining cardiac anatomy, functional echocardiography may be used to assess cardiac function over time. Flow in the superior vena cava provides an excellent assessment of the blood flow to the upper body and has been used to assess response to therapeutic interventions to reverse shock.

Near-infrared spectroscopy (NIRS) may help with assessing the peripheral perfusion and cerebral oxygenation. Although the utilization of this device in the management of shock has not been studied extensively in neonates, it is used quite commonly in postoperative cardiac patients to measure adequate oxygen delivery, end organ perfusion, and response to therapeutic interventions.

V. TREATMENT. Treatment for shock involves addressing the underlying etiology and managing its cardiovascular and systemic effects. Fluids, inotropes, vasopressors, and hydrocortisone replacement are used to treat shock in the neonate.

  A. **Fluid therapy.** The initial approach is usually to administer crystalloids such as normal saline. An infusion of 10 to 20 mL/kg isotonic saline solution is used to treat suspected hypovolemia. If the shock is due to anemia with or without blood loss, then red blood cell transfusions or fresh frozen plasma for DIC may be better alternatives to normal saline. Use of albumin solutions has been proposed as an alternative to normal saline infusion as they may improve intravascular oncotic pressures, but there is no evidence that they are superior to normal saline. When managing shock, it is important to give sufficient volume to stabilize the cardiovascular system and improve cardiac output. In this regard, measurement of central venous pressure (CVP) may help management, especially in term or late preterm infants. CVP is measured using a catheter with its tip in the right atrium or the intrathoracic superior vena cava. In many neonates, maintaining CVP at 5 to 8 mm Hg with volume infusions is associated with an improved cardiac output. If CVP exceeds 5 to 8 mm Hg, additional volume replacement will usually not be helpful. CVP is influenced by noncardiac factors such as mechanical ventilator pressures and by cardiac factors such as tricuspid valve function. Both factors may affect the interpretation and usefulness of CVP measurements.

  B. **Supportive treatment.** Correction of negative inotropic factors such as hypoxia, acidosis, hypoglycemia, and other metabolic derangements will improve cardiac output. In addition, hypocalcemia frequently occurs in infants with circulatory failure, especially in settings of large amounts of volume replacement. In this setting, administration of calcium frequently produces a positive inotropic effect. Calcium gluconate 10% (100 mg/kg) can be infused slowly if ionized calcium levels are low.

C. Medications

1. **Inotropes** are used to improve cardiac function and include the following (Table 36.1):

   a. **Sympathomimetic amines** are commonly used in infants. The advantages include rapidity of onset, ability to control dosage, and ultra short half-life.

   i. **Dopamine** activates receptors in a dose-dependent manner. At low doses (0.5 to 2 µg/kg/minute), dopamine stimulates peripheral dopamine receptors and increases renal, mesenteric, and coronary blood flow with little effect on cardiac output. In intermediate doses (5 to 9 µg/kg/minute), dopamine has positive inotropic and chronotropic effects. The increase in myocardial contractility depends in part on myocardial norepinephrine stores.

   ii. **Dobutamine** is a synthetic catecholamine with relatively cardioselective inotropic effects. In doses of 5 to 15 µg/kg/minute, dobutamine increases cardiac output with little effect on heart rate. Dobutamine can decrease SVR and is often used with dopamine to improve cardiac output in cases of decreased myocardial function as its inotropic effects, unlike those of dopamine, are independent of norepinephrine stores. However, because hypotension is a result of decreased SVR in the majority of nonasphyxiated newborns, dopamine remains the first-line pressor therapy in newborns.

   iii. **Epinephrine** has potent inotropic and chronotropic effects in the 0.05 to 0.3 µg/kg/minute doses. At these doses, it has greater β2-adrenergic effects in the peripheral vasculature with little α-adrenergic effect resulting in lower SVR. It is not a first-line drug in newborns; however, it may be effective in patients who do not respond to dopamine. Epinephrine is an effective adjunct therapy to dopamine because cardiac norepinephrine stores are readily depleted with prolonged and high-rate dopamine infusions.

   b. **Milrinone** is a phosphodiesterase-III inhibitor that enhances intracellular cyclic adenosine monophosphate (cAMP) content preferentially in the myocardium leading to increase in cardiac contractility. It improves diastolic myocardial function more readily than dobutamine. Milrinone also lowers pulmonary vascular resistance (PVR) and SVR by increasing cAMP levels in vascular smooth muscle often necessitating the use of volume and dopamine (see Appendix A for dosage).

2. **Vasopressor therapy** is used to increase SVR and improve BP which will restore perfusion to vital organs. Such medications include the following:

   a. **Dopamine** in high doses (10 to 20 µg/kg/minute) causes vasoconstriction by releasing norepinephrine from sympathetic vesicles as well as acting directly on α-adrenergic receptors. Neonates have reduced releasable stores of norepinephrine. Dopamine-resistant shock commonly responds to **norepinephrine** or high-dose **epinephrine**. Norepinephrine may be the preferred agent in shock associated with SVR.

b. Vasopressin has primarily been studied in adults for the treatment of shock, with limited experience in neonates. It is a hormone that is primarily involved in the postnatal regulation of fluid homeostasis but also plays a significant role in maintaining vascular tone. Vasopressin deficiency may occur in catecholamine-resistant hypotension in the evolution of sepsis and hence its reported efficacy in vasodilatory shock. There is insufficient data for the use of vasopressin in neonates. It is not routinely used to treat shock in the infants but may be a therapeutic option to consider in the setting of abnormal peripheral vasoregulation. A proposed benefit of vasopressin therapy may be its inhibitory action on NO-induced increases in the second messenger cyclic guanosine monophosphate (cGMP), a potent vasodilatory signal that predominates in the setting of sepsis from the increased endotoxin/inflammation-induced NO synthesis (usual dose of vasopressin is 0.0002 to 0.006 µg/kg/minute).

3. **Hydrocortisone replacement.** Corticosteroids may be useful in infants with hypotension refractory to volume expansion and vasopressors, especially among premature infants. Hydrocortisone stabilizes BP through multiple mechanisms. It induces the expression of the cardiovascular adrenergic receptors that are downregulated by prolonged use of sympathomimetic agents and also inhibits catecholamine metabolism. After hydrocortisone administration, there is a rapid increase in intracellular calcium availability, resulting in enhanced responsiveness to adrenergic agents. The BP response is evident as early as 2 hours after hydrocortisone treatment. For refractory hypotension, hydrocortisone can be used at a dose of 1 mg/kg. If efficacy is noted, the dose can be repeated every 8 hours for 2 to 3 days. Occasionally, hypotension will recur after stopping corticosteroid therapy, requiring a longer duration of therapy with a slow dosage wean.

VI. TYPICAL CLINICAL SCENARIOS OF SHOCK IN THE NEONATE AND THEIR MANAGEMENT

A. **Very low birth weight (VLBW) neonate in the immediate postnatal period**

1. Physiology includes poor vasomotor tone, immature myocardium that is more sensitive to changes in afterload, and dysregulated NO production.

2. What level of BP defines hypotension in the VLBW is unclear. In general, a mean BP that equals the baby's gestational age in weeks is considered adequate if there is adequate perfusion and urine output. Pressor therapy has been associated with worse outcomes in ELBW infants, but it remains uncertain if this is due to the hypotension itself or its therapy.

3. Recommended therapy is dopamine and judicious use of volume if hypovolemia is suspected. It is important not to give large-volume infusions due to their association with increased risk of bronchopulmonary dysplasia and intraventricular hemorrhage reported in premature infants. Hydrocortisone may be considered for dopamine-resistant hypotension.

B. Perinatal depression in preterm or full-term neonate

1. Physiology involves the release of endogenous catecholamines leading to normal or increased SVR clinically manifested by pallor, mottled appearance, and poor perfusion and myocardial dysfunction. The baby is likely to be euvolemic and may have associated pulmonary hypertension.

2. Recommended therapy is dopamine with or without dobutamine up to 10 μg/kg/minute. Milrinone can be considered to provide afterload reduction and inotropic effects without risk of further myocardial injury due to excess catecholamine exposure. Some infants may manifest vasodilatory shock and would benefit from increased doses of dopamine. The patient's skin color and perfusion on physical examination can be used to guide therapy.

C. Septic shock

1. Physiology involves relative hypovolemia, myocardial dysfunction, peripheral vasodilation, and increased pulmonary pressures secondary to acidosis and hypoxia.

2. Therapy includes volume resuscitation with crystalloid (10 to 30 mL/kg) which should be repeated as needed and administration of dopamine 5 to 20 μg/kg/minute with or without epinephrine 0.05 to 0.3 μg/kg/minute. A cardiac echocardiogram can be obtained to evaluate cardiac function, superior vena cava flow, cardiac output, and intracardiac shunting. Consider extracorporeal membrane oxygenation (ECMO) in infants >34 weeks' gestation if they do not respond to these interventions.

D. Preterm neonate with patent ductus arteriosus

1. Physiology includes ductal "steal" compromising vital organ perfusion and increase in left-to-right shunt with increased risk of pulmonary hemorrhage.

2. Recommended therapy includes avoiding high-dose dopamine (>10 μg/kg/minute) as its use will further increase left-to-right shunting and reduce vital organ perfusion. Use dobutamine to enhance cardiac inotropy. Target ventilation management to increase PVR by increasing positive end-expiratory pressure (PEEP), maintaining permissive hypercarbia, and avoiding hyperoxygenation.

E. Preterm neonates with "pressor-resistant" hypotension

1. A proportion of VLBW infants become dependent on medium to high doses of vasopressors (usually dopamine) beyond the first postnatal days. Etiologies include relative cortisol deficiency, adrenal insufficiency, and downregulation of adrenergic receptors.

2. Consider low-dose hydrocortisone (1 to 3 mg/kg/day for 2 to 5 days in three divided doses); some centers routinely measure a serum cortisol level prior to treatment, but there is poor correlation with cortisol levels and the degree of hypotension in VLBW infants. Studies support the efficacy of hydrocortisone in raising BP within 2 hours of administration, yet the long-term neurologic effects of this treatment in the VLBW infant remain to be investigated. Due to a published report of possible

increased incidence of intestinal perforation in infants who have been treated with indomethacin who are also treated with hydrocortisone, the concurrent use of these drugs cannot be recommended until larger trials are conducted.

Suggested Readings

Carcillo JA. A synopsis of 2007 ACCM clinical practice parameters for hemodynamic support of term newborn and infant septic shock. *Early Hum Dev* 2014;90(suppl 1):S45–S47.

Dempsey EM, Barrington KJ. Evaluation and treatment of hypotension in the preterm infant. *Clin Perinatol* 2009;36:75–85.

Giesinger RE, McNamara PJ. Hemodynamic instability in the critically ill neonate: an approach to cardiovascular support based on disease pathophysiology. *Semin Perinatol* 2016;40(3):174–188.

Seri I, Noori S. Diagnosis and treatment of neonatal hypotension outside the transitional period. *Early Hum Dev* 2005;81:405–411.

Short BL, Van Meurs K, Evans JR, et al. Summary proceedings from the cardiology group on cardiovascular instability in preterm infants. *Pediatrics* 2006;117:S34–S39.

41 Cardiac Disorders

John P. Breinholt

KEY POINTS

- The incidence of congenital heart disease is 0.6% to 0.8% of all live births.
- The most serious congenital heart lesions are usually symptomatic in the newborn period.
- Prompt recognition and treatment of critical congenital heart disease can be lifesaving.

I. **INTRODUCTION.** Pediatric cardiology is a relatively young field. In an early 20th century textbook of medicine, Dr. William Osler dismissed congenital heart disease as "limited clinical interest as in a large proportion of cases the anomaly is not compatible with life, and in others, nothing can be done to remedy the defect or even relieve the symptoms." This would change dramatically in 1938, when Dr. Robert Gross successfully ligated a patent ductus arteriosus (PDA) in a 7-year-old girl at Children's Hospital, Boston. In the years since, the capabilities of medical therapy, procedural, and surgical interventions have improved dramatically, with the ability to treat increasingly complex diseases and defects with decreasing morbidity and mortality.

   In critical congenital heart disease, patient outcomes are dependent on (i) early and accurate identification of the cardiac lesion and (ii) evaluation and treatment of secondary organ damage. Therefore, an important mantle of responsibility rests on the neonatologists and pediatricians who often first evaluate and manage these patients. Thereafter, a multidisciplinary team of several subspecialty services is frequently required to avoid the deleterious effects of the cardiac disease on the heart, lung, and brain. Such effects include failure to thrive, increased infection risk, pulmonary vascular disease, cognitive developmental delay, and neurologic deficits. This chapter is an overview of the initial evaluation and management, by neonatologists and pediatricians, of neonates and infants suspected of having congenital heart disease. Additional details about specific heart defects and conditions can be found in current textbooks of pediatric cardiology and pediatric cardiac surgery.

II. **INCIDENCE AND SURVIVAL.** The reported incidence of congenital heart defects in live born infants varies between 0.6% and 0.8% of live births, resulting in 25,000 to 35,000 infants with congenital heart disease each year in the United States alone. This incidence has remained constant over the past several decades. Some reports indicate as high as 1.2% incidence that may be due to inclusion of minor defects that will resolve spontaneously, but are identified by improvements in diagnostic modalities, and the inclusion of such findings as bicuspid aortic valve without stenosis or insufficiency but indicate a higher risk of developing disease later in life. Data from large population studies suggest that approximately 1 per 110 live births have congenital heart disease, and approximately 25% of congenital heart defects are considered critical congenital heart disease, requiring intervention in the first year of life. Most of these infants with congenital heart disease are identified by the end of the neonatal period. The most common congenital heart lesions presenting in the first weeks of life are summarized in Table 41.1. Advances in diagnostic imaging, cardiac

Table 41.1. Top Five Diagnoses Presenting at Different Ages*

Diagnosis	Percentage of Patients
Age on admission: 0–6 d (n = 537)	
D-Transposition of great arteries	19
Hypoplastic left ventricle	14
Tetralogy of Fallot	8
Coarctation of aorta	7
Ventricular septal defect	3
Others	49
Age on admission: 7–13 d (n = 195)	
Coarctation of aorta	16
Ventricular septal defect	14
Hypoplastic left ventricle	8
D-Transposition of great arteries	7
Tetralogy of Fallot	7
Others	48
Age on admission: 14–28 d (n = 177)	
Ventricular septal defect	16
Coarctation of aorta	12
Tetralogy of Fallot	7
D-Transposition of great arteries	7
Patent ductus arteriosus	5
Others	53

*Reprinted with permission from Flanagan MF, Yeager SB, Weindling SN. Cardiac disease. In: MacDonald MG, Mullett MD, Seshia MMK, eds. *Avery's Neonatology: Pathophysiology and Management of the Newborn.* 6th ed. Philadelphia, PA: Lippincott Williams & Wilkins; 2005.

surgery, and intensive care have reduced the operative risks of many complex lesions; the hospital mortality following all forms of neonatal cardiac surgery has significantly decreased in the past decade.

III. CLINICAL PRESENTATIONS OF CONGENITAL HEART DISEASE IN THE NEONATE.

The timing of presentation is dependent on three primary elements: (i) the type and severity of the congenital defect; (ii) alterations in the cardiovascular physiology secondary to the effects of the transitional circulation, principally **closure of the ductus arteriosus** and the decrease **in pulmonary vascular resistance**; and (iii) any *in utero* effects of the defect.

Overall, cardiac emergencies are uncommon in children. Nevertheless, more serious cardiac disease and symptoms are more likely to present earlier in life. The first 72 hours are particularly important because many of the most severe and acutely life-threatening lesions present in this time frame.

A. **Parallel, nonmixing circulations.** The primary diagnosis of this description is D-transposition of the great arteries (D-TGA). D-TGA is defined as the aorta arising from the morphologically right ventricle, wherein the systemic venous blood returns to the right cardiac chambers and returns to the systemic arterial system without passing through the pulmonary vasculature. The pulmonary artery arises from the morphologically left ventricle, leading to the fully oxygen-saturated blood from the pulmonary venous system returning to the left cardiac chambers, and then returning to the pulmonary vasculature. As such, the two circulations work in parallel, with oxygen-saturated blood not reaching the systemic circulation.

The two locations where oxygen-saturated blood can enter the systemic circulation are (i) the PDA and (ii) the patent foramen ovale (PFO). As the PDA closes as part of the transitional circulatory changes, the sole source of oxygenated blood becomes the PFO, which commonly becomes increasingly restrictive. Without intervention, the neonate will become increasingly cyanotic and develop a metabolic acidosis, and subsequent circulatory shock.

Palliative interventions are urgent to prevent this clinical presentation. These include initiation of a prostaglandin E_1 (PGE_1) infusion that maintains patency of the ductus arteriosus. Frequently, this is insufficient, or becomes insufficient, and a balloon atrial septostomy is necessary via cardiac catheterization techniques. These interventions allow time to stabilize the patient in anticipation of neonatal reparative surgery via the arterial switch procedure.

B. **Critically obstructed left heart lesions.** This group of cardiac defects includes those in which patency of the ductus arteriosus is necessary to maintain systemic blood flow. As a result of the expected ductal constriction and closure, the neonate will become acidotic and develop cardiogenic shock. Some of these lesions can present later in life; however, those that present in the first 72 hours are of a more severe nature.

1. **Hypoplastic left heart syndrome.** This defect comprises underdevelopment of left heart structures including the mitral and aortic valve (either stenotic or atretic), small or absent left ventricular chamber, and hypoplasia of the ascending aorta, including coarctation.

2. **Critical aortic valve stenosis.** In its most severe form, systemic output is dependent on the PDA because sufficient blood flow does not cross

the aortic valve to sustain the body. Less severe forms can be monitored beyond the neonatal period and may not require intervention for months or years.

3. Coarctation of the aorta. The most common site of coarctation is near the ductus arteriosus, and as the ductus arteriosus closes, the inadequate systemic output manifests. Again, less severe forms may not be discovered until months or years after the neonatal period. Those requiring early and urgent intervention are those with the most severe disease.

4. Interrupted aortic arch. In this lesion, there is absence of continuity between the ascending and descending aorta. The different types are distinguished by the location of discontinuity relative to the head and neck vessels. Without the PDA, there is no blood flow to the lower body.

C. Critically obstructed right heart lesions. This group of cardiac defects includes those in which patency of the ductus arteriosus is necessary to maintain pulmonary blood flow. As a result, the neonate will become cyanotic without appropriate intervention. Milder forms of these lesions may present later in life; however, those that present in the first 72 hours are of a more severe nature.

1. Pulmonary atresia (PA). This defect occurs as a result of the pulmonary valve not achieving patency during fetal life. As a result, pulmonary blood flow is entirely dependent on the ductus arteriosus. This lesion presents in multiple forms:

a. PA with intact ventricular septum. In this variant, blood flow in the right ventricle has no outlet other than via tricuspid regurgitation and subsequent right-to-left shunt across the foramen ovale. The high pressure generated in the right ventricle, in the absence of outflow, is correlated with coronary artery fistulas that can be dependent on the high pressure in the ventricle for coronary blood flow. This presents an independent risk factor for this disease.

b. PA with ventricular septal defect. In this variant, systemic venous blood entering the right ventricle will mix with pulmonary venous blood entering the left ventricle and enter the systemic circulation via the aortic valve.

c. PA with major aortopulmonary collateral arteries (MAPCAs). This variant is *not* dependent on ductal circulation for pulmonary blood flow. Native pulmonary arteries may or may not be present and are uniformly hypoplastic. Collateral vessels form off the descending aorta and provide pulmonary blood flow.

2. Critical pulmonary valve stenosis. In its most severe form, pulmonary blood flow is dependent on the PDA because sufficient blood does not cross the pulmonary valve to provide effective pulmonary blood flow. Less severe forms can be monitored beyond the neonatal period and may not require intervention for months or years.

3. Ebstein's anomaly. This disease is a product of distal displacement of the tricuspid valve into the right ventricle. The result is a large right atrium with an "atrialized" right ventricle and a limited, functional right ventricular (RV) chamber. In its severe form, the tricuspid valve displacement can cause an outflow tract obstruction, requiring a PDA.

Milder forms have been found incidentally in adulthood and may not require intervention.

D. **Total anomalous pulmonary venous return (TAPVR).** Anomalous pulmonary venous connections can present similar to a large left-to-right shunt, similar to an atrial septal defect, however, in its obstructed form, represents a surgical emergency. Obstructed TAPVR has an initial clinical manifestation similar to pulmonary hypertension but should be considered when traditional pulmonary hypertension therapies are ineffective. There is no medical management that will improve this condition. There are some reports of interventional cardiologists placing percutaneous stents to relieve the obstruction, but this is a palliative intervention meant to allow time for somatic growth, or for a critically ill patient to recover prior to undergoing surgery.

Without acute intervention, many of the heart lesions described earlier can have significant morbidity and mortality. Fortunately, currently, many diagnoses are made prenatally due to improvements in ultrasound technology and the availability of fetal echocardiography. In the absence of prenatal diagnoses, these and other forms of heart disease present in the neonatal period that, although not requiring short-term intervention, require early recognition for proper therapy.

Important clinical findings should alert the clinician to the possibility of congenital heart disease. Key findings that require additional evaluation include (i) cyanosis, (ii) congestive heart failure (CHF), (iii) cardiovascular collapse or shock, (iv) heart murmur, and (v) arrhythmia.

IV. CLINICAL MANIFESTATIONS OF CONGENITAL HEART DISEASE

A. **Cyanosis**

1. **Clinical findings.** Cyanosis (bluish tinge of the skin and mucous membranes) is a common presenting sign of congenital heart disease in the neonate. In the setting of congenital heart disease, cyanosis is an indication of hypoxemia or decreased arterial oxygen saturation. However, depending on the underlying skin complexion, clinically apparent cyanosis is usually not visible until there is >3 g/dL of **desaturated** hemoglobin in the arterial system. Therefore, the degree of visible cyanosis depends on both the severity of hypoxemia (which determines the percentage of oxygen saturation) as well as the hemoglobin concentration. For example, consider two infants with similar degrees of hypoxemia—each having an arterial oxygen saturation of 85%. The polycythemic newborn (hemoglobin of 22 g/dL) will have 3.3 g/dL (15% of 22 g/dL) desaturated hemoglobin and have more visibly apparent cyanosis than the anemic infant (hemoglobin of 10 g/dL) who will only have 1.5 g/dL (15% of 10 g/dL) desaturated hemoglobin. Also, there are a few instances when cyanosis is associated with normal arterial oxygen saturation. True central cyanosis should be a generalized finding (i.e., not acrocyanosis, blueness of the hands and feet only, which is a normal finding in a neonate) and can often best be appreciated in the mucous membranes.

Because determining cyanosis by visual inspection can be challenging for the reasons mentioned, adding routine pre- and postductal extremity pulse oximetry has been proposed as an additional screening test in the first 48 hours of life. A 2009 prospective study in Sweden demonstrated an improved total detection rate of ductal-dependent circulation to 92%. Importantly, the combination of physical exam and pulse oximetry screening demonstrated better sensitivity than either screen alone. In 2011, the U.S. Secretary of Health and Human Services recommended that critical congenital heart defects be added to the U.S. Recommended Uniform Screening Panel for newborns. Implementation of this would entail pulse oximetry screening after 24 hours of life, with further evaluation by echocardiogram for oxygen saturations below 95%. Multiple states have included it in their screening mandates, with additional studies to validate its clinical and cost-effectiveness underway.

2. **Differential diagnosis.** Differentiation of cardiac from respiratory causes of cyanosis in the neonatal intensive care unit (NICU) is a common problem. Pulmonary disorders are frequently the cause of cyanosis in the newborn due to intrapulmonary right-to-left shunting. Primary lung disease (pneumonia, hyaline membrane disease, pulmonary arteriovenous malformations, etc.), pneumothorax, airway obstruction, extrinsic compression of the lungs (congenital diaphragmatic hernia, pleural effusions, etc.), and central nervous system abnormalities may produce varying degrees of hypoxemia manifesting as cyanosis in the neonate. For a more complete differential diagnosis of pulmonary causes of cyanosis in the neonate, see Chapters 33 to 38. Finally, clinical cyanosis may occur in an infant without hypoxemia in the setting of methemoglobinemia or pronounced polycythemia. Table 41.2 summarizes the differential diagnosis of cyanosis in the neonate.

B. **Congestive heart failure**

1. **Clinical findings.** CHF in the neonate (or in a patient of any age) is a **clinical** diagnosis made based on the presence of certain signs and symptoms rather than on radiographic or laboratory findings, which may corroborate the diagnosis. Signs and symptoms of CHF occur when the heart is unable to meet the metabolic demands of the tissues. Clinical findings are frequently due to homeostatic mechanisms attempting to compensate for this imbalance. In early stages, the neonate may be tachypneic and tachycardic with an increased respiratory effort, rales, hepatomegaly, and delayed capillary refill. In contrast to adults, edema is rarely seen. Diaphoresis, feeding difficulties, and growth failure may be present. Diaphoresis during feeding is a common scenario that this symptom manifests. Finally, CHF may present acutely with cardiorespiratory collapse, particularly in "left-sided" lesions (see section VI.A). *Hydrops fetalis* is an extreme form of intrauterine CHF (see Chapter 5).

2. **Differential diagnosis.** The age when CHF develops depends on the physiologic effects of the responsible lesion. When heart failure develops in the first weeks of life, the differential diagnosis includes (i) a structural lesion causing severe pressure and/or volume overload, (ii) a primary myocardial lesion causing myocardial dysfunction, or (iii) arrhythmia. Table 41.3 summarizes the differential diagnoses of CHF in the neonate.

Table 41.2. Differential Diagnosis of Cyanosis in the Neonate

Primary cardiac lesions

Decreased pulmonary blood flow, intracardiac right-to-left shunt

Critical pulmonary stenosis

Tricuspid atresia

Pulmonary atresia/intact ventricular septum

Tetralogy of Fallot

Ebstein anomaly

Total anomalous pulmonary venous connection with obstruction

Normal or increased pulmonary blood flow, intracardiac mixing

Hypoplastic left heart syndrome

Transposition of the great arteries

Truncus arteriosus

Tetralogy of Fallot/pulmonary atresia

Complete common atrioventricular canal

Total anomalous pulmonary venous connection without obstruction

Other single-ventricle complexes

Pulmonary lesions (intrapulmonary right-to-left shunt) (see Chapters 32–38)

Primary parenchymal lung disease

Aspiration syndromes (e.g., meconium and blood)

Respiratory distress syndrome

Pneumonia

Airway obstruction

Choanal stenosis or atresia

Pierre Robin syndrome

Tracheal stenosis

Pulmonary sling

Absent pulmonary valve syndrome

(continued)

Table 41.2. *(Continued)*

Extrinsic compression of the lungs
Pneumothorax
Pulmonary interstitial or lobar emphysema
Chylothorax or other pleural effusions
Congenital diaphragmatic hernia
Thoracic dystrophies or dysplasia
Hypoventilation
Central nervous system lesions
Neuromuscular diseases
Sedation
Sepsis
Pulmonary arteriovenous malformations
Persistent pulmonary hypertension (see Chapter 36)
Cyanosis with normal PO$_2$
Methemoglobinemia
Polycythemia* (see Chapter 46)

PO$_2$, partial pressure of oxygen.
*In the case of polycythemia, these infants have plethora and venous congestion in the distal extremities, which gives the appearance of distal cyanosis; these infants actually are not hypoxemic (see text).

C. **Heart murmur.** Heart murmurs are not uncommonly heard when examining neonates. It is estimated that >50% of children have a murmur at some point during childhood, with the majority presenting in the neonatal period. Murmurs heard in newborns in the first days of life are often associated with structural heart disease of some type, and therefore may need further evaluation, particularly if there are any other associated clinical symptoms. Nevertheless, it is not uncommon for an innocent murmur to be heard during the transition from fetal circulation, specifically the closing of the PDA. Other transient murmurs may be heard, including a very small muscular ventricular septal defect that is closing or peripheral branch pulmonary artery stenosis that is due to blood flow turbulence at the pulmonary artery branches that disappears as the branches grow.

Pathologic murmurs tend to appear at characteristic ages. Semilunar valve stenosis (systolic ejection murmurs) and atrioventricular valvular insufficiency (systolic regurgitant murmurs) tend to be noted very shortly

Table 41.3. Differential Diagnosis of Congestive Heart Failure in the Neonate

Pressure overload

  Aortic stenosis

  Coarctation of the aorta

Volume overload

  Left-to-right shunt at level of great vessels

    Patent ductus arteriosus

    Aorticopulmonary window

    Truncus arteriosus

    Tetralogy of Fallot, pulmonary atresia with multiple aorticopulmonary collaterals

  Left-to-right shunt at level of ventricles

    Ventricular septal defect

    Common atrioventricular canal

    Single ventricle without pulmonary stenosis (includes hypoplastic left heart syndrome)

  Arteriovenous malformations

Combined pressure and volume overload

  Interrupted aortic arch

  Coarctation of the aorta with ventricular septal defect

  Aortic stenosis with ventricular septal defect

Myocardial dysfunction

  Primary

    Cardiomyopathies

      Inborn errors of metabolism

      Genetic

    Myocarditis

(continued)

Table 41.3. *(Continued)*
Secondary
Sustained tachyarrhythmias
Perinatal asphyxia
Sepsis
Severe intrauterine valvular obstruction (e.g., aortic stenosis)
Premature closure of the ductus arteriosus

after birth, on the first day of life. In contrast, murmurs due to left-to-right shunt lesions (a ventricular septal defect murmur or continuous PDA murmur) may not be heard until the second to fourth week of life, when the pulmonary vascular resistance has decreased and the left-to-right shunt increases. Therefore, the **age of the patient** when the murmur is first noted and the **character of the murmur** provide important clues to the nature of the malformation.

D. **Arrhythmias.** See section IX (Arrhythmias) of this chapter for a detailed description of the identification and management of the neonate with an arrhythmia.

E. **Fetal echocardiography.** It is increasingly common for infants to be born with a diagnosis of probable congenital heart disease due to the widespread use of obstetric ultrasonography and fetal echocardiography. This may be quite valuable to the team of physicians caring for mother and baby, guiding plans for prenatal care, site and timing of delivery, as well as immediate perinatal care of the infant. The recommended timing for fetal echocardiography is 18 to 20 weeks' gestation, although reasonable images can be obtained as early as 16 weeks, and transvaginal ultrasonography may be used for diagnostic purposes in fetuses in the first trimester. Indications for fetal echocardiography are summarized in Table 41.4. It is important to note, however, that most cases of prenatally diagnosed congenital heart disease occur in pregnancies without known risk factors. Most severe forms of congenital heart disease can be accurately diagnosed by fetal echocardiography. Coarctation of the aorta, small ventricular and atrial septal defects, TAPVR, and mild aortic or pulmonary stenosis are abnormalities that may be missed by fetal echocardiography. It is important to consider that the expected PDA can mask a coarctation, and the fetal circulation requires a PFO for survival that can make the presence of an atrial septal defect uncertain. In general, in complex congenital heart disease, the main abnormality is noted; however, the full extent of cardiac malformation may be better determined on postnatal examinations.

Fetal tachyarrhythmias or bradyarrhythmias (intermittent or persistent) may be detected on routine obstetric screening ultrasound examinations; this should prompt more complete fetal echocardiography to rule

Table 41.4. Indications for Fetal Echocardiography

Fetus-related indications

Suspected congenital heart disease on screening ultrasonography

Fetal chromosomal anomaly

Fetal extracardiac anatomic anomaly

Fetal cardiac arrhythmia

  Persistent bradycardia

  Persistent tachycardia

  Irregular rhythm

Nonimmune hydrops fetalis

Mother-related indications

Congenital heart disease

Maternal metabolic disease

  Diabetes mellitus

  Phenylketonuria

Maternal rheumatic disease (such as systemic lupus erythematosus)

Maternal environmental exposures

  Alcohol

  Cardiac teratogenic medications

    Amphetamines

    Anticonvulsants

      Phenytoin

      Trimethadione

      Carbamazepine

      Valproate

    Isotretinoin

    Lithium carbonate

  Maternal viral infection

    Rubella

(continued)

Table 41.4. *(Continued)*
Family-related indications
Previous child or parent with congenital heart disease
Previous child or parent with genetic disease associated with congenital heart disease

out associated structural heart disease, assess fetal ventricular function, and further define the arrhythmia.

Fetal echocardiography has allowed for improved understanding of the *in utero* evolution of some forms of congenital heart disease. This, in turn, has led to the development of fetal cardiac intervention. Several institutions have begun intervening in semilunar valve stenosis, as well as select other defects. This progress represents a promising new method of treatment for congenital heart disease, however, further research is needed to assess outcomes.

V. EVALUATION OF THE NEONATE WITH SUSPECTED CONGENITAL HEART DISEASE.
The most time-sensitive presentation of the neonate with congenital heart disease is circulatory collapse. In this scenario, emergency treatment of circulatory shock should precede cardiac diagnostic studies. Low cardiac output should generate a suspicion for congenital heart disease.

A. Initial evaluation

1. **Physical examination.** The physical examination should extend beyond the heart. Inexperienced examiners frequently focus solely on the presence or absence of cardiac murmurs, but many other findings can guide diagnostic decision making.

   a. **Inspection**. Cyanosis may first be apparent on inspection of the mucous membranes and/or nail beds (see section IV.A.1). Mottling of the skin and/or an ashen, gray color are important clues to severe cardiovascular compromise and incipient shock. While observing the infant, particular attention should be paid to the pattern of respiration including the work of breathing and use of accessory muscles.

   b. **Palpation.** Palpation of the **distal extremities** with attention to temperature and capillary refill is imperative. Although cool extremities with delayed capillary refill would indicate a suspicion for sepsis, it should also raise suspicion of congenital heart disease. While palpating the distal extremities, note the presence and character of the distal pulses. Diminished or absent distal pulses are suggestive of aortic arch obstruction. Palpation of the *precordium* may provide important information suggesting congenital heart disease. A precordial thrill may be present in the setting of at least moderate pulmonary or aortic outflow obstruction. A restrictive ventricular septal defect with low RV pressure could also generate a thrill; however, it is less likely in the early neonatal period. A hyperdynamic precordium suggests a significant left-to-right shunt.

c. Auscultation. This part of the exam should be performed systematically and not be rushed to identify heart murmurs. Many severe congenital heart defects will not have a murmur in the neonatal period. First, listen to the heart rate to determine if it is regular. Second, listen carefully to the heart sounds. The second heart sound is important because its split indicates the presence of two semilunar valves. Hearing this can be difficult in neonates that have fast heart rates. However, the presence of a S3 or S4 is more obvious and more indicative of a neonate in crisis. Distinguishing them may be difficult, but the presence of either is abnormal and should prompt further study and consultation. A systolic ejection click suggests aortic or pulmonary valve stenosis.

The presence and intensity of systolic murmurs suggest the type and severity of the underlying anatomic diagnosis. When associated with pathology, they are associated with (i) semilunar valve or outflow tract stenosis, (ii) shunting through a septal defect, or (iii) atrioventricular valve regurgitation. Diastolic murmurs are **always** indicative of cardiovascular pathology. For a more complete description of auscultation of the heart, refer to the cardiology texts from the chapter reference list.

A careful search for other anomalies is essential because congenital heart disease is accompanied by at least one extracardiac malformation in 25% of these patients. Table 41.5 summarizes malformation and chromosomal syndromes commonly associated with congenital heart disease.

2. **Four-extremity blood pressure.** Measurement of blood pressure should be taken in bilateral upper and lower extremities. The lower extremities should be equivalent because both are located distal to any aortic arch obstruction. A difference between leg blood pressures is likely due to sampling and not indicative of disease. Automated blood pressure cuffs are most commonly used today, but in a small neonate with pulses that are difficult to palpate, manual blood pressure measurement with Doppler amplification may be necessary for an accurate measurement. A systolic pressure that is 10–15 mm Hg higher in the upper body compared to the lower body is abnormal and suggests coarctation of the aorta, aortic arch hypoplasia, or interrupted aortic arch. It should be noted that a systolic blood pressure gradient is quite specific for an arch abnormality but not sensitive; a systolic blood pressure gradient will not be present in the neonate with an arch abnormality in whom the ductus arteriosus is patent and nonrestrictive. Therefore, the lack of a systolic blood pressure gradient in newborn does **not** conclusively rule out coarctation or other arch abnormalities, but the presence of a significant systolic pressure gradient is diagnostic of an aortic arch abnormality.

3. **Pulse oximetry.** Multiple studies indicate improved detection of congenital heart disease with the implementation of routine pulse oximetry screening. As such, many countries include this as part of the neonatal evaluation. The primary approach includes pre- and postductal extremity pulse oximetry measurement >24 hours after birth. Values <95% would result in further evaluation with echocardiography. Some investigators suggest that the threshold may need to be adjusted for patients born at altitude.

Table 41.5. Chromosomal Anomalies, Syndromes, and Associations Commonly Associated with Congenital Heart Disease

	Approximate Incidence or Mode of Inheritance	Extracardiac Features	Cardiac Features
Chromosomal anomalies			
Trisomy 13 (Patau syndrome)	1/5,000	SGA; facies (midfacial hypoplasia, cleft lip and palate, microphthalmia coloboma, low-set ears); brain anomalies (microcephaly holoprosencephaly); aplasia cutis congenita of scalp; polydactyly	≥80% have cardiac defects, VSD most common
Trisomy 18 (Edward syndrome)	1/3,000 (female:male = 3:1)	SGA; facies (dolichocephaly, prominent occiput, short palpebral fissures, low-set posteriorly rotated ears, small mandible); short sternum; rocker bottom feet; overlapping fingers with "clenched fists"	≥95% have cardiac defects, VSD most common (sometimes multiple); redundant valvular tissue with regurgitation often affecting more than one valve (polyvalvular disease)
Trisomy 21 (Down syndrome)	1/660	Facies (brachycephaly, flattened occiput, midfacial hypoplasia, mandibular prognathism, upslanting palpebral fissures, epicanthal folds, Brushfield spots, large tongue); simian creases, clinodactyly with short fifth finger; pronounced hypotonia	40%–50% have cardiac defects, CAVC, VSD most common, also TOF, ASD, PDA; complex congenital heart disease is very rare
45,X (Turner syndrome)	1/2,500	Lymphedema of hands, feet; short stature; short-webbed neck; facies (triangular with downslanting palpebral fissures, low-set ears); shield chest	25%–45% have cardiac defects, coarctation, bicuspid aortic valve most common

(continued)

Table 41.5. Chromosomal Anomalies, Syndromes, and Associations Commonly Associated with Congenital Heart Disease *(Continued)*

	Approximate Incidence or Mode of Inheritance	Extracardiac Features	Cardiac Features
Single-gene defects			
Noonan syndrome	AD	Facies (hypertelorism, epicanthal folds, downslanting palpebral fissures, ptosis); low-set ears; short webbed neck with low hairline; shield chest, cryptorchidism in men	50% have cardiac defect, usually pulmonary valve stenosis, also ASD, hypertrophic CM
Holt-Oram syndrome	AD	Spectrum of upper limb and shoulder girdle anomalies	≥50% have cardiac defect, usually ASD or VSD
Alagille syndrome	AD	Cholestasis; facies (micrognathism, broad forehead, deep-set eyes); vertebral anomalies, ophthalmologic abnormalities	Cardiac findings in 90%. Peripheral pulmonic stenosis is most common.
Gene deletion syndromes			
Williams syndrome (deletion 7q11)	1/7,500	SGA, FTT; facies ("elfin" with short palpebral fissures, periorbital fullness or puffiness, flat nasal bridge, stellate iris, long philtrum, prominent lips); fussy infants with poor feeding, friendly personality later in childhood; characteristic mental deficiency (motor more reduced than verbal performance)	50%–70% have cardiac defect, most commonly supravalvular aortic stenosis; other arterial stenoses also occur, including PPS, CoA, renal artery, and coronary artery stenoses.
DiGeorge syndrome (deletion 22q11)	1/6,000	Thymic hypoplasia/aplasia; parathyroid hypoplasia/aplasia; cleft palate or velopharyngeal incompetence	IAA and conotruncal malformations including truncus, TOF

Associations

VACTERL	Vertebral defects, anal atresia, cardiac defects, TE fistula, radial and renal anomalies, limb defects	Approximately 50% have cardiac defect, most commonly VSD.
CHARGE	Coloboma, heart defects, choanal atresia, growth and mental deficiency, genital hypoplasia (in men), ear anomalies and/or deafness	50%–70% have cardiac defect, most commonly conotruncal anomalies (TOF, DORV, truncus arteriosus)

SGA, small for gestational age; VSD, ventricular septal defect; CAVC, complete atrioventricular canal; TOF, tetralogy of Fallot; ASD, atrial septal defect; PDA, patent ductus arteriosus; AD, autosomal dominant; CM, cardiomyopathy; FTT, failure to thrive; PPS, peripheral pulmonary stenosis; CoA, coarctation of the aorta; IAA, interrupted aortic arch; TE, tracheoesophageal; DORV, double outlet right ventricle.

4. **Chest x-ray.** A frontal and lateral view (if possible) of the chest should be obtained. In infants, particularly newborns, the size of the heart may be difficult to determine due to an overlying thymus. Nevertheless, useful information can be gained from the chest x-ray. In addition to heart size, notation should be made of visceral and cardiac situs (dextrocardia and *situs inversus* are frequently accompanied by congenital heart disease). The aortic arch side (right or left) often can be determined; a right-sided aortic arch is associated with congenital heart disease in >90% of patients. Dark or poorly perfused lung fields suggests decreased pulmonary blood flow, whereas diffusely opaque lung fields may represent increased pulmonary blood flow or significant left atrial hypertension.

5. **Electrocardiogram (ECG).** The neonatal ECG reflects the hemodynamic relations that existed *in utero*; therefore, the normal ECG is notable for RV predominance. As many forms of congenital heart disease have minimal prenatal hemodynamic effects, the ECG is frequently "normal for age" despite significant structural pathology (e.g., transposition of the great arteries, tetralogy of Fallot). Throughout the neonatal period, infancy, and childhood, the ECG will evolve due to the expected changes in physiology and the resulting changes in chamber size and thickness that occur. Because most findings on a neonate's ECG would be abnormal in an older child or adult, it is essential to refer to age-specific charts of normal values for most ECG parameters. Refer to Tables 41.6 and 41.7 for normal ECG values in term and premature neonates.

   When interpreting an ECG, the following determinations should be made: (i) rate and rhythm; (ii) P, QRS, and T axes; (iii) intracardiac conduction intervals; (iv) evidence for chamber enlargement or hypertrophy; (v) evidence for pericardial disease, ischemia, infarction, or electrolyte abnormalities; and (vi) if the ECG pattern fits with the clinical picture. When the ECG is abnormal, one should also consider incorrect lead placement; a simple confirmation of lead placement may be done by comparing QRS complexes in limb lead I and precordial lead V_6—each should have a similar morphology if the limb leads have been properly placed. The ECG of the premature infant is somewhat different from that of the term infant (Table 41.7).

6. **Hyperoxia test.** In **all** neonates with suspected critical congenital heart disease (not just those who are cyanotic), a hyperoxia test should be considered. **This single test is perhaps the most sensitive and specific tool in the initial evaluation of the neonate with suspected disease.** In sites with timely access to echocardiography, a complete hyperoxia test may not need to be performed; however, it is important to appreciate that this can be a valuable test when echocardiography is not quickly available.

   To investigate the possibility of a fixed, intracardiac right-to-left shunt, the arterial oxygen tension should be measured in room air (if tolerated) followed by repeat measurements with the patient receiving 100% inspired oxygen (the "hyperoxia test"). If possible, the arterial partial pressure of oxygen (PO_2) should be measured directly through arterial puncture, although properly applied transcutaneous oxygen monitor (TCOM) values for PO_2 are also acceptable. **Pulse oximetry cannot be used** for documentation; in a neonate given 100% inspired

Table 41.6. ECG Standards in Newborns

Measure	Age (Days)			
	0–1	**1–3**	**3–7**	**7–30**
Term infants				
Heart rate (bpm)	122 (99–147)	123 (97–148)	128 (100–160)	148 (114–177)
QRS axis (degrees)	135 (91–185)	134 (93–188)	133 (92–185)	108 (78–152)
PR interval, II (s)	0.11 (0.08–0.14)	0.11 (0.09–0.13)	0.10 (0.08–0.13)	0.10 (0.08–0.13)
QRS duration (s)	0.05 (0.03–0.07)	0.05 (0.03–0.06)	0.05 (0.03–0.06)	0.05 (0.03–0.08)
V_1, R amplitude (mm)	13.5 (6.5–23.7)	14.8 (7.0–24.2)	12.8 (5.5–21.5)	10.5 (4.5–18.1)
V_1, S amplitude (mm)	8.5 (1.0–18.5)	9.5 (1.5–19.0)	6.8 (1.0–15.0)	4.0 (0.5–9.7)
V_6, R amplitude (mm)	4.5 (0.5–9.5)	4.8 (0.5–9.5)	5.1 (1.0–10.5)	7.6 (2.6–13.5)
V_6, S amplitude (mm)	3.5 (0.2–7.9)	3.2 (0.2–7.6)	3.7 (0.2–8.0)	3.2 (0.2–3.2)

(continued)

Table 41.6. ECG Standards in Newborns *(Continued)*

Measure	Age (Days)			
	0–1	**1–3**	**3–7**	**7–30**
Preterm infants				
Heart rate (bpm)	141 (109–173)	150 (127–182)	164 (134–200)	170 (133–200)
QRS axis (degrees)	127 (75–194)	121 (75–195)	117 (75–165)	80 (17–171)
PR interval (s)	0.10 (0.09–0.10)	0.10 (0.09–1.10)	0.10 (0.09–0.10)	0.10 (0.09–0.10)
QRS duration (s)	0.04	0.04	0.04	0.04
V_1, R amplitude (mm)	6.5 (2.0–12.6)	7.4 (2.6–14.9)	8.7 (3.8–16.9)	13.0 (6.2–21.6)
V_1, S amplitude (mm)	6.8 (0.6–17.6)	6.5 (1.0–16.0)	6.8 (0.0–15.0)	6.2 (1.2–14.0)
V_6, R amplitude (mm)	11.4 (3.5–21.3)	11.9 (5.0–20.8)	12.3 (4.0–20.5)	15.0 (8.3–21.0)
V_6, S amplitude (mm)	15.0 (2.5–26.5)	13.5 (2.6–26.0)	14.0 (3.0–25.0)	14.0 (3.1–26.3)

Source: Davignon A, Rautaharja P, Boiselle E, et al. Normal ECG standards for infants and children. *Pediatr Cardiol* 1980;1(2):123–131; Sreenivasan VV, Fisher BJ, Liebman J, et al. Longitudinal study of the standard electrocardiogram in the healthy premature infant during the first year of life. *Am J Cardiol* 1973;31(1):57–63.

Table 41.7. ECG Findings in Premature Infants (Compared to Term Infants)
Rate
Slightly higher resting rate with greater activity-related and circadian variation (sinus bradycardia to 70, with sleep not uncommon)
Intracardiac conduction
PR and QRS duration slightly shorter
Maximum QT_c <0.44 s (longer than for term infants, QT_c <0.40 s)
QRS complex
QRS axis in frontal plane more leftward with decreasing gestational age
QRS amplitude lower (possibly due to less ventricular mass)
Less right ventricular predominance in precordial chest leads
Source: Reproduced with permission from Thomaidis C, Varlamis G, Karamperis S. Comparative study of the electrocardiograms of healthy fullterm and premature newborns. *Acta Paediatr Scand* 1988;77(5):653–657.

oxygen, a value of 100% oxygen saturation may be obtained with an arterial PO_2 ranging from 80 torr (abnormal) to 680 torr (normal, see section IV.A.1).

Measurements should be made (by arterial blood gas or TCOM) at both "preductal" and "postductal" sites and the exact site of PO_2 measurement must be recorded because some congenital malformations with desaturated blood flow entering the descending aorta through the ductus arteriosus may result in "differential cyanosis" (as seen in persistent pulmonary hypertension of the newborn). Markedly higher oxygen content in the upper versus the lower part of the body can be an important diagnostic clue to such lesions, including all forms of critical aortic arch obstruction or left ventricular outflow obstruction. There are also the rare cases of "reverse differential cyanosis" with elevated lower body saturation and lower upper body saturation. This occurs only in children with transposition of the great arteries with an abnormal pulmonary artery to aortic shunt due to coarctation, interruption of the aortic arch, or suprasystemic pulmonary vascular resistance ("persistent fetal circulation").

When a patient breathes 100% oxygen, an arterial PO_2 of >250 torr in both upper and lower extremities virtually eliminates critical structural cyanotic heart disease (a "passed" hyperoxia test). An arterial PO_2 of <100 in the absence of clear-cut lung disease (a "failed" hyperoxia test) is most likely due to intracardiac right-to-left shunting and is virtually diagnostic of cyanotic congenital heart disease. Patients who have an arterial PO_2 between 100 and 250 **may** have structural heart disease with complete intracardiac mixing and greatly increased pulmonary blood flow, as is occasionally seen with single-ventricle complexes such as hypoplastic left heart syndrome. **The neonate who "fails" a hyperoxia test is very likely to have congenital heart disease involving ductal-dependent systemic or pulmonary blood flow and should receive PGE$_1$ until anatomic definition can be accomplished** (see section V.B.2).

B. **Stabilization and transport.** On the basis of the initial evaluation, if an infant has been identified as likely to have congenital heart disease, further medical management must be planned as well as arrangements made for a definitive anatomic diagnosis. This may involve transport of the neonate to another medical center where a pediatric cardiologist is available.

1. **Initial resuscitation.** For the neonate who presents with evidence of decreased cardiac output or shock, initial attention is devoted to the basics of advanced life support. A stable airway must be established and maintained as well as adequate ventilation. Reliable vascular access is essential, optimally including an arterial line. In the neonate, this can most reliably be accomplished through the umbilical vessels. Volume resuscitation, inotropic support, and correction of metabolic acidosis are required with the goal of improving cardiac output and tissue perfusion (see Chapter 40).

2. **PGE$_1$.** The neonate who "fails" a hyperoxia test (or has an equivocal result in addition to other signs or symptoms of congenital heart disease), as well as the neonate who presents in shock within the first 3 weeks of life, is highly likely to have congenital heart disease. These neonates will most likely have congenital lesions resulting in ductal-dependent systemic or pulmonary blood flow or have a PDA that aids in intercirculatory mixing.

PGE$_1$, administered as a continuous intravenous (IV) infusion, has important side effects that must be anticipated. PGE$_1$ causes apnea in 10% to 12% of neonates, usually within the first 6 hours of administration. Therefore, the infant who will be transferred to another institution while receiving PGE$_1$ should be intubated for maintenance of a stable airway before leaving the referring hospital. In infants who will not require transport, intubation may not be required but continuous cardiorespiratory monitoring is essential. In addition, PGE$_1$ typically causes peripheral vasodilation and subsequent hypotension in many infants. A separate IV line should be secured for volume administration in any infant receiving PGE$_1$, especially those who require transport.

Specific information regarding other adverse reactions, dose, and administration of PGE$_1$ is in section VIII.A.

The need to begin a PGE$_1$ infusion cannot be overemphasized in any neonate in whom congenital heart disease is strongly suspected (i.e., a failed hyperoxia test and/or severe, acute CHF). In the neonate with ductal-dependent pulmonary blood flow, oxygen saturation will typically improve and the pulmonary blood flow will remain secure until an anatomic diagnosis and plans for surgery are made. In neonates with transposition of the great arteries, maintenance of a patent ductus improves intercirculatory mixing. Most important, **neonates who present in shock in the first few weeks of life have duct-dependent**

systemic blood flow until proved otherwise; resuscitation will not be successful unless the ductus arteriosus is opened. In these cases, it is appropriate to begin an infusion of PGE_1 even **before** a precise anatomic diagnosis can be made by echocardiography.

It is prudent to remeasure arterial blood gases and reassess perfusion, vital signs, and acid–base status within 15 to 30 minutes of starting a PGE_1 infusion. Rarely, a patient's clinical status may worsen after beginning PGE_1. This is usually due to lesions with left atrial hypertension: hypoplastic left heart syndrome with a restrictive PFO, infradiaphragmatic TAPVR, mitral atresia with a restrictive PFO, transposition of the great arteries with intact ventricular septum and a restrictive PFO, and some cases of Ebstein anomaly (see section VI.B.5). In these lesions, deterioration on PGE_1 is often a helpful diagnostic finding, and **urgent** plans for echocardiography and possible interventional catheterization or surgery should be made.

3. **Inotropic agents.** Continuous infusions of inotropic agents, usually the sympathomimetic amines, can improve myocardial performance as well as perfusion of vital organs and the periphery. Care should be taken to replete intravascular volume before institution of vasoactive agents. **Dopamine** is a precursor of norepinephrine and stimulates β_1, dopaminergic, and α-adrenergic receptors in a dose-dependent manner. Dopamine can be expected to increase mean arterial pressure, improve ventricular function, and improve urine output with a low incidence of side effects at doses <10 µg/kg/minute. **Dobutamine** is an analog of dopamine, with predominantly β_1 effects and relatively weak β_2 and α-receptor stimulating activity. In comparison with dopamine, dobutamine lacks renal vasodilating properties, has less chronotropic effect (in adult patients), and does not depend on norepinephrine release from peripheral nerves for its effect. There are few published data available concerning the use of dobutamine in neonates, although clinical experience has been favorable. A combination of low-dose dopamine (up to 5 µg/kg/minute) and dobutamine may be used to minimize the potential peripheral vasoconstriction induced by high doses of dopamine while maximizing the dopaminergic effects on the renal circulation. See section VIII.B for details of administration of inotropic agents and additional pharmacologic agents (see Chapter 40).

4. **Transport.** After initial stabilization, the neonate with suspected congenital heart disease often needs to be transferred to an institution that provides subspecialty care in pediatric cardiology and cardiac surgery. A successful transport actually involves two transitions of care for the neonate: (i) from the referring hospital staff to the transport team and (ii) from the transport team staff to the accepting hospital staff. The need for accurate, detailed, and complete communication of information between all of these teams cannot be overemphasized. If possible, the pediatric cardiologist who will be caring for the patient should be included in the discussions of care while the neonate is still at the referring hospital.

Reliable **vascular access** should be secured for the neonate receiving continuous infusions of PGE_1 or inotropic agents. Umbilical lines placed for resuscitation and stabilization should be left in place for transport; the neonate with congenital heart disease may potentially require cardiac catheterization through this route. The umbilical venous catheter should be at the inferior vena cava (IVC)—right atrial junction to ensure that access to the heart via this route is possible.

Particular attention should be paid to the patient's airway and respiratory effort before transport. In general, all neonates receiving a PGE_1 infusion should be **intubated for transport** (see section V.B.2). Neonates with probable or definite congenital heart disease will most likely require surgical or interventional catheterization management during the hospitalization; therefore, it is likely that they will be intubated at some point. All intubated patients should have gastric decompression by nasogastric or orogastric tube.

Acid–base status and oxygen delivery should be checked with an arterial blood gas before transport. Supplemental oxygen at or near 100% is often **not** the inspired oxygen concentration of choice for the neonate with congenital heart disease (see section VI for details of lesion-specific care). This management decision for transport is particularly important for those infants with duct-dependent systemic blood flow and complete intracardiac mixing with single-ventricle physiology and emphasizes the need to consult with a pediatric cardiologist before transport to achieve optimal intratransport patient care.

Finally, it is important to remember in neonates that **hypotension** is a late finding in shock. Therefore, other signs of incipient decompensation, such as persistent tachycardia and poor tissue perfusion, are important to note and treat before transport. Before leaving the referring hospital, the patient's current hemodynamic status (distal perfusion, heart rate, systemic blood pressure, acid–base status, etc.) should be reassessed and relayed to the receiving hospital team.

C. Diagnosis confirmation

1. **Echocardiography.** Two-dimensional echocardiography, supplemented with Doppler and color Doppler has become the primary diagnostic tool for anatomic definition in pediatric cardiology. Echocardiography provides information about the structure and function of the heart and great vessels in a timely fashion. Although not an invasive test *per se*, a complete echocardiogram on a newborn suspected of having congenital heart disease may take an hour or more to perform and may therefore not be well tolerated by a sick and/or premature newborn. Temperature instability due to exposure during this extended time of examination may be a problem in the neonate. Extension of the neck for suprasternal notch views of the aortic arch may be problematic, particularly in the neonate with respiratory distress or with a tenuous airway. Therefore, in sick neonates, **close monitoring by a medical staff person other** than the one performing the echocardiogram is essential, with attention to vital signs, respiratory status, temperature, etc.

2. **Cardiac catheterization**
   a. Indications (Table 41.8). Neonatal cardiac catheterization has changed a great deal in its focus. In the current era, cardiac catheterization is rarely necessary for anatomic definition of intracardiac structures

Table 41.8. Indications for Neonatal Catheterization

Interventions

Therapeutic

  Balloon atrial septostomy

  Balloon pulmonary valvuloplasty

  Balloon aortic valvuloplasty*

  Balloon angioplasty of native coarctation of the aorta*

  Coil embolization of abnormal vascular communications

  Radiofrequency perforation of the atretic pulmonary valve*

  Device closure of the patent ductus arteriosus*

  Stent implant in the ductus arteriosus*

Diagnostic

  Endomyocardial biopsy

Anatomic definition (not visualized by echocardiography)

Coronary arteries

  Pulmonary atresia/intact ventricular septum

  Transposition of the great arteries

  Tetralogy of Fallot

Aortic to pulmonary artery collateral vessels

  Tetralogy of Fallot

  Pulmonary atresia

Distal pulmonary artery anatomy

Hemodynamic measurements

*These interventions have alternative surgical options, and utilization is based on institutional experience.

(although catheterization is still necessary for definition of the distal pulmonary arteries, aortopulmonary collaterals, and certain types of coronary artery anomalies) or for physiologic assessment as Doppler technology has assumed an increasingly important role in this regard. Increasingly, catheterization is performed for catheter-directed therapy of congenital lesions. See Figure 41.1 for normal newborn oxygen saturation and pressure measurements obtained during cardiac catheterization.

Normal Newborn

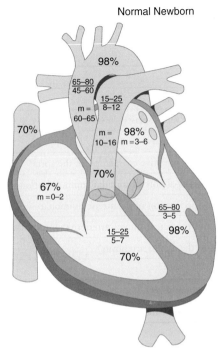

Figure 41.1. Typical hemodynamic measurements obtained at cardiac catheterization in a newborn, term infant without congenital or acquired heart disease. In this (and subsequent diagrams), oxygen saturations are shown as percentages, and typical hemodynamic pressure measurements in mm Hg are shown. In this example, the transition from fetal to infant physiology is complete; the pulmonary vascular resistance has fallen, the ductus arteriosus has closed, and there is no significant shunt at the foramen ovale. m, mean value.

b. Interventional catheterization. Since the first balloon dilation of the pulmonary artery reported by Kan in 1982, balloon valvuloplasty has become the procedure of choice in many types of valvar lesions, even extending to critical lesions in the neonate. Balloon valvuloplasty is considered the initial treatment of choice for both pulmonary and aortic stenosis, with >90% immediate success rate in the neonate. The application of balloon dilation of native coarctation of the aorta is controversial (see the subsequent text) and is typically utilized in select circumstances when surgery is contraindicated or high risk. The recent introduction of biodegradable stents for coronary artery applications may provide an attractive alternative to surgery for coarctation when these products become available in larger sizes. Other neonatal catheterization procedures include balloon atrial septostomy, radiofrequency (RF) perforation of the pulmonary valve in pulmonary atresia with intact ventricular septum, and closure of the persistent ductus arteriosus.

c. Preparation for catheterization. Catheterization in the neonate is not without its attendant risks; young age, small size, and interventional procedures are risk factors for complications. With appropriate anticipatory care, complications can be minimized. In addition to basic medical stabilization (see section V.B), specific attention to airway management is crucial. Sedation and analgesia are necessary but will depress the respiratory drive in the neonate. In most centers, neonatal catheterization will utilize intubation and mechanical ventilation, especially if an intervention is contemplated.

Supervision of the neonate undergoing catheterization should also include periodic evaluation of the patient's body temperature, acid–base status, serum glucose, and monitoring of blood loss. All infants undergoing interventional catheterization should have 10 to 25 mL/kg packed red blood cells (PRBCs) typed and cross-matched **in the catheterization laboratory** during the procedure. IV lines are recommended in the upper extremities or head (because the lower body will be draped and inaccessible during the case) in order to provide unobstructed access for medications, volume infusions, etc. Finally, the neonate may have the catheterization performed through umbilical vessels that were previously used for the administration of fluid, glucose, PGE_1, inotropic agents, or blood administration. Therefore, a peripheral line should be started and medications changed to that site before transfer of the neonate to the cardiac catheterization laboratory.

Consultation with the pediatric cardiologist who will be performing the case beforehand will help clarify these issues and allow the infant to be well prepared and monitored during the case.

VI. "LESION-SPECIFIC" CARE FOLLOWING ANATOMIC DIAGNOSIS

A. **Duct-dependent systemic blood flow.** Commonly referred to as **left-sided obstructive lesions**, this group of lesions includes a spectrum of hypoplasia of left-sided structures of the heart ranging from isolated coarctation of the aorta to hypoplastic left heart syndrome. These infants typically present in cardiovascular collapse as the ductus arteriosus closes, with resultant systemic hypoperfusion; they may also present more insidiously with symptoms of CHF (see section IV.B). Although all infants with significant left-sided lesions and duct-dependent systemic blood flow require prostaglandin-induced patency of the ductus arteriosus as part of the initial management, additional care varies somewhat with each lesion.

1. **Aortic stenosis** (Fig. 41.2). Morphologic abnormalities of the aortic valve may range from a bicuspid, nonobstructive, functionally normal valve to a unicuspid, markedly deformed and severely obstructive valve, which greatly limits systemic cardiac output from the left ventricle. By convention, "severe" aortic stenosis is defined as a mean systolic gradient from left ventricle to ascending aorta of 40–50 mm Hg. "Critical" aortic stenosis results from severe anatomic obstruction with accompanying left ventricular failure and/or shock, regardless of the measured gradient. Patients with critical aortic stenosis have severe obstruction present *in utero* (usually due to a unicuspid, "platelike" valve), with resultant left ventricular hypertrophy and, frequently, endocardial fibroelastosis.

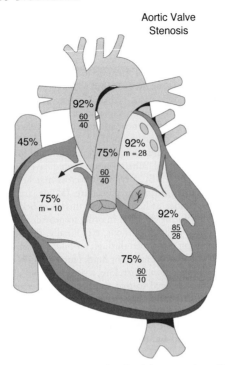

Figure 41.2. Critical aortic valve stenosis with a closed ductus arteriosus. Typical anatomic and hemodynamic findings include (i) a morphologically abnormal, stenotic valve; (ii) poststenotic dilatation of the ascending aorta; (iii) elevated left ventricular end diastolic pressure and left atrial pressures contributing to pulmonary edema (mild pulmonary venous and arterial desaturation); (iv) a left-to-right shunt at the atrial level (note increase in oxygen saturation from superior vena cava to right atrium); (v) pulmonary artery hypertension (also secondary to the elevated left atrial pressure); and (vi) only a modest (25 mm Hg) gradient across valve. The low measured gradient (despite severe anatomic obstruction) across the aortic valve is due to a severely limited cardiac output, as evidenced by the low mixed venous oxygen saturation (45%) in the superior vena cava. m, mean value.

Associated left-sided abnormalities such as mitral valve disease and co-arctation are not uncommon. Following closure of the ductus, the left ventricle must supply all of the systemic cardiac output. In cases of severe myocardial dysfunction, clinical CHF or shock will become apparent.

Initial management of the severely affected infant includes treatment of shock, stable vascular access, airway management and mechanical ventilation, sedation and muscle paralysis, inotropic support, and institution of PGE_1. Positive end-expiratory pressure (PEEP) is helpful to overcome pulmonary venous desaturation from pulmonary edema secondary to left atrial hypertension. For a patient with critical aortic stenosis to benefit from a PGE_1 infusion, there must be a small PFO to allow effective systemic blood flow (pulmonary venous return) to cross the atrial septum and ultimately enter the systemic vascular bed through the ductus. Inspired oxygen should be limited to a fractional concentration of inspired oxygen (FiO$_2$) of 0.5 to 0.6 unless severe hypoxemia is present.

Following anatomic definition of left ventricular size, mitral valve, and aortic arch anatomy by echocardiography, cardiac catheterization or surgery should be performed as soon as possible to perform aortic valvotomy. With either type of therapy, patient outcome will depend largely on (i) the degree of relief of the obstruction, (ii) the degree of aortic regurgitation, (iii) associated cardiac lesions (especially left ventricular size), and (iv) the severity of end-organ dysfunction secondary to the initial presentation (e.g., necrotizing enterocolitis or renal failure). All patients with aortic stenosis will require lifelong follow-up because stenosis frequently recurs. Multiple procedures in childhood are possible, if not likely.

2. **Coarctation of the aorta** (Fig. 41.3) is an anatomic narrowing of the descending aorta, most commonly at the site of insertion of the ductus arteriosus (i.e., "juxtaductal"). Additional cardiac abnormalities are common, including bicuspid aortic valve (present in 80% of patients) and ventricular septal defect (present in 40% of patients). In addition, hypoplasia or obstruction of other left-sided structures including the mitral valve, the left ventricle, and the aortic valve are not uncommon and must be evaluated during the initial echocardiographic evaluation.

In utero, systemic blood flow to the lower body is through the PDA. Following ductal closure in the newborn with a critical coarctation, the left ventricle must suddenly generate adequate pressure and volume to pump the entire cardiac output past a significant point of obstruction. This sudden pressure load may be poorly tolerated by the neonatal myocardium, and the neonate may become rapidly and critically ill because of lower body hypoperfusion.

As in critical aortic stenosis, initial management of the severely affected infant includes treatment of shock, stable vascular access, airway management and mechanical ventilation, moderate supplemental oxygen, sedation and muscle paralysis, inotropic support, and institution of PGE$_1$. PEEP is helpful to overcome pulmonary venous desaturation from pulmonary edema secondary to left atrial hypertension. In some infants, PGE$_1$ is unsuccessful in opening the ductus arteriosus.

In infants with symptomatic coarctation, surgical repair is performed as soon as the infant has been resuscitated and medically stabilized. Usually the procedure is performed through a left lateral thoracotomy incision. In infants with symptomatic coarctation and a large, coexisting ventricular septal defect, consideration is given to repair both defects in the initial procedure through a median sternotomy. Alternatively, a pulmonary artery band may be placed at the time of coarctation repair to protect from excessive pulmonary blood flow until the ventricular septal defect can be addressed at a later age. Balloon dilation of native coarctation is controversial because of the high incidence of restenosis and aneurysm formation, especially given the safe and effective surgical alternative.

3. **Interrupted aortic arch** (Fig. 41.4) consists of atresia of a segment of the aortic arch. There are three anatomic subtypes of interrupted aortic arch based on the location of the interruption: distal to the left

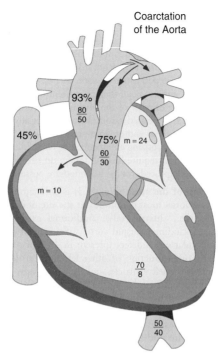

Coarctation
of the Aorta

93%
80/50

45%

75% m = 24
60/30

m = 10

70/8

50/40

Figure 41.3. Coarctation of the aorta in a critically ill neonate with a nearly closed ductus arteriosus. Typical anatomic and hemodynamic findings include (i) "juxtaductal" site of the coarctation, (ii) a bicommissural aortic valve (seen in 80% of patients with coarctation), (iii) narrow pulse pressure in the descending aorta and lower body, and (iv) a bidirectional shunt at the ductus arteriosus. As in critical aortic stenosis (see Fig. 41.2), there is an elevated left atrial pressure, pulmonary edema, a left-to-right shunt at the atrial level, pulmonary artery hypertension, and only a moderate (30 mm Hg) gradient across the arch obstruction. The low measured gradient (despite severe anatomic obstruction) across the aortic arch is due to low cardiac output. m, mean value.

subclavian artery (type A), between the left subclavian artery and the left carotid artery (type B), and between the innominate artery and the left carotid artery (type C). Type B is the most common variety. More than 99% of these patients have a ventricular septal defect; abnormalities of the aortic valve and narrowed subaortic regions are associated anomalies.

Infants with interrupted aortic arch are completely dependent on a PDA for lower body blood flow and, therefore, become critically ill when the ductus closes. Immediate management is similar to that described for coarctation (see section VI.A.2); PGE_1 infusion is essential. All other resuscitative measures will be ineffective if blood flow to the lower body is not restored. Oxygen saturations should be measured in the upper body; pulse oximetry readings in the lower body are reflective of the pulmonary artery oxygen saturation and are typically lower than

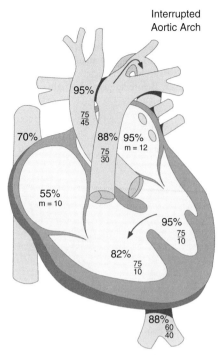

Figure 41.4. Interrupted aortic arch with restrictive patent ductus arteriosus. Typical anatomic and hemodynamic findings include (i) atresia of a segment of the aortic arch between the left subclavian artery and the left common carotid (the most common type of interrupted aortic arch—break "type B"), (ii) a posterior malalignment of the conal septum resulting in a large ventricular septal defect and a narrow subaortic area, (iii) a bicuspid aortic valve occurs in 60% of patients, (iv) systemic pressure in the right ventricle and pulmonary artery (due to the large, nonrestrictive ventricular septal defect), (v) increased oxygen saturation in the pulmonary artery due to left-to-right shunting at the ventricular level, (vi) "differential cyanosis" with a lower oxygen saturation in the descending aorta due to a right-to-left shunt at the patent ductus. Note the lower blood pressure in the descending aorta due to constriction of the ductus; opening the ductus with prostaglandin E_1 (PGE_1) results in equal upper and lower extremity blood pressures but continued "differential cyanosis." m, mean value.

that distributed to the central nervous system and coronary arteries. High concentrations of inspired oxygen may result in low pulmonary vascular resistance, a large left-to-right shunt, and a "run-off" during diastole from the lower body to the pulmonary circulation. Inspired oxygen levels should therefore be minimized, aiming for normal (95%) oxygen saturations in the **upper** body.

Surgical reconstruction should be performed as soon as metabolic acidosis (if present) has resolved, end-organ dysfunction is improving, and the patient is hemodynamically stable. The repair typically entails a corrective approach through a median sternotomy, with arch reconstruction (usually an end-to-end anastomosis) and closure of the ventricular septal defect.

4. **Hypoplastic left heart syndrome** (Fig. 41.5A and Fig. 41.5B) represents a heterogeneous group of anatomic abnormalities in which there is a small-to-absent left ventricle with hypoplastic to atretic mitral and aortic valves. Before surgery, the right ventricle supplies both the

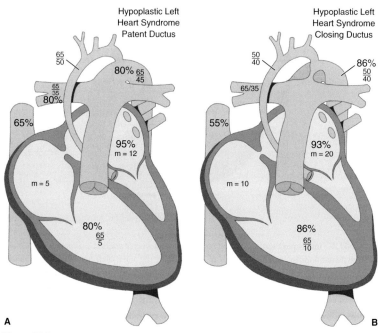

Figure 41.5. **A:** Hypoplastic left heart syndrome in a 24-hour-old patient with falling pulmonary vascular resistance and a nonrestrictive ductus arteriosus. Typical anatomic and hemodynamic findings include (i) atresia or hypoplasia of the left ventricle, mitral, and aortic valves; (ii) a diminutive ascending aorta and transverse aortic arch, usually with an associated coarctation; (iii) coronary blood flow is usually *retrograde* from the ductus arteriosus through the tiny ascending aorta; (iv) systemic arterial oxygen saturation (in FiO$_2$ of 0.21) of 80%, reflecting relatively balanced systemic and pulmonary blood flows—the pulmonary artery and aortic saturations are equal (see text); (v) pulmonary hypertension secondary to the nonrestrictive ductus arteriosus; (vi) minimal left atrial hypertension; and (vii) normal systemic cardiac output (note superior vena cava oxygen saturation of 65%) and blood pressure (65/45 mm Hg). **B:** Acute circulatory collapse following constriction of the ductus arteriosus in hypoplastic left heart syndrome. These neonates are typically in shock with poor perfusion, tachycardia, acidosis, and in respiratory distress. The anatomic features are similar to those in Figure 41.5A, with the exception of the narrowed ductus arteriosus. Note (i) the low cardiac output (as evidenced by the low mixed venous oxygen saturation in the superior vena cava of 55%); (ii) narrow pulse pressure; (iii) elevated atrial and ventricular end-diastolic pressure—elevated left atrial pressure may cause pulmonary edema (note left atrial saturation of 93%); and (iv) significantly increased pulmonary blood flow, as reflected in an arterial oxygen saturation (in FiO$_2$ of 0.21) of 86%. m, mean value.

pulmonary and systemic blood flows (through the PDA) with the proportion of cardiac output going to either circuit dependent on the relative resistances of these vascular beds.

As the pulmonary vascular resistance begins to fall (see Fig. 41.5A), blood flow is preferentially directed to the pulmonary circulation at the expense of the systemic circulation. As systemic blood flow decreases, stroke volume and heart rate increase as a mechanism to preserve systemic cardiac output. The right ventricle becomes progressively volume overloaded with mildly elevated end-diastolic and left atrial pressures. The infant may be tachypneic or in respiratory distress, and hepatomegaly may develop. The greater proportion of pulmonary venous return in the mixed ventricular blood results in mildly decreased systemic arterial oxygen saturation (80%), and visible cyanosis may be mild or absent. Not infrequently, these infants are discharged from the nursery as normal newborns. A goal of neonatal pulse oximetry screening is to detect this desaturation before discharge.

At this point, the continued fall in pulmonary vascular resistance results in a progressive increase in pulmonary blood flow and relative decrease in systemic cardiac output. As the total RV output is limited by heart rate and stroke volume, there is the onset of clinically apparent CHF, RV dilation and dysfunction, progressive tricuspid regurgitation, poor peripheral perfusion with metabolic acidosis, decreased urine output, and pulmonary edema. Arterial oxygen saturation approaches 90%.

Alternatively, a sudden deterioration takes place with rapidly progressive CHF and shock as the ductus arteriosus constricts (see Fig. 41.5B). There is decreased systemic perfusion and increased pulmonary blood flow, which is largely independent of the pulmonary vascular resistance. The peripheral pulses are weak to absent. Renal, hepatic, coronary, and central nervous system perfusion is compromised, possibly resulting in acute tubular necrosis, necrotizing enterocolitis, or cerebral infarction or hemorrhage. A vicious cycle may also result from inadequate retrograde perfusion of the ascending aorta (coronary blood supply), with further myocardial dysfunction and continued compromise of coronary blood flow. The pulmonary to systemic flow ratio approaches infinity as systemic blood flow nears zero. Therefore, one has the paradoxical presentation of profound metabolic acidosis in the face of a relatively high PO_2 (70 to 100 mm Hg).

The arterial blood gas may represent the single best indicator of hemodynamic stability. Low arterial saturation (75% to 80%) with normal pH indicates an acceptable balance of systemic and pulmonary blood flow with adequate peripheral perfusion, whereas elevated oxygen saturation (>90%) with acidosis represents significantly increased pulmonary and decreased systemic flow with probable myocardial dysfunction and secondary effects on other organ systems.

Resuscitation of these neonates involves pharmacologic maintenance of ductal patency with PGE_1 and ventilatory maneuvers to **increase** pulmonary resistance. In our experience, a mild respiratory acidosis (e.g., pH 7.35) is appropriate for most of these infants. It is important to note that **hyperventilation and/or supplemental oxygen**

is usually of no significant benefit and may be harmful by causing excessive pulmonary vasodilation and pulmonary blood flow at the expense of the systemic blood flow.

Hypotension in these infants is more frequently caused by increased pulmonary blood flow (at the expense of systemic flow) rather than intrinsic myocardial dysfunction. Although small-to-moderate doses of inotropic agents are frequently beneficial, **large doses of inotropic agents may have a deleterious effect**, depending on the relative effects on the systemic and pulmonary vascular beds. Preferential selective elevations of systemic vascular tone will secondarily increase pulmonary blood flow, and careful monitoring of mean arterial blood pressure and arterial oxygen saturation is warranted.

Similar to the patient with critical aortic stenosis, in order for the neonate with hypoplastic left heart syndrome to benefit from a PGE_1 infusion, there must be at least a small PFO to allow for effective systemic blood flow (pulmonary venous return) to cross the atrial septum and ultimately enter the systemic vascular bed through the ductus arteriosus. An infant with hypoplastic left heart syndrome and a severely restrictive or absent PFO will be critically ill with profound cyanosis (oxygen saturation <60% to 65%) and will not improve after the institution of PGE_1. **In these neonates, emergent balloon dilation of the atrial septum, or balloon atrial septostomy, may be necessary.**

Medical therapy may be briefly palliative; however, surgical therapy is necessary for survival of infants with hypoplastic left heart syndrome. After a period of medical stabilization and support to allow for recovery of ischemic organ system injury (particularly of the kidneys, liver, central nervous system, and the heart), surgical relief of left-sided obstruction is required. Surgical intervention involves either staged reconstruction (with a neonatal Norwood procedure followed by the Glenn and Fontan operations later in infancy and childhood, respectively) or neonatal cardiac transplantation. Recent results from both reconstructive surgery and transplantation have vastly improved the outlook for infants born with this previously 100% fatal condition.

B. **Duct-dependent pulmonary blood flow.** This underlying physiology is shared by a diverse group of lesions with the common finding of restricted pulmonary blood flow due to severe pulmonary stenosis or pulmonary atresia. Closure of the ductus arteriosus results in marked cyanosis.

1. **Pulmonary stenosis** (Fig. 41.6) with obstruction to pulmonary blood flow may occur at several levels: (i) within the body of the right ventricle, (ii) at the pulmonary valve (as pictured in Fig. 41.6), and (iii) in the peripheral pulmonary arteries. Pulmonary valve stenosis with an intact ventricular septum is the second most common form of congenital heart disease; "critical" obstruction occurs more rarely. Grading of the degree of pulmonary stenosis is similar to that of aortic stenosis (see section VI.A.1) with severe pulmonary stenosis defined as a peak systolic gradient from right ventricle to pulmonary artery of 60 mm Hg or more. By convention, "critical" pulmonary stenosis is defined as severe valvular obstruction with associated hypoxemia due to a right-to-left

Pulmonary Valve
Stenosis

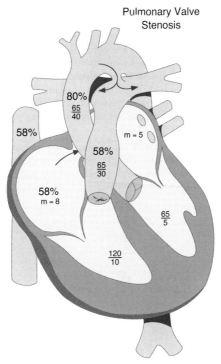

Figure 41.6. Critical pulmonary valve stenosis in a neonate with a nonrestrictive patent ductus arteriosus while receiving prostaglandin E_1 (PGE$_1$). Typical anatomic and hemodynamic findings include (i) thickened, stenotic pulmonary valve; (ii) poststenotic dilatation of the main pulmonary artery with normal-sized branch pulmonary arteries; (iii) right ventricular hypertrophy with suprasystemic pressure; (iv) a right-to-left shunt at the atrial level through the patent foramen ovale with systemic desaturation (80%); (v) suprasystemic right ventricular (RV) pressure with a 55 mm Hg peak systolic ejection gradient; (vi) systemic pulmonary artery pressure (due to the nonrestrictive patent ductus); and (vii) pulmonary blood flow through the patent ductus arteriosus. m, mean value.

shunt at the foramen ovale. Critical pulmonary stenosis may be associated with hypoplasia of the right ventricle and/or tricuspid valve and significant RV hypertrophy. The pressure in the right ventricle is often higher than the left ventricular pressure (i.e., suprasystemic) in order to eject blood through the severe narrowing. Due to the longstanding (*in utero*) increased RV pressure, there is typically a hypertrophied, non-compliant right ventricle with a resultant increase in right atrial filling pressure. When right atrial pressure exceeds left atrial pressure, a right-to-left shunt at the foramen ovale results in cyanosis and hypoxemia. There may be associated RV dysfunction and/or tricuspid regurgitation.

After initial stabilization of the patient and definitive diagnosis by echocardiography, transcatheter balloon valvotomy is the treatment of choice for this lesion. Surgical valvotomy is a rare alternative. Despite successful relief of the obstruction during catheterization, cyanosis is usually not completely relieved but rather resolves gradually over the first weeks of life as the right ventricle becomes more compliant, tricuspid regurgitation lessens, and there is less right-to-left shunting at the atrial level. Due to subvalvular outflow tract hypertrophy and persistence of a dynamic obstructive pattern, short-term treatment with a β-blocker is sometimes employed. Successful balloon valvuloplasty is associated with excellent clinical results among patients; the need for repeat procedures is <10%.

2. **Pulmonary atresia with intact ventricular septum** (Fig. 41.7) is comparable to hypoplastic left heart syndrome in that there is atresia of the pulmonary valve with varying degrees of RV and tricuspid valve hypoplasia. Perhaps the most important associated anomaly is the presence of

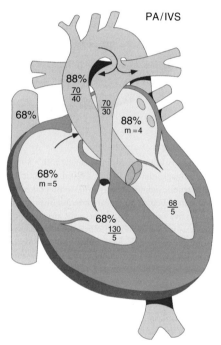

Figure 41.7. Pulmonary atresia (PA) with intact ventricular septum (IVS) in a neonate with a nonrestrictive patent ductus arteriosus while receiving prostaglandin E_1 (PGE$_1$). Typical anatomic and hemodynamic findings include (i) hypertrophied, hypoplastic right ventricle; (ii) hypoplastic tricuspid valve and pulmonary annulus; (iii) atresia of the pulmonary valve with no antegrade flow; (iv) suprasystemic right ventricular pressure; (v) pulmonary blood flow through the patent ductus; and (vi) right-to-left shunt at the atrial level with systemic desaturation. Many patients have significant coronary abnormalities with sinusoidal or fistulous connections to the hypertensive right ventricle or significant coronary stenoses (not shown). m, mean value.

coronary artery–myocardial–RV sinusoidal connections. The coronary arteries may be very abnormal, including areas of stenoses or atresia. Myocardial perfusion therefore may be dependent on the hypertensive right ventricle to supply the distal coronary arteries (RV-dependent coronary arteries). Surgical relief of the pulmonary atresia in this patient subset (with a RV-to-pulmonary artery connection) could lead to myocardial infarction and death because blood would flow preferentially to the pulmonary arteries instead of the distal coronary segments that are dependent on the previously hypertensive right ventricle. The presence of sinusoidal connections between the right ventricle and the coronary arteries is associated with poorer long-term survival. Because there is no outlet of the right ventricle, there is typically suprasystemic pressure in the right ventricle and some tricuspid regurgitation. There is an obligatory right-to-left shunt at the atrial level, and pulmonary blood flow is entirely dependent on a PDA.

Although the cornerstone of initial management is PGE_1 infusion to maintain ductal patency, a more permanent and reliable form of pulmonary blood flow must be created for the infant to survive. Surgical management is often preceded by catheterization to define the coronary artery anatomy. In patients without significant coronary abnormalities, pulmonary blood flow is established by creating an outflow for the right ventricle. In the setting of a "platelike" atresia where a well-formed outflow is present, with a mobile but imperforate valve plate, a catheter can be placed in the outflow tract and an RF wire can be used to perforate the valve, followed by balloon pulmonary valvuloplasty. Thus, the atresia is addressed and some patients may avoid neonatal surgical intervention. Alternatively, surgical pulmonary valvotomy and/or RV outflow tract augmentation can be performed. If additional patient growth is desired prior to surgical intervention, or if pulmonary valvotomy (catheter- or surgical-based) is insufficient, a systemic-to-pulmonary artery shunt (most often a Blalock-Taussig shunt) is constructed to augment pulmonary blood flow. In patients who undergo RF perforation of the valve and require additional pulmonary blood flow, stent implantation in the ductus arteriosus has been used to provide additional pulmonary blood flow. In patients with RV-dependent coronary arteries, a systemic-to-pulmonary artery shunt is the typical procedure performed.

3. **Tricuspid atresia** (Fig. 41.8) involves absence of the tricuspid valve and therefore no direct communication from right atrium to right ventricle. The right ventricle may be severely hypoplastic or absent. More than 90% of patients have an associated ventricular septal defect, allowing blood to pass from the left ventricle to the RV outflow and pulmonary arteries. Most patients have some form of additional pulmonary stenosis. In 70% of cases, the great arteries are normally aligned with the ventricles; however, in the remaining 30%, the great arteries are transposed. An atrial level communication is necessary for blood to travel right to left because no source of right-sided inflow is present; right-sided outflow is derived from the left-heart. In patients with normally related great arteries, pulmonary blood flow is derived from the right ventricle;

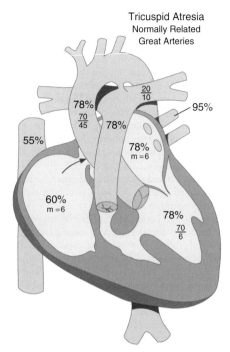

Figure 41.8. Tricuspid atresia with normally related great arteries and a small patent ductus arteriosus. Typical anatomic and hemodynamic findings include (i) atresia of the tricuspid valve; (ii) hypoplasia of the right ventricle; (iii) restriction to pulmonary blood flow at two levels: a (usually) small ventricular septal defect and a stenotic pulmonary valve; (iv) all systemic venous return must pass through the patent foramen ovale to reach the left ventricle; (v) complete mixing at the left atrial level, with systemic oxygen saturation of 78% (in FiO_2 of 0.21), suggesting balanced systemic and pulmonary blood flow ("single ventricle physiology"—see text). m, mean value.

if the right ventricle (or its connection with the left ventricle through a ventricular septal defect) is severely diminutive, the pulmonary blood flow may be ductal-dependent; closure of the ductus arteriosus leads to profound hypoxemia and acidosis.

Immediate medical management is primarily aimed at maintenance of adequate pulmonary blood flow. In the usual case of severe pulmonary stenosis and limited pulmonary blood flow, PGE_1 infusion maintains pulmonary blood flow through the ductus arteriosus. Surgical creation of a more permanent source of pulmonary blood flow (usually a Blalock-Taussig shunt) is undertaken as soon as possible. More complex cases (e.g., with transposition) may require more extensive palliative procedures. Patients with adequate pulmonary blood flow, with a normal pulmonary valve and adequate pulmonary arteries, may develop hypoxemia in the subsequent weeks to months if the ventricular septal defect becomes smaller, thus restricting pulmonary blood flow.

Tetralogy of
Fallot

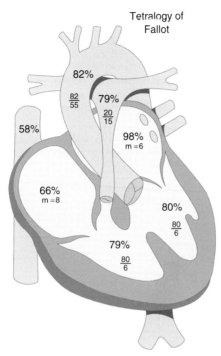

Figure 41.9. Tetralogy of Fallot. Typical anatomic and hemodynamic findings include (i) an anteriorly displaced infundibular septum, resulting in subpulmonary stenosis, a large ventricular septal defect, and overriding of the aorta over the muscular septum; (ii) hypoplasia of the pulmonary valve, main, and branch pulmonary arteries; (iii) equal right and left ventricular pressures; and (iv) a right-to-left shunt at ventricular level, with a systemic oxygen saturation of 82%.

4. **Tetralogy of Fallot** (Fig. 41.9) consists of RV outflow obstruction, a ventricular septal defect (anterior malalignment type), "overriding" of the aorta over the ventricular septum, and hypertrophy of the right ventricle. There is a wide spectrum of anatomic variation encompassing these findings, depending particularly on the site and severity of the RV outflow obstruction. The severely cyanotic neonate with tetralogy of Fallot most likely has severe RV outflow tract obstruction and a large right-to-left shunt at the ventricular level through the large ventricular septal defect. Pulmonary blood flow may be ductal-dependent.

Immediate medical management involves establishing adequate pulmonary blood flow, usually with PGE_1 infusion, although balloon dilation of the RV outflow tract has been used. Detailed anatomic definition particularly regarding coronary artery anatomy, the presence of additional ventricular septal defects, and the sources of pulmonary blood flow (systemic to pulmonary collateral vessels) is necessary before surgical intervention. If echocardiography is not able to fully show these details, then diagnostic catheterization is performed.

Surgical repair of the **asymptomatic** child with tetralogy of Fallot is usually recommended within the first 6 months of life. The **symptomatic** (i.e., severely cyanotic) neonate should have operative intervention. The decision whether to perform complete repair versus placement of a systemic-to-pulmonary artery shunt is dependent on the institution. Other interventions include stent implant in the ductus arteriosus to simulate a systemic-to-pulmonary artery shunt, or in the case of a severely hypoplastic pulmonary annulus, stent implant in the RV outflow tract has been employed.

5. **Ebstein anomaly** (Figs. 41.10A and 41.10B) is an uncommon and challenging anatomic lesion when it presents in the neonatal period.

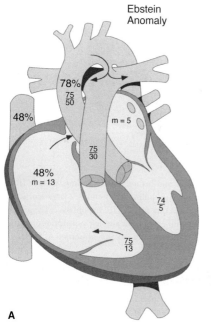

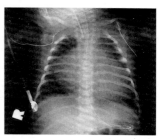

A   B

Figure 41.10. A: Ebstein anomaly (with large nonrestrictive ductus arteriosus). Typical anatomic and hemodynamic findings include (i) inferior displacement of the tricuspid valve into the right ventricle, which may also cause subpulmonary obstruction; (ii) diminutive muscular right ventricle; (iii) marked enlargement of the right atrium due to "atrialized" portion of right ventricle as well as tricuspid regurgitation; (iv) right-to-left shunting at the atrial level (note arterial oxygen saturation of 78%); (v) a left-to-right shunt and pulmonary hypertension secondary to a large patent ductus arteriosus supplying the pulmonary blood flow; and (vi) low cardiac output (note low mixed venous oxygen saturation in the superior vena cava). **B:** Chest radiograph in a neonate with severe Ebstein anomaly and no significant pulmonary blood flow from the ductus arteriosus. The cardiomegaly is due to marked dilation of the right atrium. The pulmonary vascular markings are diminished due to the decreased pulmonary blood flow. Hypoplasia of the lungs is common due to the large heart causing a "space-occupying lesion." m, mean value.

Anatomically, there is apical displacement of the tricuspid valve into the body of the right ventricle. The tricuspid valve is frequently regurgitant resulting in marked right atrial enlargement and a large right-to-left shunt at the atrial level; there is little forward flow out the RV outflow tract into the pulmonary circulation, often resulting in functional pulmonary atresia. The prognosis for neonates presenting with profound cyanosis due to Ebstein anomaly is very poor. Surgical options are limited and generally reserved for the severely symptomatic child. Further complicating the medical condition, Ebstein anomaly is often associated with Wolff-Parkinson-White (WPW) syndrome and supraventricular tachycardia (SVT).

Medical management is aimed at supporting the neonate through the initial period of transitional circulation. Because of elevated pulmonary vascular resistance, pulmonary blood flow may be severely limited with profound hypoxemia and acidosis as a result. Medical treatment includes treatment of pulmonary hypertension with oxygen, alkalosis, and inhaled nitric oxide (iNO) (see Chapter 36). If there is total pulmonary valve atresia, PGE_1 is used to maintain patency of the ductus arteriosus. However, the presence of pulmonary regurgitation makes the clinical management more complex. If the RV pressure is high (>20), the goal is to avoid PGE_1 and close the ductus (pharmacologically or surgically) to promote antegrade flow across the pulmonary valve. If the RV pressure is low then the RV may not be able to eject antegrade. This is the group with the worst prognosis (pulmonary regurgitation and low RV pressure). An important contributor to the high mortality rate in the neonate with severe Ebstein anomaly is the associated pulmonary hypoplasia that is present (due to the massively enlarged right heart *in utero*, see Fig. 41.10B).

C. **Parallel circulation/transposition of the great arteries** (Fig. 41.11). **Transposition of the great arteries** is defined as an aorta arising from the morphologic right ventricle and the pulmonary artery from the morphologic left ventricle. Approximately one-half of all patients with transposition have an associated ventricular septal defect.

In the usual arrangement, this creates a situation of "parallel circulations" with systemic venous return being pumped through the aorta back to the systemic circulation and pulmonary venous return being pumped through the pulmonary artery to the pulmonary circulation. Following separation from the placenta, neonates with transposition are dependent on mixing between the parallel systemic and pulmonary circulations in order for them to survive. In patients with an intact ventricular septum, this communication exists through the PDA and the PFO. These patients are usually clinically cyanotic within the first hours of life leading to their early diagnosis. Those infants with an associated ventricular septal defect typically have somewhat improved mixing between the systemic and pulmonary circulations and may not be as severely cyanotic.

In neonates with transposition of the great arteries and an intact ventricular septum, a very low arterial PaO_2 (15 to 20 torr) with high $PaCO_2$ (despite adequate chest motion and ventilation) and metabolic acidosis are markers for severely decreased effective pulmonary blood flow and need

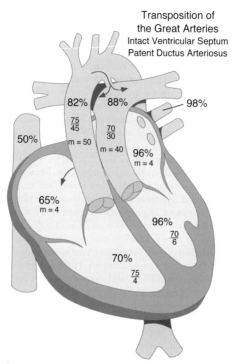

Figure 41.11. Transposition of the great arteries with an intact ventricular septum, a large patent ductus arteriosus (on prostaglandin E_1 [PGE_1]) and atrial septal defect (status postballoon atrial septostomy). Note the following: (i) the aorta arises from the anatomic right ventricle and the pulmonary artery from the anatomic left ventricle; (ii) "transposition physiology," with a higher oxygen saturation in the pulmonary artery than in the aorta; (iii) "mixing" between the parallel circulations (see text) at the atrial (after balloon atrial septostomy) and ductal levels; (iv) shunting from the left atrium to the right atrium through the atrial septal defect (not shown) with equalization of atrial pressures; (v) shunting from the aorta to the pulmonary artery through the ductus arteriosus; (vi) pulmonary hypertension due to a large ductus arteriosus. m, mean value.

urgent attention. The initial management of the severely hypoxemic patient with transposition includes (i) **ensure adequate mixing** between the two parallel circuits and (ii) **maximize mixed venous oxygen saturation**.

In patients who do not respond with an increased arterial oxygen saturation by opening of the ductus arteriosus with PGE_1 infusion (usually these neonates have very restrictive atrial defects and/or pulmonary hypertension), **the foramen ovale should be emergently enlarged by balloon atrial septostomy**. Hyperventilation and treatment with sodium bicarbonate are important maneuvers to promote alkalosis, lower pulmonary vascular resistance, and increase pulmonary blood flow (which increases atrial mixing following septostomy). A respiratory acidosis is particularly unfavorable.

In transposition of the great arteries, most of the systemic blood flow is recirculated systemic venous return. In the presence of poor mixing, much can be gained by increasing the mixed venous oxygen saturation, which is the **major determinant of systemic arterial oxygen saturation**. These maneuvers include (i) decreasing the whole body oxygen consumption (muscle relaxants, sedation, mechanical ventilation) and (ii) improving oxygen delivery (increase cardiac output with inotropic agents, increase oxygen-carrying capacity by treating anemia). Coexisting causes of pulmonary venous desaturation (e.g., pneumothorax) should also be sought and treated. Increasing the FiO_2 to 100% will have little effect on the arterial PO_2, unless it serves to lower pulmonary vascular resistance and increase pulmonary blood flow.

In the current era, definitive management is surgical correction with an arterial switch operation in the early neonatal period. If severe hypoxemia persists despite medical management, mechanical support with extracorporeal membrane oxygenation (ECMO) or an urgent arterial switch operation may be indicated.

D. **Lesions with complete intracardiac mixing**

1. **Truncus arteriosus** (Fig. 41.12) consists of a single great artery arising from the heart, which gives rise to (in order) the coronary arteries, the pulmonary arteries, and the brachiocephalic arteries. The truncal valve is often anatomically abnormal (only 50% are tricuspid) and is frequently thickened, stenotic, and/or regurgitant. A coexisting ventricular septal defect is present in >98% of cases. The aortic arch is right-sided in approximately one-third of cases; other arch anomalies such as hypoplasia, coarctation, and interruption are seen in 10% of cases. Extracardiac anomalies are present in 20% to 40% of cases. Thirty-five percent of patients with truncus arteriosus have a chromosome 22q11 deletion, detectable by fluorescence *in situ* hybridization (FISH) testing.

   The overwhelming majority of infants with truncus arteriosus present with symptoms of CHF in the first weeks of life. The infants may be somewhat cyanotic, but CHF symptoms and signs usually dominate. The pulmonary blood flow is increased, with significant pulmonary hypertension common. The natural history of truncus arteriosus is quite bleak. Left unrepaired, only 15% to 30% survive the first year of life. Furthermore, in survivors of the immediate neonatal period, the occurrence of accelerated irreversible pulmonary vascular disease is common, making surgical repair in the neonatal period (or as soon as the diagnosis is made) the treatment of choice. "Medical management" of heart failure would be considered only a temporizing measure until surgical correction can be accomplished.

2. **Total anomalous pulmonary venous connection** (Figs. 41.13A and 41.13B) occurs when all pulmonary veins drain into the systemic venous system with complete mixing of pulmonary and systemic venous return, usually in the right atrium. The systemic blood flow is therefore dependent on an obligate shunt through the PFO into the left heart. The anomalous connections of the pulmonary veins may be (i) supracardiac (usually into a vertical vein posterior to the left atrium that connects to

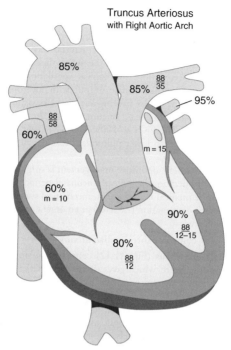

Figure 41.12. Truncus arteriosus (with right aortic arch). Typical anatomic and hemodynamic findings include (i) a single artery arises from the conotruncus giving rise to coronary arteries (not shown), pulmonary arteries, and brachiocephalic vessels; (ii) abnormal truncal valve (quadricuspid shown) with stenosis and/or regurgitation common; (iii) right-sided aortic arch (occurs in ~30% of cases); (iv) large conoventricular ventricular septal defect; (v) pulmonary artery hypertension with a large left-to-right shunt (note superior vena cava oxygen saturation of 60% and pulmonary artery oxygen saturation of 85%); and (vi) complete mixing (of the systemic and pulmonary venous return) occurs at the great vessel level. m, mean value.

the left innominate vein and the superior vena cava), (ii) cardiac (usually to the right atrium or coronary sinus), (iii) infradiaphragmatic (usually into the portal system), or (iv) mixed drainage.

In patients with total connection below the diaphragm, the pathway is frequently obstructed with severely limited pulmonary blood flow, pulmonary hypertension, and profound cyanosis. This form of total anomalous pulmonary venous connection is a surgical emergency, with minimal beneficial effects from medical management. Although PGE$_1$ will maintain ductal patency, the limitation of pulmonary blood flow in these patients is **not** due to limited antegrade flow into the pulmonary circuit but rather due to outflow obstruction at the pulmonary veins. In the current era of prostaglandin, ventilatory support, and advanced medical intensive care, obstructed total anomalous pulmonary venous connection represents one of the few remaining lesions that require

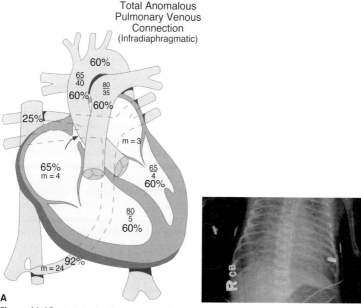

Figure 41.13. A: Infradiaphragmatic total anomalous pulmonary venous connection. Note the following: (i) pulmonary venous confluence does not connect with the left atrium but descends to connect with the portal circulation below the diaphragm. This connection is frequently severely obstructed; (ii) obstruction to pulmonary venous return results in significantly elevated pulmonary venous pressures, decreased pulmonary blood flow, pulmonary edema, and pulmonary venous desaturation (92%); (iii) systemic to suprasystemic pressure in the pulmonary artery (in the absence of a patent ductus arteriosus, pulmonary artery pressures may exceed systemic pressures when severe pulmonary venous obstruction is present); (iv) all systemic blood flow must be derived through a right-to-left shunt at the foramen ovale; and (v) nearly equal oxygen saturations in all chambers of the heart (i.e., complete mixing at right atrial level), with severe hypoxemia (systemic oxygen saturation 60%) and low cardiac output (mixed venous oxygen saturation 25%). **B:** Chest radiograph in a 16-hour-old neonate with severe infradiaphragmatic obstruction to pulmonary venous return. Note the pulmonary edema, small heart, and hyperinflated lungs (on mechanical ventilation). Despite high inflating and positive end-expiratory pressures and an FiO_2 of 1, the arterial blood gas revealed a pH of 7.02, arterial carbon dioxide tension ($PaCO_2$) of 84, and an arterial oxygen tension (PaO_2) of 23 torr. Emergent surgical management is indicated. m, mean value.

emergent, "middle of the night" surgical intervention. Early recognition of the problem (see Fig. 41.13B) and prompt surgical intervention (surgical anastomosis of the pulmonary venous confluence to the left atrium) are necessary in order for the infant to survive. Patients with a mild degree of obstruction typically have minimal symptoms, with many neonates escaping recognition until later in infancy when they present with signs and symptoms of CHF.

3. Complex single ventricles. There are multiple complex anomalies that share the common physiology of complete mixing of the systemic and pulmonary venous return, frequently with anomalous connections of the systemic and/or pulmonary veins and with obstruction to one of the great vessels (usually the pulmonary artery). In cases with associated polysplenia or asplenia and abnormalities of visceral situs, the term *heterotaxy syndrome* is frequently applied. Physiologically, systemic blood flow and pulmonary blood flow is determined by the balance of anatomic and/ or vascular resistance in the systemic and pulmonary circulations. In the well-balanced single ventricle, the oxygen saturation in the pulmonary artery and the aorta will be essentially the same (usually in the high 70% to low 80% range) with a normal pH on arterial blood gas ("single ventricle physiology"). It is beyond the scope of this chapter to define this heterogeneous group of patients further, although all will fail a hyperoxia test, most have significantly abnormal ECGs, and the diagnosis of complex congenital heart disease is rarely in doubt (even before anatomic confirmation with echocardiography). As there is complete mixing of venous return and essentially a single pumping chamber, initial management is similar to that described for hypoplastic left heart syndrome or pulmonary atresia with ventricular septal defect (see section VI.A.4).

E. Left-to-right shunt lesions. For the most part, infants with pure left-to-right shunt lesions are not diagnosed because of severe systemic illness but rather due to the finding of a murmur or symptoms of CHF usually occurring in the late neonatal period or beyond. The lesion of this group most likely to require attention in the neonatal nursery is that of a PDA.

1. PDA is not particularly common in term newborns and rarely causes CHF. However, the frequency that a premature neonate will develop a hemodynamically significant left-to-right shunt through a PDA is inversely proportional to advancing gestational age and weight (see Chapter 13).

The typical presentation of a PDA begins with a harsh systolic ejection murmur heard over the entire precordium but loudest at the left upper sternal border and left infraclavicular areas. As the pulmonary vascular resistance decreases, the intensity of the murmur increases and later becomes continuous (i.e., extends through the second heart sound). The peripheral pulses increase in amplitude ("bounding pulses"), the pulse pressure widens to >25 mm Hg, the precordial impulse becomes hyperdynamic, and the patient's respiratory status deteriorates (manifesting as tachypnea or apnea, carbon dioxide retention, and an increasing mechanical ventilation requirement). Serial chest x-rays show an increase in heart size, and the lungs may appear more radiopaque.

It is important to remember that this typical progression of clinical signs is **not specific** only for a hemodynamically significant PDA. Other lesions may produce bounding pulses, a hyperdynamic precordium, and cardiac enlargement (e.g., an arteriovenous fistula or an aortopulmonary window). Generally, however, the clinical assessment of a premature infant with the typical findings of a hemodynamically significant ductus arteriosus is adequate to guide therapeutic decisions. If the diagnosis is in doubt, an echocardiogram will clarify the anatomic diagnosis.

Initial medical management includes increased ventilatory support, fluid restriction, and diuretic therapy. In symptomatic patients, indomethacin or ibuprofen may be used for pharmacologic closure of PDA in the premature neonate and is effective in approximately 80% of cases. Birth weight does not affect the efficacy of medical therapy, and there is no increase in complications associated with surgery after unsuccessful medical therapy. Adverse reactions to indomethacin and ibuprofen include transient oliguria, electrolyte abnormalities, decreased platelet function, and hypoglycemia. Contraindications to use of indomethacin and ibuprofen as well as dosing information are noted in Appendix A.

Surgical ligation may be considered in neonates in whom one or more courses of pharmacologic therapy fail to close the symptomatic PDA. However, indications for pharmacologic or surgical closure of a PDA in extremely low birth weight infants (ELBW) vary from institution to institution and are controversial. Although presence of a PDA is associated with the development of bronchopulmonary dysplasia (BPD) in ELBW infants, studies show that early or later closure of the PDA does not improve outcomes in these infants (see Chapter 13).

2. **Complete atrioventricular canal** (Fig. 41.14) consists of a combination of defects in the (i) endocardial portion of the atrial septum; (ii) the inlet portion of the ventricular septum; and (iii) a common, single atrioventricular valve. Because of the large net left-to-right shunt, which increases as the pulmonary vascular resistance falls, these infants typically present early in life with CHF. There may be some degree of cyanosis as well, particularly in the immediate neonatal period before the pulmonary vascular resistance has fallen. In the absence of associated RV outflow tract obstruction, pulmonary artery pressures are at systemic levels; pulmonary vascular resistance is frequently elevated, particularly in patients with trisomy 21.

Approximately 70% of infants with complete atrioventricular canal have trisomy 21; phenotypic findings of trisomy 21 often lead to evaluation of the patient for possible congenital heart disease (see Table 41.5). In the immediate neonatal period, these infants may have an equivocal hyperoxia test because there may be some right-to-left shunting through the large intracardiac connections. Symptoms of congestive failure ensue during the first weeks of life as the pulmonary vascular resistance falls and the patient develops an increasing left-to-right shunt. These patients have a characteristic ECG finding of a "superior axis" (QRS axis from 0 to 180 degrees; see Fig. 41.15) which can be a useful clue for the presence of congenital heart disease in an infant with trisomy 21.

Most patients with complete atrioventricular canal will require medical treatment for symptomatic CHF, although prolonged medical therapy in patients with failure to thrive and symptomatic heart failure is not warranted. Complete surgical repair is undertaken electively at approximately 4 to 6 months of age, with earlier repair in symptomatic patients.

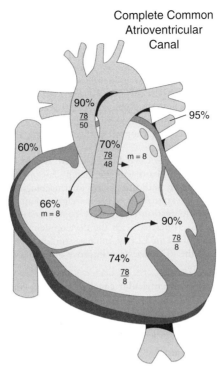

Complete Common
Atrioventricular
Canal

Figure 41.14. Complete common atrioventricular canal. Typical anatomic and hemodynamic findings include (i) large atrial and ventricular septal defects of the endocardial cushion type; (ii) single, atrioventricular valve; (iii) pulmonary artery hypertension (due to large ventricular septal defect); and (iv) bidirectional shunting (with mild hypoxemia) at atrial and ventricular level when pulmonary vascular resistance is elevated in the initial neonatal period. With subsequent fall in pulmonary vascular resistance, the shunt becomes predominantly left-to-right with symptoms of congestive heart failure. m, mean value.

3. **Ventricular septal defect** is the most common cause of CHF after the initial neonatal period. Moderate-to-large ventricular septal defects become hemodynamically significant as the pulmonary vascular resistance decreases and pulmonary blood flow increases due to a left-to-right shunt across the defect. Because this usually takes 2 to 4 weeks to develop, term neonates with ventricular septal defect and symptoms of CHF should be investigated for coexisting anatomic abnormalities, such as left ventricular outflow tract obstruction, coarctation of the aorta, or PDA. Premature infants, who have a lower initial pulmonary vascular resistance, may develop clinical symptoms of heart failure earlier or require longer mechanical ventilation compared with term infants.

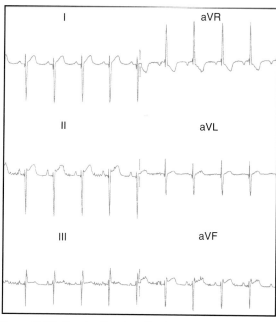

Figure 41.15. Superior ("northwest") axis as seen on the electrocardiogram (only frontal plane leads shown) in a newborn with complete atrioventricular canal. Note the initial upward deflection of the QRS complex (and subsequent predominantly negative deflection) in leads I and aVF. A superior axis (0 to 180 degrees) is present in 95% of patients with endocardial cushion defects.

Ventricular septal defects may occur anywhere in the ventricular septum and are usually classified by their location (Fig. 41.16). Defects in the membranous septum are the most common type. The diagnosis of ventricular septal defect is usually initially suspected on physical examination of the infant; echocardiography confirms the diagnosis and localizes the defect in the ventricular septum. Because a large number (as many as 90% depending on the anatomic type and size) of ventricular septal defects may close spontaneously in the first few months of life, surgery is usually deferred beyond the neonatal period. In large series, only 15% of all patients with ventricular septal defects ever become clinically symptomatic. Medical management of CHF typically includes diuretics and caloric supplementation. Digoxin is used in some institutions. Growth failure is the most common symptom of CHF not fully compensated by medical management. When it occurs, failure to thrive is an indication for surgical repair of the defect.

F. **Cardiac surgery in the neonate.** In the past, because of the perceived high risk of open-heart surgery early in life, critically ill neonates were mostly subjected to palliative procedures or prolonged medical management.

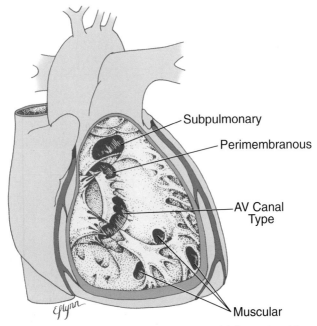

Subpulmonary

Perimembranous

AV Canal
Type

Muscular

Figure 41.16. Diagram of types of ventricular septal defects as viewed from the right ventricle. AV, arteriovenous. (From Fyler DC, ed. *Nadas' Pediatric Cardiology.* St. Louis, MO: Mosby; 1992.)

The unrepaired circulation and residual hemodynamic abnormalities frequently resulted in secondary problems of the heart, lungs, brain, as well as more nonspecific problems of failure to thrive, frequent hospitalizations, and infections. In addition, there are difficult-to-quantitate psychologic burdens to the family of a chronically ill infant.

Low birth weight should not be considered an absolute contraindication for surgical repair. In one series, prolonged medical therapy in low birth weight infants to achieve further weight gain in the presence of a significant hemodynamic burden did not improve the survival rate, and prolonged intensive care management was associated with nosocomial complications. We believe that the symptomatic neonate with congenital heart disease should be repaired as early as possible to prevent the secondary sequelae of the congenital lesion on the heart, lungs, and brain.

Recently, improvements in surgical techniques, cardiopulmonary bypass, and intensive care of the neonate and infant have resulted in significant improvements in surgical mortality and quality of life in the survivors. It is beyond the scope of this chapter to describe the multiple surgical procedures currently employed in the management of congenital heart disease; the reader is referred to Table 41.9 and general texts of cardiac surgery.

Table 41.9. Common Neonatal Operations and Their Early Sequelae

Lesion	Surgical Repair (Eponym)	Early Postoperative Sequelae	
		Common	Rare
Corrective procedures TGA	Arterial switch procedure (Jatene) **1.** Division and reanastomosis of PA to RV and aorta to LV (anatomically correct ventricles) **2.** Translocation of coronary arteries **3.** Closure of septal defects if present	Transient decrease in cardiac output 6–12 hours after surgery	Coronary ostial stenosis or occlusion/sudden death Hemidiaphragm paresis Chylothorax
	Atrial switch procedure (Senning or Mustard) **1.** Intra-atrial baffling of systemic venous return to LV (to PA) and pulmonary venous return to RV (to AO) **2.** Closure of septal defects if present	Supraventricular tachycardia Sick sinus syndrome Tricuspid regurgitation	Pulmonary or systemic venous obstruction
TOF	**1.** Patch closure of VSD through ventriculotomy or right atrium **2.** Enlargement of RVOT with infundibular patch or muscle bundle resection **3.** ± Pulmonary valvotomy **4.** ± Transannular RV to PA patch **5.** ± RV to PA conduit	Pulmonary regurgitation (if transannular patch, valvotomy, or nonvalved conduit) Transient RV dysfunction Right-to-left shunt through PFO, usually resolves postoperatively as RV function improves	Residual left-to-right shunt at VSD patch Residual RVOT obstruction Junctional ectopic tachycardia Complete heart block

(continued)

Table 41.9. Common Neonatal Operations and Their Early Sequelae *(Continued)*

Lesion	Surgical Repair (Eponym)	Early Postoperative Sequelae	
		Common	Rare
CoA	Resection with end-to-end anastomosis, or subclavian flap (Waldhausen), or patch augmentation	Systemic hypertension Absent left-arm pulse (if Waldhausen)	Ileus Hemidiaphragm paresis Vocal cord paresis Chylothorax
PDA	Ligation (± division) of PDA using open thoracotomy and direct visualization or video-assisted thoracoscopic visualization, or device occlusion via cardiac catheterization.	—	Hemidiaphragm paresis Vocal cord paresis Chylothorax Interruption of left PA or descending aorta
TAPVC	1. Reanastomosis of pulmonary venous confluence to posterior aspect of left atrium 2. Division of connecting vein	Pulmonary hypertension Transient low cardiac output	Residual pulmonary venous obstruction
Truncus arteriosus	1. Closure of VSD: baffling LV to truncus (neoaorta) 2. Removal of PAs from truncus 3. Conduit placement from RV to PAs	Reactive pulmonary hypertension Transient RV dysfunction with right-to-left shunt through PFO Hypocalcemia (DiGeorge syndrome)	Truncal valve stenosis or regurgitation Residual VSD Complete heart block

Palliative procedure			
HLHS*	Stage I (Norwood) 1. Connection of main PA to aorta with reconstruction of aortic arch 2. Systemic-to-pulmonary shunt 3. Atrial septectomy	Low systemic cardiac output due to excessive pulmonary blood flow	Aortic arch obstruction Restrictive atrial septal defect
Complex lesions with decreased pulmonary blood flow*	Systemic-to-pulmonary shunt (using prosthetic tube = modified Blalock-Taussig shunt; using subclavian artery = classic Blalock-Taussig shunt)	Excessive pulmonary blood flow and mild congestive heart failure	Hemidiaphragm paresis Vocal cord paralysis Chylothorax Seroma
Complex lesions with excessive pulmonary blood flow*	Ligation of main PA, creation of systemic-to-pulmonary shunt PA band (prosthetic or Silastic constriction of main PA)		PA distortion Aneurysm of main PA

TGA, transposition of the great arteries; PA, pulmonary artery; RV, right ventricle; LV, left ventricle; AO, aorta; TOF, tetralogy of Fallot; VSD, ventricular septal defect; RVOT, right ventricular outflow tract; PFO, patent foramen ovale; CoA, coarctation of the aorta; PDA, patent ductus arteriosus; TAPVC, total anomalous pulmonary venous connection; HLHS, hypoplastic left heart syndrome.

*In patients with a single ventricle, the goal is to separate pulmonary and systemic venous return, rerouting systemic venous blood directly to pulmonary arteries (Fontan operation), although this is done in late infancy or early childhood.

Source: Adapted from Warnovsky G, Erickson LC, Wessel DL. Cardiac emergencies. In: May HL, ed. *Emergency Medicine.* Boston, MA: Little, Brown and Company; 1992.

VII. ACQUIRED HEART DISEASE

A. **Myocarditis** may occur in the neonate as an isolated illness or as a component of a generalized illness with associated hepatitis and/or encephalitis. Myocarditis is usually the result of a viral infection (coxsackie virus, adenovirus, parvovirus, and varicella are most common), although other infectious agents such as bacteria and fungi as well as noninfectious conditions such as autoimmune diseases also may cause myocarditis. Although the clinical presentation (and in some cases, endomyocardial biopsy) makes the diagnosis, specific identification of the etiologic agent may not be made in most cases.

   The infant with acute myocarditis presents with signs and symptoms of CHF (see section IV.B.1) and/or arrhythmia (see section IX). The course of the illness is frequently fulminant and fatal; however, full recovery of ventricular function may occur if the infant can be supported and survive the acute illness. Supportive care including supplemental oxygen, diuretics, inotropic agents, afterload reduction, and mechanical ventilation is frequently used. In severe cases, mechanical support of the myocardium with ECMO or ventricular assist devices can be considered. Care should be used when administering digoxin due to the potential for the potentiation of arrhythmias or complete heart block (CHB).

B. **Transient myocardial ischemia** with myocardial dysfunction may occur in any neonate with a history of perinatal asphyxia. Myocardial dysfunction may be associated with maternal autoimmune disease such as systemic lupus erythematosus. A tricuspid or mitral regurgitant murmur is often heard. An elevated serum creatine kinase MB fraction or cardiac troponin level may be helpful in determining the presence of myocardial damage. Supportive treatment is dictated by the severity of myocardial dysfunction.

C. **Hypertrophic and dilated cardiomyopathies** represent a rare and multifactorial complex of diseases, complete discussion of which is beyond the scope of this chapter. The differential diagnoses includes primary diseases (e.g., genetic causes as well as metabolic, storage, and neuromuscular disorders) or secondary diseases (e.g., end-stage infection, ischemic, endocrine, nutritional, drugs). The reader is referred to texts of pediatric cardiology for more complete discussion.

   The most common hypertrophic cardiomyopathy presenting in neonates is that type seen in **infants born to diabetic mothers**. Echocardiographically and hemodynamically, these infants are indistinguishable from patients with other types of hypertrophic cardiomyopathy. They are different in one important respect: Their cardiomyopathy will completely resolve in 6 to 12 months. Noting a systolic ejection murmur, with or without CHF, in the infant of a diabetic mother, should raise the question of congenital heart disease including hypertrophic cardiomyopathy. Treatment is supportive, addressing the infant's particular CHF symptoms. Propranolol has been used successfully in some patients with severe obstruction. Most patients require no specific care and no long-term cardiac follow-up (see Chapter 2).

VIII. PHARMACOLOGY

A. **PGE₁.** PGE₁ has been used since the late 1970s to pharmacologically maintain patency of the ductus arteriosus in patients with duct-dependent systemic or pulmonary blood flow. PGE_1 must be administered as a continuous parenteral infusion. The usual starting dose is 0.05 to 0.1 µg/kg/minute. Once a therapeutic effect has been achieved, the dose may often be decreased to as low as 0.025 µg/kg/minute without loss of therapeutic effect. The response to PGE_1 is often immediate if patency of the ductus arteriosus is important for the hemodynamic state of the infant. Failure to respond to PGE_1 may mean that the initial diagnosis was incorrect, the ductus arteriosus is unresponsive to PGE_1 (usually only in an older infant), or the ductus is absent. The infusion site has no significant effect on the ductal response to PGE_1. Adverse reactions to PGE_1 include apnea (10% to 12%), fever (14%), cutaneous flushing (10%), bradycardia (7%), seizures (4%), tachycardia (3%), cardiac arrest (1%), and edema (1%). See Table 41.10 for recommended mixing and dosing protocol for PGE_1.

B. **Sympathomimetic amine infusions** are the mainstay of pharmacologic therapies aimed at improving cardiac output and are discussed in detail elsewhere in this book (see Chapter 40). Catecholamines, endogenous (dopamine, epinephrine) or synthetic (dobutamine, isoproterenol), achieve an effect by stimulating myocardial and vascular adrenergic receptors. These agents must be given as a continuous parenteral infusion. They may be given in combination to the critically ill neonate in an effort to maximize the positive effects of each agent while minimizing the negative effects. While receiving catecholamine infusions, patients should be closely monitored, usually with an electrocardiographic monitor and an arterial catheter. Before beginning sympathomimetic amine infusions, intravascular volume should be repleted if necessary, although this may further compromise a congenital lesion with coexisting volume overload. Adverse reactions to catecholamine infusions include tachycardia (which increases myocardial oxygen consumption), atrial and ventricular arrhythmias, and increased afterload due to peripheral vasoconstriction (which may decrease cardiac output). See Table 41.11 for recommended mixing and dosing of the sympathomimetic amines.

Table 41.10. Suggested Preparation of Prostaglandin E_1

Add 1 Ampule (500 µg/1 mL) to	Concentration (µg/mL)	mL/hour × Weight (kg), Needed to Infuse 0.1 µg/kg/minute
200 mL	2.5	2.4
100 mL*	5.0	1.2
50 mL	10.0	0.6

*Usually the most convenient dilution, provides one-fourth of maintenance fluid requirement. Usually mix in dextrose-containing solution for newborns.
Source: Adapted from Warnovsky G, Erickson LC, Wessel DL. Cardiac emergencies. In: May HL, ed. *Emergency Medicine*. Boston, MA: Little, Brown and Company; 1992.

Table 41.11. Sympathomimetic Amines		
Drug	**Usual Dose (μg/kg/minute)**	**Effect**
Dopamine	1–5	↑ Urine output, ↑ HR (slightly), ↑ contractility
	6–10	↑ HR, ↑ contractility, ↑ BP
	11–20	↑ HR, ↑ contractility, ↑ SVR, ↑ BP
Dobutamine	1–20	↑ HR (slightly), ↑ contractility, ↓ SVR
Epinephrine	0.05–0.50	↑ HR, ↑ contractility, ↑ SVR, ↑ BP
Isoproterenol	0.05–1.00	↑ HR, ↑ contractility, ↓ SVR, ↓ PVR

These infusions may be mixed in intravenous solutions containing dextrose and/or saline. For neonates, dextrose-containing solutions with or without salt should usually be chosen. Calculation for convenient preparation of intravenous infusions:

$$6 \times \frac{\text{desired dose (μg/kg/minute)}}{\text{desired rate (mL/hour)}} \times \text{weight (kg)} = \frac{\text{mg drug}}{100 \text{ mL fluid}}$$

HR, heart rate; BP, blood pressure; SVR, systemic vascular resistance; PVR, pulmonary vascular resistance.

C. Afterload-reducing agents

1. **Phosphodiesterase inhibitors** such as **milrinone** are **bipyridine** compounds that selectively inhibit cyclic nucleotide phosphodiesterase. These nonglycosidic and nonsympathomimetic agents exert their effect on cardiac performance by increasing cyclic adenosine monophosphate (cAMP) in the myocardial and vascular muscle, but do so independently of β-receptors. cAMP promotes improved contraction through calcium regulation through two mechanisms: (i) activation of protein kinase (which catalyzes the transfer of phosphate groups from adenosine triphosphate [ATP]) leading to faster calcium entry through the calcium channels and (ii) activation of calcium pumps in the sarcoplasmic reticulum resulting in release of calcium.

   There are three major effects of phosphodiesterase inhibitors: (i) increased inotropy, with increased contractility and cardiac output as a result of cAMP-mediated increase in transsarcolemmal calcium flux; (ii) vasodilatation, with increase in arteriolar and venous capacitance as a result of cAMP-mediated increase in uptake of calcium and decrease in calcium available for contraction; and (iii) increased lusitropy, or improved relaxation properties during diastole.

   Indications for use include low cardiac output with myocardial dysfunction and elevated systemic vascular resistance (SVR) not accompanied by severe hypotension. Side effects have been minimal and are typically the need for volume infusions (5 to 10 mL/kg) following loading dose administration. As such, many institutions avoid loading dose administration and start the infusion at the desired dosing. See Appendix A for dosing information.

The use of phosphodiesterase inhibitors after cardiac surgery in the pediatric patient population has been shown to increase cardiac index and decrease SVR without a significant increase in heart rate. Phosphodiesterase inhibitors are frequently the second-line drug (after dopamine) in the treatment of low cardiac output in neonates, infants, and children following cardiopulmonary bypass.

2. **Other vasodilators** improve low cardiac output principally by decreasing impedance to ventricular ejection; these effects are especially helpful after cardiac surgery in children and in adults when SVR is particularly elevated.

Sodium nitroprusside is the most widely used afterload-reducing agent. It acts as a nitric oxide donor, increasing intracellular cyclic guanosine monophosphate (cGMP), which effects relaxation of vascular smooth muscle in both arterioles and veins. The overall effect is a decrease in atrial filling pressure and SVR with a concomitant increase in cardiac output. The vasodilatory effects of nitroprusside occur within minutes with IV administration. The principal metabolites of sodium nitroprusside are thiocyanate and cyanide; thiocyanate toxicity is unusual in children with normal hepatic and renal function, and monitoring of cyanide and thiocyanate concentrations in children may not be correlated with clinical signs of toxicity.

In neonates with low cardiac output, there may be an increase in urine output and improvement in perfusion with institution of nitroprusside, but there can also be a significant drop in blood pressure necessitating care in its use.

Many other agents have been used as arterial and venous vasodilators to treat hypertension, reduce ventricular afterload and SVR, and improve cardiac output. A second nitrovasodilator, **nitroglycerine**, principally **a venous dilator**, also has rapid onset of action and a short half-life (~2 minutes). Tolerance may develop after several days of continuous infusion. Nitroglycerine is used extensively in adult cardiac units for patients with ischemic heart disease; experience in pediatric patients is more limited. **Hydralazine** is more typically used for acute hypertension; its relatively long half-life limits its use in postoperative patients with labile hemodynamics. The angiotensin-converting enzyme inhibitor **enalapril** similarly has a relatively long half-life (2 to 4 hours) that limits its use in the acute setting. **β-Blockers** (e.g., propranolol, esmolol, labetalol), although excellent in reducing blood pressure, may have deleterious effects on ventricular function. **Calcium channel blockers** (e.g., verapamil) may cause acute and severe hypotension and bradycardia in the neonate and should **rarely be used**. All intravenous vasodilators must be used cautiously in patients with moderate-to-severe lung disease; their use has been associated with increased intrapulmonary shunting and acute reductions of PaO_2.

D. **Digoxin** (see Appendix A) remains important for the treatment of CHF and arrhythmia. A "digitalizing dose" (with a total dose of 30 μg/kg in 24 hours for term infants and 20 μg/kg in 24 hours for premature infants) is usually only used for treatment of arrhythmias or severe heart failure. One-half of this **total digitalizing dose (TDD)** may be given IV, intramuscular (IM), or oral (PO), followed by one-fourth of the TDD every 8 to 12 hours for the remaining two doses. An initial maintenance dose of one-fourth to one-third of the TDD (range 5 to 10 μg/kg/day) may then be adjusted according to the patient's clinical response, renal function, and tolerance for the drug (see Appendix A for further details). Infants with mild symptoms, primary myocardial disease, renal dysfunction, or the potential for atrioventricular block may be digitalized using only the maintenance dose (omitting the loading dose). The maintenance dose is divided into equal twice-daily doses, 12 hours apart.

Digoxin toxicity most commonly manifests with gastrointestinal upset, somnolence, and sinus bradycardia. More severe digoxin toxicity may cause high-grade atrioventricular block and ventricular ectopy. Infants suspected of having digoxin toxicity should have a digoxin level drawn and further doses withheld. The therapeutic level is <1.5 ng/mL, with probable toxicity occurring at levels >4.0 ng/mL. In infants particularly, however, digoxin levels do not always correlate well with therapeutic efficacy or with toxicity.

Digoxin toxicity in neonates is usually manageable by withholding further doses until the signs of toxicity resolve and by correcting electrolyte abnormalities (such as hypokalemia), which can potentiate toxic effects. Severe ventricular arrhythmias associated with digoxin toxicity may be managed with phenytoin, 2 to 4 mg/kg over 5 minutes, or lidocaine, 1 mg/kg loading dose, followed by an infusion at 1 to 2 mg/kg/hour. Atrioventricular block is usually unresponsive to atropine. Severe bradycardia may be refractory to these therapies and require temporary cardiac pacing.

The use of digoxin-specific antibody Fab (antigen-binding fragments) preparation (Digibind; Burroughs Wellcome Fund, Research Triangle Park, NC) is reserved for those patients with evidence of severe digoxin intoxication and clinical symptoms of refractory arrhythmia and/or atrioventricular block; in these patients, it is quite effective. Calculation of the Digibind dose in milligrams is as follows: (serum digoxin concentration in nanograms per milliliter $\times$ 5.6 $\times$ the body weight in kilograms/1,000) $\times$ 64. The dose is given as a one-time IV infusion. A second dose of Digibind may be given to those patients who continue to have clinical evidence of residual toxicity.

E. **Diuretics** (see Appendix A) are frequently used in patients with CHF, often in combination with digoxin. **Furosemide**, 1 to 2 mg/kg/dose, usually results in a brisk diuresis within an hour of administration. If no response is noted in an hour, a second dose (double the first dose) may be given. Chronic use of furosemide may produce urinary tract stones as a result of its calciuric effects. A more potent diuretic effect may be achieved using a combination of a thiazide and a "loop" diuretic such as furosemide. Combination diuretic therapy may be complicated by hyponatremia and hypokalemia. Oral or intravenous potassium supplementation (3 to 4 mEq/kg/day) or an aldosterone antagonist usually should accompany the use of thiazide and/or "loop" diuretics to avoid excessive potassium wasting. It is important to carefully monitor serum potassium and sodium levels when beginning or changing the dose of diuretic medications. When changing from an effective parenteral to oral dose of furosemide, the dose should be increased by 50% to 80%. Furosemide may increase the nephro- and ototoxicity of concurrently used aminoglycoside antibiotics. Detailed discussion of alternative diuretics (e.g., chlorothiazide, spironolactone) is found elsewhere in the text (see Appendix A).

IX. ARRHYTHMIAS

A. **Initial evaluation.** When evaluating any infant with an arrhythmia, it is essential to simultaneously assess the electrophysiology and hemodynamic status. If the baby is poorly perfused and/or hypotensive, reliable IV access should be secured and a level of resuscitation employed appropriate for the degree of illness. As always, **emergency treatment of shock should precede definitive diagnosis**. It should be emphasized, however, that there is **rarely** a situation in which it is justified to omit a 12-lead ECG from the evaluation of an infant with an arrhythmia, the exceptions being ventricular fibrillation or torsade de pointes with accompanying hemodynamic instability. These arrhythmias frequently require immediate defibrillation but are extremely rare arrhythmias in neonates and young infants.

In nearly all circumstances, appropriate therapy (short and long term) depends on an accurate electrophysiologic diagnosis. Determination of the mechanism of a rhythm disturbance is most often made from a 12-lead ECG in the abnormal rhythm compared to the patient's baseline 12-lead ECG in sinus rhythm. Although rhythm strips generated from a cardiac monitor can be helpful supportive evidence of the final diagnosis, they are typically **not** diagnostic and should **not** be the only documentation of arrhythmia if at all possible.

The three broad categories for arrhythmias in neonates are (i) tachyarrhythmias, (ii) bradyarrhythmias, and (iii) irregular rhythms. An algorithm for approaching the differential diagnosis of tachyarrhythmias can be consulted (Fig. 41.17) in most cases. When analyzing the ECG for the mechanism of arrhythmia, a stepwise approach should be taken in three main areas: (i) **rate** (variable, too fast, or too slow), (ii) **rhythm** (regular or irregular, paroxysmal or gradual), and (iii) **QRS morphology**.

B. **Differential diagnosis and initial management in the hemodynamically stable patient**

1. **Narrow QRS complex tachycardias**

   a. **SVTs** are the most common symptomatic arrhythmias in all children, including neonates. SVTs usually have (i) a rate >200 beats per minute, frequently "fixed" with no beat-to-beat variation in rate; (ii) rapid onset and termination (in reentrant rhythms); and (iii) normal ventricular complexes on the surface ECG. The infant may initially be asymptomatic, but later may become irritable, fussy, and refuse feedings. CHF usually does not develop before 24 hours of continuous SVT; however, heart failure is seen in 20% of patients after 36 hours and in 50% after 48 hours.

   SVT in the neonate is almost always "reentrant," involving either an accessory atrioventricular pathway and the atrioventricular node or

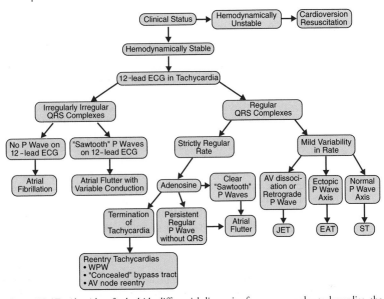

Figure 41.17. Algorithm for bedside differential diagnosis of narrow complex tachycardias, the most common type of arrhythmia in neonates. Note that, regardless of the mechanism of tachycardia, if the patient is hemodynamically unstable, immediate measures to resuscitate the infant including cardioversion are required. Also, treatment with adenosine is helpful therapeutically as well as diagnostically. In general, tachycardias that terminate (even briefly) after adenosine are of the reentry type. ECG, electrocardiogram; AV, atrioventricular; JET, junctional ectopic tachycardia; EAT, ectopic atrial tachycardia; ST, sinus tachycardia; WPW, Wolff-Parkinson-White syndrome.

due to atrial flutter. Approximately half of these patients will manifest preexcitation (delta wave) on the ECG when not in tachycardia (WPW syndrome; see Fig. 41.18). Less commonly, the reentrant circuit may be within the atrium itself (atrial flutter) or within the atrioventricular (AV) node (AV node reentrant tachycardia). Patients with SVT may have associated structural heart disease (10% to 15%); evaluation for structural heart disease should be considered in all neonates with SVT. Another rare cause of SVTs in a neonate is ectopic atrial tachycardia in which the distinguishing features are an abnormal P wave axis, normal QRS axis, and significant variability in the overall rate.

Long-term medical therapy for SVT in the neonate is based on the underlying electrophysiologic diagnosis. **β-Blocker therapy** is the initial therapy of choice in patients with SVT. **Propranolol** is used as the initial and chronic drug therapy for patients with SVT due to WPW syndrome, to avoid the potential facilitation of antegrade (atrioventricular) conduction through the accessory pathway. Treatment with propranolol may be associated with apnea and hypoglycemia; therefore, neonates started on propranolol, especially premature infants, should be

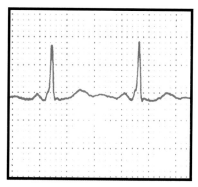

Figure 41.18. Wolff-Parkinson-White syndrome. Note the characteristic "slurred" initial QRS deflection and short PR interval that can occur in any lead; lead I only pictured here.

observed on a continuous cardiac monitor and have serial serum glucose evaluated for 1 to 2 days. If the patient is successfully maintained in sinus rhythm, it typically is continued for 6 to 12 months.

Digoxin is also commonly used in non-WPW syndrome SVT without CHF. Digoxin is avoided in WPW syndrome because of its potential for enhancing antegrade conduction across the accessory pathway. Vagal maneuvers (ice in a plastic bag applied to the face to elicit the "diving reflex") may be tried in stable neonates. Direct pressure over the eyes should be avoided.

The addition or substitution of other antiarrhythmic drugs such as amiodarone alone or in combination may be necessary and should be done only in consultation with a pediatric cardiologist. In neonates, **verapamil should only rarely be used** because it has been associated with sudden death in this patient population.

In utero **SVT** may be suspected when a very rapid fetal heart rate is noted by the obstetrician during prenatal care. The diagnosis is confirmed by fetal echocardiography. At that time, an initial search for congenital heart disease and fetal hydrops may be made. *In utero* treatment of the immature fetus with SVT may be accomplished by treatment of the mother with antiarrhythmic drugs that cross the placenta. Digoxin, flecainide, and other antiarrhythmic drugs have been successful therapies. Failure to control the fetal SVT in the presence of fetal hydrops is an indication for delivery. Cesarean delivery of an infant in persistent SVT may be necessary because the fetal heart rate will not be a reliable indicator of fetal distress.

b. Sinus tachycardia in the neonate is defined as persistent heart rate >2 standard deviations above the mean for age with normal ECG complexes including a normal P-wave morphology and axis. Sinus tachycardia is common and occurs particularly in response to systemic events such as anemia, stress, fever, high levels of circulating catecholamines, hypovolemia, and xanthine (e.g., aminophylline) toxicity. An important clue to the existence of sinus tachycardia, in addition to its normal ECG morphology, is that the rate is not fixed but rather will vary by 10% to 20% over time. Medical management consists of identifying and treating the underlying cause.

2. **Wide-complex tachycardia**

   a. **Ventricular tachycardia** in the neonate is relatively rare and is usually associated with severe medical illnesses including hypoxemia, shock, electrolyte disturbances, digoxin toxicity, and catecholamine toxicity. It may rarely be due to an abnormality of the electrical conducting system of the heart such as prolonged QT_c syndrome and intramyocardial tumors. This ECG pattern may be simulated by SVT in patients with WPW syndrome in whom there is antegrade conduction through the anomalous pathway (SVT with "aberrancy"). Ventricular tachycardia is a potentially unstable rhythm commonly with hemodynamic consequences. The underlying cause should be rapidly sought and treated. The hemodynamically stable patient should be treated with a lidocaine bolus, 1 to 2 mg/kg, followed by a lidocaine infusion, 20 to 50 μg/kg/minute. Direct current cardioversion (starting dose to 1 to 2 J/kg) should be used if the patient is hemodynamically compromised, although will frequently be ineffective in the presence of acidosis. If a severe acidosis (pH <7.2) is present, it should be treated with hyperventilation and/or sodium bicarbonate before cardioversion. Phenytoin, 2 to 4 mg/kg, may be effective if the arrhythmia is due to digoxin toxicity (see section VIII.D).

   b. **Ventricular fibrillation** in the neonate is almost always an agonal (preterminal) arrhythmia. There is a coarse, irregular pattern on ECG with no identifiable QRS complexes. There are no peripheral pulses or heart sounds on examination. Cardiopulmonary resuscitation should be instituted and defibrillation (starting dose 1 to 2 J/kg) performed. A bolus of lidocaine, 1 mg/kg, followed by a lidocaine infusion should be started. Once the infant has been resuscitated, the underlying problems should be evaluated and treated.

3. **Bradycardia**

   a. **Sinus bradycardia** in the neonate is not uncommon especially during sleep or during vagal maneuvers, such as bowel movements. If the infant's perfusion and blood pressure are normal, transient bradycardia is not of major concern. Persistent sinus bradycardia may be secondary to hypoxemia, acidosis, and elevated intracranial pressure. Finally, a stable sinus bradycardia may occur with digoxin toxicity, hypothyroidism, or sinus node dysfunction (usually a complication of cardiac surgery).

   b. **Heart block**

      i. **First-degree atrioventricular block** occurs when the PR interval is >0.16 seconds. In the neonate, first-degree atrioventricular block may be due to a nonspecific conduction disturbance, medications (e.g., digoxin), myocarditis, hypothyroidism, or associated with certain types of congenital heart disease (e.g., complete atrioventricular canal or ventricular inversion). No specific treatment is generally indicated.

ii. Second-degree atrioventricular block. Second-degree atrioventricular block refers to **intermittent** failure of conduction of the atrial impulse to the ventricles. Two types have been described: (i) Mobitz I (Wenckebach phenomenon) and (ii) Mobitz II (intermittent failure to conduct P waves, with a constant PR interval). Second-degree atrioventricular block may occur with SVT, digitalis toxicity, or a nonspecific conduction disturbance. No specific treatment is usually necessary other than diagnosis and treatment of the underlying cause.

iii. CHB refers to **complete** absence of conduction of any atrial activity to the ventricles. CHB typically has a slow, constant ventricular rate that is independent of the atrial rate. CHB is frequently detected *in utero* as fetal bradycardia. Although CHB may be secondary to surgical trauma, **congenital** CHB falls into two main categories. The most common causes include (i) anatomic defects (ventricular inversion and complete atrioventricular canal) and (ii) fetal exposure to maternal antibodies related to systemic rheumatologic disease such as lupus erythematosus. The presence of CHB without structural heart disease should alert the clinician to investigate the mother for rheumatologic disease. In cases of *in utero* CHB caused by maternal antibodies related to lupus erythematosus, the prognosis may be poor. If there is a high risk of developing CHB (previous fetus with CHB, miscarriage, abnormal fetal echocardiography), treatment in pregnancy with dexamethasone, azathioprine, IV gamma globulin, or plasmapheresis should be considered.

Symptoms related to CHB are related both to the severity of the associated cardiac malformation (when present) and the degree of bradycardia. Fortunately, the fetus with CHB adapts well by increasing stroke volume and will usually come to term without difficulty. Infants with isolated congenital CHB usually have a heart rate >50 beats per minute, are asymptomatic, and grow normally.

4. **Irregular rhythms**

   a. **Premature atrial contractions (PACs; see Fig. 41.19)** are common in neonates, are usually benign, and do not require specific therapy. Most PACs result in a normal QRS morphology (see Fig. 41.19A), distinguishing them from premature ventricular contractions (PVCs). If the PAC occurs while the atrioventricular node is partially repolarized, an aberrantly conducted ventricular depolarization pattern may be observed on the surface ECG (see Fig. 41.19B). If the premature beat occurs when the atrioventricular node is refractory (i.e., early in the cardiac cycle, occurring soon after the normal sinus beat), the impulse will not be conducted to the ventricle ("blocked") and may therefore give the appearance of a marked sinus bradycardia (see Fig. 41.19C).

   b. **PVCs** (Fig. 41.20) are "wide QRS complex" beats that occur when a ventricular focus stimulates a spontaneous beat before the normally conducted sinus beat. Isolated PVCs are not uncommon in the normal neonate and do not generally require treatment. Although PVCs frequently

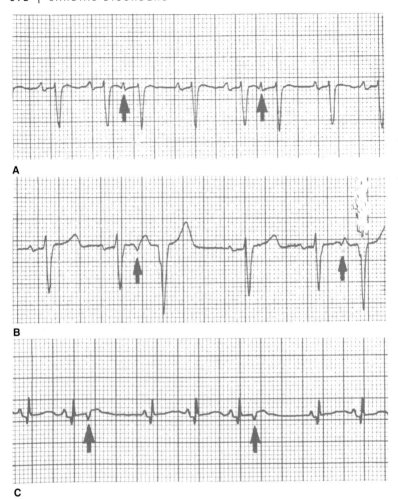

A

B

C

Figure 41.19. Premature atrial contractions (*arrows*) causing **(A)** early ventricular depolarization with a normal QRS complex. **B:** Early ventricular depolarization with "aberration" of the QRS complex. **C:** Block at the atrioventricular node. (From Fyler DC, ed. *Nadas' Pediatric Cardiology*. St. Louis, MO: Mosby; 1992.)

occur sporadically, they occasionally are grouped, such as every other beat (bigeminy; see Fig. 41.20A), every third beat (trigeminy), and so on. These more frequent PVCs are typically no more worrisome than isolated PVCs, although their greater frequency usually prompts a more extensive diagnostic workup. PVCs may be caused by digoxin toxicity, hypoxemia, electrolyte disturbances, catecholamine, or xanthine toxicity. PVCs occurring in groups of two or more (i.e., couplets, triplets, etc.;

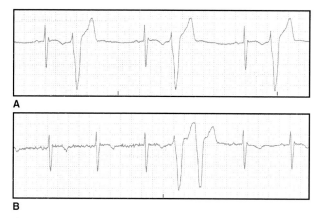

Figure 41.20. Premature ventricular contractions (PVCs). **A:** PVCs alternating with normal sinus beats (ventricular bigeminy) are usually not indicative of significant pathology. **B:** Paired PVCs ("couplet") are a potentially more serious rhythm and require further investigation.

see Fig. 41.20B) are pathologic and "high grade"; they may be a marker for myocarditis or myocardial dysfunction, and further evaluation should be strongly considered.

C. **Emergency treatment in the hemodynamically compromised patient.** With all therapies described in the following, it is important to have easily accessible resuscitation equipment available before proceeding with these antiarrhythmic interventions. It is important to have an ECG machine attached to the patient to document the conversion to sinus rhythm, where possible. Reliance on bedside monitors frequently loses the opportunity to provide important diagnostic information regarding the arrhythmia.

1. **Tachycardia**

   a. **Adenosine.** Adenosine has become the drug of choice for acute management. Adenosine transiently blocks AV node conduction, allowing termination of rapid reentrant rhythms involving the AV node. It must be given by very rapid IV push because its half-life is 10 seconds or less. Due to this short half-life, adenosine is a relatively safe medication; however, it has been reported to cause transient AV block severe enough to require pacing (albeit briefly), so it should be used with caution and in consultation with a pediatric cardiologist. Adenosine, by virtue of its acute action on the AV node, is frequently **diagnostic** as well. Patients who respond with abrupt termination of the SVT have reentrant tachycardias involving the AV node; those with SVT due to atrial flutter will have acute AV block and easily visible flutter waves with reappearance of SVT in 10 to 15 seconds.

   b. **Cardioversion.** In the hemodynamically unstable patient, **first** line therapy is synchronized direct current cardioversion. The energy should start at 1 J/kg and be increased by a factor of 2 if unsuccessful. Care should be taken to avoid skin burns and arcing of the current outside the body by only using electrical transmission gel with the paddles. Paddle position should be anterior–posterior if possible.

c. Transesophageal pacing. When available, esophageal overdrive pacing is an effective maneuver for terminating tachyarrhythmias. The close proximity of the left atrium to the distal esophagus allows electrical impulses generated in the esophagus to be transmitted to atrial tissue; burst pacing may then terminate reentrant tachyarrhythmias.

2. **Bradycardia.** Therapeutic options for treating a symptomatic bradyarrhythmia are more limited. A transvenous pacemaker is a temporary measure in severely symptomatic neonates while preparing for placement of permanent epicardial pacemaker leads; however, transvenous pacing in a small neonate is technically difficult and frequently requires fluoroscopy. A number of transcutaneous pacemakers (Zoll) are available, but long-term use must be avoided due to cutaneous burns. An isoproterenol infusion may temporarily increase the ventricular rate and cardiac output in an infant with CHF. The treatment of choice for sinus node dysfunction is transesophageal pacing at an appropriate rate, but this can only be accomplished with intact atrioventricular conduction and is not effective in patients with CHB. For the infant with transient bradycardia (due to increased vagal tone), IV atropine may be used.

Suggested Readings

Allen HD, Gutgesell HP, Clark EB, et al. *Moss and Adams' Heart Disease in Infants, Children, and Adolescents Including the Fetus and Young Adult.* 6th ed. Philadelphia, PA: Lippincott Williams & Wilkins; 2001.

Aranda JV, Thomas R. Systematic review: intravenous Ibuprofen in preterm newborns. *Semin Perinatol* 2006;30(3):114–120.

Burkhardt BE, Stiller B, Grohmann J. Stenting of the obstructed ductus venosus as emergency and bridging strategy in a very low birth weight infant with infradiaphragmatic total anomalous pulmonary venous connection. *Catheter Cardiovasc Interv* 2014;84(5):820–823.

Dohlen G, Chaturvedi RR, Benson LN, et al. Stenting of the right ventricular outflow tract in the symptomatic infant with tetralogy of Fallot. *Heart* 2009;95:142–147.

Gewillig M, Boshoff DE, Dens J, et al. Stenting the neonatal arterial duct in duct-dependent pulmonary circulation: new techniques, better results. *J Am Coll Cardiol* 2004;43:107–112.

Hoffman JIE, Kaplan S. The incidence of congenital heart disease. *J Am Coll Cardiol* 2002;39(12):1890–1900.

Jonas RA. *Comprehensive Surgical Management of Congenital Heart Disease.* London, United Kingdom: Arnold; 2004.

Keane JF, Lock JE, Fyler DC. *Nadas' Pediatric Cardiology.* 2nd ed. Philadelphia, PA: WB Saunders; 2006.

Kovalchin JP, Silverman NH. The impact of fetal echocardiography. *Pediatr Cardiol* 2004;25(3):299–306.

Liske MR, Greeley CS, Law DJ, et al. Report of the Tennessee Task Force on Screening Newborn Infants for Critical Congenital Heart Disease. *Pediatrics* 2006;118(4):e1250–e1256.

Mai CT, Riehle-Colarusso T, O'Halloran A, et al. Selected birth defects data from population-based birth defects surveillance programs in the United States, 2005–2009: featuring critical congenital heart defects targeted for pulse oximetry screening. *Birth Defects Res A Clin Mol Teratol* 2012;94(12): 970–983.

Mavroudis C, Backer C. *Pediatric Cardiac Surgery*. 3rd ed. Philadelphia, PA: Mosby; 2003.

Rein AJ, Omokhodion SI, Nir A. Significance of a cardiac murmur as the sole clinical sign in the newborn. *Clin Pediatr* 2000;39(9):511–520.

Saar P, Hermann W, Müller-Ladner U. Connective tissue diseases and pregnancy. *Rheumatology* 2006;45(suppl 3):iii30–iii32.

Shah SS, Ohlsson A. Ibuprofen for the prevention of patent ductus arteriosus in preterm and/or low birth weight infants. *Cochrane Database Syst Rev* 2006;(1):CD004113.

Tworetzky W, Wilkins-Haug L, Jennings RW, et al. Balloon dilation of severe aortic stenosis in the fetus: potential for prevention of hypoplastic left heart syndrome: candidate selection, technique, and results of successful intervention. *Circulation* 2004;110(15):2125–2131.

Zahn EM, Nevin P, Simmons C, et al. A novel technique for transcatheter patent ductus arteriosus closure in extremely preterm infants using commercially available technology. *Catheter Cardiovasc Interv* 2015;85:240–248.

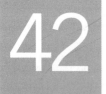

42 Blood Products Used in the Newborn

Steven R. Sloan

KEY POINTS

- Blood components should be transfused when clinically indicated to promote oxygen delivery and coagulation.
- Immunocompromised patients such as those with congenital immune deficiencies or very low weight infants are at risk for transfusion-associated graft-versus-host disease and require irradiated red blood cell (RBC) and platelet units.
- Neonates at risk for cytomegalovirus (CMV) should receive blood components that are CMV safe. Blood from donors lacking antibodies to CMV and leukoreduced blood components are CMV safe.
- Risks of transfusion-transmitted infections are very low, with the highest current risks being due to bacterial contamination of platelets.

I. WHOLE BLOOD AND BLOOD COMPONENT TRANSFUSIONS

A. General principles. There are six types of blood components including packed red blood cells (RBCs), platelets, frozen plasma, fresh frozen plasma (FFP), cryoprecipitate (CRYO), and granulocytes. In some cases, whole blood, usually in the form of reconstituted whole blood, is used. However, in most cases, blood components are preferred because each component has specific optimal storage conditions and component therapy maximizes the use of blood donations. Other blood products include those used for hematopoietic stem cell transplants, such as umbilical cord blood (UCB), and derivatives purified from blood, such as intravenous immunoglobulin (IVIG).

B. Side effects

1. **Infectious diseases.** A variety of infectious diseases can be transmitted by blood transfusion. In the United States, HIV, hepatitis B virus, hepatitis C virus, syphilis, human T-lymphotropic virus types I or II (HTLV I/II), Chagas disease, and West Nile virus are screened for by medical history questionnaires and laboratory tests. Medical history questionnaires alone are used to screen for other diseases such as malaria, babesiosis, and Zika virus, although tests are being developed for babesiosis and Zika virus. The risk of acquiring a transfusion-transmitted infectious disease is very low and too low to accurately measure but has

Table 42.1. Current Infectious Disease Risks from Blood Transfusions

Pathogen	Risk per Unit
Human immunodeficiency virus (HIV)	1 in 2,135,000
Hepatitis C virus (HCV)	1 in 1,935,000
Hepatitis A virus	1 in 1,000,000
Hepatitis B virus (HBV)	1 in 205,000–488,000
West Nile virus (WNV)	none
Parvovirus B19	1 in 10,000

Source: From Stramer SL. Current risks of transfusion-transmitted agents: a review. *Arch Pathol Lab Med* 2007;131(5):702–707.

been calculated in the United States and are shown in Table 42.1. The risks vary depending on the prevalence of the disease and the testing performed and thus differ in other countries.

Cytomegalovirus (CMV) can also be transmitted by blood, but this is rare if the blood is leukoreduced and/or it tests negative for antibodies to CMV. Animal studies suggest that variant Creutzfeldt-Jakob disease (vCJD) can also be transmitted by blood transfusion, and a few probable cases of transfusion-transmitted vCJD in humans have been reported.

C. **Special considerations**

1. **Directed or designated donor blood.** Blood donated by family members or friends for specific patients is commonly known as directed or designated donor blood. Directed donations have a small increase in rate of infectious disease transmission. Additionally, in a case of hemolytic disease of the newborn or neonatal alloimmune thrombocytopenia, the neonate's blood contains maternal antibodies that are directed against paternally inherited antigens on blood cells. In these cases, paternal relatives' blood may carry the same antigens rendering their blood incompatible with the baby. Finally, directed donor blood from relatives can induce an immune response against human leukocyte antigen (HLA) and other antigens against those relatives. This would complicate future therapy if the relatives were to be considered as donors of other tissue for the patient later in life. For these reasons, some medical centers do not offer directed donor blood.

2. **Leukoreduction and irradiation.** Whole blood, platelets, and red blood cells (RBCs) can be leukoreduced by filtration and/or irradiated to reduce the incidence of specific complications.

3. **Leukoreduction.** Leukoreduction filters remove approximately 99.9% of the white blood cells from RBCs and platelets. In addition, most

platelets collected by apheresis are leukoreduced even without additional filtration. Benefits of leukoreduction include the following:

a. Decreased rate of febrile transfusion reactions

b. Decreased rate of CMV transmission to a negligible rate

c. Potential to reduce a possible immunomodulatory effect of blood transfusions

d. Decreased immunization to antigens on leukocytes such as HLA. This has only been shown for some oncology patients, and its importance for neonates is unknown.

Neonates, especially premature infants, often receive leukoreduced blood components to decrease CMV transmission.

4. Irradiation. Transfusion-associated graft-versus-host disease (TA-GVHD) occurs when transfused lymphocytes mount an immune response against the patient and the patient is unable to destroy the transfused lymphocytes. Irradiation of the blood component prevents proliferation of lymphocytes and thus prevents TA-GVHD. Some premature infants and children with certain congenital immunodeficiencies are at risk for TA-GVHD. Additionally, recipients of blood from first-degree relatives are at risk for TA-GVHD. Hence, these directed donor units must be irradiated.

II. PACKED RED BLOOD CELLS

A. General principles

1. Mechanism. RBCs provide oxygen carrying capacity for patients whose blood lacks sufficient oxygen carrying capacity due to anemia, hemorrhage, or a hemoglobinopathy. Transfusion for hemoglobinopathies is unusual in the neonatal period when most patients will have significant amounts of fetal hemoglobin.

Several types of RBC units are available that vary in the preservatives added. Chemical additives delay storage damage to RBCs allowing for extended storage times. The types of units that are currently available in the United States are as follows:

a. Anticoagulant-preservative solution units. These units contain approximately 250 mL of a concentrated solution of RBCs. The hematocrit of these units is usually 70% to 80%. In addition, these units contain 62 mg of sodium, 222 mg of citrate, and 46 mg of phosphate. Three types of units are currently approved for use in the United States. These are as follows:

  i. CPD. This contains 773 mg of dextrose and has a 21-day shelf life.

  ii. CP2D. This contains 1,546 mg of dextrose and has a 21-day shelf life.

  iii. CPDA-1. This contains 965 mg of dextrose and 8.2 mg of adenine and has a 35-day shelf life. This is the most widely used of the anticoagulant-preservative solution units but is infrequently used because most RBC units are stored in additives.

b. Additive solution units. Most RBC units used in the United States are additive units. Four additive solutions are currently approved for use

Table 42.2. Glucose (Dextrose) Concentrations in Red Blood Cell Additive Solutions (mM)

AS-1*	AS-3*	AS-5*	AS-7*	SAGM	MAP	PAGGSM
111	55	45	80	45	40	47

*U.S. Food and Drug Administration (FDA)-approved for use in the United States.
AS, additive solution; SAGM, saline, adenine, glucose, mannitol; MAP, mitogen-activated protein; PAGGSM, phosphate-adenine-glucose-guanosine-saline-mannitol.

in the United States. Each of these units contains approximately 350 mL, has an average hematocrit of 50% to 60%, and has a 42-day shelf life. Neonatologists should be aware of the glucose concentrations in these units (Table 42.2) as this can significantly impact neonatal glucose homeostasis.

2. **Several changes occur in RBCs during storage:**
   a. The pH decreases from 7.4 to 7.55 to pH 6.5 to 6.6 at the time of expiration.
   b. Potassium is released from the RBCs. The initial plasma K+ concentration is approximately 4.2 mM and increases to 78.5 mM in CPDA-1 units at day 35 and 45 to 50 mM in additive solution units on day 42. CPDA-1 units contain about one-third the supernatant volume as additive units, so the total amount of extracellular potassium is similar in all units of the same age.
   c. 2,3-Diphosphoglycerol (2,3-DPG) levels drop rapidly during the first 2 weeks of storage. This increases the affinity of the hemoglobin for oxygen and decreases its efficiency in delivering oxygen to tissue. The 2,3-DPG levels replenish over several hours after being transfused.

3. **Toxicity.** Although there are theoretical concerns that mannitol may cause a rapid diuresis and adenine may be a nephrotoxin in the premature infant, case reports and case series have found no risk associated with additive solution units. Although some hospitals still attempt to avoid additive solution units for neonates, the constituents of additives are not present in high enough concentrations to cause harm.

B. **Indications/contraindications.** RBC transfusions are indicated for neonates who have signs or symptoms of hypoxia or who require an exchange transfusion (see Chapter 45). One study suggests that RBC transfusions in premature infants help neurologic development. However, the opposite result has been seen in another study, and this question is one of active investigation. At this point, RBC transfusion triggers for premature infants should be based on how severely ill the patient is and may range from 8 to 10 g/dL hemoglobin (Hb) for healthy infants to as high as 15 g/dL for premature infants requiring substantial oxygen support.

C. **Dosing and administration.** The usual dose for a simple transfusion is 5 to 15 mL/kg transfused at a rate of approximately 5 mL/kg/hour. This may be adjusted depending on the severity of the anemia and/or the patient's ability to tolerate increases in intravascular volume.

D. Side effects

1. **Acute transfusion reactions**

   a. Acute hemolytic transfusion reactions. These reactions are usually due to incompatibility of donor RBCs with antibodies in the patient's plasma. The antibodies usually responsible for acute hemolytic transfusion reactions are isohemagglutinins (anti-A, anti-B). These reactions are rare in neonates who do not make isohemagglutinins until they are 4 to 6 months old. However, maternal isohemagglutinins can be present in the neonatal circulation.

   i. **Symptoms.** Possible symptoms include hypotension, fever, tachycardia, infusion site pain, and hematuria.

   ii. **Treatment.** Administer fluids and furosemide to protect kidneys. If necessary, treat hypotension with pressors and use hemostatic agents for bleeding; may need to transfuse compatible RBCs.

   b. Allergic transfusion reactions. These are unusual in neonates. Allergic reactions are due to antibodies in the patient's plasma that react with proteins in donor plasma.

   i. **Symptoms.** Mild allergic reactions are characterized by hives and possibly wheezing. More severe reactions can present as anaphylaxis.

   ii. **Treatment.** These reactions can be treated with antihistamines, bronchodilators, and corticosteroids as needed. These reactions are usually specific to individual donors. If they are serious or reoccur, RBCs and platelets can be washed.

   c. Volume overload. Blood components have high oncotic pressure, and rapid infusion can cause excessive intravascular volume. This can cause a sudden deterioration of vital signs. Chronically anemic neonates can be especially susceptible to volume overload from transfusions.

   d. Hypocalcemia. Rapid infusion of components, especially FFP, can cause transient hypocalcemia secondary to transfusion of citrate. This can cause hypotension.

   e. Hypothermia. Cool blood can cause hypothermia. Transfusion through blood warmers can prevent this.

   f. Transfusion-associated acute lung injury (TRALI). This is often due to antibodies in donor plasma that react with the patient's histocompatibility (HLA) antigens. These reactions present as respiratory compromise and are more likely to occur with blood components containing significant amounts of plasma such as platelets or FFP. Blood centers now minimize collections of these products from female donors who developed anti-HLA antibodies during pregnancies. This has substantially decreased the incidence of these reactions.

   g. Hyperkalemia. Extracellular potassium concentrations are insignificant for simple transfusions of 5 to 20 mL/kg. However, transfusion-associated hyperkalemia has been reported secondary to large transfusions such as exchange transfusions or transfusions for major surgery. Ideally, fresher RBC units can be provided for these transfusions. If fresh RBCs are unavailable, washing blood will reduce the extracellular potassium concentration.

h. Febrile nonhemolytic transfusion reactions are usually due to cytokines released from leukocytes in the donor unit. These occur less frequently from transfusions of leukoreduced units.

i. Bacterial contamination can occur but is rare with RBC transfusions.

j. TA-GVHD. Lymphocytes from donor blood components can mount an immune response against the patient. Patients are at risk if they are unable to mount immune responses against the transfused lymphocytes. Such patients include premature infants, infants with congenital immune deficiencies, and patients sharing HLA types with blood donors as often occurs when people donate blood for relatives. TA-GVHD can be prevented by irradiation. Leukoreduction filters do not remove enough lymphocytes to prevent TA-GVHD.

k. Necrotizing enterocolitis is likely NOT due to transfusions despite multiple reports of a temporal association. Anemia itself, not transfusions, is likely in the causative pathway of necrotizing enterocolitis.

E. Special considerations. Donor exposures can be minimized by reserving a fresh unit of RBCs for a neonate at his or her first transfusion. Subsequent transfusions can utilize aliquots of that unit until it is depleted or expires. This is useful for premature infants who are expected to require multiple simple transfusions for anemia of prematurity.

III. FRESH FROZEN PLASMA, THAWED PLASMA

A. General principles. The two frozen plasma products that are most frequently available are FFP and thawed plasma. Both components are used to administer all clotting factors. The contents are as follows:

1. Each component has approximately 1 unit/mL of each coagulation factor except that thawed plasma may have approximately two-thirds the levels of the least stable factors: factors V and VIII.

2. 160 to 170 mEq/L sodium and 3.5 to 5.5 mEq/L potassium

3. All plasma proteins including albumin and antibodies

4. 1,440 g sodium citrate

B. Indications. FFP and thawed plasma are indicated to correct coagulopathies due to factor deficiencies. Although plasma contains proteins and albumins, these components are not indicated for intravascular volume expansion or for antibody replacement because other components are safer for those indications (see Chapter 43).

C. Dosing and administration. Ten to 20 mL/kg is usually an adequate dose, and this may need to be repeated every 8 to 12 hours depending on the clinical situation.

D. Side effects. Many of the side effects of RBC transfusion can also occur with plasma transfusions, with some differences in the risk profile for plasma:

1. Hyperkalemia will not occur.

2. TRALI is more likely because plasma products contain more antibodies that can cause TRALI.

3. Acute hemolytic reactions involving hemolysis of transfused RBCs is extremely unlikely. However, if the plasma contains incompatible antibodies (e.g., group O plasma transfused to a group A patient), an acute hemolytic reaction could theoretically occur. For this reason, transfused plasma should be compatible with the patient's blood group.

4. **Citrate-induced hypocalcemia** is a risk with plasma infusions. The amount of citrate is unlikely to cause transient hypocalcemia in most situations, but this can happen with rapid infusions of large amounts of plasma.

IV. PLATELETS

A. **General principles.** Platelets can be prepared from whole blood donations or collected by apheresis. If they are collected by apheresis, an aliquot is obtained for a neonatal transfusion. Often only a portion of a whole blood–derived platelet unit is transfused to neonates, but most blood banks do not aliquot whole blood–derived platelets.

B. **Contents.** Each unit of whole blood–derived platelets contains at least 5×10^{10} platelets in approximately 50 mL of anticoagulated plasma including proteins and electrolytes. Because platelets are stored at room temperature for up to 5 days, there may be relatively low levels of the least stable coagulation factors V and VIII.

C. **Indications.** No good studies exist, but neonatal intensive care unit (NICU) patients at increased risk for intracranial hemorrhage should probably be maintained at a platelet count of 50,000 to 100,000 platelets/mm^3. For additional information, see Chapter 47.

D. **Dosing and administration.** A dose of approximately 5 mL/kg should raise the platelet count by approximately 30,000/mm^3.

E. **Side effects.** The side effects of FFP transfusions can also occur with platelet transfusions. Additionally:

1. Platelets are more likely to be contaminated with bacteria causing septic reactions because platelets are stored at room temperature. For this reason, blood banks in the United States test units for bacteria or treat platelet units to inactivate bacteria.

2. Inventory issues can limit the ability to match ABO types of platelets and patients. ABO incompatible plasma in a platelet unit can rarely cause a hemolytic transfusion reaction. For this reason, some blood banks remove plasma from platelet units containing antibodies that are incompatible with the patient or avoid platelets with high titers of these antibodies.

F. **Special considerations.** Platelets can be concentrated by centrifugation resulting in a volume of 15 to 20 mL and then need to be resuspended. Some units are not successfully resuspended, and even if the platelet product appears acceptable, the platelets may have been activated and may not properly function in the patient.

V. GRANULOCYTES

A. **Indications** (see Chapter 49). Granulocyte transfusions are a controversial therapy that may benefit patients with severe neutropenia or dysfunctional neutrophils and a bacterial or fungal infection not responding to antimicrobial therapy. Most granulocytes are given to patients who are neutropenic secondary to hematopoietic progenitor cell (HPC) transplants. However, septic infants with chronic granulomatous disease also may benefit from granulocyte transfusions. Granulocyte transfusions are a temporary therapy until the patient starts producing neutrophils or until another curative therapy can be instituted.

B. **Dosing and administration.** 10 to 15 mL/kg. This may need to be repeated every 12 to 24 hours.

C. **Side effects.** In addition to all the potential adverse effects associated with RBC transfusions, granulocyte transfusions can cause pulmonary symptoms and must be administered slowly to minimize the chances of severe reactions. Additionally, granulocytes can transmit CMV. Hence, donors should be serologically negative for CMV if the patient is at risk for CMV disease.

D. **Special considerations.** Granulocyte collections need to be specially scheduled, and the granulocytes should be transfused as soon as possible after collection and no later than 24 hours after the collection.

VI. WHOLE BLOOD

A. **General principles.** Whole blood contains RBCs and plasma clotting factors. Few units are stored as whole blood. Whole blood can be reconstituted from a unit of RBCs and FFP.

B. **Indications.** Whole blood is usually used for neonatal exchange transfusions. It also may be used as a substitute for blood components in priming circuits for extracorporeal membrane oxygenation (ECMO) or cardiopulmonary bypass, but this may cause increased fluid retention and longer postoperative recovery times. Whole blood may be useful for neonates immediately following disconnection from a cardiopulmonary bypass circuit for cardiac surgery.

C. **Side effects.** All of the adverse effects of individual blood components can occur with whole blood.

D. **Special considerations.** Whole blood should be transfused when it is relatively fresh because whole blood is stored at 1° to 6°C and coagulation factors decay at this temperature. When used just after cardiopulmonary bypass, the blood should be no more than 2 to 3 days old. When used in other situations, the whole blood should be no more than 5 to 7 days old.

Platelets in whole blood will be cleared rapidly following transfusion, and reconstituted whole blood lacks significant quantities of platelets.

VII. INTRAVENOUS IMMUNOGLOBULIN

A. **General principles.** IVIG is a concentrated purified solution of immunoglobulins with stabilizers such as sucrose. Most products contain over 90% immunoglobulin G (IgG) with small amounts of immunoglobulin M (IgM) and immunoglobulin A (IgA). Several brands of IVIG are available.

B. **Indications.** IVIG can have an immunosuppressive effect that is useful for alloimmune disorders such as neonatal alloimmune thrombocytopenia and possibly alloimmune hemolytic anemia. Both of these disorders are due to maternal antibodies to antigens on the neonate's cells (see Chapters 26 and 47).

IVIG can also be used to replace immunoglobulins for patients who are deficient in immunoglobulins as occurs with some congenital immuno-deficiency syndromes.

Some studies have attempted to determine whether IVIG is useful as a prophylaxis or treatment for neonatal sepsis. Results from these studies are mixed, and not enough evidence exists for routine use of IVIG for general sepsis (see Chapter 49).

1. **Hyperimmune immunoglobulins.** High titer disease-specific immu-noglobulins are available for several infectious agents including varicella zoster virus and respiratory syncytial virus. These immunoglobulins may be useful for infants at high risk for these infections.

C. **Dosing and administration.** IVIG (non–disease-specific) is usually given at a dose of 500–1000 mg/kg. Doses for the disease-specific immunoglobu-lins should follow manufacturer's recommendations.

D. **Side effects.** Rare complications include transient tachycardia or hyperten-sion. Because of the purification processes, current IVIG has a negligible risk of transmitting infectious diseases.

VIII. UMBILICAL CORD BLOOD

A. **General principles.** UCB is the only blood that is derived from neonatal blood. UCB contains HPCs and is used for HPC transplants. UCB can be used for autologous transplants in which the patient receives the same blood that he or she donated or can be used for allogeneic transplants in which the UCB is infused into an individual who did not donate the UCB.

B. **UCB donations.** UCB is collected from the placenta and umbilical cord immediately following delivery and clamping of the umbilical cord. If the mother and baby are healthy, the cord blood can be collected without any impact on the neonate.

UCB can be collected for processing, freezing, and storage by private UCB banks which charge families for this service. A UCB unit stored in a private bank may be used by the neonate that donated the UCB or by other people designated by the family. The UCB has a very low chance of being needed by the neonate because he or she would only be able to use the UCB if he or she were to develop a malignancy for which an autolo-gous transplant is indicated when he or she is a child. A single UCB unit has an insufficient dose for transplants for adolescents or adults, although approaches to expand the cells in the cord blood are under investigation.

UCB can be processed, frozen, and stored by a public UCB bank. Such banks do not charge for this service. A UCB unit in a public bank is available for any patient who could use it and can be a valuable source of stem cells for a child with a malignancy or for a child with some congenital hematologic diseases.

C. Dosing and administration. An entire cord blood is used for younger children, and two cord bloods or a single expanded cord blood may be used for transplants to larger patients. Cord bloods are usually infused into central veins as part of a hematopoietic cell transplant protocol.

D. Side effects. All of the side effects for other blood components can occur for UCB transplants. However, the plasma content is low and TRALI is unlikely. Because UCB cannot be leukoreduced, febrile reactions are more common than with other blood components. Because UCB cannot be irradiated and patients are immunosuppressed, the risk of GVHD is significant.

Suggested Readings

Del Vecchio A, Motta M, Radicioni M, et al. A consistent approach to platelet transfusion in the NICU. *J Matern Fetal Neonatal Med* 2012;25(suppl 5):93–96.

Ferrer-Marin F, Stanworth S, Josephson C, et al. Distinct differences in platelet production and function between neonates and adults: implications for platelet transfusion practice. *Transfusion* 2013;53:2814–2821.

Kelly AM, Williamson LM. Neonatal transfusion. *Early Hum Dev* 2013;89:855–860.

Whyte RK. Neurodevelopmental outcome of extremely low-birth-weight infants randomly assigned to restrictive or liberal hemoglobin thresholds for blood transfusion. *Semin Perinatol* 2012;36:290–293.

43

Bleeding
Stacy E. Croteau

KEY POINTS

- Normal levels of pro- and anticoagulant proteins are age-dependent. The physiologic balance of pro- and anticoagulant proteins and platelet function differs in the neonate compared to the older child or adult. Despite this "developmental hemostasis," the *healthy* neonate is not predisposed to hemorrhage or thrombosis.
- Cord blood samples may be sent for coagulation testing; venipuncture blood draw is the method of choice if cord blood samples are not obtained. Heel sticks and arterial draws should be avoided.
- One-third of patients with severe hemophilia have *de novo* mutations, so family history alone cannot exclude the diagnosis.
- Vitamin K is essential for normal production of several coagulation factors. Lack of administration to neonates increases their risk for severe bleeding over the first several days to weeks of life.

I. ETIOLOGY

A. Deficient clotting factors

1. **Transitory deficiencies** of the procoagulant vitamin K–dependent factors II, VII, IX, and X and anticoagulant proteins C and S are characteristic of the newborn period and may be accentuated by the following:

a. **The administration of total parenteral alimentation or antibiotics or the lack of administration of vitamin K** to premature infants

b. **Term infants may develop vitamin K deficiency** by day 2 or 3 if they are not supplemented with vitamin K parenterally because of negligible stores and inadequate intake.

c. Liver disease may interfere with the production of clotting factors by the liver.

d. **Transplacental exposure to certain drugs can cause bleeding in the first 24 hours of life.**

   i. Phenytoin (Dilantin), phenobarbital, and salicylates interfere with the effect of vitamin K on clotting factor synthesis.

   ii. Warfarin and related compounds given to the mother interfere with the synthesis of vitamin K–dependent clotting factors by

This is a revision of a chapter from the seventh edition by Ellis J. Neufeld.

both the maternal and fetal livers; bleeding may not be immediately reversed by administration of vitamin K.

2. Disturbances of clotting

    a. Disseminated intravascular coagulation (DIC) may be due to infection, shock, anoxia, necrotizing enterocolitis (NEC), renal vein thrombosis (RVT), or the use of vascular catheters.

    b. Extracorporeal membrane oxygenation (ECMO) in neonates with critical cardiopulmonary disease is a special case of coagulopathy related to consumption of clotting factors in the bypass circuit plus therapeutic anticoagulation (see Chapter 39).

3. Inherited abnormalities of clotting factors

    a. X-linked (expressed predominantly in males; affected females should raise concern of Turner syndrome, partial X deletions, or nonrandom X chromosome inactivation). **One-third of patients with severe hemophilia have "new mutations," so family history alone cannot exclude the diagnosis.**

        i. Factor VIII levels are decreased in the newborn with hemophilia A (1 in 5,000 males).

        ii. Hemophilia B, or Christmas disease, is due to a deficiency of factor IX (1 in 25,000 males).

    b. Autosomal dominant (expressed in boys and girls with one parent affected)

        i. Von Willebrand disease (VWD) is caused by decreased levels or functional activity of von Willebrand factor (VWF), which acts as a carrier for factor VIII and plays a role in platelet aggregation. VWD is the most common inherited coagulation defect (up to 1% of the population as assayed by levels). Neonatal levels of VWF are elevated in normal neonates compared to older children and nonpregnant adults because of maternal estrogen.

        ii. Dysfibrinogenemia (very rare) is due to fibrinogen structural mutations.

    c. Autosomal recessive (occurs in both boys and girls born to carrier parents). In order of frequency, deficiencies of factors XI, VII, V, X, II, fibrinogen, and factor XIII are all encoded by autosomal genes. Factor XII is a special case because deficiency causes prolonged partial thromboplastin time (PTT) but never bleeding. Combined factors V and VIII deficiency is caused by a transport gene mutation, not mutations of the factor V and factor VIII genes.

        i. Severe factor VII or factor XIII deficiency can present as intracranial hemorrhage in neonates. Bleeding from the umbilical stump is also a feature of factor XIII deficiency.

        ii. Factor XI deficiency is incompletely recessive because heterozygotes may have unpredictable bleeding problems with surgery or trauma.

        iii. VWD type III (rare, complete absence of VWF)

B. Platelet problems (see Chapter 47)

    1. Qualitative disorders include hereditary conditions (e.g., storage pool defects, Glanzmann thrombasthenia, Bernard-Soulier syndrome, platelet-type VWD) and transient disorders that result from maternal use of antiplatelet agents.

2. **Quantitative disorders** include the following:

a. Immune thrombocytopenia (maternal idiopathic thrombocytopenic purpura [ITP] or neonatal alloimmune thrombocytopenia [NAIT])

b. Maternal preeclampsia or Hemolysis, elevated liver enzymes, and low platelets (HELLP) syndrome (see Chapter 3) or severe uteroplacental vascular insufficiency

c. DIC

d. **Inherited marrow failure syndromes, including Fanconi anemia** and congenital amegakaryocytic thrombocytopenia

e. **Congenital** leukemia

f. Inherited thrombocytopenia syndromes, including gray-platelet syndrome and the macrothrombocytopenias (e.g., MYH9-related disorders, May-Hegglin syndrome)

g. Consumption of platelets, i.e., catheter-related thrombosis, RVT, NEC, or vascular anomalies, such as Kasabach-Merritt phenomenon (KMP) from kaposiform hemangioendothelioma or tufted angioma

h. Heparin-induced thrombocytopenia (HIT) results from antibody development to the complex of heparin with platelet factor IV. It is probably rare in neonates, although the antibody can be detected by enzyme-linked immunosorbent assay (ELISA) after cardiac surgery.

C. **Other potential causes of bleeding**

1. **Vascular** anomalies may cause central nervous system, gastrointestinal (GI), or pulmonary hemorrhage.

2. **Trauma** (see Chapter 6)

a. Rupture of spleen or liver associated with breech delivery

b. Retroperitoneal or intraperitoneal bleeding may present as scrotal ecchymosis.

c. Subdural hematoma, cephalohematoma, or subgaleal hemorrhage (the latter may be associated with vacuum extraction)

II. DIAGNOSTIC WORKUP OF THE BLEEDING INFANT

A. **History**

1. Family history of excessive bleeding or clotting

2. Maternal medications (e.g., aspirin, phenytoin)

3. Pregnancy and birth history

4. Maternal history of a prior infant with a bleeding disorder

5. Illness, medication, anomalies, or procedures performed on the infant

B. **Examination**

The crucial decision in diagnosing and managing the bleeding infant is determining whether the infant is sick or well (Table 43.1).

1. **Sick infant.** Consider DIC, viral or bacterial infection, or liver disease. Hypoxic/ischemic injury may lead to DIC.

2. **Well infant.** Consider vitamin K deficiency, isolated clotting factor deficiencies, or immune thrombocytopenia. Maternal blood in the infant's GI tract will not cause symptoms in the infant.

Table 43.1. Differential Diagnosis of Bleeding in the Neonate

Clinical Evaluation	Laboratory Studies			Likely Diagnosis
	Platelets	**PT**	**PTT**	
"Sick"	D−	I+	I+	DIC
	D−	N	N	Platelet consumption (infection, necrotizing enterocolitis, renal vein thrombosis, KMP)
	N	I+	I+	Liver disease
	N	N	N	Compromised vascular integrity associated with hypoxia, prematurity, acidosis, hyperosmolality
"Healthy"	D−	N	N	Immune thrombocytopenia, occult infection, thrombosis, bone marrow hypoplasia (rare), or bone marrow infiltrative disease
	N	I+	I+	Hemorrhagic disease of newborn (vitamin K deficiency)
	N	N	I+	Hereditary clotting factor deficiencies
	N	N	N	Bleeding due to local factors (trauma, anatomic abnormalities), qualitative platelet abnormalities (rare), factor XIII deficiency (rare), von Willebrand disease

PT, prothrombin time; PTT, partial thromboplastin time; D−, decreased; I+, increased; DIC, disseminated intravascular coagulation; N, normal; KMP, Kasabach-Merritt phenomenon. *Source*: Modified from Glader BE, Amylon MO. Bleeding disorders in the newborn infant. In: Taeusch HW, Ballard RA, Avery ME, eds. *Diseases of the Newborn*. Philadelphia, PA: WB Saunders; 1991.

3. **Petechiae, small superficial ecchymosis, or mucosal bleeding** suggests a platelet problem or von Willebrand disease.

4. **Large bruises** suggest deficiency of clotting factors, DIC, liver disease, or vitamin K deficiency.

5. **Enlarged spleen** suggests possible congenital infection or erythroblastosis.

6. **Jaundice** suggests infection, liver disease, or resorption of a large hematoma.

7. **Abnormal retinal findings** suggest infection (see Chapter 48).

C. Laboratory tests

Cord blood samples may be sent for coagulation testing if there is a suspicion for an inherited bleeding disorder at birth. Heel sticks and arterial draws should be avoided in patients at risk for a bleeding diathesis; venipuncture blood draw is the method of choice if cord blood samples are not obtained (Table 43.2).

1. The Apt test is used to rule out maternal blood. If the infant is well and only "GI bleeding" is noted, an Apt test is performed on gastric aspirate or stool to rule out the presence of maternal blood swallowed during labor or delivery or from a bleeding breast. A breast pump can be used to collect milk to confirm the presence of blood in the milk, or the infant's stomach can be aspirated before and after breastfeeding.

a. Procedure. Mix one part bloody stool or vomitus with five parts water; centrifuge it and separate the clear pink supernatant (hemolysate); add 1 mL of sodium hydroxide 1% (0.25 M) to 4 mL of hemolysate.

Table 43.2. Normal Values for Laboratory Screening Tests in the Neonate

Laboratory Test	Premature Infant Having Received Vitamin K	Term Infant Having Received Vitamin K	Child 1–2 Months of Age
Platelet count/μL	150,000–400,000	150,000–400,000	150,000–400,000
PT (seconds)*	14–22	13–20	12–14
PTT (seconds)*	35–55	30–45	25–35
Fibrinogen (mg/dL)	150–300	150–300	150–300

PT, prothrombin time; PTT, partial thromboplastin time.
*Normal values may vary from laboratory to laboratory, depending on the particular reagents employed. In full-term infants who have received vitamin K, the PT and PTT values generally fall within the normal "adult" range by several days (PT) to several weeks (PTT) of age. Small premature infants (under 1,500 g) tend to have longer PT and PTT than larger babies. In infants with hematocrit levels >60%, the ratio of blood to anticoagulant (sodium citrate 3.8%) in tubes should be 19:1 rather than the usual ratio of 9:1; otherwise, spurious results will be obtained because the amount of anticoagulant solution is calculated for a specific volume of plasma. Blood drawn from heparinized catheters should not be used. The best results are obtained when blood from a clean venipuncture is allowed to drip directly into the tube from the needle or scalp vein set. Factor levels II, VII, IX, and X are decreased. Three-day-old full-term baby not receiving vitamin K has levels similar to a premature baby. Factor XI and XII levels are lower in preterm infants than in term infants and account for prolonged PTT. Fibrinogen, factor V, and factor VIII are normal in premature and term infants. Factor XIII is variable.
Source: Data from normal laboratory values at the Hematology Laboratory, The Children's Hospital, Boston; Alpers JB, Lafonet MT, eds. Laboratory Handbook. Boston, MA: The Children's Hospital; 1984.

b. Result. Hemoglobin A (HbA) changes from pink to yellow brown (maternal blood); hemoglobin F (HbF) stays pink (fetal blood).

2. **Peripheral blood smear** is used to assess the number, size, and granulation of platelets and the presence of fragmented red blood cells (RBCs) as seen in DIC. Large platelets reflect either a congenital macrothrombocytopenia or young platelets, suggesting an immune-mediated or destructive thrombocytopenia.

3. **Platelet count**
   Significant bleeding from thrombocytopenia **is a greater risk with platelet counts ≤20,000 to 30,000/mm³**; however, bleeding with platelet counts up to 50,000 platelets/mm³ may be seen with NAIT. These alloantibodies against the platelet antigen HPA1 (also known as PLA1) interfere with platelet surface fibrinogen receptor, glycoprotein IIb to IIIa causing functional impairment (see Chapter 47).

4. **PT** is a test of the "extrinsic" clotting system, integrating activation of factor X by factor VII and tissue factor. Factor Xa, with factor Va as a cofactor, activates prothrombin (factor II) to form thrombin. Thrombin cleaves fibrinogen to fibrin.

5. **PTT** is a test of the "intrinsic" clotting system and of the activation of factor X by factors XII, XI, IX, and VIII as well as the downstream factors of the common coagulation pathway (factor V, prothrombin, and fibrinogen).

6. **Fibrinogen** can be measured on the same sample used for PT and PTT. It may be decreased in liver disease and consumptive states. The usual functional assay is low in dysfibrinogenemia.

7. **D-Dimer assays** measure degradation products of fibrin found in the plasma. D-Dimers are derivatives of cross-linked fibrin generated by the action of plasmin on fibrin clot. Normal levels vary by specific assay used (hospital-lab dependent). Levels are increased in patients with liver disease who have problems clearing fibrin split products, thromboembolism, and DIC. False-positive elevation in D-dimers are common in the intensive care unit setting because trivial clotting from catheter tips and other causes give positive results in this sensitive assay.

8. **Specific factor assays and von Willebrand panel** for patients with positive family history **can be measured in cord blood or by venipuncture after birth**. Age-specific norms must be used.

9. **Bleeding time is discouraged in all patients but especially in neonates.** This test measures response to a standardized razor blade cut. The apparatus is not well suited to infants and should never be used. Prolongation is not predictive of surgical bleeding.

10. Platelet function analysis using instruments such as the PFA100 may be useful as a screening test for VWD or platelet dysfunction in some settings, but confirmatory assays are required for positive tests. Because functional platelet assays are best drawn through large bore needles, if possible, assessment later in infancy or in affected family members is preferable to testing neonates.

III. TREATMENT OF NEONATES WITH ABNORMAL COAGULATION LABS WITHOUT CLINICAL BLEEDING.
In general, we treat *clinically ill* infants or infants weighing <1,500 g with fresh frozen plasma (FFP; 10 mL/kg) if the PT or PTT or both are ≥2 times normal for age and with platelets (10 to 15 mL/kg) (see section IV.C) if the platelet count is ≤20,000/mm^3 (see Chapter 42). This will vary with the clinical situations, trend of the laboratory values, impending surgery, and so forth. Some neonates will receive platelets if their platelet count is <50,000/mm^3, particularly in NAIT. In rare cases such as KMP, attempt at correction of the platelet count in the absence of bleeding can actually cause enlargement of the underlying vascular anomaly and worsening of symptoms.

IV. TREATMENT OF BLEEDING

A. Replacement therapies

1. **Vitamin K$_1$ (Aquamephyton).** An intravenous (IV) or intramuscular (IM) dose of 1 mg is administered in case the infant was not given vitamin K at birth. Infants receiving total parenteral nutrition and infants receiving antibiotics for more than 2 weeks should be given at least 0.5 mg of vitamin K$_1$ (IM or IV) weekly to prevent vitamin K depletion. If bleeding is minimal, vitamin K (rather than FFP) should be given for prolonged PT and PTT due to vitamin K deficiency. FFP should be reserved for significant or emergent bleeding; correction using vitamin K can take 12 to 48 hours.

2. **FFP and cryoprecipitate** (see Chapter 42). FFP (10 mL/kg) is given intravenously for active bleeding and is repeated every 8 to 12 hours as needed. A drip of 1 mL/kg/hour is an alternative, particularly if fluid balance is an issue. FFP replaces all the clotting factors; however, 10 mL/kg of FFP will transiently raise the factor levels approximately to 20% of adult control, so specific factor deficiencies should be treated with factor concentrate when available. Cryoprecipitate contains only factor VIII, VWF, fibrinogen, and factor XIII. Cryoprecipitate is the most practical source of fibrinogen or factor XIII for neonates until a specific diagnosis is made.

3. **Platelets** (see Chapter 47). In the absence of platelet destruction (such as DIC, immune destruction, or sepsis), 1 unit of random donor platelets should raise the platelet count by 50,000 to 100,000/mm^3 in a neonate. The platelet count will drop over 3 to 5 days unless platelet production increases. For alloimmune platelet destruction, either maternal platelets or platelets from a known platelet-compatible donor should be used if available. In the setting of bleeding, random donor platelets can be used.

4. **Fresh whole blood** (see Chapters 42 and 45). Whole blood is no longer available at most institutions. Initial transfusion may be 10 mL/kg but should be tailored to the clinical situation. Reconstituted components (FFP, packed red blood cell [PRBC], cryoprecipitate, and platelets) are more flexible and readily dosed than fresh whole blood.

5. **Clotting factor concentrates** (see Chapter 42). Factor concentrates are available for factors VIII, IX, VII, and XIII. When there is a known deficiency of factor VIII or IX, the plasma concentration should be raised to normal adult levels (50% to 100% of pooled normal control plasma, or 0.5 to 1.0 unit/mL) to stop serious bleeding. Factor VIII or IX concentrates should be used if the diagnosis is clear. If severe VWD is considered, a VWF-containing, plasma-derived factor VIII concentrate should be used. Recombinant VWF concentrate was recently licensed in the United States but has not been investigated in the neonatal setting.

B. **Treatment of specific disorders**

1. **DIC.** The infant typically appears ill and may have petechiae, GI hemorrhage, oozing from venipuncture sites, signs of infection, asphyxia, or hypoxia. The platelet count is decreased; PT and PTT are increased. Fibrinogen is decreased, and D-dimers are increased. Fragmented RBCs are seen on the blood smear. Treatment involves the following steps:

   a. **Identify and treat the underlying cause** (e.g., sepsis, NEC, herpes). This is **always** the most important factor in treatment of DIC.

   b. **Confirm that vitamin K$_1$ has been given.**

   c. **Administer platelets and FFP** as needed to keep the platelet count ≥50,000/mL and to control bleeding. FFP contains anticoagulant proteins, which may slow down or stop ongoing consumption.

   d. **For persistent bleeding** consider the following:
      i. Exchange transfusion with fresh citrated whole blood or reconstituted whole blood (PRBCs, platelets, FFP)
      ii. Continued transfusion with platelets, PRBCs, and FFP as needed particularly if exchange is not possible.
      iii. Administration of cryoprecipitate (1 to 2 units per 10 kg) for hypofibrinogenemia

   e. For consumptive coagulopathy secondary to large vessel thrombosis without concurrent bleeding, consider treatment with unfractionated heparin (UFH) infusion **without a bolus** (e.g., 20 to 25 units/kg/hour as a continuous infusion) to maintain a UFH level of 0.35 to 0.7 units/mL. Check levels 4 hours after initiation and 4 hours after each infusion rate change. Administer platelets and FFP after heparin initiation to maintain platelet counts ≥50,000/mL and provide antithrombin and anticoagulant proteins essential to heparin function. Anticoagulation is generally contraindicated in the presence of intracranial hemorrhage. When DIC manifests as both bleeding and thrombosis concurrently, heparinization is complicated; consult an expert immediately (see Chapter 44).

2. **Hemorrhagic disease of the newborn (HDN)** occurs in 1 out of every 200 to 400 neonates not given vitamin K prophylaxis.

   a. In the healthy infant, **HDN may occur when the infant is not given vitamin K**. The infant may have been born in a busy delivery room, at home, or transferred from elsewhere. Bleeding and bruising may occur after the infant is 48 hours old. The platelet level is normal, and PT and PTT are prolonged. If there is active bleeding, 10 mL/kg of FFP and an IV dose of 1 mg of vitamin K are given.

   b. **If the mother has been treated with phenytoin (Dilantin), primidone (Mysoline), methsuximide (Celontin), or phenobarbital, the**

infant may be vitamin K deficient and bleed during the first 24 hours. The mother should receive 10 mg of vitamin K_1 IM 24 hours before delivery. The usual dose of vitamin K_1 (1 mg) should be given to the infant postpartum and repeated in 24 hours. The newborn should have PT, PTT, and platelet counts monitored if any signs of bleeding occur. Infuse FFP for bleeding.

c. Delayed HDN from vitamin K deficiency can occur at 4 to 12 weeks of age. Although blood tests show that breastfed infants are at potential risk for HDN, HDN has not been reported in infants who received IM vitamin K at birth. Vitamin K_1, 1 mg/week orally for the first 3 months of life for breastfed infants, may prevent late HDN. Infants receiving broad-spectrum antibiotics or infants with malabsorption (liver disease, cystic fibrosis) are at greater risk for vitamin K deficiency and hemorrhagic disease.

Suggested Readings

Andrew M, Paes B, Johnston M. Development of the hemostatic system in the neonate and young infant. *Am J Pediatr Hematol Oncol* 1990;12:95–104.

Arnold PD. Coagulation and the surgical neonate. *Paediatr Anaesth* 2014;24:89–97.

Avila ML, Shah V, Brandão LR. Systematic review on heparin-induced thrombocytopenia in children: a call to action. *J Thromb Haemost* 2013;11:660–669.

Kenet G, Chan AK, Soucie JM, et al. Bleeding disorders in neonates. *Haemophilia* 2010;16(suppl 5);168–175.

Peterson JA, McFarland JG, Curtis BR, et al. Neonatal alloimmune thrombocytopenia: pathogenesis, diagnosis and management. *Br J Haematol* 2013;161: 3–14.

Revel-Vilk S. The conundrum of neonatal coagulopathy. *Hematology Am Soc Hematol Educ Program* 2012;2012:450–454.

Neonatal Thrombosis

Katherine A. Sparger and Munish Gupta

KEY POINTS

- Neonatal thrombosis is a rare but significant cause of neonatal morbidity and mortality.
- The presence of an intravascular catheter is the single most important risk factor for neonatal thrombosis and is associated with the vast majority of thrombotic events. Renal vein thrombosis is the most common cause of non–catheter-associated thrombosis in neonates and can result in long-term renal impairment.
- It is generally recommended that neonates with clinically significant thrombosis should undergo a thrombophilia evaluation. The frequency and contribution of inherited and acquired prothrombotic states to thromboembolic events in neonates remains poorly understood.
- Unfractionated heparin and low molecular weight heparin (e.g., enoxaparin) are first-line therapies for the treatment of neonates with clinically significant thrombosis.
- Thrombolysis with tissue plasminogen activator (tPA) can be considered for organ-, limb-, or life-threatening thrombosis, although associated risks must be carefully weighed.

I. PHYSIOLOGY

A. **Physiology of thrombosis**

1. **Thrombin is the primary procoagulant protein**, converting fibrinogen into a fibrin clot. The intrinsic and extrinsic pathways of the coagulation cascade result in formation of active thrombin from prothrombin.

2. **Inhibitors of coagulation** include antithrombin, heparin cofactors, protein C, protein S, α2-macroglobulin, and tissue factor pathway inhibitor. Antithrombin activity is potentiated by heparin.

3. **Plasmin is the primary fibrinolytic enzyme**, degrading fibrin in a reaction that produces fibrin degradation products and D-dimers. Plasmin is formed from plasminogen by numerous enzymes, most important of which is tPA.

4. In neonates, factors affecting blood flow, blood composition (leading to hypercoagulability), and vascular endothelial integrity can all contribute to thrombus formation.

B. Unique physiologic characteristics of hemostasis in neonates

1. *In utero*, coagulation proteins are synthesized by the fetus as early as 10 weeks gestational age and do not cross the placenta.

2. Both thrombogenic and fibrinolytic pathways are altered in the neonate compared with the older child and adult, resulting in increased vulnerability to both hemorrhage and pathologic thrombosis. Under normal physiologic conditions, however, the hemostatic system in preterm and term newborns is in balance, and healthy neonates do not clinically demonstrate hypercoagulable or bleeding tendencies.

3. Concentrations of most procoagulant proteins, particularly vitamin K–dependent coagulation factors, are reduced in neonates compared with adult values; levels of some procoagulant factors such as factor VIII and fibrinogen are typically normal or even increased. Compared to adults, neonates have a decreased ability to generate thrombin, and values for the prothrombin time (PT) and the activated partial thromboplastin time (PTT) are prolonged.

4. Concentrations of most antithrombotic and fibrinolytic proteins are also reduced, including protein C, protein S, plasminogen, and antithrombin, although α2-macroglobulin concentration is increased. Thrombin inhibition by plasmin is diminished compared with adult plasma.

5. Platelet number and life span appear to be similar to that of adults. The bleeding time, an overall assessment of platelet function and interaction with vascular endothelium, is shorter in neonates than in adults, suggesting more rapid platelet adhesion and aggregation.

II. EPIDEMIOLOGY AND RISK FACTORS

A. Epidemiology

1. Thrombosis occurs more frequently in the neonatal period than at any other age in childhood.

2. The presence of an **indwelling vascular catheter** is the single greatest risk factor for arterial or venous thrombosis. Indwelling catheters are responsible for more than 80% of venous and 90% of arterial thrombotic complications.

3. Autopsy studies show 20% to 65% of infants who expire with an umbilical venous catheter (UVC) in place are found to have a thrombus associated with the catheter. Venography suggests asymptomatic thrombi are present in 30% of newborns with a UVC.

4. Umbilical arterial catheterization (UAC) appears to result in severe symptomatic vessel obstruction requiring intervention in approximately 1% of patients. Asymptomatic catheter-associated thrombi have been found in 3% to 59% of cases by autopsy and 10% to 90% of cases by angiography or ultrasound.

5. **Multiple maternal, perinatal, and neonatal risk factors are thought to contribute to thrombotic events in newborns.** Maternal factors

include infertility, oligohydramnios, preeclampsia, diabetes, intrauterine growth restriction (IUGR), prolonged rupture of membranes, chorio-amnionitis, and autoimmune and prothrombotic disorders. Perinatal risk factors include emergent cesarean section or instrumented delivery and fetal heart rate abnormalities. Neonatal risk factors include congenital heart disease, sepsis, birth asphyxia, respiratory distress syndrome, dehydration, polycythemia, congenital nephritic/nephrotic syndrome, necrotizing enterocolitis, pulmonary hypertension, and prothrombotic disorders.

6. Infants undergoing surgery involving the vascular system, including repair of congenital heart disease, are at increased risk for thrombotic complications. Diagnostic or interventional catheterizations also increase the risk of thrombosis.

7. **Renal vein thrombosis** is the most common type of non–catheter-related pathologic thrombosis in newborns.

8. Registries from Canada, Germany, The Netherlands, and Italy have described series of cases of neonatal thrombosis.

   a. Incidence of clinically significant thrombosis among infants in neonatal intensive care units (NICUs) was reported as 2.4 per 1,000 NICU admissions in Canada, 6.8 per 1,000 NICU admissions in The Netherlands, and 5.8 and 6.6 per 1,000 NICU admissions at two large centers in Italy. Incidence among live births was estimated at 5.1 per 100,000 births in Germany, 14.5 per 10,000 neonates in The Netherlands, and 3.4 and 6.5 per 10,000 live births at the Italian centers.

   b. Three series examined both venous and arterial thromboses. Among all thrombotic events, the percentage of renal vein thrombosis ranged from 19% to 44%, other venous thrombosis ranged from 33% to 40%, and arterial thrombosis from 24% to 34%.

   c. Excluding cases of renal vein thrombosis, 67%, 89%, and 94% of venous thromboses were found to be associated with indwelling central lines in three series.

   d. Mortality was rare and generally restricted to very premature infants or infants with large arterial or intracardiac thromboses.

B. Inherited hypercoagulable states

1. **Inherited prothrombotic disorders** are characterized by positive family history, early age of onset, recurrent disease, and unusual or multiple locations of thromboembolic events. Although it is estimated that a genetic risk factor can be identified in 10% to 50% of children with thrombosis, the incidence of these disorders in newborns with thrombosis is not well known.

2. Important inherited prothrombotic disorders include the following:

   a. Deficiencies of protein C, protein S, and antithrombin appear to have the largest increase in relative risk for thromboembolic disease but are relatively rare.

   b. Activated protein C resistance, including factor V Leiden mutation and prothrombin G20210A mutation, have a high incidence, particularly in certain populations, but appear to have low risk of thrombosis in neonates.

    c. **Hyperhomocysteinemia, increased lipoprotein (a) levels, and poly-morphism in the methylene tetrahydrofolate reductase (MTHFR) gene** are relatively common, but their significance in neonatal thrombosis is still poorly understood.

3. Multiple other defects in the anticoagulation, fibrinolytic, and antifi-brinolytic pathways have been identified, including abnormalities in thrombomodulin, tissue factor pathway inhibitor, fibrinogen, plasmino-gen, tPA, and plasminogen-activator inhibitors. The frequency and im-portance of these defects in neonatal thrombosis is poorly understood.

4. The incidence of thrombosis in patients heterozygous for most inherited thrombophilias is small; however, increasing evidence suggests that the presence of a second risk factor substantially increases the risk for throm-bosis. This second risk factor can be an acquired clinical condition or another inherited defect. Patients with single defects for inherited pro-thrombotic disorders rarely present in neonatal period, unless another pathologic event occurs.

5. Patients who are homozygous for a single defect or double heterozy-gotes for different defects can present in the neonatal period, often with significant illness due to thrombosis. The classic presentation of homo-zygous prothrombotic disorders is **purpura fulminans** associated with homozygous protein C or S deficiency, which presents within hours or days of birth, often with evidence of *in utero* cerebral damage.

6. Overall, the importance of inherited thrombophilias as independent risk factors for neonatal thrombosis is still undetermined. It appears that the absolute risk of thrombosis in the neonatal period in all patients with an inherited non-homozygous thrombophilia is low. Among neonates with thrombotic disease, however, the incidence of an inherited thrombo-philia appears to be substantially increased compared to that of the gen-eral population, and evaluation for thrombophilia should be considered.

C. **Acquired thrombophilias**

1. Newborns can acquire significant coagulation factor deficiencies due to placental transfer of maternal antiphospholipid antibodies, including lupus anticoagulant and anticardiolipin antibodies.

2. These neonates can present with significant thrombosis, including pur-pura fulminans.

3. Mothers should potentially be screened for the presence of autoimmune antibodies as part of a thrombophilia evaluation for neonates presenting with clinically significant thrombosis.

III. SPECIFIC CLINICAL CONDITIONS

A. **Venous thromboembolic disorders**

    1. **General considerations**

        a. Most venous thrombosis occur secondary to **central venous lines (CVLs)**. Spontaneous (i.e., non–catheter-related) venous thrombosis can occur in renal veins, adrenal veins, superior or inferior vena cava, portal vein, hepatic veins, and the venous system of the brain.

b. Spontaneous venous thrombi usually occur in the presence of another risk factor. Less than 1% of clinically significant venous thromboembolic events in neonates are idiopathic.

c. Thrombosis of the **sinovenous system of the brain** is an important cause of neonatal cerebral infarction.

d. Surgical repair of complex congenital heart disease has been associated with an increased risk of thrombosis, particularly of the superior vena cava.

e. It is likely that the frequency of pulmonary embolism in sick neonates is underestimated because signs and symptoms would be similar to other common neonatal pulmonary diseases.

f. Short-term complications of venous catheter–associated thrombosis include loss of access, pulmonary embolism, superior vena cava syndrome, and specific organ impairment.

g. Long-term complications of venous thrombosis are poorly understood. Inferior vena cava thrombosis, if extensive, can be associated with a high rate of persistent partial obstruction and symptoms such as leg edema, abdominal pain, lower extremity thrombophlebitis, varicose veins, and leg ulcers. Other complications can include chylothorax, portal hypertension, and embolism.

2. **Catheter-associated venous thrombosis**
   a. **Signs and symptoms**
      i. The most common initial sign of catheter-related thrombosis is usually difficulty infusing through or withdrawing from the line.
      ii. Additional signs of venous obstruction include swelling of the extremities, head and neck, or distended superficial veins.
      iii. The onset of thrombocytopenia in the presence of a CVL also raises the suspicion of thrombosis.
   b. **Diagnosis**
      i. **Ultrasound with Doppler** is diagnostic in most cases of significant venous thrombosis. In smaller infants or low-flow states; however, ultrasound may not provide sufficient information about the size of the thrombus, and a significant false-negative rate has been documented.
      ii. Contrast studies, including a radiographic line study or venography through peripheral vessels, may assist with the diagnosis of catheter-associated thrombosis. However, these studies are rarely performed secondary to improvements in ultrasound technology and associated risks in neonates.
   c. **Prevention of catheter-associated venous thrombosis**
      i. Unfractionated heparin 0.5 U/mL is added to all compatible infusions through CVLs.
      ii. UVCs should be removed as soon as clinically feasible and should not remain in place for longer than 10 to 14 days. A peripherally inserted central catheter (PICC) line is typically placed if the anticipated need for central access is >7 days.
   d. **Management of catheter-associated venous thrombosis**
      i. **Nonfunctioning CVL.** If fluid can no longer be easily infused through the catheter, remove the catheter unless the CVL is

absolutely necessary. If continued central access through the catheter is judged to be clinically necessary, however, clearance of the blockage with thrombolytic agents (e.g., tPA) can be considered.

ii. Local obstruction. If a small occlusive catheter-related thrombosis is documented, a low-dose infusion of thrombolytic agent through the catheter can be considered for localized site-directed thrombolytic therapy. If infusion through the catheter is not possible, the CVL should be removed and heparin therapy considered.

iii. Extensive venous thrombosis. It is currently recommended that UVCs and CVLs associated with confirmed extensive thrombosis by ultrasound be left in place for 3 to 5 days of therapeutic anticoagulation and subsequently removed in order to reduce the risk of paradoxical emboli. Systemic thrombolytic therapy should be reserved for extensive non–catheter-related organ-, limb-, or life-threatening venous thrombosis.

3. Renal vein thrombosis

a. Renal vein thrombosis occurs primarily in newborns and young infants and most often presents in the first week of life. A significant proportion of cases appear to result from *in utero* thrombus formation.

b. Affected neonates are usually term and often large for gestational age. There is an increased incidence among infants of diabetic mothers, and males are more often affected than females. A recent review demonstrated bilateral renal vein thrombus formation in up to 30% of cases.

c. Additional risk factors include perinatal asphyxia, hypotension, polycythemia, increased blood viscosity, and cyanotic congenital heart disease.

d. Presenting symptoms in the neonatal period include flank mass, hematuria, proteinuria, thrombocytopenia, and renal dysfunction. The diagnosis is made by ultrasound with Doppler interrogation. Coagulation studies may be prolonged, and fibrin degradation products are usually increased.

e. Complications can include hypertension, renal failure, adrenal hemorrhage, extension of the thrombus into the inferior vena cava, and death.

f. Retrospective studies have demonstrated that 43% to 67% of neonates with renal vein thrombosis had at least one or more prothrombotic risk factors. A thrombophilia evaluation of infants with renal vein thrombosis is warranted.

g. Management is generally based on the extent of thrombosis.

i. Unilateral renal vein thrombosis without significant renal dysfunction or extension into the inferior vena cava is often managed with supportive care and close radiologic monitoring.

ii. Unilateral renal vein thrombosis with renal dysfunction or extension into the inferior vena cava and bilateral renal vein thrombosis should be considered for therapeutic anticoagulation with unfractionated heparin or LMWH for a total duration of 6 weeks to 3 months. Note that dosing of LMWH may need to be reduced in patients with renal insufficiency.

iii. Bilateral renal vein thrombosis with significant renal dysfunction should be considered for thrombolysis with tPA followed by anticoagulation with unfractionated heparin or LMWH.

4. Portal vein thrombosis

a. Portal vein thrombosis is primarily associated with sepsis, omphalitis, exchange transfusion, and the presence of a UVC.

b. Diagnosis is made by ultrasound with Doppler, and reversal of portal flow is an indication of severity.

c. Spontaneous resolution is common (30% to 70% of cases); however, portal vein thrombosis can be associated with later development of portal hypertension.

d. There are currently no data to suggest that anticoagulation decreases the time to resolution or the risk of developing portal hypertension.

5. Cerebral sinovenous thrombosis

a. Thrombosis of the sinovenous system of the brain is an important cause of neonatal cerebral infarction and is associated with significant morbidity including epilepsy, cerebral palsy, and cognitive impairment in 10% to 80% of cases. Reported mortality rates range between 2% and 24%.

b. Major presenting clinical features of cerebral sinovenous thrombosis in neonates include seizures, lethargy, irritability, and poor feeding. The majority of cases present within the first day to week of life.

c. The superior sagittal sinus, transverse sinuses, and straight sinus are most commonly affected.

d. Hemorrhagic infarction is a frequent complication of sinovenous thrombosis and noted in 50% to 60% of cases on initial imaging.

e. The majority of cases of neonatal sinovenous thrombosis are associated with maternal conditions including preeclampsia, diabetes, and chorioamnionitis as well as acute systemic illness in the neonate.

f. Inherited thrombophilias have been reported in 15% to 20% of neonates with sinovenous thrombosis.

g. Ultrasound and computed tomography (CT) scan can identify sinovenous thrombosis, but magnetic resonance imaging (MRI) with venography is the imaging modality of choice for optimal detection of sinovenous thrombosis and associated cerebral injury.

h. Data on management remains limited. In general, neonates with cerebral sinovenous thrombosis without associated hemorrhage should be considered for anticoagulation therapy initially with unfractionated heparin or LMWH and subsequently LMWH for a total of 6 weeks to 3 months. If significant hemorrhage is present, anticoagulation should be reserved for cases with propagation of the thrombus.

B. Aortic or clinically significant arterial thrombosis

1. General considerations

a. Spontaneous arterial thrombi in the absence of a vascular catheter are unusual but may occur in ill neonates. Potential locations include the aortic arch, descending aorta, left pulmonary artery, and iliac arteries.

b. Acute complications of catheter-related and spontaneous arterial thrombi depend on location and can include renal failure, hypertension, intestinal necrosis, peripheral gangrene, other organ failure, and death.

c. Thrombosis of cerebral arteries is an important cause of neonatal cerebral infarction.

d. Long-term effects of symptomatic and asymptomatic arterial thrombi are not well studied but may include increased risk for atherosclerosis and chronic renal hypertension.

2. Aortic thrombosis

a. Signs and symptoms

i. An initial sign is often isolated dysfunction of the UAC.

ii. Mild clinical signs include microscopic or gross hematuria in absence of transfusions or hemolysis, hypertension, and intermittent decreased perfusion or color change of the lower extremities.

iii. Strong clinical signs include persistent lower extremity color change or decreased perfusion, blood pressure differential between upper and lower extremities, decrease or loss of lower extremity pulses, oliguria despite adequate intravascular volume, signs of necrotizing enterocolitis, or congestive heart failure.

b. Diagnosis

i. Ultrasound with Doppler flow imaging should be performed in all cases of suspected aortic thrombosis. If signs of thrombosis are mild and resolve promptly after removal of the arterial catheter, an ultrasound may not be necessary. Ultrasound is diagnostic in most cases, although a significant false-negative rate has been documented.

ii. Historically, radiographic **contrast studies** were performed if ultrasound was inconclusive. These studies are generally no longer recommended in neonates because of the associated risks.

iii. Echocardiogram should be considered if there is concern for the presence of thrombus within the heart, aortic arch, or proximal aorta or if there is evidence of congestive heart failure.

c. Prevention of catheter-associated arterial thrombosis

i. Unfractionated heparin 0.5 to 1 U/mL is added to all compatible infusions through arterial catheters in order to prolong patency. This has not been shown to decrease the risk of associated thrombosis.

ii. A review of the literature suggests **"high" umbilical arterial lines** (tip in descending aorta below left subclavian artery and above diaphragm) are preferable to "low" lines (tip below renal arteries and above aortic bifurcation), with fewer clinically evident ischemic complications and trend toward a decreased incidence of associated thrombi. No difference was noted in the incidence of serious complications including necrotizing enterocolitis and renal dysfunction.

iii. Consider placing a **peripheral arterial line** rather than an umbilical arterial line in infants weighing >1,500 g.

iv. Monitor carefully for clinical evidence of thrombus formation when a UAC is present, including serial evaluations of lower extremity color, pulses, and perfusion; concordance of upper and lower extremity blood pressures; hypertension; decreased urine output; urine for microscopic or gross hematuria; and waveform dampening with difficulty flushing or withdrawing blood.

v. UACs should be removed as soon as clinically feasible. It is generally recommended that UACs remain in place for no longer than

5 to 7 days. If necessary, a peripheral arterial line should be placed if continued arterial access is needed.

d. Management of aortic and clinically significant arterial thrombosis

    i. Minor aortic thrombi with mild symptoms can often be managed with prompt removal of the UAC, resulting in rapid resolution of symptoms.

    ii. For **large but nonocclusive thrombi** that are not accompanied by signs of significant clinical compromise, the arterial catheter should be removed and anticoagulation with unfractionated heparin or LMWH considered. Close follow-up with serial ultrasound imaging is indicated.

    iii. Large occlusive aortic thrombi or thrombi accompanied by signs of significant clinical compromise should be managed aggressively. If the catheter is still present and patent, consider local thrombolytic therapy through the catheter. If the catheter has already been removed or is obstructed, consider systemic thrombolytic therapy. The catheter should be removed if still in place and obstructed.

    iv. Surgical thrombectomy is generally not indicated with the exception of life- or limb-threatening thrombosis because the associated mortality and morbidity in neonates are considered to exceed that of current medical management. Some recent experience suggests thrombectomy and subsequent vascular reconstruction may have utility in significant peripheral arterial thrombosis, although experience is limited.

3. Peripheral arterial thrombosis

a. Although rare, congenital occlusions of large peripheral arteries are seen and can present with symptoms ranging from a poorly perfused pulseless extremity to a black necrotic limb, depending on the duration and timing of the occlusion. Common symptoms include decreased perfusion, decreased pulses, and pallor. Embolic phenomena may manifest as skin lesions or petechiae. The diagnosis can often be made by Doppler flow ultrasound.

b. Peripheral arterial catheters are rarely associated with significant thrombosis. Poor perfusion to the distal extremity is frequently seen and usually resolves with prompt removal of the arterial line. Unfractionated heparin 0.5 to 1 U/mL at 1 to 2 mL/hour is generally infused continuously through all peripheral arterial lines. Treatment of significant thrombosis or persistently compromised extremity perfusion associated with a peripheral catheter should consist of heparin anticoagulation and consideration of systemic thrombolysis for extensive lesions. Close follow-up with serial ultrasound imaging is indicated.

IV. DIAGNOSTIC CONSIDERATIONS

A. Ultrasound with Doppler flow analysis is the most commonly used diagnostic modality. Advantages include relative ease of performance, non-invasiveness, and ability to perform sequential scans to assess progression of thrombosis or response to treatment.

B. Although uncommonly used, **radiographic line study and venography** can aid in diagnosis. Imaging after injection of contrast material through a central catheter can be diagnostic for catheter-associated thrombi, although a line study will not provide information on thrombosis proximal to catheter tip. Venography with injection of contrast through peripheral vessels may be necessary when other diagnostic methods fail to demonstrate the extent and severity of thrombosis; upper extremity and upper chest venous thromboses can be particularly difficult to visualize by ultrasound.

V. MANAGEMENT

A. Evaluation for thrombophilia

1. Consider evaluating for congenital or acquired thrombophilias in neonates with severe or unusual manifestations of thrombosis or with positive family histories of thrombosis. The benefit of evaluation in infants with known risk factors such as indwelling central catheters is uncertain.

2. Initial evaluation should include consideration of deficiencies of protein C, protein S, and antithrombin, presence of activated protein C resistance, factor V Leiden mutation, prothrombin G20210A mutation, and passage of maternal antiphospholipid antibodies.
   a. Protein C, protein S, and antithrombin deficiencies can be evaluated by measurement of antigen or activity levels. Results of testing of neonates should be compared with standard gestational age–based reference ranges because normal physiologic values can be as low as 15% to 20% of adult values. In addition, levels will be physiologically depressed in the presence of active thrombosis and may be difficult to interpret. It is generally recommended that levels be rechecked 2 to 3 months after the acute thrombotic episode. As an alternative to or in conjunction with testing of the neonate, parents can be tested for carrier status by measurement of protein C, protein S, and antithrombin levels.
   b. Factor V Leiden, prothrombin G20210A, and MTHFR mutations can be assayed by specific genetic tests in the neonate. Parents can be tested for carrier status.
   c. Autoimmune antibodies, including an antiphospholipid antibody panel, anticardiolipin, and lupus anticoagulant levels, can be checked in the mother.

3. If the given testing is negative, subsequent specialized laboratory evaluation includes abnormalities or deficiencies of homocysteine, lipoprotein (a), plasminogen, and fibrinogen. Very rarely seen are abnormalities or deficiencies of heparin cofactor II, thrombomodulin, plasminogen activator inhibitor-1, platelet aggregation, and tPA.

B. General considerations

1. Precautions

a. It is important to note that recommendations and dosing regimens for anticoagulant and thrombolytic therapies in neonates are largely based on findings from adult and pediatric studies. Small neonatal cohort studies and case series have further informed expert consensus.

b. Watchful waiting is a reasonable option for thrombotic events that are not organ-, limb-, and life-threatening. Clinicians must carefully weigh the risks and benefits of anticoagulation and thrombolytic therapies for clinically significant thrombotic events in a high-risk neonatal population.

c. Practically, it is important to avoid procedures such as intramuscular injections and arterial punctures and limit physical manipulation of the patient (i.e., no physical therapy) during anticoagulant or thrombolytic therapy. It is similarly important to avoid indomethacin or other antiplatelet drugs during therapy.

d. Monitor clinical status carefully for signs of hemorrhage, particularly internal and intracranial hemorrhage.

2. **Guidelines for choice of therapy**

a. Small asymptomatic nonocclusive arterial or venous thrombi related to catheters can often be treated with catheter removal and supportive care alone.

b. Large or occlusive arterial or venous thrombi can be treated with anticoagulation with unfractionated heparin or LMWH. Usually, relatively short courses of anticoagulation are sufficient, but occasionally, long-term treatment may be necessary.

c. In cases of massive arterial or venous thrombi with significant clinical compromise, treatment with local or systemic thrombolysis should be considered.

3. **Contraindications to anticoagulation and thrombolytic therapy**

a. In general, **absolute contraindications** include central nervous system surgery or ischemia within past 10 days, invasive procedures within past 3 days, seizures within past 48 hours, and active bleeding.

b. In general, **relative contraindications** include platelet count $<50,000/\mu L$ or $<100,000/\mu L$ in critically ill neonates, fibrinogen level <100 mg/dL, international normalized ratio (INR) >2, severe coagulopathy, and hypertension.

C. **Unfractionated heparin**

1. **General considerations**

a. Term newborns generally have faster clearance of heparin and lower antithrombin levels compared with adults. These factors generally result in a relative increase in the heparin dose required to achieve therapeutic levels in neonates. There is also significant variability in heparin dosage requirements between patients.

b. If possible, unfractionated heparin should be infused through a dedicated intravenous (IV) line not used for any other medications or fluids.

c. Prior to starting heparin therapy, a baseline complete blood count (CBC), PT, and PTT should be obtained and monitored serially during the course of treatment. Heparin-induced thrombocytopenia (HIT), secondary to heparin-associated antiplatelet antibodies, is an extremely rare complication of heparin therapy in neonates.

d. Adjustment of the unfractionated heparin infusion rate is based on clinical response, serial evaluation of thrombus (usually by ultrasound), and monitoring of laboratory parameters.

e. Use of PTT to monitor heparin effect is problematic in neonates due to significant variability of coagulation factor concentrations and baseline prolongation of the PTT. **Heparin activity level** is generally considered to be a more reliable marker. Therapeutic heparin activity for treatment of most thromboembolic events is considered to be an antifactor Xa level of 0.35 to 0.7 U/mL or a heparin level by protamine titration of 0.2 to 0.4 U/mL. Most laboratories report heparin activity levels as an antifactor Xa level.

f. Heparin activity is dependent on the presence of antithrombin. Consider administration of fresh frozen plasma (10 mL/kg) when effective anticoagulation with unfractionated heparin is difficult to achieve. Administration of antithrombin concentrate can also be considered, although evidence for its use in neonates is limited.

    i. Antithrombin levels can be measured directly to aid in therapy, although administration of exogenous antithrombin can increase sensitivity to heparin even in patients with near-normal antithrombin levels.

    ii. Note that measurement of heparin activity levels, unlike measurement of PTT, is independent of the presence of antithrombin. Therefore, measured heparin activity levels may be therapeutic even though effective anticoagulation has not been achieved due to antithrombin deficiency.

2. Dosing guidelines

    a. Standard unfractionated heparin is given as an initial bolus of 75 U/kg IV, followed by a continuous infusion that is begun at 28 U/kg/hour. In premature infants under 37 weeks' gestation, lower dosing of 25 to 50 U/kg bolus followed by 15 to 20 U/kg/hour can be considered.

    b. Heparin activity levels and/or PTT should be measured 4 hours after initial bolus and 4 hours after each change in infusion dose and every 24 hours once a therapeutic infusion dose has been achieved (Table 44.1).

3. Duration of therapy. Anticoagulation with unfractionated heparin may continue up to 10 to 14 days. Oral anticoagulants are generally not recommended in neonates. If long-term anticoagulation is needed, consult hematology and consider transitioning to LMWH.

4. Reversal of anticoagulation

    a. Termination of the unfractionated heparin infusion will quickly reverse anticoagulation effects of heparin therapy and is usually sufficient.

    b. If rapid reversal is necessary, protamine sulfate may be given IV. Protamine can be given in a concentration of 10 mg/mL at a rate not to exceed 5 mg/minute. Hypersensitivity can occur in patients who have received protamine-containing insulin or previous protamine therapy.

    c. Dosing. Based on total amount of heparin received in last 2 hours as shown in Table 44.2.

D. Low molecular weight heparin

    1. General considerations

        a. In recent years, LMWH, specifically enoxaparin (Lovenox), has become the anticoagulant of choice for neonates based on growing experience as well as evidence of safety and efficacy in this patient population.

Table 44.1. Unfractionated Heparin Dosage Monitoring and Adjustment

PTT (second)*	Heparin Activity (U/mL)	Bolus (U/kg)	Hold	Rate	Recheck
<50	0–0.2	50	—	+10%	4 hours
50–59	0.21–0.34	0	—	+10%	4 hours
60–85	0.35–0.7	0	—	—	24 hours
86–95	0.71–0.8	0	—	−10%	4 hours
96–120	0.81–1.0	0	30 minutes	−10%	4 hours
>120	>1	0	60 minutes	−15%	4 hours

*Partial thromboplastin time (PTT) values may vary by laboratory depending on reagents used. Generally, PTT values of 1.5 to 2.5 × the baseline normal for a given laboratory correspond to heparin activity levels of 0.35 to 0.7 U/mL.
Source: Adapted from Monagle P, Chan AK, Goldenberg NA, et al. Antithrombotic therapy in neonates and children: Antithrombotic Therapy and Prevention of Thrombosis, 9th ed: American College of Chest Physicians Evidence-Based Clinical Practice Guidelines. *Chest* 2012;141(2 suppl):e737S–e801S.

b. Several **advantages of LMWHs** over standard unfractionated heparin exist: more predictable pharmacokinetics, decreased need for laboratory monitoring, decreased need for dedicated venous access, subcutaneous twice daily (BID) dosing, reduced risk of HIT, and possible reduced risk of bleeding at recommended dosages.

Table 44.2. Protamine Dosage to Reverse Heparin Therapy (Based on Total Amount of Unfractionated Heparin Received in Prior 2 Hours)

Time Since Last Heparin Dose (minutes)	Protamine Dose (mg/100 U Heparin Received)
<30	1.0
30–60	0.5–0.75
60–120	0.375–0.5
>120	0.25–0.375

Maximum dosage is 50 mg. Maximum infusion rate is 5 mg/minute of 10 mg/mL solution.
Source: Adapted from Monagle P, Chan AK, Goldenberg NA, et al. Antithrombotic therapy in neonates and children: Antithrombotic Therapy and Prevention of Thrombosis, 9th ed: American College of Chest Physicians Evidence-Based Clinical Practice Guidelines. *Chest* 2012;141(2 suppl):e737S–e801S.

c. Therapeutic dosage of LMWH is titrated to antifactor Xa levels. **Target antifactor Xa levels** for the treatment of most thromboembolic events are 0.50 to 1.0 U/mL, measured 4 to 6 hours after a subcutaneous injection. In patients at particularly high risk for bleeding, target levels of 0.4 to 0.6 U/mL can be considered. When used for prophylaxis, target levels are 0.1 to 0.4 U/mL. After therapeutic levels have been achieved for 24 to 48 hours, levels should be followed at least weekly along with a CBC as thrombocytopenia can occur.

d. Infants younger than 2 months of age have a higher dose requirement than older children. In addition, some studies suggest higher initial doses for preterm infants. Dosage requirements to maintain target levels in preterm infants may be quite variable.

e. Several different LMWHs are available, and the dosages are not interchangeable. **Enoxaparin (Lovenox)** has the most widespread pediatric usage.

f. Cases of severe bleeding, including hematoma formation at injection sites, gastrointestinal bleeding, and intracranial hemorrhage have been reported in rare cases in association with LMWH usage in neonates and should be monitored for closely.

2. Dosing guidelines (Tables 44.3 and 44.4)

3. Reversal of anticoagulation

a. Termination of subcutaneous injections usually is sufficient to reverse anticoagulation when clinically necessary.

b. If rapid reversal is needed, protamine sulfate can be given within 3 to 4 hours of last injection, although protamine may not completely reverse anticoagulant effects. Administer 1 mg protamine sulfate per 1 mg LMWH given in last injection.

E. Thrombolysis

1. General considerations

a. Thrombolytic agents act by converting endogenous plasminogen to plasmin. Plasminogen levels in neonates are reduced compared with adult values, and thus, effectiveness of thrombolytic agents may be diminished. Cotreatment with plasminogen with the administration of fresh frozen plasma can increase thrombolytic effect of these agents.

Table 44.3. Initial Dosing of Enoxaparin, Age-Dependent (in mg/kg/dose SQ)

Age	Initial Treatment Dose	Initial Prophylactic Dose
<2 months	1.5 q12h	0.75 q12h
>2 months	1.0 q12h	0.5 q12h

Initial dose of 2 mg/kg every 12 hours can be considered in preterm infants. SQ, subcutaneous. *Source*: Adapted from Truven Health Analytics. Micromedex NeoFax Essentials. https://itunes.apple.com/us/app/thomson-reuters-neofax-essentials/id460060130?mt=8; and Monagle P, Chan AK, Goldenberg NA, et al. Antithrombotic therapy in neonates and children: Antithrombotic Therapy and Prevention of Thrombosis, 9th ed: American College of Chest Physicians Evidence-Based Clinical Practice Guidelines. *Chest* 2012;141(2 suppl):e737S–e801S.

Table 44.4. Monitoring and Dosage Adjustment of Enoxaparin Based on Antifactor Xa Level Measured 4 Hours after Dose of Enoxaparin

Antifactor Xa Level (U/mL)	Hold Dose	Dose Change	Repeat Anti-Xa Level
<0.35	—	+25%	4 hours after next dose
0.35–0.49	—	+10%	4 hours after next dose
0.5–1.0	—	—	24 hours
1.1–1.5	—	−20%	Before next dose
1.6–2.0	3 h	−30%	Before next dose and then 4 hours after next dose
>2.0	Until level is 0.5 U/mL	−40%	Before next dose; if level not <0.5 U/mL, repeat q12h

Source: Adapted from Monagle P, Chan AK, Goldenberg NA, et al. Antithrombotic therapy in neonates and children: Antithrombotic Therapy and Prevention of Thrombosis, 9th ed: American College of Chest Physicians Evidence-Based Clinical Practice Guidelines. *Chest* 2012;141(2 suppl):e737S–e801S.

b. Indications include massive arterial or venous thrombosis with evidence of organ dysfunction, compromised limb viability, or life-threatening thrombosis. Thrombolytic agents can also be used to restore patency of occluded central vascular catheters. Local infusions of low-dose thrombolytic agents can also be used for small to moderate occlusive thrombosis near a central catheter.

c. Minimal data exist in newborn populations regarding all aspects of thrombolytic therapy, including appropriate indications, safety, efficacy, choice of agent, duration of therapy, use of heparin, and monitoring guidelines. Recommendations for use are generally based on small series, case reports, and expert consensus which overall suggest that thrombolytic therapy in neonates can be effective with limited significant complications.

d. Consider evaluating all patients for intraventricular hemorrhage prior to initiating thrombolytic therapy.

2. **Treatment guidelines**
   a. **Preparation for thrombolytic therapy**
   - i. Place sign at head of bed indicating thrombolytic therapy.
   - ii. Have topical thrombin available in unit refrigerator.
   - iii. Notify blood bank to ensure availability of cryoprecipitate.
   - iv. Notify pharmacy to ensure availability of amino caproic acid (Amicar).
   - v. Obtain good venous access. Consider need for mode of access to allow frequent blood draws to minimize need for phlebotomy.
   - vi. Consider hematology consult.

   b. **Thrombolysis can be achieved by local, site-directed administration of thrombolytic agents in low doses** directly onto or near a thrombosis via a central catheter or by **systemic** administration of thrombolytic agents in higher doses. Local therapy is generally limited to small or moderate-sized thromboses. Minimal data exist supporting one method over the other.

c. Recombinant tPA is the thrombolytic agent of choice for neonates. Streptokinase and urokinase have also been used in newborns, but tPA is preferred (although significantly more expensive) due to better clot lysis, less risk for allergic reactions, and shortest half-life.

d. Obtain a baseline CBC, PT, PTT, and fibrinogen level prior to initiating therapy.

e. Monitor PT, PTT, and fibrinogen every 4 hours initially and then at least every 12 to 24 hours. Monitor hematocrit and platelet count every 12 to 24 hours. Monitor thrombosis by imaging every 6 to 24 hours.

f. Expect fibrinogen to decrease by 20% to 50%. If no decrease in fibrinogen is seen, obtain D-dimers or fibrinogen split products to show evidence that a thrombolytic state has been achieved.

g. Maintain fibrinogen level above 100 mg/dL and **platelet count above 50,000 to 100,000** to minimize the risks of clinical bleeding. Administer cryoprecipitate 10 mL/kg (or 1 U/5 kg) or platelets 10 mL/kg as needed. If fibrinogen level drops below 100, decrease the dose of thrombolytic agent by 25%.

h. If no improvement in clinical condition or thrombosis size is seen after initiating therapy, and if fibrinogen levels remain high, **consider giving fresh frozen plasma 10 mL/kg**, which may correct deficiencies of plasminogen and other thrombolytic factors.

i. Duration of therapy. Thrombolytic therapy is usually provided for a brief period, (i.e., 6 to 12 hours), but longer durations can be used for refractory thromboses with appropriate monitoring. Overall, therapy should balance resolution of the thrombus and improvement in clinical status against signs of clinical bleeding.

j. Concomitant unfractionated heparin therapy, usually without the loading bolus dose, should be initiated during or immediately after completion of thrombolytic therapy.

3. Dosing (Tables 44.5 and 44.6)

Table 44.5. Systemic Thrombolytic Therapy

Agent	Load	Infusion	Notes
tPA	None	0.1–0.6 mg/ kg/hour for 6 hours	Duration usually 6 hours; can continue for 12 hours or repeat after 24 hours, although lysis of clot will continue for hours after infusion stops. Lower dose appears to be as effective as higher dose.

Consider concomitant unfractionated heparin therapy at 5 to 20 U/kg/hour without bolus dose. Optimal duration of therapy is uncertain and can be individualized based on clinical response. tPA, tissue plasminogen activator.

Table 44.6. Local Site-Directed Thrombolytic Therapy

Agent	Infusion	Notes
tPA	0.01–0.05 mg/kg/hour	Duration of therapy is based on clinical response. Systemic thrombolysis has been reported at doses of 0.05 mg/kg/hour.

Monitor laboratory studies similar to systemic treatment. tPA, tissue plasminogen activator

4. Treatment of bleeding during thrombolytic therapy

a. For localized bleeding, apply pressure, administer topical thrombin, and provide supportive care. Thrombolytic therapy does not necessarily need to be stopped if bleeding is controlled.

b. For severe bleeding, stop the infusion and administer cryoprecipitate (1 U/5 kg).

c. In the setting of life-threatening bleeding, stop the infusion, give cryoprecipitate, and infuse amino caproic acid (Amicar) (at usual dose of 100 mg/kg IV every 6 hours) after consulting hematology.

5. Postthrombolytic therapy. Consider initiating unfractionated heparin without the initial loading dose or LMWH. Consider discontinuing heparin if no reaccumulation of the thrombus occurs after 24 to 48 hours.

F. **Treatment of central catheter obstruction**

1. **Treatment guidelines**

a. Central catheters may become occluded because of thrombus or chemical precipitate often secondary to parenteral nutrition.

b. Nonfunctioning central catheters should be removed whenever possible, unless continued access through the catheter is absolutely medically necessary.

c. tPA may be used for thrombosis, and hydrochloric acid (HCl) may be attempted for chemical blockage.

d. General procedure

i. Instill chosen agent at volume needed to fill catheter (up to 1 to 2 mL) with gentle pressure. Agent should not be forced if resistance is too high. If instillation is difficult, a three-way stopcock can be used to create a vacuum in the catheter: Attach catheter, 10-mL empty syringe, and 1-mL syringe containing agent to the stopcock. Create vacuum by gently drawing back several milliliters in the 10-mL syringe while the stopcock is off to the 1-mL syringe. While holding pressure, turn stopcock off to the 10-mL syringe and allow vacuum in catheter to draw in infusate from the 1-mL syringe.

ii. Use of HCl for central catheter clearance in neonates is based on limited clinical data and experience and should be performed with caution. Suggested volumes to use range from 0.1 mL to 1 mL of

Table 44.7. Local Instillation of Agents for Catheter Blockage

Agent	Dosing
tPA	0.5 mg/lumen diluted in NS to volume needed to fill line, to max 3 mL
HCl	0.1 M, 0.1–1 mL/lumen

tPA, tissue plasminogen activator; NS, normal saline; HCl, hydrochloric acid.

0.1 molar solution. Because severe tissue damage may result from peripheral administration or extravasation of HCl, consultation with a surgeon prior to HCl use should be considered.

    iii. Wait 1 to 2 hours for tPA agents and 30 to 60 minutes for HCl and attempt to withdraw fluid through the catheter.

    iv. If unsuccessful, previous steps can be repeated once.

    v. If clearance of catheter is not successful after two attempts, the catheter should be removed.

  e. Low-dose continuous infusion of thrombolytic agents can be considered for local thrombosis occluding catheter tip (see preceding text).

2. Dosing guidelines (Table 44.7)

Suggested Readings

Monagle P, Chan AK, Goldenberg NA, et al. Antithrombotic therapy in neonates and children: Antithrombotic Therapy and Prevention of Thrombosis, 9th ed: American College of Chest Physicians Evidence-Based Clinical Practice Guidelines. *Chest* 2012;141(2 suppl):e737S–e801S.

Park CK, Paes BA, Nagel K, et al; and the Thrombosis and Hemostasis in Newborns (THiN) Group. Neonatal central venous catheter thrombosis: diagnosis, management, and outcome. *Blood Coagul Fibrinolysis* 2014;25:97–106.

Rashish G, Paes BA, Nagel K, et al. Spontaneous neonatal arterial thromboembolism: infants at risk, diagnosis, treatment, and outcomes. *Blood Coagul Fibrinolysis* 2013;24:787–797.

Saxonhouse MA. Thrombosis in the neonatal intensive care unit. *Clin Perinatol* 2015;42:651–673.

Saxonhouse MA, Manco-Johnson MJ. The evaluation and management of neonatal coagulation disorders. *Semin Perinatol* 2009;33:52–65.

Anemia

Asimenia I. Angelidou and Helen A. Christou

KEY POINTS

- A postnatal fall in hemoglobin is physiologically expected in all infants due to suppression of erythropoietin production in the relatively hyperoxic extrauterine environment reaching nadir between 8 and 12 weeks of age. The degree of anemia, as well as the nadir period, is more dramatic in preterm infants.
- Infant growth and development are likely affected by hemoglobin levels, but current evidence is inconclusive regarding optimal hematocrit (Hct)/hemoglobin target levels.
- Enteral iron supplementation of 2 to 4 mg/kg/day in the preterm infant leads to higher hemoglobin levels, improves iron stores, and lowers the risk of iron deficiency anemia, but its effect on neurodevelopment remains unclear. Erythropoiesis-stimulating agents are not routinely recommended because they are of limited benefit in reducing the number and volume of transfusions in preterm infants once strict transfusion criteria are used. However, their use may be associated with improved neurodevelopmental outcomes, and this is being addressed in ongoing clinical trials in preterm infants.
- An association between red blood cell (RBC) transfusions and necrotizing enterocolitis (NEC) has been reported in observational studies, but randomized controlled trials do not support a causal relationship.

I. **HEMATOLOGIC PHYSIOLOGY OF THE NEWBORN.** Significant **changes occur in the red blood cell (RBC)** mass of an infant during the neonatal period and ensuing months. The evaluation of anemia must take into account this developmental process as well as the infant's physiologic needs.

A. Normal development: The physiologic anemia of infancy

1. *In utero*, the fetal aortic oxygen saturation is 45%, erythropoietin levels are high, and RBC production is rapid. The fetal liver is the major site of erythropoietin production.

2. After birth, the oxygen saturation is 95%, and erythropoietin is undetectable. RBC production by day 7 is <1/10th the level *in utero*. Reticulocyte counts are low, and the hemoglobin level falls (Table 45.1).

3. Despite dropping hemoglobin levels, the ratio of hemoglobin A to hemoglobin F increases, and the levels of 2,3-diphosphoglycerate (2,3-DPG)

Table 45.1. Hemoglobin Changes in Babies in the First Year of Life

Week	Hemoglobin Level		
	Term Babies	Premature Babies (1,200–2,500 g)	Small Premature Babies (<1,200 g)
0	17.0	16.4	16.0
1	18.8	16.0	14.8
3	15.9	13.5	13.4
6	12.7	10.7	9.7
10	11.4	9.8	8.5
20	12.0	10.4	9.0
50	12.0	11.5	11.0

Source: From Glader B, Naiman JL. Erythrocyte disorders in infancy. In: Taeusch HW, Ballard RA, Avery ME, eds. *Diseases of the Newborn*. Philadelphia, PA: WB Saunders; 1991.

(which interacts with hemoglobin A to decrease its affinity for oxygen, thereby enhancing oxygen release to the tissues) are high. As a result, oxygen delivery to the tissues actually increases. This physiologic "anemia" is not a functional anemia in that oxygen delivery to the tissues is adequate. Iron from degraded RBCs is stored.

4. At 8 to 12 weeks, hemoglobin levels reach their nadir (Table 45.2), oxygen delivery to the tissues is impaired, renal erythropoietin production is stimulated, and RBC production increases.

Table 45.2. Hemoglobin Nadir in Babies in the First Year of Life

Maturity of Baby at Birth	Hemoglobin Level at Nadir	Time of Nadir (week)
Term babies	9.5–11.0	6–12
Premature babies (1,200–2,500 g)	8.0–10.0	5–10
Small premature babies (<1,200 g)	6.5–9.0	4–8

Source: From Glader B, Naiman JL. Erythrocyte disorders in infancy. In: Taeusch HW, Ballard RA, Avery ME, eds. *Diseases of the Newborn*. Philadelphia, PA: WB Saunders; 1991.

5. Infants who have received transfusions in the neonatal period have lower nadirs than normal because of their higher percentage of hemoglobin A.

6. During this period of active erythropoiesis, iron stores are rapidly utilized. Iron stores are sufficient for 15 to 20 weeks in term infants. After this time, the hemoglobin level decreases if iron is not supplied.

B. **Anemia of prematurity** is an exaggeration of the normal physiologic anemia (see Tables 45.1 and 45.2).

1. RBC mass and iron stores are decreased because of low birth weight; however, hemoglobin concentrations are similar in preterm and term infants.

2. The hemoglobin nadir is reached earlier than in the term infant because of the following:
   a. RBC survival is decreased in comparison with the term infant.
   b. There is a relatively more rapid rate of growth in premature babies than in term infants. For example, a premature infant gaining 150 g per week requires approximately a 12 mL per week increase in total blood volume.
   c. Many preterm infants have reduced red cell mass and iron stores because of iatrogenic phlebotomy for laboratory tests. This has been somewhat ameliorated with the use of microtechniques.
   d. Vitamin E deficiency is common in small premature infants, unless the vitamin is supplied exogenously.

3. The hemoglobin nadir in premature babies is lower than in term infants because erythropoietin is produced by the term infant at a hemoglobin level of 10 to 11 g/dL but is produced by the premature infant at a hemoglobin level of 7 to 9 g/dL.

4. Iron administration before the age of 10 to 14 weeks does not increase the nadir of the hemoglobin level or diminish its rate of reduction. However, this iron is stored for later use.

5. Once the nadir is reached, RBC production is stimulated, and iron stores are rapidly depleted because less iron is stored in the premature infant than in the term infant.

II. ETIOLOGY OF ANEMIA IN THE NEONATE

A. **Blood loss** is manifested by a decreased or normal Hct, increased or normal reticulocyte count, and a normal bilirubin level (unless the hemorrhage is retained). If blood loss is recent (e.g., at delivery), the Hct and reticulocyte count may be normal, and the infant may be in shock. The Hct will fall later because of hemodilution. If the bleeding is chronic, the Hct will be low, the reticulocyte count up, and the baby normovolemic.

1. **Obstetric causes of blood loss**, including the following malformations of placenta and cord:
   a. Abruptio placentae
   b. Placenta previa
   c. Incision of placenta at cesarean section
   d. Rupture of anomalous vessels (e.g., vasa previa, velamentous insertion of cord, or rupture of communicating vessels in a multilobed placenta)

e. Hematoma of cord caused by varices or aneurysm

f. Rupture of cord (more common in short cords and in dysmature cords)

2. Occult blood loss

a. Fetomaternal bleeding may be chronic or acute. It occurs in 8% of all pregnancies, and in 1% of pregnancies, the volume may be as large as 40 mL. The diagnosis of this problem is by Kleihauer-Betke stain of maternal smear for fetal cells. Chronic fetal-to-maternal transfusion is suggested by a reticulocyte count >10%. Many conditions may predispose to this type of bleeding:

    i. Placental malformations—chorioangioma or choriocarcinoma

    ii. Obstetric procedures—traumatic amniocentesis, external cephalic version, internal cephalic version, breech delivery

    iii. Spontaneous fetomaternal bleeding

b. Fetoplacental bleeding

    i. Chorioangioma or choriocarcinoma with placental hematoma

    ii. Cesarean section, with infant held above the placenta

    iii. Tight nuchal cord or occult cord prolapse

c. Twin-to-twin transfusion

d. Twin anemia polycythemia sequence (TAPS), an uncommon form of chronic inter-twin transfusion between monochorionic twins characterized by large inter-twin hemoglobin differences in the absence of amniotic fluid discordance.

3. Bleeding in the neonatal period may be due to the following causes:

a. Intracranial bleeding associated with the following:

    i. Prematurity

    ii. Second twin

    iii. Breech delivery

    iv. Rapid delivery

    v. Hypoxia

b. Massive cephalohematoma, subgaleal hemorrhage, or hemorrhagic caput succedaneum

c. Retroperitoneal bleeding

d. Ruptured liver or spleen

e. Adrenal or renal hemorrhage

f. Gastrointestinal bleeding (maternal blood swallowed from delivery or breast should be ruled out by the Apt test) (see Chapter 43)

    i. Peptic ulcer

    ii. NEC

    iii. Nasogastric catheter

g. Bleeding from umbilicus

4. Iatrogenic causes. Excessive blood loss may result from blood sampling with inadequate replacement.

B. Hemolysis is manifested by a decreased Hct, increased reticulocyte count, and an increased bilirubin level.

1. Immune hemolysis (see Chapter 26)

a. Rh incompatibility

b. ABO incompatibility

c. Minor blood group incompatibility (e.g., c, E, Kell, Duffy)

d. Maternal disease (e.g., lupus), autoimmune hemolytic disease, rheumatoid arthritis (positive direct Coombs test in mother and newborn, no antibody to common red cell antigen Rh, AB, etc.), or drugs

2. Hereditary RBC disorders

a. RBC membrane defects such as spherocytosis, elliptocytosis, or stomatocytosis

b. Metabolic defects—glucose-6-phosphate dehydrogenase (G6PD) deficiency (significant neonatal hemolysis due to G6PD deficiency is usually seen only in Mediterranean or Asian G6PD-deficient men; blacks in the United States have a 10% incidence of G6PD deficiency but rarely have significant neonatal problems unless an infection or drug is operative), pyruvate-kinase deficiency, 5'-nucleotidase deficiency, and glucose-phosphate isomerase deficiency

c. Hemoglobinopathies

i. α- and γ-Thalassemia syndromes

ii. α- and γ-Chain structural abnormalities

3. Acquired hemolysis

a. Infection—bacterial or viral

b. Disseminated intravascular coagulation

c. Vitamin E deficiency and other nutritional anemias

d. Microangiopathic hemolytic anemia, hemangioma, renal artery stenosis, and severe coarctation of the aorta

C. Diminished RBC production is manifested by a decreased Hct, decreased reticulocyte count, and normal bilirubin level.

1. Diamond-Blackfan syndrome

2. Congenital leukemia or other tumor

3. Infections, especially rubella and parvovirus (see Chapters 48 and 49)

4. Osteopetrosis, leading to inadequate erythropoiesis

5. Drug-induced suppression of RBC production

6. Physiologic anemia or anemia of prematurity (see sections I.A and I.B)

III. DIAGNOSTIC APPROACH TO ANEMIA IN THE NEWBORN (Table 45.3)

A. The **family history** should include questions about anemia, jaundice, gallstones, and splenectomy.

B. The **obstetric history** should be evaluated.

C. The **physical examination** may reveal an associated abnormality and provide clues to the origin of the anemia.

1. Acute blood loss leads to shock, with cyanosis, poor perfusion, and acidosis.

2. Chronic blood loss produces pallor, but the infant may exhibit only mild symptoms of respiratory distress or irritability.

3. Chronic hemolysis is associated with pallor, jaundice, and hepatosplenomegaly.

Table 45.3. Classification of Anemia in the Newborn

Reticulocytes	Bilirubin	Coombs Test	RBC Morphology	Diagnostic Possibilities
Normal or ↓	Normal	Negative	Normal	Physiologic anemia of infancy or pre-maturity; congenital hypoplastic anemia; other causes of decreased production
Normal or ↑	Normal	Negative	Normal	Acute hemorrhage (fetomaternal, placental, umbilical cord, or internal hemorrhage)
↑	↑	Positive	Hypochromic microcytes	Chronic fetomaternal hemorrhage
			Spherocytes	Immune hemolysis (blood group incompatibility or maternal autoantibody)
Normal or ↑	↑	Negative	Spherocytes	Hereditary spherocytosis
			Elliptocytes	Hereditary elliptocytosis
			Hypochromic microcytes	α- or γ-Thalassemia syndrome
			Spiculated RBCs	Pyruvate-kinase deficiency
			Schistocytes and RBC fragments	Disseminated intravascular coagulation; other microangiopathic processes
			Bite cells (Heinz bodies with supravital stain)	Glucose-6-phosphate dehydrogenase deficiency
			Normal	Infections; enclosed hemorrhage (cephalohematoma)

RBC, red blood cell; ↓, decreased; ↑, increased.
Source: Adapted from the work of Dr. Glader Bertil, director of Division of Hematology-Oncology, Children's Hospital at Stanford, California, 1991.

D. **Complete blood cell count.** Capillary blood Hct is 3.7% to 2.7% higher than venous Hct. Warming the foot reduced the difference from 3.9% to 1.9%.

E. **Reticulocyte count** (elevated with chronic blood loss and hemolysis, depressed with infection and production defect)

F. **Blood smear** (see Table 45.3)

G. **Coombs test and bilirubin level**

H. **Apt test** (see Chapter 43) on gastrointestinal blood of uncertain origin

I. **Kleihauer-Betke preparation** of the mother's blood. A 50-mL loss of fetal blood into the maternal circulation will show up as 1% fetal cells in the maternal circulation.

J. **Ultrasound of abdomen and head**

K. **Parental testing**—complete blood cell count, smear, and RBC indices are useful screening studies. Osmotic fragility testing and RBC enzyme levels (e.g., G6PD, pyruvate kinase) may be helpful in selected cases.

L. **Studies for infection** (toxoplasmosis, other, rubella, cytomegalovirus, and herpes simplex [TORCH]; see Chapters 48 and 49)

M. **Bone marrow** (rarely used except in cases of bone marrow failure from hypoplasia or tumor)

IV. THERAPY

A. **Transfusion** (see Chapter 42). Neonatal transfusion practices have changed dramatically in the last 30 years. According to the premature infants in need of transfusion (PINT) study published in 2006 by Kirpalani et al, a liberal practice using higher hemoglobin thresholds to transfuse extremely low birth weight (ELBW) infants resulted in more infants receiving transfusions but conferred little benefit, whereas a restrictive transfusion strategy was not associated with adverse outcomes. A follow-up study in 2009, the PINT outcome study (PINTOS), addressing neurodevelopmental outcomes at 18 to 21 months corrected gestational age, showed that all adverse outcomes (death or serious neurodevelopmental disability, cerebral palsy, cognitive delay, severe hearing, or visual deficit) were more frequent in the restrictive group, but the difference did not reach statistical significance. We must also consider the possible adverse effects of transfusion on neurodevelopment which may result from circulation of proinflammatory mediators from stored red cells or the resulting depression of erythropoietin. It still remains unclear at which physiologic threshold hemoglobin levels become low enough to threaten the growth and development of the infant brain in chronic anemia of prematurity. Table 45.4 summarizes the transfusion thresholds described in a 2011 Cochrane Review.

1. **Indications for transfusion.** The decision to transfuse must be made in consideration of the infant's condition and physiologic needs.
   a. Infants with significant respiratory disease or congenital heart disease (e.g., large left-to-right shunt) may need their Hct maintained above 40%. Transfusion with adult RBCs provides the added benefit of lowered

Table 45.4. Suggested Hemoglobin Levels and Hematocrit Thresholds for Transfusing Infants with Anemia of Prematurity

Postnatal Age	Respiratory Support	No Respiratory Support
Week 1	11.5 (35)	10.0 (30)
Week 2	10.0 (30)	8.5 (25)
Week 3 and older	8.5 (25)	7.5 (23)

Data presented as hemoglobin (g/dL) (hematocrit %). Respiratory support is defined as FiO_2 >25% or the need for mechanical increase in airway pressure
Source: Adapted from Whyte R, Kirpalani H. Low versus high haemoglobin concentration threshold for blood transfusion for preventing morbidity and mortality in very low birth weight infants. *Cochrane Database Syst Rev* 2011;(11):CD000512.

hemoglobin oxygen affinity, which augments oxygen delivery to tissues. Blood should be fresh (3 to 7 days old) to ensure adequate 2,3-DPG levels.

b. Healthy, asymptomatic newborns will self-correct a mild anemia, provided that iron intake is adequate.

c. Infants with ABO incompatibility who do not have an exchange transfusion may have protracted hemolysis and may require a transfusion several weeks after birth. This may be ameliorated with the use of intravenous immunoglobulin (IVIG). If they do not have enough hemolysis to require treatment with phototherapy, they will usually not become anemic enough to need a transfusion (see Chapter 26).

d. Premature babies may be quite comfortable with hemoglobin levels of 6.5 to 7.0 mg/dL. The level itself is not an indication for transfusion. Growing premature infants may manifest a need for transfusion by exhibiting poor weight gain, apnea, tachypnea, or poor feeding. Sick infants (e.g., with sepsis, pneumonia, or bronchopulmonary dysplasia) may require increased oxygen-carrying capacities and therefore need transfusion. Transfusion guidelines are shown in Table 45.5. Despite efforts to adopt uniform transfusion criteria, significant variation in transfusion practices among neonatal intensive care units (NICUs) has been reported.

e. An association between RBC transfusions and late-onset or transfusion-associated NEC, also referred to as transfusion-related acute gut injury (TRAGI), has been reported in observational studies and the proposed mechanisms relate to variability in splanchnic tissue oxygenation in combination with the lower average tissue oxygenation in preterm infants. However, data from randomized controlled trials (RCTs) do not support a causal relationship between RBC transfusions and NEC, and it has been suggested that significant anemia and the pretransfusion Hct may play a role in transfusion-associated NEC.

Table 45.5. Transfusion Guidelines for Premature Infants

1. Asymptomatic infants with Hct ≤18% (hemoglobin ≤6 g/dL) and reticulocytes <100, 000 cells/μL (<2%)

2. Infants with Hct ≤20% (hemoglobin ≤7 g/dL) on supplemental oxygen who are not requiring mechanical ventilation but have one or more of the following:

a. ≥24 hours of tachycardia (heart rate >180 bpm) or tachypnea (respiratory rate >80 breaths per minute)

b. A doubling oxygen requirement from the previous 48 hours

c. Acute metabolic acidosis (pH <7.20) or lactate ≥2.5 mEq/L

d. Weight gain of <10 g/kg/day for 4 days while receiving ≥120 kcal/kg/day

e. If the infant will undergo major surgery within 72 hours

3. Infants with Hct ≤25% (hemoglobin ≤8 g/dL) requiring minimal mechanical ventilation, defined as MAP ≤8 cm H_2O by CPAP or conventional ventilation, or MAP <14 on high-frequency ventilation, and/or FiO_2 ≤0.40

4. Infants with Hct ≤30% (hemoglobin ≤10 g/dL) requiring moderate or significant mechanical ventilation, defined as MAP >8 cm H_2O on conventional ventilation, or MAP >14 on high-frequency ventilation, and/or FiO_2 >0.40

5. A transfusion should be considered if acute blood loss of ≥10% associated with symptoms of decreased oxygen delivery occurs, or if significant hemorrhage of ≥20% total blood volume occurs.

Hct, hematocrit; bpm, beats per minute; MAP, mean airway pressure; CPAP, continuous positive airway pressure.
Source: Data from Bishara N, Ohls RK. Current controversies in the management of the anemia of prematurity. *Semin Perinatol* 2009;33(1):29–34.

2. Blood products and methods of transfusion (see Chapter 42)

a. Packed RBCs. The volume of transfusion may be calculated as follows:

$$\frac{\text{Weight in kilogram} \times \text{blood volume per kilogram} \times (\text{Hct desired} - \text{Hct observed})}{\text{Hct of blood to be given}} = \frac{\text{volume of}}{\text{transfusion}}$$

The average newborn blood volume is 80 mL/kg; the Hct of packed RBCs is 60% to 80% and should be checked before transfusion. We generally transfuse 15 to 20 mL/kg; larger volumes may need to be divided in more than one aliquots.

b. Whole blood is indicated when there is acute blood loss.

c. Isovolemic transfusion with high Hct-packed RBCs may be required for severely anemic infants, when routine transfusion of the volume of packed RBCs necessary to correct the anemia would result in circulatory overload (see Chapter 26).

d. Irradiated RBCs are recommended in premature infants weighing <1,200 g. Premature infants may be unable to reject foreign lymphocytes in transfused blood. **We use irradiated blood for all neonatal transfusions. Leukocyte depletion** with third-generation transfusion filters has substantially reduced the risk of exposure to foreign lymphocytes and cytomegalovirus (CMV). However, blood from CMV-negative donors for neonatal transfusion is preferable.

e. Directed-donor transfusion is requested by many families. Irradiation of directed-donor cells is especially important, given the human leukocyte antigen (HLA) compatibility among first-degree relatives and the enhanced potential for foreign lymphocyte engraftment.

f. Because of concern for multiple exposure risk associated with repeated transfusions in ELBW infants, **we recommend transfusing stored RBCs from a single unit reserved for an infant**.

B. Prophylaxis

1. Term infants. According to the 2010 American Academy of Pediatrics (AAP) recommendation, breastfed infants should be started on iron supplementation at the age of 4 months. Nonbreastfed infants should be sent home from the hospital on iron-fortified formula (2 mg/kg/day).

2. Premature infants (preventing or ameliorating the anemia of prematurity). The following is a description of our usual nutritional management of premature infants from the point of view of providing RBC substrates and preventing additional destruction:

a. Iron supplementation in the preterm infant introduced between 4 and 6 weeks of age at the onset of reticulocytosis, leads to higher hemoglobin levels, improves iron stores, and lowers the risk of iron deficiency anemia after the first 6 months of life. Early (up to 3 weeks of age) versus late (4 weeks to 60 days) commencement of iron supplementation did not result in differences in cognitive outcome, but an increased rate of abnormal neurologic exam at 5 years of age was noted in the late iron group. It remains unclear whether iron supplementation in preterm and low birth weight infants has long-term benefits in terms of neurodevelopmental outcome and growth. We routinely supplement iron in premature infants at a dose of 2 to 4 mg of elemental iron/kg/day once full enteral feeding is achieved (see Chapter 21). There is no discernible hematologic benefit in exceeding "standard" doses of iron; in fact, excess exogenous iron can contribute to oxidative injury in preterm babies.

b. Mother's milk or formulas similar to mother's milk in that they are low in linoleic acid are used to maintain a low content of polyunsaturated fatty acids in the RBCs.

c. Vitamin E (5 to 25 IU of water-soluble form) is given daily until the baby is 38 to 40 weeks' postconceptional age (this is usually stopped at discharge from the hospital).

d. These infants should be followed up carefully, and additional iron supplementation may be required.

e. Methods and hazards of transfusion are described in Chapter 42.

f. Recombinant human erythropoietin (rh-EPO) has been evaluated as a promising measure in ameliorating anemia of prematurity. Studies in which we participated showed that rh-EPO stimulates red cell production and may decrease the frequency and volume of RBC transfusions administered to premature infants. However, many studies have shown that erythropoietin treatment is of limited benefit in reducing the number or volume of transfusions once strict transfusion criteria are instituted. A trend for increased risk for retinopathy of prematurity (ROP) with both early (first week of life) and late (beyond first week of life) erythropoietin (EPO) use was reported in some studies, but recent meta-analyses found no statistically significant differences in stage 3 or greater ROP between EPO and placebo groups. Currently, we do not routinely use EPO prophylaxis for anemia, although there may be utility in exploring this option for families who withhold consent to transfusion of blood products. Complementary strategies to reduce phlebotomy losses and the use of conservative standardized transfusion criteria have contributed to significant reductions in transfusions.

Beyond erythropoiesis, there seems to be a beneficial effect of erythropoiesis-stimulating agents in neurodevelopmental outcomes of preterm infants. An RCT comparing erythropoiesis-stimulating agents with placebo showed improvement in cognitive outcomes at 18 to 22 months corrected age in the treated preterm infants. Ongoing randomized controlled studies are evaluating this approach further.

Suggested Readings

Bishara N, Ohls RK. Current controversies in the management of the anemia of prematurity. *Semin Perinatol* 2009;33(1):29–34.

Kirpalani H, Whyte RK, Andersen C, et al. The premature infants in need of transfusion (PINT) study: a randomized, controlled trial of a restrictive (low) versus liberal (high) transfusion threshold for extremely low birth weight infants. *J Pediatr* 2006;149(3):301–307.

Kirpalani H, Zupancic JA. Do transfusions cause necrotizing enterocolitis? The complementary role of randomized trials and observational studies. *Semin Perinatol* 2012;36(4):269–276.

Mills RJ, Davies MW. Enteral iron supplementation in preterm and low birth weight infants. *Cochrane Database Syst Rev* 2012;(3):CD005095.

Ohls RK, Kamath-Rayne BD, Christensen RD, et al. Cognitive outcomes of preterm infants randomized to darbepoetin, erythropoietin, or placebo. *Pediatrics* 2014;133(6):1023–1030.

46 Polycythemia

Deirdre O'Reilly

KEY POINTS

- Polycythemia and hyperviscosity of the blood in newborns may lead to symptoms such as hypoglycemia, poor feeding, and irritability; yet, most newborns with polycythemia are asymptomatic.
- Partial exchange transfusion to reduce hematocrit should be considered for newborns with levels >65%.
- Partial exchange transfusion will likely treat symptoms if they are present but has not been shown to affect neurodevelopmental outcome.

As the central venous hematocrit rises, there is increased viscosity and decreased blood flow. When the hematocrit increases to >60%, there is decreased oxygen delivery (Fig. 46.1). Newborns have larger, irregularly shaped red blood cells (RBC) with different membrane characteristics than the RBCs of adults. As viscosity increases, there is impairment of tissue oxygenation and decreased glucose in plasma, leading to increased risk of microthrombus formation. If these events occur in the cerebral cortex, kidneys, or adrenal glands, significant damage may result. Hypoxia and acidosis increase viscosity and deformity further. Poor perfusion increases the possibility of thrombosis.

I. DEFINITIONS

A. **Polycythemia** is defined as venous hematocrit of at least 65%. Hematocrit measurements vary greatly with site of sample, and capillary hematocrit may be up to 20% higher than venous. Hematocrit initially rises after birth from placental transfer of RBCs and then decreases to baseline by approximately 24 hours. The mean venous hematocrit of term infants is 53% in cord blood, 60% at 2 hours of age, 57% at 6 hours of age, and 52% at 12 to 18 hours of age.

B. **Hyperviscosity** is defined as viscosity >2 standard deviations greater than the mean. Blood viscosity, as described by Poiseuille, is the ratio of shear stress to shear rate and is dependent on such factors as the pressure gradient along the vessel, radius, length, and flow. The relationship between hematocrit and viscosity is nearly linear below a hematocrit of 60%, but viscosity increases exponentially at a hematocrit of 70% or greater (Fig. 46.1).

Other factors affect blood viscosity, including plasma proteins such as fibrinogen, local blood flow, and pH. The hyperviscosity syndrome is usually seen only in infants with venous hematocrits above 60%.

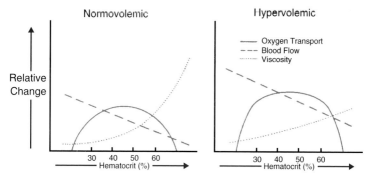

Figure 46.1. Effect of hematocrit on viscosity, blood flow, and oxygen transport. (Adapted from Glader B, Naiman JL. Erythrocyte disorders in infancy. In: Taeusch HW, Ballard RA, Avery ME, eds. *Diseases of the Newborn*. Philadelphia, PA: WB Saunders; 1991.)

II. INCIDENCE. The incidence of polycythemia is 1% to 5% in term newborns. Polycythemia is increased in babies that have intrauterine growth restriction (IUGR), are small for gestational age (SGA), and are born postterm.

III. CAUSES OF POLYCYTHEMIA

A. **Placental red cell transfusion**

1. **Delayed cord clamping** may occur either intentionally or in unattended deliveries.

   a. When the cord is clamped within 1 minute after birth, the blood volume of the infant is approximately 80 mL/kg.

   b. When the cord is clamped 2 minutes after delivery, the blood volume of the infant is 90 mL/kg.

   c. In newborns with polycythemia, blood volume per kilogram of body weight varies inversely in relation to birth weight (Fig. 46.2).

2. **Cord stripping** (thereby pushing more blood into the infant)

3. **Holding the baby below the mother at delivery**

4. **Maternal-to-fetal transfusion** is diagnosed with the Kleihauer-Betke stain technique of acid elution to detect maternal cells in the circulation of the newborn (see Chapter 45).

5. **Twin-to-twin transfusion** (see Chapter 11)

6. **Forceful uterine contractions before cord clamping**

B. **Placental insufficiency (increased fetal erythropoiesis secondary to chronic intrauterine hypoxia)**

1. SGA and IUGR infants

2. Maternal hypertension syndromes (preeclampsia, renal disease, etc.)

3. Postterm infants

4. Infants born to mothers with chronic hypoxia (heart disease, pulmonary disease)

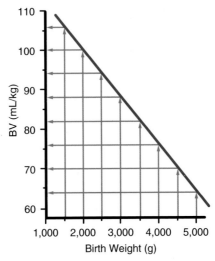

Figure 46.2. Nomogram designed for clinical use, correlating blood volume per kilogram with birth weight in polycythemic neonates. BV, blood volume. (From Rawlings JS, Pettett G, Wiswell T, et al. Estimated blood volumes in polycythemic neonates as a function of birth weight. *J Pediatr* 1982; 101:594–599.)

    5. Pregnancy at high altitude

    6. Maternal smoking

C. Other conditions

    1. Infants of diabetic mothers (increased erythropoiesis)

    2. Some large for gestational age (LGA) babies

    3. Infants with congenital adrenal hyperplasia, Beckwith-Wiedemann syndrome, neonatal thyrotoxicosis, congenital hypothyroidism, trisomy 21, trisomy 13, trisomy 18

    4. Drugs (maternal use of propranolol)

    5. Dehydration of infant

    6. Sepsis (increase in fibrinogen, lower RBC deformability)

IV. CLINICAL FINDINGS. Most infants with polycythemia are asymptomatic. Clinical symptoms, syndromes, and laboratory abnormalities that have been described in association with polycythemia include the following:

    A. Central nervous system (CNS). Poor feeding, lethargy, hypotonia, apnea, tremors, jitteriness, seizures, cerebral venous thrombosis

B. **Cardiorespiratory.** Cyanosis, tachypnea, heart murmur, congestive heart failure, cardiomegaly, elevated pulmonary vascular resistance, prominent vascular markings on chest x-ray

C. **Renal.** Decreased glomerular filtration, decreased sodium excretion, renal vein thrombosis, hematuria, proteinuria

D. **Other.** Other thrombosis, thrombocytopenia, poor feeding, increased jaundice, persistent hypoglycemia, hypocalcemia, testicular infarcts, necrotizing enterocolitis (NEC), priapism, disseminated intravascular coagulation

> **All of these symptoms may be associated with polycythemia and hyperviscosity but may not be caused by it. They are common symptoms in many neonatal disorders.**

V. SCREENING. The routine screening of all newborns for polycythemia/hyperviscosity has been advocated by some authors. The timing and site of blood sampling alter the hematocrit value. We do not routinely screen well term newborns for this syndrome because there are few data showing that treatment of asymptomatic patients with partial exchange transfusion is beneficial in the long term.

VI. DIAGNOSIS. The capillary blood or peripheral venous hematocrit level should be determined in any baby who appears plethoric, who has any predisposing cause of polycythemia, who has any of the symptoms mentioned in section IV, or who is not well for any reason.

A. Warming the heel before drawing blood for a capillary hematocrit determination will give a better correlation with the peripheral venous or central hematocrit. If the capillary blood hematocrit is above 65%, the peripheral venous hematocrit should be determined.

B. Few hospitals are equipped to measure blood viscosity. If the equipment is available, the test should be done because some infants with venous hematocrits under 65% will have hyperviscous blood.

VII. MANAGEMENT

A. Once other causes of illness have been considered and excluded (e.g., sepsis, pneumonia, hypoglycemia), any child with symptoms that could be due to hyperviscosity should be considered for **partial exchange transfusion if the peripheral venous hematocrit is >65%.**

B. **Asymptomatic infants** with a peripheral venous hematocrit between 60% and 70% **can usually be managed by increasing fluid intake and repeating the hematocrit in 4 to 6 hours**.

C. Many neonatologists perform an **exchange transfusion when the peripheral venous hematocrit is >70% in the absence of symptoms, but this is a controversial** issue.

D. The following formula can be used to calculate the exchange with 5% albumin or normal saline that will bring the hematocrit from 50% to 60%. In infants with polycythemia, the blood volume varies inversely with the birth weight (Fig. 46.2). **Usually, we take the blood from the umbilical vein and replace it with 5% albumin or normal saline in a peripheral vein.** Because randomized trials show no advantage with albumin, and there is less chance of infection, nonhuman products, such as saline, are preferred. There are many methods of exchange (see Chapter 26).

Volume of exchange in mL

$$= \frac{(\text{blood volume/kg} \times \text{weight in kg}) \times (\text{observed hematocrit} - \text{desired hematocrit})}{\text{observed hematocrit}}$$

Example: A 3-kg infant, hematocrit 75%, blood volume 80 mL/kg—to bring hematocrit to 50%:

$$\text{Volume of exchange (in mL)} = \frac{(80 \text{ mL} \times 3 \text{ kg}) \times (75 - 50)}{75}$$
$$= \frac{240 \text{ mL} \times 25}{75}$$
$$= 80\text{-mL exchange}$$

The total volume exchanged is usually 15 to 20 mL/kg of body weight. This will depend on the observed hematocrit. (Blood volume may be up to 100 mL/kg in polycythemic infants.)

VIII. OUTCOME

A. **Infants with polycythemia and hyperviscosity who have decreased cerebral blood flow velocity and increased vascular resistance develop normal cerebral blood flow following partial exchange transfusion.** They also have improvement in systemic blood flow and oxygen transport.

B. **The long-term neurologic outcome** in infants with asymptomatic polycythemia/hyperviscosity, whether treated or untreated, **remains controversial**.

1. One trial with small numbers of randomized patients showed decreased IQ scores in school-age children who had neonatal hyperviscosity syndrome, in both treated and untreated newborns.

2. Another retrospective study, with small numbers of patients, showed no difference in the neurologic outcome of patients with asymptomatic neonatal polycythemia, including both treated and untreated newborns.

3. A small prospective study showed no difference at follow-up between control infants and those with hyperviscosity, between those with symptomatic and those with asymptomatic hyperviscosity, and between asymptomatic infants treated with partial exchange transfusion and those who were observed. Analysis revealed that other perinatal risk factors and race, rather than polycythemia or partial exchange transfusion, significantly influenced the long-term outcome.

4. An increased incidence of NEC following partial exchange transfusions by umbilical vein has been reported. NEC was not seen in one retrospective analysis of 185 term polycythemic babies given partial exchange

transfusions with removal of blood from the umbilical vein and reinfusion of a commercial plasma substitute through peripheral veins.

5. A larger prospective, randomized clinical trial comparing partial exchange transfusion with symptomatic care (increased fluid intake, etc.) equally balanced for risk factors and the etiologies of the polycythemia will be necessary to give guidelines for treatment of the asymptomatic newborn with polycythemia/hyperviscosity.

6. Partial exchange transfusion will lower hematocrit, decrease viscosity, and reverse many of the physiologic abnormalities associated with polycythemia/hyperviscosity but has not been shown to significantly change the long-term outcome of these infants.

Suggested Readings

Ozek E, Soll R, Schimmel MS. Partial exchange transfusion to prevent neurodevelopmental disability in infants with polycythemia. *Cochrane Database Syst Rev* 2010;(1):CD005089.

Sarkar S, Rosenkrantz TS. Neonatal polycythemia and hyperviscosity. *Semin Fetal Neonatal Med* 2008;13:248–255.

Vlug RD, Lopriore E, Janssen M, et al. Thrombocytopenia in neonates with polycythemia: incidence, risk factors and clinical outcome. *Expert Rev Hematol* 2015;8(1):123–129.

47 Thrombocytopenia

Emöke Deschmann, Matthew Saxonhouse, and
Martha Sola-Visner

KEY POINTS

- The most common cause of mild-to-moderate, early-onset thrombocytopenia in well-appearing neonates is placental insufficiency, frequently manifesting as small for gestational status at birth. This thrombocytopenia resolves spontaneously, usually within 10 days, and carries good prognosis. Thrombocytopenia in sick infants is usually associated with sepsis or necrotizing enterocolitis (NEC) and requires prompt intervention.

- Neonates with severe thrombocytopenia in the first day of life, particularly if well appearing, should be screened for neonatal alloimmune thrombocytopenia (NAIT). Random-donor platelet transfusions (± intravenous immunoglobulin [IVIG]) represent the first line of therapy for these infants, unless human platelet antigen (HPA)-1b1b and 5a5a platelets are maintained in the blood bank inventory and are immediately available for use (as is the case in some European countries). In those cases, these platelets are the preferred first-line treatment.

- There is significant worldwide variability in platelet transfusion thresholds used in the neonatal intensive care unit (NICU). The only randomized controlled trial to date evaluating infants $<1,500$ g during the first week of life showed no differences in the frequency or severity of intraventricular hemorrhages between neonates transfused for platelet counts $<60 \times 10^3/\mu L$ versus $<150 \times 10^3/\mu L$. Thus, there is no evidence that platelet transfusions given to nonbleeding infants with moderate thrombocytopenia (platelet counts 60 to $150 \times 10^3/\mu L$) are of any benefit.

- The risk of bleeding in thrombocytopenic neonates is multifactorial and is not related to the severity of the thrombocytopenia. Current evidence suggests that gestational age <28 weeks, postnatal age <10 days, and a diagnosis of NEC are more important predictors of bleeding than the platelet count itself.

- The Platelets for Neonatal Transfusion—Study 2 (PlaNeT-2) is a prospective randomized multicenter study comparing the safety and efficacy of $25 \times 10^3/\mu L$ versus $50 \times 10^3/\mu L$ as platelet transfusion thresholds in thrombocytopenic NICU patients. The study is currently actively enrolling patients in several European countries.

I. INTRODUCTION. Neonatal thrombocytopenia is traditionally defined as a platelet count of $<150 \times 10^3/\mu L$ and is classified as mild (100 to 149 $\times$ $10^3/\mu L$), moderate (50 to 99 $\times$ $10^3/\mu L$), or severe ($<50 \times 10^3/\mu L$). However, platelet counts in the 100 to 149 $\times$ $10^3/\mu L$ range are somewhat more common among neonates than adults. The most recent and largest study on neonatal platelet counts demonstrated that platelet counts at birth increase with advancing gestational age. Importantly, while the mean platelet count was $\geq 200 \times$ $10^3/\mu L$ even in the most preterm infants, the 5th percentile was $104 \times 10^3/\mu L$ for those ≤ 32 weeks' gestation, and $123 \times 10^3/\mu L$ for late-preterm and term neonates. These findings suggest that different definitions of thrombocytopenia may be applied to preterm infants. For that reason, careful follow-up and expectant management in an otherwise healthy-appearing neonate with mild, transient thrombocytopenia is an acceptable approach, although lack of quick resolution, worsening of thrombocytopenia, or changes in clinical condition should prompt further evaluation.

The incidence of thrombocytopenia in neonates varies significantly, depending on the population studied. Specifically, while the *overall* incidence of neonatal thrombocytopenia is relatively low (0.7% to 0.9%), the incidence among neonates admitted to the NICU is rather high (18% to 35%). Within the NICU, mean platelet counts are lower among preterm neonates than among neonates born at or near term, and the incidence of thrombocytopenia is inversely correlated to the gestational age, reaching approximately 70% among neonates born with a weight $<1,000$ g.

II. APPROACH TO THE THROMBOCYTOPENIC NEONATE. When evaluating a thrombocytopenic neonate, the first step to narrow the differential diagnosis is to classify the thrombocytopenia as either **early onset (within the first 72 hours of life)** or **late onset (after 72 hours of life)**, and to determine whether the infant is clinically ill or well. Importantly, infection/sepsis should always be considered near the top of the differential diagnosis (regardless of the time of presentation and the infant's appearance) because any delay in diagnosis and treatment can have life-threatening consequences.

A. **Early-onset thrombocytopenia** (Fig. 47.1). The most frequent cause of early-onset thrombocytopenia in a well-appearing neonate is placental insufficiency, as occurs in infants born to mothers with pregnancy-induced hypertension/preeclampsia or diabetes and in those with intrauterine growth restriction (IUGR). This thrombocytopenia is always mild to moderate, presents immediately or shortly after birth, and resolves within 7 to 10 days. If an infant with a prenatal history consistent with placental insufficiency and mild-to-moderate thrombocytopenia remains clinically stable and the platelet count normalizes within 10 days, no further evaluation is necessary. However, if the thrombocytopenia becomes severe and/or persists >10 days, further investigation is necessary.

Severe early-onset thrombocytopenia in an otherwise healthy infant should trigger suspicion for an immune-mediated thrombocytopenia, either autoimmune (i.e., the mother is also thrombocytopenic) or alloimmune (the mother has a normal platelet count). These varieties of thrombocytopenia

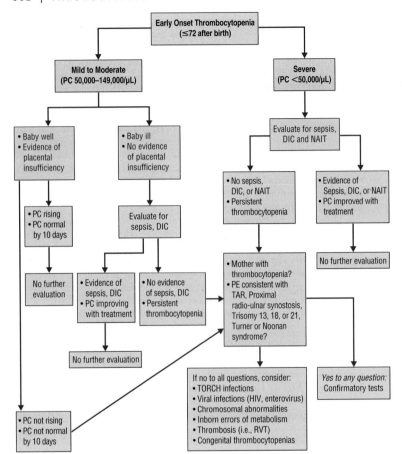

Figure 47.1. Guidelines for the evaluation of neonates with early-onset thrombocytopenia (≤72 hours of life). PC, platelet count; DIC, disseminated intravascular coagulation; NAIT, neonatal alloimmune thrombocytopenia; PE, physical examination; TAR, thrombocytopenia-absent radius; TORCH, toxoplasmosis, other, rubella, cytomegalovirus, and herpes simplex; RVT, renal vein thrombosis.

are discussed in detail in the following text. Early-onset thrombocytopenia of any severity in an *ill-appearing* term or preterm neonate should prompt evaluation for sepsis, congenital viral or parasitic infections, or disseminated intravascular coagulation (DIC). DIC is most frequently associated with sepsis but can also be secondary to birth asphyxia.

In addition to these considerations, the affected neonate should be carefully examined for any radial abnormalities (suggestive of thrombocytopenia-absent radius [TAR] syndrome, amegakaryocytic thrombocytopenia with radioulnar synostosis [ATRUS], or Fanconi anemia). Although thrombocytopenia associated with Fanconi almost always presents later (during childhood), neonatal cases have been reported. In these patients, thumb abnormalities are frequently found, and chromosomal fragility testing is nearly always diagnostic. If the infant has radial abnormalities with normal-appearing thumbs, TAR syndrome should be considered. The platelet count is usually $<50 \times 10^3/\mu L$, and the white cell count is elevated in $>90\%$ of TAR syndrome patients, sometimes exceeding $100 \times 10^3/\mu L$ and mimicking congenital leukemia. Infants that survive the first year of life generally do well because the platelet count then spontaneously improves to low-normal levels that are maintained through life. The inability to rotate the forearm on physical examination, in the presence of severe early-onset thrombocytopenia, suggests the rare diagnosis of congenital amegakaryocytic thrombocytopenia with proximal radioulnar synostosis. Radiologic examination of the upper extremities in these infants confirms the proximal synostosis of the radial and ulnar bones. Other genetic disorders associated with early-onset thrombocytopenia include trisomy 21, trisomy 18, trisomy 13, Turner syndrome, Noonan syndrome, and Jacobsen syndrome. Cases of Noonan syndrome presenting with mild dysmorphic features and very severe neonatal thrombocytopenia (mimicking congenital amegakaryocytic thrombocytopenia) have been recently described. The presence of hepato- or splenomegaly is suggestive of a viral infection, although it can also be seen in hemophagocytic syndrome and liver failure from different etiologies. Other diagnoses, such as renal vein thrombosis, Kasabach-Merritt syndrome, and inborn errors of metabolism (mainly propionic acidemia and methylmalonic acidemia), should be considered and evaluated for based on specific clinical indications (i.e., hematuria in renal vein thrombosis, presence of a vascular tumor in Kasabach-Merritt syndrome).

B. **Late-onset thrombocytopenia** (Fig. 47.2)**.** The most common causes of thrombocytopenia of any severity presenting after 72 hours of life are sepsis (bacterial or fungal) and necrotizing enterocolitis (NEC). Affected infants are usually ill appearing and have other signs suggestive of sepsis and/or NEC. However, thrombocytopenia can be the first presenting sign of these processes and can precede clinical deterioration. Appropriate treatment (i.e., antibiotics, supportive respiratory and cardiovascular care, bowel rest in case of NEC, and surgery in case of surgical NEC) usually improves the platelet count in 1 to 2 weeks, although in some infants, the thrombocytopenia persists for several weeks. The reasons underlying this prolonged thrombocytopenia are unclear.

If bacterial/fungal sepsis and NEC are ruled out, viral infections such as herpes simplex virus, cytomegalovirus (CMV), or enterovirus should be considered. These are frequently accompanied by abnormal liver enzymes. If the infant has or has recently had a central venous or arterial catheter, thromboses should be part of the differential diagnosis. Finally, drug-induced thrombocytopenia should be considered if the infant is clinically well and is receiving heparin, antibiotics (penicillins, ciprofloxacin, cephalosporins, metronidazole, vancomycin, and rifampin), indomethacin, famotidine, cimetidine, phenobarbital, or phenytoin, among others. Other less common causes of late-onset thrombocytopenia include inborn errors of metabolism and Fanconi anemia (rare).

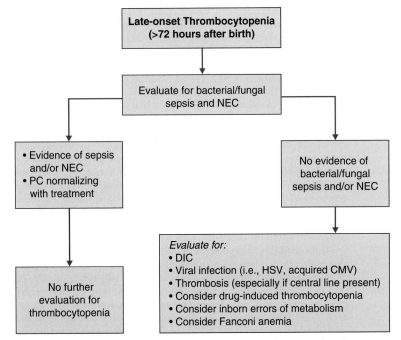

Figure 47.2. Guidelines for the evaluation of neonates with late-onset thrombocytopenia (>72 hours of life). NEC, necrotizing enterocolitis; PC, platelet count; DIC, disseminated intravascular coagulation; HSV, herpes simplex virus; CMV, cytomegalovirus.

Novel tools to evaluate platelet production and aid in the evaluation of thrombocytopenia have been recently developed and are likely to become widely available to clinicians in the near future. Among those, the immature platelet fraction (IPF) measures the percentage of newly released platelets (<24 hours). The IPF can be measured in a standard hematologic cell counter (Sysmex 2100 XE or XN Hematology Analyzer) as part of the complete cell count and can help differentiate thrombocytopenias associated with decreased platelet production from those with increased platelet destruction, in a manner similar to the use of reticulocyte counts to evaluate anemia. Recent studies have shown the usefulness of the IPF to evaluate mechanisms of thrombocytopenia and to predict platelet recovery in neonates. The IPF should be particularly helpful to guide the diagnostic evaluation of infants with thrombocytopenia of unclear etiology.

III. IMMUNE THROMBOCYTOPENIA. Immune thrombocytopenia occurs due to the passive transfer of antibodies from the maternal to the fetal circulation. There are two distinct types of immune-mediated thrombocytopenia: (i) neonatal alloimmune thrombocytopenia (NAIT) and (ii) autoimmune thrombocytopenia. In NAIT, the antibody is produced in the mother against a specific human platelet antigen (HPA) present in the fetus but absent in the mother. The antigen is inherited from the father of the fetus. The anti-HPA antibody produced in the maternal serum crosses the placenta and reaches the fetal circulation, leading to platelet destruction, inhibition of megakaryocyte development, and thrombocytopenia. In autoimmune thrombocytopenia, the antibody is directed against an antigen on the mother's own platelets (autoantibody) as well as on the baby's platelets. The maternal autoantibody also crosses the placenta, resulting in destruction of fetal platelets and thrombocytopenia.

A. **NAIT.** NAIT should be considered in any neonate who presents with severe thrombocytopenia at birth or shortly thereafter, particularly in the absence of other risk factors, clinical signs, or abnormalities in the physical exam. In a study of more than 200 neonates with thrombocytopenia, using a platelet count $<50 \times 10^3/\mu L$ in the first day of life as a screening indicator identified 90% of the patients with NAIT. In addition, the combination of severe neonatal thrombocytopenia with a parenchymal (rather than intraventricular) intracranial hemorrhage (ICH) is highly suggestive of NAIT.

   Laboratory investigation. When NAIT is suspected, blood should be collected from the mother and father and submitted for confirmatory testing (if accessible). The initial antigen screening should include HPA 1, 3, and 5. This evaluation should identify approximately 90% of cases of NAIT. However, if the diagnosis is strongly suspected and the initial evaluation is negative, further testing should be undertaken for HPA 9 and 15 (and HPA 4 if the parents are of Asian descent). If positive, these tests will reveal an antibody in the mother's plasma directed against the specific platelet antigen in the father. If blood cannot be collected from the parents in a timely fashion, neonatal serum may be screened for the presence of antiplatelet antibodies. However, a low antibody concentration in the neonate coupled with binding of the antibodies to the infant's platelets can lead to false-negative results. It is still uncertain if there is any correlation between the affinity of the antibodies and the severity of disease. Due to the complexity of testing, evaluations should be performed in an experienced reference laboratory that has a large number of typed controls available for antibody detection and the appropriate DNA-based technology to type multiple antigens.

   Brain imaging studies (cranial ultrasound) should be performed as soon as NAIT is suspected, regardless of the presence or absence of neurologic manifestations, because findings from these studies will dictate the aggressiveness of the treatment regimen for the affected infant and for the mother's future pregnancies. The clinical course of NAIT is short in most cases, often resolving almost entirely within 2 weeks. However, to confirm the diagnosis, it is important to follow the platelet count frequently until a normal count is achieved.

   Management. The management of NAIT differs depending on the specific clinical scenario:

   1. Suspected NAIT in an unknown pregnancy
   2. Known case of NAIT

3. Antenatal management of pregnant woman with previous history of NAIT.
   a. ***Management of the neonate with suspected NAIT in an unknown pregnancy***. Based on recent data demonstrating that a large proportion of infants with NAIT respond to **random-donor platelet transfusions, this is now considered the first line of therapy for infants in whom NAIT is suspected**.

      i. If the patient is clinically stable and does not have evidence of an ICH, platelets are usually given when the platelet count is $<30 \times 10^3$/mL, although this is arbitrary. In the case of a preterm infant, or a clinically unstable infant (i.e., respiratory distress, infection), a platelet transfusion is usually given when the platelet count falls below 50×10^3/mL during the first week of life (Table 47.1). In addition to platelets, if the diagnosis of NAIT is confirmed or strongly suspected, intravenous immune globulin (IVIG) (1 g/kg/day for up to 2 consecutive days) may be infused to increase the patient's own platelets and potentially to protect the transfused platelets. Because in NAIT, the platelet count usually falls after birth, IVIG may be infused when the platelet count is between 30 and 50×10^3/mL to try to prevent a further drop.

      ii. If the patient has evidence of an ICH, the goal is to maintain a platelet count $>100 \times 10^3$/mL, but this may be challenging in neonates with NAIT. In all of these scenarios, it is important to keep in mind that some infants with NAIT fail to respond to random-donor platelets and IVIG. For that reason, the blood bank

Table 47.1. Guidelines for Platelet Transfusion

Platelet Count ($\times 10^3$/μL)	Guidelines
<30	*Transfuse all*
30–49	*Transfuse if:* ■ BW $<1,500$ g and ≤ 7 days old ■ Clinically unstable ■ Recent diagnosis of NEC ■ Concurrent coagulopathy ■ Previous major hemorrhage (i.e., grade 3 or 4 IVH) ■ Prior to surgical procedure ■ Postoperative period (72 hours)
50–100	*Transfuse if:* ■ Active bleeding ■ NAIT with intracranial bleed ■ Before or after neurosurgical procedures

BW, birth weight; NEC, necrotizing enterocolitis; IVH, intraventricular hemorrhage; NAIT, neonatal alloimmune thrombocytopenia.

should be immediately alerted about any infant with suspected NAIT, and arrangements should be made to secure a source of antigen-negative platelets (either from HPA-1b1b and 5a5a donors, which should be compatible in >90% of cases, or from the mother) as soon as possible if there is no response to the initial therapies. If maternal platelets are used, they need to be concentrated to decrease the amount of antiplatelet antibodies (present in the mother's plasma) infused into the infant. Platelets can also be washed to eliminate the plasma, but this induces more damage to the platelets than concentrating them. Of note, in some European countries, HPA-1b1b and 5a5a platelets are maintained in the blood bank inventory and are immediately available for use. In those cases, these are preferable to random-donor platelets and/ or IVIG and should be the first line of therapy.

    iii. Methylprednisolone (1 mg/kg BID for 3 to 5 days) has also been used in individual case reports and small series but should only be considered in exceptional circumstances when the infant does not respond to random platelets and IVIG, and antigen-matched platelets are not readily available. We don't routinely use or recommend the use of steroids.

    b. Management of the neonate with known NAIT. When a neonate is born to a mother who had a previous pregnancy affected by confirmed NAIT, genotypically matched platelets (e.g., HPA-1b1b platelets) should be available in the blood bank at the time of delivery and should be the first line of therapy if the infant is thrombocytopenic.

    c. Antenatal management of pregnant women with previous history of NAIT. Mothers who delivered an infant with NAIT should be followed in high-risk obstetric clinics during all future pregnancies. The intensity of prenatal treatment will be based on the severity of the thrombocytopenia and the presence or absence of ICH in the previously affected fetus. This is particularly important to assess the risk of developing an ICH in the current pregnancy and to minimize this risk. Current recommendations involve maternal treatment with IVIG (1 to 2 g/kg/ week) ± steroids (0.5 to 1.0 mg/kg/day prednisone), starting at 12 or at 20 to 26 weeks of gestation, depending on whether the previously affected fetus suffered an ICH, and if so, at what time during pregnancy. Most recent studies showed that the combination of IVIG and steroids is the most efficient treatment. Regarding mode of delivery, elective cesarean section is recommended in most countries, regardless of ICH status, to avoid ICH.

B. Autoimmune thrombocytopenia. The diagnosis of neonatal autoimmune thrombocytopenia should be considered in any neonate who has early-onset thrombocytopenia and a maternal history of either immune thrombocytopenic purpura (ITP) or an autoimmune disease (with or without thrombocytopenia). A retrospective study of obstetric patients who had ITP (including a high number of mothers who had thrombocytopenia during their pregnancies) demonstrated a relatively high incidence of affected babies: Twenty-five percent of neonates exhibited thrombocytopenia at birth; the thrombocytopenia was severe in 9%, and 15% received treatment for it.

Other large studies confirmed an incidence of severe neonatal thrombocytopenia in this population ranging from 8.9% to 14.7%, with ICH occurring in 0.0% to 1.5% of affected neonates. Based on these data, it is recommended that all neonates born to mothers who have autoimmune diseases undergo a screening platelet count at or shortly after birth. If the platelet count is normal, no further evaluation is necessary. If the infant has mild thrombocytopenia, however, the platelet count should be repeated in 2 to 3 days, because it usually reaches the nadir between days 2 and 5 after birth. If the platelet count is $<30 \times 10^3/\mu L$, IVIG (1 g/kg, repeated if necessary) is the first line of therapy. Random-donor platelets, in addition to IVIG, should be provided if the infant has evidence of active bleeding, although some authors give them in addition to IVIG when the platelet count is $<30 \times 10^3/\mu L$ and provide IVIG alone for platelet counts between 30 and $50 \times 10^3/\mu L$. Cranial imaging (cranial ultrasound) should be obtained in all infants with platelet counts $<50 \times 10^3/\mu L$ to evaluate for ICH. Importantly, neonatal thrombocytopenia secondary to maternal ITP may last for weeks to months and requires long-term monitoring and sometimes a second dose of IVIG at 4 to 6 weeks of life.

Maternal management. Even if the mother has true ITP, it appears that fetal hemorrhage *in utero* is very rare, compared with the small but definite risk of such hemorrhage in alloimmune thrombocytopenia. Because of that, treatment of ITP during pregnancy is mostly based on the risk of maternal hemorrhage. A small prospective randomized trial of low-dose betamethasone (1.5 mg/day orally) failed to prevent thrombocytopenia in newborns. IVIG given prenatally to the mother with ITP has also not been clearly shown to affect the fetal platelet count.

There is in general little correlation between fetal platelet counts and either maternal platelet counts, platelet antibody levels, or history of maternal splenectomy. However, attempts to measure the fetal platelet count before delivery are not recommended due to the risk associated with such attempts. In regard to the mode of delivery, there is no evidence that cesarean section is safer for the fetus with thrombocytopenia than uncomplicated vaginal delivery. Given this fact, combined with the difficulty predicting severe thrombocytopenia in neonates and the very low risk of serious hemorrhage, the 2010 International Consensus Report on the Investigation and Management of Primary Immune Thrombocytopenia concluded that the mode of delivery in ITP patients should be determined by purely obstetric indications. However, interventions that increase the risk of bleeding in the fetus should be avoided, such as vacuum or forceps delivery.

IV. PLATELET TRANSFUSIONS IN THE NICU.

Recent studies have shown that there is great variability in neonatal transfusion practices in the United States and worldwide. To a large extent, this is attributable to the paucity of scientific evidence in the field. Only one randomized trial has compared different platelet transfusion thresholds in neonates, and it was limited to very low birth weight (VLBW) infants in the first week of life, excluding patients with severe thrombocytopenia (platelet count $<50 \times 10^3/\mu L$). This study found no differences in the incidence or severity of intraventricular hemorrhages (IVHs) between a group of neonates transfused for any platelet count $<150 \times 10^3/\mu L$ and a group transfused only for counts below $60 \times 10^3/\mu L$. Based on these findings, the investigators concluded that transfusing VLBW infants with platelet counts 60 to $150 \times 10^3/\mu L$ does not reduce the risk of IVH. In the contemporary prospective multicenter observational PlaNeT-1 study, platelet transfusions were administered at a median platelet count of $27 \times 10^3/\mu L$. In a secondary analysis, the temporal association between platelet transfusions and minor bleeding was assessed. This analysis showed that neonates had 21% fewer bleeding events during the 12 hours following a platelet transfusion, compared with the 12 hours prior to transfusion. However, these findings should be interpreted with caution, partly because of the study design (observational study being prone to confounders and lacking a control group), and because these results were part of a secondary analysis. A more recent analysis by von Lindern et al compared bleeding outcomes in NICUs that used liberal transfusion thresholds versus NICUs that used restrictive transfusion thresholds. The study found no significant differences in bleeding outcomes between units.

The relationship between degree of thrombocytopenia and bleeding risk has been assessed in a number of neonatal studies. The PlaNeT-1 study found that 9% of thrombocytopenic neonates experienced clinically significant bleeding (most commonly intracranial). Eighty-seven percent of these hemorrhages occurred during the first 2 weeks of life, and 87% were in neonates <28 weeks' gestation. A secondary analysis found that a lower nadir platelet count was associated with only a slightly increased number of bleeding events. Importantly, the strongest predictors of hemorrhage were gestational age <28 weeks, postnatal age <10 days, and a diagnosis of NEC, suggesting that factors other than the platelet count are the most important determinants of bleeding risk.

Based on this limited evidence, we currently propose administering platelet transfusions to neonates according to the criteria shown in Table 47.1.

There is more consensus in regard to the platelet product that should be transfused. Most experts agree that neonates should receive 10 to 15 mL/kg of a standard platelet suspension, either a platelet concentrate ("random-donor platelets") or apheresis platelets. Each random-donor platelet unit has approximately 50 mL of volume and contains approximately 10×10^9 platelets per 10 mL. There is no need to pool more than one random-donor unit for a neonatal transfusion, a practice that only increases donor exposures and induces platelet activation, without any benefit. Two additional important considerations in neonatology are the prevention of transfusion-transmitted CMV infections and graft versus host disease (GVHD). Most blood banks provide either CMV-negative or leukoreduced products to neonates, both of which significantly reduce (but do not eliminate) the risk of transfusion-transmitted CMV. Transfusion of CMV-negative and leukoreduced blood products effectively prevents transmission of CMV to VLBW infants. GVHD is effectively prevented by irradiating cellular blood products prior to transfusion. Of note, most neonatal cases of GVHD have been reported in neonates with underlying immunodeficiencies, receiving intrauterine or large volume transfusions (i.e., double exchange transfusions), or receiving blood products from a first-degree relative. These are all absolute indications for irradiating blood products.

When making platelet transfusion decisions, it is important for neonatologists to be aware of the risks associated with these transfusions. In the case of platelet suspensions, the risk of bacterial contamination is higher than the combined risk of all viral infections for which platelets are routinely tested. In addition, platelet transfusions can induce transfusion-associated lung injury (TRALI), a process characterized by the onset of hypoxemia and bilateral pulmonary infiltrates within 6 hours of a transfusion. Given that neonates have frequent episodes of respiratory decompensation due to different causes, TRALI is likely to be underrecognized in the NICU. Several recent publications have also shown a strong association between the number of platelet transfusions and the mortality rate among NICU patients. It is unclear from these studies whether this association simply reflects sicker patients receiving more platelets or whether platelet transfusions adversely affect outcomes. Nevertheless, while we await for data from well-designed randomized controlled studies (the ongoing PlaNeT-2 trial is comparing 25 vs. $50 \times 10^3/\mu L$ as platelet transfusion thresholds in neonates), platelet transfusion decisions in neonates should be made thoughtfully, carefully balancing the risks and benefits in each individual patient.

Suggested Readings

Andrew M, Vegh P, Caco C, et al. A randomized, controlled trial of platelet transfusions in thrombocytopenic premature infants. *J Pediatr* 1993;123(2): 285–291.

Bussel JB, Sola-Visner MC. Current approaches to the evaluation and management of the fetus and neonate with immune thrombocytopenia. *Semin Perinatol* 2009;33(1):35–42.

Cremer M, Solar-Visner MC, Roll S, et al. Platelet transfusions in neonates: practices in the United States vary significantly from those in Austria, Germany, and Switzerland. *Transfusion* 2011;51(12):2634–2641.

Stanworth SJ, Clarke P, Watts T, et al. Prospective, observational study of outcomes in neonates with severe thrombocytopenia. *Pediatrics* 2009;124(5): e826–e834.

von Lindern JS, Hulzebos CV, Bos AF, et al. Thrombocytopenia and intraventricular haemorrhage in very premature infants: a tale of two cities. *Arch Dis Child Fetal Neonatal Ed* 2012;97(5):F348–F352.

Wiedmeier SE, Henry E, Sola-Visner MC, et al. Platelet reference ranges for neonates, defined using data from over 47,000 patients in a multihospital healthcare system. *J Perinatol* 2009;29(2):130–136.

48 Viral Infections

Sallie R. Permar

KEY POINTS

- Vertically transmitted (mother to child) viral infections of the fetus and newborn can generally be divided into three distinct categories by transmission modes—congenital, peripartum, and postnatal infections.

- Although classically the congenital infections have gone by the acronym TORCH (T = toxoplasmosis, O = other, R = rubella, C = cytomegalovirus, H = herpes simplex virus), the concept of obtaining "TORCH titers" for diagnostics in an infant is out of date with current viral diagnostic testing platforms.

- When congenital or perinatal infections are suspected, the diagnosis of each of the possible infectious agents should be considered separately and the appropriate most rapid diagnostic test is requested in order to implement therapy as quickly as possible.

- Congenital cytomegalovirus (CMV) infection is the most common congenital infection and a leading cause of birth defects and pediatric disabilities.

- Neonatal herpes simplex virus (HSV) infection is associated with a high risk of infant death and lifelong disabilities, yet the disease can be considerably ameliorated with early use of acyclovir in suspected cases.

- Pediatric HIV-1 infections have been markedly reduced through the use of maternal and/or infant antiretroviral treatment (ART), yet break through infections and incomplete access/adherence to antiretroviral therapy impede global elimination of vertical HIV-1 transmission.

- Infant infection after exposure to a hepatitis B surface antigen (HBsAg)-positive mother can be avoided through a combination of active (hepatitis B vaccine) and passive hepatitis B immune globulin (HBIG) immunization of the infant.

I. INTRODUCTION. Vertically transmitted (mother to child) viral infections of the fetus and newborn can generally be divided into three distinct categories by transmission modes. The first is **congenital infections**, which can be transmitted to the fetus via the placenta *in utero*. The second category is **peripartum infections**, which are acquired intrapartum or during the delivery. The final category is **postnatal infections**, viruses transmitted in the postpartum period, commonly via breast milk feeding. Classifying these infections into congenital and perinatal categories highlights aspects of their pathogenesis in the fetus and newborn infant. When these infections occur in older children or adults, they are typically benign. However, if the host is immunocompromised or if the immune system is not yet developed, such as in the neonate, clinical symptoms may be quite severe or even fatal. Congenital infections can have manifestations that can lead to spontaneous fetal loss, or become clinically apparent antenatally by ultrasonography or when the infant is born, whereas perinatal infections may not become clinically obvious until after the first few weeks of life.

Although classically the congenital infections have gone by the acronym TORCH (T = toxoplasmosis, O = other, R = rubella, C = cytomegalovirus, H = herpes simplex virus), the concept of obtaining "TORCH titers" for diagnostics in an infant is out of date with current viral diagnostic testing platforms. When congenital or perinatal infections are suspected, the diagnosis of each of the possible infectious agents should be considered separately and the appropriate most rapid diagnostic test is requested in order to implement therapy as quickly as possible. Useless information is often obtained when the diagnosis is attempted by drawing a single serum sample to be sent for measurement of "TORCH" titers. These immunoglobulin G (IgG) antibodies are acquired by passive transmission to the fetus and merely reflect the maternal serostatus. Pathogen-specific immunoglobulin M (IgM) antibodies do reflect fetal/infant infection status but with variable sensitivity and specificity. The following discussion is divided by pathogen as to the usual timing of acquisition of infection (congenital or peripartum or postnatal) and in approximate order of prevalence. A summary of the diagnostic evaluations for separate viral infections is shown in Table 48.1.

II. CYTOMEGALOVIRUS (CMV) (CONGENITAL, PERIPARTUM, AND POSTNATAL).

CMV is a double-stranded enveloped DNA virus that results lifelong infection. It is a member of the herpesvirus family, is highly species-specific, and derives its name from the histopathologic appearance of infected cells, which have abundant cytoplasm and both intranuclear and cytoplasmic inclusions. The highly common rate of congenital infection following maternal infection and its resulting brain damage and birth defects has led the Institute of Medicine to name the development of a CMV vaccine as a top priority.

A. Epidemiology. CMV is present in saliva, urine, genital secretions, breast milk, and blood/blood products of infected persons and can be transmitted by exposure to any of these sources. Primary infection (acute infection) is usually asymptomatic in older infants, children, and adults but may manifest with mononucleosis-like symptoms, including a prolonged fever and a mild hepatitis. Latent infection is asymptomatic unless the host becomes immunocompromised. CMV infection is very common, with seroprevalence in the United States between 50% and 85% by age 40 years. Approximately 40% of pregnant women in the United States are infected, which is in contrast to over 90% seropositivity in underdeveloped nations. Yet, the U.S. seroprevalence rates are highly dependent on race distribution and geography, with Southeastern

Table 48.1. Diagnostic Techniques for Diagnosis of Perinatal Infections

Pathogen	Test of Choice	Sensitivity	Expense	Turnaround
HSV	PCR of skin lesion, blood, or CSF	High	Moderate	Hours
Parvovirus	PCR blood	High	Moderate	Hours*
Parvovirus	IgM	Moderate	Low	Days
CMV	PCR urine/saliva	High	Moderate	Hours*
CMV	Spin-enhanced urine culture (shell vial)	High	Moderate	Days
HIV	DNA PCR of blood if mother known HIV-infected	High	High	Hours*
HIV	RNA PCR of plasma if mother not treated	High	Moderate	Hours*
HBV	HBsAg of blood	High	Low	Hours
HBV	DNA PCR of blood	High	Moderate	Hours*
HCV	RNA PCR of plasma <12 months	High	Moderate	Hours*
HCV	RIBA or ELISA >15 months	High	Low	Hours*
VZV	PCR of skin lesion	Moderate	Moderate	Hours
HEV	RNA PCR blood or CSF	High	Moderate	Hours*
HEV	Culture urine, oro-pharynx, stool	Moderate	High	Days
Rubella	Culture urine	Moderate	High	Many days
RSV	PCR of nasopharyn-geal secretions	Moderate	Moderate	Hours

HSV, herpes simplex virus; PCR, polymerase chain reaction; CSF, cerebrospinal fluid; IgM, immunoglobulin M; CMV, cytomegalovirus; HBV, hepatitis B virus; HBsAg, hepatitis B surface antigen; HCV, hepatitis C virus; RIBA, recombinant immunoblot assay; ELISA, enzyme-linked immunosorbent assay; VZV, varicella-zoster virus; HEV, hepatitis E virus; RSV, respiratory syncytial virus.
*PCRs in general are done within a half day but often are a send-out test to a central lab requiring days to ship and retrieve data.

states having higher seroprevalence rates compared to the rest of the country and Latin and African American women demonstrating the highest preconception seroimmunity. Primary CMV infection occurs in approximately 1% of pregnant women, likely via sexual transmission or exposure to mucosal fluid of CMV-infected toddlers who shed high amounts of the virus. Primary maternal infection is a high-risk setting for the infant, with a fetal transmission rate of 30% to 40%. This high fetal transmission rate in primary infection is in contrast to the 1% to 2% transmission rate in women infected with CMV prior to pregnancy. In this setting, virus is transmitted following maternal virus reactivation or reinfection. Approximately half of congenital infections are due to primary maternal CMV infection during pregnancy. Although transmission in the setting of nonprimary maternal infection can result in hearing loss, congenital CMV infection in the setting of no preexisting immunity disproportionately contributes to the symptomatic infections. The risk of transmission to the fetus as a function of gestational age is uncertain, but infection during early gestation likely carries a higher risk of severe fetal disease.

Congenital CMV occurs in approximately 1% of all live births in the United States and is the leading infectious cause of sensorineural hearing loss (SNHL), developmental delay, and occasional childhood death. In fact, CMV contributes to more cases of childhood deafness than that of *Haemophilus influenzae* bacterial meningitis in the prevaccine era. Annually, 30,000 to 40,000 CMV-infected infants are born in the United States (at least 1 in 150 live births), with 10% presenting with symptomatic disease at birth. Additionally, 10% to 15% of the asymptomatic neonates will develop significant sequelae in the first year of life, most commonly hearing loss. Therefore, over 5,000 infants are severely affected or die from CMV infection in the United States each year (1 in 750 live births). Congenital CMV infection is more common among HIV-exposed infants, and coinfected infants may have more rapid progression of HIV-1 disease. Therefore, screening for congenital CMV infection in HIV-exposed infants is advised.

Finally, only in unique settings can perinatal or postnatal transmission of CMV lead to neonatal disease, including postnatal infection of very low birth weight preterm infants and children with congenital immunodeficiencies, such as severe combined immunodeficiency (SCID). In the neonatal intensive care unit, many postnatal CMV infections were previously caused by transfusion of CMV seropositive blood products, which has mainly been eliminated through the use of seronegative and leukoreduced blood products. Currently, postnatal transmission via breast milk feeding is the most common mode of infection in preterm infants, which can lead to a sepsis-like illness, pneumonitis, and enteritis. The impact of this infection on long-term outcome and neurodevelopment is an area of ongoing investigation.

B. Clinical disease in congenital infection may present at birth or may manifest with symptoms later in infancy. Only very low birth weight preterm infants (<1,500 g) or immunosuppressed infants will have symptomatic disease from peripartum or postnatal CMV acquisition.

1. **Congenital symptomatic CMV disease** can present as an acute **fulminant** infection involving multiple organ systems with as high as 30% mortality. **Signs** include petechiae or purpura (79%), hepatosplenomegaly (HSM) (74%), jaundice (63%), pneumonitis, and/or "blueberry muffin spots" reflecting extramedullary hematopoiesis. **Laboratory abnormalities** include elevated hepatic transaminases and bilirubin levels (as much as half conjugated), anemia, and thrombocytopenia. Hyperbilirubinemia may be present at birth or develop over time and can persists beyond the period of physiologic jaundice. Approximately one-third of these infants are preterm, and one-third has intrauterine growth restriction (IUGR) and microcephaly.

   A second early presentation includes infants who are symptomatic, most commonly with SNHL but without life-threatening complications. These babies may also have IUGR or disproportionate microcephaly (48%) with or without intracranial calcifications. These calcifications may occur anywhere in the brain but are classically found in the periventricular area. Other findings of central nervous system (CNS) disease can include ventricular dilatation, cortical atrophy, and migrational disorders such as lissencephaly, pachygyria, and demyelination as well as chorioretinitis in approximately 10% to 15% of infants. Babies with CNS manifestations almost always have developmental abnormalities and neurologic dysfunction. These range from mild learning and language disability or mild hearing loss to IQ scores below 50, motor abnormalities, deafness, and visual problems. Because SNHL is the most common sequela of CMV infection (60% in symptomatic and 5% in asymptomatic infants at birth), any infant failing the newborn hearing screen also should be screened for CMV infection. Conversely, infants with documented congenital CMV infection should be assessed for hearing loss as neonates and throughout the first 2 years of life.

2. **Asymptomatic congenital infection** at birth in 5% to 15% of neonates can manifest as **late disease** in infancy, throughout the first 2 years of life. Abnormalities include developmental abnormalities, hearing loss, seizures, mental retardation, motor spasticity, and acquired microcephaly.

3. **Peripartum and postnatally acquired CMV infection** may occur (i) from intrapartum exposure to the virus within the maternal genital tract, (ii) from postnatal exposure to infected breast milk, (iii) from exposure to infected blood or blood products, or (iv) nosocomially through urine or saliva. The time from infection to disease presentation varies from 4 to 12 weeks. Almost all term infants who are infected perinatally and postnatally remain asymptomatic, with the exception of severely immunocompromised infants. Although long-term developmental and neurologic abnormalities are rarely seen, an acute infection syndrome including neutropenia, anemia, thrombocytopenia, and hepatosplenomegaly can occur in preterm infants. Data suggest that all infants regardless of gestational age should have hearing testing over the first 2 years of life if documented to have acquired CMV.

4. **CMV pneumonitis.** CMV has been associated with pneumonitis occurring primarily in preterm infants <4 months old. Symptoms and radiographic findings in CMV pneumonitis are similar to those seen in afebrile pneumonia of other causes in neonates and young infants, including *Chlamydia trachomatis*, *Ureaplasma urealyticum*, and respiratory syncytial virus (RSV). Symptoms include tachypnea, cough, coryza, and nasal congestion. Intercostal retractions and hypoxemia may be present, and apnea may occur. Radiographically, there is hyperinflation, diffusely increased pulmonary markings, thickened bronchial walls, and focal atelectasis. A small number of infants may have symptoms that are severe enough to require mechanical ventilation or require an increased level of respiratory support. Long-term sequela include recurrent pulmonary problems, including wheezing, bronchopulmonary dysplasia (defined as prolonged oxygen dependence), and, in some cases, repeated hospitalizations for respiratory distress. Whether this presentation reflects congenital or perinatal CMV infection is unclear. Conversely, merely finding CMV in respiratory secretions of a preterm infant does not prove causality because CMV is present in saliva of infected infants.

5. **Transfusion-acquired CMV infection.** In the past, significant morbidity and mortality could occur in newborn infants receiving CMV-infected blood or blood products. Because both the cellular and humoral maternal immune systems are helpful in preventing infection or in ameliorating clinical disease, those most severely affected were preterm, low birth weight infants born to CMV-seronegative women. Mortality was estimated to be 20% in very low birth weight infants. Symptoms typically developed 4 to 12 weeks after transfusion; lasted for 2 to 3 weeks; and consisted of respiratory distress, pallor, and hepatosplenomegaly. Hematologic abnormalities were also seen, including hemolysis, thrombocytopenia, and atypical lymphocytosis. Transfusion-acquired CMV is now rare in the United States, prevented by using blood/blood products from CMV-seronegative donors or filtered, leukoreduced products (see Chapter 42).

C. **Diagnosis.** CMV infection should be suspected in any infant having typical symptoms of infection or if there is a maternal history of seroconversion or a mononucleosis-like, febrile illness in pregnancy or ultrasound findings consistent with CMV infection (i.e., echogenic bowel, intracranial calcifications). The diagnosis is made if CMV is identified in amniotic fluid or urine, saliva, blood, or respiratory secretions of the infant and defined as *congenital* infection if found in the infant within the first 3 weeks of life and as *peripartum* or *postnatal* infection if negative in the first 3 weeks and positive after 4 weeks of life. Depending on when the fetus or infant infection occurred, blood is the earliest specimen to become positive and is highly specific for congenital disease when CMV is detected in blood of a newborn; however, not all congenitally infected infants are viremic at birth. Thus, detection of CMV shedding in urine or saliva provides the highest sensitivity for diagnosis. A negative viral test from blood cannot rule out CMV infection, but a negative urine or saliva test in an untreated infant symptomatic for

4 weeks or more does rule out infection. There are three rapid diagnostic techniques:

1. **CMV polymerase chain reaction (PCR).** CMV may be detected by PCR in urine, saliva, or blood. The sensitivity and specificity of using this test for diagnosis is quite high for urine and saliva, but a negative PCR in blood does not rule out infection. Saliva is a preferred specimen in infants due to ease of collection. In fact, a CMV PCR testing platform based on dried saliva "spots" on filter paper has been validated as highly sensitive and specific and may be amenable to being added to the current newborn screening tests that utilize dried blood spots.

2. **Spin-enhanced or "shell vial" culture.** Virus can be isolated from saliva and in high titer from urine. Depending on local laboratory specifications, the specimen is collected as fluid or with a Dacron swab, inoculated into viral transport medium, then inoculated into viral tissue culture medium containing a coverslip on which tissue culture cells (MRC5) have been grown and incubated. Viable CMV infects the cells, which are then lysed and stained with antibody to CMV antigens. Virus can be detected with high sensitivity and specificity within 24 to 72 hours of inoculation. It is much more rapid than standard tissue culture, which may take from 2 to 6 weeks for replication and identification. A negative result generally rules out CMV infection except in infants who may have acquired infection within the prior 2 to 3 weeks.

3. **CMV antigen.** Peripheral blood can be centrifuged and the buffy coat spread on a slide. The neutrophils are then lysed and stained with an antibody to CMV pp65 antigen. Positive results confirm CMV infection and viremia; however, negative results do not rule out CMV infection. This test only used to follow efficacy of therapy and may be replaced by quantitative blood PCR tests.

4. **CMV IgG and IgM.** The determination of serum antibody titers to CMV has limited usefulness for the neonate, although negative IgG titers in both maternal and infant sera are sufficient to exclude congenital CMV infection. A positive IgM during pregnancy without the detection of CMV-specific IgG should be repeated to look for a new seroconversion, whereas a positive IgM in the presence of IgG should be further assessed with a CMV IgG avidity assay. Low maternal CMV IgG avidity would indicate recent infection and therefore the infant should be tested for CMV and followed closely after birth. The interpretation of a positive IgG titer in the newborn is complicated by the presence of transplacentally derived maternal IgG. Uninfected infants usually show a decline in IgG within 1 month and have no detectable titer by 4 to 12 months, whereas infected infants will continue to produce IgG. Tests for CMV-specific IgM have limited specificity but may help in the diagnosis of an infant infection.

If the diagnosis of congenital CMV infection is made, the newborn should have a thorough physical and neurologic examination, a head ultrasound of the brain, potentially followed by magnetic resonance imaging (MRI) scan of the brain, an ophthalmologic examination, and repeated hearing tests. Laboratory evaluation should include a complete blood count, liver function tests, and, preferably, cerebrospinal fluid (CSF) examination. In CMV-infected infants with symptomatic disease, approximately 90% with abnormal brain imaging will have CNS sequelae. However, about 30% of infants with normal brain imaging will also have sequelae. Infants with evidence of neurologic involvement should be considered as candidates for antiviral treatment.

D. Treatment. Ganciclovir and the oral prodrug, valganciclovir, have been effective in the treatment of and prophylaxis against dissemination of CMV in immunocompromised patients and infants. The earliest studies of infants with symptomatic CMV disease showed a strong trend toward efficacy in the IV ganciclovir-treated infants as assessed by stabilization or improvement of SNHL. Further studies indicated that extended treatment of symptomatic infants with valganciclovir for 6 months showed improvements in hearing loss and developmental delay over 6 weeks of treatment. The primary reported toxicity of valganciclovir treatment is mild neutropenia. Yet, the occurrence of neutropenia was equally common between 6 weeks and 6 months of age in infants who received the prolonged or short course of valganciclovir—indicating that the viral infection, as opposed to the drug treatment, is the primary contributor to the observed neutropenia. Families should be advised that although evidence is increasing as to ganciclovir's ability to improve long-term neurologic outcomes, there is a potential for future reproductive system effects because testicular atrophy and gonadal tumors were found in some animals treated with pharmacologic doses of ganciclovir. Moreover, the efficacy of initiating treatment at >1 month of age in symptomatic infection is not known, demonstrating the importance of early diagnosis. Finally, although the treatment of postnatally acquired CMV infection is recommended in highly immunosuppressed infants, the effectiveness of treatment of symptomatic postnatal CMV infection in preterm infants to ameliorate the disease course or improve long-term outcome is unknown. Thus, treatment should be recommended and supervised by a pediatric infectious disease specialist.

E. Prevention

1. **Screening.** Because only about 1% of women acquire primary CMV infection during pregnancy and there are no currently available prevention strategies in pregnant women that have been shown to be effective in randomized trials, screening for women at risk for seroconversion is generally not recommended. Isolation of virus from the cervix or urine of pregnant women cannot be used to predict fetal infection. In cases of documented primary maternal infection or seroconversion, quantitative PCR testing of amniotic fluid can determine whether the fetus acquired infection. However, counseling about a positive finding of fetal infection is difficult because approximately 80% of infected fetuses will only have mild or asymptomatic disease. Some investigators have found that higher CMV viral loads from the amniotic fluid tended to correlate with abnormal neurodevelopmental outcome. One case-control study suggested a protective benefit against severe neonatal disease by administering hyperimmune CMV immunoglobulin

antenatally to women with low affinity antibody to CMV, yet a subsequent randomized controlled trial did not demonstrate benefit in preventing congenital infection. Yet, pregnant women, and particularly those that are exposed to toddlers, can be counseled to reduce their CMV acquisition risk. The Centers for Disease Control and Prevention (CDC) recommends that (i) pregnant women practice hand washing with soap and water after contact with diapers or oral secretions; do not share food, utensils, toothbrushes, and pacifiers with children; and avoid saliva when kissing a child; (ii) pregnant women who develop a mononucleosis-like illness during pregnancy should be evaluated for CMV infection and counseled about risks to the unborn child; (iii) antibody testing can confirm prior CMV infection; (iv) the benefits of breastfeeding outweigh the minimal risk of acquiring CMV; (v) there is no need to screen for CMV or exclude CMV-excreting children from schools or institutions.

2. **Immunization.** Passive immunization with hyperimmune anti-CMV immunoglobulin and active immunization with a live-attenuated CMV vaccine represent attractive therapies for prophylaxis against congenital CMV infections. However, data from clinical trials have not shown adequate efficacy of either of these approaches with current passive and active vaccine products. Two live-attenuated CMV vaccines have been developed, but their efficacy has not been clearly established. A subunit vaccine consisting of the major immunodominant glycoprotein present on the surface of the virus, glycoprotein B (gB), was studied for the prevention of maternal CMV acquisition following delivery, yet was only 50% efficacious in preventing CMV acquisition. Ongoing vaccine development has focused on distinct glycoprotein complexes and the elicitation of both humoral and cellular immunity, holding promising eventual development of a maternal CMV vaccine that will eliminate congenital CMV transmission, much like that of the rubella virus vaccine.

3. **Breast milk feeding.** Although breast milk is a common source for postnatal CMV infection in the newborn, symptomatic infection is rare in term infants. In this setting, protection against disseminated disease may be provided by transplacentally derived maternal IgG or antibody in breast milk. However, there may be insufficient transplacental IgG to provide adequate protection in preterm infants. For mothers of extremely premature and low birth weight infants known to be CMV seropositive, freezing breast milk will reduce the titer of CMV but will not eliminate active virus. At present, there is no recommended method of minimizing the risk of exposure to CMV in breast milk for preterm infants; maternal breast milk is the preferred enteral nutrition in preterm infants. Methods to reduce acquisition of CMV via breast milk feeding for preterm infants is needed to eliminate this risk for preterm infants.

4. **Environmental restrictions.** Day care centers and hospitals are potential high-risk environments for acquiring CMV infection. Not surprisingly, a number of studies confirmed an increased risk of infection in day care workers. However, there does not appear to be an increased

risk of infection in hospital personnel, indicating that hand hygiene and infection control measures practiced in hospital settings are sufficient to control the spread of CMV to workers. Unfortunately, such control may be difficult to achieve in day care centers. Good hand-washing technique should be suggested to pregnant women with children in day care settings and with children attending day care, especially if the women are known to be seronegative. The determination of CMV susceptibility of these women by serology may be useful for counseling.

5. **Transfusion product restrictions.** The risk of transfusion-acquired CMV infection in the neonate has been almost eliminated by the use of CMV antibody-negative donors, by freezing packed red blood cells (PRBCs) in glycerol, or by removing the white blood cells. It is particularly important to use blood from one of these sources in preterm, low birth weight infants (see Chapter 42).

III. HERPES SIMPLEX VIRUS (HSV: PERINATAL).
HSV, a lifelong infection, is a double-stranded, enveloped DNA virus with two virologically distinct types: types 1 and 2. HSV-2 was previously the primary cause of genital lesions, yet HSV-1 has become the predominant virus type in genital lesions of young women. Both types produce clinically indistinguishable neonatal syndromes. The virus can cause localized disease of the infant's skin, eye, or mouth (SEM) or may disseminate by cell-to-cell contiguous spread or viremia. After adsorption and penetration into host cells, viral replication proceeds, resulting in cellular swelling, hemorrhagic necrosis, formation of intranuclear inclusions, cytolysis, and cell death.

A. **Epidemiology.** Acquisition of HSV results in lifelong disease, with periodic virus reactivation and mucosal shedding. At least 80% of the U.S. population is infected with HSV type 1 by the fifth decade of life, the cause of recurrent orolabial disease and an increasing cause of genital disease. According to the 2005 to 2008 National Health and Nutrition Examination Survey, the overall seroprevalence of HSV-1 and -2 in the United States in 19- to 49-year-olds is 54% and 16%, respectively. Women without prior exposure to HSV have a 4% chance of primary infection during pregnancy and a 2% chance of a nonprimary acute infection with either HSV-1 or -2 (previously infected with the alternate HSV type). The majority of these new HSV acquisitions will be asymptomatic.

Infection in the newborn occurs as a result of direct exposure to the virus, most commonly in the perinatal period from maternal genital disease or asymptomatic virus shedding. In one study, the characteristic ulcerations of the genitalia were present only in two-thirds of the genital tracts from which HSV could be isolated. It is estimated that up to 0.4% of all women presenting for delivery are shedding virus, and more than 1% of all women with a history of recurrent HSV infection asymptomatically shed HSV at delivery. Yet, **it is critical to recognize that most mothers of infants with neonatal HSV do not have a history of HSV outbreaks**. Approximately 30% to 50% of infants will acquire HSV infection if maternal primary infection occurs near delivery, whereas <1% of infants are infected if born to a woman with preexisting immunity (recurrent disease). Additionally, one-third of infants born to mothers with newly acquired HSV-2 or -1, although already infected with the other HSV type (nonprimary, first episode defined by detection of virus in the maternal genital tract at the time of delivery but no IgG response for the type-specific HSV identified), may acquire HSV infection. This may be due to protective maternal type-specific antibodies in the infant's serum or the birth canal. The overall incidence of newborn infection with HSV is estimated to be 1 in 3,000 to 1 in 20,000 (or 200 to 1,333 infants per year) in the United States.

B. **Transmission**

1. **Intrapartum transmission** is the most common cause of neonatal HSV infection. It is primarily associated with active shedding of virus from the cervix or vulva at the time of delivery. Up to 90% of newborn infections occur as a result of intrapartum transmission. Maternal immunity and the related amount and duration of maternal virus shedding are major determinates of peripartum transmission. Transmission risks are greatest with primary maternal infection during pregnancy, with nonprimary acute infection with HSV-1 or -2 being the next highest risk setting. In fact, when maternal antibody is present, the risk of acquisition of HSV, even for the newborn exposed to HSV in the birth canal, is much lower than that of primary maternal infection. The exact mechanism of action of maternal antibody in preventing perinatal infection is not known, but transplacentally acquired antibody is associated with reduced risk of severe newborn disease following perinatal HSV exposure. The risk of intrapartum infection increases with ruptured membranes, especially when ruptured longer than 4 hours. Finally, direct methods for fetal monitoring, such as with scalp electrodes, increase the risk of fetal transmission in the setting of active shedding. It is best to avoid these techniques if possible in women with a history of recurrent infection or suspected primary HSV disease.

2. **Antenatal transmission.** *In utero* infection with HSV has been documented but is uncommon. Spontaneous abortion has occurred with primary maternal infection before 20 weeks' gestation, but the true risk to the fetus of early-trimester primary infection is not known. Fetal infections may occur by either transplacental or ascending routes and have been documented in the setting of both primary and, rarely, recurrent maternal disease. There may be a wide range of clinical manifestations, from localized skin or eye involvement to multiorgan disease and congenital malformations. Chorioretinitis, microcephaly, and hydranencephaly may be found in these small numbers of congenitally infected patients.

3. **Postnatal transmission.** A small percentage of neonatal HSV infections result from postnatal HSV exposure (~10%). Potential sources include symptomatic and asymptomatic oropharyngeal shedding by either parent, hospital personnel, or other contacts, and maternal breast lesions. Measures to minimize exposure from these sources are discussed in the following text.

C. **Clinical manifestations.** The morbidity and mortality of neonatal HSV best correlates with three categories of disease. These are (i) infections localized to the SEM, (ii) encephalitis with or without localized mucocutaneous disease, and (iii) disseminated infection with multiple organ involvement.

1. **SEM infection.** Approximately 50% of infants with HSV have disease localized to the skin, eye, or mucocutaneous membranes. Vesicles typically appear on the sixth to ninth day of neonatal life. A cluster of vesicles often develops on the presenting part of the body, where extended direct contact with virus may occur. Vesicles occur in 90% of infants with localized mucocutaneous infection, and recurrent disease is common. Significant morbidity can occur in these infants despite the absence of signs of disseminated disease at the time of diagnosis. Up to 10% of infants later show neurologic impairment, and infants with keratoconjunctivitis can develop chorioretinitis, cataracts, and retinopathy. Thus, ophthalmologic and neurologic follow-up is important in all infants with mucocutaneous HSV. Infants with three or more recurrences of vesicles, likely reflecting poor immunologic control of virus replication, have an increased risk of neurologic complications.

2. **CNS infection.** Approximately one-third of neonates with HSV present with encephalitis in the absence of disseminated disease, and as many as 60% of these infants do not have mucocutaneous vesicles. These infants usually become symptomatic at 10 to 14 days of life with lethargy, seizures, temperature instability, and hypotonia. In the setting of disseminated disease, HSV is thought to invade the CNS from hematogenous spread. However, CNS infection in the absence of disseminated disease can occur, most often in infants having transplacentally derived viral-neutralizing antibodies, which may protect against widespread dissemination but not influence intraneuronal viral replication. Mortality is high without treatment and is approximately 15% with treatment. Late treatment is associated with increased mortality, highlighting the need for early treatment when neonatal HSV infection is suspected. Approximately two-thirds of surviving infants have impaired neurodevelopment. Long-term sequelae from acute HSV encephalitis include microcephaly, hydranencephaly, porencephalic cysts, spasticity, blindness, deafness, chorioretinitis, and learning disabilities.

3. **Disseminated infection.** This is the most severe form of neonatal HSV infection. It accounts for approximately 22% of all infants with neonatal HSV infection and can result in mortality for over half. Pneumonitis and fulminant hepatitis are associated with greater mortality. Symptoms usually begin within the first week of neonatal life. The liver, adrenals, and other visceral organs are usually involved. Approximately two-thirds of infants also have encephalitis. Clinical findings include seizures, shock, respiratory distress, disseminated intravascular coagulation (DIC), and respiratory failure. A typical vesicular rash may be absent in as many as 20% of infants. Forty percent of the infants who survive have long-term morbidity.

D. **Diagnosis.** HSV infection should be considered in the differential diagnosis of ill neonates with a variety of clinical presentations. These include CNS abnormalities, fever, shock, DIC, and/or hepatitis. HSV also should be considered in infants with respiratory distress without an obvious bacterial cause or a clinical course and findings consistent with prematurity.

The possibility of concomitant HSV infection with other commonly encountered problems of the preterm infant should be considered. **Viral isolation** or **PCR detection of viral DNA** in the appropriate clinical setting remains critical to the diagnosis. For the infant with mucocutaneous lesions, tissue should be scraped from vesicles, placed in the appropriate viral transport medium, and promptly processed for culture and/or PCR by a diagnostic virology laboratory. Virus also can be isolated or detected from the oropharynx and nasopharynx, conjunctivae, stool, urine, and CSF. In the absence of a vesicular rash, viral isolation or detection from these sites may aid in the diagnosis of disseminated HSV or HSV encephalitis. With encephalitis, an elevated CSF protein level and pleocytosis are often seen, but initial values may be within normal limits. Therefore, serial CSF examinations may be very important. Electroencephalography and computed tomography (CT)/MRI are also useful in the diagnosis of HSV encephalitis. Viral isolation from CSF is reported to be successful in as many as 40% of cases, and rates of detection in CSF by PCR may reach close to 100%. Combined HSV-1 and -2 serology is of little value, because many women are infected with HSV-1 and because these tests usually have a relatively slow turnaround time; however, obtaining type-specific antibody (HSV-1 or -2) has an 80% to 98% sensitivity and >96% specificity for identifying previous maternal infection and, thus, will assist in assessing infant risk of acquiring HSV. Infant HSV-specific IgM detection is not useful. Laboratory abnormalities seen with disseminated disease include elevated hepatic transaminase levels, direct hyperbilirubinemia, neutropenia, thrombocytopenia, and coagulopathy. A diffuse interstitial pattern is usually observed on radiographs of infants with HSV pneumonitis.

E. **Treatment.** Antiviral therapy (acyclovir, a nucleoside analog that selectively inhibits HSV replication) is highly efficacious in this setting, but the timing of therapy is critical. Treatment is indicated for all forms of neonatal HSV disease. Initial antiviral studies were carried out with vidarabine, which reduced morbidity and mortality of HSV-infected neonates. Mortality with encephalitis was reduced from 50% to 15% and in disseminated disease from 90% to 70%. Later studies found that acyclovir is as efficacious as vidarabine for the treatment of neonatal HSV. Furthermore, acyclovir is a selective inhibitor of viral replication with minimal side effects on the host and can be administered in relatively small volumes over short infusion times. Recommendations include treating infants with disease limited to the SEM disease with 20 mg acyclovir per kilogram every 8 hours for 14 days, and those with CNS or disseminated disease for at least 21 days, or longer if the CSF PCR remains positive. Infants with ocular involvement should have an ophthalmologic evaluation and treatment with topical ophthalmic antiviral agents in addition to parenteral therapy. Oral therapy such as with valacyclovir is not recommended for initial treatment. Yet, oral acyclovir suppressive therapy following initial acute treatment at a dose of 300 mg/ m^2/dose three times a day for 6 months of life was beneficial in improving the developmental outcome for infants with neonatal HSV infection. Other reports have demonstrated good outcomes in perinatally infected infants treated with suppressive therapy with higher doses of oral acyclovir for up to 2 years of life.

F. Prevention

1. **Pregnancy strategies.** Pregnant women known to be HSV-seronegative (or seronegative for HSV-1 or -2) should avoid genital sexual intercourse with a known HSV-seropositive partner in the third trimester. For women who do acquire primary HSV during pregnancy or have recurrent outbreaks, several trials have shown efficacy and safety of treating pregnant women with clinically symptomatic primary HSV infection with a 10-day course of acyclovir (oral therapy or IV if more severe disease) and its subsequent reduction in cesarean section. It is also recommended that women with HSV-2 be tested for HIV because HSV-2 seropositive persons have a twofold greater risk for acquisition of HIV than those who are seronegative for HSV-2.

2. **Delivery strategies.** Cesarean section is recommended for women with active genital lesions or prodromal symptoms at the time of delivery. The principal problem in developing antenatal strategies for the prevention of HSV transmission is the inability to identify maternal shedding of virus at the time of delivery. Viral identification requires isolation in tissue culture or PCR, so any attempt to identify women who may be shedding HSV at delivery would require antenatal cervical sampling and rapid turnaround with virus detection. Unfortunately, such screening cultures taken before labor fail to predict active excretion at delivery. Until more rapid HSV detection techniques are available, the only clear recommendation that can be made is to deliver infants by cesarean section if genital lesions are present at the start of labor. The efficacy of this approach may diminish when membranes are ruptured beyond 4 hours. Nevertheless, it is generally recommended that cesarean section be considered even with membrane rupture of longer durations. For women with a history of prior genital herpes, careful examination should be performed to determine whether lesions are present when labor commences. If lesions are observed, cesarean section should be offered. If no lesions are identified, vaginal delivery is appropriate, but a cervical swab should be obtained for culture and/or PCR and obtain maternal serology to determine if a new acquisition of a nonprimary infection with HSV-1 or -2 has occurred. Women with known clinical disease or serologic evidence of primary or nonprimary first-episode infection can be offered acyclovir near term until delivery, enabling a vaginal delivery if there are no visible lesions, but the impact of this strategy on prevention of neonatal disease is not established.

3. **Management of the newborn at risk for HSV** (Table 48.2). At this time, there are no data to support the prophylactic use of antiviral agents or immunoglobulin to prevent transmission to the newborn infant. Infants inadvertently delivered vaginally in the setting of cervical lesions should be isolated from other infants in the nursery, and swabs should be obtained from the oropharynx/nasopharynx, conjunctivae, and anus for viral detection at 12 to 24 hours of age. If the mother has no prior history of HSV, initiate acyclovir treatment while awaiting the laboratory results. If the mother can be identified as having recurrent infection, the risk of neonatal infection rate is low, and parents should be

Table 48.2. Management of the Child Born to a Woman with Active Genital Herpes Simplex Virus (HSV) Infection

Maternal primary or nonprimary first-episode infection (HSV PCR or culture of genital lesion positive, type-specific HSV-1 or -2 IgG negative)

- Consider offering an elective cesarean section, regardless of lesion status at delivery, or if membranes ruptured <4 hours.

- Swab infant's conjunctivae, nasopharynx, and anus for PCR and culture to determine exposure to HSV.
  - □ Collect blood HSV PCR, serum ALT.
  - □ Collect CSF for HSV PCR, cell count, and chemistries.
  - □ Initiation of acyclovir while pending laboratory results or if signs of neonatal HSV

- Treat with acyclovir if PCR or culture positive or signs of neonatal HSV (60 mg/kg/day in 3 divided doses × 14 [SEM] or 21 [disseminated/CNS]).

- If primary or nonprimary first-episode infection of the mother is confirmed, yet no signs of virus positive, some experts recommend 10 days of acyclovir treatment.

Recurrent infection, active at delivery (HSV PCR or culture of genital lesion positive, type-specific HSV IgG positive)

- Swab infant's conjunctivae, nasopharynx, and anus for PCR and culture to determine exposure to HSV.
  - □ Collect blood for HSV PCR.

- Treat with acyclovir if PCR or culture positive or signs of HSV infection.

PCR, polymerase chain reaction; IgG, immunoglobulin G; ALT, alanine aminotransferase; CSF, cerebrospinal fluid; SEM, skin, eye, or mouth; CNS, central nervous system.

instructed to consult their pediatrician if a rash or other clinical changes (lethargy, tachypnea, poor feeding) develop. Weekly pediatric follow-up during the first month is recommended. If the mother is found to have either recent primary or nonprimary, first-episode infection and a genital lesion, it is recommended by some experts to treat the infant for 10 days of acyclovir even without symptomatology or detection of virus in the infant. Infants with a positive culture or PCR from any site or the evolution of clinical symptomatology should immediately have cultures repeated and antiviral therapy started. Before starting acyclovir therapy, the infant should have conjunctival, nasopharyngeal, anal swabs for culture/PCR, plasma viral load, and a CSF evaluation for pleocytosis and HSV DNA PCR. Evidence of dissemination should be evaluated with hepatitic transaminases, blood counts and coagulation tests for hematologic and clotting disorders, and a chest radiograph if respiratory symptoms develop.

4. Postnatal strategies. Infants and mothers with HSV lesions should be in contact isolation. Careful hand washing and preventing the infant from having direct contact with any lesions on the caregivers should be emphasized. Breastfeeding should be avoided if there are breast lesions, and women with oral HSV should wear a mask while breastfeeding. Hospital personnel with orolabial HSV infection represent a low risk to the newborn, although the use of face masks should be recommended if active lesions are present. Of course, hand washing or use of gloves should again be emphasized. The exception to these guidelines is nursery personnel with herpetic whitlows. Because they have a high risk of viral shedding, and as transmission can occur despite the use of gloves, these individuals should not care for newborns.

IV. PARVOVIRUS B19 (CONGENITAL).

Parvoviruses are small, unenveloped single-stranded DNA viruses. Humans are the only known host. The cellular receptor for parvovirus B19 is the P blood group antigen, which is found on erythrocytes, erythroblasts, megakaryocytes, endothelial cells, placenta, and fetal liver and heart cells. This tissue specificity correlates with sites of clinical abnormalities (which are usually anemia with or without thrombocytopenia and sometimes fetal myocarditis). Lack of the P antigen is extremely rare, but these persons are resistant to infection with parvovirus.

A. **Epidemiology.** Parvovirus transmission results after contact with respiratory secretions, blood/blood products, or by vertical transmission. Cases can occur sporadically or in outbreak settings (especially in schools in late winter and early spring). Secondary spread occurs in at least half of susceptible household contacts. Infection is very common, such that 90% of elderly persons are seropositive. The prevalence of infection increases throughout childhood, such that approximately half of women of childbearing age are immune and the other half are susceptible to primary infection. The annual seroconversion rate in these women is 1.5%; however, because assessment of parvovirus infection status is not part of routine prenatal testing and because clinical infection is often asymptomatic, the rate of fetal infection in women who seroconvert during pregnancy is unknown. Women who are parents of young children, elementary school teachers, or childcare workers may be at greatest risk for exposure. Unfortunately, the time of greatest transmissibility of parvovirus is before the onset of symptoms or rash. Additionally, 50% of contagious contacts may not have a rash, and 20% may be asymptomatic. The incubation period is usually 4 to 14 days but can be as long as 21 days. Rash and joint symptoms occur 2 to 3 weeks after infection. The virus is usually spread by means of respiratory secretions, which clear in patients with typical erythema infectiosum at or shortly after the onset of rash. The epidemiology of community outbreaks of erythema infectiosum suggests that the risk of infection to susceptible schoolteachers is approximately 19% (compared with 50% for household contacts). This would lower the risk of B19 fetal disease in pregnant schoolteachers to <1%. Therefore, special precautions are not necessary in this setting. In fact, there is likely to be widespread unapparent infection in both adults and children, providing a constant background exposure rate that cannot be altered.

The overall rate of vertical transmission of parvovirus from the mother with primary infection to her fetus is approximately 30%. The risk of fetal loss (3% to 6%) is greatest when maternal infection occurs in the first half of pregnancy. Fetal death usually occurs within 6 weeks of maternal infection. The risk of fetal hydrops is approximately 1%. Therefore, parvovirus B19 could be the cause of as many as 1,400 cases of fetal death or hydrops fetalis each year in the United States.

B. Transmission is from mothers to fetuses antenatally and therefore falls in the category of congenital infections.

C. Clinical manifestations

1. **Disease in children.** Parvovirus B19 has been associated with a variety of rashes, including the typical "slapped cheek" rash of erythema infectiosum (fifth disease). In approximately 60% of school-age children with erythema infectiosum, fever occurs 1 to 4 days before the facial rash appears. Associated symptoms include myalgias, upper respiratory or gastrointestinal symptoms, and malaise, but these symptoms generally resolve with the appearance of the rash. The rash is usually macular, progresses to the extremities and trunk, and may involve the palms and soles. The rash may be pruritic and may recur. These children are likely most infectious before the onset of fever or rash. In group settings such as classrooms, the appearance of one clinically symptomatic child could reinforce the need for good hand-washing practices among potentially seronegative pregnant women.

2. **Disease in adults.** The typical school-age presentation of erythema infectiosum can occur in adults, but arthralgias and arthritis are more common. As many as 60% of adults with parvovirus B19 infection may have acute joint swelling, most commonly involving peripheral joints (symmetrically). Rash and joint symptoms occur 2 to 3 weeks after infection. Arthritis may persist for years and may be associated with the development of rheumatoid arthritis.

3. **Less common manifestations of parvovirus B19 infection**
   a. Infection in patients with severe anemia or immunosuppression. Parvovirus B19 has been identified as a cause of persistent and profound anemia in patients with rapid red blood cell turnover, including those with sickle cell (SC) disease, hemoglobin (Hb) SC disease, thalassemia, hereditary spherocytosis, and cellular enzyme deficits, such as pyruvate kinase deficiency. Parvovirus B19 also has been associated with acute and chronic red blood cell aplasia in immunosuppressed patients.
   b. Fetal infection. Although parvovirus B19 has genotypic variation, no antigenic variation between isolates has been demonstrated. Parvoviruses tend to infect rapidly dividing cells and can be transmitted across the placenta, posing a potential threat to the fetus. Based primarily on the demonstration of viral DNA in fetal tissue samples, parvovirus B19 has been implicated in approximately 10% of cases of fetal nonimmune hydrops. The presumed pathogenic sequence is as follows: maternal primary infection → transplacental transfer of B19 virus → infection of red blood cell precursors → arrested red blood cell production → severe anemia (Hb <8 g/dL) → congestive heart failure → edema.

Furthermore, B19 DNA has been detected in cardiac tissues from aborted fetuses. B19 may cause fetal myocarditis which can contribute to the development of hydrops. Finally, fetal hepatitis with severe liver disease has been documented. Although there have been rare case reports of infants with fetal anomalies and parvovirus infection, it is unlikely that parvovirus causes fetal anomalies. Hence, therapeutic abortion should not be recommended in women infected with parvovirus during pregnancy. Rather, the pregnancy should be followed carefully by frequent examination and ultrasonography for signs of fetal involvement.

D. **Diagnosis.** Parvovirus B19 will not grow in standard tissue cultures because humans are the only host. Determination of serum IgG and IgM levels is the most practical test. Serum B19 IgG is absent in susceptible hosts, and IgM appears by day 3 of an acute infection. Serum IgM may be detected in as many as 90% of patients with acute B19 infection, and serum levels begin to fall by the second to third month after infection. Serum IgG appears a few days after IgM and may persist for years. Serum or plasma can also be assessed for viral DNA by PCR and defines recent infection. Viral antigens may be directly detected in tissues by radioimmunoassay, enzyme-linked immunosorbent assay (ELISA), immunofluorescence, *in situ* nucleic acid hybridization, or PCR. These techniques may be valuable for certain clinical settings, such as the examination of tissues from fetuses with nonimmune hydrops or determination of infection (PCR).

E. **Treatment.** Treatment is generally supportive. Intravenous immunoglobulin (IVIG) has been used with reported success in a limited number of patients with severe hematologic disorders related to persistent parvovirus infection. The rationale for this therapy stems from the observations that (i) the primary immune response to B19 infection is the production of specific IgM and IgG, (ii) the appearance of systemic antibody coincides with the resolution of clinical symptoms, and (iii) specific antibody prevents infection. However, no controlled studies have been performed to establish the efficacy of IVIG prophylaxis or therapy for B19 infections. There are no recommendations for use of IVIG in pregnancy. In the carefully followed pregnancy in which hydrops fetalis is worsening, intrauterine blood transfusions may be considered, especially if the fetal Hb is <8 g/dL. The risk/benefit of this procedure to the mother and fetus should be assessed because some hydropic fetuses will improve without intervention. In some cases, if there is also fetal myocardiopathy secondary to parvovirus infection, the cardiac function may be inadequate to handle transfusion. Attempts to identify other causes of fetal hydrops are obviously important (see Chapter 26).

F. **Prevention.** The three groups of pregnant women of interest when considering the potential risk of fetal parvovirus disease are (i) those exposed to an infected household contact, (ii) school teachers, and (iii) health care providers. In each, the measurement of serum IgG and IgM levels may be useful to determine who is at risk or acutely infected after B19 exposure. The risk of fetal B19 disease is small for asymptomatic pregnant women in communities where outbreaks of erythema infectiosum occur. In this setting, no special diagnostic tests or precautions may be indicated. However, household contacts with erythema infectiosum patient place pregnant women at increased risk for acute B19 infection. The estimated risk of B19 infection in a susceptible adult with a household contact is approximately 50%. Considering an estimated risk of 5% for severe fetal disease with acute maternal B19 infection, the risk of hydrops fetalis is approximately 2.5% for susceptible pregnant women exposed to an infected household contact during the first 18 weeks of gestation. Management of these women may include the following:

1. **Determination of susceptibility of acute infection** by serum IgG and IgM and PCR

2. In susceptible or acutely infected women, **serial fetal ultrasonography** to monitor fetal growth and the possible evolution of hydrops

3. Serial determinations of **maternal serum alpha-fetoprotein (AFP)** (AFP may rise up to 4 weeks before ultrasonography evidence of fetal hydrops), although this use is of uncertain value.

4. Determination of **fetal IgM or DNA PCR** by percutaneous umbilical blood sampling (PUBS). The utility of this is questionable given the relatively high risk–benefit ratio at present, especially because it is unclear that obstetric management will be altered by results. It may be useful to confirm B19 etiology when hydrops fetalis is present.

Considering the high prevalence of B19, the low risk of severe fetal disease, and the fact that attempts to avoid potential high-risk settings only reduce but do not eliminate exposure; exclusion of pregnant school teachers from the workplace is not recommended. A similar approach may be taken for pregnant health care providers where the principal exposure will be from infected children presenting to the emergency room or physician's office. However, in the majority of cases, the typical rash of erythema infectiosum may already be present, at which time infectivity is low. Furthermore, precautions directed at minimizing exposure to respiratory secretions may be taken to decrease the risk of transmission. Particular care should be exercised on pediatric wards where there are immunocompromised patients or patients with hemolytic anemias in whom B19 disease is suspected. These patients may shed virus well beyond the period of initial clinical symptoms, particularly when presenting with aplastic crisis. In this setting, there may be a significant risk for the spread of B19 to susceptible health care workers or other patients at risk for B19-induced aplastic crisis. To minimize this risk, patients with aplastic crises from B19 infections should be maintained on contact precautions, masks should be worn for close contact, and pregnant health care providers should not care for these patients.

V. HIV (CONGENITAL AND PERINATAL). HIV is a retrovirus and the causative agent of lifelong infection and AIDS, for which there is no cure. The virus binds to the host $CD4^+$ cell and a chemokine coreceptor, and the viral core enters the host cell cytoplasm. The virus uses reverse transcriptase to synthesize DNA from its viral RNA, and this viral DNA integrates into the host genome. On cell activation, the viral DNA is transcribed to RNA, and viral proteins are synthesized. The virion acquires its outer envelope coat on budding from the host cell surface and is then infectious for other $CD4^+$ cells. The genome consists of the three genes found in all retroviruses (*gag, pol, env*), along with at least six additional genes, including gp120, which is necessary for the binding of virus to target cells. When HIV-infected lymphocytes are activated, such as in intercurrent illnesses, many virions may be transcribed, and the cell can be lysed or apoptosis enhanced, each resulting in host cell death. Because $CD4^+$ T lymphocytes are central to developing an appropriate immune response to almost all pathogens, the host with $CD4^+$ T cell counts below 200/μL is highly susceptible to opportunistic infections and malignancies which define the AIDS.

A. **Epidemiology.** HIV-1 is the principal cause of HIV infection and perinatal HIV infections in the United States and throughout the world. A related virus, HIV-2, has a more benign clinical course and is primarily geographically limited to Western Africa.

1. **Domestically**, the Center for Disease Control and Prevention reports that there are currently 1.2 million people living with HIV-1 in the United States. Although the transmission rate has decreased by nearly two-thirds from its peak, the annual new infection rate of approximately 50,000 has been relatively unchanged since the late 1990s. Of these new infections, certain groups have disproportionately high infection rates, including men who have sex with men (MSM) and African Americans. Remarkably, one in seven HIV-infected individuals is unaware of their transmission status, thwarting efforts to further reduce transmission. The decreased death rate in recent years is in large part attributed to access to more potent antiretroviral therapies available since 1996. In the year 2012, there were about 13,700 deaths in individuals with AIDS.

   Approximately 23% of those living with HIV infection in the United States are **women**, most of childbearing age, with higher rates in African American women. For 85% of these women, the leading risk behavior is heterosexual contact with a known HIV-infected person or unknown risk behavior (presumably heterosexual contact with a person of unknown positive status). Yet, in 2011, only 45% of HIV-infected women were engaged in care and only 32% had achieved viral remission. Whereas enormous successes in reduction of mother-to-child transmission have been realized with introduction of antiretroviral prophylaxis and treatment—zidovudine in 1994 and potent antiretrovirals in 1996—it is estimated that 100 to 200 infants still acquire perinatal HIV infection yearly. The vast majority of these infected infants are born to women who were unaware of their diagnosis or presented late for prenatal care. The CDC currently recommends routine antenatal "opt-out" HIV testing, which has been shown to be far more effective in identifying HIV-infected persons than systems in which written informed consent is required. At present, >90% of HIV-infected pregnant women receive antiretroviral therapy at or before delivery.

2. **Globally**, the World Health Organization (WHO) estimated that by the end of 2014, there were 36.9 million persons living with HIV (17.4 million women and 2.6 million children younger than 15 years). New HIV infections were estimated in 2014 to be 2 million, including 220,000 children. AIDS-related deaths in 2014 were 1.2 million (150,000 in children). All of these numbers are much improved from the peak of the epidemic, reflecting the global response to HIV prevention

and treatment access. Currently, approximately 67% of HIV-infected women receive antiretroviral regimens during pregnancy in countries of high HIV prevalence, and it is recommended that these women stay on treatment throughout the breastfeeding period and beyond. Yet, adherence and maintenance in care postpartum has been problematic. Although breastfeeding has been found to increase the rate of perinatal transmission by up to 14%, formula feeding is associated with high rates of morbidity and mortality from malnutrition and other infections in some areas, including respiratory and gastrointestinal infections. It has been demonstrated that exclusive breastfeeding in the first 6 months of life has a lower risk of HIV-1 acquisition compared to mixed feeding. Moreover, maternal treatment with antiretroviral has been shown to considerably reduce postpartum HIV transmission. Therefore, in areas where formula feeding is unsafe or unfeasible, the WHO recommends exclusive breastfeeding for the first 6 months of life and continued breastfeeding until 1 year of life while the mother continues on ART. In areas of high HIV prevalence, acute maternal infection during pregnancy or breastfeeding is a very high-risk setting for infant HIV acquisition and a scenario that is not addressed by antiretroviral-based prevention strategies. Moreover, the rising incidence of HIV infection in young women in some countries of high HIV prevalence is especially challenging for further reductions in infant HIV acquisition, suggesting that only the development of a universal HIV vaccine administered in infancy will completely eliminate pediatric HIV infections. Unquestionably, HIV has posed one of the most serious and challenging health problems of the late 20th and early 21st centuries. Although there are still many remaining challenges of implementation, access, adherence, and monitoring, significant progress is being made.

B. **Transmission.** There are three principal routes for HIV transmission: sexual contact, parenteral inoculation, and maternal–fetal or maternal–newborn transfer.

  1. **Sexual contact.** This remains the principal mode of transmission of HIV in the United States and worldwide. Both semen and vaginal secretions have been found to contain HIV. The principal risk behavior for 85% of mothers of children reported with AIDS is heterosexual contact.

  2. **Parenteral inoculation.** Parenteral transmission of HIV results from the direct inoculation of infected blood or blood products. The groups affected have been intravenous drug users and patients receiving transfusions or factor concentrates. Screening of blood donors for risk factors for infection, universal HIV antibody and viral testing of donated blood, and the special preparation of clotting factor to eliminate the risk of viral contamination have greatly reduced the incidence of transfusion-acquired HIV. The most likely reason for false-negative HIV serology is the seronegative window that occurs between the time of initial infection and the production of antiviral antibody. The odds of transfusion-acquired HIV infection from the transfusion of a single unit of tested blood have been estimated to be from 1:250,000 to 1:150,000.

  3. **Congenital and perinatal transmission.** More than 92% of pediatric AIDS cases have resulted from maternal blood exposure antenatally,

at birth, or postnatally through breast milk. The rate of transmission of HIV from untreated infected mothers to their fetuses and newborn infants has been estimated to be between 15% and 40%. HIV has been isolated from cord blood specimens, and products of conception have demonstrated HIV infection as early as 14 to 20 weeks' gestation; however, it is believed that most of the infection is transmitted in late third trimester or at delivery. The mechanism of transplacental transfer of HIV is not known, but HIV can infect trophoblast and placental macrophage cell lines. Neither infection nor quantity of virus present in the placenta correlates with congenital infection. This may suggest that the placenta in general acts as a protective barrier to transmission or conversely as a focus of potential transmission. In a study of 100 sets of twins delivered to HIV-infected mothers, twin A was infected in 50% delivered vaginally and 38% delivered by cesarean. Twin B was infected in 19% of both vaginal and cesarean deliveries. This study as well as the Women and Infants Transmission study and a meta-analysis of transmission studies suggests that intrapartum infection occurs as a correlate of duration of ruptured membranes and that elective (without onset of labor) cesarean section deliveries may be preventive, primarily if the maternal HIV viral load is not controlled at delivery.

C. **Clinical disease.** In untreated patients, CD4$^+$ cell loss progresses, with the median duration of the asymptomatic phase being approximately 10 years in adults. After this phase, the patient becomes symptomatic, generally with opportunistic infections, especially tuberculosis, and death occurs within 5 years.

1. **HIV infection in infants** manifests with an initially high viral load, which declines over the first 5 years of life as the immune system develops. Current U.S. and WHO guidelines suggest treating all infants diagnosed with HIV infection in the first year of life so that the immune system can develop normally, and many experts continue treatment to assure suppression of HIV. Although previous algorithms of when to initiate treatment in HIV-infected children were based on clinical course and CD4$^+$ T-cell percentages, it is now recommended that all infected children be treated with combination antiretroviral treatment (cART) from diagnosis. In fact, use of highly potent antiretroviral regimens has been associated with long-term viral remission off therapy in at least one infant, the "Mississippi baby," who remained without evidence of viral replication off therapy for nearly 2 years, providing hope that future HIV remission or cure can be achieved with additional treatment agents to reduce the size of the latent virus reservoir. Willingness of the care provider to assure the infant or child receives every dose every day is a critical component of success.

2. **HIV in pregnancy.** HIV-infected pregnant women should receive closely monitored prenatal care, including being screened for other sexually transmitted diseases (gonorrhea, herpes, chlamydia, hepatitis B and C, and syphilis), as well as tested for infection with CMV and toxoplasmosis. The mother should also have a tuberculin skin test and, when appropriate, be offered hepatitis B, pneumococcal, and influenza vaccines. If not already on ART, a triple drug regimen should be initiated as soon as possible in pregnancy with the goal of complete virologic control

well prior to delivery. Generally, drug regimens used in nonpregnant individuals are similar to those recommended in pregnancy. Exceptions to these recommendations include efavirenz, which has shown teratogenic effects in animal studies; the combination of didanosine and stavudine, which has been associated with rare cases of maternal hepatic steatosis and death; and nevirapine, which has resulted in fulminant hepatitis in women with higher $CD4^+$ lymphocyte counts. Therefore, these agents should be used cautiously in pregnancy. Recently, the ongoing international Promoting Mother-Infant Survival Everywhere (PROMISE) study reported that triple drug therapy with lamivudine, zidovudine, and ritonavir-boosted lopinavir (the lamivudine combination) or tenofovir, emtricitabine, and ritonavir-boosted lopinavir (the tenofovir combination) reduced transmission detected at 2 weeks of age to 0.5%, significantly lower than that of a two-drug regimen. Yet, both regimens were associated with a higher risk of infant prematurity, and the tenofovir-containing arm demonstrated a higher risk of death, raising concerns on the safety of these regimens in areas of limited health care resources to adequately care for preterm infants.

Currently in the United States, the rate of vertical transmission is <2% in women who are diagnosed and take antiretroviral therapy before delivery. This makes perinatal transmission of HIV an essentially preventable disease when women have antenatal counseling and testing and receive antiretroviral therapy for themselves and their infants. HIV testing, although no longer requiring consent, is not a mandatory component of antenatal care; hence, every obstetric provider and pediatrician should offer testing and counseling to all pregnant women so they may consider therapeutic options for themselves and prophylactic options for their fetuses. *Pneumocystis jirovecii* and possibly *Mycobacterium avium intracellulare* prophylaxis also should be considered in pregnancy.

3. **HIV infection in children.** Most pediatric AIDS cases occur in infants and young children, reflecting the preponderance of congenital and perinatally acquired infections. Where HIV infection is undiagnosed, 50% of pediatric AIDS cases are reported in the first year of life, and approximately 80% are reported by the age of 3. Of these patients, HIV-related symptoms occur in >80% in the first year of life (median age at onset of symptoms is 9 months). It is estimated that 20% of untreated infants with congenital/perinatal HIV infection will die within the first year of life, and 60% will have severe symptomatic disease by the age of 18 months. These patients are defined as "rapid progressors." These statistics reflect only pediatric AIDS cases reported to the CDC and may reflect only the part of the spectrum of disease that is identified. Statistics are also heavily influenced by the natural disease progression in untreated children. It is possible that many infected children are undiagnosed and remain asymptomatic for years. Children should be prescribed antiretroviral regimens based on the goal of maintaining a CD4+ lymphocyte percentage of >15%, and many experts would suggest 25%, along with a moderately low or suppressed HIV viral load. In developed countries, pediatric HIV infection should be considered a treatable chronic infection, not a disease with a limited life span or poor quality of life.

The clinical presentation differs in children compared with adults. The HIV-infected newborn is usually asymptomatic but may present with lymphadenopathy and/or hepatosplenomegaly. Generally, the infant infected peripartum does not develop signs or symptoms until after the first 2 weeks of life. These include lymphadenopathy and hepatosplenomegaly (as in adults), poor weight gain as might be found in chronic viral infection, and occasionally, neuromotor abnormalities or encephalopathy. Before antiretroviral therapy was available to children, 50% to 90% of HIV-infected children had CNS involvement characterized by an encephalopathy that was often clinically devastating. Although the clinical presentation may vary, developmental delay or loss of developmental milestones and diminished cognitive function are common features. Not infrequently, an infant is diagnosed with AIDS between the ages of 2 and 6 months when he or she presents with *P. jirovecii* pneumonia. This is an interstitial pneumonia often without auscultatory findings. Patients present with low-grade fever, tachypnea, and often, tachycardia. Progressive hypoxia ensues and may result in mortality as high as 90%. This is the AIDS-defining illness at presentation in 37% of pediatric patients, with a peak incidence at the age of 4 months. Treatment is intravenous trimethoprim-sulfamethoxazole and steroids. Prophylaxis to prevent such life-threatening possibilities is of course preferable to acquisition of disease. It is now recommended by the Public Health Service that all HIV-infected infants be started on *P. jirovecii* pneumonia prophylaxis at the age of 1 month. A second condition, possibly unique to pediatric AIDS, is the development of chronic interstitial lung disease, referred to as *lymphoid interstitial pneumonitis* (LIP). LIP is characterized by a diffuse lymphocytic and plasma cell infiltrate. The clinical course of LIP is quite variable but may be progressive, resulting in marked respiratory distress (tachypnea, retractions, wheezing, and hypoxemia). There is an association with Epstein-Barr virus infection, but the significance of this is uncertain. After the initial presentation, the prognosis appears to be more favorable for children with symptomatic HIV infection when the AIDS-defining illness is LIP. In addition to LIP, recurrent bacterial infections are a frequent feature of pediatric AIDS, owing in part to the early occurrence of B cell dysfunction with dysfunctional hypergammaglobulinemia. Both focal and disseminated infections are encountered, with sepsis being most common. The organism usually isolated from the bloodstream is *Streptococcus pneumoniae*, but a variety of other bacteria have been recovered, especially from hospitalized patients. Pneumococcal disease is less common now that conjugated pneumococcal vaccines are standard of care for infants in the first 6 months of life. Other manifestations of HIV infection that may be more common in children are parotitis and cardiac dysfunction. Older children present with the more typical AIDS-defining opportunistic infections when the $CD4^+$ T-cell count wanes.

D. Diagnosis. The diagnosis of HIV infection in adults is made by the detection of specific antibody by an ELISA with confirmation by Western blot analysis. Infants who are DNA PCR or high-level RNA PCR positive in the first 3 days of life are considered to have been infected *in utero*; infants who test negative in the first 3 days and positive for HIV thereafter are considered to have peripartum-acquired HIV. This differentiation is relevant because offering potent antiretroviral therapy at the time of delivery, even in undiagnosed and/or untreated mothers, may be highly effective in reducing vertical transmission. Rapid diagnostic testing for HIV in previously untested women at presentation for delivery with institution of prophylactic therapy has been shown to reduce transmission. On the basis of this kind of information, investigators are targeting the intrapartum interval to offer potent, rapidly active preventive treatments such as antiretroviral therapy (especially using nevirapine). Intrapartum transmission is likely to account for at least 50% of HIV infections in infants. Testing should be offered to anyone engaging in risk behaviors for HIV transmission and for all pregnant women.

Serology is of limited value in diagnosing vertically transmitted HIV infection in infants <15 months old because maternal IgG crosses the placenta and can persist in infants throughout the first year or more of life. In the presence of an AIDS-defining illness and a positive antibody test, the diagnosis is made even if the infant is <15 months of age. However, the picture is less clear in infants with minimal or no symptomatology. Therefore, viral detection tests must be used to identify infected infants born to HIV-seropositive mothers. These include the following:

1. PCR to detect viral DNA in peripheral blood cells
2. PCR for viral RNA in plasma, or viral load

   The mainstay of early viral diagnostic testing of the infant born to an HIV-infected mother remains HIV PCR to detect both viral RNA and DNA, with a DNA test often recommended to avoid possible issues of delayed/cleared RNA viremia in the setting of maternal or infant prophylactic ART. The blood samples for these tests should be collected in anticoagulant, but not heparin, to avoid interference with PCR. Older tests of viral culture and p24 antigen detection are generally no longer done. Culture is sensitive and specific but is expensive, technically difficult, and may require weeks before results are obtained. The p24 antigen assay suffers from a lack of sensitivity, particularly in infants, and can be replaced by acid-dissociated p24 antigen detection, which has a much greater sensitivity. The importance of obtaining an early diagnosis is clear: to provide even very young infants the benefit of ART, which is hoped to reduce viral load and possibly prevent or reduce the latent viral burden at tissue sites, including the CNS, as well as to maintain normal numbers of $CD4^+$ T cells throughout immunologic development.

E. **Treatment.** The major part of the management of HIV infection is ART. Recent studies have confirmed that this should be offered to all infected patients regardless of $CD4^+$ T-cell count to improve the long-term outcome and reduce transmission to uninfected individuals. At present, there is no cure for HIV infection, but the goal of ART is to suppress the HIV viral load and to maintain or reconstitute $CD4^+$ T-cell numbers. Generally, these agents are of four classes:

1. Nucleoside or nucleotide analog reverse transcriptase inhibitors (NRTIs) (e.g., zidovudine/AZT). These agents prevent viral RNA from being reverse-transcribed to DNA; therefore, infection of cells can be aborted.

2. Nonnucleoside analog reverse transcriptase inhibitors (NNRTIs) (e.g., nevirapine). These agents also act to prevent reverse transcription but at a slightly different site on the enzyme. They are generally more potent than the NRTIs, but resistance can develop rapidly if the viral load is not controlled.

3. Protease inhibitors (PIs) act to prevent processing of viral proteins. These agents are quite potent but are highly protein bound, and therefore, little crosses the placenta, making these excellent agents to treat maternal viral load but limit exposure of the fetus.

4. Integrase inhibitors act to prevent virion production and are increasingly a component of antiretroviral therapy. Generally, although initial prophylaxis regimens of infants born to HIV-infected mothers often include zidovudine with or without nevirapine (NRTI and NNRTI, respectively), initial therapy of an infected infant should include two NRTIs and either a PI or an NNRTI—often zidovudine/lamivudine or emtricitabine/lopinavir boosted ritonavir.

Other possible therapies being investigated include other sites of action in the retroviral life cycle such as fusion inhibitors, viral entry inhibitors, and immune-based therapies. The combination ART regimen that was used in the "Mississippi baby" who was born to a viremic mother and infected peripartum but achieved a unique long-term remission when the child was lost to follow-up and stopped treatment, included zidovudine (2 mg/kg every 6 hours), zidovudine (4 mg/kg twice daily), nevirapine (2 mg/kg twice daily), and the nevirapine later switched to ritonavir-boosted lopinavir at 1 week of age (prior to the U.S. Food and Drug Administration [FDA] warning against beginning ritonavir-boosted lopinavir before 14 days of age due to cases of heart block). Thus, this early, aggressive treatment regimen and similar regimens are being evaluated for its ability to result in this type of remission for other perinatally infected infants.

Optimization of nutrition, routine immunizations, prophylaxis against opportunistic infections (most notably *P. jirovecii*) and the prompt recognition and treatment of HIV-related complications (e.g., opportunistic infections, cardiac dysfunction) are paramount to the improvement in the longevity and the quality of life for HIV-infected patients. In the newborn, special attention should be given to the possibility of congenitally and perinatally transmitted pathogens, such as tuberculosis, CMV, toxoplasmosis, and sexually transmitted diseases, which may have a relatively high prevalence in HIV-infected adults.

F. Prevention. In this chapter, we will only focus on prevention strategies to reduce **maternal-to-child transmission** both in the United States and globally.

1. Domestically, efforts to prevent mother-to-child transmission of HIV have been highly successful in the United States. Combined information from the randomized Pediatric AIDS Clinical Trials Group studies PACTG 076 and PACTG 185, found that HIV-infected pregnant women who received zidovudine antenatally, intrapartum intravenously at 2 mg/kg for the first hour of labor followed by 1 mg/kg/hour until delivery, and to their infants orally at 2 mg/kg every 6 hours for the first

6 weeks of life, had a markedly lower transmission compared to placebo recipients (8.3% of the infants in the zidovudine-receiving group were infected vs. 25.5% in the placebo group for 076). Therefore, since 1994, it has been the standard of care to offer the 076 algorithm as a backbone of antiretroviral regimens for pregnant women. With the development of highly active cART and its recommended use throughout pregnancy, the recommendation for intrapartum zidovudine has been modified to include only women with HIV viral load $>1,000$ copies/mL, unknown viral load, or problems with adherence; yet, the infant prophylaxis regimen is continued to be recommended for all HIV-exposed infants. Elective cesarean section (before onset of labor) can further reduce transmission if the HIV viral load remains $>1,000$ copies/mL. There is no added benefit to elective cesarean if the HIV viral load is suppressed below this value. Several studies have shown that higher maternal viral load, along with lower $CD4^+$ T-cell counts, is a strong correlate of vertical transmission; therefore, it is imperative to treat pregnant women with an optimized antiretroviral regimen to suppress viral load. Resistance testing should also be performed even for women who have never been treated because it is estimated that as many as 15% of previously untreated persons will have an HIV isolate that has resistance to one or more antiretrovirals. It is advised that care of HIV-infected pregnant women be offered in concert with obstetricians, internists, and pediatricians with experience taking care of HIV-infected patients for optimal outcome. Current standard of care in the United States is to suppress maternal viral load to nondetectable levels during pregnancy (and after pregnancy to optimize maternal health) using combinations of the approved agents to treat HIV infection and are safe for use during pregnancy. The rate of vertical transmission is $<1\%$ for women with a nondetectable viral load.

Occasionally, mothers learn for the first time that they are HIV infected during their pregnancy. The appropriate social support network must be effectively in place to achieve the best pregnancy outcome possible, optimization of the mother–baby pair is key in effecting the best possible outcome.

Any instrumentation, including fetal scalp electrodes and pH sampling, during the intrapartum period that would expose the fetus to maternal blood and secretions should be avoided in HIV-positive women. Postpartum, the mother should be advised to avoid allowing her infant to contact her blood or secretions. Breastfeeding is contraindicated for HIV-infected women in the United States due to the relative safety of alternative feeding and reliable availability of formula and clean water.

2. **Globally**, there has also been significant progress in limiting perinatal HIV infection. A trial in Uganda (HIVNET 012) offered a single dose of nevirapine to HIV-infected women in labor and followed this with a single dose of nevirapine at 3 days of life to the infants. The rate of perinatal transmission was markedly reduced in the nevirapine arm. Nevirapine was found to readily cross the placenta, and with the two-dose regimen for the mother–infant pair, the nevirapine level in the infant's blood is above the level needed to reduce HIV viral load

for at least a week. However, by 18 months of age, the infant mortality in the nevirapine-treated group equaled that in the other group, most likely because of HIV transmission from breastfeeding. Several studies later established that continuing maternal ART and/or infant antiretroviral prophylaxis during the breastfeeding period significantly reduced postnatal HIV transmission. Although exclusive breastfeeding and early weaning at 6 months of age when feasible and safe was a suggested strategy to reduce breast milk transmission, the suggested weaning period was extended to after 12 months of age after several studies showed an increase in malnutrition and diarrheal illness after rapid weaning at 6 months of age. WHO 2013 guidelines for treatment of pregnant women, dubbed "option B+," recommends that HIV-seropositive women be offered antenatal treatment with a triple antiretroviral regimen as soon as the infection is diagnosed, continue the treatment intrapartum, throughout the period of breastfeeding and beyond, while providing the infant prophylaxis with daily nevirapine until 6 weeks of age. Additional recommendations include that each country should decide whether HIV-seropositive women should exclusively formula feed their infants or breastfeed with concomitant antiretroviral therapy based on the risks of formula feeding (malnutrition, unclean water, increased risk of other infections). If breastfeeding is recommended, women should be counseled to exclusively breastfeed for the first 6 months with complementary foods added at 6 months and weaning at 12 months, if adequate nutrition is available and safe for the baby at that time. In studies of women in endemic areas who were not HIV infected at the time of delivery but who seroconverted postpartum, some infants seroconverted almost simultaneously with their mothers. It may be that infants whose mothers acquire primary HIV infection during lactation are at a higher risk for acquisition of HIV exposure through breast milk than are those exposed to virus in a chronically infected mother, and this mode of transmission likely accounts for a large proportion of the ongoing infant HIV transmission. Therefore, pursuit of a universally protective HIV vaccine for infants to provide immunity during the breastfeeding period, and potentially allowing for late boosting of immunity prior to sexual debut, remains an important endeavor to ending pediatric HIV.

VI. HEPATITIS. Acute viral hepatitis is defined by the following clinical criteria: (i) symptoms consistent with viral hepatitis, (ii) elevation of serum aminotransaminase levels to >2.5 times the upper limit of normal, and (iii) the absence of other causes of liver disease. At least five agents have been identified as causes of viral hepatitis: hepatitis A virus (HAV), hepatitis B virus (HBV), hepatitis D virus (HDV), hepatitis C virus (HCV) (formerly posttransfusion non-A, non-B hepatitis virus [NANB]), and hepatitis E virus (HEV) (enteric, epidemic NANB hepatitis virus). Very few suspected cases of perinatal transmission of HAV have been reported and is generally not considered to be vertically transmitted, thus will not be discussed further. HDV, also referred to as the delta agent, is a defective virus that requires coinfection or superinfection with HBV. HDV is coated with hepatitis B surface antigen (HBsAg). Specific antibodies to HDV can be detected in infected individuals, but there is no known therapy to prevent infection in exposed HBsAg-positive patients. For the newborn, therapy directed at the prevention of HBV infection should also prevent HDV infection because coinfection is required.

A. HBV (congenital and peripartum). This DNA virus is one of the most common causes of acute and chronic hepatitis worldwide. The virus has a major surface antigen (HBsAg), a core antigen, a regulatory X protein, and the viral polymerase soluble e antigen (hepatitis B e antigen [HBeAg]). The hepatocellular cytotoxicity in HBV is related to the host immune response as opposed to the virus itself. The virus is highly transmissible via contact with blood and/or body fluids of infected individuals.

   1. Epidemiology. In endemic populations, the carrier state is high, and perinatal transmission is a common event. The risk of chronic HBV infection is inversely proportional to age, with a 90% carriage rate following infection in neonates. The overall incidence of HBV infections in the United States is relatively low. Approximately 19,000 acute infections occur yearly, with <1% resulting in death from fulminate disease. The incubation period for HBV infection is approximately 120 days (range 45 to 160 days). **High-risk groups for HBV infection** in the United States include the following:

   a. Persons born in endemic areas. Alaskan natives and Pacific Islanders and natives of China, Southeast Asia, most of Africa, parts of the Middle East, and the Amazon basin; descendants of individuals from endemic areas

   b. Persons with high-risk behavior. MSM, intravenous drug use, and multiple sex partners

   c. Close contacts with HBV-infected persons (sex partners, family members)

   d. Selected patient populations, particularly those receiving multiple blood or blood product transfusions

   e. Selected occupational groups, including health care providers

   2. Transmission occurs by percutaneous or permucosal routes from infected blood or body fluids. The transmission of HBV from infected mothers to their newborns is thought to result primarily from exposure to maternal blood at the time of delivery. Transplacental transfer accounts for <4% of all cases and has been reported to occur in Taiwan, but this has not been reported in other parts of the world, including the United States. There is a high chronic carrier rate in Taiwan that may be related to the transplacental transfer observed in that country. When acute maternal HBV infection occurs during the first and second trimesters of pregnancy, there is generally little risk to the newborns because antigenemia is usually cleared by term and anti-HBV antibodies are present. Acute maternal HBV infection during late pregnancy or near the time of delivery, however, may result in up to 90% transmission rate in the absence of any prophylaxis and is most common in women who have both HBsAg and HBeAg detected in blood, indicating high plasma HBV DNA level.

   3. Clinical disease with chronic active hepatitis is seen in approximately 25% of the 1 million individuals who are chronic carriers. Symptoms include anorexia, malaise, nausea, vomiting, abdominal pain, and jaundice. Patients with chronic active hepatitis are at increased risk for developing cirrhosis and hepatocellular carcinoma, and approximately 5,000 of these patients die each year in the United States from HBV-related hepatic complications (primarily cirrhosis).

4. **Diagnosis.** The diagnosis is made by specific serology and by the detection of viral antigens. The specific tests are as follows:

   a. HBsAg determination. Usually found 1 to 2 months after exposure and lasts a variable period of time

   b. Anti-hepatitis B surface antigen (anti-HBs). Appears after resolution of infection or immunization and provides long-term immunity

   c. Anti-hepatitis B core antigen (anti-HBc). Present with all HBV infections and lasts for an indefinite period of time

   d. Anti-HBc IgM. Appears early in infection, is detectable for 4 to 6 months after infection, and is a good marker for acute or recent infection

   e. Hepatitis B e antigen (HBeAg). Present in both acute and chronic infections and correlates with viral replication and high infectivity

   f. Anti-hepatitis B e antigen (anti-HBe). Develops with resolution of viral replication and correlates with reduction in infectivity. Infectivity correlates best with HBeAg positivity, but any patient positive for HBsAg is potentially infectious. Acute infection can be diagnosed by the presence of clinical symptoms and a positive HBsAg or anti-HBc IgM. The chronic carrier state is defined as the presence of HBsAg on two occasions, 6 months apart, or the presence of HBsAg without anti-HBc IgM.

5. **Treatment.** Treatments such as lamivudine, tenofovir, or etanercept may be suggested by infectious disease specialists to further reduce the possibility of transmission, especially in women with higher HBV viral loads. However, there is no specific therapy for infants with acute HBV infection.

6. **Prevention.** The principal strategy for the prevention of neonatal HBV disease has been to use a combination of passive and active immunoprophylaxis for **newborns** at high risk for infection, as well as routine active neonatal immunization to protect against postnatal exposure (Table 48.3). High-risk infants born to HBsAg-positive mothers should

Table 48.3. Doses of Hepatitis B Vaccines in Neonates*

	Active Immunization: Either		Passive Immunization HBIG
	Recombivax HB (Merck)	Engerix-B (SmithKline Beecham)	
Infants of HBsAg-negative mothers	5 μg (0.5 mL)	10 μg (0.5 mL)	—
Infants of HBsAg-positive mothers	5 μg (0.5 mL)	10 μg (0.5 mL)	0.5 mL

HBIG, hepatitis B immune globulin; HBsAg = hepatitis B surface antigen.
*Both vaccine regimens use a three-dose schedule.

receive HBV hyperimmune globulin (hepatitis B immune globulin [HBIG]) and active HBV vaccination within 12 hours of life. Universal immunization severely reduced the chronic carrier state in Taiwan and is now routinely recommended for all U.S. infants born to all HBsAg-positive and HBsAg-negative mothers, with three doses administered before the age of 18 months. Certain high-risk populations, such as Alaskan natives, Pacific Islanders, and infants of immigrant mothers from areas where HBV is endemic, should receive the three-dose series by the age of 6 to 9 months. The recommended schedule begun during the newborn period; the second dose is given 1 to 2 months later; and the third dose is given at the age of 6 months for infants of mothers with HBsAg-positive or unknown status and between 6 and 18 months for infants of mothers with negative HBsAg status. The preterm infant born to an HBsAg-positive mother should be started on the immunization series and given treatment with HBIG immediately (see Table 48.3). The *Red Book: Report of the Committee on Infectious Diseases* by the American Academy of Pediatrics is the best source for dosing based on gestational age and birth weight. Other methods of disease control have been considered; these include delivery by cesarean section. In one study in Taiwan, cesarean delivery in conjunction with maternal immunization dramatically reduced the incidence of perinatally acquired HBV from highly infective mothers. These results are promising and may offer a potential adjunctive therapy for very high-risk situations (e.g., HBsAg/Hbe-positive women).

It is recommended that all pregnant women be screened for HBsAg. Screening should be done early in gestation. If the test result is negative, no further evaluation is recommended unless there is a potential exposure history. When there is any concern about a possible infectious contact, development of acute hepatitis, or high-risk behavior in a non-immunized woman, testing should be repeated at the time of delivery. If the mother has emigrated from an endemic area, HBIG also should be considered unless the mother is known to be HBsAg negative. Postnatal transmission of HBV by the fecal–oral route probably occurs, but the risk appears to be small. Nevertheless, this possibility adds further support to the need for the immunization of infants born to HBsAg-positive women. Another potential route of infection is by means of breast milk. This mode of transmission appears to be very uncommon in developed countries; there has been no documented increase in the risk of HBV transmission by breastfeeding mothers who are HBsAg positive. This is true despite HBsAg being detected in breast milk. The risk of postnatal infection via breastfeeding is certain to be negligible in infants who have received HBIG and hepatitis vaccine.

Prevention of nosocomial spread from HBsAg-positive infants in the nursery is minimized if nursery personnel wear gloves and gowns when caring for infected infants. Of course, with current precautions, the risk of exposure to blood and body secretions already should be minimized. Immunization of health care workers is also strongly recommended, but if exposure should occur in a nonimmunized person, blood samples should be sent for hepatitis serology and HBIG administered as soon as possible unless the individual is known to be anti-HBs positive.

This should apply to personnel having close contact without appropriate precautions, as well as those exposed parenterally (e.g., from a contaminated needle).

B. HCV (congenital and peripartum). Hepatitis C is the agent responsible for most non-A, non-B hepatitis in transfusion or organ transplant recipients and is a single-strand RNA virus related to the *Flavivirus* family. Like HBV, most hepatotoxicity that results from HCV is due to the cellular immune response against virus-infected cells.

1. **Epidemiology.** Six HCV subtypes have been characterized based on sequence heterogeneity of the viral genome. HCV is found worldwide, and different subtypes have been identified from the same area. Subtype 1 is the most common in the United States and has a poorer prognosis than other subtypes.

   a. Horizontal transmission. Injection drug use is now the most common risk behavior of infection. In addition to injection drug users and transfusion recipients, dialysis patients and sexual partners of HCV-infected persons may also be infected, but 50% of identified persons are unable to define a risk factor.

   b. Vertical transmission. Overall rate of transmission is approximately 5% from known hepatitis C–infected women to their infants. The transmission rate may well be much higher and may approach 70% when the pregnant mother has a high viral load. HCV is transmitted at a higher frequency if the mother is also HIV infected, but this has not been assessed in women with a controlled HIV viral load and low HCV viral load. The mode of transmission is also unknown. Detection of HCV by RNA PCR in cord blood would suggest that at least in some cases, *in utero* transmission occurs, yet by 18 months, some of these infants may become blood PCR negative. There is also a case report of one infant having been infected with an HCV strain different from all maternal strains at the time of delivery, suggesting *in utero* transmission. Conversely, PCR-negative infants at birth may develop PCR positivity later in infancy, suggesting perinatal infection. One study found 50% of vaginal samples collected at 30 weeks' gestation from HCV-positive mothers contain HCV, suggesting the possibility of infection by passage through the birth canal. The potential risk of breastfeeding is not well defined. HCV has been detected in breast milk by PCR, but vertical transmission rates in breastfed and bottle-fed infants are similar. The CDC currently states that maternal HCV infection is not a contraindication to breastfeeding. The decision to breastfeed should be discussed with the mother on an individual basis.

2. **Clinical manifestations.** HCV accounts for 20% to 40% of viral hepatitis in the United States. The incubation period is 40 to 90 days after exposure, and manifestations often present insidiously. Serum transaminase levels may fluctuate or remain chronically elevated for as long as 1 year. Chronic disease may result in as many as 60% of community-acquired HCV infections. Cirrhosis may result in as many as 20% of chronic disease cases but may be less likely in pediatric patients.

3. **Diagnosis.** ELISA detects antibodies to three proteins (c100–3, c22–3, and c33c) that are components of HCV. This test may be able to detect

infection as early as 2 weeks after exposure. Another serologic assay with even greater sensitivity is the radioimmunoblot assay, which detects antibodies to the three antigens detected by the ELISA and a fourth antigen, 5–5-1. Infants born to HCV-infected mothers will show evidence of passively acquired maternal antibody; therefore, to determine infection in the infant, RNA PCR, which detects the viral genome itself, must be performed. This assay can detect viremia within 1 week of infection in adults. In adults, approximately 70% of samples with detectable antibody will also be positive by PCR. Persons who have had an acute infection that resolves will become antibody negative. Infants born to known seropositive women should be tested for HCV RNA by PCR at 1 to 2 months of age and again at 1 year of life because up to 30% of infections in infants can spontaneously resolve. If both are negative, the infant is likely uninfected; if the PCR is negative, but infants should be tested for anti-HCV antibodies at 18 months to confirm the absence of infection.

4. **Treatment.** Although only treatment with α-interferon and ribavirin is approved for use in children, newer direct antiviral agents have proved highly efficacious in the treatment of chronic HCV infection in adults and would likely be recommended for symptomatic infection in children. Although none of these agents have been approved in pregnancy, they may be beneficial in the future to eliminate perinatal transmission.

5. **Prevention.** Blood products are routinely screened for antibody to HCV. Presence of the antibody likely also indicates presence of virus, and the unit is discarded if antibody is positive. **Thus, there is *no* benefit to intravenous IVIG given to the exposed infant or to the needle-stick recipient because products containing antibody are excluded from the lot**. Postexposure prophylaxis with antiviral agents is not currently recommended.

C. **HEV.** Enterically transmitted NANB viral hepatitis (HEV) is a single-stranded RNA virus that is similar to a calcivirus. It is primarily spread by fecal-contaminated water supplies, yet there are several case reports of vertical transmission of HEV. Epidemics have been documented in parts of Asia, Africa, and Mexico, and shellfish have been implicated as sources of infection. Incubation is 15 to 60 days. The clinical picture in infected individuals is similar to that of HAV infection, with fever, malaise, jaundice, abdominal pain, and arthralgia. HEV infection has an unusually high incidence of mortality in pregnant women. Treatment is supportive. The efficacy of immunoglobulin prophylaxis against this form of hepatitis is unknown, but because the infection is not endemic in the United States, commercial preparations in the United States would not be expected to be helpful.

D. **Hepatitis G virus (HGV).** HGV is a single-stranded RNA virus in the *Flaviviridae* family that shares 27% homology with HCV. HGV can be found worldwide and is found in approximately 1.5% of blood donors in the United States. Coinfection with HBV or HCV may be as much as 20%, suggesting common routes of transmission, such as transfusion or organ transplantation. Transplacental transmission is probably rare and may be associated with higher maternal viral loads. HGV is diagnosed by RNA PCR in research settings, and there is no current treatment or prophylactic therapy.

VII. VARICELLA-ZOSTER VIRUS (VZV: CONGENITAL OR PERIPARTUM).

The causative agent of varicella (chickenpox) is a DNA virus and a member of the herpesvirus family. The same agent is responsible for herpes zoster (shingles); hence, this virus is referred to as VZV. Chickenpox results from primary VZV infection, following which the virus may remain latent in sensory nerve ganglia. Zoster results from reactivation of latent virus later in life or if the host becomes immunosuppressed.

A. **Epidemiology.** Before the use of varicella vaccine, there were approximately 3 million cases of varicella yearly in the United States, most occurring in school-age children. Most adults have antibodies to VZV, indicating prior infection, even when there is thought to be no history of chickenpox. It follows that varicella is an uncommon occurrence in pregnancy. The precise incidence of gestational varicella is uncertain but is certainly less than it was before widespread use of varicella vaccine. There are recommendations to immunize nonimmune adults at risk for infection unless they are pregnant. Alternatively, zoster is primarily a disease of adults. The incidence of zoster in pregnancy is also unknown, but the disease is likely to be uncommon as well. The overall estimated risk of the congenital varicella syndrome following maternal infection is low, with only 0.4% in the first 12 weeks of pregnancy, and 2% from 13 to 20 weeks' gestation. It is primarily seen with gestational varicella but may rarely occur with maternal zoster.

The primary mode of transmission of VZV is through respiratory droplets from patients with chickenpox. Spread through contact with vesicular lesions also can occur. Typically, individuals with chickenpox are contagious from 1 to 2 days before and 5 days after the onset of rash. Conventionally, a patient is no longer considered contagious when all vesicular lesions have dried and crusted over. The incubation period for primary disease extends from 10 to 21 days, with most infections occurring between 13 and 17 days. Transplacental transfer of VZV may take place, presumably secondary to maternal viremia, but its frequency is unknown. Varicella occurs in approximately 25% of newborns whose mothers developed varicella within the peripartum period. The onset of disease usually occurs 13 to 15 days after the onset of maternal rash. The greatest risk of severe infant disease is seen when maternal varicella occurs in the 5 days before or 2 days after delivery. In these cases, there is insufficient time for the fetus to acquire transplacentally derived VZV-specific antibodies. Symptoms generally begin 5 to 10 days after delivery, and the expected mortality is high, approximately 30%. When *in utero* transmission of VZV occurs before the peripartum period, there is no obvious clinical impact in most fetuses; however, congenital varicella syndrome can occur.

B. **Clinical manifestations**

1. **Congenital varicella syndrome.** There is a strong association between gestational varicella and a spectrum of congenital defects comprising a unique syndrome. Characteristic findings include skin lesions, ocular defects, limb abnormalities, CNS abnormalities, IUGR, and fetal demise or early death. The syndrome most commonly occurs with maternal VZV infection between weeks 7 and 20 of gestation.

2. **Zoster.** Zoster is uncommon in young infants but may occur as a consequence of *in utero* fetal infection with VZV. Similarly, children who develop zoster but have no history of varicella most likely acquired VZV *in utero*. Zoster in childhood is usually self-limiting, with only symptomatic therapy indicated in otherwise healthy children.

3. **Postnatal varicella.** Varicella acquired in the newborn period as a result of postnatal exposure is generally a mild disease likely due to the presence of maternal antibodies against the virus. Rarely, severe disseminated disease occurs in newborns exposed shortly after birth following an acute maternal infection. In these instances, treatment with acyclovir may be beneficial. Varicella has been detected in breast milk by PCR; therefore, it may be prudent to defer breastfeeding at least during the period of time in which the mother is likely to be viremic and/or infectious.

C. **Diagnosis.** Infants with congenital varicella resulting from *in utero* infection occurring before the peripartum period do not shed virus, and the determination of VZV-specific antibodies is often confounded by the presence of maternal antibodies. Therefore, the diagnosis is made on the basis of clinical findings and maternal history. With neonatal disease, the presence of a typical vesicular rash and a maternal history of peripartum varicella or postpartum exposure are all that is required to make the diagnosis. Laboratory confirmation can be made by (i) culture of vesicular fluid, although the sensitivity of this method is not optimal because the virus is quite labile; (ii) demonstration of a fourfold rise in VZV antibody titer by the fluorescent antibody to membrane antigen assay or by ELISA; and (iii) antigen can also be detected from cells at the base of a vesicle by immunofluorescent antibody or PCR detection. The latter is sensitive, specific, and rapid and should be the preferred method of diagnosis when vesicles are present. The confirmation of VZV in a lesion should then be followed by measurement of VZV plasma viral load to have a baseline for following the effect of therapy, if implemented.

D. **Treatment.** Infants with congenital infection, resulting from *in utero* transmission before the peripartum period, are unlikely to have active viral disease, so antiviral therapy is not indicated. However, infants with perinatal varicella acquired from maternal infection near the time of delivery are at risk for severe disease. In this setting, therapy with acyclovir is generally recommended. Data are not available on the most efficacious and safe dose of acyclovir for the treatment of neonatal varicella, but minimal toxicity has been shown with the administration of 60 mg/kg divided every 8 hours for the treatment of neonatal HSV infection. For exposures, including maternal infection between 5 days prior to and 2 days following delivery, VariZIG, a hyperimmune gammaglobulin product, should be administered within 96 hours of exposure. Alternatively, if VariZIG is unavailable, IVIG at a dose of 400 mg/kg may be given as postexposure prophylaxis because it will contain anti-VZV antibodies.

E. **Prevention**

1. **Vaccination** of women who are not immune to varicella should decrease the incidence of congenital and perinatal varicella. Women should not receive the vaccine if they are pregnant or in the 3 months before pregnancy.

If this inadvertently occurs, the women should be enrolled in the National Registry. Additionally, acyclovir should also be considered for seronegative women exposed to varicella during pregnancy beginning 7 to 9 days postexposure and continuing 7 days. Women who acquire primary varicella during pregnancy should be treated with acyclovir for their own health as well as to prevent fetal infection.

2. **Management of varicella in the nursery.** The risk of horizontal spread of varicella following exposure in the nursery appears to be low, possibly because of a combination of factors, including (i) passive protection resulting from transplacentally derived antibody in infants born to varicella-immune mothers and (ii) brief exposure with a lack of intimate contact. Nevertheless, nursery outbreaks do occur, so steps should be taken to minimize the risk of nosocomial spread. The infected infant should be isolated in a separate room, and visitors and caregivers should be limited to individuals with a history of varicella. A gown should be worn on entering the room, and good hand-washing technique should be used. Bedding and other materials should be bagged and sterilized. VariZIG can be given to all other exposed neonates, but this can be withheld from full-term infants whose mothers have a history of varicella. Neonates at <28 weeks' gestation should be given VariZIG or IVIG postexposure regardless of maternal status. Exposed personnel without a history of varicella and unknown immunization status should be tested for VZV antibodies. In the regular nursery, all exposed infants will ordinarily be discharged home before they could become infectious. Occasionally, an exposed infant needs to remain in the nursery for more than the incubation period of 8 days, and in this circumstance, isolation may be required. In the neonatal intensive care unit, exposed neonates are generally cohorted and isolated from new admissions within 8 days of exposure. If there is antepartum exposure within 21 days of hospital admission for a mother without a history of varicella, the mother and infant should be discharged as soon as possible from the hospital. If the exposure occurred 6 days or less before admission, and the mother is discharged within 48 hours, no further action is required. Otherwise, mothers hospitalized between 8 and 21 days after exposure should be kept isolated from the nursery and other patients. Personnel without a history of varicella should be kept from contact with a potentially infectious mother. If such an individual is inadvertently exposed, serologic testing should be performed to determine susceptibility, and further contact should be avoided until immunity is proved. If the mother at risk for infection has not developed varicella 48 hours after the staff member was exposed, no further action is required. Alternatively, if a susceptible staff member is exposed to any individual with active varicella lesions or in whom a varicella rash erupts within 48 hours of the exposure, contact with any patients should be restricted for that staff member from day 8 to day 21 after exposure. Personnel without a history of varicella should have serologic testing, and if not immune, they should be vaccinated. For mothers in whom varicella has occurred in the 21 days before delivery, if there were resolution of the infectious stage before hospitalization, maternal isolation is not required. The newborn

should be isolated from other infants (room in with mother). If the mother has active varicella lesions on admission to the hospital, isolate the mother and administer VariZIG to the newborn if maternal disease began <5 days before delivery or within 2 days postpartum (not 100% effective and may consider acyclovir in addition). The infant should be isolated from the mother until she is no longer infectious. If other neonates were exposed, VariZIG may be administered; these infants may require isolation if they are still hospitalized by day 8 after exposure.

VIII. ENTEROVIRUSES (CONGENITAL). The *enteroviruses* are RNA viruses belonging to the *Picornaviridae* family. They are classified into four major groups: coxsackieviruses group A, coxsackieviruses group B, *echoviruses*, and polioviruses. All four groups cause disease in the neonate. Infections occur throughout the year, with a peak incidence between July and November. The viruses are shed from the upper respiratory and gastrointestinal tracts. In most children and adults, infections are asymptomatic or produce a nonspecific febrile illness.

A. **Epidemiology.** Most infections in newborns are caused by coxsackieviruses B and *echoviruses*. The mode of transmission appears to be primarily transplacental, although this is less well understood for *echoviruses*. Clinical manifestations are most commonly seen with transmission in the perinatal period.

B. **Clinical manifestations.** Symptoms in the newborn often appear within the first week postpartum. Clinical presentations vary from a mild nonspecific febrile illness to severe life-threatening disease. There are three major clinical presentations in neonates with enterovirus infections. Approximately 50% have meningoencephalitis, 25% have myocarditis, and 25% have a sepsis-like illness, which can result in fulminant hepatic failure. The mortality (approximately 10%) is lowest for the group with meningoencephalitis. With myocarditis, there is a mortality of approximately 50%. The mortality from the sepsis-like illness is essentially 100%. Most (70%) of severe enteroviral infections in neonates are caused by *echovirus* 11.

C. **Diagnosis.** The primary task in symptomatic enterovirus infections is differentiating between viral and bacterial sepsis and meningitis. In almost all cases, presumptive therapy for possible bacterial disease must be initiated. Obtaining a careful history of a recent maternal viral illness, as well as that of other family members, particularly young siblings, and especially during the summer and fall months, may be helpful. The principal diagnostic laboratory aid generally available at this time is viral culture or PCR. Material for cultures should be obtained from the nose, throat, stool, blood, urine, and CSF and from blood, urine, stool, or CSF for PCR. Usually, evidence of viral growth can be detected within 1 week, although a longer time is required in some cases.

D. **Treatment.** In general, treatment of symptomatic enteroviral disease in the newborn is supportive only. There are no approved specific antiviral agents known to be effective against *enteroviruses*. However, protection against severe neonatal disease appears to correlate with the presence of specific transplacentally derived antibody. Furthermore, the administration of immune serum globulin appears to be beneficial in patients with agammaglobulinemia who have chronic enteroviral infection. Given these observations, it has been recommended that high-dose immune serum globulin be given to infants with severe, life-threatening enterovirus infections. It may also be beneficial to delay the time of delivery if acute maternal enteroviral infection is suspected, provided there are no maternal or fetal contraindications. This is done to allow transplacental passage of maternal antibody. The clinical presentation in infants with a sepsis-like syndrome frequently evolves into shock, fulminant hepatitis with hepatocellular necrosis, and DIC. In the initial stages of treatment, broad-spectrum antibiotic therapy is indicated for possible bacterial sepsis. Later, with the recognition of progressive viral disease, some form of antibiotic prophylaxis to suppress intestinal flora may be helpful. Neomycin (25 mg/kg every 6 hours) has been recommended. Drugs designed to prevent attachment of *enterovirus* to the host cell (e.g., pleconaril) are under study for neonatal enteroviral sepsis but not clinically available.

IX. RUBELLA (CONGENITAL). This human-specific RNA virus is a member of the Togavirus family. It causes a mild self-limiting infection in susceptible children and adults, but its effects on the fetus can be devastating.

A. Epidemiology. Before widespread immunization beginning in 1969, rubella was a common childhood illness: 85% of the population was immune by late adolescence and approximately 100% by ages 35 to 40 years. Epidemics occurred every 6 to 9 years, with pandemics arising with a greater and more variable cycle. During pandemics, susceptible women were at significant risk for exposure to rubella, resulting in a high number of fetal infections. A worldwide epidemic from 1963 to 1965 accounted for an estimated 11,000 fetal deaths and 20,000 cases of congenital rubella syndrome (CRS). The relative risk of fetal transmission and the development of CRS as a function of gestational age have been studied. With maternal infection in the first 12 weeks of gestation, the rate of fetal infection was 81%. The rate dropped to 54% for weeks 13 to 16, 36% for weeks 17 to 22, and 30% for weeks 23 to 30. During the last 10 weeks of gestation, the rate of fetal infection again rose: 60% for weeks 31 to 36 and 100% for weeks 36 and beyond. Fetal infection can occur at any time during pregnancy, but early-gestation infection may result in multiple organ anomalies. When maternofetal transmission occurred during the first 10 weeks of gestation, 100% of the infected fetuses had cardiac defects and deafness. Deafness was found in one-third of fetuses infected at 13 to 16 weeks, but no abnormalities were found when fetal infection occurred beyond the 20th week of gestation. There are also case reports of vertical transmission with maternal reinfection. Introduction of the highly effective rubella vaccine in 1969 dramatically reduced the number of cases of CRS to <1 case per year by the year 2000, and the remaining cases were primarily in immigrant population. In fact, rubella was declared eliminated in the United States in 2004 and in the Americas in 2015. However, rubella continues to be endemic in many parts of the world where the rubella vaccine is not universal, resulting in ongoing cases of CRS.

B. Clinical manifestations. Classically, CRS is characterized by the constellation of cataracts, SNHL, and congenital heart disease. The most common cardiac defects are patent ductus arteriosus and pulmonary artery stenosis. Common early features of CRS are IUGR, retinopathy, microphthalmia, meningoencephalitis, electroencephalographic abnormalities, hypotonia, dermatoglyphic abnormalities, hepatosplenomegaly, thrombocytopenic purpura, radiographic bone lucencies, and diabetes mellitus. The onset of some of the abnormalities of CRS may be delayed months to years. Many additional rare complications have been described, including myocarditis, glaucoma, microcephaly, chronic progressive panencephalitis, hepatitis, anemia, hypogammaglobulinemia, thymic hypoplasia, thyroid abnormalities, cryptorchidism, and polycystic kidney disease. A 20-year follow-up study of 125 patients with congenital rubella from the 1960s epidemic found ocular disease to be the most common disorder (78%), followed by sensorineural hearing deficits (66%), psychomotor retardation (62%), cardiac abnormalities (58%), and mental retardation (42%).

C. Diagnosis

1. **Maternal infection.** The diagnosis of acute rubella in pregnancy requires serologic testing. This is necessary because the clinical symptoms of rubella are nonspecific and can be seen with infection by other viral agents (e.g., *enteroviruses*, measles, and human parvovirus). Furthermore, a large number of individuals may have subclinical infection. Several sensitive and specific assays exist for the detection of rubella-specific antibody. Viral isolation from the nose, throat, and/or urine is possible, but this is costly and not practical in most instances. **Symptoms** typically begin 2 to 3 weeks after exposure and include malaise, low-grade fever, headache, mild coryza, and conjunctivitis occurring 1 to 5 days before the onset of rash. The rash is a salmon-pink macular or maculopapular exanthem that begins on the face and behind the ears and spreads downward over 1 to 2 days. The rash disappears in 5 to 7 days from onset, and posterior cervical lymphadenopathy is common. Approximately one-third of women may have arthralgias without arthritis. In women suspected of having acute rubella infection, confirmation can be made by demonstrating a fourfold or higher rise in serum IgG titers when measured at the time of symptoms and approximately 2 weeks later. When there is uncertainty about the interpretation of assay results, advice should be obtained from the laboratory running the test and an infectious diseases consultation.

2. **Recognized or suspected maternal exposure.** Any individual known to have been immunized with rubella vaccine after his or her first birthday is generally considered immune. However, it is best to determine immunity by measuring rubella-specific IgG, which has become a standard of practice in obstetric care. If a woman exposed to rubella is known to be seropositive, she is immune, and the fetus is considered not to be at risk for infection. If the exposed woman is known to be seronegative, a serum sample should be obtained 3 to 4 weeks after exposure for determination of titer. A negative titer indicates that no infection has occurred, whereas a positive titer indicates infection. Women with an uncertain immune status and a known exposure to rubella should have serum samples obtained as soon as possible after exposure. If this is done within 7 to 10 days of exposure, and the titer is positive, the patient is

rubella immune and no further testing is required. If the first titer is negative or was determined on serum taken more than 7 to 10 days after exposure, repeat testing (~3 weeks later) and careful clinical follow-up are necessary. When both the immune status and the time of exposure are uncertain, serum samples for titer determination should be obtained 3 weeks apart. If both titers are negative, no infection has occurred. Alternatively, infection is confirmed if seroconversion or a fourfold increase in titer is observed. Further testing and close clinical follow-up are required if titer results are inconclusive. In this situation, specific IgM determination may be helpful. It should be emphasized that all serum samples should be tested simultaneously by the same laboratory when one is determining changes in titers with time.

3. **Congenital rubella infection**
   a. Antenatal diagnosis. The risk of severe fetal anomalies is highest with acute maternal rubella infection during the first 16 weeks of gestation. However, not all early-gestation infections result in adverse pregnancy outcomes. Approximately 20% of fetuses may not be infected when maternal rubella occurs in the first 12 weeks of gestation, and as many as 45% of fetuses may not be infected when maternal rubella occurs closer to 16 weeks of gestation. Unfortunately, there is no foolproof method of determining infected from uninfected fetuses early in pregnancy, but *in utero* diagnosis is being investigated. One method that has been used with some success is the determination of specific IgM in fetal blood obtained by percutaneous umbilical cord blood sampling. Direct detection of rubella antigen and RNA in a chorionic villous biopsy specimen also has been used successfully. Although these techniques offer promise, their use may be limited by sensitivity and specificity or the lack of widespread availability.
   b. Postnatal diagnosis. Guidelines for the establishment of congenital rubella infection or CRS in neonates have been summarized by the CDC. The diagnosis of congenital infection is made by one of the following:
      i. **Isolation of rubella virus** (oropharynx, urine). Notify the laboratory in advance because special culture medium needs to be prepared.
      ii. **Detection of rubella-specific IgM** in cord or neonatal blood
      iii. **Persistent rubella-specific titers over time** (i.e., no decline in titer as expected for transplacentally derived maternal IgG). If, in addition, there are congenital defects, the diagnosis of CRS is made.

D. **Treatment.** There is no specific therapy for either maternal or congenital rubella infection. Maternal disease is almost always mild and self-limiting. If primary maternal infection occurs during the first 5 months of pregnancy, termination options should be discussed with the mother. More than half of newborns with congenital rubella may be asymptomatic at birth. If infection is known to have occurred beyond the 20th week of gestation, it is unlikely that any abnormalities will develop, and parents should be reassured. Nevertheless, hearing evaluations should be repeated during childhood. Closer follow-up is required if early-gestation infection is suspected or the timing of infection is unknown. This is true for asymptomatic infants as well as those with obvious CRS. The principal reason for close follow-up is to identify delayed-onset abnormalities or progressive disorders, such as glaucoma. Unfortunately, there is no specific therapy to halt the progression of most of the complications of CRS.

E. **Prevention.** The primary means of prevention of CRS is by immunization of all susceptible persons. Immunization is recommended for all nonimmune individuals 12 months or older. Documentation of maternal immunity is an important aspect of good obstetric management. When a susceptible woman is identified, she should be reassured of the low risk of contracting rubella, but she should also be counseled to avoid contact with anyone known to have acute or recent rubella infection. Individuals with postnatal infection typically shed virus for 1 week before and 1 week after the onset of rash. On the other hand, infants with congenital infection may shed virus for many months, and contact should be avoided during the first year. Unfortunately, once exposure has occurred, little can be done to alter the chances of maternal and subsequently fetal disease. Although hyperimmune globulin has not been shown to diminish the risk of maternal rubella following exposure or the rate of fetal transmission, it should be given in large doses to any woman who is exposed to rubella and who does not wish to terminate her pregnancy. The lack of proven efficacy must be emphasized in these cases. Susceptible women who do not become infected should be immunized soon after pregnancy. There have been reports of acute arthritis occurring in women immunized in the immediate postpartum period, and a small percentage of these women developed chronic joint or neurologic abnormalities or viremia. Vaccine-strain virus also may be shed in breast milk and transmitted to breastfed infants, some of whom may develop chronic viremia. Immunization during pregnancy is not recommended because of the theoretical risk to the fetus, and conception should be avoided for 3 months after immunization. Inadvertent immunizations during pregnancy have occurred, and fetal infection has been documented in a small percentage of these pregnancies; however, no cases of CRS have been identified. In fact, the rubella registry at the CDC has been closed, with the following conclusions: The number of inadvertent immunizations during pregnancy is too small to be able to state with certainty that no adverse pregnancy outcomes will occur, but these would appear to be very uncommon. Therefore, it is still recommended that immunization not be carried out during pregnancy, but when this has occurred, reassurance of little risk to the fetus can be given.

X. RSV (NEONATAL).
RSV is an enveloped RNA paramyxovirus that is the leading cause of bronchiolitis and severe or even fatal lower respiratory tract disease, especially in preterm infants. Conditions that increase the risk of severe disease include cyanotic or complicated congenital heart disease, pulmonary hypertension, chronic lung disease, and immunocompromised states.

A. **Epidemiology.** Humans are the only source of infection, spread by respiratory secretions as droplets or fomites, which can survive on environmental surfaces for hours. Spread by hospital workers to infants occurs, especially in the winter and early spring months in temperate climates. Viral shedding is 3 to 8 days, but in very young infants may take weeks. The incubation period is 2 to 8 days.

B. Diagnosis. Rapid diagnosis is made by PCR or immunofluorescent antigen testing of respiratory secretions. This test can have up to 95% sensitivity and is quite specific. Viral culture usually requires 3 to 5 days.

C. Treatment. Treatment is largely supportive, with hydration, supplemental oxygen, and mechanical ventilation as needed. Controversy exists as to whether nebulized bronchodilator therapy is beneficial. Ribavirin has been marketed for treatment of infants with RSV infection because it does have *in vitro* activity; however, efficacy has never been repeatedly proven in randomized trials. This makes the risk of ribavirin (aerosol route, potentially toxic side effects to health care personnel, and high cost) important to consider on a case-by-case basis. The use of anti-RSV monoclonal antibody, palivizumab, may be considered for treatment in consultation with an infectious disease specialist for the most severely affected, immunocompromised infants but has not shown much efficacy in this setting.

D. Prevention. Palivizumab (Synagis), a humanized mouse monoclonal antibody given intramuscularly, has been approved by the FDA for prevention of RSV disease in children younger than 2 years of age with chronic lung disease or who were <35 weeks' gestation. Palivizumab is easy to administer, has a low volume, and is given just before and monthly throughout the RSV season (typically mid-November to March/April). Because the drug is costly and its protection incomplete, the American Academy of Pediatrics has made the following recommendations regarding which high-risk infants should receive palivizumab, last updated in 2014:

1. **Infants who have required therapy for chronic lung disease born <32 weeks' gestation** during their first year of life, and for a second season if they continue to need respiratory support up to 6 months prior to the next RSV season

2. **Infants who are born at <29 weeks' gestation** without chronic lung disease during their first year of life

3. **Children** who are 24 months of age or younger with hemodynamically significant acyanotic **congenital heart disease**, including those receiving medications to control congestive heart failure, have severe pulmonary hypertension, or receive a heart transplant

4. **Infants with anatomic pulmonary abnormalities of the airway or neuromuscular disorder** during their first year of life

5. **Severely immunocompromised infants (such as SCID)** up to 24 months of age

6. **Infants with symptomatic cystic fibrosis** with evidence of chronic lung disease (CLD) or nutritional compromise in the first 2 years of life

    If an RSV outbreak is documented in a high-risk unit (e.g., pediatric intensive care unit), primary emphasis should be placed on proper infection-control practices. The need for and efficacy of antibody prophylaxis in these situations has not been documented. Each unit should evaluate the risk to its exposed infants and decide on the need for treatment. If the patient stays hospitalized, this may only require one dose. Palivizumab does not interfere with the routine immunization schedule.

E. Antibody preparations are not recommended for the following:

1. Healthy preterm babies >29 weeks' gestation without other risk factors

2. Patients with hemodynamically insignificant heart disease

3. Infants with lesions adequately corrected by surgery, unless they continue to require medication for congestive heart failure

Future anti-RSV monoclonal antibodies with longer half-lives may be made available in the United States at a lower price point than the current product and be comparable to the current costs of vaccines. Therefore, the recommendations may change once new monoclonal antibody prevention products are available. There is also considerable ongoing effort to develop RSV vaccines that can elicit potent neutralizing antibody responses in pregnant women and young infants.

Suggested Readings

American Academy of Pediatrics, Committee on Infectious Diseases. *2015 Red Book: Report of the Committee on Infectious Diseases*. 30th ed. Elk Grove Village, IL: American Academy of Pediatrics; 2015.

Kimberlin DW, Baley J; Committee on Infectious Diseases, Committee on Fetus and Newborn. Guidance on management of asymptomatic neonates born to women with active genital herpes lesions. *Pediatrics* 2013;131(2): 383–386. doi:10.1542/peds.2012-3217.

Kimberlin DW, Jester PM, Sánchez PJ, et al. Valganciclovir for symptomatic congenital cytomegalovirus disease. *N Engl J Med* 2015;372(10):933–943. doi:10.1056/NEJMoa1404599.

Mofenson LM. Antiretroviral drugs to prevent breastfeeding HIV transmission. *Antiviral Ther* 2010;15:537–553.

Suggested Websites

Joint United Nations Programme on HIV/AIDS. Global report: UNAIDS report on the AIDS epidemic 2013. **http://www.unaids.org/sites/default/files/media_asset/UNAIDS_Global_Report_2013_en_1.pdf**. Accessed June 16, 2016.

Panel on Antiretroviral Therapy and Medical Management of HIV-Infected Children. Guidelines for the use of antiretroviral agents in pediatric HIV infection. **http://aidsinfo.nih.gov/contentfiles/lvguidelines/pediatricguidelines.pdf**. Accessed August 10, 2015.

Panel on Treatment of HIV-Infected Pregnant Women and Prevention of Perinatal Transmission. Recommendations for use of antiretroviral drugs in pregnant HIV-1-infected women for maternal health and interventions to reduce perinatal HIV transmission in the United States. **http://aidsinfo.nih.gov/contentfiles/lvguidelines/PerinatalGL.pdf**. Accessed August 10, 2015.

49 Bacterial and Fungal Infections

Karen M. Puopolo

KEY POINTS

- Risk factors for neonatal early-onset sepsis (EOS) include prematurity, documented maternal colonization with group B *Streptococcus* (GBS), intrapartum fever and other signs of chorioamnionitis, and prolonged rupture of membranes; risk is modified by the administration of intrapartum antibiotics.

- Empiric antibiotic therapy includes broad coverage for organisms known to cause EOS, usually a β-lactam antibiotic and an aminoglycoside. The most common microbial causes of EOS include GBS, *Escherichia coli*, viridans streptococci, *Enterococcus*, and a variety of *Enterobacteriaceae* such as *Klebsiella* and *Haemophilus* spp.

- Risk for neonatal late-onset sepsis (LOS) increases with lower gestational age and birth weight and with longer duration of central venous access, mechanical ventilation, and use of total parenteral nutrition.

- Empiric antibiotic therapy for LOS should be tailored to the local microbiology of infection, which may include different relative contributions of coagulase-negative staphylococci, methicillin-sensitive and methicillin-resistant *Staphylococcus aureus*, β-lactam-resistant gram-negative organisms, and *Candida* spp.

I. BACTERIAL SEPSIS AND MENINGITIS

A. Introduction. Bacterial sepsis and meningitis continue to be major causes of morbidity and mortality in newborns, particularly in premature infants. Although improvements in neonatal intensive care have decreased the impact of early-onset sepsis (EOS) in term infants, preterm infants remain at high risk for both EOS and its sequelae. Very low birth weight (VLBW) infants are also at risk for late-onset (hospital acquired) sepsis. Neonatal survivors of sepsis can have severe neurologic sequelae due to central nervous system (CNS) infection as well as from secondary hypoxemia resulting from septic shock, persistent pulmonary hypertension, and severe parenchymal lung disease.

B. Epidemiology of EOS. The overall incidence of EOS has decreased significantly since the Centers for Disease Control and Prevention (CDC) first published recommendations for intrapartum antibiotic prophylaxis (IAP) against group B *Streptococcus* (GBS) in 1996. Studies conducted afterward showed the overall incidence of EOS to be ≤1 case per 1,000 live births. The incidence is twice as high among moderately premature infants compared to term infants and highest among VLBW (<1,500 g) infants with recent reports ranging from 10 to 15 cases/1,000 VLBW births.

C. **Risk factors for EOS.** The pathogenesis of EOS is that of ascending colonization of the maternal genital tract and uterine compartment with gastrointestinal and genitourinary flora, and subsequent transition to invasive infection of the fetus or newborn. Maternal and infant characteristics associated with the development of EOS have been most rigorously studied with respect to GBS EOS. Maternal factors predictive of GBS disease include documented maternal GBS colonization, intrapartum fever (>38°C) and other signs of chorioamnionitis, and prolonged rupture of membranes (ROM) (>18 hours). Neonatal risk factors include prematurity (<37 weeks' gestation) and low birth weight (BW) (<2,500 g). These factors are modified by the administration of intrapartum antibiotics.

D. **Clinical presentation of EOS.** Early-onset disease can manifest as asymptomatic bacteremia, generalized sepsis, pneumonia, and/or meningitis. The clinical signs of EOS are usually apparent in the first hours of life; >90% of infants are symptomatic by 24 hours of age. Respiratory distress is the most common presenting symptom. Respiratory symptoms can range in severity from mild tachypnea and grunting, with or without a supplemental oxygen requirement, to respiratory failure. Persistent pulmonary hypertension of the newborn (PPHN) can also accompany sepsis. Other less specific signs of sepsis include irritability, lethargy, temperature instability, poor perfusion, and hypotension. Disseminated intravascular coagulation (DIC) with purpura and petechiae can occur in more severe septic shock. Gastrointestinal symptoms can include poor feeding, vomiting, and ileus. Meningitis may present with seizure activity, apnea, and depressed sensorium but may complicate sepsis without specific neurologic symptoms, underscoring the importance of the lumbar puncture (LP) in the evaluation of sepsis.

   Other diagnoses to be considered in the immediate newborn period in the infant with signs of sepsis include transient tachypnea of the newborn, meconium aspiration syndrome, intracranial hemorrhage, congenital viral disease, and congenital cyanotic heart disease. In infants presenting at more than 24 hours of age, closure of the ductus arteriosus in the setting of a ductal-dependent cardiac anomaly (such as critical coarctation of the aorta or hypoplastic left heart syndrome) can mimic sepsis. Other diagnoses that should be considered in the infant presenting beyond the first few hours of life with a sepsis-like picture include bowel obstruction, necrotizing enterocolitis (NEC), and inborn errors of metabolism.

E. **Evaluation of the symptomatic infant for EOS. Laboratory evaluation** of the symptomatic infant suspected of EOS includes at minimum a complete blood count (**CBC**) with differential and blood culture. Other laboratory abnormalities can include hyperglycemia and metabolic acidosis. Thrombocytopenia as well as evidence of DIC (elevated prothrombin time [PT], partial thromboplastin time [PTT], and international normalized ratio [INR]; decreased fibrinogen) can be found in more severely ill infants, particularly those born preterm. For infants with a strong clinical suspicion of sepsis, **an LP for cerebrospinal fluid (CSF) cell count, protein and**

glucose concentration, Gram stain, and culture should be performed before the administration of antibiotics if the infant is clinically stable. The LP may be deferred until after the institution of antibiotic therapy if the infant is clinically unstable, or if later culture results or clinical course demonstrates that sepsis was present.

Infants with respiratory symptoms should have a **chest radiograph** as well as other indicated evaluation such as arterial blood gas measurement. Radiographic abnormalities caused by retained fetal lung fluid or atelectasis usually resolve within 48 hours. **Neonatal pneumonia** will present with persistent focal or diffuse radiographic abnormalities and variable degrees of respiratory distress. Neonatal pneumonia (particularly that caused by GBS) can be accompanied by primary or secondary surfactant deficiency.

F. **Treatment of EOS. Empiric antibiotic therapy** includes broad coverage for organisms known to cause EOS, usually a β-lactam antibiotic and an aminoglycoside. In our institutions, we use ampicillin and gentamicin as initial therapy. We add a third-generation cephalosporin (cefotaxime or ceftazidime) to the empiric treatment of critically ill infants for whom there is a strong clinical suspicion for sepsis to optimize therapy for ampicillin-resistant enteric gram-negative organisms, primarily ampicillin-resistant *Escherichia coli* (see Table 49.1 for treatment recommendations). **Supportive treatments for sepsis** include the use of mechanical ventilation, exogenous surfactant therapy for pneumonia and respiratory distress syndrome (RDS), volume and pressor support for hypotension and poor perfusion, sodium bicarbonate for metabolic acidosis, and anticonvulsants for seizures. **Echocardiography** may be of benefit in the severely ill, cyanotic infant to determine if significant pulmonary hypertension or cardiac failure is present: Infants born at ≥34 weeks with symptomatic pulmonary hypertension may benefit from treatment with inhaled nitric oxide (**iNO**). Extracorporeal membrane oxygenation (**ECMO**) can be offered to infants ≥34 weeks if respiratory and circulatory failure occurs despite all conventional measures of intensive care. ECMO is not generally available to infants <34 weeks' gestation.

A variety of **adjunctive immunotherapies** for sepsis have been trialed since the 1980s to address deficits in immunoglobulin and neutrophil number and function. Double-volume exchange transfusions, granulocyte infusions, the administration of intravenous immunoglobulin (IVIG), and treatment with granulocyte-colony stimulating factor (G-CSF) and granulocyte macrophage-colony stimulating factor (GM-CSF) have all been investigated with variable results.

1. **Double-volume exchange transfusion and granulocyte infusion.** Both of these approaches to replete neutrophils in neutropenic septic infants have been studied in small numbers of infants. Both present significant risks, including graft-versus-host disease; blood-group sensitization; and transmission of infections such as cytomegalovirus (CMV), HIV, and viral hepatitis. We do not currently use either of these treatments in the treatment of early- or late-onset sepsis (LOS).

2. **IVIG.** The use of IVIG in the acute treatment of neonatal sepsis has been studied in several small trials, with mixed results. A definitive trial including 3,493 infants was conducted in nine countries from 2001 to 2007. This was a randomized, placebo-controlled trial of IVIG

Table 49.1. Suggested Antibiotic Regimens for Sepsis and Meningitis*

Organism	Antibiotic	Bacteremia	Meningitis
GBS	Ampicillin or penicillin G	10 days	14–21 days
Escherichia coli	Cefotaxime or ampicillin and gentamicin	10–14 days	21 days
CONS	Vancomycin	7 days	14 days
Klebsiella, Serratia[†]	Cefotaxime or meropenem and gentamicin	10–14 days	21 days
Enterobacter, Citrobacter[‡]	Cefepime or meropenem and gentamicin	10–14 days	21 days
Enterococcus[**]	Ampicillin or vancomycin and gentamicin	10 days	21 days
Listeria	Ampicillin and gentamicin	10–14 days	14–21 days
Pseudomonas	Ceftazidime or piperacillin/ tazobactam and gentamicin or tobramycin	14 days	21 days
Staphylococcus aureus[‡‡]	Nafcillin	10–14 days	21 days
MRSA	Vancomycin	10–14 days	21 days

GBS, group B *Streptococcus*; CONS, coagulase-negative staphylococci; MRSA, methicillin-resistant *Staphylococcus aureus*.

*All treatment courses are counted from the first documented negative blood culture and assumed that antibiotic sensitivity data are available for the organisms. In late-onset infections, all treatment courses assume central catheters have been removed. With CONS infections, the clinician may choose to retain the catheter during antibiotic treatment, but if repeated cultures remain positive, the catheters must be removed. Many infectious disease specialists recommend repeat lumbar punctures at the completion of therapy for meningitis to ensure eradication of the infection.

[†]The spread of plasmid-borne extended-spectrum β-lactamases (ESBL) among enteric pathogens such as *E. coli, Klebsiella*, and *Serratia* is an increasing clinical problem. ESBL-containing organisms can be effectively treated with cefepime or meropenem. Reports of carbapenemase-producing organisms are of concern and infection with these requires consultation with an infectious disease specialist.

[‡]*Enterobacter* and *Citrobacter* spp. have inducible, chromosomally encoded cephalosporinases. Cephalosporins other than the fourth-generation cefepime should not be used to treat infections with these organisms **even if** initial *in vitro* antibiotic sensitivity data suggest sensitivity to third-generation cephalosporins such as cefotaxime. There are some reports in the literature of cefepime-resistant *Enterobacter*.

[**]Enterococci are resistant to all cephalosporins. Ampicillin-resistant strains of enterococci are common in hospitals and require treatment with vancomycin. Treatment of vancomycin-resistant strains (VRE) requires consultation with an infectious disease specialist.

[‡‡]Uncomplicated methicillin-sensitive *S. aureus* and MRSA bacteremias may be treated for only 10 days if central catheters have been removed. Persistent bacteremias can require treatment for 3–4 weeks. Bacteremias complicated by deep infections such as osteomyelitis or infectious arthritis often require surgical drainage and treatment for up to 6 weeks. The use of additional agents such as linezolid, daptomycin, and rifampin to eradicate persistent *S. aureus* infection or to treat vancomycin-intermediate *Staphylococcus aureus* (VISA) and vancomycin-resistant *Staphylococcus aureus* (VRSA) strains requires consultation with an infectious disease specialist.

administration to infants with suspected or proven sepsis. The administration of IVIG resulted in no change in the primary outcome of death or major disability at 2 years of age, nor any change in a number of secondary outcomes, including second episodes of sepsis. IVIG is not recommended for treatment of neonatal sepsis.

3. **Cytokines.** Recombinant G-CSF and GM-CSF have been shown to restore neutrophil levels in small studies of neutropenic growth-restricted infants, ventilator-dependent neutropenic infants born to mothers with preeclampsia, and in neutropenic infants with sepsis. A rise in the absolute neutrophil count (ANC) above 1,500/mm^3 occurred in 24 to 48 hours. To date, nine randomized, controlled trials of recombinant colony-stimulating factors have been reported, all enrolling small numbers of infants. Assessment of these trials is complicated by the use of different preparations, dosages, and durations of therapy as well as variable enrollment criteria. None of the trials included neurodevelopmental follow-up. These studies suggest that G-CSF may result in lower mortality among neutropenic, septic VLBW infants, but overall, there is currently insufficient evidence to support the routine use of these preparations in the acute treatment of neonatal sepsis.

4. **Activated protein C (APC) and pentoxifylline.** Both of these immunomodulatory preparations have been studied in adults with severe sepsis. Both are active in preventing the microvascular complications of sepsis, by promoting fibrinolysis (APC) and improving endothelial cell function (pentoxifylline), and both decrease the production of tumor necrosis factor (TNF). APC has not been studied in neonates in randomized trials and has been withdrawn from clinical production due to safety concerns in adult patients. Pentoxifylline has been studied in a small number of preterm infants with LOS with potential improvement in mortality. Neither medication can be recommended for use in neonates without further study.

G. **Evaluation of the asymptomatic infant at risk for EOS.** There are a number of clinical factors that place infants at risk for EOS. These factors also identify a group of asymptomatic infants who may have colonization or bacteremia that places them at risk for the development of symptomatic EOS. These infants include those born to mothers who have received inadequate IAP for GBS (see subsequent text) and those born to mothers with suspected chorioamnionitis. Blood cultures are the definitive determination of bacteremia. A number of laboratory tests have been evaluated for their ability to predict which of the at-risk infants will go on to develop symptomatic or culture-proven sepsis, but no single test has adequate sensitivity and specificity.

1. **Blood culture.** With advances in the development of computer-assisted, continuous-read culture systems, most blood cultures will be positive within 24 to 36 hours of incubation if organisms are present. Most institutions, including ours, empirically treat infants for sepsis for a minimum of 48 hours with the assumption that true positive cultures will turn positive within that period. At least 1 mL (and up to 3 mL) of blood should be placed in most pediatric blood culture bottles. The use of two culture bottles for each sepsis evaluation aids in the distinction

of true bacteremia versus contaminants. Depending on the clinical scenario, one aerobic and one anaerobic culture bottle is optimal, despite the fact that most blood culture systems do not provide pediatric-specific anaerobic culture bottles. Certain organisms causing EOS (such as *Bacteroides fragilis*) will only grow under anaerobic conditions; 5% to 10% of culture-proven EOS in preterm infants is due to strictly anaerobic species when anaerobic blood culture is performed. NEC may also be complicated by anaerobic bacteremia. Additionally, GBS, staphylococci, and many gram-negative organisms grow in a facultative fashion, and the use of two culture bottles increases the likelihood of detecting low-level bacteremia with these organisms.

2. **White blood cell (WBC).** The WBC and differential is readily available and commonly used to evaluate both symptomatic and asymptomatic infants at risk for sepsis. Interpretation of neonatal WBC has been compromised by the impact of differences mediated by gestational age, postnatal age, mode of delivery, and maternal conditions. Maternal fever, neonatal asphyxia, meconium aspiration syndrome, pneumothorax, and hemolytic disease have all been associated with neutrophilia; maternal pregnancy-induced hypertension and preeclampsia are associated with neonatal neutropenia as well as thrombocytopenia.

   One finding common to all published neonatal WBC data is the "roller coaster" shape of the WBC and ANC and immature to total neutrophil ratio (I/T) curves in the first 72 hours of life. This suggests that optimal interpretation of WBC data to predict EOS should account for the natural rise and fall in WBC during this period. Recent studies support the use of CBC only after the first few hours of life, when placed in the proper clinical context and used as part of an algorithm to evaluate infants for sepsis risk. The WBC and ANC are most predictive of infection when these values were low (WBC <5,000 and ANC <1,000). An elevated WBC (>20,000) is neither worrisome nor reassuring in neonates. The I/T ratio is most informative if measured at 1 to 4 hours after birth, with low values (<0.15) reassuring, while elevated values (>0.3) are weakly associated with EOS. The combination of low ANC and elevated I/T ratio is the most predictive combination of WBC indices for EOS.

   Although studies demonstrate that no component of the WBC is very sensitive among term and late preterm infants for the prediction of sepsis, there are little data to guide interpretation of the WBC among VLBW infants at risk for EOS. The WBC and its components may be of more value in the VLBW infant and/or in the evaluation of late-onset infection, especially if interpreted in relation to values obtained prior to the concern for infection.

3. **C-reactive protein (CRP).** CRP is a nonspecific marker of inflammation or tissue necrosis. Elevations in CRP are found in bacterial sepsis and meningitis. A single determination of CRP at birth lacks both sensitivity and specificity for infection. Serial CRP determinations at the time of blood culture, 12 to 24 hours and 48 hours later, have been used to manage infants at risk for LOS. Some centers use serial CRP measurements to determine length of antibiotic treatment for infants

with culture-negative clinical sepsis, despite the absence of data to support the efficacy of this practice.

4. **Cytokine measurements.** Advances in the understanding of the immune responses to infection and in the measurement of small peptide molecules have allowed investigation into the utility of these inflammatory molecules in predicting infection in neonates at risk. Serum levels of interleukin-6, interleukin-8, interleukin-10, interleukin-1 β, G-CSF, TNF-α, and procalcitonin (PCT), as well as measurements of inflammatory cell-surface markers such as CD64, have been variably correlated with culture-proven, clinical, and viral sepsis. The need for serial measurements and the availability of the specific assays so far limit the use of cytokine markers in diagnosing neonatal infection. PCT is increasingly available in clinical settings and correlates with bacterial infection; however, there is a natural rise in PCT levels in the hours after birth for all infants, normal ranges vary with gestational age, and like CRP, PCT levels rise in response to noninfectious inflammatory signals. In addition, most studies of biomarkers have been performed on infants who are symptomatic and being evaluated for sepsis. None of these has yet proven useful in predicting infection in initially well-appearing infants.

5. **Other strategies. Urine latex particle agglutination testing for GBS** remains available at some institutions; we do not use this test due to very poor predictive value. Latex particle testing of CSF for both GBS and *E. coli* K1 can be of use in evaluating CSF after the institution of antibiotic treatment.

6. **LP.** The use of routine LP in the evaluation of **asymptomatic neonates** at risk for EOS remains controversial. A retrospective review of 13,495 infants born at all gestational ages from 150 neonatal intensive care units (NICUs) on whom an LP was performed found 46 cases of culture-proven GBS meningitis. In 9 out of 46 cases, the accompanying blood culture was sterile. Another retrospective study of CSF taken from a population of 169,849 infants identified 8 infants with culture-positive CSF but with negative blood cultures and no CNS symptoms. In both studies, the authors concluded that the selective use of LP in the evaluation of EOS might lead to missed diagnoses of meningitis. However, in both studies, infants were not all evaluated for sepsis in the absence of symptoms, and the subjects were drawn from large numbers of hospitals with likely disparate culture systems. Another study reviewed the results of sepsis evaluations in a population of 24,452 infants from a single institution. This study found 11 cases of meningitis, all in symptomatic infants; 10 of 11 corresponding blood cultures were positive for the same organism. No cases of meningitis were found in 3,423 asymptomatic infants evaluated with LP.

Current national guidelines from the United States and Great Britain for evaluation of infants at risk for EOS endorse the selective use of LP when there is strong clinical suspicion for sepsis and/or specifically for meningitis. We do not perform LPs for the evaluation of **asymptomatic term infants** at risk for EOS. **It is our current policy to perform LPs only** on (i) infants with positive blood cultures and (ii) symptomatic infants with a high risk for EOS whose condition is stable enough to tolerate LP and (iii) infants with negative blood cultures who are treated empirically for the clinical diagnosis of sepsis.

When LPs are performed after the administration of antibiotics, a clinical evaluation of the presence of meningitis is made, taking into account the blood culture results, the CSF cell count, protein, and glucose levels as well as the clinical scenario. We recommend sending two separate CSF samples for cell count from the same LP in these circumstances to account for the role of possible fluctuation in CSF cell count measurements. Interpretation of CSF WBC values can be challenging. **Normal CSF WBC counts** in term, noninfected infants are variable, with most studies reporting a mean of <20 cells/mm^3, with ranges of up to 90 cells, and widely varying levels of polymorphonuclear cells on the differential. One recent study assessed CSF parameters among neonate without bacterial or viral blood or CSF infection, in CSF samples with <500 red blood cell (RBC)/mm^3. This study reported a mean CSF WBC 3/mm^3 with an upper reference limit of 14 cells; no significant differences were found between term and preterm infants. Another study of culture-proven early-onset meningitis demonstrated only 80% sensitivity and specificity for CSF WBC values >20. The presence of blood in the CSF, due to subarachnoid or intraventricular hemorrhage, or to blood contamination of CSF samples by "traumatic" LPs, can yield abnormal cell counts that may be due to the presence of blood in the CSF rather than true infection. Adjustment of the WBC in "traumatic" LP results (those with >500 RBC/mm^3) using different algorithms has not been shown to substantially improve the sensitivity and specificity of the WBC in predicting culture-confirmed meningitis.

H. Algorithm for the evaluation of the infant born at ≥35 weeks' gestation at risk for EOS. Assessing risk of EOS among term and late preterm infants is a common clinical task in birth centers. Depending on the local structure of neonatal care, EOS evaluation may be performed by pediatric residents, community pediatricians, newborn hospitalists, midwives, and/or neonatal intensive care specialists. The use of an algorithm to guide assessment can ensure consistency among caregivers. An example of such an algorithm which has been used at the Brigham and Women's Hospital (BWH) is shown in Figure 49.1. Algorithms should (i) establish criteria for EOS evaluation based on established risk factors for EOS, (ii) specify laboratory testing standards, and (iii) provide guidance for empiric administration of antibiotics. At our institutions, EOS risk assessment is informed by guidelines set forth by the CDC 2010 GBS prevention guidelines and the American Academy of Pediatrics. Risk factors used to identify newborns at risk for EOS include maternal intrapartum fever ≥38°C and other signs of chorioamnionitis, gestational age <37 weeks, inadequate indicated GBS prophylaxis, and premature and/or prolonged duration of ROM. A total WBC <5,000 or an I/T ratio >0.3 is used to guide treatment decisions in the evaluation of the well-appearing infant at risk for sepsis. A single CBC determination is used in most cases to avoid multiple blood draws from otherwise asymptomatic infants; as noted earlier, WBC values may have better predictive value when performed after 1 hour of age. These guidelines are based on a delivery service for which a screening-based approach to GBS

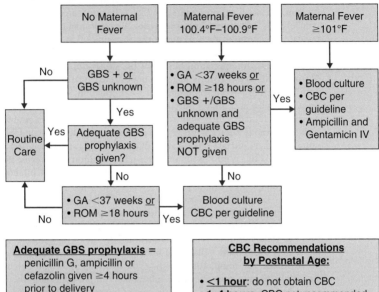

**Guidelines for the Management of Asymptomatic Infants
Born at ≥35 weeks Gestation at Risk for Early-Onset Sepsis**

Adequate GBS prophylaxis =
penicillin G, ampicillin or
cefazolin given ≥4 hours
prior to delivery

Inadequate GBS prophylaxis =
any antibiotic given <4 hours
prior to delivery or any other
antibiotic for any duration

**CBC Recommendations
by Postnatal Age:**

• **≤1 hour**: do not obtain CBC
• **1–4 hours**: CBC not recommended.
  If obtained, repeat at 6–12 hours to
  guide treatment decisions.
• **>4 hours**: obtain CBC with blood
  culture

Following values should raise concern
for infection:
  • WBC <5000
  • ANC <2000
  • I/T ratio ≥0.3

ADDITIONAL NOTES

1. Chorioamnionitis is an obstetrical clinical diagnosis made on the basis of
   clinical findings, laboratory data and fever. If obstetrical staff diagnose
   chorioamnionitis, the infant should be evaluated for sepsis and receive
   empiric antibiotic treatment.
2. Maternal fever that occurs within one hour of delivery should be treated like
   intrapartum fever.
3. Women with a previous infant with GBS disease should receive intrapartum
   GBS prophylaxis.
4. Blood cultures should consist of aerobic and anaerobic bottles with minimum
   1 mL blood in each bottle.

Figure 49.1. Algorithm for sepsis evaluations in at-risk asymptomatic infants ≥35 weeks' gestation.

prophylaxis has been in place since 1996 and for which the vast majority of vaginal deliveries involve epidural placement (which alone can cause low-grade intrapartum fever).

EOS algorithms based on risk factor threshold values are limited by an inability to account for interactions between risk factors and do not utilize the full value of information that falls just below or well above threshold values. A recent study used a cohort of >600,000 infants born ≥34 weeks' gestation to develop a multivariate predictive model of sepsis risk using established risk factors. This model provides estimates of individual infant EOS risk using only objective clinical data available at the time of birth, combined with the infant's clinical condition in the first 6 hours of life. The model provides as Sepsis Risk Score and is available as a web-based calculator at https://www.dor.kaiser.org/external/DORExternal/research/infectionprobabilitycalculator.aspx and http://newbornsepsiscalculator.org. The care recommendations provided are those used in a large integrated health care system in the United States and may not be universally appropriate. The Sepsis Risk Score is best used considering the local incidence of EOS and local structure of newborn care.

I. **Specific organisms causing EOS.** The bacterial species responsible for EOS vary by locality and time period. In the United States since the 1980s, GBS has been the leading cause of neonatal EOS. Despite the implementation of IAP against GBS, it remains the leading cause of EOS in term infants. However, coincident with the increased use of IAP for GBS, gram-negative enteric bacteria have become the leading cause of EOS in preterm infants. Enteric bacilli causing EOS include *E. coli*, other *Enterobacteriaceae* (*Klebsiella, Pseudomonas, Haemophilus*, and *Enterobacter* spp.) and the anaerobe *B. fragilis.* Less common organisms that can cause serious early-onset disease include *Listeria monocytogenes* and *Citrobacter diversus.* Staphylococci and enterococci can be found in EOS but are more commonly causes of nosocomial sepsis and are discussed under that heading in the subsequent text. Fungal species can cause EOS primarily in preterm infants; this is also discussed separately in the subsequent text.

1. **GBS.** GBS (*Streptococcus agalactiae*) frequently colonizes the human genital and gastrointestinal tracts and the upper respiratory tract in young infants. In addition to causing neonatal disease, GBS is a frequent cause of urinary tract infection (UTI), chorioamnionitis, postpartum endometritis, and bacteremia in pregnant women. There is some evidence suggesting that vaginal colonization with a high inoculum of GBS during pregnancy contributes to premature birth.

a. **Microbiology.** GBS are facultative diplococci that are easily cultivated in selective laboratory media. GBS are primarily identified by the Lancefield group B carbohydrate antigen and are further subtyped into 10 distinct serotypes (types Ia, Ib, II–IX) by analysis of capsular polysaccharide composition. Most neonatal diseases in the United States are currently caused by types Ia, Ib, II, III, and V GBS. Type III GBS are associated with the development of meningitis and are commonly a cause of late-onset GBS disease.

b. **Pathogenesis.** Neonatal GBS infection is acquired *in utero* or during passage through the birth canal. Because not all women are colonized with GBS, documented colonization with GBS is the strongest predictor of GBS EOS. Approximately 20% to 30% of American women are colonized with GBS at any given time. A longitudinal study of GBS colonization in a cohort of primarily young, sexually active women demonstrated that 45% of initially GBS-negative women acquired colonization at some time over a 12-month period. In the absence of IAP, approximately 50% of infants born to mothers colonized with GBS are found to be colonized with this organism at birth. Approximately 1% to 2% of all colonized infants develop invasive GBS disease, with clinical factors such as gestational age and duration of ROM contributing to risk for any individual infant (see subsequent text). Lack of maternally derived, protective capsular polysaccharide-specific antibody is associated with the development of invasive GBS disease. Other factors predisposing the newborn to GBS disease are less well understood, but relative deficiencies in complement, neutrophil function, and innate immunity may be important.

c. Clinical risk factors for GBS EOS (Table 49.2). GBS bacteriuria during pregnancy is associated with heavy colonization of the rectovaginal tract and is considered a significant risk factor for EOS. Black race and maternal age <20 years are associated with higher rates of GBS EOS, although it is not entirely clear whether this reflects only higher rates of GBS colonization in these populations. Multiple gestation is **not** an independent risk factor for GBS EOS.

d. Prevention of GBS infection. Multiple trials have demonstrated that the use of intrapartum penicillin or ampicillin significantly reduces the rate of neonatal colonization with GBS and the incidence of early-onset GBS disease. IAP for the prevention of GBS EOS can be administered to pregnant women during labor based on (i) specific risk factors for

Table 49.2. Risk Factors for Early-Onset Group B _Streptococcus_ (GBS) Sepsis in the Absence of Intrapartum Antibiotic Prophylaxis

Risk Factor	Odds Ratio (95% CI)
Maternal GBS colonization	204 (100–419)
BW <1,000 g	24.8 (12.2–50.2)
BW <2,500 g	7.37 (4.48–12.1)
Prolonged ROM >18 hours	7.28 (4.42–12.0)
Chorioamnionitis	6.42 (2.32–17.8)
Intrapartum fever >37.5°C	4.05 (2.17–7.56)

CI, confidence interval; BW, birth weight; ROM, rupture of membranes.
Source: Data from Benitz WE, Gould JB, Druzin MML. Risk factors for early-onset group B streptococcal sepsis: estimation of odds ratios by critical literature review. _Pediatrics_ 1999;103(6):e77.

carly onset GBS infection or (ii) the results of antepartum screening of pregnant women for GBS colonization. Beginning in 1996, the CDC issued guidelines recommending the use of IAP to prevent neonatal GBS EOS. The most recent CDC guidelines were published in 2010 (http://www.cdc.gov/groupbstrep/guidelines/guidelines.html). These guidelines recommend universal screening of pregnant women for GBS by recto-vaginal culture at 35 to 37 weeks' gestation and management of IAP based on screening results. Pregnant women with documented GBS bacteriuria during pregnancy or who previously delivered an infant who developed invasive GBS disease need not be screened because these women should be given IAP **regardless of current GBS colonization status**. IAP is also recommended for all women who present in preterm labor with unknown GBS status. For women in labor at $\geq$37 weeks' gestation with unknown GBS status, IAP is recommended if intrapartum maternal fever $\geq$100.5°F occurs, or if duration of ROM is $\geq$18 hours prior to delivery. The 2010 guidelines provide recommendations for the management of neonates at risk for EOS; recommendations for antibiotic choices for GBS IAP; specific recommendations for mothers who experience preterm labor and premature ROM; expanded laboratory methods for the detection of GBS including use of alternate culture-based detection methods; and for the first time, endorsed intrapartum nucleic acid amplification testing (NAAT) as an alternative to culture-based detection of maternal GBS colonization.

Penicillin and ampicillin are the recommended antibiotics for GBS IAP. The document addresses the challenges to providing adequate IAP to the roughly 10% of women who report penicillin allergy. There is no data directly supporting the efficacy of any antibiotic other than penicillin, ampicillin, or cefazolin for GBS IAP. Because a significant proportion of GBS isolates (15% to 40%) are resistant to macrolide antibiotics, it is recommended that any GBS isolates identified on screening of penicillin-allergic women be tested for antibiotic susceptibility including specific testing for inducible clindamycin resistance. For the woman with a non–life-threatening penicillin allergy, cefazolin is the recommended antibiotic for IAP. If a woman has a documented history of anaphylactic penicillin or cephalosporin allergy (including urticaria, angioedema, and/or respiratory distress), clindamycin is recommended if the colonizing isolate is fully susceptible to this antibiotic; otherwise, vancomycin is the recommended agent. For the purpose of infant management, however, the 2010 guideline does not consider the administration of clindamycin or vancomycin to constitute fully adequate IAP.

e. Current status of GBS EOS. CDC active surveillance data for the United States in 2014 demonstrates that the overall incidence of GBS EOS has fallen to 0.24 cases per 1,000 live births (compared to 1.7 cases per 1,000 live births in 1993). There is ongoing racial disparity with the incidence among black infants roughly three times that of white infants. Approximately one-quarter of all GBS EOS now occurs among infants born at <37 weeks' gestation. We evaluated the reasons for persistent GBS EOS despite the use of a screening-based approach to IAP at the BWH. We found that most GBS EOS in term infants now occurs in infants born to women with **negative** antepartum screens for GBS colonization. Subsequent CDC multistate surveillance studies from 2003 to 2004 found that 61% of GBS disease among term infants occurred in infants born to mother who screened GBS negative. These "false-negative" screens may be due to improper culture technique or acquisition of GBS between the time of culture and start of labor.

Bacterial culture remains the CDC-recommended standard for detection of maternal GBS colonization. The 2010 revision includes recommendations for the use of chromogenic GBS detection media and for the use of direct broth detection methods by latex agglutination, probe detection, or NAAT methods. These approaches may shorten the time to GBS identification. In 2002, the U.S. Food and Drug Administration (FDA) approved the first **PCR-based** rapid NAAT diagnostic for detection of maternal GBS colonization directly from vaginal/rectal swab specimens. Different kits are commercially available, and the 2010 guideline endorses the optional use of these NAATs for the management of women whose GBS status is unknown at the time of delivery. Recent data demonstrates that NAATs are more sensitive than antenatal culture in predicting intrapartum GBS status, but real-time use is compromised by a 10% incidence of nonresults due to technical issues. Due to the costs and technicalities of providing continuous support for a real-time PCR-based diagnostic, as well as the inherent time delay in an intrapartum diagnostic, most obstetric services continue to rely on antenatal culture-based screening programs.

f. Evaluation of infants after maternal GBS IAP. The 2010 CDC guidelines include a recommended algorithm for the evaluation of infants born to mothers exposed to IAP. As in prior versions, the algorithm recommends a full diagnostic evaluation (CBC with white cell differential, LP, CSF, blood cultures, and chest radiograph) and empiric antibiotic therapy for any infant with clinical signs of infection. For asymptomatic infants, a limited evaluation including CBC with differential and blood culture and empiric antibiotic therapy is recommended if there were intrapartum signs of maternal chorioamnionitis. The CBC with differential may be delayed until 6 to 12 hours after birth for optimal predictive value. **Only the administration of penicillin, ampicillin, or cefazolin ≥4 hours prior to delivery constitutes adequate IAP. If GBS IAP was indicated but not adequately administered, the revised guideline recommends limited diagnostic evaluation only if other risk factors for EOS are present (gestational age <37 weeks and/or ROM ≥18 hours).**

g. Treatment of infants with invasive GBS disease. When GBS is identified as the sole causative organism in EOS, empiric antibiotic treatment should be narrowed to ampicillin (200 to 300 mg/kg/day) or penicillin G (250,000 to 450,000 U/kg/day) alone, with the higher dosing reserved for cases complicated by meningitis. The total duration of therapy should be at least 10 days for sepsis without a focus, 14 to 21 days for meningitis, and 28 days for osteomyelitis. Bone and joint infections that involve the hip or shoulder require surgical drainage in addition to antibiotic therapy.

h. Recurrent GBS infection. Recurrent GBS infections are infrequent, with reported incidences ranging from 1% to 6%. Infants usually fail to have a specific antibody response after infection with GBS, and GBS can be isolated from mucosal surfaces of infants even after appropriate antibiotic treatment for invasive disease. Occasionally, reinfection with a new strain of GBS occurs. Treatment of recurrent GBS infections is the same as for primary infection except that susceptibility testing of the GBS strain to penicillin is recommended if not routinely performed. Rifampin, which eliminates colonization in other infections such as meningococcal disease, does not reliably eradicate mucous membrane colonization with GBS. In addition, neither maternal GBS IAP nor neonatal antibiotic administration prevents the development of primary late-onset GBS disease (infection occurring ≥7 days of life).

2. ***E. coli* and other enteric gram-negative bacilli.** With the implementation of IAP against GBS, an **increasing proportion** of EOS cases are caused by gram-negative organisms. Whether GBS IAP policies are contributing to an absolute increase in the **incidence** of EOS caused by gram-negative organisms, and in particular, of ampicillin-resistant gram-negative organisms, is a matter of ongoing controversy. Single centers report variable findings, but most experts agree that there is no evidence of an increase in non-GBS EOS among term infants. **However, increases in non-GBS EOS and ampicillin-resistant EOS are reported in among VLBW infants.** In a report from the National Institute of Child Health and Human Development (NICHD) from 2006 to 2009, 78% of *E. coli* EOS among VLBW infants were resistant to ampicillin. Trends in the microbiology of EOS likely vary to some extent by institution and may be influenced by local obstetrical practices as well as by local variation in indigenous bacterial flora.

   a. Microbiology and pathogenesis. *E. coli* are aerobic gram-negative rods found universally in the human intestinal tract and commonly in the human vagina and urinary tract. There are hundreds of different lipopoly-saccharide (LPS), flagellar, and capsular antigenic types of *E. coli*, but EOS *E. coli* infections, particularly those complicated by meningitis, are primarily due to strains with the K1-type polysaccharide capsule. *E. coli* with the K1 antigen are resistant to the bactericidal effect of normal human serum; strains that possess both a complete LPS and K1 capsule have been shown to specifically evade both complement-mediated bacteriolysis and neutrophil-mediated killing. The K1 antigen has been shown to be a primary factor in the development of meningitis in a rat model of *E. coli* infection. The K1 capsule is a poor immunogen and despite widespread carriage of this strain in the population, there is usually little protective maternal antibody available to the infant. In addition to the K1 antigen, surface fimbriae, or pili, have been associated with adherence to vaginal and uroepithelial surfaces and may also function as a virulence mechanism in EOS.

   b. Treatment. When there is a strong clinical suspicion for sepsis in a critically ill infant, the possibility of ampicillin-resistant *E. coli* must be considered. The addition of a third-generation cephalosporin such as cefotaxime or ceftazidime is recommended in this setting. *E. coli* bacteremia should be treated with a total of 14 days of antibiotic according to the identified sensitivities. *E. coli* meningitis is treated with a 21-day course of cefotaxime as indicated by sensitivities (see Appendix A).

3. ***L. monocytogenes*.** Although uncommon, *L. monocytogenes* deserves special note due to its unique role in pregnancy. *L. monocytogenes* are

gram-positive, β-hemolytic, motile bacteria that frequently cause disease in animals, and most commonly infect humans through the ingestion of contaminated food. These bacteria do not cause significant disease in immunocompetent adults but can cause severe illness in the elderly, in immunocompromised patients, in pregnant women and their fetuses, and in newborns. There is human epidemiologic evidence and evidence in animal models of listeriosis that indicate that *L. monocytogenes* is particularly virulent in pregnancy. The bacteria readily invades the placenta and can infect the developing fetus either by ascending infection, direct tissue invasion, or hematogenous spread, causing spontaneous abortion or preterm labor and delivery, and often fulminant early-onset disease. Like GBS, *L. monocytogenes* can also cause late-onset neonatal infection, the pathogenesis of which is not fully understood. Over 90% of late-onset infections are complicated by meningitis.

Listeriosis is a reportable disease, and CDC data for the United States in 2013 revealed an overall incidence of 0.26 cases/100,000 population, with most cases occurring among persons ≥65 years old. The true incidence of listeriosis in pregnancy is difficult to determine because many cases are undiagnosed when they result in spontaneous abortion of the previable fetus. In 2013, 11% of cases reported to CDC active surveillance were associated with pregnancy. Hispanic ethnicity was found in one-third of cases. Fetal death was associated with 21% of reported cases, whereas 3% of reported cases resulted in death of a live-born infant. Nationally, the frequency of neonatal EOS among live births caused by *Listeria* is estimated to be approximately 2 cases per 100,000 live births.

Listeriosis can result from ingestion of contaminated food such as soft cheeses, deli meat, or hot dogs. A large outbreak in 2011 was associated with cantaloupe from a single site. Although frequently associated with unpasteurized food products, an outbreak in 2008 in Massachusetts was notable in that the source of infection was pasteurized milk produced a single dairy, highlighting the potential for postpasteurization contamination of processed foods with *Listeria*. Infection in pregnant woman may not be recognized or may cause a mild febrile illness with or without gastrointestinal symptoms before resulting in pregnancy loss or preterm labor.

a. Microbiology and pathogenesis. *L. monocytogenes* are distinguished from other gram-positive rods by tumbling motility that is most prominent at room temperature. The organisms can be gram-variable and, depending on growth stage, can also appear cocci-like, and can therefore be initially misdiagnosed on a Gram stain. *L. monocytogenes* is an intracellular pathogen that can invade cells as well as persist in phagocytic cells (monocytes, macrophages). *Listeria* possess a variety of virulence factors, including surface proteins that promote cellular invasion, and enzymes (listeriolysin O, phospholipase) that enhance the ability of the organism to persist intracellularly. On pathologic examination of tissues infected with *Listeria*, miliary granulomas and areas of necrosis and suppuration are seen. The liver is prominently involved. Both T cell–mediated killing as well as immunoglobulin M (IgM) complement–mediated killing is involved in host response to listeriosis. Deficiencies in both of these arms of the newborn immune system may contribute to the virulence of

L. monocytogenes in the neonate; similarly, it is hypothesized that local downregulation of the immune response in the pregnant uterus may account for proliferation of the bacteria in the placenta.

b. Treatment. EOS due to *L. monocytogenes* is treated with ampicillin and gentamicin for 14 days; meningitis is treated for 21 days. *L. monocytogenes* is resistant to cephalosporins. In the case of meningitis, it is recommended that LPs be repeated daily until sterilization of the CSF is achieved. Additional therapy with rifampin or trimethoprim-sulfamethoxazole as well as cerebral imaging is recommended if the organism persists in the CSF for longer than 2 days. *L. monocytogenes* can persist in the stool of preterm infants even after adequate systemic treatment of the infection; thus, proper infection control measures must be observed to prevent nosocomial spread of the organism.

4. **Other organisms responsible for EOS.** Bacteria causing EOS vary with time and locality. Beyond GBS and *E. coli*, there are a number of pathogens that cause EOS in the United States in the era of IAP for GBS. Viridans streptococci (species such as *Streptococcus mitis*, *Streptococcus oralis*, and *Streptococcus sanguis*, which are part of the oral flora), enterococci, and *S. aureus* are next in frequency. *Listeria*, a variety of gram-negative organisms (*Klebsiella*, *Haemophilus*, *Enterobacter*, and *Pseudomonas* spp.) and the anaerobe *B. fragilis* cause most of the remaining infections. Gram-negative organisms, especially *E. coli* and *Klebsiella*, predominate in some Asian and South American countries.

J. **LOS.** Late-onset neonatal sepsis is defined as occurring from 8 to 90 days of life. LOS can be divided into two distinct entities: disease occurring in otherwise healthy term infants in the community and disease affecting premature infants in the NICU. The latter is often referred to as hospital-acquired sepsis because the risk factors for LOS in premature infants are related to the necessities of their care (i.e., the presence of central lines) and the bacteria that cause LOS are often acquired in the NICU. For epidemiologic purposes, LOS infections occurring in VLBW infants in the NICU are defined as those occurring at >72 hours of life.

This section is primarily devoted to LOS in the NICU population, but disease in otherwise **healthy term and near-term infants** deserves mention. In these infants, LOS is largely caused by GBS and gram-negative species such as *E. coli* and *Klebsiella* spp. Causes of bacteremia in older infants (such as *Streptococcus pneumoniae* and *Neisseria meningitidis*) occur less frequently. The **risk factors for late-onset GBS disease** are not as well defined as for early-onset disease but like early-onset disease are related to prematurity, colonization of the infant from maternal and community (or less commonly, hospital) sources, gestational age, and lack of maternally derived protective antibody. The use of IAP for GBS has had no significant impact on the rate of GBS LOS; the incidence of GBS LOS was reported to be 0.27 cases per 1,000 live births in 2013. Preterm infants account for a disproportionate number of GBS late-onset infections, with approximately 50% of late-onset GBS cases occurring in infants born at <37 weeks' gestation, with a median gestational age of 30 weeks among the preterm cases. GBS LOS is more often complicated by meningitis than early-onset disease and is predominantly caused by polysaccharide serotype III strains.

Although mortality from GBS LOS is low (1% to 5% in term and preterm infants, respectively), sequelae in survivors of GBS meningitis can be severe. A recent study of GBS meningitis occurring in infants born at ≥36 weeks' gestation from 1998 to 2006 revealed that a quarter of all infants died or survived with significant neurologic impairment.

Gram-negative bacteremia is often associated with UTI. Different series report 20% to 30% of UTIs in infants <1 month of age are complicated by bacteremia. Mortality is low if promptly treated, and sequelae are few unless meningitis occurs. *L. monocytogenes* can also cause late-onset disease, with onset commonly by 30 days of life and can account for up to 20% of LOS in some centers. Late-onset listeriosis is frequently complicated by meningitis, but unlike late-onset GBS meningitis, the morbidity and long-term sequelae are infrequent if the disease is diagnosed and treated in timely fashion.

Term infants with LOS generally present with fever and/or poor feeding and lethargy to the private pediatrician or emergency department. Evaluation in the infant younger than 3 months old in most centers includes at minimum a CBC; urinalysis; CSF cell count; glucose and protein; and cultures of blood, urine, and CSF. Infants under 1 month are generally hospitalized for empiric intravenous (IV) therapy that includes coverage for GBS, *Listeria*, and gram-negative organisms (commonly ampicillin and cefotaxime); over 1 month, management varies in different centers.

K. **Epidemiology of LOS in premature infants.** Most LOS occurs in the NICU among low BW infants. The NICHD Neonatal Research Network (NRN) data from 2008 to 2012 revealed that 24% of their VLBW cohort (BW <1,500 g and gestational age 22 to 28 weeks) had at least one episode of blood culture–proven sepsis beyond 3 days of life. There was considerable variability with gestational age in the incidence of LOS, ranging from 46% at 23 weeks to 12% at 28 weeks' birth gestation among the 20 NICHD network centers. NICHD network LOS data from 1998 to 2000 demonstrated overall mortality from LOS was 18% of infected infants versus 7% of uninfected infants. The mortality among infants with gram-negative infections was about 40% and 30% with fungal infections.

L. **Risk factors for LOS.** A number of clinical factors are associated with an increased risk of LOS (Table 49.3). The incidence of LOS is inversely related to BW. The risk of developing LOS associated with central catheters, parenteral nutrition, and mechanical ventilation are all increased with longer duration of these therapies.

M. **Microbiology of LOS.** Nearly half of cases of LOS are caused by coagulase-negative staphylococci (CONS). In the NICHD study, 22% of cases of LOS were caused by other gram-positive organisms (*S. aureus*, *Enterococcus*, GBS), 18% by gram-negative organisms (*E. coli*, *Klebsiella*, *Pseudomonas*, *Enterobacter*, and *Serratia*), and 12% by fungal species (*Candida albicans* and *Candida parapsilosis*). The distribution of organisms causing LOS may vary significantly at individual centers. Awareness of local variation in the microbiology of LOS is important in choosing empiric antibiotic therapy for the acutely ill infant in whom LOS is suspected.

1. **CONS.** CONS are a heterogeneous group of gram-positive organisms with a structure similar to *S. aureus*, but these organisms lack protein A

Table 49.3. Risk Factors for Late-Onset Sepsis in Infants with Birth Weight <1,500 g

Birth weight <750 g
Presence of central venous catheters (umbilical, percutaneous, and tunneled)
Delayed enteral feeding
Prolonged hyperalimentation
Mechanical ventilation
Complications of prematurity
Patent ductus arteriosus
Bronchopulmonary dysplasia
Necrotizing enterocolitis

Source: Data from Stoll BJ, Hansen N, Fanaroff AA, et al. Late-onset sepsis in very low birth weight neonates: the experience of the NICHD Neonatal Research Network. *Pediatrics* 2002;110(2, pt 1):285–291; Makhoul IR, Sujov P, Smolkin T, et al. Epidemiological, clinical, and microbiological characteristics of late-onset sepsis among very low birth weight infants in Israel: a national survey. *Pediatrics* 2002;109(1):34–39.

and have different cell wall components. *Staphylococcus epidermidis* is the primary cause of NICU disease. CONS universally colonize the skin of NICU patients. They are believed to cause bacteremia by first colonizing the surfaces of central catheters. A polysaccharide surface adhesin (PSA), as well as several other surface components, have been implicated in adherence to and colonization of the catheter surface; subsequent biofilm and slime production inhibit the ability of the host to eliminate the organism. Most CONS are resistant to penicillin, semisynthetic penicillins, and gentamicin, and empiric treatment for LOS in the NICU usually includes vancomycin. CONS disease is rarely fatal even to the VLBW infant and rarely, if ever, causes meningitis or site-specific disease. However, CONS disease can cause systemic instability resulting in temporary cessation of enteral feeding and/or escalation of ventilatory support and is associated with prolonged hospitalization and poorer neurodevelopmental outcome.

2. **S. aureus.** *S. aureus* is an encapsulated gram-positive organism that elaborates multiple adhesins, virulence-associated enzymes, and toxins to cause a wide range of serious disease, including bacteremia, meningitis, cellulitis, omphalitis, osteomyelitis, and arthritis. *S. aureus* is distinguished from CONS by the production of coagulase and by the presence of protein A, a component of the cell wall that contributes to virulence by binding to the Fc portion of immunoglobulin G (IgG) antibody and blocking opsonization. LOS caused by *S. aureus* can result in significant morbidity. Disease is frequently complicated by focal site infections (soft tissue, bone, and joint infections are commonly observed

in neonates) and marked by persistent bacteremia despite antibiotic administration. Joint infections often require open surgical drainage and can lead to joint destruction and permanent disability. The treatment of methicillin-sensitive *S. aureus* (MSSA) requires the use of semisynthetic penicillins such as nafcillin or oxacillin.

Methicillin-resistant *S. aureus* (MRSA) is an increasingly recognized pathogen in NICUs. An NICHD NRN study of infants born with BW 400 to 1,500 g between 2006 and 2008 reveals that 3.7% had a late-onset infection due to *S. aureus*; roughly one-third of these infections were due to MRSA. Mortality was high in this study, occurring in approximately 25% of infants infected with either MSSA or MRSA. Resistance to semisynthetic penicillins is mediated by chromosomal acquisition of the *mecA* gene, found on different types of staphylococcal chromosomal cassette *mec* (SCC*mecA*) elements. The *mecA* gene encodes a modified penicillin-binding protein (PBP) with a low affinity for methicillin. Once acquired, the modified PBP replaces similar proteins on the bacterial cell membrane and results in resistance to all β-lactam antibiotics. The emergence of MRSA infections in NICUs appears to track the increase in these infections in both general hospital settings and in the community. MRSA isolates can be grouped as hospital associated (HA-MRSA) or community associated (CA-MRSA) in origin. Uniform resistance to all common antibiotics except for vancomycin characterizes HA-MRSA and most HA-MRSA carry SCC*mec* type II or III. Community-acquired isolates are usually resistant only to β-lactam antibiotics and erythromycin and usually carry SCC*mec* type IV or V. Distinguishing between the two types of organisms can be important for determining the source of epidemic outbreaks of MRSA disease within individual units as well as for developing effective infection control measures. Whatever the source of the organism, however, it can be rapidly spread within the NICU by nosocomial transmission on the hands of caregivers. Infection control measures including identification of colonized infants by routine surveillance and cohorting and isolation of colonized infants may be required to prevent spread and persistence of the organism. MRSA infections usually require treatment with **vancomycin**. As with MSSA, MRSA infections can be complicated by deep tissue involvement and persistent bacteremia that may require surgical debridement for resolution. Although it cannot be used as a single agent, rifampin can be a helpful adjunctive therapy for persistent MRSA infection. Consultation with an infectious disease specialist is recommended regarding the utility of adding newer gram-positive antibiotics (the oxazolidinone antibiotic linezolid or the lipopeptide antibiotic daptomycin) to eradicate persistent MRSA bacteremia.

3. **Enterococci.** Formerly categorized as members of Group D streptococci, both *Enterococcus faecalis* and *Enterococcus faecium* cause LOS in premature infants. These organisms are associated with indwelling catheters; they are encapsulated organisms that produce both biofilm and slime and can adhere to and persist on catheter surfaces as described in the preceding text for CONS. Although disease can be complicated by meningitis and is sometimes associated with NEC, enterococcal LOS is associated with low overall mortality. Enterococci are resistant to cephalosporins and may be

resistant to penicillin G and ampicillin; treatment requires the synergistic effect of an aminoglycoside with ampicillin or vancomycin. Vancomycin-resistant enterococci (VRE) present a significant problem in adult intensive care settings, and outbreaks have occurred in NICUs as well. Linezolid, daptomycin, and quinupristin/dalfopristin (Synercid) have variable activity against VRE. Linezolid is approved for use in neonates and is effective against vancomycin-resistant *E. faecalis* and *E. faecium*. VRE of *faecium* origin can be treated with quinupristin/dalfopristin but this combination is not effective against *E. faecalis*. Treatment decisions should be made in consultation with infectious diseases experts. VRE outbreaks may also require the institution of infection control measures (surveillance to identify colonized infants, isolation and cohorting of those colonized) to control spread and persistence of the organism.

4. **Gram-negative organisms.** LOS caused by gram-negative organisms is complicated by a 40% mortality rate in the NICHD cohort. *E. coli* was discussed under EOS (see section I.I.2).

a. *Pseudomonas aeruginosa.* Mortality associated with *P. aeruginosa* sepsis in low BW infants is high (76% in the NICHD cohort). A number of bacterial factors, including LPS, mucoid capsule, adhesins, invasins, and toxins (notably exotoxin A) contribute to its extreme virulence in premature infants as well as in debilitated adults and burn victims. Both LPS and the mucoid capsule help the organism avoid opsonization and secreted proteases inactivate complement, cytokines, and immunoglobulin. The lipid A moiety of LPS (endotoxin) causes the typical aspects of gram-negative septicemia (i.e., hypotension, DIC). Exotoxin A is antigenically distinct from diphtheria toxin but acts by the same mechanism: adenovirus death protein (ADP)-ribosylation of eukaryotic elongation factor 2 results in inhibition of protein synthesis and cell death. *P. aeruginosa* is present in the intestinal tract of approximately 5% of healthy adults but colonizes premature infants at much higher rates due to nosocomial acquisition of the bacteria. Selection of the bacteria, likely due to the resistance of *Pseudomonas* to most common antibiotics, also plays a role in colonization; prolonged exposure to IV antibiotics is an identified risk factor for LOS with *Pseudomonas*. *Pseudomonas* can be found in environmental reservoirs in intensive care units (ICUs) (i.e., sinks, respiratory equipment), and outbreaks of nosocomial disease have been linked to both environmental sources and spread by the hands of health care workers.

Treatment requires a combination of two agents active against *Pseudomonas*, such as ceftazidime, piperacillin/tazobactam, gentamicin, or tobramycin. Generally, a β-lactam–based antibiotic combined with an aminoglycoside is preferred; however, both extended-spectrum β-lactamases (ESBL) and constitutive AmpC-type β-lactamases are emerging in pseudomonal species (see subsequent text), and treatment must be guided by isolate antibiotic sensitivity testing. A survey of neonatologists' practices in the treatment of LOS reveals that the most common antibiotics empirically used are vancomycin and gentamicin. When an infant presents as severely ill or when the infant becomes acutely sicker during or after standard antibiotic treatment, consideration should be given to empiric coverage for *Pseudomonas* until blood culture results are available.

b. *Enterobacter* **spp.** Like *E. coli*, *Enterobacter* spp. are LPS-containing, gram-negative rods that are normal constituents of colonic flora that can cause overwhelming sepsis in low BW infants. The most common isolates are *Enterobacter cloacae* and *Enterobacter aerogenes*. *Enterobacter sakazakii* has received publicity due to outbreaks of disease caused by contamination of powdered infant formulas with this organism. Although *Enterobacter* spp. account for <5% of total infections in NICHD and our local data, there are multiple reports of epidemic outbreaks of cephalosporin-resistant *Enterobacter* in NICUs. *Enterobacter* spp. contain chromosomally encoded, inducible β-lactamases (AmpC-encoded cephalosporinases), and treatment with third-generation cephalosporins, even if the initial isolate appears to be sensitive, can result in the emergence of cephalosporin-resistant organisms. In addition, stably derepressed, high-level constitutive AmpC-producing strains of *Enterobacter*, *Citrobacter*, and *Serratia* have been reported. The fourth-generation cephalosporin cefepime is relatively stable against AmpC-type β-lactamases. ESBLs (discussed in the subsequent text) have also been reported in *Enterobacter* spp. Given the increasing concern about cephalosporin resistance among infectious disease experts, cefepime or meropenem and gentamicin is usually recommended for treatment of infections caused by *Enterobacter* spp. Infection control measures and restriction of cephalosporin use can be effective in controlling outbreaks of resistant organisms.

N. Symptoms and evaluation of LOS. Lethargy, an increase in the number or severity of apneic spells, feeding intolerance, temperature instability, and/or an increase in ventilatory support all may be early signs of LOS—or may be part of the variability in the course of the VLBW infant. The difficulty in distinguishing between these two in part explains the frequency of evaluation for LOS; in one NICHD study, 62% of VLBW infants had at least one blood culture drawn after day of life 3. With mild symptoms and a low suspicion for the presence of sepsis, it is reasonable to draw a CBC with differential, ± CRP, and a blood culture and wait for the results of the tests (while monitoring the infant's symptoms closely) before beginning empiric antibiotic therapy. If laboratory tests are abnormal or the infant's status worsens, empiric antibiotic therapy should be started. If the suspicion for sepsis is still low, and/or the clinical impression is that a CONS infection is likely, it is not unreasonable to obtain a blood culture only. Ideally, CSF culture should also be obtained before antibiotic therapy, both to guide empiric therapy and to ensure proper follow-up (such as renal imaging if a UTI is present). A study of late-onset infection in VLBW infants underscores the importance of **performing an LP in the evaluation of LOS** in this population. Two-thirds of a cohort of over 9,000 infants had one or more blood cultures drawn after 72 hours of life; one-third had an LP. Culture-proven meningitis was diagnosed in 134 infants (5% of those on whom an LP was performed) and in 45 out of 134 cases, the coincident blood culture was negative. Urine cultures should also be considered prior to beginning empiric antibiotic therapy, particularly for older infants without central venous access. Urine cultures should be obtained by catheterization or ultrasound-guided suprapubic aspiration (SPA) in VLBW infants; cultures of urine obtained by other means are likely to contain contaminant species.

If a previously well, convalescing premature infant presents primarily with increased apnea with or without upper respiratory infection (URI) symptoms, consideration should be given to a viral source of infection as well. Tracheal or nasal aspirate should be sent for rapid analysis and culture to rule out respiratory syncytial virus (RSV), parainfluenzae, and influenzae A and B if seasonally appropriate.

O. **Treatment of LOS.** Table 49.1 lists suggested antibiotic regimens for selected organisms. Note that for many antibiotics, dosing is dependent on gestational and postnatal age (see Appendix A). A study of **central line removal** in culture-proven LOS demonstrated that bacteremic infants experience fewer complications of infection if central lines are removed promptly upon identification of a positive culture. This was particularly true for infections caused by *S. aureus* and gram-negative organisms.

Esbls are plasmid-encoded bacterial enzymes that confer resistance to a variety of penicillins and cephalosporins. Esbls are distinguished from the generally chromosomally encoded AmpC-type enzymes by sensitivity to clavulanate. Nosocomial gram-negative pathogens that commonly colonize and cause disease in VLBW infants (such as *E. coli, Enterobacter, Klebsiella, Pseudomonas,* and *Serratia*) are increasingly found to harbor these resistance enzymes. ESBL organisms have become a significant problem in adult ICUs. Multiple international reports document an increasing impact of ESBL-producing organisms in NICUs. The magnitude of the problem in American NICUs is limited to case reports of outbreaks, primarily with ESBL-containing *Klebsiella* spp. Risk factors for acquiring ESBL organisms include low gestational age and use of third-generation cephalosporins. Current recommendations to control outbreaks of these organisms include restriction of third-generation cephalosporin use and the same infection control measures (routine surveillance for colonization, cohorting, and isolation of colonized infants) as are needed for control of MRSA. Treatment of ESBL infections should ideally include consultation with infectious disease specialists; carbapenems, cefepime, and piperacillin/tazobactam are currently most effective, with increasing rates of coresistance reported for aminoglycosides and fluoroquinolones.

Carbapenemase-producing organisms and other multidrug-resistant organisms (MDROs) have been recently recognized in hospital settings. Carbapenem resistance can occur in gram-negative organisms either by the acquisition of specific enzymes or by reduced carbapenem influx caused by the loss of outer membrane protein porins in ESBL organisms. In the United States, most carbapenemase-producing organisms contain the transposon-mediated *Klebsiella pneumoniae* carbapenemase (KPC), but other enzymes such as the New Delhi metallo-β-lactamase (NDM) and the Verona integron-encoded metallo-β-lactamase (VIM) are common outside the United States. Early recognition of these organisms is critical, both for proper individual treatment and to prevent nosocomial spread. Laboratory standards for identification of carbapenem-resistant *Enterobacteriaceae* (CRE) organisms include reduced susceptibility to meropenem, imipenem, or doripenem using breakpoints defined in 2012 clinical laboratory standards and resistance to all third-generation cephalosporins. Current treatment of infections with most carbapenemase-producing organisms requires the use of the polymyxin B, an antibiotic with significant toxicity. Recent reports of hospital-acquired infections by extensively drug-resistant *Acinetobacter baumannii* raise the specter of infection with organisms for which no effective treatment exists, underscoring the importance of good infection control practices and responsible use of antibiotics in all intensive care settings.

P. **Prevention of LOS.** In addition to significant mortality, LOS is associated with prolonged hospitalization and overall poorer outcome in VLBW infants compared to those that remain uninfected. A number of strategies to lower rates of LOS have been studied. These include administration of specific medications and biologics for infection prophylaxis, antibiotic restriction and surveillance policies to prevent antibiotic-resistant infections, and "bundled" implementation of multiple care practices to prevent central line–associated bloodstream infections (CLABSI).

1. **IVIG.** Multiple studies have been conducted using prophylactic administration of IVIG to address the relative deficiency of immunoglobulin in low BW infants and prevent LOS. A meta-analysis of these demonstrated no significant decrease in mortality or other serious outcomes and is generally not recommended.

2. **G-CSF.** G-CSF has been shown to resolve preeclampsia-associated neutropenia and may thereby decrease the rate of LOS in this population of infants. One trial of GM-CSF in premature neonates with the clinical diagnosis of early-onset disease did not improve mortality but was associated with acquiring fewer nosocomial infections over the subsequent 2 weeks.

3. **Prophylactic vancomycin.** A meta-analysis of several trials of low-dose vancomycin administration to VLBW infants demonstrated that the administration of prophylactic vancomycin reduced the incidence of both total LOS- and CONS-associated infections but did not improve mortality or length of hospitalization. Prophylactic vancomycin IV lock solution has been studied with some success in decreasing CONS infection. Antibiotic-impregnated catheters are not currently available for VLBW infants. There is concern that widespread use of vancomycin in these ways will lead to the increased emergence of vancomycin-resistant organisms.

4. **Probiotics.** Several clinical trials have evaluated the administration of probiotic formulations in the prevention of both LOS and NEC. A recent meta-analysis of 10 randomized, placebo-controlled trials (most published since 2010) concluded that probiotic administration significantly reduced the risk of death or NEC among VLBW infants but found no significant effect on the incidence of LOS. The bacterial formulations and doses used varied among the studies; all included some form of *Lactobacillus* or *Bifidobacterium* spp. Some experts feel this evidence is strong enough to offer probiotic formulations to all VLBW infants without further placebo-controlled trials. Others argue that the lack of standardized, regulated probiotic products and the relative lack of data among infants with BW <1,000 g suggest that further study is required.

5. **Lactoferrin.** Lactoferrin is the major whey protein in both human and cow's milk. Present in high concentration in human colostrum, lactoferrin is important to innate immune defense against microbial pathogens, acting by sequestering iron and by impacting microbial membrane integrity. One randomized, placebo-controlled trial of oral administration of bovine lactoferrin with or without a *Lactobacillus* probiotic preparation demonstrated a 70% reduction in the incidence of LOS among VLBW infants. Several large ongoing trials are ongoing in 2015 that may better inform the full value of this protein in LOS prevention.

6. **Establishment of early enteral feedings** in VLBW infants may have the greatest effect on reducing LOS by reducing exposure to parenteral nutrition and allowing for decreased use of central catheters. **Breast milk** feeding may also help decrease nosocomial infection rates among VLBW infants, both by its numerous infection-protective properties (i.e., secretory immunoglobulin A [IgA], lactoferrin, lysozyme) and by aiding in the establishment of enteral feeds. Systematic review of studies of the human milk feeding and risk of LOS have not been able to rigorously establish that human milk prevents LOS among VLBW infants, but multiple small studies support the role of human milk in preventing NEC. Human milk feeding may impact the risk of LOS by decreasing the time to full enteral feeding and thus decreasing the duration of central venous access and use of total parenteral nutrition (TPN).

7. **Antibiotic restriction.** Limitation of the use of broad-spectrum antibiotics in neonatal, pediatric, and adult ICUs has been inconsistently associated with decrease rates of patient colonization with antibiotic-resistant organisms. Cycling of antibiotics used for empiric treatment has not been successful in preventing neonatal LOS or impacting colonization patterns. **However, the widespread emergence of MRSA, VRE, and multidrug-resistant gram-negative organisms has led to an increased awareness of the risk of empiric use of vancomycin and third-generation cephalosporins among infectious diseases experts.** Some studies suggest that substitution of oxacillin for vancomycin in the empiric treatment of LOS is not likely to cause significant morbidity in VLBW infants because of the low virulence of the organism and may decrease the acquisition and spread of VRE and other antibiotic-resistant organisms.

8. **Surveillance practices.** A concern over emergence of MRSA, VRE, and multidrug-resistant gram-negative organisms has led to increased interest in the effect of ongoing surveillance to detect neonatal colonization. Multiple reports document the combined use of bacterial surveillance cultures, cohorting, isolation, and in some cases, attempts at decolonization to control the outbreaks of infection with specific pathogens within NICUs. The impact of ongoing, longitudinal surveillance practices is less certain. We have shown that ongoing use of a weekly MRSA surveillance program in our NICU may help prevent patient-to-patient spread of MRSA but did not completely eliminated introduction of MRSA into the NICU, likely due to the prevalence of this pathogen in the general population. Surveillance programs must be accompanied by strict hand hygiene practices for optimal impact, including reinforcement of hand-washing policies; routine use of waterless hand disinfectants; and

restriction of artificial fingernails, natural nails over 1/4-inch length, nail polish; and wearing of rings, watches, and bracelets in the NICU setting.

9. **Implementation of recommended best practices to prevent CLABSI.** Most bloodstream infections that occur in VLBW infants are associated with the presence of central venous catheters. CLABSI are defined as culture-proven bloodstream infections occurring in the presence of a central catheter for which there is no other obvious source of infection (i.e., perinatal exposures in EOS or perforated bowel in NEC). The recognition of significant inter-NICU variation in the incidence of these infections has led to efforts to define optimal care practices associated with lower rates of infection.

Multiple resources are now available to guide optimal care practices for the prevention of CLABSI. The basic components of CLABSI prevention bundles are shown in Table 49.4. The **California Perinatal Quality Care Collaborative (CPQCC)** summarizes and

---

Table 49.4. Components of Neonatal CLABSI Prevention

Hand Hygiene

- Before and after any patient contact
- Before and after donning gloves
- Before central line placement or adjustment

Central Line Care Practices

- Maximal barrier precautions/sterile procedure for insertion
- Formalized daily use and dressing maintenance procedures
- Preparation of parenteral fluids in pharmacy under laminar flow hood
- Standards for timing of administration set changes
- Daily review of central line necessity

Diagnostic Criteria and Reporting Practices

- Optimize practices for obtaining and interpreting blood culture results
- Collect accurate data to determine CLABSI per 1,000 line days
- Communicate CLABSI data and trends to local caregivers
- Benchmark local data against appropriate national standards

Source: Data from Bowles S, Pettit J, Mickas N, et al. *Neonatal Hospital-Acquired Infection Prevention.* https://www.cpqcc.org/sites/default/files/2007HAIToolkit.pdf; O'Grady NP, Alexander M, Dellinger EP, et al. Guidelines for the prevention of intravascular catheter-related infections. The Hospital Infection Control Practices Advisory Committee, Center for Disease Control and Prevention, U.S. *Pediatrics* 2002;110(5):e51.

provides critical review of evidence-based practices for neonatal infection prevention in their toolkit, **"Neonatal Hospital-Acquired Infection Prevention,"** available at http://www.cpqcc.org.

II. ANAEROBIC BACTERIAL INFECTIONS. Anaerobic bacteria comprise a significant portion of the oral, vaginal, and gastrointestinal flora. Although many anaerobes are of low virulence, a few anaerobic organisms can cause both EOS and LOS. These organisms include *Bacteroides* spp. (primarily *B. fragilis*), *Peptostreptococcus*, and *Clostridium perfringens*. NEC and/or bowel perforation can be complicated by anaerobic sepsis alone or in a polymicrobial infection. In addition to bacteremia, *B. fragilis* can cause abdominal abscesses, meningitis, omphalitis, cellulitis at the site of fetal scalp monitors, endocarditis, osteomyelitis, and arthritis in the neonate.

A. **Treatment of anaerobic infections.** Bacteremia and/or meningitis are treated with IV antibiotics; abscesses and other focal infections often require surgical drainage. *B. fragilis* is a gram-negative rod, and although oral *Bacteroides* spp. are sensitive to penicillin, *B. fragilis* usually requires treatment with drugs such as metronidazole, clindamycin, cefoxitin, or imipenem. Occasional strains of *B. fragilis* are also resistant to cefoxitin and/or imipenem; as many as one-fourth of all strain in the United States are now resistant to clindamycin. Most other cephalosporins and vancomycin are ineffective against *B. fragilis*. *Peptostreptococcus* and *Clostridia* are gram-positive organisms that are sensitive to penicillin G. NEC and intestinal perforations are treated with ampicillin, gentamicin, and clindamycin (or metronidazole) to provide coverage for the spectrum of organisms that can complicate these illnesses.

B. **Neonatal tetanus.** This syndrome is caused by the effect of a neurotoxin produced by the anaerobic bacterium *Clostridium tetani*. Infection can occur by invasion of the umbilical cord due to unsanitary childbirth or cord care practices. It has historically been a significant cause of neonatal mortality in developing countries. An estimated 787,000 deaths due to neonatal tetanus occurred worldwide in 1988. The World Health Organization (WHO) has set multiple target dates for neonatal tetanus worldwide elimination since 1989. Elimination has been achieved in many developing countries, but neonatal tetanus persists in remote and poverty-ridden regions, associated with lack of adequate maternal tetanus toxoid immunization and unsanitary delivery settings. WHO estimates 49,000 deaths occurred worldwide from neonatal tetanus in 2013. This disease is virtually nonexistent in the United States due to maternal immunization and good infection control practices; only one case was reported to the CDC from 2001 to 2008. Infected infants develop hypertonia and muscle spasms including trismus and consequent inability to feed. Treatment consists of the administration of tetanus immunoglobulin (TIG) (500 U intramuscular [IM]) and penicillin G (100,000 U/kg/day divided every 4 to 6 hours for 7 to 10 days) or metronidazole (30 mg/kg/day divided every 6 hours) as well as supportive care with mechanical ventilation, sedatives, and muscle relaxants. IVIG may be given if TIG is not available. Neonatal tetanus does not result in immunity to tetanus, and infants require standard tetanus immunizations after recovery.

III. FUNGAL INFECTIONS

A. Mucocutaneous candidiasis. Fungal infections in the well-term infant are generally limited to mucocutaneous disease involving *C. albicans. Candida* spp. are normal commensal flora beyond the neonatal period and rarely cause serious disease in the immunocompetent host. Immaturity of host defenses and colonization with *Candida* before complete establishment of normal intestinal flora probably contribute to the pathogenicity of *Candida* in the neonate. Oral and gastrointestinal colonization with *Candida* occurs before the development of oral candidiasis (thrush) or diaper dermatitis. *Candida* can be acquired through the birth canal or through the hands or breast of the mother. Nosocomial transmission in the nursery setting has been documented, such as transmission from feeding bottles and pacifiers.

Oral candidiasis in the young infant is treated with a nonabsorbable oral antifungal medication, which has the advantages of little systemic toxicity and concomitant treatment of the intestinal tract. **Nystatin** oral suspension (100,000 U/mL) is standard treatment (1 mL is applied to each side of the mouth every 6 hours for a minimum of 10 to 14 days). Ideally, treatment is continued for several days after lesions resolve. Fluconazole (6 mg/kg IV or orally (PO) once followed by 3 mg/kg IV/PO each day) can be used for severe oral candidiasis if nystatin oral therapy is not effective. Systemic **fluconazole** is also highly effective in treating chronic mucocutaneous candidiasis in the immunocompromised host. Infants with chronic, severe thrush refractory to treatment should be evaluated for an underlying congenital or acquired immunodeficiency.

Oral candidiasis in the **breastfed infant** is often associated with superficial or ductal candidiasis in the mother's breast. Concurrent treatment of both the mother and infant is necessary to eliminate continual cross-infection. Breastfeeding of term infants can continue during treatment. Mothers with breast ductal candidiasis who are providing expressed breast milk for VLBW infants should be advised to withhold expressed milk until treatment has been instituted. *Candida* can be difficult to detect in breast milk because lactoferrin inhibits the growth of *Candida* in culture. Freezing does not eliminate *Candida* from expressed breast milk.

Candidal diaper dermatitis is effectively treated with topical agents such as 2% nystatin ointment, 2% miconazole ointment, or 1% clotrimazole cream. Concomitant treatment with oral nystatin to eliminate intestinal colonization is often recommended but not well studied. It is reasonable to use simultaneous oral and topical therapy for refractory candidal diaper dermatitis.

B. Systemic candidiasis. Systemic candidiasis is a serious form of nosocomial infection in VLBW infants. Data on late-onset candidal sepsis from the NICHD NRN showed that 9% of a cohort of 1,515 infants with BW <1,000 g developed candidal sepsis or meningitis, primarily caused by *C. albicans* and *C. parapsilosis*. One-third of these infants died. Invasive candidiasis is associated with overall poorer neurodevelopmental outcomes and higher rates of threshold retinopathy of prematurity, compared to matched VLBW control infants. Gastrointestinal tract colonization of the low BW infants often precedes invasive infection, and **risk factors for colonization and invasive disease** are similar. The most significant epidemiologic factors specific to candidal LOS in the NICHD cohort studies were BW <1,000 g, presence of central catheter, delay in enteral feeding, and days of broad-spectrum antibiotic exposure. Other clinical factors included in a recent clinical predictive model for invasive candidiasis in the BW <1,000 g population include the presence of candidal diaper dermatitis, vaginal delivery, lower gestational age, and significant hypoglycemia and thrombocytopenia. The use of H_2 blockers or systemic steroids have also been identified as independent risk factor for the development of invasive fungal infection.

1. **Microbiology.** Disseminated candidiasis is primarily caused by *C. albicans* and *C. parapsilosis* in preterm infants, but infection with *Candida tropicalis, Candida lusitaniae, Candida guilliermondii, Candida glabrata*, and *Candida krusei* are reported less frequently in neonates. The pathogenicity of *C. albicans* is associated with the variable production of a number of toxins, including an endotoxin. *C. albicans* can be acquired perinatally as well as postnatally. *C. parapsilosis* has emerged as the second most common cause of disseminated neonatal candidiasis in recent years. Studies suggest that *C. parapsilosis* is primarily a nosocomial pathogen in that it is acquired at a later age than *C. albicans* and is associated with colonization of health care workers' hands. In NICHD studies, fungal species (primarily *C. albicans* vs. *C. parapsilosis*) did not independently predict death or later neurodevelopmental impairment, and a delay in removal of central catheters was associated with higher mortality rates from *Candida* LOS regardless of species.

2. **Clinical manifestations.** Candidiasis due to *in utero* infection can occur. Congenital cutaneous candidiasis can present with severe, widespread, and desquamating skin involvement. Pulmonary candidiasis can occur in isolation or with disseminated infection and presents as a severe pneumonia. Most cases of systemic candidiasis, however, present as LOS in VLBW infants, most often after the second or third week of life. The initial clinical features of **late-onset invasive candidiasis** are often non-specific and can include lethargy, increased apnea or need for increased ventilatory support, poor perfusion, feeding intolerance, and hyperglycemia. Both the total WBC and the differential can be normal early in the course of infection, and although thrombocytopenia is a consistent feature, it is not universally found at presentation. The clinical picture is initially difficult to distinguish from sepsis caused by CONS infection and contrasts with the abrupt onset of septic shock that often accompanies LOS caused by gram-negative organisms. Candidemia can be complicated by meningitis and brain abscess as well as end-organ involvement of the kidneys, heart, joints, and eyes (endophthalmitis). The fatality rate of disseminated candidiasis is high relative to that found in CONS infections and increases in the presence of CNS involvement.

3. **Diagnosis.** *Candida* can be cultured from standard pediatric blood culture systems; the time to identification of a positive culture is usually by 48 hours, although late identification (beyond 72 hours) does occur more frequently than with bacterial species. Specialized fungal isolator tubes can aid in the identification of fungal infection if it is suspected by allowing for direct culture on selective media but are not necessary to identify candidemia. Both fungal culture and fungal staining (KOH preparation) of urine obtained by SPA can be helpful in making the

diagnosis of systemic candidiasis. Specimens obtained by bag urine collection or bladder catheterization are difficult to interpret because they can be readily contaminated with colonizing species. We have obtained urine by SPA from VLBW infants under bedside ultrasound guidance for maximal safety. Before the initiation of antifungal therapy, CSF should be obtained for cell count and fungal culture.

4. **Treatment.** Systemic candidiasis is treated with **amphotericin B**, 0.5 to 1.0 mg/kg/day for durations of 7 to 14 days after a documented negative blood culture if the infection is considered to be catheter associated and the catheter has been promptly removed. Otherwise, recommended length of treatment for neonatal candidemia is 3 weeks and for longer periods if specific end-organ infection is present. All common strains of Candida other than some strains of *C. lusitaniae*, *C. glabrata*, and *C. krusei* are sensitive to amphotericin. This medication is associated with a variety of dose-dependent immediate and delayed toxicities in older children and adults and can cause phlebitis at the site of infusion. Febrile reactions to the infusion do not usually occur in the low BW infant (although renal and electrolyte disturbances can occur), and we start infants at the higher 1 mg/kg dose from the beginning of treatment. The medication is given over 2 hours to minimize the risk of seizures and arrhythmias during the infusion. There is increased experience in VLBW babies with **liposomal preparations of amphotericin B** and this formulation can be used for invasive candidiasis if urinary tract and CNS involvement are excluded. Doses of 5 mg/kg/day can be used without toxicity, and the medication can be given over 2 hours with less irritation at the site of infusion. There is some concern that liposomal preparations are less effective in neonates. CNS disease can be treated with nonliposomal amphotericin alone; an additional second agent, commonly **5-fluorocytosine (flucytosine 5-FC) (50 to 150 mg/kg/day) or fluconazole (6 mg/kg/day) should be added only if initial therapy with amphotericin is not effective**. Flucytosine achieves good CNS penetration, and appears to be safe in infants, but is only available for enteral administration, limiting its utility in sick VLBW infants. Bone marrow and liver toxicity has occurred in adults and correlates with elevated serum levels of the medication. Serum levels can be monitored (40 to 60 μg/mL is desirable.) Fluconazole is safe for use in infants and can be successfully used for primary treatment of candidemia. It should not be used until candidal speciation is completed because *C. krusei* and *C. glabrata* are frequently resistant to fluconazole.

   Removal of central catheters in place when candidemia is identified is essential to the eradication of the infection. Delayed catheter removal is associated with persistent candidemia and increased mortality.

   Further evaluation of the infant with invasive candidiasis should include renal and brain ultrasonography to rule out fungal abscess formation and ophthalmologic examination to rule out endophthalmitis. In infants who are persistently fungemic despite catheter removal and appropriate therapy, an echocardiogram to rule out endocarditis or vegetation formation is warranted.

5. **Prevention.** Minimizing use of broad-spectrum antibiotics (particularly cephalosporins and carbapenems) and H_2 blockers may be helpful in

preventing disseminated candidiasis. The CDC recommends changing infusions of lipid suspensions every 12 hours to minimize microbial contamination; solutions of parenteral nutrition and lipid mixtures should be changed every 24 hours. Several randomized, placebo-controlled trials of **prophylactic fluconazole administration** to prevent invasive fungal infection in VLBW infants have been published since 2001. All the trials demonstrated decreased rates of colonization with fungal species, and most also demonstrated decreased rates of invasive fungal infection. Initial concerns that widespread implementation of a fluconazole prophylaxis regimen would result in colonization or infection with less fluconazole-sensitive *Candida* spp. have not been born out. One study of the impact of fluconazole prophylaxis on long-term neurodevelopmental outcome revealed no safety concerns. However, there is no evidence that fluconazole prophylaxis impacts overall mortality or neurodevelopmental outcome. A recent randomized trial of 361 infants with BW <750 g treated with fluconazole prophylaxis for 42 days demonstrated a statistically significant decrease in invasive fungal disease (from 9% in the placebo group to 3% in the treatment group) but no impact on the combined outcome of death or candidiasis and no impact on neurodevelopmental outcome. In light of these findings, individual NICUs should balance the potentially severe consequences of invasive fungal infection (in the NICHD cohort, 73% of infants with LOS fungal sepsis died or survived with significant neurodevelopmental impairment) as well as the frequency of LOS fungal infection in an individual NICU in making a decision to implement a fluconazole prophylaxis policy. Targeted use of fluconazole prophylaxis in infants with multiple risk factors—for example, those with BW <1,000 g receiving long-term broad-spectrum antibiotics—may be the optimal course, rather than use determined by a BW alone.

IV. FOCAL BACTERIAL INFECTIONS

A. **Skin infections.** The newborn may develop a variety of rashes associated with both systemic and focal bacterial disease. Responsible organisms include all of the usual causes of EOS (GBS, enteric gram-negative rods, and anaerobes) as well as gram-positive organisms that specifically colonize the skin—staphylococci and other streptococci. Colonization of the newborn skin occurs with organisms acquired from vaginal flora as well as from the environment. **Sepsis** can be accompanied by skin manifestations such as maculopapular rashes, erythema multiforme, and petechiae or purpura. **Localized infections** can arise in any site of traumatized skin: in the scalp at lesions caused by intrapartum fetal monitors or blood gas samples, in the penis and surrounding tissues due to circumcision, in the extremities at sites of venipuncture or IV placement, and in the umbilical stump (omphalitis). Generalized pustular skin infections can occur due to *S. aureus*, occasionally in epidemic fashion; focal abscesses can be caused by MRSA.

1. **Cellulitis** usually occurs at traumatized skin sites as noted in the preceding text. Localized erythema and/or drainage in a term infant (e.g., at a scalp electrode site) can be treated with careful washing and local antisepsis with antibiotic ointment (bacitracin or mupirocin ointment)

and close monitoring. Cellulitis at sites of IV access or venipuncture in premature infants must be addressed in a more aggressive fashion due to the risk of local and systemic spread, particularly in the VLBW infant. If the premature infant with a localized cellulitis is well appearing, a CBC and blood culture should be obtained and IV antibiotics administered to provide coverage primarily for skin flora (i.e., oxacillin or nafcillin and gentamicin). If MRSA is a concern in a particular setting, vancomycin should be substituted for nafcillin. If blood cultures are negative, the infant can be treated for a total of 5 to 7 days with resolution of the cellulitis. If an organism grows from the blood culture, an LP should be performed to rule out meningitis and careful physical examination should be performed to rule out accompanying osteomyelitis or septic arthritis. Therapy is guided by the organism identified (see Tables 49.1 and 49.2).

2. **Pustulosis.** Infectious pustulosis is usually caused by *S. aureus* and must be distinguished from the benign neonatal rash erythema toxicum and transient pustular melanosis. The pustules are most commonly found in the axillae, groin, and periumbilical area; both erythema toxicum and transient pustular melanosis have a more generalized distribution. Lesions can be unroofed after cleansing in sterile fashion with Betadine or 4% chlorhexidine, and contents aspirated and analyzed by Gram stain and culture. Gram stain of infectious pustules will reveal neutrophils and gram-positive cocci, whereas Wright stain of erythema toxicum lesions will reveal predominantly eosinophils and no (or a few contaminating) organisms. Gram stain of transient pustular melanosis lesions will reveal neutrophils but no organisms. Cultures of the benign rashes will be sterile or grow contaminating organisms such as *S. epidermidis*. Treatment of pustulosis caused by *S. aureus* is tailored to the degree of involvement and condition of the infant. A few lesions in a healthy term infant may be treated with topical mupirocin and oral therapy with medications such as amoxicillin/clavulanate, dicloxacillin, clindamycin, or cephalexin depending on organism antibiotic sensitivity. More extensive lesions, systemic illness, or pustulosis occurring in the premature infant requires IV therapy with nafcillin or oxacillin.

Some strains of *S. aureus* produce toxins that can cause **bullous lesions or scalded skin syndrome.** The cutaneous changes are due to local and systemic spread of toxin. Although blood cultures may be negative, IV antibiotics should be given (nafcillin or oxacillin) until the progression of disease stops and skin lesions are healing.

Pediatricians who diagnose infectious pustulosis in an infant under 2 weeks of age should report the case to the birth hospital; **epidemic outbreaks due to nosocomial acquisition in newborn nurseries** are often recognized in this way because the rash may not occur until after hospital discharge. This has become particularly important with the emergence of MRSA infections among infants <1 month in the community. When such outbreaks are recognized in the nursery or NICU, hospital infection control experts should be consulted. Appropriate steps may include surveillance cultures of staff members and newborns and cohorting of colonized infants.

3. Omphalitis. Omphalitis is characterized by erythema and/or induration of the periumbilical area with purulent discharge from the umbilical stump. The infection can progress to widespread abdominal wall cellulitis or necrotizing fasciitis; complications such as peritonitis, umbilical arteritis or phlebitis, hepatic vein thrombosis, and hepatic abscess have all been described. Responsible organisms include both gram-positive and gram-negative species. Treatment consists of a full sepsis evaluation (CBC, blood culture, LP) and empiric IV therapy with oxacillin or nafcillin and gentamicin. With serious disease progression, broader spectrum gram-negative coverage with a cephalosporin or piperacillin/tazobactam should be considered. As noted in section II.A, invasion of the umbilical stump by *C. tetani* under conditions of poor sanitation can result in neonatal tetanus in the infant of an unimmunized mother.

B. Conjunctivitis (ophthalmia neonatorum). This condition refers to inflammation of the conjunctiva within the first month of life. Causative agents include topical medications (chemical conjunctivitis), bacteria, and herpes simplex viruses. Chemical conjunctivitis is most commonly seen with silver nitrate eye prophylaxis, requires no specific treatment, and usually resolves within 48 hours. Bacterial causes include *Neisseria gonorrhoeae*; *Chlamydia trachomatis*; as well as staphylococci, streptococci, and gram-negative organisms. In the United States, where routine birth prophylaxis against ophthalmia neonatorum is practiced, the incidence of this disease is very low. In developing countries in the absence of prophylaxis, the incidence is 20% to 25% and remains a major cause of blindness.

1. Prophylaxis against infectious conjunctivitis. One percent silver nitrate solution (1 to 2 drops to each eye), 0.5% erythromycin ophthalmic ointment or 1% tetracycline ointment (1-cm strip to each eye), and 2.5% povidone-iodine solution (1 drop to each eye) administered within 1 hour of birth are all effective in the prevention of ophthalmia neonatorum. In a trial comparing the use of these three agents conducted in Kenya, povidone-iodine was shown to be slightly more effective against both *C. trachomatis* and other causes of infectious conjunctivitis, and equally effective against *N. gonorrhoeae* and *S. aureus*. Povidone-iodine was associated with less noninfectious conjunctivitis and is less costly than the other two agents; in addition, this agent is not associated with the development of bacterial resistance. However, an ophthalmic preparation of povidone-iodine solution is not currently available in the United States. In our institution, where most mothers receive prenatal care and the incidences of chlamydia and gonorrhea are low, we use erythromycin ointment. Silver nitrate or povidone-iodine is the preferred agent in areas where the incidence of penicillinase-producing *N. gonorrhoeae* is high.

2. *N. gonorrhoeae*. Pregnant women should be screened for *N. gonorrhoeae* as part of routine prenatal care. High-risk women or women without prenatal care should be screened at delivery. If a mother is known to have untreated *N. gonorrhoeae* infection, the infant should receive **ceftriaxone 25 to 50 mg/kg IV or IM (not to exceed 125 mg)**.

Gonococcal conjunctivitis presents with chemosis, lid edema, and purulent exudate beginning 1 to 4 days after birth. Clouding of the cornea or pan-ophthalmitis can occur. Gram stain and culture of conjunctival scrapings will confirm the diagnosis. The treatment of infants with un-complicated gonococcal conjunctivitis requires only a single dose of cef-triaxone (25 to 50 mg/kg IV or IM, not to exceed 125 mg). Additional topical treatment is unnecessary. However, infants with gonococcal conjunctivitis should be hospitalized and screened for invasive disease (i.e., sepsis, meningitis, arthritis). Scalp abscesses can result from internal fetal monitoring. Treatment of these complications is ceftriaxone (25 to 50 mg/kg/day IV or IM every 24 hours) or cefotaxime (25 mg/kg IV or IM every 12 hours) for 7 days (10 to 14 days for meningitis). The infant and mother should be screened for coincident chlamydial infection.

3. ***C. trachomatis.*** Pregnant women should be screened for ***C. trachomatis*** as part of routine prenatal care. Prophylaxis for infants born to moth-ers with untreated chlamydial infection is not indicated. Chlamydial conjunctivitis is the most common identified cause of infectious con-junctivitis in the United States. It presents with variable degrees of inflammation, yellow discharge, and eyelid swelling 5 to 14 days after birth. Conjunctival scarring can occur, although the cornea is usually not involved. DNA hybridization tests or shell vial culture are used to detect *Chlamydia* in conjunctival specimens. NAATs are commer-cially available and more sensitive than direct hybridization or culture methods and have largely replaced other methods in clinical practice. However, use of NAATs for nongenital specimens may be done with local verification of clinical laboratory standards because they are not currently FDA approved for detecting chlamydia in conjunctival speci-mens. Chlamydial conjunctivitis is treated with oral **erythromycin base or ethylsuccinate 40 mg/kg/day divided into four doses for 14 days**. Topical treatment alone is not adequate and is unnecessary when sys-temic therapy is given. An association of oral erythromycin therapy and infantile hypertrophic pyloric stenosis has been reported in infants younger than 6 weeks. Infants should be monitored for this condition. The efficacy of treatment is approximately 80%, and infants must be evaluated for treatment failure and the need for a second course of treat-ment. Infants should also be evaluated for the concomitant presence of chlamydial pneumonia. The treatment for pneumonia is the same as for conjunctivitis, in addition to necessary supportive respiratory care.

4. **Other bacterial conjunctivitis.** Other causes are generally diagnosed by culture of eye exudate. *S. aureus*, *E. coli*, and *Haemophilus influenzae* can cause conjunctivitis that is usually easily treated with local ophthalmic ointments (erythromycin or gentamicin) without complication. Very se-vere cases caused by *H. influenzae* may require parenteral treatment and evaluation for sepsis and meningitis. *P. aeruginosa* can cause a rare and devastating form of conjunctivitis that requires parenteral treatment.

C. **Pneumonia.** The diagnosis of **neonatal pneumonia** is challenging. It is dif-ficult to distinguish primary (occurring from birth) neonatal bacterial pneu-monia clinically from sepsis with respiratory compromise, or radiographically from other causes of respiratory distress (hyaline membrane disease, retained fetal lung fluid, meconium aspiration, amniotic fluid aspiration). Persis-tent focal opacifications on chest radiograph due to neonatal pneumonia are uncommon, and their presence should prompt some consideration of noninfectious causes of focal lung opacification (such as congenital cystic lesions or pulmonary sequestration). The causes of neonatal bacterial pneumonia are the same as for EOS, and antibiotic treatment is generally the same as for sepsis. The infant's baseline risk of infection, radiographic and laboratory studies, and most important, the clinical progression must all be taken into account when making the diagnosis of neonatal pneumonia.

The diagnosis of **nosocomial, or ventilator-associated pneumonia** in neonates who are ventilator dependent due to chronic lung disease or other illness, is equally challenging. Culture of tracheal secretions in infants who are chronically ventilated can yield a variety of organisms, including all the causes of EOS and LOS as well as (often antibiotic resistant) gram-negative organisms that are endemic within a particular NICU. A distinction must be made between colonization of the airway and true tracheitis or pneumonia. Culture results must be taken together with the infant's respiratory and systemic condition, as well as radiographic and laboratory studies when making the diagnosis of nosocomial pneumonia.

Ureaplasma urealyticum deserves mention with respect to chronically ventilated infants. This mycoplasmal organism frequently colonizes the vagina of pregnant women and has been associated with chorioamnionitis, spontaneous abortion and premature delivery, and infection of the premature infant. Infection with *Ureaplasma* has been studied as a contributing factor to the development of chronic lung disease, but the role of the organism and the value of diagnosis and treatment are unclear and controversial. *Ureaplasma* requires special culture conditions and will grow within 2 to 5 days. PCR-based diagnostics have been developed but are not widely available. It will not be identified on routine bacterial culture. It is sensitive to erythromycin, but is difficult to eradicate, and few data are available on the dosing, treatment duration, and efficacy of treatment when this organism is found in tracheal secretions. There is no current evidence to support the use of *Ureaplasma* treatment to prevent bronchopulmonary dysplasia (BPD).

D. UTI. UTIs may occur secondary to bacteremia, or bacteremia may occur secondary to primary UTI. UTI is a common cause of infection among febrile infants <3 months of age. The incidence is highest among uncircumcised males. Among community infants who present with febrile UTI, the prevalence of high-grade (grade 5) vesicoureteral reflux (VUR) diagnosed on subsequent vesicourethrocytogram (VCUG) is approximately 1%. The incidence of UTI among VLBW infants in the NICU is much less well documented. Evaluation for infection in this population often excludes urine culture, focusing on central line, pulmonary, and GI sources of infection.

The most common causative organisms are gram-negative, such as *E. coli*, but enterococci and staphylococci can also cause UTI, especially among VLBW NICU infants. Culture of urine is not routinely recommended as part of the evaluation for EOS but is an essential part of the evaluation for LOS (see section I.N). The most common presenting symptoms in term and older preterm infants are fever, lethargy, and poor feeding; younger preterm infants will present as for LOS. Diagnosis is made by urinalysis and urine culture. Culture of urine obtained from a bag collection or diaper is of little value because it will commonly be contaminated with skin and fecal flora. Specimens should be obtained by bladder catheterization or SPA with sterile technique. Ultrasound guidance can be useful in performing SPA in the VLBW infant. Empiric treatment in term and preterm infants is as for LOS (see section I.J); antibiotic choice and treatment duration is guided by blood, urine, and CSF culture results. If the urine culture **alone** is positive in a term infant, treatment is completed with oral therapy once the infant is afebrile. Treatment duration in the absence of a positive blood or CSF culture is 10 to 14 days.

The American Academy of Pediatrics recommends that infants with UTI undergo renal ultrasound after a first episode of UTI. VCUG imaging to identify any underlying anatomic or functional abnormalities (i.e., VUR) that may have contributed to the development of the UTI is recommended if the renal ultrasound is abnormal, or after a second episode of UTI. Traditionally, infants have received UTI prophylaxis with amoxicillin (10 to 20 mg/kg once per day) after completing UTI treatment until imaging studies are performed and have continued with prophylaxis if VUR is documented. Several recent meta-analyses have found little to no value in antibiotic prophylaxis for low-grade VUR, although it remains widely used and is recommended only for high-grade (grade 5) VUR.

E. **Osteomyelitis and septic arthritis.** These focal infections are rare in newborns and may result from hematogenous seeding in the setting of bacteremia, or direct extension from a skin source of infection. The most common organisms are *S. aureus*, GBS, and gram-negative organisms including *N. gonorrhoeae.* Symptoms include localized erythema, swelling, and apparent pain or lack of spontaneous movement of the involved extremity. The hip, knee, and wrist are commonly involved in septic arthritis, and the femur, humerus, tibia, radius, and maxilla are the most common bone sites of infection. The evaluation should be as for sepsis, including blood, urine, and CSF culture, and culture of any purulent skin lesions. Needle aspiration of an infected joint is sometimes possible, and plain film and ultrasound can aid in diagnosis. Empiric treatment is with nafcillin or oxacillin and gentamicin, and/or vancomycin if MRSA is a concern, and is later tailored to any identified organisms. Joint infections commonly require surgical drainage; material can be sent for Gram stain and culture at surgery. Duration of therapy is 3 to 4 weeks. Significant disability can result from joint or growth plate damage.

Suggested Readings

Benjamin DK Jr, Hudak ML, Duara S, et al. Effect of fluconazole prophylaxis on candidiasis and mortality in premature infants: a randomized clinical trial. *JAMA* 2014;311(17):1742–1749.

Bizzarro MJ, Sabo B, Noonan M, et al. A quality improvement initiative to reduce central line-associated bloodstream infections in a neonatal intensive care unit. *Infect Control Hosp Epidemiol* 2010;31(3):241–248.

Escobar GJ, Puopolo KM, Wi S, et al. Stratification of risk of early-onset sepsis in newborns ≥ 34 weeks' gestation. *Pediatrics* 2014;133(1):30–36.

Isenberg SJ, Apt L, Wood M. A controlled trial of povidone-iodine as prophylaxis against ophthalmia neonatorum. *N Engl J Med* 1995;332(9):562–566.

Kaufman D, Boyle R, Hazen KC, et al. Fluconazole prophylaxis against fungal colonization and infection in preterm infants. *N Engl J Med* 2001;345(23):1660–1666.

Newman TB, Puopolo KM, Wi S, et al. Interpreting complete blood counts soon after birth in newborns at risk for sepsis. *Pediatrics* 2010;126(5):903–909.

Olsen R, Greisen G, Schrøder M, et al. Prophylactic probiotics for preterm infants: a systematic review and meta-analysis of observational studies. *Neonatology* 2016;109:105–112.

Stoll BJ, Hansen N, Fanaroff AA, et al. Late-onset sepsis in very low birth weight neonates: the experience of the NICHD Neonatal Research Network. *Pediatrics* 2002;110(2, pt 1):285–291.

Weston EJ, Pondo T, Lewis MM, et al. The burden of invasive early-onset neonatal sepsis in the United States, 2005–2008. *Pediatr Infect Dis J* 2011;30: 937–941.

50 Congenital Toxoplasmosis

Galit Holzmann-Pazgal

KEY POINTS

- Toxoplasmosis can be acquired without exposure to cats via ingestion of infected oocysts in contaminated food or water or tissue cysts in undercooked/raw meat.
- In the United States, 500 to 5,000 infants are born with congenital toxoplasmosis annually.
- The risk of intrauterine infection increases with gestational age, but the effects on the fetus are more severe with fetal infection occurring earlier in gestation.
- Congenital toxoplasmosis can occur secondary to acute maternal infection during pregnancy and also due to reactivation of prior infection in an immunocompromised mother.
- Treatment of congenital toxoplasmosis for 1-year duration has been associated with prevention of sequela and improved outcomes.

I. **EPIDEMIOLOGY.** *Toxoplasma gondii*, an obligate, intracellular protozoan parasite, is an important human pathogen, especially for the fetus, newborn, and immunocompromised patient.

  A. **Transmission.** *T. gondii* exists in three infectious forms: tachyzoite, tissue cysts containing bradyzoites, and oocysts containing sporozoites. The tachyzoite is the form responsible for symptoms during acute infection, whereas the tissue cyst is responsible for latent infection. The only definitive host of *T. gondii* is the cat. When infected, cats are usually asymptomatic. Intermediate hosts include all warm-blooded animals and humans. Tissue cysts form in the intermediate host, particularly in brain, eye, and muscle. The cysts are infectious. Cats are infected by ingesting cysts from an infected intermediate host, ultimately shedding oocysts from their intestinal lumen into the environment. Cats can shed up to 10 million oocysts a day for 20 to 24 days following initial infection. Sporulated oocysts remain infective in soil for up to 18 months. Other animals become infected by ingesting the oocysts resulting in tissue cysts containing viable organisms predominantly in muscle and brain.

  T. gondii infection can be acquired via ingestion of infected oocysts from the environment (contaminated food or water), ingestion of tissue cysts from raw or undercooked meat (most common in developed world), or via transplacental transmission (congenital infection). Risk factors associated with acute infection in the United States include eating raw ground beef and lamb; eating locally produced, cured, dried, or smoked meat; working with meat; drinking unpasteurized goat's milk; and having three or more kittens. Raw oysters and clams have also been associated with transmission. Untreated water has been reported to be the source of major outbreaks around the world. The prevalence of *T. gondii* varies broadly among different countries and geographic areas. The presence of serum antibodies to *T. gondii* increases with age. 22.5% of people ≥ 12 years of age in the United States have been infected with *T. gondii*.

The reported prevalence of *T. gondii* antibodies in women of child-bearing age ranges from 10% to 80% worldwide. Women without antibodies are at risk for acute toxoplasmosis during pregnancy.

Seroconversion during pregnancy also varies by geographic location. Rates range from 1.5% in France, a high-prevalence country, to 0.17% in Norway, a low-prevalence country. Incidence of maternal seroconversion during pregnancy in the United States is estimated at 0.2% to 1%. The rate of mother-to-child transmission in the United States is 50% to 60% for mothers not treated during pregnancy and 25% to 30% for those treated.

B. Incidence. The reported incidence of congenital toxoplasmosis in the United States has decreased during the last 20 years from a high of 20 per 10,000 to 1 per 10,000. In the United States, an estimated 500 to 5,000 infants are born each year with congenital toxoplasmosis.

II. PATHOPHYSIOLOGY

A. Postnatal infection. Normal children and adults are susceptible to acute infection if they lack specific antibody to the organism. Both humoral and cell-mediated immunity are important in the control of infection. The majority of *T. gondii* infections in immunocompetent hosts are asymptomatic. Possible mild symptoms include lymphadenopathy, malaise, fever, and headache. More severe symptoms such as encephalitis, myocarditis, pneumonia, and hepatitis are less common. Chorioretinitis has also been reported in postnatally acquired cases. In immunocompetent hosts, infection with *T. gondii* imparts lifelong immunity.

B. Congenital infection. Congenital infection is most commonly secondary to acute maternal infection during pregnancy and less commonly due to reactivation of previous infection in an immunocompromised mother. It should also be considered in women infected within 3 months prior to conception. Parasitemia in the mother leads to placental invasion by the parasite and subsequent passage into the fetal circulation and tissues resulting in fetal infection.

The risk of intrauterine infection increases with gestational age. One analysis demonstrated the risk of transmission to the fetus to be 6% at 13 weeks, 40% at 26 weeks, and 72% at 36 weeks. However, the effects on the fetus are more severe with maternal infection occurring earlier in pregnancy. Sixty-one percent of infants will have clinical manifestations when seroconversion occurs at 13 weeks' gestation in contrast to about 9% at 36 weeks. Infection early in pregnancy may result in intrauterine fetal demise and spontaneous abortion. Nearly all infants infected during the third trimester will be asymptomatic accounting for 67% to 80% of prenatally infected infants.

Immunocompetent women with prior toxoplasma infection are protected from transmitting infection to the fetus. Immunocompromised pregnant patients previously infected with *T. gondii* may transmit infection to the fetus if their immune system is unable to suppress the parasite (i.e., HIV infection, lymphoma, immunosuppressive therapy).

III. MATERNAL/FETAL INFECTION

A. Clinical manifestations

1. Maternal infection is asymptomatic in more than 90% of women. However, symptoms can include fatigue, painless lymphadenopathy, and chorioretinitis.

2. Fetal findings on ultrasound (US) include hydrocephalus, brain, splenic and hepatic calcifications, hepatosplenomegaly, and ascites.

B. Diagnosis

1. **Recommended maternal tests**
   a. Screening: serum immunoglobulin M (IgM) and immunoglobulin G (IgG)
   i. Detection and quantification of antibodies in pregnant women can determine if and potentially when infection has occurred. Serology performed earlier in pregnancy (i.e., first trimester) is more helpful in determining if infection was acquired during pregnancy than serology drawn after 18 weeks' gestation.
   ii. Toxoplasma IgG and IgM: Initial testing can be done at a non-reference commercial lab. Negative results or positive IgG and negative IgM (old infection) should be reliable to rule out infection during current pregnancy if done before the third trimester. A positive or equivocal IgM should be confirmed at reference laboratory (Palo Alto Medical Foundation Toxoplasma Serology Laboratory. www.pamf.org/serology.
   iii. IgM can be positive 2 weeks after infection and peaks in 1 month. It typically becomes negative within 6 to 9 months but can persist for more than a year. A reference lab can help determine if a patient with a positive IgM acquired infection recently or in the distant past.
   b. Confirmatory testing of a positive or equivocal IgM test at a reference laboratory: IgG, IgM, IgA, and IgE
   A series of IgG tests can help differentiate acute versus remote infection.
   i. Toxoplasma IgG avidity test used in conjunction with differential agglutination (AC/HS) test. High avidity antibodies develop at least 12 to 16 weeks after infection. If positive during the first months of pregnancy, they would indicate that infection

occurred prior to conception. AC/HS compares IgG titers for sera against formalin (HS) versus acetone (AC) fixed tachyzoites. AC antigens detect acute IgG antibodies formed only during the acute stage of infection.

ii. Immunoglobulin A (IgA) and immunoglobulin E (IgE) antibodies become undetectable earlier than IgM antibodies.

2. Fetal testing

a. US is recommended monthly in women suspected of having acute infection acquired during or just before gestation. Fetal abnormalities detected include hydrocephalus, brain, splenic and hepatic calcifications, splenomegaly, and ascites.

b. Amniotic fluid polymerase chain reaction (PCR) is recommended to diagnose fetal infection in cases when there is serologic evidence of acute infection or infection acquired during pregnancy cannot be ruled out, there is evidence of fetal abnormality on US, or pregnant woman is significantly immunocompromised with risk of reactivation. The optimal time for performance of an amniotic fluid PCR is at 18 weeks' gestation or later. Gestational age at time of maternal infection significantly influences the sensitivity and negative predictive value of the PCR testing. Sensitivity of PCR testing is greatest when maternal infection occurs between 17 and 21 weeks (93% sensitive) as opposed to earlier. High parasite DNA levels can be found in cases in which infection occurred earlier in gestation or sequelae are more severe. A negative amniotic fluid PCR does not rule out fetal infection with exception if maternal infection occurred at <7 weeks (100% negative predictive value [NPV]) because the accuracy range is wide and parasite transmission from the mother to the fetus may be delayed.

C. Treatment. For maternal infection confirmed or suspected to have occurred at <18 weeks' gestation, treatment with spiramycin is recommended in an effort to prevent placental transmission of toxoplasmosis. For mothers with confirmed or acquired infection at ≥18 weeks' gestation or those with positive amniotic fluid PCR or abnormal US findings of congenital toxoplasmosis, treatment with pyrimethamine, sulfadiazine, and folinic acid is recommended in an effort to prevent and treat fetal infection. Treatment should be instituted for mothers with acute infections and immunocompromised mothers with evidence of distant infection.

1. Spiramycin can potentially prevent placental transmission of toxoplasma but does not cross the placenta so will not treat the fetus. There is some controversy to its efficacy because no clearly designed prospective trials have been performed. Incidence of congenital infection was decreased by up to 60% in some retrospective studies. This macrolide antibiotic reduces or delays vertical transmission to the fetus through high placental drug levels. Spiramycin should be continued until delivery in patients with negative amniotic fluid PCR because of the theoretical risk of fetal transmission occurring later in pregnancy from maternal infection acquired earlier in gestation. Spiramycin is available in the United States as an Investigational New Drug through the U.S. Food and Drug Administration.

2. **Pyrimethamine, sulfadiazine, and folinic acid.** This drug combination is used in an effort to treat fetal infection and/or prevent transmission to the fetus when maternal infection occurred at ≥18 weeks' gestation. Pyrimethamine has teratogenic potential and should not be used prior to 18 weeks' gestation. It can cause bone marrow suppression, so patients should have complete blood count (CBC) monitoring during therapy.

3. For women with infection acquired ≥6 months before gestation, no treatment is recommended with exception of women who are immunosuppressed.

IV. NEONATAL INFECTION

A. **Clinical manifestations. There are four recognized patterns of presentation for congenital toxoplasmosis.**

1. **Subclinical/asymptomatic infection.** Most infants with congenital toxoplasmosis (70% to 90%) do not have overt signs of infection at birth. If untreated, a large proportion will later demonstrate visual, central nervous system (CNS) deficits, including hearing impairment, learning disabilities, or mental retardation several months to years later.

2. **Neonatal symptomatic disease.** Signs of congenital disease at birth include maculopapular rash, lymphadenopathy, hepatosplenomegaly, jaundice, pneumonitis, diarrhea, hypothermia, petechiae, and thrombocytopenia. CNS disease symptoms include cerebral calcifications, hydrocephalus, seizures, cerebrospinal fluid (CSF) abnormalities, meningoencephalitis, and chorioretinitis.

3. **Delayed onset** is most often seen with premature infants and occurs within the first 3 months of age. It can behave like neonatal symptomatic disease.

4. **Sequelae or relapse in infancy through adolescence of a previously untreated infection.** Chorioretinitis develops in up to 85% of adolescents/young adults with previously untreated congenital infection.

B. **Differential diagnosis.** The clinical and laboratory findings are common to congenital infections caused by rubella, cytomegalovirus, syphilis, neonatal herpes simplex virus, HIV, and lymphocytic choriomeningitis virus (LCMV). Other disorders to be considered include hepatitis B, varicella, bacterial sepsis, hemolytic diseases, metabolic disorders, immune thrombocytopenia, histiocytosis, and congenital leukemia.

C. **Diagnosis.** All neonates suspected of having congenital toxoplasmosis based on symptoms, maternal acute *T. gondii* infection during pregnancy, or maternal HIV with a history of chronic *T. gondii* infection should be evaluated. Diagnosis may be made by serology, PCR, and less commonly by pathology. Currently, the vast majority of states in the United States do not screen or report congenital toxoplasmosis.

1. **IgG, IgM, IgA.** Testing should be performed in a reference laboratory with special expertise in toxoplasma serologic assays (i.e., Palo Alto Medical Foundation Toxoplasma Serology Laboratory). Sabin-Feldman

dye test (IgG), IgM immunosorbent agglutination assay (ISAGA), and IgA enzyme–linked immunosorbent assay (ELISA) should be obtained from the infant. In addition, serologic testing should also be performed in the mother after birth in an effort to determine if she could have been infected during gestation.

a. IgG appears within 1 to 2 weeks, peaks at 1 to 2 months, and persists throughout life. Transplacental IgG antibody disappears by 6 to 12 months of age. A positive IgG at 12 months of age is diagnostic of congenital toxoplasmosis.

b. Positive IgM or IgA antibody at least 10 days after birth is also diagnostic. Data from the Palo Alto Medical Foundation Toxoplasma Serology Laboratory database demonstrated that in infants with untreated congenital toxoplasmosis, IgM was positive 86.6% of the time, IgA 77.4% of the time, and when both IgM and IgA were taken into consideration, 93.3% were positive.

c. In congenital toxoplasmosis, antibody production varies significantly and is affected by treatment.

2. PCR. Blood, CSF, and urine should be tested in infants with suspected infection. A positive PCR is diagnostic of infection. When CSF PCR results were combined with IgM and IgA antibody results for diagnosis of congenital toxoplasmosis, sensitivity for diagnosis was increased. Ideally, samples should be obtained prior to starting therapy.

3. **Other** tests. CSF cell count. CSF eosinophilia and/or elevated protein can be seen.

4. Pathologic findings. *T. gondii* specific immunoperoxidase staining can be performed on any tissue. Presence of extracellular antigens and surrounding inflammatory response are diagnostic.

5. Ophthalmology exam at birth and every 3 months until 18 months of age followed by every 6 to 12 months until 18 years old

6. Screening for hearing loss with auditory brainstem response or otoacoustic emissions by 3 months of age. Full audiologic evaluation by 24 months of age.

7. Routine labs. Abnormal CBC, liver enzymes, and bilirubin levels can also be seen with disseminated disease.

8. Brain imaging. Head computed tomography (CT) scan without contrast is the preferred study. One study reported a clear relationship between the lesions on CT scan, neurologic signs, and the date of maternal infection.

a. CT scan may detect calcifications not seen by ultrasonography. They may be single or multiple.

b. Hydrocephalus is usually due to periaqueductal obstruction. Massive hydrocephalus may develop in as quickly as 1 week.

9. Multidisciplinary consultation is usually helpful for patient management. Specialty consultation is typically required from the following:

a. Infectious diseases

b. Ophthalmology

c. Neurosurgery

d. Neurodevelopmental pediatrics

D. Treatment

1. Medications. Combination therapy for 1-year duration has been associated with decreased incidence of neurologic, cognitive, auditory and retinal sequelae; resolution of acute symptoms; and improved outcomes. Patients should be weighed weekly and dosing adjusted accordingly. Monitoring for toxicity should occur weekly as well. Improved outcomes occur if infants are treated in the first year of life. Infected newborns who are not treated or who receive short courses of treatment have poor outcomes including high risk of developing new chorioretinal lesions later in life along with other long-term sequelae.

   a. Pyrimethamine 2 mg/kg once daily for 2 days, then 1 mg/kg once daily for 6 months, then 1 mg/kg three times a week (every other day) to complete 1 year of therapy

   b. Sulfadiazine 50 mg/kg every 12 hours for 1 year

   c. Folinic acid 10 mg three times a week, administered until 1 week after completing pyrimethamine

   d. Prednisone (0.5 mg/kg every 12 hours) may be added if CSF protein exceeds 1 g/dL or active chorioretinitis with lesions very close to macula.

2. Adverse events

   a. Most common adverse effect of pyrimethamine (a dihydrofolate reductase inhibitor) is neutropenia. Also possible are thrombocytopenia and anemia. CBC should be monitored weekly. Temporary cessation of pyrimethamine may be necessary if absolute neutrophil count (ANC) falls below 500.

   b. Adverse effects of sulfadiazine include hemolysis in infants with glucose-6-phosphate dehydrogenase (G6PD) deficiency, bone marrow suppression, renal failure, and hypersensitivity. Alternative therapy for infants who develop allergy to sulfadiazine includes clindamycin.

   c. The same treatment regimen is recommended for infants born to mothers infected with both HIV and *T. gondii*. However, combining these agents with antiretrovirals such as zidovudine may increase bone marrow toxicity.

3. Ventricular shunting for hydrocephalus is recommended when necessary.

V. OUTCOMES. The National Collaborative Congenital Toxoplasmosis (NCCT) study has reported outcomes in a series of children with congenital infection. Treatment for 1-year duration significantly improved outcomes for many congenitally infected children. All children who died had severe infection at birth.

A. Chorioretinitis. Ninety-one percent of children with asymptomatic or mild neurologic disease at birth did not develop new eye lesions after treatment. Sixty-four percent of children with moderate or severe neurologic disease at birth did not develop new or recurrent lesions. With treatment, chorioretinitis usually resolved within 1 to 2 weeks and did not relapse during therapy. Relapse after treatment may occur, often during adolescence. Visual impairment is a prominent sequela, even with treatment, in 85% of patients who had severe disease at birth and 15% of neonates with mild or asymptomatic disease.

B. Neurologic outcomes. All neurologically asymptomatic or mildly affected patients at birth who were treated for 1 year had normal cognitive function, neurologic function, and hearing. More than 72% of those with moderate to severe neurologic disease who were treated for 1 year had normal cognitive or neurologic outcomes, and none had hearing loss.

C. These outcomes are significantly improved as compared to previous studies of untreated patients or patients treated for short duration.

Suggested Readings

American Academy of Pediatrics. Toxoplasmosis. In: Kimberlin DW, Brady MT, Jackson MA, et al., eds. *Red Book: 2015 Report of the Committee on Infectious Diseases*. 30th ed. Elk Grove Village, IL: American Academy of Pediatrics; 2015:787–795.

Boyer K, Hill D, Mui E, et al. Unrecognized ingestion of *Toxoplasma gondii* oocysts leads to congenital toxoplasmosis and causes epidemics in North America. *Clin Infect Dis* 2011;53:1081–1089.

Dannemann BR, Vaughan WC, Thulliez P, et al. Differential agglutination test for diagnosis of recently acquired infection with *Toxoplasma gondii*. *J Clin Microbiol* 1990;28:1928–1933.

McLeod R, Boyer K, Karrison T, et al. Outcome of treatment for congenital toxoplasmosis, 1981–2004: the National Collaborative Chicago-based, Congenital Toxoplasmosis Study. *Clin Infect Dis* 2006;42:1383–1394.

Moncada PA, Montoya JG. Toxoplasmosis in the fetus and newborn: an update on prevalence, diagnosis and treatment. *Expert Rev Anti Infect Ther* 2012;10: 815–828.

Montoya JG, Remington JS. Management of *Toxoplasma gondii* infection during pregnancy. *Clin Infect Dis* 2008;47:554–566.

Olariu TR, Remington JS, McLeod R, et al. Severe congenital toxoplasmosis in the United States: clinical and serologic findings in untreated infants. *Pediatr Infect Dis J* 2011;30:1056–1061.

Olariu TR, Remington JS, Montoya JG. Polymerase chain reaction in cerebrospinal fluid for the diagnosis of congenital toxoplasmosis. *Pediatr Infect Dis J* 2014;33:566–570.

Tenter AM, Heckertoh AR, Weiss LM. *Toxoplasma gondii*: from animals to humans. *Int J Parasitol* 2000;30:1217–1258.

Wong SY, Remington JS. Toxoplasmosis in pregnancy. *Clin Infect Dis* 1994;18: 853–862.

Online Resources

Centers for Disease Control and Prevention. **http://www.cdc.gov/parasites/ toxoplasmosis/epi.html**. Accessed July 2015.

Toxoplasma Serology Laboratory at the Palo Alto Medical Foundation Research Institute, Ames Bldg, 795 El Camino Real, Palo Alto, CA 94301-2302 (Tel: [650] 853-4828, Fax [650] 614-3292; Email: toxolab@pamf.org; Web: **http://www.pamf.org/serology/**)

51 Syphilis
Gloria Heresi

KEY POINTS

- Prevention of congenital syphilis depends on the identification and adequate treatment of pregnant women with syphilis.
- Trends in congenital syphilis usually follow trends in primary and secondary syphilis among women, with a lag of 1 to 2 years.
- The most important risk factors for congenital syphilis are lack of prenatal health care and maternal illicit drug use.
- Women with syphilis should be tested for HIV and other sexually transmitted diseases (STDs).
- Centers for Disease Control and Prevention (CDC) 2011 reaffirmed that nontreponemal tests be used to screen for syphilis and that treponemal testing be used to confirm syphilis.
- Parenteral Penicillin G remains the preferred drug for prevention and treatment of congenital syphilis.

I. **INTRODUCTION.** Syphilis is a sexually transmitted infection caused by the spirochete *Treponema pallidum*. Pregnant women with syphilis can transmit it through the placenta to the fetus or at birth to the neonate. Congenital infection can have severe consequences to the fetus and newborn including perinatal death, premature delivery, low birth weight, congenital anomalies, active congenital syphilis, and/or long-term sequela such as deafness and neurologic impairment. Prevention of congenital syphilis depends on the identification and adequate treatment of pregnant women with syphilis.

II. **CLINICAL CLASSIFICATION**

A. **Congenital syphilis** results from transplacental passage of *T. pallidum* or contact with infectious lesions during birth. The risk of transmission to the fetus correlates largely with the duration of maternal infection—the more recent the maternal infection, the more likely transmission to the fetus. During the primary and secondary stages of syphilis, the likelihood of transmission from an untreated woman to her fetus is extremely high, approaching 100%. After the secondary stage, the likelihood of transmission to the fetus declines steadily until it reaches approximately 10% to 30% in late latency. Transplacental transmission of *T. pallidum* can occur throughout pregnancy.

1. **Clinical presentation.** Congenital infection may result in stillbirth, hydrops fetalis, prematurity, or a wide spectrum of symptoms and signs. Most affected infants will be asymptomatic at birth, but clinical signs

usually develop within the first 3 months of life. The most common signs of early congenital syphilis (<2 years old) include hepatosplenomegaly, rash, condylomata lata, watery nasal discharge (snuffles), jaundice, anemia or edema, and skeletal abnormalities (osteochondritis, periostitis, pseudoparalysis). Late congenital syphilis in an untreated older child (>2 years old) may have stigmata with bony changes (frontal bossing, short maxilla, high palatal arch, Hutchinson teeth, saddle nose), interstitial keratitis, and sensorineural deafness, among others.

2. **Case definition.** The Centers for Disease Control and Prevention (CDC) 2015 case definition for congenital syphilis includes the following:
   Laboratory criteria for diagnosis
   Demonstration of *T. pallidum* by darkfield microscopy, polymerase chain reaction (PCR), or immunohistochemical (IHC) test, or special stains of specimens from lesions, placenta, umbilical cord, or autopsy material.

3. **Case classification**
   Probable
   Infant whose mother had untreated or inadequately treated syphilis at delivery, regardless of signs in the infant, or an
   a. Infant or child who has a reactive nontreponemal test for syphilis (venereal disease research laboratory [VDRL], rapid plasma reagin [RPR] or equivalent) and any one of the following:
   b. Any evidence of congenital syphilis on physical examination
   c. Any evidence of congenital syphilis on radiographs of long bones
   d. A reactive cerebrospinal fluid (CSF) VDRL test
   e. An elevated CSF cell count or protein (without other cause)
   Confirmed
   Case that is laboratory confirmed

4. **Differential diagnosis**
   Symptoms and signs of congenital syphilis in neonates are similar to those of other neonatal infections, including toxoplasmosis, herpes simplex, cytomegalovirus, rubella, and neonatal sepsis. Clinical data from mother, physical findings, and laboratory tests can help to make the diagnosis.

B. **Maternal infection** can be divided into three stages.

1. First stage or primary syphilis is manifested by one or more chancres (painless indurated ulcers) at the site of inoculation, typically the genitalia, anus, or mouth. It is often accompanied by regional lymphadenopathy. Lesions appear around 3 weeks after exposure and heal spontaneously in a few weeks.

2. Second stage or secondary syphilis is a disseminated process that occurs in around 25% of untreated patients, 3 to 6 weeks after the appearance of the chancre. The secondary stage is characterized by a polymorphic rash, most commonly maculopapular, generalized, and involving the palms and soles, sparing the face. Sore throat, fever, headache, diffuse lymphadenopathy, myalgias, arthralgias, alopecia, condylomata lata, and mucous membrane plaques may also be present. The symptoms resolve without treatment in 3 to 12 weeks, leaving the person completely asymptomatic. A latent period follows. Most women present at this stage.
   a. Latent syphilis is defined as "the period after infection" when patients are seroreactive but demonstrate no clinical manifestations of disease.

b. Early latent syphilis refers to infection <1 year.
c. Late latent syphilis if initial infection is >1 year or indeterminate.

3. Tertiary stage or tertiary syphilis usually occurs 4 to 12 years after the secondary stage in about one-third of untreated patients and is characterized by gummata, cardiovascular syphilis, especially inflammation of the great vessels, or neurosyphilis. These lesions are thought to be due to a pronounced immunologic reaction.

Neurosyphilis may occur at any stage of the disease especially in HIV patients and in neonates with congenital syphilis. Early manifestations include syphilitic meningitis, uveitis, and neurovascular disease. Late manifestations include dementia, posterior column disease (tabes dorsalis), and seizures, among others.

III. EPIDEMIOLOGY. Trends in congenital syphilis usually follow trends in primary and secondary syphilis among women, with a lag of 1 to 2 years.

CDC reported that the rate of primary and secondary syphilis among women declined 95.4% (from 17.3 to 0.8 cases per 100,000 females) during 1990 to 2004. And the rate of congenital syphilis declined by 92.4% (from a peak of 107.6 cases to 8.2 cases per 100,000 live births) during 1991 to 2005. Rates of both female primary and secondary and congenital syphilis increased during 2005 to 2008. During 2008 to 2012, rates of both female primary and secondary and congenital syphilis declined (from 1.5 to 0.9 cases per 100,000 population and from 10.5 to 8.4 cases per 100,000 live births, respectively). Rates of primary and secondary syphilis in women remained unchanged (0.9 cases), but rates of congenital syphilis increased (to 8.7 cases) during 2013.

The most important risk factors for congenital syphilis are lack of prenatal health care and maternal illicit drug use, particularly cocaine. Clinical scenarios that contribute to the occurrence of congenital syphilis include lack of prenatal care; no serologic test for syphilis (STS) performed during pregnancy; a negative STS in the first trimester, without repeat test later in pregnancy; a negative maternal STS around the time of delivery in a woman who was recently infected with syphilis but had not converted her STS yet; laboratory error in reporting STS results; delay in treatment of a pregnant woman identified as having syphilis; and failure of treatment in an infected pregnant woman.

IV. DIAGNOSIS OF SYPHILIS. Effective prevention and detection of congenital syphilis depends on the identification of syphilis in pregnant women and, therefore, on the routine serologic screening of pregnant women during the first prenatal visit. CDC recommends additional testing at 28 weeks' gestation and again at delivery for women who are at increased risk or live in communities with increased prevalence for syphilis infection. Routine screening of newborn sera or umbilical cord blood is not recommended because it does not prevent symptomatic congenital syphilis. No mother or newborn infant should leave the hospital without maternal serologic status having been documented at least once during pregnancy, and preferably again at delivery.

A. Serologic tests for syphilis

1. Nontreponemal tests include the RPR card test, the VDRL slide test, the unheated serum reagin (USR), and the toluidine red unheated serum test (TRUST). These tests measure antibody directed against a lipoidal antigen from *T. pallidum* and/or its interaction with host tissues. These antibodies give quantitative results, allowing establishment of a baseline titer, which allows evaluation of recent infection and response to treatment. Titers usually rise with each new infection and fall after effective treatment. A sustained fourfold decrease in titer of the nontreponemal test with treatment demonstrates adequate therapy; a similar increase after treatment suggests reinfection.

Nontreponemal tests will be positive in approximately 80% of cases of primary syphilis, nearly 100% of cases of secondary syphilis, and 75% of cases of latent and tertiary syphilis. In secondary syphilis, the RPR or VDRL test result is usually positive in a titer >1:16. In the first attack of primary syphilis, the RPR or VDRL test will usually become nonreactive 1 year after treatment, whereas in secondary syphilis, the test will usually become nonreactive approximately 2 years after treatment. In latent or tertiary syphilis, the RPR or VDRL test may become nonreactive 4 or 5 years after treatment or may never turn completely nonreactive. A cause of false-negative nontreponemal tests is the prozone phenomenon, a negative or weakly positive reaction that occurs with very high antibody concentrations. In this case, dilution of the serum will result in a positive test.

In 1% of cases, a positive RPR or VDRL result is not caused by syphilis. This has been called a biologic false-positive (BFP) reaction and is probably related to tissue damage from various causes. Rarely, BFPs are seen as a result of pregnancy alone. Patients with BFPs usually have low titers (1:8 or less) and nonreactive treponemal tests. Patients with systemic lupus erythematosus may have a positive RPR or VDRL test result. The titer is usually 1:8 or less. Nontreponemal test results may be falsely negative in early primary syphilis, latent acquired syphilis of long duration, and late congenital syphilis.

A reactive nontreponemal test positive in patients with classical symptoms indicates a presumptive diagnosis; however, any positive nontreponemal test should be confirmed by one of the specific treponemal test to exclude a false-positive test result.

2. **Treponemal tests** include the fluorescent treponemal antibody absorption test (FTA-ABS), the *T. pallidum* particle agglutination (TP-PA) test, and enzyme immunoassay (EIA). Although these tests are more specific than nontreponemal tests, they are also more expensive and labor-intensive and are therefore not used for screening. Rather, they are used to confirm positive nontreponemal tests. The treponemal tests correlate poorly with disease activity and usually remain positive for life, even after successful therapy, and therefore should not be used to assess treatment response.

In populations of low disease prevalence, treponemal tests can be used for screening, utilizing a rapid test or EIA format. Then, all positive patients would either be treated presumptively because the serious consequences of untreated infection far outweigh the effect of overtreatment or have a follow-up RPR or VDRL to determine if they have active infection before treatment. This "reverse sequence screening" approach is associated with high rates of false-positive results, and in 2011, the CDC reaffirmed that nontreponemal tests be used to screen for syphilis and that treponemal testing be used to confirm syphilis as the cause of nontreponemal reactivity. False-positive treponemal tests occur occasionally, particularly in other spirochetal diseases such as Lyme disease, yaws, pinta, leptospirosis, and rat-bite fever; nontreponemal tests should be negative in these situations. Also, in some cases where antibodies to DNA are present, such as in systemic lupus erythematosus, rheumatoid arthritis, polyarteritis, and other autoimmune diseases, a false-positive FTA-ABS test result may occur.

B. Neurosyphilis. CSF abnormalities in patients with neurosyphilis include increased protein concentration, increased white blood cell (WBC) count, and/or a reactive CSF VDRL test. The CSF VDRL is highly specific but is insensitive. Therefore, a positive CSF VDRL test result is diagnostic of neurosyphilis, but a negative CSF VDRL test result does not exclude neurosyphilis. The FTA-ABS test is recommended by some experts for CSF testing because it is more sensitive than the VDRL test; however, contamination with blood during the lumbar puncture may result in a false-positive CSF FTA-ABS test result. A negative CSF FTA-ABS test result is good evidence against neurosyphilis. The RPR test should not be used for CSF testing.

V. EVALUATION AND TREATMENT OF INFANTS FOR CONGENITAL SYPHILIS.

No newborn should be discharged from the hospital until the mother's serologic syphilis status has been determined at least once during pregnancy and also at delivery. Screening of newborn serum or cord blood in place of screening maternal blood is not recommended because of potential false-negative results.

A. Any infant born to a mother with a reactive nontreponemal test confirmed by a treponemal test should be evaluated with the following:

1. Complete physical examination looking for evidence of congenital syphilis.

2. Quantitative nontreponemal test (RPR or VDRL). This test should be performed on infant serum. The infant's titer should begin to fall by 3 months and become nonreactive by 6 months if the antibody is passively acquired. If the baby was infected, the titer will not fall and may rise. The tests may be negative at birth if the infection was acquired late in pregnancy. In this case, repeating the test later will confirm the diagnosis.

3. Pathologic examination of the placenta or umbilical cord using specific fluorescent antitreponemal antibody staining, if available

4. Darkfield microscopic examination or direct fluorescent antibody staining of any suspicious lesions or body fluids (e.g., nasal discharge)

   The diagnosis and treatment approach to infants being evaluated for congenital syphilis depends on (i) identification of maternal syphilis, (ii) adequacy of maternal therapy, (iii) maternal serologic response to therapy, (iv) comparison of maternal and infant serologic titers, and (v) the findings on the infant's physical examination.

B. CDC recommends classifying infants evaluated for congenital syphilis into one of the following four scenarios:

1. **Scenario one**
   a. Proven or highly probable disease
   i. Abnormal physical examination consistent with congenital syphilis
   ii. Nontreponemal titer that is fourfold higher than the mother's titer, i.e., mother's titer 1:2 or 1:4, neonate 1:8 or 1:16. (Note: The absence of a fourfold or greater titer does not exclude congenital syphilis.)
   iii. A positive darkfield test or PCR of lesions or body fluids
   b. Recommended evaluation
   i. CSF analysis for VDRL, cell count, and protein concentration. In the neonatal period, interpretation of CSF values may be difficult. Normal values of protein and WBC are higher in preterm infants and in first month of life in neonates. Values up to 25 WBC/mm^3 and 150 mg protein/dL may be normal.
   ii. Complete blood count (CBC) with differential and platelet count
   iii. Other tests as clinically indicated, including long-bone radiographs, chest radiograph, liver function tests, neuroimaging, ophthalmologic examination, and auditory brainstem response
   c. Recommended regimens
   i. Aqueous crystalline penicillin G 100,000 to 150,000 units/kg/day IV, administered as 50,000 units/kg/dose every 12 hours during the first 7 days of life and every 8 hours thereafter for a total of 10 days
   ii. Penicillin G procaine 50,000 units/kg/dose IM in a single dose daily for 10 days

2. **Scenario two**
   a. Possible congenital syphilis. Any neonate who has a normal physical examination and a serum quantitative nontreponemal serologic titer equal to or less than fourfold the maternal titer and one of the following:
   i. Maternal treatment not given, inadequately treated, or has no documentation of having received treatment.
   ii. Mother was treated with erythromycin or any other nonpenicillin G regimen.
   iii. Maternal treatment administered <4 weeks before delivery.
   b. Recommended evaluation
   i. CSF analysis for VDRL, cell count, and protein
   ii. CBC with differential and platelet count
   iii. Long-bone radiographs
   c. Recommended regimens
   i. Aqueous crystalline penicillin G 100,000 to 150,000 units/kg/day intravenous (IV), administered as 50,000 units/kg/dose every 12 hours during the first 7 days of life and every 8 hours thereafter for a total of 10 days
   ii. Penicillin G procaine 50,000 units/kg/dose intramuscular (IM) in a single dose daily for 10 days
   iii. Penicillin G benzathine 50,000 units/kg/dose IM in a single dose
   The penicillin benzathine can be given if the complete evaluation is normal (CBC with differential and platelets, CSF analysis with

VDRL, cell count and protein concentration, and long-bone radiographs) and follow-up is certain. If any part of the infant's evaluation is abnormal or not interpretable (e.g., CSF sample contaminated with blood), or if follow-up is not certain, then the full 10-day course of penicillin G should be given.

3. Scenario three
   a. Congenital syphilis less likely. Neonates who have a normal physical examination and a serum quantitative nontreponemal titer the same as or less than fourfold the maternal titer and both of the following are true:
      i. Mother was treated during pregnancy with a penicillin regimen appropriate for the stage of infection and >4 weeks before delivery.
      ii. No evidence of maternal reinfection or relapse.
   b. Recommended evaluation
      i. Such infants require no further evaluation.
   c. Recommended regimen
      i. Penicillin G benzathine 50,000 units/kg/dose IM in a single dose
      ii. Another approach involves not treating the infant but provide a close follow-up every 2 to 3 months for 6 months for infants whose mother's nontreponemal titers decrease at least fourfold after proper therapy for early syphilis or remained stable for low titer, latent syphilis (RPR <1:4).

4. Scenario four
   a. Congenital syphilis unlikely. Any neonate who has a normal physical examination and a serum quantitative nontreponemal serologic titer equal or less than fourfold the maternal titer and both of the following:
      i. Adequate maternal treatment before pregnancy
      ii. Maternal nontreponemal titer remained low and stable (serofast) before and during pregnancy and at delivery (VDRL <1:2 or RPR <1:4).
   b. Recommended evaluation
      i. No evaluation is recommended.
   c. Recommended regimen
      i. No treatment is required; however, some experts recommend a single dose of penicillin G benzathine 50,000 units/kg IM, particularly if follow-up is uncertain.

C. Evaluation and treatment of infants and children older than 1 month. Infants and children identified as having a reactive STS should be examined thoroughly and have maternal serology and treatment records reviewed to determine if the child has congenital or acquired syphilis. Any infant or child at risk for congenital syphilis should receive a full evaluation and testing for HIV infection.

   1. Recommended evaluation
      a. CSF analysis for VDRL, cell count, and protein concentration
      b. CBC with differential and platelet count
      c. Other tests as clinically indicated, including long-bone radiographs, chest radiograph, liver function tests, cranial ultrasonography, ophthalmologic examination, and auditory brainstem responses

2. Recommended treatment
  a. Aqueous crystalline penicillin G 200,000 to 300,000 units/kg/day IV, administered as 50,000 units/kg every 4 to 6 hours for 10 days. If the infant or child has no clinical manifestations of congenital syphilis and the evaluation (including the CSF examination) is normal, treatment with up to 3 weekly doses of penicillin G benzathine, 50,000 units/kg IM can be considered. Some experts also suggest administering a single dose of penicillin G benzathine 50,000 units/kg IM following the 10-day course of IV therapy.

VI. SCREENING AND TREATMENT OF PREGNANT WOMEN FOR SYPHILIS

A. All pregnant women should be screened early in pregnancy for syphilis with a nontreponemal STS. Testing should be performed at the first prenatal visit and, in high-risk populations, should also be repeated at the beginning of third trimester (28 to 32 weeks') gestation if at high risk and at delivery. When a woman presents in labor with no history of prenatal care or if results of previous testing are unknown, an STS should be performed at delivery, and the infant should not be discharged from the hospital until the test results are known. In women at very high risk, consideration should be given to a repeat STS 1 month postpartum to capture the rare patient who was infected just before delivery but had not yet seroconverted. All positive nontreponemal STS in pregnant women should be confirmed with a treponemal test.

B. Pregnant women with a reactive nontreponemal STS confirmed by a reactive treponemal STS should be treated regardless of stage of pregnancy unless previous adequate treatment is clearly documented and follow-up nontreponemal titers have declined at least fourfold. Treatment depends on the stage of infection:

  1. Primary and secondary syphilis. Penicillin G benzathine 2.4 million units IM in a single dose. Some experts recommend a second dose of 2.4 million units IM 1 week after the first dose.

  2. Early latent syphilis (without neurosyphilis). Treatment is the same as in primary and secondary syphilis.

  3. Late latent syphilis (without neurosyphilis). Penicillin G benzathine 2.4 million units administered as three single doses at 1-week intervals

  4. Tertiary syphilis (without neurosyphilis). Penicillin G benzathine 7.2 million units administered as three doses of 2.4 million units IM at 1-week interval

  5. Neurosyphilis. Aqueous crystalline penicillin G 18 to 24 million units daily administered as 3 to 4 million units IV every 4 hours for 10 to 14 days. If compliance can be assured, an alternative regimen of penicillin G procaine 2.4 million units IM daily plus probenecid 500 mg orally four times a day for 10 to 14 days may be used. At the end of these therapies, some experts recommend penicillin G benzathine 2.4 million units IM weekly for up to 3 weeks.

  6. Penicillin-allergic patients. There are no proven alternatives to penicillin for the prevention of congenital syphilis. If an infected pregnant woman has a history of penicillin allergy, she may be skin-tested against the major and minor penicillin determinants. If these test results are negative, penicillin may be given under medical supervision. If the test results are positive or unavailable, the patient should be desensitized and then given penicillin. Desensitization should be done in consultation with an expert and in a facility where emergency treatment is available.

7. **Human immunodeficiency virus (HIV)-infected pregnant women** should receive the same treatment as HIV-negative pregnant women, except that treatment for primary and secondary syphilis and early latent syphilis may be extended to 3 weekly doses of benzathine penicillin G 2.4 million units IM per week.

8. Adequate treatment for pregnant women is defined as "completion of a penicillin-based regimen," in accordance with CDC treatment guidelines, appropriate for stage of infection, initiated 30 or more days before delivery.

9. **The Jarisch-Herxheimer reaction**—the occurrence of fever, chills, headache, myalgias, and exacerbation of cutaneous lesions—may occur after treatment of pregnant women for syphilis. Fetal distress, premature labor, and stillbirth are rare but possible. Patients should be made aware of the possibility of such reactions, but concern about such complications should not delay treatment.

10. If a mother is treated for syphilis in pregnancy, monthly follow-up should be provided. A sustained fourfold decrease in nontreponemal titer should be seen with successful treatment.

    All patients with syphilis should be evaluated for other sexually transmitted diseases, such as chlamydia, gonorrhea, hepatitis B, and HIV.

VII. FOLLOW-UP OF INFANTS TREATED FOR CONGENITAL SYPHILIS.

All neonates with reactive nontreponemal tests should receive careful follow-up examinations and nontreponemal titer every 2 to 3 months until the test becomes nonreactive. In the neonate who was not treated because unlikely infected or infected but adequately treated, nontreponemal antibody titers should decline by age 3 months and be nonreactive by age 6 months. At 6 months, if the nontreponemal test is nonreactive, no further evaluation or treatment is needed. Treated neonates that exhibit persistent nontreponemal test titers by 6 to 12 months should be reevaluated through CSF examination and managed in consultation with an expert. Retreatment with a 10-day course of a penicillin G regimen may be indicated. Neonates whose initial CSF evaluations are abnormal should undergo a repeat lumbar puncture approximately every 6 months until the results are normal. A reactive CSF VDRL test or abnormal CSF indices that persist and cannot be attributed to other ongoing illness requires retreatment for possible neurosyphilis and should be managed in consultation with an expert.

VIII. INFECTION CONTROL

A. **Isolation of hospitalized patient.** *Red Book 2015* recommends standard precautions for all patients, including infants with suspected or proven congenital syphilis. Gloves should be worn when caring for patients with congenital, primary, and secondary syphilis with skin and mucous membranes lesions until 24 hours of treatment has been completed because moist open lesions, secretions, and possible blood are contagious in all patients with syphilis.

B. Control measures. All people, who have had close unprotected contact with a patient with early congenital syphilis before identification of the disease or during first 24 hours of therapy, should be examined clinically for the presence of lesions 2 to 3 weeks after contact. Serologic testing should be performed and repeated 3 months after contact or sooner if symptoms occur. Infants and their mothers at risk for syphilis or are infected with syphilis should be evaluated for other sexually transmitted diseases such as hepatitis B, gonorrhea, chlamydia, and HIV.

C. Assistance and guidance in syphilis testing and treatment are available from the CDC, Atlanta, Georgia, and state health departments.

Suggested Readings

American Academy of Pediatrics. Syphilis. In: Kimberlin DW, Brady MT, Jackson MA, et al, eds. *Red Book: 2015 Report of the Committee on Infectious Diseases*. 30th ed. Elk Grove Village, IL: American Academy of Pediatrics; 2015: 755–768.

Centers for Disease Control and Prevention. National Notifiable Diseases Surveillance system (NNDSS). Congenital syphilis (*Treponema pallidum*) 2015 case definition. http://wwwn.cdc.gov/nndss/conditions/congenital-syphilis/case-definition/2015/. Accessed October 15, 2015.

Centers for Disease Control and Prevention. Sexually transmitted diseases treatment guidelines, 2015. *Morb Mortal Wkly Rep* 2015;64(RR-03):1–137.

Wolff T, Shelton E, Sessions C, et al. Screening for syphilis infection in pregnant women: evidence for the U.S. Preventive Services Task Force reaffirmation recommendation statement. *Ann Intern Med* 2009;150:710–716.

52

Tuberculosis

Heather Y. Highsmith and Jeffrey R. Starke

KEY POINTS

- The World Health Organization (WHO) estimates that 600,000 children develop tuberculosis (TB) disease a year, causing 74,000 deaths in HIV-uninfected children.

- TB infection is determined through use of either the Mantoux tuberculin skin test (TST) or an interferon gamma release assay (IGRA).

- True congenital TB with transmission from the mother to the fetus *in utero* is quite rare but can occur in several ways: hematogenous spread through the umbilical vein, aspiration of infected amniotic fluid, or ingestion of other infected materials.

- The clinical signs and symptoms of congenital TB vary in relation to the intensity of transmission as well as the site of disease.

I. **EPIDEMIOLOGY AND INCIDENCE.** *Mycobacterium tuberculosis* is the etiologic agent that cases tuberculosis (TB). The organism produces a spectrum of clinical entities that have differing diagnostic and management approaches. Prior to any discussion about TB, it is helpful to define these entities at the outset (Table 52.1).

Over one-third of the world's population is infected with *M. tuberculosis*. Each year, at least 9 million people develop TB disease, and almost 2 million people die as a result. The World Health Organization (WHO) estimates that 600,000 children develop TB disease a year, causing 74,000 deaths in HIV-uninfected children (there are no estimates for HIV-infected children, who likely have the majority of the deaths).

In the early 20th century, TB was a common entity in the United States. The advent of effective anti-TB medications in the 1950s resulted in a declining TB prevalence until the mid-1980s. At that time, a decline in public health services, the HIV epidemic, an increase in immigration from high-prevalence countries, and increased transmission in congregate settings caused a sudden upsurge in cases (20% increase overall and 40% increase among children). This surge peaked in 1992 at 26,673 reported annual cases. Once increased strategic public health were enacted in the early 1990s, the incidence subsequently decreased to only 9,582 cases in 2013.

In the United States, most TB-infected patients are found in certain high-risk groups, as listed in Table 52.2. Over 60% of TB cases in the United States occur in foreign-born individuals. Foreign-born individuals are screened and treated only for TB disease before they immigrate; treatment of TB infection

Table 52.1. Definitions

Tuberculosis exposure	Occurs when an individual has had contact with a case of contagious tuberculosis disease in the past 3 months. An exposed individual may or may not have infection or disease.
Tuberculosis infection	Occurs when an individual has a positive tuberculin skin test result (defined in Table 52.2) or a positive interferon gamma release assay result (defined in the text), a normal physical exam, and a chest radiograph that is either normal or shows evidence of healed calcifications. An untreated infected individual can develop tuberculosis disease in the near or distant future.
Tuberculosis disease	Occurs when an evident illness (signs, symptoms, and/or radiographic changes) is caused by *Mycobacterium tuberculosis*.
Congenital tuberculosis disease	Occurs when a neonate is infected with *M. tuberculosis in utero* or during delivery and develops disease afterward. This is determined by having a positive acid-fast bacillus stain or culture from the neonate, with exclusion of possible postnatal transmission, and either lesions in the first week of life, primary hepatic complex or caseating hepatic granulomas, or tuberculosis infection of the placenta or maternal genital tract.
Postnatally acquired tuberculosis disease	Occurs when an infant is infected after delivery, either through inhalation of *M. tuberculosis* from a contagious caregiver or ingestion of *M. tuberculosis* via infected breast or cow milk, and develops signs, symptoms, and/or radiographic evidence of tuberculosis disease.

Table 52.2. Groups at High Risk for Tuberculosis Infection

Foreign-born person from high-prevalence countries
Individuals who travel to high-prevalence countries
Inmates of correctional facilities
Illicit drug users
Migrant families
Homeless persons

requires that they enter into care after arrival in the United States, which can be difficult due to lack of insurance and a medical home. Persons traveling to the United States on visitors' visas receive no TB screening. Thus, many foreign-born women are at risk for developing TB disease after arrival in the United States. For many young women, their first health care visit after arrival is during their pregnancy or at labor and delivery, and this may be the best opportunity to diagnose and manage their TB infection or disease.

II. TRANSMISSION AND PATHOGENESIS.

Transmission of *M. tuberculosis* most commonly occurs when an individual expectorates infectious droplet nuclei, which may remain airborne for hours. An individual whose sputum is acid-fast bacillus (AFB) smear positive is the most likely to be infectious. Individuals who are AFB smear negative but culture positive are less infectious than those who are AFB smear positive, but many can still transmit the organism. Fomites and other secretions rarely cause transmission.

Children with pulmonary TB usually do not produce a cough effective enough to expectorate the droplet nuclei necessary to spread the disease, and they usually have a low burden of organisms; hence, childhood TB is often called "pauci-bacillary disease." As a result, children rarely infect others. However, adolescents with reactivation pulmonary disease or children who have hallmarks of adult-type disease (cavitary lung lesions with an effective cough) may be contagious. In addition, children with true congenital TB often have a large pulmonary burden of organisms and may transmit infection to health care workers, especially if they are intubated. Within 2 weeks of starting effective treatment, a patient of any age with drug-susceptible TB usually becomes noncontagious, but a patient with multidrug-resistant TB (MDR-TB) may remain infectious for weeks to months after starting treatment.

Once the droplet nuclei are inhaled, *M. tuberculosis* bacilli land in the alveoli where they multiply freely or are consumed by alveolar macrophages. In some individuals, the immune system is able to clear the infection without treatment. In others, *M. tuberculosis* subverts the alveolar macrophages' attempts at its degradation and instead replicates inside macrophages for several weeks. As the bacilli multiply, they frequently are carried into regional lymph nodes by alveolar macrophages and can spread hematogenously to other sites, including but not limited to the vertebrae, peritoneum, meninges, liver, spleen, lymph nodes, and genitourinary tract. Most patients are asymptomatic during this time and usually have no radiologic evidence of disease. The exception to this occurs in infants, who are at much higher risk for progressing rapidly to symptomatic disease due to their immature immune system. Although healthy adults infected with *M. tuberculosis* have a 5% to 10% of developing TB disease within their lifetime, the majority who do so—including pregnant women—develop disease within the first 1 to 2 years after infection. Infants and toddlers who are infected but untreated have a 40% chance of developing disease within 6 to 9 months. The risk to both the mother and the child is greatest when the mother has been infected recently. Any condition that depresses cell-mediated immunity (HIV infection, diabetes mellitus, poor nutritional status, or high-dose corticosteroids) increases the risk of progression to from infection to disease in adults and children.

In young children, the organisms tend to spread to the regional hilar and mediastinal lymph nodes, which then enlarge if inflammation is intense. The lymph nodes can compress or erode into the bronchi, frequently resulting in a distal atelectasis or parenchymal infection, causing the so-called "collapse-consolidation" lesion. However, the hallmark of childhood TB is intrathoracic lymphadenopathy with or without subsequent parenchymal disease.

A. **Tuberculosis infection.** TB infection is defined as having evidence of an immune response to *M. tuberculosis*–related antigens. **TB infection is determined through use of either the Mantoux tuberculin skin test (TST) or an interferon gamma release assay (IGRA).**

1. **The TST** is a delayed-type hypersensitivity test to determine if the patient reacts to a purified protein derivative (PPD) of *M. tuberculosis*. The delayed-type hypersensitivity typically develops 3 to 9 weeks after the TB infection occurs; the TST will be negative before this time. The PPD is placed subcutaneously, typically on the left volar forearm. After 48 to 72 hours, the area is examined for any induration and the amount of induration is measured and recorded. A TST is interpreted as positive depending on the measurement of the induration as well as risk factors that the patient may have (see Table 52.3).

2. **IGRAs** are blood tests that detect the production of interferon-gamma, a chemical routinely released by immune cells as they combat TB organisms. The IGRAs include positive and negative controls, and because there is no "gold standard" for TB infection, their thresholds for positivity have been determined from studies in adults who have culture-positive TB disease. These tests help to determine if someone has been infected with *M. tuberculosis*, but they do not differentiate between infection and disease. There are two IGRAs approved for clinical use in the United States: QuantiFERON Gold-TB test (QIAGEN, Germantown, Maryland) and the T-SPOT.TB test (Oxford Immunotec, Abingdon, United Kingdom). Although PPD contains hundreds of mycobacterial antigens, the IGRA tests utilize only two or three that are specific for *M. tuberculosis*. The IGRAs do not cross-react with *Mycobacterium* bovis-BCG (the organism used in TB vaccines) or *Mycobacterium avium* complex, the most common environmental nontuberculous mycobacterium. Because these two organisms are responsible for most false-positive TST results, the IGRAs are more specific than the TST. An additional advantage of the IGRAs is that they require only one provider visit to take blood. However, they require specific laboratory capacities and are more expensive than the TST. Although the IGRAs are more specific for infection by *M. tuberculosis* than TSTs, they appear to offer no increased sensitivity. IGRAs can be used to diagnose TB infection in both adults and children, except in children <2 years of age; the American Academy of Pediatrics currently recommends against using IGRAs in children under 2 years of age because there are limited data regarding reliability of a negative test result, and a false-negative result has important implications because these children are more prone to rapidly advance to severe disease.

III. **MATERNAL TUBERCULOSIS.** There are few studies in the modern era that examine the impact of pregnancy on TB and of TB on pregnancy. The majority of literature predates the 1960s. Prior to the availability of anti-TB

Table 52.3. Definitions of Positive Tuberculin Skin Test

≥5 mm Induration	10 mm–14 mm Induration	≥15 mm Induration
HIV-positive persons	Persons who immigrated from a high-prevalence country in the past 5 years	Persons with no risk factors for tuberculosis disease
Recent contacts of contagious tuberculosis disease cases	Injection drug users	
Individuals with chest radiographic changes suggestive of prior tuberculosis disease	Residents and employees of the following high-risk congregate settings: ■ Prisons/jails ■ Nursing homes/long-term care facilities for the elderly ■ Hospitals and other health care facilities ■ Residential facilities for HIV/AIDS patients ■ Homeless shelters	
Organ transplant or otherwise immunosuppressed patients (receiving the equivalent of 15 mg/day of prednisone or more)	Mycobacteriology laboratory personnel	
	Persons with any of the following high-risk clinical conditions: ■ Silicosis ■ Diabetes mellitus ■ Chronic renal failure ■ Hematologic disorders (e.g., leukemia and lymphoma) ■ Carcinoma of the head, neck, or lung ■ Weight loss (>10% ideal body weight) ■ Gastrectomy/jejunoileal bypass ■ Children <4 years old ■ Any infant, child, or adolescent in contact with a high-risk adult	

medications, TB disease had a poor prognosis for both the fetus and the mother. Now, with effective therapy, the mother with TB can be cured and the fetus or child spared from disease. Providers should screen all pregnant women for risk factors of TB infection or disease at an early prenatal visit, and questionnaires have been developed to aid this screening. Women belonging to high-risk groups, such as those listed in Table 52.2, or contacts to a current or previous TB case, should be tested with a TST or an IGRA. There is strong evidence that pregnancy does not alter the response to the TST and that the TST does not adversely affect the woman or the fetus. Similarly, the IGRA results do not appear to be affected by pregnancy.

A. **Management of maternal TB infection.** If a pregnant woman has a positive TST as defined in Table 52.2, or a positive IGRA, she should undergo an evaluation for TB disease, which includes a complete medical history and physical exam and a chest radiograph with abdominal shielding. The chest radiograph should not be deferred until after delivery because the fetus can be protected and the outcome for the mother and the baby usually is worse if TB disease goes undetected during the pregnancy. Once TB disease is excluded, the timing of treatment of TB infection in the mother is considered. If the mother likely has been infected recently, or is immunocompromised in any way, treatment of the mother's TB infection should be started during the pregnancy. If the woman does not belong to these highest risk groups, some experts recommend that her treatment wait until after the child is delivered. The most common treatment of TB infection for the pregnant woman is 300 mg of isoniazid (INH) taken daily. Because INH is known to cause a peripheral neuropathy due to depletion of vitamin B_6 (pyridoxine) and there is increased vitamin B_6 (pyridoxine)

   1. **When the pregnant woman has TB infection**, it is recommended that the remainder of the household and extended family be investigated for TB infection and disease. The purpose is to find, diagnose, and treat a potentially infectious individual that the child could be exposed to, thereby minimizing risk of transmission of the organism to the infant and others. However, if this has not occurred by the time of delivery, the child's discharge to home should not be held up while this is occurring unless a symptomatic family member is identified. Although the local health departments are typically responsible for contact tracing when a case of TB disease is found, due to inadequate resources, most do not provide this service when the pregnant woman has only TB infection, and this investigation is left to other health care providers. When the mother is undergoing treatment for TB infection and no current case of TB disease is found, her infant does not need to be treated for TB infection or disease.

B. **Management of maternal TB disease** (Fig. 52.1)

   1. **Symptoms.** If a pregnant woman is found to have a positive TST or IGRA, the clinical evaluation for TB disease should include a history and thorough physical examination. Patients with pulmonary TB usually complain of some combination of fever, cough, weight loss, fatigue, or less frequently, hemoptysis. However, pregnant women can have

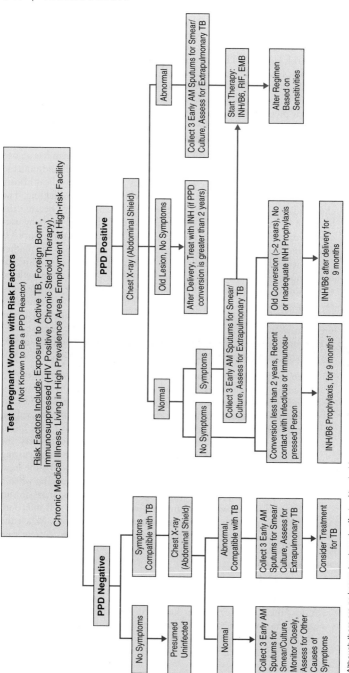

Figure 52.1. Diagnosis and treatment of tuberculosis in the pregnant woman. PPD, purified protein derivative; TB, tuberculosis; INH, isoniazid; RIF, rifampin; EMB, ethambutol.

†Although there are no known teratogenic effects of isoniazid, some experts recommend waiting until the 2nd trimester before initiating treatment for tuberculosis infection.

relatively fewer symptoms than might be suggested by the extent of disease in the chest radiograph. Extrapulmonary TB can occur almost anywhere in the body, but the most common sites are the cervical or supraclavicular lymph nodes, bones and joints, peritoneum, meninges, or genitourinary system. The most common "symptom" of female genitourinary TB is difficulty conceiving, but abnormal patterns of menstrual bleeding also occur commonly. Extrapulmonary TB rates are increased in HIV-coinfected patients.

Maternal TB disease portends negative effects on the fetus. Mothers with untreated TB disease are more likely to have infants who are premature or are small for gestational age. They are also more likely to have stillbirths.

2. **Radiographic findings.** A chest radiograph, performed with abdominal shielding to protect the fetus, should be obtained for every pregnant woman with untreated TB infection to rule out pulmonary TB disease even if she is asymptomatic. Radiographic findings consistent with TB disease include focal or multinodular infiltrates, cavitation, decreased expansion of the upper lobes of the lung, and hilar or mediastinal adenopathy. Although most adults with pulmonary TB have lesions in the apexes of the upper lobes, pregnant women have an increased tendency to have lesions in other lung areas, presenting with a somewhat "atypical" radiographic picture.

3. **Culture.** Any pregnant woman suspected of having pulmonary TB disease will need microbiologic evaluation, which usually consists of three early morning sputum samples that are stained for acid-fast bacteria and cultured for mycobacteria. Due to the slow growth of the *M. tuberculosis*, up to 6 weeks may be required to detect the organism on solid media, and drug susceptibility testing takes several weeks longer. If liquid media are used, as is common in modern laboratories, the organism is more often detected within 2 to 3 weeks. If extrapulmonary disease is suspected, appropriate samples, including tissue biopsy of the affected sites if no secretion or excretion is available, should be obtained and sent for AFB stain and mycobacterial culture. In some centers, a molecular diagnostic technique is available to assist with diagnosis. GeneXpert MTB/RIF (Cepheid, Sunnydale, California) is a nested real-time PCR that tests for *M. tuberculosis* DNA as well as the genetic material that confers resistance to the first-line drug rifampin (RIF). GeneXpert is less sensitive than culture but yields results within 2 to 3 hours. The sensitivity improves in instances of AFB smear positive disease.

4. **Treatment**
   a. **Nonpregnant adults.** When TB disease is suspected in nonpregnant adults, initial therapy consists of four drugs: INH, RIF, pyrazinamide (PZA), and ethambutol (EMB). If the patient is found to have drug-susceptible disease, EMB can be removed from the regimen at that time. The other drugs are continued for 2 months as an induction period. After 2 months, PZA is then removed from the regimen, but INH and RIF are continued for another 4 months in a continuation phase. This gives a total length of therapy of 6 months. If drug resistance is found,

it is recommended that an expert in TB treatment be consulted. If there are extrapulmonary manifestations or the patient does not respond quickly to standard treatment, the treatment course may need to be prolonged. All TB disease treatment regimens should be administered via direct observation of therapy (DOT), an intervention where medications are administered to the patient by a health care professional or trained third-party member, often a local health department employee, who observes and documents that the patient ingests each dose of medication.

b. Pregnant women. Treatment in pregnant women differs in that the initial regimen often includes only INH, RIF, and EMB. PZA is often excluded because there is a smaller amount of data on PZA's safety during pregnancy. Some experts do not recommend its routine use in pregnant women, although the WHO recommends its use in pregnancy. Pyridoxine is added to prevent the peripheral neuropathy associated with INH use during pregnancy, as mentioned earlier. The three first-line drugs are considered relatively safe for the fetus, and the risks of poorly treated disease far outweigh the risks of treatment. Other anti-TB drugs that are contraindicated for pregnant women include kanamycin, amikacin, capreomycin (hearing loss), and the fluoroquinolones (inadequate safety data). If drug resistance is found that requires use of medications with unknown or adverse fetal effects, consultation with a TB expert is recommended.

c. Other considerations. Anti-TB medications are present in small amounts in breast milk, on average about 5% to 10% of serum concentrations. Treatment of TB infection or disease in the mother is not a contraindication to breastfeeding. Because breast milk also has very low concentrations of pyridoxine, it is recommended to give pyridoxine to any breastfeeding infant who is taking INH or whose mother is taking the drug.

Pregnant women with pulmonary TB disease may be contagious via the airborne route. While hospitalized, all patients suspected of having pulmonary TB disease should be placed initially in airborne isolation in a negative air pressure room. All staff should wear fit-tested N95 respirator masks. Most hospitals will require that a patient remain in isolation until there have been three consecutive negative early morning AFB sputum smears. If a patient is found to have MDR-TB, the patient should be isolated for the entire hospital stay.

In all instances of *suspected* TB disease, the local health department should be notified promptly to start a contact investigation aimed at finding newly infected individuals as well as others who may have TB disease so that they can be treated and stop transmission to others.

IV. TUBERCULOSIS OF THE FETUS OR NEWBORN

A. Congenital tuberculosis

1. **Pathogenesis.** True congenital TB with transmission from the mother to the fetus *in utero* is quite rare but can occur in several ways: hematogenous spread through the umbilical vein, aspiration of infected amniotic fluid, or ingestion of other infected materials. If the mother has TB disease or is infected during pregnancy, the organisms may disseminate

hematogenously to the placenta and from there, may spread to the fetus via the umbilical vein. However, placental infection does not guarantee transmission to the fetus; likewise, the absence of organisms in the placenta does not ensure that the child remains uninfected. The usual deposits of hematogenous spread follow the path of the umbilical vein. The liver is frequently infected, where a primary focus develops within periportal lymph nodes. The organisms may spread beyond the liver and into the main systemic circulation by the patent foramen ovale or into the pulmonary circulation via the right ventricle. Multiple sites may be seeded initially or seeded secondary to the initial hepatic or pulmonary foci. The definitive lesion of congenital TB is the hepatic primary complex with caseating hepatic granulomas. Congenital TB may disseminate to include bone marrow infiltration; osteomyelitis; mesenteric lymphadenitis; and tubercles and granulomas of the adrenal glands, GI tract, spleen, kidneys, meninges, and skin.

If the placenta develops a caseous lesion that ruptures into the amniotic fluid, the fetus can inhale or ingest the organisms that can spread to the middle ear and cause disease via the Eustachian tube as the fetus swallows. Primary foci may be found in the lungs or in the gastrointestinal tract. The disease can then secondarily disseminate to other organ systems. Rarely, the dissemination can be swift and massive, and the child will present with a sepsis-like syndrome.

2. **Symptoms.** The clinical signs and symptoms of congenital TB vary in relation to the intensity of transmission as well as the site of disease. Occasionally, symptoms are noted at birth, but they more commonly begin at 1 to 3 weeks of life because the organisms are obligate aerobes and thrive best in the oxygen-rich postnatal environment. The initial presentation is very similar to sepsis or a congenital infection and should be suspected if an ill neonate does not respond to empiric antimicrobials and has an otherwise unrevealing evaluation. Hepatosplenomegaly and respiratory distress are the two most common signs and symptoms, followed by fever.

3. **Radiographic findings.** Chest radiography is usually abnormal, with half of neonates having a miliary disease pattern (but this pattern may not develop for several days to weeks of illness). Other neonates have adenopathy and parenchymal infiltrates.

4. **Additional considerations.** All neonates suspected of having congenital TB should be placed in airborne isolation while the evaluation is in process because confirmed cases often have extensive pulmonary involvement; there have been case reports of transmission of *M. tuberculosis* from a congenitally infected patient to a health care worker, but not directly to other neonates, with the exception of transmission due to contaminated respiratory equipment. The congenitally infected neonate's family members should also be screened with radiography because they may have subclinical but radiographic signs of TB disease that has not yet been diagnosed.

Investigation of congenital TB should include assessment of the mother's risk factors for TB, and suspicion should be high if the mother has had an otherwise unexplained pneumonia, bronchitis, meningeal disease, unusual pattern of uterine bleeding, or endometritis before, during, or after pregnancy. The placenta should be examined by a pathologist and should be cultured for *M. tuberculosis*. If the placenta is not available, the mother should be examined and consideration be given to performing a uterine dilation and curettage because endometrial specimens often yield positive culture results. The infant should be evaluated for microbiologic confirmation of disease by AFB smear and culture of body fluids or tissues, including gastric aspirates, middle ear fluid, bone marrow, tissue biopsy, and tracheal aspirates. The cerebrospinal fluid (CSF) should also be examined because TB meningitis occurs in one-third of congenital TB cases.

V. POSTNATAL TRANSMISSION OF *MYCOBACTERIUM TUBERCULOSIS*.

Persons with TB infection are not contagious, so there is no risk to the infant if the mother has TB infection without disease. Occasionally, an infant will be exposed postnatally to a visitor or caregiver with TB disease, including the child's mother, another household contact, or even a nursery worker. Recommended management in these scenarios includes evaluating the neonate for clinical evidence of TB disease with a physical examination and chest radiography (posteroanterior and lateral views). Infants with postnatal acquisition of *M. tuberculosis* frequently have the same symptoms as congenitally infected neonates. However, they typically present later, at the age of 1 to 4 months, and lack the primary hepatic focus seen in congenital TB. If an infant has evidence of TB disease, the same clinical evaluation, isolation precautions, and treatment as used for suspected congenital TB should occur.

VI. TREATMENT OF NEONATAL TUBERCULOSIS DISEASE.

Once the diagnosis of congenital or postnatal TB is *suspected*, treatment should be initiated promptly. Due to the rarity of these conditions, the data regarding the pharmacokinetics of anti-TB drugs in neonates are limited. INH, RIF, PZA, and either EMB or an aminoglycoside such as amikacin comprise the initial suggested regimen. Neonates and infants have a high risk of developing disseminated disease or meningitis, so amikacin is often used instead of EMB due to its bactericidal activity and better central nervous system (CNS) penetration across inflamed meninges. If the organism is susceptible to first-line medications, the initial four-drug regimen should be continued for the first 2 months of therapy, followed by treatment with INH and RIF for an additional 7 to 10 months, a total duration of treatment of 9 to 12 months. If TB meningitis is suspected, 2 mg/kg/day of prednisone (or equivalent corticosteroid) should be administered for the first 4 to 6 weeks with a slow taper to prevent development of hydrocephalus or infarcts caused by vasculitis. Neonatal TB always should be managed with the help of an expert in TB.

A. **Prognosis.** The prognosis of neonatal TB disease—particularly true congenital TB—is guarded, and the mortality rate, even with effective treatment, is 25% to 50%. The diagnosis and institution of effective treatment are often delayed because congenital TB is rare, the mother's TB disease has not been diagnosed, and confirming the disease in the neonate and the mother can be difficult. Pulmonary damage in the infant can be extensive resulting in atelectasis or a bronchiolitis obliterans–like picture. Infants often suffer from growth delay, even when usually adequate calories are taken, because of the energy requirements created by the disease. Electrolyte disturbances are common, particularly hyponatremia caused by the inappropriate secretion of antidiuretic hormone or renal salt wasting. A variety of neurologic complications can occur when TB meningitis is present, including hearing loss, visual impairments, global developmental delay, seizures, hemiparesis, and cognitive abnormalities.

VII. MANAGEMENT OF AN EXPOSED NEONATE. The American Academy of Pediatrics' 2015 *Red Book* includes recommendations for the management of a neonate or infant exposed to a contact with TB infection or TB disease and are as follows:

A. **Mother (or household contact) has evidence of TB infection and a normal chest radiograph findings.** If the mother or household contact is asymptomatic, no separation is required. The mother usually is a candidate for treatment of TB infection after the initial postpartum period. The newborn infant needs no special evaluation or therapy. Because of the young infant's exquisite susceptibility, and because the mother's positive TST or IGRA result could be a marker of an unrecognized case of contagious TB within the household, other household members should have a TST or IGRA and further evaluation if positive; however, this evaluation should not delay the infant's discharge from the hospital. The mother can breastfeed her child.

B. **Mother (or household contact) has clinical signs and symptoms and/or abnormal findings on chest radiograph consistent with TB disease.** Cases of suspected or proven TB disease in mothers (or household contacts) should be reported immediately to the local health department, and investigation of all household members should start as soon as possible. If the mother has possible TB disease, the infant should be evaluated for congenital TB, and the mother should be tested for HIV infection. If the mother has an abnormal chest radiograph, she and the infant should be separated until she has been evaluated, and if TB disease is suspected, until she and her infant are receiving appropriate anti-TB therapy. Once the infant is receiving INH, separation is not necessary unless the mother (or household contact) has possible MDR-TB disease or has poor adherence to treatment, and DOT is not possible. If the mother is suspected of having MDR-TB disease, an expert in TB disease treatment should be consulted. When the mother and child are together, the mother should wear a mask and must be willing to adhere to all appropriate infection-control measures. Usually, contact between a potentially contagious mother and her infant should be brief and occur in a very well-ventilated room. Women with drug-susceptible TB disease who have been treated appropriately for 2 or more weeks and who are not considered contagious can breastfeed.

Once congenital TB is excluded, INH is given until the infant is 3 or 4 months of age (some experts recommend 6 months of age), when a TST should be performed. If the TST result is positive, the infant should be reassessed for TB disease. If TB disease is excluded in an infant with a positive TST result, INH alone should be continued for a total of 9 months.

The infant should be evaluated monthly during treatment for signs of illness or poor growth. If the TST result is negative at 3 to 4 months of age and the mother (or household contact) has good adherence and response to treatment and is no longer contagious, INH should be discontinued.

C. **Mother (or household contact) has a positive TST or IGRA and abnormal findings on chest radiography but no evidence of TB disease.** If the chest radiograph of the mother (or household contact) appears abnormal but is not suggestive of TB disease and the history, physical examination, and sputum smear indicate no evidence of TB disease, the infant can be assumed to be at low risk for *M. tuberculosis* infection and need not be separated from the mother (or the household contact). The mother and her infant should receive follow-up care, and the mother should be treated for TB infection. Other household members should have a TST or IGRA and further evaluation.

VIII. BACILLE CALMETTE-GUÉRIN VACCINATION (BCG). BCG vaccines are among the oldest vaccines worldwide. They are attenuated strains of *Mycobacterium bovis*, a close relative of *M. tuberculosis*. The original BCG strain created at the Pasteur Institute has been lost, but early on it was sent to several different laboratories which have each maintained their own strain. As a result of the different methods or propagation used at these laboratories, there are many BCG strains that differ significantly in important properties. The preponderance of evidence indicates that BCG vaccination prevents 60% to 90% of disseminated TB disease and TB meningitis in infants and young children. There is inconsistent evidence that the vaccine prevents pulmonary disease in older persons. The BCG vaccines remain in use in most high burden countries.

Within the United States, the use of BCG vaccine is very limited. The Centers for Disease Control and Prevention currently recommends considering BCG vaccination for children with a negative TST who cannot be separated from an untreated or "ineffectively treated" adult with TB disease, or an MDR-TB case, as defined by resistance to at least INH and RIF.

The vaccine is typically given intradermally and produces a pustule at the injection site before leading to a permanent scar. Possible adverse reactions include local ulceration and regional lymphadenitis. These adverse events are not necessarily immediate. In normal hosts, these events may take weeks to months to develop and resolve. In immunocompromised hosts, the lesions may take years to develop and resolve. Severely immunocompromised individuals can develop disseminated disease from the BCG vaccine. As a result, BCG is not recommended for HIV-infected or exposed children; patients with congenital immunodeficiency or malignancy; or patients on immune-modulating drugs such as corticosteroids, chemotherapy, or radiation. All adverse events should be reported to the disease manufacturer.

It should be noted that after BCG immunization, the child may develop a positive reaction to a TST. Some studies have shown that the majority of children who received a BCG vaccine in infancy will have a negative TST at 5 to 10 years of age. However, the BCG vaccines do not induce a positive IGRA test result. (Tables 52.4 and 52.5)

Table 52.4. Commonly Used Medications for Treatment of Tuberculosis Disease

Drug and Dosage Forms	Activity	Dosage	Maximum Dose	Pregnancy Category	Side Effects	Other
Isoniazid (INH) Scored tablets: 100 mg 300 mg Intravenous solution	Bactericidal	10–15 mg/ kg/day Or 20–30 mg/kg/ dose twice weekly after 2 months of treatment	300 mg	C	Peripheral neuropathy Mild transaminitis Hepatitis Hypersensitivity	Requires pyridoxine supplementation (25–50 mg/day) if the patient has any of the following: 1. Breastfed, pregnant, or lactating 2. Nutritional deficiencies 3. Symptomatic HIV infection 4. Meat and milk deficient diet
Rifampin (RIF) Capsules: 150 mg 300 mg Intravenous solution	Bactericidal	10–20 mg/kg/ day (same dose when given twice weekly)	600 mg	C	Vomiting Hepatitis Influenza-like reaction Thrombocytopenia Pruritus	Discolors urine and other secretions an orange color Causes oral contraceptives to be ineffective

(continued)

Table 52.4. Commonly Used Medications for Treatment of Tuberculosis Disease *(Continued)*

Drug and Dosage Forms	Activity	Dosage	Maximum Dose	Pregnancy Category	Side Effects	Other
Pyrazinamide (PZA) Scored tablets: 500 mg	Bactericidal	30–40 mg/kg/day Or 50 mg/kg/dose twice weekly	2 g	C	Hepatitis Hyperuricemia Arthralgia GI upset	Hyperuricemia and arthralgias most prominent in adolescents and adults
Ethambutol (EMB) Tablets: 100 mg 400 mg	Bacteriostatic (except at high doses)	15–25 mg/kg/day	2.5 g	C	Optic neuritis Decreased red-green color discrimination GI disturbances Hypersensitivity	Does not cross blood–brain barrier well, thus not recommended for TB meningitis treatment
Amikacin Intravenous solution		15–30 mg/kg IV or IM	1 g	D —	Auditory and vestibular toxicities Nephrotoxicity	Can be used in place of ethambutol in TB meningitis treatment

GI, gastrointestinal; IV, intravenous; IM, intramuscular; TB, tuberculosis.

Table 52.5. Key Summary Points

Tuberculosis in the United States is most common among people born or with frequent travel to high-prevalence countries.

The presenting signs and symptoms of neonatal tuberculosis include a sepsis-like episode that does not respond to empiric antibiotics or a presentation consistent with congenital infection for which no other cause can be found.

Diagnostic criteria for congenital tuberculosis:
1. Proved tuberculous lesions such as positive stain or culture
2. One of the following:
   a. Lesions in the first week of life
   b. Primary hepatic complex or caseating hepatic granulomas
   c. Tuberculosis infection of the placenta or maternal genital tract
   d. Exclusion of the possibility of postnatal transmission

All neonates suspected of having congenital tuberculosis should be put in air-borne isolation, and all visitors should be screened for tuberculosis disease.

The health department should be notified of all suspected tuberculosis disease cases in order to start a contact investigation.

The neonate with possible congenital tuberculosis should be evaluated for disseminated disease and meningitis.

Treatment should always include the following:
- Rifampin
- Isoniazid
- Pyrazinamide
- An aminoglycoside should be used if tuberculous meningitis is suspected. If CSF evaluation is negative for meningitis, then ethambutol can be used.
- Pyridoxine should be added if the patient is exclusively taking breast milk.

Therapy should be tailored based on the patient or the mother's drug susceptibility testing.

All treatment should be administered by directly observed therapy (DOT).

CSF, cerebrospinal fluid.

Suggested Readings

American Academy of Pediatrics. Tuberculosis. In: Kimberlin D, Brady M, Jackson M, et al., eds. *Red Book: 2015 Report of the Committee on Infectious Diseases.* 30th ed. Elk Grove Village, IL: American Academy of Pediatrics; 2015:805.

Cantwell M, Shehab Z, Costello A, et al. Brief report: congenital tuberculosis. *N Engl J Med* 1994;330(15):1051–1054.

Centers for Disease Control and Prevention. Slide sets—epidemiology of pediatric tuberculosis in the United States, 1993–2013. http://www.cdc.gov/tb/publications/slidesets/pediatricTB/default.htm. Updated April 2014. Accessed August 7, 2015.

Mazade MA, Evans EM, Starke JR, et al. Congenital tuberculosis presenting as sepsis syndrome: case report and review of the literature. *Pediatr Infect Dis J* 2001;20(4):439–442.

Starke J; and the Committee on Infectious Diseases. Interferon-γ release assays for diagnosis of tuberculosis infection and disease in children. *Pediatrics* 2014;134(6):e1763–e1773.

Starke J, Cruz A. Tuberculosis. In: *Remington and Klein's Infectious Diseases of the Fetus and Newborn Infant.* 7th ed. Philadelphia, PA: Elsevier Saunders; 2011:577.

53 Lyme Disease

Norma Pérez

KEY POINTS

- No evidence of congenital Lyme borreliosis syndrome
- Pregnant females who develop Lyme disease should be treated.
- No evidence that *Borrelia burgdorferi* is transmitted in human milk
- Prevention of Lyme disease is best by avoiding tick-infested areas, use of tick repellents, and surveillance for tick attachment with immediate removal.

I. **LYME DISEASE** (Lyme borreliosis) is the most commonly reported vector-borne disease in the United States. The causative organism is the spirochete *Borrelia burgdorferi* sensu stricto, which is transmitted to humans through the bite of the *Ixodes* tick. In the United States, the cases of Lyme disease correlate with the distribution of the infected tick vector: *Ixodes scapularis* in the East and Midwest and *Ixodes pacificus* in the West. Most cases in the United States are clustered in the northeast New England states but extend down the Atlantic coast to Virginia, in the Midwest in Wisconsin and Minnesota, or with less frequency in the west in northern California. Lyme disease also occurs in eastern Canada, Europe, China, Japan, and Russia. In Eurasia, there are two additional genotypes (*Borrelia afzelii* and *Borrelia garinii*) that cause Lyme disease but with a variation in the clinical presentation. In the United States, humans are most likely to be infected in the summer months of June through August. The incubation period from tick bite to the appearance of skin lesion(s) ranges from 1 to 32 days with a median of 11 days.

The clinical manifestations of Lyme disease are generally divided into three stages: early localized, early disseminated, and late disease. In the **early localized** stage, an annular, erythematous, nonpruritic lesion known as *erythema migrans* presents at the site of a tick bite, usually within 1 to 2 weeks. Over several days, the lesion enlarges to 5 cm or more in diameter and occasionally develops central clearing providing the classic "bulls-eye" appearance. The early localized stage may present with or without constitutional symptoms such as malaise, headache, neck stiffness, myalgia, and arthralgia. Patients with **early disseminated** disease commonly present with multiple erythema migrans lesions due to spirochetemia, weeks to months after the initial tick bite. These lesions are typically smaller than the primary solitary lesion seen in early localized disease. Other manifestations of early disseminated disease may include neurologic involvement (lymphocytic meningitis, cranial nerve palsy—especially cranial nerve VII—and peripheral radiculopathy), carditis (atrioventricular block and myocardial dysfunction), and ocular manifestations (conjunctivitis, optic neuritis, keratitis, and uveitis). Patients may also have mild constitutional symptoms during this stage. **Late disseminated** disease occurs months to years after the onset of infection, typically in a patient without a history of early localized or early disseminated Lyme disease. The most common manifestation is recurrent pauciarticular arthritis of large joints with few cases presenting with encephalopathy, encephalitis, or polyneuropathy.

Early case reports and case series have documented that transplacental transmission of *B. burgdorferi* was possible and raised concerns about a potential congenital Lyme disease syndrome analogous to that seen with other spirochetal infections such as syphilis. A wide variety of clinical manifestations were noted, with most initial concerns being focused on congenital cardiac malformations and fetal death. However, epidemiologic studies and literature reviews have not supported an association between congenital infection and adverse fetal or neonatal outcomes. A prospective study of 2,014 pregnant women living in an endemic area had Lyme serology during their first prenatal visit and at delivery. Results showed no association between seropositivity or history of tick bite during pregnancy and congenital malformations, low birth weight, premature delivery, or fetal death. A report by the same authors compared 2,504 infants born in an endemic region to 2,507 delivered in a nonendemic region. This study showed a significant increase in the rate of congenital cardiac malformations in the endemic compared with the nonendemic region, but notably, no association within the endemic region between seropositivity and cardiac malformation. Similarly, in a retrospective case control study of 796 children with congenital heart disease and 704 control children, there was no association between cardiac anomalies and clinical evidence of Lyme disease during pregnancy. Although these studies were limited by the low prevalence of Lyme disease, it appears from available evidence that any increased risk for adverse neonatal effects of prenatal Lyme borreliosis are likely to be small.

There is no evidence that *B. burgdorferi* is transmitted in human milk.

II. DIAGNOSIS. Early Lyme disease is a clinical diagnosis made upon the recognition of the classic erythema migrans lesion in patients living in or visiting a Lyme disease endemic area. As such, no serologic testing is indicated in this scenario. However, the spectrum of clinical symptoms may be variable, especially when erythema migrans goes unrecognized. To date, there is no accepted syndrome of congenital Lyme borreliosis. Serologic testing is only indicated when all of the following are present: (i) there is a recent history of living or traveling to an endemic Lyme disease area, (ii) there is a risk factor for tick exposure, and (iii) symptoms are consistent with either early disseminated or late Lyme disease as described earlier. Standard serologic testing in these scenarios entails a two-tier assay using either an enzyme-linked immunosorbent assay (ELISA or EIA) or immunofluorescence assay (IFA) to detect immunoglobulin M (IgM) and immunoglobulin G (IgG) antibodies against *B. burgdorferi*. The IgM antibodies are detected 1 to 2 weeks after the appearance of erythema migrans and may be negative for patients with isolated erythema migrans, those who are pregnant, or those who have been treated early. In addition, false-positive EIA and IFA results can occur secondary to cross-reaction with other borrelial, spirochetal, bacterial, and viral infections as well as autoimmune diseases.

Therefore, positive or equivocal EIA or IFA test results should be confirmed with Western immunoblot as the second-tier test. The presence of at least two IgM bands (23/24, 39, and 41 kDa polypeptides) or five IgG bands (18, 23/24, 28, 30, 39, 41, 45, 60, 66, and 93 kDa polypeptides) is considered a positive immunoblot result. Caution must be taken when interpreting results due to laboratory reporting variability. A new serologic test, VlsE C6 peptide ELISA, which measure IgG to the variable major protein-like sequence-expressed sixth variant region, is now licensed and commercially available. VlsE C6 is being further studied as a potential for either single or concomitant use with current serologic testing modalities. If central nervous system involvement is suspected, spinal fluid serology should also be obtained. Polymerase chain reaction (PCR) for detection of *B. burgdorferi* in either cerebrospinal fluid (CSF) or synovial fluid can be used as adjunct for diagnostic purposes in seropositive patients with clinical symptoms suspicious of Lyme disease only if done in a reliable laboratory. False-positive PCR testing is common, and PCR results will not differentiate between active or previous infection.

III. TREATMENT OF MOTHERS AND THE NEWBORN. Patients known to have Lyme disease or who are suspected of having Lyme disease during pregnancy should be treated. The treatment is the same as for nonpregnant persons except that doxycycline is contraindicated.

A. Isolation. Standard isolation precautions are recommended.

B. Tick bite. Prophylactic treatment of tick bites with a single dose of doxycycline in endemic areas is not generally recommended. The Infectious Diseases Society of America recommends prophylactic treatment within 72 hours of tick removal in nonpregnant/nonlactating individuals older than 8 years old, with identified prolonged duration of an adult or nymph *Ixodes scapularis* tick attachment (>36 hours) based on engorgement and where local rates of tick infection with *B. burgdorferi* are ≥20%.

C. Early localized Lyme disease. Amoxicillin 500 mg PO TID for adults; 50 mg/kg/day divided TID PO (maximum 500 mg per dose) for children for 14 to 21 days or cefuroxime axetil 500 mg PO BID for adults; 30 mg/kg/day divided BID PO (maximum 500 mg per dose) for 14 to 21 days for children. For penicillin-allergic patients, azithromycin, erythromycin, and clarithromycin are alternatives; however, macrolides appear to be less effective, and these patients should therefore be closely followed up.

D. Early disseminated or late disseminated Lyme disease. Ceftriaxone 2 g intravenous (IV) once daily for adults; 50 to 75 mg/kg IV once daily (maximum 2 g per dose) for children or cefotaxime 2 g IV every 8 hours for adults; 150 to 200 mg/kg/day in three divided doses (maximum 6 g per day) for children. Alternatively, penicillin G 18 to 24 million units IV every day divided every 4 hours for adults; 200,000 to 400,000 units/kg/day divided every 4 hours (maximum 18 to 24 million units per day) in children. Length of therapy with any of these regimens is from 14 to 28 days depending on clinical response and severity of illness. Patients with isolated cranial nerve palsy, first- or second-degree heart block, or arthritis without neurologic manifestations may be treated with oral therapy as for localized early Lyme disease. Jarich-Herxheimer reaction (an acute febrile reaction accompanied by headache, myalgia, and an aggravated clinical picture lasting <24 hours) can occur when therapy is initiated. Symptomatic treatment, use of nonsteroidal anti-inflammatory drugs (NSAIDs), and continuation of the antimicrobial agent are recommended.

E. **Newborn of mother with confirmed Lyme disease in pregnancy.** The relative risk of fetal transmission as a function of severity of maternal disease during pregnancy, the timing of acquisition of Lyme disease during pregnancy, or the choice of antibiotic and route of administration used to treat maternal Lyme during pregnancy is not known. Similarly, data are lacking on the optimal therapy for the newborn infant with symptoms concerning for Lyme disease. In one report, a 38-week fetus born to a mother who developed acute Lyme disease one week before delivery developed petechiae and a vesicular rash that resolved with the IV administration of penicillin G for 10 days. If an infant is thought to have Lyme disease, treatment with penicillin, cefotaxime, or ceftriaxone IV should be given for 14 to 21 days after studies are taken from blood and spinal fluid. If a mother was treated for Lyme disease with erythromycin during pregnancy, consideration should be given to treatment of the infant based on clinical presentation.

F. **Prevention of Lyme disease.** A recombinant vaccine against the outer surface protein of *B. burgdorferi* was licensed by the U.S. Food and Drug Administration (FDA) in 1998 for individuals between 15 and 70 years of age. It was not recommended for use in pregnant women. The vaccine was withdrawn from the market in 2002 by the manufacturer owing to lack of demand. In the absence of a vaccine, prevention rests on avoidance of tick-infested areas, use of appropriate tick and insect repellents, and careful examination for and removal of ticks as soon as possible after attachment. Persons with acute infection should not donate blood, but persons who have been treated for Lyme disease can be considered for blood donation. Routine screening of pregnant women whether living in endemic or nonendemic areas is not recommended.

Suggested Readings

American Academy of Pediatrics Committee on Infectious Diseases. Prevention of Lyme disease. *Pediatrics* 2000;105:142–147.

American Academy of Pediatrics. Lyme disease. In: Kimberlin DW, Brady MT, Jackson MA, et al, eds. *Red book: 2015 Report of the Committee on Infectious Diseases.* 30th ed. Elk Grove Village, IL: American Academy of Pediatrics; 2015:516–525.

Elliott DJ, Eppes SC, Klein JD. Teratogen update: Lyme disease. *Teratology* 2001;64:276–281.

Mylonas I. Borreliosis during pregnancy: a risk for the unborn child? *Vector Borne Zoonotic Dis* 2011;11:891–898.

Silver HM. Lyme disease during pregnancy. *Infect Dis Clin North Am* 1997;11: 93–97.

Strobino BA, Abid S, Gewitz M. Maternal Lyme disease and congenital heart disease: a case-control study in an endemic area. *Am J Obstet Gynecol* 1999;180:711–716.

Strobino BA, Williams CL, Abid S, et al. Lyme disease and pregnancy outcome: a prospective study of two thousand prenatal patients. *Am J Obstet Gynecol* 1993;169:367–374.

Williams CL, Strobino BA, Weinstein A, et al. Maternal Lyme disease and congenital malformations: a cord blood serosurvey in endemic and control areas. *Paediatr Perinat Epidemiol* 1995;9:320–330.

Wormser GP, Dattwyler RJ, Shapiro ED, et al. The clinical assessment, treatment, and prevention of Lyme disease, human granulocytic anaplasmosis, and babesiosis: clinical practice guidelines by the Infectious Diseases Society of America. *Clin Infect Dis* 2006;43:1089–1134.

54

Intracranial Hemorrhage and White Matter Injury/Periventricular Leukomalacia

Janet S. Soul

KEY POINTS

- A large intracranial hemorrhage (ICH) of any type is an emergency that requires prompt stabilization with volume replacement pressors and respiratory support, as needed, and urgent neuroimaging.
- Due to radiation exposure, computed tomography (CT) scanning should be reserved for URGENT situations in which magnetic resonance imaging (MRI) is not available.
- Neurosurgical consultation should be obtained for large ICH with mass effect, particularly if there are signs of brainstem dysfunction and/or increased intracranial pressure.
- Seizures are common but may be subclinical, so electroencephalogram (EEG) monitoring should be obtained for newborns with significant intraventricular, parenchymal, subarachnoid, or subdural hemorrhage.

OVERVIEW

The incidence of intracranial hemorrhage (ICH) varies from 2% to >30% in newborns, depending on gestational age (GA) at birth and the type of ICH. Bleeding within the skull can occur in the following:

1. External to the brain into the epidural, subdural, or subarachnoid spaces

2. Into the parenchyma of the cerebrum or cerebellum

3. Into the ventricles from the subependymal germinal matrix or choroid plexus (Table 54.1)

The incidence, pathogenesis, clinical presentation, diagnosis, management, and prognosis of ICH varies according to the ICH location and size and the newborn's GA.[1,2] There is often a combination of two or more types of ICH because an ICH in one location often extends into an adjacent compartment; for example, extension of a parenchymal hemorrhage into the subarachnoid space or ventricles, such as a thalamic hemorrhagic infarction with associated intraventricular hemorrhage.

Table 54.1. Neonatal ICH by Location

Type (Location) of Hemorrhage	Principal Source of ICH	Relative Incidence in PT versus T
1. Subdural and epidural hemorrhage	1° > 2°	T > PT
2. Subarachnoid hemorrhage (SAH)	2° > 1°*	Unknown*
3. Intraparenchymal hemorrhage		
Cerebral	2° > 1°	PT > T
Cerebellar	2° > 1°?	PT > T
4. Germinal matrix/intraventricular hemorrhage	1° > 2°	PT > T

*True incidence unknown, small 1° SAH may be more common than is recognized in both PT and T newborns.
ICH, intracranial hemorrhage; PT, preterm; T, term.

Diagnosis usually depends on clinical suspicion when a newborn presents with typical neurologic signs, such as seizures, irritability, depressed level of consciousness, and/or focal neurologic deficits referable to either the cerebrum or brainstem. Diagnosis is confirmed with an appropriate neuroimaging study. Magnetic resonance imaging (MRI) is the optimal imaging modality for almost all types of ICH, but ultrasound (US) is typically preferred for premature newborns and critically ill newborns who are not stable for transport to MRI. To avoid exposure of newborns to the ionizing radiation associated with computed tomography (CT), CT scan should be used only for emergent imaging studies when neither MRI nor US is available/possible. The American Academy of Neurology (AAN) practice parameter states that all newborns with a birth GA of <30 weeks should undergo routine cranial ultrasound (CUS) between 7 and 14 days and optimally repeated between 36 and 40 weeks' postmenstrual age.[3] Our local practice is to obtain a CUS on every newborn with a birth GA of <32 weeks and birth weight <1,500 g.

Management varies according to the size and location of the ICH and the presenting neurologic signs. In general, only very large hemorrhages with clinical signs require surgical intervention for removal of the ICH itself. With a large ICH, pressor support or volume replacement (with normal saline, albumin, or packed red blood cells) may be required because of significant blood loss. More commonly, management is focused on treating complications such as seizures or the development of posthemorrhagic hydrocephalus. In general, although a large ICH is more likely to result in greater morbidity or mortality than a small one, the presence and severity of parenchymal injury, whether due to hemorrhage, infarction, or other neuropathology, is usually the best predictor of outcome.

Table 54.1 illustrates neonatal ICH by location, and whether each ICH type is predominantly primary[1] or secondary[2] source of bleeding, and the relative incidence in preterm or term newborns.

I. SUBDURAL HEMORRHAGE AND EPIDURAL HEMORRHAGE

A. **Etiology and pathogenesis.** The pathogenesis of subdural hemorrhage (SDH) relates to rupture of the draining veins and sinuses of the brain that occupy the subdural space. Vertical molding, fronto-occipital elongation, and torsional forces acting on the head during delivery may provoke laceration of dural leaflets of either the tentorium cerebelli or the falx cerebri. These lacerations can result in rupture of the vein of Galen, inferior sagittal sinus, straight sinus and/or transverse sinus, and usually result in posterior fossa SDH. Breech presentation also predisposes to occipital osteodiastasis, a depressed fracture of the occipital bone or bones, which may lead to direct laceration of the cerebellum or rupture of the occipital sinus. Clinically significant SDH in the posterior fossa can result from trauma in the full-term newborn, although small, inconsequential SDH ("parturitional SDH") is fairly common in uncomplicated deliveries (the true incidence in apparently well newborns is unknown). SDH in the supratentorial space usually results from rupture of the bridging, superficial veins over the cerebral convexity. Other risk factors for SDH include factors that increase the likelihood of significant forces on the newborn's head, such as large head size, rigid pelvis (e.g., in a primiparous or older multiparous mother), nonvertex presentation (breech, face, etc.), very rapid or prolonged labor or delivery, difficult instrumented delivery, or rarely, a bleeding diathesis. Postnatally, SDH and epidural hemorrhage (EH) are almost always due to direct head trauma or shaking; hence, nonaccidental injury needs to be suspected in cases of acute presentation of SDH or EH beyond the perinatal period. However, care should be taken not to confuse an old chronic effusion from a birth-related ICH with an acute postnatally acquired ICH. Careful interpretation of neuroimaging studies, particularly MRI, should help distinguish acute SDH or EH from chronic effusion.

B. **Clinical presentation.** When the accumulation of blood is rapid and large, as occurs with rupture of large veins or sinuses, the presentation follows shortly after birth and evolves rapidly. This is particularly true in infratentorial SDH where compression of the brainstem may result in nuchal rigidity or opisthotonus, obtundation or coma, apnea, other abnormal respiratory patterns, and unreactive pupils and/or abnormal extraocular movements. With increased intracranial pressure (ICP), there may be a bulging fontanelle and/or widely split sutures. With large hemorrhage, there may be systemic signs of hypovolemia and anemia. When the sources of hemorrhage are small veins, there may be few clinical signs for up to a week, at which time either the hematoma attains a critical size, imposes on the brain parenchyma, and produces neurologic signs or hydrocephalus develops. Seizures may occur in neonates with SDH, particularly with SDH over the cerebral convexity. With cerebral convexity SDH, there may also be subtle focal cerebral signs and mild disturbances of consciousness, such as irritability. Subarachnoid hemorrhage probably coexists in the majority of cases of neonatal SDH, as demonstrated by a cerebrospinal fluid (CSF) exam.[4] Finally, a chronic subdural effusion may gradually develop over months, presenting as abnormally rapid head growth, with the occipitofrontal circumference (OFC) crossing percentiles in the first weeks to months after birth.

C. **Diagnosis.** The diagnosis should be suspected on the basis of history and clinical signs and confirmed with a neuroimaging study. MRI is the study of choice for diagnosing SDH or EH, but CT may be used for acute emergencies if MRI cannot be obtained quickly, e.g., an unstable newborn with elevated ICP who may require neurosurgical intervention.[3] Although CUS may be valuable in evaluating the sick newborn at the bedside, **US imaging of structures adjacent to bone (i.e., the subdural space) is often inadequate.** MRI has proven to be quite sensitive to small hemorrhage and can help establish timing of ICH. MRI is also superior for detecting other lesions, such as contusion, thromboembolic infarction, or hypoxic-ischemic injury that may result from severe hypovolemia/anemia or other risk factors for parenchymal lesions. **When there is clinical suspicion of a large SDH, a lumbar puncture (LP) should not be performed until after neuroimaging is obtained.** An LP may be contraindicated if there is a large hemorrhage within the posterior fossa or supratentorial compartment. If a small SDH is found, an LP should be performed to rule out infection in the newborn with seizures, depressed mental status, or other systemic signs of illness because small SDH are often clinically silent.

D. **Management and prognosis.** Most newborns with SDH do not require surgical intervention and can be managed with supportive care and treatment of any accompanying seizures. Newborns with rapid evolution of a large infratentorial SDH require prompt stabilization with volume replacement (fluid and/or blood products), pressors, and respiratory support, as needed. An urgent head CT and neurosurgical consultation should be obtained in any newborn with signs of progressive brainstem dysfunction (i.e., coma, apnea, cranial nerve dysfunction), opisthotonus, or tense, bulging fontanelle. Open surgical evacuation of the clot is the usual management for the minority of newborns with large SDH in any location accompanied by such severe neurologic abnormalities or obstructive hydrocephalus. When the clinical picture is stable and no deterioration in neurologic function or unmanageable increase in ICP exists, supportive care and serial CT examinations instead of surgical intervention should be utilized in the management of posterior fossa SDH.[5] Laboratory testing to rule out sepsis or a bleeding diathesis should be considered with large SDH, particularly if there is no history of trauma or other risk factor for large SDH. The newborn should be monitored for the development of hydrocephalus, which can occur in a delayed fashion following SDH. Finally, chronic subdural effusions may occur rarely and can present weeks to months later with abnormally increased head growth. The outcome for newborns with nonsurgical SDH is usually good, provided there is no other significant neurologic injury or disease. The prognosis is also good for cases in which prompt surgical evacuation of the hematoma is successful and there is no other parenchymal injury.

E. **Epidural hemorrhage.** EH is uncommon in newborns compared with older infants and children. EH appears to be correlated with trauma (e.g., difficult instrumented delivery), and a large cephalohematoma or skull fracture was found in about half the reported cases of EH. Removal or aspiration of the hemorrhage was performed in the majority of reported cases, and the prognosis was quite good except when other ICH or parenchymal pathology was present. Similar to SDH, a small EH does not necessarily require surgical treatment but should still be monitored carefully with serial imaging to ensure there is no progressive enlargement of the EH or other hemorrhage or brain injury.

II. SUBARACHNOID HEMORRHAGE

A. Etiology and pathogenesis. Subarachnoid hemorrhage (SAH) is a common form of ICH among newborns, although the true incidence of small SAH remains unknown. Primary SAH (i.e., SAH not due to extension from ICH in an adjacent compartment) is probably frequent but clinically insignificant. In these cases, SAH may go unrecognized because of a lack of clinical signs. For example, hemorrhagic or xanthochromic CSF may be the only indication of such a hemorrhage in newborns who undergo a CSF exam to rule out sepsis. Small SAH probably results from the normal "trauma" associated with the birth process. The source of bleeding is usually ruptured bridging veins of the subarachnoid space or ruptured small leptomeningeal vessels. This is quite different from SAH in adults, where the source of bleeding is usually arterial and therefore produces a much more emergent clinical syndrome. SAH should be distinguished from subarachnoid extension of blood from a germinal matrix hemorrhage/intraventricular hemorrhage (GMH/IVH), which occurs most commonly in the preterm newborn. SAH may also result from extension of SDH or a cerebral contusion (parenchymal hemorrhage). Finally, subpial hemorrhage is a focal subtype of SAH that occurs mostly in term newborns and is likely caused by local trauma resulting in venous compression or occlusion in the setting of a vaginal delivery (often instrumented).[6]

B. Clinical presentation. As with other forms of ICH, clinical suspicion of SAH may result because of blood loss or neurologic dysfunction. Only rarely is the blood volume loss large enough to provoke catastrophic results. More often, neurologic signs manifest as seizures, irritability, or other mild alteration of mental status, particularly with SAH or subpial hemorrhage occurring over the cerebral convexities. Small SAH may not result in any overt clinical signs except seizures in an otherwise well-appearing baby. In these circumstances, the seizures may be misdiagnosed as abnormal movements or other clinical events.

C. Diagnosis. Seizures, irritability, lethargy, or focal neurologic signs should prompt investigation to determine whether there is a SAH (or other ICH). The diagnosis is best established with a brain MRI scan, or by LP, to confirm or diagnose small SAH. CT scans may be adequate to diagnose SAH but as in the case of SDH/EH, an MRI is preferred because of the lack of radiation and to determine if there is any other parenchymal pathology. For example, SAH may occur in the setting of hypoxic-ischemic brain injury or meningoencephalitis, pathologies which are better detected by MRI than CT or US. CUS is not sensitive for the detection of small SAH so should be used only if the patient is too unstable for transport to MRI/CT.

D. Management and prognosis. Management of SAH usually requires only symptomatic therapy, such as anticonvulsant therapy for seizures (see Chapter 56) and nasogastric feeds or intravenous fluids if the newborn is too lethargic to feed orally. The majority of newborns with small

SAH do well with no recognized sequelae. In rare cases, a very large SAH will cause a catastrophic presentation with profound depression of mental status, seizures, and/or brainstem signs. In such cases, blood transfusions and cardiovascular support should be provided as needed, and neurosurgical intervention may be required. It is important to establish by MRI whether there is coexisting hypoxia-ischemia or other significant neuropathology that will be the crucial determinant of a poor neurologic prognosis because a surgical procedure may not improve outcome if there is extensive brain injury in addition to the SAH. Occasionally, hydrocephalus will develop after a moderate-to-large SAH, and thus, follow-up CUS scans should be performed in such newborns, particularly if there are signs of increased ICP or abnormally rapid head growth.

III. INTRAPARENCHYMAL HEMORRHAGE

A. Etiology and pathogenesis

1. **Primary cerebral hemorrhage** is uncommon in all newborns, whereas cerebellar hemorrhage is found in 5% to 10% of autopsy specimens in the premature newborn. An intracerebral hemorrhage may occur rarely as a primary event related to rupture of an arteriovenous malformation or aneurysm, from a coagulation disturbance (e.g., hemophilia, thrombocytopenia), or from an unknown cause. More commonly, cerebral intraparenchymal hemorrhage (IPH) occurs as a secondary event, such as hemorrhage into a region of hypoxic-ischemic brain injury. From the venous side of the cerebral circulation, IPH may occur as a result of venous infarction (because venous infarctions are typically hemorrhagic) either in relation to a large GMH/IVH (preterm > term; see section IV) or as a result of sinus venous thrombosis (term > preterm). From the arterial side, bleeding may occur secondarily into an arterial embolic infarction or into areas of hypoxic-ischemic brain injury from global hypoxia-ischemia (term > preterm). Occasionally, there may be hemorrhage that occurs secondarily within an area of necrotic periventricular leukomalacia (PVL) (preterm > term). IPH may be found occasionally in newborns undergoing extracorporeal membrane oxygenation (ECMO) therapy. Finally, cerebral IPH may occur as an extension of a large ICH in another compartment, such as large SAH or SDH, as rarely occurs with significant trauma or coagulation disturbance, and it may sometimes be difficult to identify the original source of hemorrhage.

2. **Intracerebellar hemorrhage** occurs more commonly in preterm than term newborns and may be missed by routine CUS because the reported incidence is higher in neuropathologic than clinical studies. The use of mastoid and posterior fontanelle views during CUS examination increases the likelihood of detection of cerebellar hemorrhage (and posterior fossa SAH), and MRI is more sensitive for the detection of small posterior fossa IPH, SAH, or SDH.[7] Intracerebellar IPH may be a primary hemorrhage or may result from venous hemorrhagic infarction or from extension of GMH/IVH or SAH (preterm > term), and small foci of cerebellar hemorrhage of unclear pathogenesis may be detected by MRI > US. It is difficult to determine the original source of cerebellar

hemorrhage by US (and sometimes MRI); hence, the proportion of primary versus secondary cerebellar hemorrhage is unclear. Cerebellar IPH rarely occurs as an extension of large SAH/SDH in the posterior fossa related to a trauma (term > preterm).

B. Clinical presentation. The presentation of IPH is similar to that of SDH, where the clinical syndrome differs depending on the size and location of the IPH. In the preterm newborn, IPH is often clinically silent in either intracranial fossa, unless the hemorrhage is quite large. In the term newborn, intracerebral hemorrhage typically presents with focal neurologic signs such as seizures, asymmetry of tone/movements, or gaze preference, along with irritability or depressed level of consciousness. A large cerebellar hemorrhage (± SDH/SAH) presents as described in section I earlier and should be managed as for a large posterior fossa SDH.

C. Diagnosis. MRI is the best imaging modality for IPH, but CUS may be used in the preterm newborn or when a rapid bedside imaging study is necessary. CT can be used for urgent evaluation when MRI is not available quickly, but the radiation exposure of CT should be avoided when possible, and CT is insensitive for detection of small posterior fossa ICH because of artifact from surrounding skull bones. MRI is superior for demonstrating the extent and age of the hemorrhage and the presence of any other parenchymal abnormality. In addition, magnetic resonance (MR) angiography/venography may be useful to demonstrate a vascular anomaly, lack of flow distal to an arterial embolus, or sinus venous thrombosis. Thus, MRI is more likely than CT or CUS to establish the etiology of the IPH and to determine accurately the long-term prognosis for the term newborn. For the preterm newborn, CUS views through the mastoid and posterior fontanelle improve the detection of hemorrhage in the posterior fossa.

D. Management and prognosis

1. Acute management of IPH is similar to that for SDH and SAH, where most small hemorrhages require only symptomatic treatment and support, whereas a large IPH with severe neurologic compromise should prompt neurosurgical intervention. It is important to diagnose and treat any coexisting pathology, such as infection or sinus venous thrombosis because these underlying conditions may cause further injury that can have a greater impact on long-term outcome than the IPH itself. A large IPH, especially in association with IVH or SAH/SDH, may cause hydrocephalus, and thus head growth and neurologic status should be monitored for days to weeks following IPH. Follow-up imaging by MRI and/or CUS should be obtained in the case of large IPH, both to establish the severity and extent of injury and to rule out hydrocephalus or remaining vascular malformation.

2. The long-term prognosis largely relates to location and size of the IPH and GA of the newborn. A small IPH may have relatively few or no long-term neurologic consequences. A large cerebral IPH may result in a lifelong seizure disorder, hemiparesis or other type of cerebral palsy (CP), feeding difficulties, and cognitive impairments ranging from learning disabilities to significant intellectual disability, depending on the location and size of parenchymal injury. Focal cerebellar hemorrhage in the term newborn often has a relatively good prognosis, although it may result in cerebellar signs of ataxia, hypotonia, tremor, nystagmus, and mild cognitive deficits. There may be only minor deficits from small, unilateral cerebellar IPH in either preterm or term newborns. In contrast, an extensive cerebellar IPH that destroys a significant portion of the cerebellum (i.e., significant bilateral cerebellar injury) in a preterm newborn may result in severe cognitive and motor disability for those newborns who survive the newborn period.[8]

IV. GERMINAL MATRIX HEMORRHAGE/INTRAVENTRICULAR HEMORRHAGE

A. Etiology and pathogenesis. GMH/IVH is found principally in the preterm newborn, where the incidence is currently 15% to 20% in newborns born at <32 weeks' GA but is uncommon in the term newborn. The etiology and pathogenesis are different for term and preterm newborns.

1. **In the term newborn**, primary IVH typically originates in the choroid plexus or in association with venous (± sinus) thrombosis and thalamic infarction and much less commonly in the small remnant of the subependymal germinal matrix. The pathogenesis of IVH in the term newborn is more likely to be related to perinatal asphyxia, venous thrombosis, trauma (i.e., from a difficult delivery), and/or other risk factors. One study suggested that IVH might occur secondary to venous hemorrhagic infarction in the thalamus in 63% of otherwise healthy term newborns with clinically significant IVH.[9] In such cases, there may be thrombosis of the internal cerebral veins, but occasionally, there may be more extensive sinovenous thrombosis.

2. **In the preterm newborn, GMH/IVH originates from the fragile involuting vessels of the subependymal germinal matrix, located in the caudothalamic groove.** There are numerous risk factors that have been identified in the etiology of IVH, including maternal factors such as infection/inflammation and hemorrhage, lack of antenatal steroids, external factors such as mode of delivery or neonatal transport to another hospital, and increasingly recognized genetic factors that predispose some newborns to IVH. These risk factors all contribute to the pathogenesis of GMH/IVH, which is largely related to intravascular, vascular, and extravascular factors (Table 54.2). The intravascular risk factors are probably the most important and are also the factors most amenable to preventive efforts.

a. The intravascular risk factors predisposing to GMH/IVH include ischemia/reperfusion, increases in cerebral blood flow (CBF), fluctuating CBF, and increases in cerebral venous pressure. Ischemia/reperfusion occurs commonly when hypotension is corrected. This scenario often occurs shortly after birth when a premature newborn may have hypovolemia or hypotension that is treated with infusion of colloid, normal saline, or hyperosmolar solutions such as sodium bicarbonate. Rapid infusions of such solutions are thought to be particularly likely to contribute to GMH/IVH. Indeed, studies of the beagle puppy model showed that ischemia/reperfusion (hypotension precipitated by blood removal followed by volume infusion) reliably produces GMH/IVH.[10]

Table 54.2. Factors in the Pathogenesis of GMH/IVH

Intravascular factors	Ischemia/reperfusion (e.g., volume infusion after hypotension)
	Fluctuating CBF (e.g., with mechanical ventilation)
	Increase in cerebral venous pressure (e.g., with high intrathoracic pressure, usually from ventilator)
	Increase in CBF (e.g., with hypertension, anemia, hypercarbia)
	Platelet dysfunction and coagulation disturbances
Vascular factors	Tenuous, involuting capillaries with large luminal diameter
Extravascular factors	Deficient vascular support
	Excessive fibrinolytic activity

GMH/IVH, germinal matrix hemorrhage/intraventricular hemorrhage; CBF, cerebral blood flow.

Briefer fluctuations in CBF has been demonstrated to be associated with GMH/IVH in preterm newborns. In one study, newborns with large fluctuations in CBF velocity by Doppler US were much more likely to develop GMH/IVH than newborns with a stable pattern of CBF velocity.[11] The large fluctuations typically occurred in newborns breathing out of synchrony with the ventilator, but such fluctuations have also been observed in newborns with large patent ductus arteriosus or hypotension, for example. Increases in cerebral venous pressure are also thought to contribute to GMH/IVH. Sources of such increases include ventilatory strategies where intrathoracic pressure is high (e.g., high continuous positive airway pressure), pneumothorax, tracheal suctioning, and both labor and delivery, where fetal head compression likely results in significantly increased venous pressure.[12] Indeed, a higher incidence of GMH/IVH is found in preterm newborns with a longer duration of labor and in those delivered vaginally compared with those delivered via cesarean section. With all of these intravascular factors related to changes in cerebral arterial and venous blood flow, the role of a **pressure-passive** cerebral circulation is likely to be important. Several studies have shown that preterm newborns, particularly asphyxiated newborns, have an impaired ability to regulate CBF in response to blood pressure changes (hence "pressure-passive").[13,14] Such impaired autoregulation puts the newborn at increased risk for rupture of the fragile germinal matrix vessels in the face of significant increases in cerebral arterial or venous pressure, and particularly when ischemia precedes such increased pressure. Sustained increases in CBF may also contribute to GMH/IVH and can be caused by seizures, hypercarbia, anemia, and hypoglycemia, which result in a compensatory increase in CBF. In addition to cerebrovascular factors affecting arterial or venous flow, impaired coagulation and platelet dysfunction are intravascular factors that can contribute to the pathogenesis or severity of GMH/IVH.

b. Vascular factors that contribute to GMH/IVH include the fragile nature of the involuting vessels of the germinal matrix. There is no muscularis mucosa and little adventitia in this area of relatively large diameter, thin-walled vessels; all of these factors make the vessels particularly susceptible to rupture.

c. Extravascular risk factors for GMH/IVH include deficient extravascular support and likely excessive fibrinolytic activity in preterm newborns (see Table 54.2).

B. **Pathogenesis of complications of GMH/IVH.** The two major complications of GMH/IVH are **periventricular hemorrhagic infarction (PVHI)** and **posthemorrhagic ventricular dilation (PVD). The risk of both complications increases with larger size of IVH.** The pathogeneses of these two complications are discussed here.

1. **PVHI** has previously been considered an extension of a large IVH, hence is often referred to as a grade IV IVH. Although this designation is still used in much of the literature, neuropathologic studies have shown that the finding of a large, often unilateral or asymmetric, hemorrhagic lesion dorsolateral to the lateral ventricle **is not an extension of the original IVH but is a separate lesion consisting of a venous hemorrhagic infarction**. Neuropathologic studies demonstrate the fan-shaped appearance of a typical hemorrhagic venous infarction in the distribution of the medullary veins that drain into the terminal vein, resulting from obstruction of flow in the terminal vein by the large ipsilateral IVH. Evidence supporting the notion of venous obstruction underlying the pathogenesis of PVHI includes the observation that PVHI occurs on the side of the larger IVH, and Doppler US studies show markedly decreased or absent flow in the terminal vein on the side of the large IVH.[15] Further neuropathologic evidence that PVHI is a separate lesion from the original IVH is that the ependymal lining of the lateral ventricle separating IVH and PVHI has been observed to remain intact in some cases, demonstrating that the IVH did not "extend" into the adjacent cerebral parenchyma. Hence, PVHI is a complication of large IVH, which is why some authors refer to it as a separate lesion rather than denoting PVHI to be a "higher" grade of IVH (i.e., a grade IV IVH). Risk factors for the development of PVHI include low GA, low Apgar scores, early life acidosis, patent ductus arteriosus, pneumothorax, pulmonary hemorrhage, and need for significant respiratory or blood pressure support.[16]

2. **Progressive PVD or posthemorrhagic hydrocephalus (PHH— terminology varies)** may occur days to weeks following the onset of GMH/IVH. Not all ventricular dilation progresses to established hydrocephalus that requires treatment; hence, the terms are used with slightly different meanings (see section IV.C.3 for clinical course of PVD). The pathogenesis of *progressive PVD* may relate in part to impaired CSF resorption and/or obstruction of the aqueduct or the foramina of

Luschka or Magendie by particulate clot.[17] However, other mechanisms likely play an important role in the pathogenesis of PVD. High levels of TGF-β1 are found in the CSF following IVH, particularly in newborns with PVD; TGF-β1 upregulates genes for extracellular matrix proteins that elaborate a "scar" which may obstruct CSF flow and/or CSF reabsorption.[17–19] In addition, restricted arterial pulsations (e.g., due to decreased intracranial compliance) have been proposed to underlie chronic hydrocephalus in hydrodynamic models of hydrocephalus.[20] The **pathogenesis of the brain injury resulting from PVD** is probably related in large part to regional hypoxia-ischemia and mechanical distension of the periventricular white matter based on animal and human studies.[21–24] In addition, the presence of non–protein-bound iron in the CSF of newborns with PVD may lead to the generation of reactive oxygen species that in turn contribute to the injury of immature oligodendrocytes in the white matter.[25] The brain injury associated with PVD is principally a bilateral cerebral white matter injury (WMI) similar to PVL with regard to both its neuropathology and long-term outcome.[24,26,27]

C. Clinical presentation

1. **GMH/IVH in the preterm newborn is usually a clinically silent syndrome** and thus is recognized only when a routine CUS is performed. The vast majority of these hemorrhages occur within 72 hours after birth, hence the use of routine CUS within 3 to 4 days after birth in many nurseries for newborns with a GA <32 weeks. Newborns with large IVH may present with full fontanelle, anemia, decreased levels of consciousness and spontaneous movements, hypotonia, abnormal eye movements, or skew deviation. Rarely, a newborn will present with a rapid and severe neurologic deterioration with full or tense fontanelle, obtundation or coma, severe hypotonia and lack of spontaneous movements, and generalized tonic posturing thought to be seizure but does not have an electrographic correlate by electroencephalogram.

2. **The term newborn with IVH typically presents with signs such as seizures, apnea, irritability or lethargy, vomiting with dehydration, or a full fontanelle.** Ventriculomegaly is often present at the time of IVH diagnosis in a term newborn. IVH may be initially unrecognized such that newborns may be discharged home after birth and then present within the first week or so after birth with the earlier-listed clinical signs.

3. **PVD may develop over days to weeks following IVH** and may present with splitting of sutures, decreased level of consciousness, increased apnea or worsening respiratory status, feeding difficulties, increasing head growth (crossing percentiles on the growth chart), bulging fontanelle, or impaired upgaze or sunsetting sign. However, PVD is often relatively asymptomatic in preterm newborns because ICP is often normal in this population, particularly with slowly progressive dilation, and the signs of PVD are relatively nonspecific. Thus, serial CUS scans are critical for diagnosis of PVD in preterm newborns with known IVH. A retrospective study of newborns with birth weight <1,500 g who developed IVH and survived at least 14 days showed that 50%

Table 54.3. Grading of GMH/IVH

Grading System	Severity of GMH/IVH	Description of Findings
Papile[29]	I	Isolated GMH (no IVH)
	II	IVH without ventricular dilatation
	III	IVH with ventricular dilatation
	IV	IVH with parenchymal hemorrhage
Volpe[2]	I	GMH with no or minimal IVH (<10% ventricular volume)
	II	IVH occupying 10%–50% of ventricular area on parasagittal view
	III	IVH occupying >50% of ventricular area on parasagittal view, usually distends lateral ventricle *(at time of IVH diagnosis)*
	Separate notation	Periventricular echodensity (location and extent)

GMH/IVH, germinal matrix hemorrhage/intraventricular hemorrhage.

of such newborns will not show ventricular dilation, 25% will develop nonprogressive ventricular dilation (or stable ventriculomegaly), and the remaining 25% will develop PVD.[28] The incidence of PVD increases with increasing severity of GMH/IVH; it is uncommon with grades I to II IVH (Table 54.3) (up to 12%) but occurs in up to 75% of newborns with grade III IVH ± PVHI. The incidence of PVD is also higher with younger GA at birth. Ventricular dilation may proceed rapidly (over a few days) or slowly (over weeks). About 40% of newborns with PVD will have spontaneous resolution of PVD without any treatment. The remaining 60% generally require medical and/or surgical therapy (~15% of this latter group does not survive).

D. **Diagnosis**

1. **The diagnosis of GMH/IVH is almost invariably made by real-time portable CUS in the premature newborn.** We obtain routine CUS studies in all newborns born at <32 weeks' GA, but the GA threshold for obtaining screening US varies from 30 to 32 weeks among different institutions. A CUS may be considered in older newborns born at >32 weeks' GA who have risk factors such as perinatal asphyxia or tension pneumothorax or who present with abnormal neurologic signs as described earlier. We perform routine CUS studies on or around days 7, 30, and 60 (or just prior to discharge) for newborns born at <32 weeks' GA (or birth weight <1,500 g). For unstable newborns in whom the

CUS may change management, we also obtain a CUS in the first few days after birth. In a very sick, very low birth weight newborn, consideration should be given to performing a first CUS within 24 hours of birth because a large IVH with/without additional intracranial pathology (e.g., PVHI) may be an important factor in considering redirection of goals of care. Also, a large IVH in very sick, very preterm newborns may require earlier follow-up CUS studies to determine whether there is rapid progressive ventricular dilation, which occurs more frequently in the smaller more preterm newborns. Newborns with GMH/IVH require more frequent CUS than newborns without GMH/IVH to monitor for complications of GMH/IVH such as PVD and PVHI and for other lesions such as PVL (see section V in the following text) or cerebellar hemorrhage. In addition, any preterm newborn who develops abnormal neurologic signs or a significant risk factor for IVH (such as pneumothorax, sepsis, sudden hypotension, or volume loss of any etiology) later in their neonatal intensive care unit (NICU) course should undergo CUS.

2. **Grading of GMH/IVH is important for determining management and prognosis.** Two systems are widely used for grading GMH/IVH as outlined in Table 54.3.[2,29] Grading of GMH/IVH should be assigned based on the earliest CUS obtained when the IVH itself is of maximal size. Notably, ventricular dilation that occurs days to weeks following GMH/IVH is **not** considered a grade III IVH if the original IVH grade was grade I or II; it represents either PVD or ventriculomegaly secondary to parenchymal volume loss. Given the variability in grading systems and in CUS interpretation, a detailed description of the CUS findings is more informative than only assigning a grade of GMH/IVH. Specifically, the description should include the following:
   a. Presence or absence of hemorrhage in the germinal matrix
   b. Laterality (or bilaterality) of the hemorrhage
   c. Presence or absence of hemorrhage in each ventricle, including volume of hemorrhage in relation to ventricle size
   d. Presence or absence of echogenicity (blood or other abnormality) in cerebral parenchyma, with specification of location and size of echogenicity
   e. Presence or absence of ventricular dilation, with measurements of ventricles when enlarged
   f. Presence or absence of any other intracranial hemorrhage (e.g., SAH) or parenchymal abnormalities

3. **In the term newborn, IVH is usually diagnosed when a CUS or MRI is performed because of seizures, apnea, or abnormal mental status. A CUS is sufficient to detect IVH**, but brain MRI is superior for the demonstration of other lesions that may be associated with IVH in full-term newborns, such as hypoxic-ischemic brain injury or thalamic hemorrhagic infarction, with or without sinus venous thrombosis, particularly when diffusion-weighted, susceptibility-weighted, and MR venography sequences are included (see Table 54.3).

E. **Management and prognosis**

1. **Prevention of GMH/IVH should be the primary goal**; the decreased incidence of GMH/IVH since the 1980s is likely related to numerous

improvements in maternal and neonatal care, although the incidence has only modestly declined further in the last decade.[30] Although antenatal administration of **glucocorticoids** has clearly been shown to decrease the incidence of GMH/IVH, antenatal phenobarbital, vitamin K, and magnesium sulfate have not been conclusively demonstrated to prevent GMH/IVH. Postnatal prevention of GMH/IVH should be directed toward minimizing risk factors outlined earlier in section IV.A. In particular, infusions of colloid or hyperosmolar solutions should be given slowly when possible, and all efforts should be directed to avoiding hypotension and large fluctuations or sustained increases in arterial blood pressure or cerebral venous pressure. Prophylactic ibuprofen and indomethacin given to close PDA have both been associated with reduced severe IVH and PVHI in some studies, but no difference was shown in long-term neurologic outcome, and these drugs are not routinely recommended solely for prevention of IVH. Elimination of CBF fluctuation related to mechanical ventilation may be achieved by administration of sedative medication. This recommendation is based on the randomized trial that showed a marked reduction in the incidence of GMH/IVH in premature newborns with fluctuating CBF who were muscle relaxed for the first 72 hours after birth, compared with newborns who were not muscle relaxed.[31] We do not routinely muscle relax our preterm newborns because of the many risks associated with this intervention but do provide sedation as needed.

2. **Management of GMH/IVH in the premature newborn largely consists of supportive care** and monitoring for and treatment of complications of GMH/IVH. An increase in the size of GMH/IVH may occur; thus, appropriate early care may prevent enlargement of the IVH. Supportive care should be directed toward maintaining stable cerebral perfusion by maintaining normal blood pressure, circulating volume, electrolytes, and blood gases. Transfusions of packed red blood cells may be required in cases of large IVH to restore normal blood volume and hematocrit. Thrombocytopenia or coagulation disturbances should be corrected.

3. **Management of IVH in the term newborn is directed at supportive care of the newborn and treatment of seizures during the acute phase.** However, as symptomatic IVH in this group of newborns is frequently large, PVD develops in many newborns and **may require serial LPs and/or eventual ventriculoperitoneal shunt placement in up to 50% of such newborns**.

4. **Management of PVD consists of careful monitoring of ventricle size by serial CUS and appropriate intervention when needed to reduce CSF accumulation, such as serial LPs to remove CSF, surgical interventions to divert CSF flow, and rarely, medications to reduce CSF production** (Fig. 54.1). The goals of therapy are to reduce ventriculomegaly and remove blood products, both of which may contribute to the pathogenesis of brain injury (see section IV.B.2) and potentially to prevent need for a permanent shunt. CSF removal has been shown to improve cerebral perfusion, metabolism, and neurophysiologic function

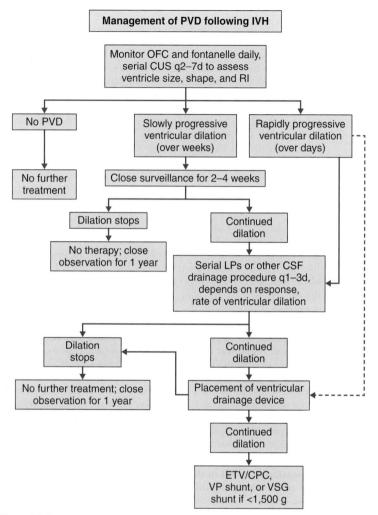

Figure 54.1. Suggested algorithm for management of posthemorrhagic ventricular dilation (PVD) following intraventricular hemorrhage (IVH). OFC, occipital-frontal circumference; CUS, cranial ultrasound; RI, resistive index; LP, lumbar puncture; CSF, cerebrospinal fluid; ETV/CPC, endoscopic third ventriculostomy combined with choroid plexus cauterization; VP, ventriculoperitoneal; VSG, ventriculosubgaleal.

in newborns with PVD.[21,32–34] Evidence from numerous animal studies and some human data suggest that earlier treatment of PVD can improve neurologic outcome,[35–38] although most human clinical trials of medications or interventions to treat PVD have not shown improved neurologic outcome. There are ongoing trials of PVD management at the time of writing, so further data may soon be available to guide management.

a. In cases of **slowly progressive PVD** (over weeks), close monitoring of clinical status (particularly OFC, fontanelle, and sutures) and ventricle size (by CUS) may be sufficient. Many such cases will have spontaneous resolution of PVD without intervention or will prove to have stable ventriculomegaly. **It is critical to determine by serial CUS which newborns have progressive dilation requiring therapy versus which newborns have stable ventriculomegaly (e.g., caused by atrophic ventriculomegaly associated with PVL).**

b. When serial CUS show persistent PVD, intervention is usually required, particularly if the newborn shows clinical signs related to the PVD (e.g., worsening clinical status, bulging fontanelle, widening sutures, abnormally rapid increase in OFC). Notably, there is currently no consensus regarding the threshold for initiating intervention or the best management strategy. One retrospective study suggested that treatment initiated before ventricle size reached the 97th percentile + 4 mm resulted in improved long-term neurologic outcome,[38] but no prospective interventional trial (drug and/or procedure) has demonstrated a clear benefit of intervention on outcome. **We typically begin therapy when progressive dilation persists for about 1 to 2 weeks in newborns with clinical signs**, although the rate of ventricular dilation and size of ventricles are assessed in each case to decide whether therapy should be initiated sooner or later. We use a combination of measures of ventricle size, rate of PVD, resistive index (RI) (see the following text), and the newborn's clinical course to decide when to initiate treatment, rather than using a single measure of ventricle size as an upper limit (e.g., 97th percentile + 4 mm).[39] Therapeutic LPs to remove CSF can be performed every 1 to 3 days (removing 10 to 15 mL of CSF per kg body weight), depending on the rate of ventricular dilation and the effectiveness of CSF removal. The opening pressure should be measured whenever possible to help guide therapy. A CUS performed before and after CSF removal is often helpful in establishing the diagnosis of PVD and determining the effect of CSF removal in decreasing ventricle size.[34] If PVD is rapidly progressive, daily taps or early surgical intervention with a subgaleal shunt or external drain may be needed.

c. Measurement of the RI can be helpful in guiding management of PVD. The RI is a measure of resistance to blood flow and may indicate when intracranial compliance is low and cerebral perfusion may be decreased. Because persistent or intermittent decreases in cerebral perfusion may result in ischemic brain injury, we use the measurement of RI to help guide treatment of PVD. **RI is obtained by measuring systolic and diastolic blood flow velocities** by Doppler US (usually in the anterior cerebral artery) and calculating the RI as given by the formula:

$$RI = \frac{(systolic - diastolic)}{systolic}$$

where "systolic" refers to systolic blood flow velocity, and "diastolic" refers to diastolic blood flow velocity. Normal RI values are <0.7 in newborns, and baseline values >0.9 to 1.0 indicate that diastolic flow to the brain is compromised. Occasionally, values of RI >1 will be recorded, due to reversal of flow during diastole, which likely puts the newborn at risk for ongoing ischemic brain injury. A significant rise in RI from baseline RI values when gentle fontanelle compression is applied may indicate hemodynamic compromise and the need to remove CSF. We typically consider a >30% increase in RI with compression compared to baseline RI, or a baseline RI >0.9, as an indication for the need for CSF removal.[40] Note that the interpretation of RI needs to take into account the presence of other conditions that can affect systolic and/or diastolic blood flow, such as a large PDA or use of high-frequency ventilation.

d. A combination of the newborn's clinical status, ventricular size and shape by serial CUS, measurement of ICP by manometry, RI by Doppler US, and response to CSF removal should be used to determine **the need for and frequency of CSF removal procedures** or other interventions to reduce intraventricular CSF volume and reduce the risk of ischemic brain injury (see Fig. 54.1).

e. If medical therapy does not successfully reduce ventricle size, and/or PVD is rapidly progressive, surgical intervention is indicated. A ventriculosubgaleal shunt (VSG), ventricular access device (reservoir), or external ventricular drain should be placed. We prefer to insert a VSG because (like a ventricular drain) it offers continuous CSF drainage and hence the potential to maintain normal ventricle size and cerebral perfusion as opposed to intermittent CSF removal by spinal or ventricular taps. A VSG may be sufficient for adequate CSF drainage into the subgaleal space for days to weeks although may provide insufficient drainage or eventually become blocked by particulate matter.[41] If there is insufficient CSF drainage by the VSG, CSF may be removed intermittently by a needle placed in the reservoir of the VSG (or ventricular access device) every 1 to 3 days, as for serial LPs. External ventricular drains are less favored by our neurosurgeons because of the risk of infection, especially if the catheter is not tunneled subcutaneously, although they do provide the ideal therapy of *continuous* (rather than intermittent) CSF drainage.

f. Acetazolamide and furosemide are carbonic anhydrase inhibitors that can be used to decrease CSF production. However, their combined use often produces electrolyte disturbances and nephrocalcinosis and may be associated with a worse long-term neurologic outcome.[42,43] For these reasons, the use of acetazolamide and furosemide together has fallen out of favor, and we rarely use these agents in our local practice. A large multicenter trial of these two agents used together showed no improvement in neurologic outcome compared with "standard therapy," although the standard therapy group was not managed according to a standardized protocol, and treatment was initiated only once the PVD was well established.[42,43] Acetazolamide could be considered for cases where intermittent CSF removal is not possible by LP, ventricular tap or surgical drainage procedure, or to reduce the frequency of intermittent CSF removal procedures, for example, in very

small or critically ill newborns in whom a surgical procedure has an un
acceptably high risk. However, the safety and efficacy of acetazolamide
monotherapy for PVD has not been demonstrated in large studies, and
pharmacotherapy alone is insufficient in most severe cases of PVD.

g. Fibrinolytic therapy alone has not been demonstrated to prevent PVD
in five separate studies of different fibrinolytic agents.[44] A pilot trial
of continuous DRainage, Irrigation and Fibrinolytic Therapy (called
"DRIFT") in 24 newborns with PVD showed a promising reduction in
the incidence of shunt surgery, mortality, and disability compared with
historical controls.[45] However, when this very intensive high-risk therapy
was tested in a larger multicenter trial, the side effects appeared to outweigh the benefit.[46] Of 34 newborns treated with DRIFT in this second
trial, 2 died and 13 received a ventriculoperitoneal (VP) shunt (44%),
whereas of the 36 newborns treated with standard therapy (lumbar or
ventricular taps), 5 died and 14 underwent a shunt placement (50%).[46]
Notably, 12 of 34 patients treated with DRIFT had a secondary IVH,
whereas only 3 of 36 in the standard therapy group had further IVH.
This second trial showed that DRIFT may have been helpful in reducing
the incidence of severe cognitive disability to a subset of newborns,[47] but
the overall risks of the therapy were greater than in the pilot trial; thus,
this therapy has not been widely adopted.

**h. If PVD has persisted for >4 weeks despite medical therapy as
described earlier, a permanent shunt will usually be needed.** However, a permanent VP shunt can usually only be placed once newborns
weigh >1,500 to 2,000 g and are stable enough to undergo this surgery.
If the newborn weighs <1,500 g, a VSG,[41] external drain, or ventricular
access device will be needed (if not already placed) until the newborn
is large enough to undergo VP shunt placement. An **endoscopic third
ventriculostomy combined with choroid plexus cauterization (ETV/
CPC)** procedure may be attempted instead of VP shunt in centers that
have the expertise for this procedure to avoid complications associated
with a permanent shunt.[48] Success of an ETV is more likely if there is no
scarring in the prepontine cistern, if the aqueduct is obstructed, and if
choroid plexus cauterization is performed.[49] Depending on these factors,
failure may occur in up to 60% of cases, usually within 6 months of the
procedure, and a VP shunt will need to be placed.

**i. Rarely, PVD will recur weeks to months later despite apparent
resolution in the neonatal period.**[50] Monitoring of head growth and
fontanelle should continue after discharge home for the first year of life.
(see Fig. 54.1)

5. **The long-term prognosis for newborns with GMH/IVH varies considerably depending on the severity of IVH, complications of IVH
or other brain lesions, the birth weight/GA, and other significant
illnesses that affect neurologic outcome.** Several studies show that
preterm newborns with grades I to II IVH have an increased risk of CP
and/or cognitive impairment compared with those without IVH.[51–53]
One study showed that >50% of adolescents born at <32 weeks'
GA had school difficulties, with IVH being a major risk factor.[54] That
being said, these cognitive impairments likely relate at least in part to

coexisting cerebral WMI (i.e., PVL, see next section), which has many of the same risk factors as GMH/IVH. Newborns with ventriculomegaly by CUS with or without GMH/IVH have been shown to be at increased risk for long-term neurologic impairments, likely because mild ventriculomegaly is a consequence of WMI that results in some cerebral atrophy.[55] It has been difficult to define the separate contributions of small GMH/IVH and cerebral WMI, especially because these lesions frequently coexist, and the latter is often missed by CUS. Newborns with grade III IVH are clearly at a higher risk for cognitive and motor impairments, although these newborns frequently have complications of IVH or other neuropathologic lesions such as PVL that likely contribute significantly to their neurologic outcome. Notably, newborns with grade III IVH and those with PVHI ("grade IV IVH") are often grouped together in outcome studies. MRI has been demonstrated to be superior to CUS in improving detection, classification, and hence, prognosis of GMH/IVH and its associated complications as well as detecting other neuropathologic lesions such as periventricular WMI.[56,57]

Newborns with the two major complications of IVH, namely PVHI and PVD, are at much higher risk for neurologic impairments than those with IVH alone. Newborns with PVD/PHH requiring significant intervention often manifest spastic diparesis and cognitive impairments due to bilateral periventricular WMI. Newborns with a localized, unilateral PVHI usually develop a spastic hemiparesis affecting the arm and leg with minimal or mild cognitive impairments.[58] Quadriparesis and significant cognitive deficits (including mental retardation) are more likely if the PVHI is extensive or bilateral, or if there is also coexisting PVL, which is common.[59] In addition to cognitive and motor impairments, newborns with severe PHH and/or PVHI are at risk for developing cerebral visual impairment and epilepsy.[59]

Outcome in term newborns with IVH relates to factors other than IVH alone because uncomplicated small IVH in this population has a favorable prognosis. This is likely related in large part to the lack of any remaining neural progenitor cells in the germinal matrix at term age that could be injured or destroyed by small GMH/IVH. Newborns with a history of trauma or perinatal asphyxia, or with neuroimaging evidence of thalamic hemorrhagic infarction, hypoxic-ischemic brain injury, or other parenchymal lesions, are at high risk for significant cognitive and/or motor deficits and epilepsy.

V. WHITE MATTER INJURY/PERIVENTRICULAR LEUKOMALACIA

A. **Etiology and pathogenesis.** PVL is a lesion found predominantly in the preterm newborn and is the neuropathologic lesion underlying much of the cognitive, motor, and sensory impairments and disabilities in children born prematurely. The true incidence of this lesion is not known, largely because detection of the mild form of this lesion is difficult using conventional neuroimaging and because the threshold for determining clinically important signal abnormality in the cerebral white matter has not been rigorously defined. WMI is a term used increasingly in place of the traditional term PVL or periventricular leukoencephalopathy, although the term PVL is still commonly used. WMI is a somewhat broader term than PVL in that it denotes the diffuse lesion of the cerebral white matter that extends beyond the periventricular regions defined in initial neuropathologic and ultrasonographic studies and is most often a noncystic lesion. The incidence of cystic PVL has declined over the years, with a rate of <1% of preterm newborns born in 2000 to 2002 with birth weight ≤1,500 g in one center.[60] An even more encompassing term, *encephalopathy of prematurity*, was proposed by Volpe[61] to include the findings of neuronal abnormalities in gray matter structures demonstrated by neuropathology and neuroimaging studies in addition to the WMI. This term is not yet in widespread use in the literature but is a term that reflects increasing evidence that premature newborns suffer a brain injury that affects many gray matter structures in addition to the cerebral white matter and altered brain development. Note that WMI with a similar imaging pattern to PVL in the preterm newborn has also been reported in newborns born at term,[62] particularly those with congenital heart disease.[63]

The **characteristic neuropathology** of PVL was first described in detail by Banker and Larroche[64] in their classic 1962 report of the histologic findings in 51 autopsy specimens. They described the classic features of PVL to include bilateral areas of focal necrosis, gliosis, and disruption of axons, with the so-called "retraction clubs and balls." The topographical distribution of the lesions was noted to be in the periventricular white matter dorsolateral to the lateral ventricles, primarily anterior to the frontal horn (at the level of the foramen of Monro) and lateral to the occipital horns. They noted that a severe "anoxic" episode occurred in 50 of 51 newborns that the lesions were consistently observed in the location of the border zone of the vascular supply and that 75% of the group had been born prematurely. They thus suggested two key features of the pathogenesis of PVL, namely, (i) hypoxia-ischemia affecting the watershed regions of the white matter and (ii) a particular vulnerability of the periventricular white matter of the premature brain. Further neuropathologic studies have extended these initial observations, demonstrating that in many cases, PVL consists of areas of both focal necrosis (which become cystic) and a diffuse white matter lesion. Neuropathology studies have demonstrated that the necrotic foci may be quite small, on the order of <1 to 5 mm,[65] hence not detectable by most imaging techniques (i.e., this does not contradict the observation of a reduced incidence of cystic PVL by imaging studies in surviving newborns). The diffuse white matter lesion consists of hypertrophic astrocytes and loss of oligodendrocytes and is followed by an overall decrease in the volume of cerebral white matter myelin. Interestingly, volumetric MRI analysis demonstrates a significant reduction in cortical and subcortical gray matter volumes (rather than white matter volume) in newborns and children born prematurely.[66–68] These MRI studies have been confirmed by recent neuropathologic studies showing that there is significant neuronal loss and gliosis in the thalamus, basal ganglia, and cerebral cortex associated with WMI in newborns born prematurely.[65,69–71] Thus, these quantitative MRI and neuropathologic data confirm the notion that PVL or WMI involves a much more diffuse destructive and developmental injury to the developing brain that involves neuronal as well as white matter abnormalities.[61]

This distinctive lesion of PVL found in the immature white matter of premature newborns likely results from the interaction of multiple pathogenetic factors. **Several major factors have been identified to date: (i) hypoxia-ischemia, (ii) intrinsic vulnerability of cerebral white matter of the premature newborn, and (iii) infection/inflammation.**[72] These three major factors will be discussed briefly as follows: First, Banker and Larroche[64] originally suggested that PVL occurred in the regions of vascular border zones in the cerebral white matter and that ischemia would thus be expected to preferentially affect these zones. Subsequent authors have further defined these zones using postmortem injection of the blood vessels to demonstrate the presence of vascular border and end zones in the periventricular white matter, where PVL is found.[73,74] It is hypothesized that these are watershed zones which are vulnerable to ischemic injury during times of vascular compromise. In addition, there is evidence to suggest the presence of a pressure-passive circulation in a subset of premature newborns, further predisposing these newborns to hypoxic-ischemic brain injury.[13,75]

Second, Banker and Larroche[64] first proposed the hypothesis that the periventricular white matter of the premature newborn may be more vulnerable to anoxia than the mature brain. A maturational vulnerability of the periventricular white matter is suggested by the finding that PVL occurs much more commonly in the premature than term newborn. Specifically, the observation that the diffuse lesion of PVL affects the oligodendrocyte (with resulting myelin loss) with relative preservation of other cellular elements suggests that the immature oligodendrocyte is the cell most vulnerable to injury. Immature oligodendrocytes are susceptible to injury and apoptotic cell death by free radical attack[76,77] and by glutamate receptor-mediated excitotoxic mechanisms.[78] Notably, apoptosis is postulated to be the mechanism of cell death by a moderate ischemic insult, as would be expected for most cases of PVL; necrosis results from severe ischemic insults.[79] Thus, there is cellular and biochemical evidence to support the original postulate that the preterm newborn's white matter displays a maturational vulnerability to hypoxic-ischemic injury that results in PVL.

Finally, epidemiologic and experimental studies suggest a role for infection and inflammation in the pathogenesis of PVL. Epidemiologic studies have shown an association between maternal infection, prolonged rupture of membranes, cord blood interleukin-6 levels, and an increased incidence of PVL,[80] leading to the hypothesis that maternal infection may be an etiologic factor in the development of PVL.[81] Experimental work has shown that certain cytokines, such as interferon-γ, have a cytotoxic effect on immature oligodendrocytes.[82] However, cytokines may also be secreted in the setting of hypoxia-ischemia (in the absence of infection). Moreover, infection and/or cytokines may lead to ischemia-reperfusion, which may cause further injury to oligodendrocytes. Thus, there are multiple pathways by which infection/inflammation might cause or contribute to the pathogenesis of PVL, and the interactions between the two pathogenetic pathways are complex based on rodent data.[83] In most cases, the pathogenesis of PVL probably involves a complex interaction of more than one of the pathogenetic mechanisms described earlier.

B. **Clinical presentation and diagnosis.** PVL is typically a clinically silent lesion evolving over days to weeks with few or no outward neurologic signs until weeks to months later when spasticity is first detected or at an even later age when children present with cognitive difficulties in school. With moderate to severe PVL, some evidence of spasticity in the lower extremities may be detected by the careful observer by term age or earlier. However, **PVL is usually diagnosed in the neonatal period by CUS or by MRI**. The evolution of echogenicity in the periventricular white matter over the first few weeks after birth, with or without echolucent cysts, is the classical description of PVL by US imaging. Ventriculomegaly due to volume loss from atrophy of the periventricular white matter is often apparent within weeks. Isolated ventriculomegaly is associated with an increased risk of CP,[55] suggesting that ventriculomegaly without radiologically detectable white matter signal abnormality may indicate the presence of PVL.

Studies correlating US and autopsy data have demonstrated that the incidence of PVL is underestimated by CUS, the technique most widely used to diagnose brain abnormalities in the preterm newborn.[84,85] MRI has been shown to be more sensitive than CUS for the detection of PVL, especially for the noncystic form of PVL.[56,57,86–88] Noncystic WMI detected by MRI in the newborn period is evident as high-signal intensity in the cerebral white matter by T2-weighted MRI and low-signal intensity by T1-weighted sequences. As for CUS studies, there is no universally accepted measure of the severity or extent of signal abnormality by MRI that defines WMI. Although it is clear that greater severity of WMI is correlated with a higher incidence of later neurodevelopmental deficits, there is a broad range of outcomes for mild, moderate, and severe WMI,[89] and the threshold for defining clinically significant WMI has not been determined. For example, one study reported diffuse excessive high-signal intensity (called DEHSI) in the white matter by MRI exam at term age in 80% of newborns born at 23 to 30 weeks' GA.[90] Although there was some correlation between this MRI finding and mild developmental delay at 18 months of age,[90] the impact of DEHSI on neurologic outcome appears to be modest, and it is unclear if DEHSI represents injury or altered development, e.g., myelination delay. The routine use of MRI scans to detect WMI or other lesions has not been recommended by practice guidelines,[3] although the clinical utility of MRI to detect brain lesions associated with prematurity is being recognized.[56,57] It is probably most useful to perform an MRI scan close to term age, if an MRI scan is to be obtained during the newborn period,[56,57] although the timing of MRI has also been debated. A brain MRI is the most useful imaging modality to confirm clinically suspected WMI in an older infant or child born prematurely who presents with cognitive, motor, and/or sensory impairments. In older infants and children, the brain MRI may show one or more of the following findings: abnormal signal within and/or decreased volume of the cerebral white matter, a thin corpus callosum, enlarged ventricles with a square appearance to the frontal horns, and/or enlarged extra-axial CSF spaces.

C. **Management.** There are currently no medications or treatments available for the specific treatment of PVL during the newborn period. Current efforts are directed at prevention based on knowledge of the various risk factors and pathogenetic mechanisms described earlier. Maintenance of normal cerebral perfusion should be attempted by careful management of systemic hemodynamics (e.g., blood pressure), intravascular volume, oxygenation and ventilation, and avoidance of sudden changes in systemic hemodynamics. It should be noted that there is controversy about the management of blood pressure in the premature newborn and that a normal blood pressure does not necessarily imply normal cerebral perfusion given the known impairments of cerebral pressure autoregulation in some premature newborns.[75] A randomized, controlled trial of targeted management of cerebral tissue oxygenation saturation (rStO2) in the first 72 hours after birth showed that near-infrared spectroscopy (NIRS) monitoring of rStO2 with specified interventions to maintain cerebral rStO2 in the range of 55% to 85% reduced by 58% the time preterm newborns spent hypoxic (mainly) or hyperoxic, with a trend to lower mortality and severe brain injury, but long-term neurologic outcome data are not yet available.[91] Avoidance and prompt treatment of infection (including prompt delivery in the setting of chorioamnionitis) may also minimize PVL, although no studies have shown conclusively any effect of such interventions. Management of PVL after discharge from the NICU is directed at identification of any cognitive, sensory or motor impairments, and appropriate therapies for any such impairments as described in the following text. Promising studies of neuroprotective strategies to prevent or minimize PVL have been tested in animal models and may be translated to humans. Clinical trials of erythropoietin (EPO) to improve neurologic outcome in preterm newborns are currently underway (NCT00413946, NCT01378273), with some early MRI data in a subset of infants that show a beneficial effect on white matter microstructure.[92,93]

D. **Prognosis. PVL is the principal cause of the cognitive, behavioral, motor, and sensory impairments found in children born at <32 weeks' GA.** There is an approximately 10% incidence of CP and up to 50% incidence of school difficulties in children born prematurely that is largely due to PVL, with PVHI being the other cerebral lesion that contributes significantly to neurologic disabilities. The incidence of neurologic impairments increases with lower GA at birth. For example, one study of extremely low birth weight newborns (<1,000 g) showed that only 30% of such children were performing at grade level without extra support at 8 years of age.[94] Similarly, the incidence of CP is much higher in children born extremely prematurely, occurring in approximately 20% of children born at ≤26 weeks' GA but in only 4% of children born at 32 weeks' GA.[52,95] Spastic diparesis is the most common form of CP in children born prematurely[52] because PVL typically affects the periventricular white matter closest to the ventricles. The axons subserving the lower extremities are located closest to the ventricle, the axons of the upper extremities are situated lateral to them, and the axons of the facial musculature are located farthest from the ventricle. Thus, PVL produces abnormal tone (usually spasticity) and weakness predominantly in the lower extremities, with the upper extremities and face demonstrating milder abnormalities. When PVL is more severe and/or widespread, quadriplegia may result. Although premature newborns can have retinopathy of prematurity affecting their vision, PVL and other cerebral lesions alone can result in strabismus, nystagmus, visual field deficits, and perceptual difficulties, which may not be recognized until school age or later.[96] In particular, the lower visual fields may be affected by PVL because the optic radiations subserving the lower visual field pass through the white matter dorsolateral to the occipital horns frequently affected by PVL.[97] Children with WMI may manifest visual perceptual defects or other higher order visual impairments that worsen their cognitive and school function, so these are particularly important to detect.[98] Because visual field deficits and other types of cerebral visual impairment can be difficult to detect, routine monitoring of visual function for early detection of these problems is important. Finally, children with severe PVL may develop epilepsy, although epilepsy is more commonly related to lesions with significant direct neuronal injury, such as PVHI.

References

1. Volpe JJ. Intracranial hemorrhage: subdural, primary subarachnoid, cerebellar, intraventricular (term infant), and miscellaneous. In: *Neurology of the Newborn*. 5th ed. Philadelphia, PA: Saunders Elsevier; 2008:483–516.

2. Volpe JJ. Intracranial hemorrhage: germinal matrix-intraventricular hemorrhage of the premature infant. In: *Neurology of the Newborn*. 5th ed. Philadelphia, PA: Saunders Elsevier; 2008:517–588.

3. Ment LR, Bada HS, Barnes P, et al. Practice parameter: neuroimaging of the neonate: report of the Quality Standards Subcommittee of the American Academy of Neurology and the Practice Committee of the Child Neurology Society. *Neurology* 2002;58(12):1726–1738.

4. Chamnanvanakij S, Rollins N, Perlman JM. Subdural hematoma in term infants. *Pediatr Neurol* 2002;26(4):301–304.

5. Perrin RG, Rutka JT, Drake JM, et al. Management and outcomes of posterior fossa subdural hematomas in neonates. *Neurosurgery* 1997;40(6):1190–1199, discussion 1199–1200.

6. Huang AH, Robertson RL. Spontaneous superficial parenchymal and leptomeningeal hemorrhage in term neonates. *AJNR Am J Neuroradiol* 2004;25(3):469–475.

7. Benders MJ, Kersbergen KJ, de Vries LS. Neuroimaging of white matter injury, intraventricular and cerebellar hemorrhage. *Clin Perinatol* 2014;41(1):69–82.

8. Bodensteiner JB, Johnsen SD. Cerebellar injury in the extremely premature infant: newly recognized but relatively common outcome. *J Child Neurol* 2005;20(2):139–142.

9. Roland EH, Flodmark O, Hill A. Thalamic hemorrhage with intraventricular hemorrhage in the full-term newborn. *Pediatrics* 1990;85(5):737–742.

10. Goddard-Finegold J, Armstrong D, Zeller RS. Intraventricular hemorrhage, following volume expansion after hypovolemic hypotension in the newborn beagle. *J Pediatr* 1982;100(5):796–799.

11. Perlman JM, McMenamin JB, Volpe JJ. Fluctuating cerebral blood-flow velocity in respiratory-distress syndrome. Relation to the development of intraventricular hemorrhage. *N Engl J Med* 1983;309(4):204–209.

12. Hill A, Perlman JM, Volpe JJ. Relationship of pneumothorax to occurrence of intraventricular hemorrhage in the premature newborn. *Pediatrics* 1982;69(2):144–149.

13. Lou H, Lassen N, Friis-Hansen B. Impaired autoregulation of cerebral blood flow in the distressed newborn infant. *J Pediatr* 1979;94(1):118–121.

14. Pryds O, Greisen G, Lou H, et al. Heterogeneity of cerebral vasoreactivity in preterm infants supported by mechanical ventilation. *J Pediatr* 1989;115:638–645.

15. Taylor GA. Effect of germinal matrix hemorrhage on terminal vein position and patency. *Pediatr Radiol* 1995;25(suppl 1):S37–S40.

16. Bassan H, Feldman HA, Limperopoulos C, et al. Periventricular hemorrhagic infarction: risk factors and neonatal outcome. *Pediatr Neurol* 2006;35(2):85–92.

17. Larroche JC. Post-haemorrhagic hydrocephalus in infancy. Anatomical study. *Biol Neonate* 1972;20(3):287–299.

18. Whitelaw A, Christie S, Pople I. Transforming growth factor-beta1: a possible signal molecule for posthemorrhagic hydrocephalus? *Pediatr Res* 1999;46(5):576–580.

19. Whitelaw A, Aquilina K. Management of posthaemorrhagic ventricular dilatation. *Arch Dis Child Fetal Neonatal Ed* 2012;97(3):F229–F233.

20. Greitz D. Radiological assessment of hydrocephalus: new theories and implications for therapy. *Neurosurg Rev* 2004;27(3):145–165.

21. Bejar R, Saugstad OD, James H, et al. Increased hypoxanthine concentrations in cerebrospinal fluid of infants with hydrocephalus. *J Pediatr* 1983;103(1):44–48.

22. da Silva M, Drake J, Lemaire C, et al. High-energy phosphate metabolism in a neonatal model of hydrocephalus before and after shunting. *J Neurosurg* 1994;81(4):544–553.

23. da Silva MC, Michowicz S, Drake JM, et al. Reduced local cerebral blood flow in periventricular white matter in experimental neonatal hydrocephalus-restoration with CSF shunting. *J Cereb Blood Flow Metab* 1995;15(6):1057–1065.

24. Del Bigio MR, Zhang YW. Cell death, axonal damage, and cell birth in the immature rat brain following induction of hydrocephalus. *Exp Neurol* 1998;154(1):157–169.

25. Savman K, Nilsson UA, Blennow M, et al. Non-protein-bound iron is elevated in cerebrospinal fluid from preterm infants with posthemorrhagic ventricular dilatation. *Pediatr Res* 2001;49(2):208–212.

26. Fukumizu M, Takashima S, Becker L. Neonatal posthemorrhagic hydrocephalus: neuropathologic and immunohistochemical studies. *Pediatr Neurol* 1995;13(3):230–234.

27. Whitelaw A, Rosengren L, Blennow M. Brain specific proteins in posthaemorrhagic ventricular dilatation. *Arch Dis Child Fetal Neonatal Ed* 2001;84(2):F90–F91.

28. Murphy BP, Inder TE, Rooks V, et al. Posthaemorrhagic ventricular dilatation in the premature infant: natural history and predictors of outcome. *Arch Dis Child Fetal Neonatal Ed* 2002;87(1):F37–F41.

29. Papile LA, Burstein J, Burstein R, et al. Incidence and evolution of subependymal and intraventricular hemorrhage: a study of infants with birth weights less than 1,500 gm. *J Pediatr* 1978;92(4):529–534.

30. Stoll BJ, Hansen NI, Bell EF, et al. Trends in care practices, morbidity, and mortality of extremely preterm neonates, 1993–2012. *JAMA* 2015;314(10): 1039–1051.

31. Perlman JM, Goodman S, Kreusser KL, et al. Reduction in intraventricular hemorrhage by elimination of fluctuating cerebral blood-flow velocity in preterm infants with respiratory distress syndrome. *N Engl J Med* 1985;312(21):1353–1357.

32. Ehle A, Sklar F. Visual evoked potentials in infants with hydrocephalus. *Neurology* 1979;29(11):1541–1544.

33. de Vries LS, Pierrat V, Minami T, et al. The role of short latency somatosensory evoked responses in infants with rapidly progressive ventricular dilatation. *Neuropediatrics* 1990;21(3):136–139.

34. Soul JS, Eichenwald E, Walter G, et al. CSF removal in infantile posthemorrhagic hydrocephalus results in significant improvement in cerebral hemodynamics. *Pediatr Res* 2004;55(5):872–876.

35. Del Bigio MR, Kanfer JN, Zhang YW. Myelination delay in the cerebral white matter of immature rats with kaolin-induced hydrocephalus is reversible. *J Neuropathol Exp Neurol* 1997;56(9):1053–1066.

36. Del Bigio MR, Crook CR, Buist R. Magnetic resonance imaging and behavioral analysis of immature rats with kaolin-induced hydrocephalus: pre- and postshunting observations. *Exp Neurol* 1997;148(1):256–264.

37. du Plessis AJ. Posthemorrhagic hydrocephalus and brain injury in the preterm infant: dilemmas in diagnosis and management. *Semin Pediatr Neurol* 1998;5(3):161–179.

38. de Vries LS, Liem KD, van Dijk K, et al. Early versus late treatment of posthaemorrhagic ventricular dilatation: results of a retrospective study from five neonatal intensive care units in The Netherlands. *Acta Paediatr* 2002;91(2):212–217.

39. Levene MI. Measurement of the growth of the lateral ventricles in preterm infants with real-time ultrasound. *Arch Dis Child* 1981;56(12):900–904.

40. Taylor GA, Madsen JR. Neonatal hydrocephalus: hemodynamic response to fontanelle compression—correlation with intracranial pressure and need for shunt placement. *Radiology* 1996;201(3):685–689.

41. Rahman S, Teo C, Morris W, et al. Ventriculosubgaleal shunt: a treatment option for progressive posthemorrhagic hydrocephalus. *Childs Nerv Syst* 1995;11(11):650–654.

42. International PHVD Drug Trial Group. International randomised controlled trial of acetazolamide and furosemide in posthaemorrhagic ventricular dilatation in infancy. *Lancet* 1998;352(9126):433–440.

43. Kennedy CR, Ayers S, Campbell MJ, et al. Randomized, controlled trial of acetazolamide and furosemide in posthemorrhagic ventricular dilation in infancy: follow-up at 1 year. *Pediatrics* 2001;108(3):597–607.

44. Haines SJ, Lapointe M. Fibrinolytic agents in the management of posthemorrhagic hydrocephalus in preterm infants: the evidence. *Childs Nerv Syst* 1999;15(5):226–234.

45. Whitelaw A, Pople I, Cherian S, et al. Phase 1 trial of prevention of hydrocephalus after intraventricular hemorrhage in newborn infants by drainage, irrigation, and fibrinolytic therapy. *Pediatrics* 2003;111(4, pt 1):759–765.

46. Whitelaw A, Evans D, Carter M, et al. Randomized clinical trial of prevention of hydrocephalus after intraventricular hemorrhage in preterm infants: brainwashing versus tapping fluid. *Pediatrics* 2007;119(5):e1071–e1078.

47. Whitelaw A, Jary S, Kmita G, et al. Randomized trial of drainage, irrigation and fibrinolytic therapy for premature infants with posthemorrhagic ventricular dilatation: developmental outcome at 2 years. *Pediatrics* 2010;125(4):e852–e858.

48. Warf BC. Endoscopic third ventriculostomy and choroid plexus cauterization for pediatric hydrocephalus. *Clin Neurosurg* 2007;54:78–82.

49. Warf BC, Kulkarni AV. Intraoperative assessment of cerebral aqueduct patency and cisternal scarring: impact on success of endoscopic third ventriculostomy in 403 African children. *J Neurosurg Pediatr* 2010;5(2):204–209.

50. Perlman JM, Lynch B, Volpe JJ. Late hydrocephalus after arrest and resolution of neonatal post- hemorrhagic hydrocephalus. *Dev Med Child Neurol* 1990;32(8):725–729.

51. Sherlock RL, Anderson PJ, Doyle LW; and the Victorian Infant Collaborative Study Group. Neurodevelopmental sequelae of intraventricular haemorrhage at 8 years of age in a regional cohort of ELBW/very preterm infants. *Early Hum Dev* 2005;81(11):909–916.

52. Ancel PY, Livinec F, Larroque B, et al. Cerebral palsy among very preterm children in relation to gestational age and neonatal ultrasound abnormalities: the EPIPAGE cohort study. *Pediatrics* 2006;117(3):828–835.

53. Patra K, Wilson-Costello D, Taylor HG, et al. Grades I-II intraventricular hemorrhage in extremely low birth weight infants: effects on neurodevelopment. *J Pediatr* 2006;149(2):169–173.

54. van de Bor M, den Ouden L. School performance in adolescents with and without periventricular-intraventricular hemorrhage in the neonatal period. *Semin Perinatol* 2004;28(4):295–303.

55. Allan WC, Vohr B, Makuch RW, et al. Antecedents of cerebral palsy in a multicenter trial of indomethacin for intraventricular hemorrhage. *Arch Pediatr Adolesc Med* 1997;151(6):580–585.

56. Kwon SH, Vasung L, Ment LR, et al. The role of neuroimaging in predicting neurodevelopmental outcomes of preterm neonates. *Clin Perinatol* 2014;41(1):257–283.

57. Hintz SR, Barnes PD, Bulas D, et al. Neuroimaging and neurodevelopmental outcome in extremely preterm infants. *Pediatrics* 2015;135(1):e32–e42.

58. de Vries LS, Groenendaal F, van Haastert IC, et al. Asymmetrical myelination of the posterior limb of the internal capsule in infants with periventricular haemorrhagic infarction: an early predictor of hemiplegia. *Neuropediatrics* 1999;30(6):314–319.

59. Bassan H, Benson CB, Limperopoulos C, et al. Ultrasonographic features and severity scoring of periventricular hemorrhagic infarction in relation to risk factors and outcome. *Pediatrics* 2006;117(6):2111–2118.

60. Hamrick SE, Miller SP, Leonard C, et al. Trends in severe brain injury and neurodevelopmental outcome in premature newborn infants: the role of cystic periventricular leukomalacia. *J Pediatr* 2004;145(5):593–599.

61. Volpe JJ. Brain injury in premature infants: a complex amalgam of destructive and developmental disturbances. *Lancet Neurol* 2009;8(1):110–124.

62. Kwong KL, Wong YC, Fong CM, et al. Magnetic resonance imaging in 122 children with spastic cerebral palsy. *Pediatr Neurol* 2004;31(3):172–176.

63. Galli KK, Zimmerman RA, Jarvik GP, et al. Periventricular leukomalacia is common after neonatal cardiac surgery. *J Thorac Cardiovasc Surg* 2004;127(3):692–704.

64. Banker B, Larroche J. Periventricular leukomalacia of infancy. A form of neonatal anoxic encephalopathy. *Arch Neurol* 1962;7:386–410.

65. Pierson CR, Folkerth RD, Billiards SS, et al. Gray matter injury associated with periventricular leukomalacia in the premature infant. *Acta Neuropathol* 2007;114(6):619–631.

66. Peterson BS, Vohr B, Staib LH, et al. Regional brain volume abnormalities and long-term cognitive outcome in preterm infants. *JAMA* 2000;284(15):1939–1947.

67. Abernethy LJ, Cooke RW, Foulder-Hughes L. Caudate and hippocampal volumes, intelligence, and motor impairment in 7-year-old children who were born preterm. *Pediatr Res* 2004;55(5):884–893.

68. Inder TE, Warfield SK, Wang H, et al. Abnormal cerebral structure is present at term in premature infants. *Pediatrics* 2005;115(2):286–294.

69. Ligam P, Haynes RL, Folkerth RD, et al. Thalamic damage in periventricular leukomalacia: novel pathologic observations relevant to cognitive deficits in survivors of prematurity. *Pediatr Res* 2009;65(5):524–529.

70. Kinney HC. The encephalopathy of prematurity: one pediatric neuropathologist's perspective. *Semin Pediatr Neurol* 2009;16(4):179–190.

71. Andiman SE, Haynes RL, Trachtenberg FL, et al. The cerebral cortex overlying periventricular leukomalacia: analysis of pyramidal neurons. *Brain Pathol* 2010;20(4):803–814.

72. Volpe JJ. Hypoxic-ischemic encephalopathy: neuropathology and pathogenesis. In: *Neurology of the Newborn*. 5th ed. Philadelphia, PA: Elsevier Saunders; 2008:347–399.

73. Takashima S, Tanaka K. Development of cerebrovascular architecture and its relationship to periventricular leukomalacia. *Arch Neurol* 1978;35(1):11–16.

74. De Reuck JL. Cerebral angioarchitecture and perinatal brain lesions in premature and full-term infants. *Acta Neurol Scand* 1984;70(6):391–395.

75. Soul JS, Hammer PE, Tsuji M, et al. Fluctuating pressure-passivity is common in the cerebral circulation of sick premature infants. *Pediatr Res* 2007;61(4):467–473.

76. Oka A, Belliveau MJ, Rosenberg PA, et al. Vulnerability of oligodendroglia to glutamate: pharmacology, mechanisms, and prevention. *J Neurosci* 1993;13(4):1441–1453.

77. Back SA, Gan X, Li Y, et al. Maturation-dependent vulnerability of oligodendrocytes to oxidative stress-induced death caused by glutathione depletion. *J Neurosci* 1998;18(16):6241–6253.

78. Follett PL, Deng W, Dai W, et al. Glutamate receptor-mediated oligodendrocyte toxicity in periventricular leukomalacia: a protective role for topiramate. *J Neurosci* 2004;24(18):4412–4420.

79. Ankarcrona M, Dypbukt JM, Bonfoco E, et al. Glutamate-induced neuronal death: a succession of necrosis or apoptosis depending on mitochondrial function. *Neuron* 1995;15(4):961–973.

80. Yoon BH, Romero R, Yang SH, et al. Interleukin-6 concentrations in umbilical cord plasma are elevated in neonates with white matter lesions associated with periventricular leukomalacia. *Am J Obstet Gynecol* 1996;174(5):1433–1440.

81. Dammann O, Leviton A. Maternal intrauterine infection, cytokines, and brain damage in the preterm newborn. *Pediatr Res* 1997;42(1):1–8.

82. Baerwald KD, Popko B. Developing and mature oligodendrocytes respond differently to the immune cytokine interferon-gamma. *J Neurosci Res* 1998;52(2):230–239.

83. Eklind S, Mallard C, Arvidsson P, et al. Lipopolysaccharide induces both a primary and a secondary phase of sensitization in the developing rat brain. *Pediatr Res* 2005;58(1):112–116.

84. Hope PL, Gould SJ, Howard S, et al. Precision of ultrasound diagnosis of pathologically verified lesions in the brains of very preterm infants. *Dev Med Child Neurol* 1988;30(4):457–471.

85. Carson SC, Hertzberg BS, Bowie JD, et al. Value of sonography in the diagnosis of intracranial hemorrhage and periventricular leukomalacia: a postmortem study of 35 cases. *AJNR Am J Neuroradiol* 1990;11(4):677–683.

86. Roelants-van Rijn AM, Groenendaal F, Beek FJ, et al. Parenchymal brain injury in the preterm infant: comparison of cranial ultrasound, MRI and neurodevelopmental outcome. *Neuropediatrics* 2001;32(2):80–89.

87. Maalouf EF, Duggan PJ, Counsell SJ, et al. Comparison of findings on cranial ultrasound and magnetic resonance imaging in preterm infants. *Pediatrics* 2001;107(4):719–727.

88. Inder TE, Anderson NJ, Spencer C, et al. White matter injury in the premature infant: a comparison between serial cranial sonographic and MR findings at term. *AJNR Am J Neuroradiol* 2003;24(5):805–809.

89. Woodward LJ, Anderson PJ, Austin NC, et al. Neonatal MRI to predict neurodevelopmental outcomes in preterm infants. *N Engl J Med* 2006;355(7):685–694.

90. Dyet LE, Kennea N, Counsell SJ, et al. Natural history of brain lesions in extremely preterm infants studied with serial magnetic resonance imaging from birth and neurodevelopmental assessment. *Pediatrics* 2006;118(2):536–548.

91. Hyttel-Sorensen S, Pellicer A, Alderliesten T, et al. Cerebral near infrared spectroscopy oximetry in extremely preterm infants: phase II randomised clinical trial. *BMJ* 2015;350:g7635.

92. Leuchter RH, Gui L, Poncet A, et al. Association between early administration of high-dose erythropoietin in preterm infants and brain MRI abnormality at term-equivalent age. *JAMA* 2014;312(8):817–824.

93. O'Gorman RL, Bucher HU, Held U, et al. Tract-based spatial statistics to assess the neuroprotective effect of early erythropoietin on white matter development in preterm infants. *Brain* 2015;138(pt 2):388–397.

94. Bowen JR, Gibson FL, Hand PJ. Educational outcome at 8 years for children who were born extremely prematurely: a controlled study. *J Paediatr Child Health* 2002;38(5):438–444.

95. Wood NS, Marlow N, Costeloe K, et al. Neurologic and developmental disability after extremely preterm birth. EPICure Study Group. *N Engl J Med* 2000;343(6):378–384.

96. Jacobson L, Ygge J, Flodmark O, et al. Visual and perceptual characteristics, ocular motility and strabismus in children with periventricular leukomalacia. *Strabismus* 2002;10(2):179–183.

97. Jacobson L, Lundin S, Flodmark O, et al. Periventricular leukomalacia causes visual impairment in preterm children. A study on the aetiologies of visual impairment in a population-based group of preterm children born 1989–95 in the county of Värmland, Sweden. *Acta Ophthalmol Scand* 1998;76(5):593–598.

98. Jacobson L, Ek U, Fernell E, et al. Visual impairment in preterm children with periventricular leukomalacia—visual, cognitive and neuropaediatric characteristics related to cerebral imaging. *Dev Med Child Neurol* 1996;38(8):724–735.

55

Perinatal Asphyxia and Hypoxic-Ischemic Encephalopathy

Anne R. Hansen and Janet S. Soul

KEY POINTS

- Therapeutic hypothermia is the only proven treatment for hypoxic-ischemic encephalopathy (HIE) and must be started with 6 hours of birth for maximal efficacy.
- Passive cooling is safe and effective in order to initiate hypothermia in the community setting with close temperature monitoring and management.
- Because seizures are often subclinical (electrographic only) and abnormal movements or posture may not be seizures, conventional electroencephalogram (EEG) remains the gold standard for diagnosing neonatal seizures, which are common in HIE.
- Careful management of ventilation, oxygenation, perfusion, metabolic state, and fluid balance are critical to optimizing outcome.

I. **PERINATAL ASPHYXIA** refers to a condition during the first and second stage of labor in which impaired gas exchange leads to fetal acidosis, hypoxemia, and hypercarbia. It is identified by fetal acidosis as measured in umbilical arterial blood. The umbilical artery pH that defines asphyxia is not the major determinant of brain injury. Although the most widely accepted definition of fetal acidosis is a pH <7.0, the likelihood of brain injury is relatively low with this degree of acidosis. The following terms may be used in evaluating a term newborn at risk for brain injury in the perinatal period:

   A. **Perinatal hypoxia, ischemia, and asphyxia.** These pathophysiologic terms describe respectively, decreased oxygen (O_2), blood flow, and gas exchange to the fetus or newborn. These terms should be reserved for circumstances when there are rigorous prenatal, perinatal, and postnatal data to support their use.

   B. **Perinatal/neonatal depression** is a clinical, descriptive term that pertains to the condition of the infant on physical examination in the immediate postnatal period, i.e., in the first hour after birth. The clinical features of infants with this condition may include depressed mental status, muscle hypotonia, and/or disturbances in spontaneous respiration and cardiovascular function.

This term makes no association with the prenatal or later postnatal (i.e., beyond the first hour) condition, physical exam, laboratory tests, imaging studies, or electroencephalograms (EEGs). After the first hour or so of life, neonatal encephalopathy is the preferred descriptive term for infants with persistently abnormal mental status and associated findings.

C. Neonatal encephalopathy is a clinical and not an etiologic term that describes an abnormal neurobehavioral state consisting of an altered level of consciousness (including hyperalert state) and usually other signs of brainstem and/or motor dysfunction. It does **not** imply a specific etiology, nor does it imply irreversible neurologic injury because it may be caused by such reversible conditions as maternal medications or hypoglycemia.

D. Hypoxic-ischemic encephalopathy (HIE) is a term that describes clinical evidence of encephalopathy as defined earlier, with objective data to support a hypoxic-ischemic (HI) mechanism as the underlying cause for the encephalopathy.

E. Hypoxic-ischemic (HI) brain injury refers to neuropathology attributable to hypoxia and/or ischemia as evidenced by neuroimaging (head ultrasonography [HUS], magnetic resonance imaging [MRI], computed tomography [CT]) or pathologic (postmortem) abnormalities. Biochemical markers of brain injury such as creatine kinase brain bound (CK-BB) and neuron specific enolase (NSE) are not used routinely in clinical practice (see section IX.B).

The diagnosis of HIE and/or HI brain injury is not a diagnosis of exclusion, but ruling out other etiologies of neurologic dysfunction is a critical part of the diagnostic evaluation. When making a diagnosis of HIE, the following information should be documented in the medical record:

1. Prenatal history: complications of pregnancy with emphasis on risk factors associated with neonatal depression, any pertinent family history

2. Perinatal history: concerns of labor and delivery including fetal heart rate (FHR) tracing, biophysical profile, sepsis risk factors, scalp and/or cord pH (specify if arterial or venous), perinatal events such as placental abruption, Apgar scores, resuscitative effort, and immediate postnatal blood gases

3. Postnatal data
   a. Admission physical exam with emphasis on neurologic exam and presence of any dysmorphic features
   b. Clinical course including presence or absence of seizures (and time of onset), oliguria, cardiorespiratory dysfunction, and treatment (e.g., need for pressor medications, ventilator support)
   c. Laboratory testing, including blood gases, electrolytes, evidence of injury to end organs other than the brain (kidney, liver, heart, lung, blood, bowel), and possible evaluation for inborn errors of metabolism
   d. Imaging studies
   e. EEG and any other neurophysiologic data (e.g., evoked potentials)
   f. Placental pathology

II. INCIDENCE. The frequency of perinatal asphyxia is approximately 1.5% of live births in developed countries with advanced obstetric/neonatal care and is inversely related to gestational age and birth weight (BW). It occurs in

0.5% of live-born newborns >36 weeks' gestation and accounts for 20% of perinatal deaths (50% if stillbirths are included). A higher incidence is noted in newborns of diabetic or toxemic mothers, those with intrauterine growth restriction, breech presentation, and newborns who are postdates.

III. ETIOLOGY. In term newborns, asphyxia can occur in the antepartum or intrapartum period as a result of impaired gas exchange across the placenta that leads to the inadequate provision of O_2 and removal of carbon dioxide (CO_2) and hydrogen (H^+) from the fetus. There is a lack of certainty regarding the timing or severity of asphyxia in many cases. Asphyxia can also occur in the postpartum period, usually secondary to pulmonary, cardiovascular, or neurologic abnormalities.

A. Factors that increase the risk of perinatal asphyxia include the following:

1. Impairment of maternal oxygenation

2. Decreased blood flow from mother to placenta

3. Decreased blood flow from placenta to fetus

4. Impaired gas exchange across the placenta or at the fetal tissue level

5. Increased fetal O_2 requirement

B. Etiologies of hypoxia-ischemia may be multiple and include the following:

1. Maternal factors: hypertension (acute or chronic), hypotension, infection (including chorioamnionitis), hypoxia from pulmonary or cardiac disorders, diabetes, maternal vascular disease, and *in utero* exposure to cocaine

2. Placental factors: abnormal placentation, abruption, infarction, fibrosis, or hydrops

3. Uterine rupture

4. Umbilical cord accidents: prolapse, entanglement, true knot, compression

5. Abnormalities of umbilical vessels

6. Fetal factors: anemia (e.g., from fetal-maternal hemorrhage), infection, cardiomyopathy, hydrops, severe cardiac/circulatory insufficiency

7. Neonatal factors: cyanotic congenital heart disease, persistent pulmonary hypertension of the newborn (PPHN), cardiomyopathy, other forms of neonatal cardiogenic and/or septic shock, respiratory failure due to meconium aspiration syndrome, neonatal pneumonia, pneumothorax, or other etiologies

IV. PATHOPHYSIOLOGY

A. Events that occur during the normal course of labor cause most babies to be born with little O_2 reserve. These include the following:

1. Decreased blood flow to placenta due to uterine contractions, some degree of cord compression, maternal dehydration, and maternal alkalosis due to hyperventilation

2. Decreased O_2 delivery to the fetus from reduced placental blood flow

3. Increased O_2 consumption in both mother and fetus

B. Hypoxia-ischemia causes a number of physiologic and biochemical alterations:

1. With **brief asphyxia**, there is a transient increase, followed by a decrease in heart rate (HR), mild elevation in blood pressure (BP), an increase in central venous pressure (CVP), and essentially no change in cardiac output (CO). This is accompanied by a redistribution of CO with an increased proportion going to the brain, heart, and adrenal glands (diving reflex). When there is severe but brief asphyxia (e.g., placental abruption then stat cesarian section), it is thought that this diversion of blood flow to vital deep nuclear structures of the brain does not occur, hence results in the typical pattern of injury to the subcortical and brainstem nuclei.

2. With **prolonged asphyxia**, there can be a loss of pressure autoregulation and/or CO_2 vasoreactivity. This, in turn, may lead to further disturbances in cerebral perfusion, particularly when there is cardiovascular involvement with hypotension and/or decreased CO. A decrease in cerebral blood flow (CBF) results in anaerobic metabolism and eventual cellular energy failure due to increased glucose utilization in the brain and a fall in the concentration of glycogen, phosphocreatine, and adenosine triphosphate (ATP). Prolonged asphyxia typically results in diffuse injury to both cortical and subcortical structures, with greater injury to neuronal populations particularly susceptible to HI insults.

C. Cellular dysfunction occurs as a result of diminished oxidative phosphorylation and ATP production. This energy failure impairs ion pump function, causing accumulation of intracellular Na^+, Cl^-, H_2O, and Ca^{2+}; extracellular K^+; and excitatory neurotransmitters (e.g., glutamate). Impaired oxidative phosphorylation can occur during the primary HI insult(s) as well as during a secondary energy failure that usually begins approximately 6 to 24 hours after the initiating insult. Cell death can be either immediate or delayed and either necrotic or apoptotic.

1. Immediate neuronal death (necrosis) can occur due to intracellular osmotic overload of Na^+ and Ca^{2+} from ion pump failure as above or excitatory neurotransmitters acting on inotropic receptors (such as the N-methyl-D-aspartate [NMDA] receptor).

2. Delayed neuronal death (apoptosis) occurs secondary to uncontrolled activation of enzymes and second messenger systems within the cell (e.g., Ca^{2+}-dependent lipases, proteases, and caspases), perturbation of mitochondrial respiratory electron chain transport, generation of free radicals and leukotrienes, generation of nitric oxide (NO) through NO synthase, and depletion of energy stores.

3. Reperfusion of previously ischemic tissue may cause further injury because it can promote the formation of excess reactive oxygen species (e.g., superoxide, hydrogen peroxide, hydroxyl, singlet oxygen), which can overwhelm the endogenous scavenger mechanisms, thereby causing damage to cellular lipids, proteins, and nucleic acids as well as to the blood–brain barrier. This may result in an influx of neutrophils that, along with activated microglia, release injurious cytokines (e.g., interleukin 1-β and tumor necrosis factor α).

V. DIAGNOSIS

A. **Perinatal assessment of risk** includes awareness of preexisting maternal or fetal problems that may predispose to perinatal asphyxia (see section III) and of changing placental and fetal conditions (see Chapter 1) ascertained by ultrasonographic examination, biophysical profile, and nonstress tests.

B. **Low Apgar scores** and need for resuscitation in the delivery room are common but nonspecific findings. Many features of the Apgar score relate to cardiovascular integrity and **not** neurologic dysfunction resulting from asphyxia.

 1. In addition to perinatal asphyxia, the differential diagnosis for a term newborn with an Apgar score ≤3 for ≥10 minutes includes depression from maternal anesthesia or analgesia, trauma, infection, cardiac or pulmonary disorders, neuromuscular, and other central nervous system (CNS) disorders or malformations.

 2. If the Apgar score is >6 by 5 minutes, perinatal asphyxia is not likely.

C. **Umbilical cord or first blood gas** determination. The specific blood gas criteria that define asphyxia causing brain damage are uncertain; however, the pH and base deficit on the cord or first blood gas is helpful for determining which infants have asphyxia that indicates need for further evaluation for the development of HIE. In the randomized clinical trials of hypothermia for neonatal HIE, severe acidosis was defined as pH ≤7.0 or base deficit ≥16 mmol/L.

D. **Clinical presentation and differential diagnosis.** HIE should be suspected in encephalopathic newborns with a history of fetal and/or neonatal distress and laboratory evidence of asphyxia. The diagnosis of HIE should not be overlooked in scenarios such as meconium aspiration, pulmonary hypertension, birth trauma, or fetal-maternal hemorrhage, where HIE may be missed because of the severity of pulmonary dysfunction, anemia, or other clinical manifestations. The diagnosis of neonatal encephalopathy includes a number of etiologies in addition to perinatal hypoxia-ischemia. Asphyxia may be suspected and HIE reasonably included in the differential diagnosis when there is:

 1. Prolonged (>1 hour) antenatal acidosis

 2. Fetal HR <60 beats per minute

 3. Apgar score ≤3 at ≥10 minutes

 4. Need for positive pressure ventilation for >1 minute or first cry delayed >5 minutes

 5. Seizures within 12 to 24 hours of birth

 6. Burst suppression or suppressed background pattern on EEG or amplitude-integrated electroencephalogram (aEEG)

VI. NEUROLOGIC SIGNS. The clinical spectrum of HIE is described as mild, moderate, or severe (Table 55.1). EEG is useful to provide objective data to grade the severity of encephalopathy.

A. **Encephalopathy.** Newborns with HIE must have abnormal consciousness by definition, whether mild, moderate, or severe. Mild encephalopathy can consist of an apparent hyperalert or jittery state, but the newborn does not respond appropriately to stimuli, and thus consciousness is abnormal. Moderate and severe encephalopathy are characterized by more impaired responses to stimuli such as light, touch, or even noxious stimuli. The background pattern detected by EEG or aEEG is useful for determining the severity of encephalopathy.

B. **Brainstem and cranial nerve abnormalities.** Newborns with HIE may have brainstem dysfunction, which may manifest as abnormal or absent brainstem reflexes, including pupillary, corneal, oculocephalic, cough, and gag reflexes. There can be abnormal eye movements such as dysconjugate gaze, gaze preference, ocular bobbing or other abnormal patterns of bilateral eye movements, or an absence of visual fixation or blink to light. Newborns may show facial weakness (usually symmetric) and have a weak or absent suck and swallow with poor feeding. They can have apnea or abnormal respiratory patterns.

C. **Motor abnormalities.** With greater severity of encephalopathy, there is generally greater hypotonia, weakness, and abnormal posture with lack of flexor tone, which is usually symmetric. With severe HIE, primitive reflexes such as the Moro or grasp reflex may be diminished. Over days to weeks, the initial hypotonia may evolve into spasticity and hyperreflexia if there is significant HI brain injury. Note that if a newborn shows significant hypertonia within the first day or so after birth, the HI insult may have occurred earlier in the antepartum period and have already resulted in established HI brain injury.

D. **Seizures** occur in up to 50% of newborns with HIE and usually start within 24 hours after the HI insult. Seizures indicate that the severity of encephalopathy is moderate or severe, not mild.

1. Seizures may be subtle, tonic, or clonic. It can sometimes be difficult to differentiate seizures from jitteriness or clonus, although the latter two are usually suppressible with firm hold of the affected limb(s).

2. Because seizures are often subclinical (electrographic only) and abnormal movements or posture may not be seizure, EEG remains the gold standard for diagnosing neonatal seizures, particularly in HIE.

3. Seizures may compromise ventilation and oxygenation, especially in newborns who are not receiving mechanical ventilation. It is important to adequately support respiration to avoid additional hypoxic injury.

E. **Increased intracranial pressure (ICP)** resulting from diffuse cerebral edema in HIE often reflects extensive cerebral necrosis rather than swelling of intact cells and indicates a poor prognosis. Treatment to reduce ICP does not affect outcome.

Table 55.1. Sarnat and Sarnat Stages of Hypoxic-Ischemic Encephalopathy*

Stage	Stage 1 (Mild)	Stage 2 (Moderate)	Stage 3 (Severe)
Level of consciousness	Hyperalert; irritable	Lethargic or obtunded	Stuporous, comatose
Neuromuscular control:	Uninhibited, overreactive	Diminished spontaneous movement	Diminished or absent spontaneous movement
Muscle tone	Normal	Mild hypotonia	Flaccid
Posture	Mild distal flexion	Strong distal flexion	Intermittent decerebration
Stretch reflexes	Overactive	Overactive, disinhibited	Decreased or absent
Segmental myoclonus	Present or absent	Present	Absent
Complex reflexes:	Normal	Suppressed	Absent
Suck	Weak	Weak or absent	Absent
Moro	Strong, low threshold	Weak, incomplete, high threshold	Absent
Oculovestibular	Normal	Overactive	Weak or absent
Tonic neck	Slight	Strong	Absent
Autonomic function:	Generalized sympathetic	Generalized parasympathetic	Both systems depressed
Pupils	Mydriasis	Miosis	Midposition, often unequal; poor light reflex
Respirations	Spontaneous	Spontaneous; occasional apnea	Periodic; apnea
Heart rate	Tachycardia	Bradycardia	Variable
Bronchial and salivary secretions	Sparse	Profuse	Variable
Gastrointestinal motility	Normal or decreased	Increased, diarrhea	Variable

(continued)

Table 55.1. *(Continued)*

Stage	Stage 1 (Mild)	Stage 2 (Moderate)	Stage 3 (Severe)
Seizures	None	Common focal or multifocal (6–24 hours of age)	Uncommon (excluding decerebration)
Electroencephalo-graphic findings	Normal (awake)	Early: generalized low voltage, slowing (continuous delta and theta)	Early: periodic pattern with isopotential phases
		Later: periodic pattern (awake); seizures focal or multifocal; 1.0–1.5 Hz spike and wave	Later: totally isopotential
Duration of symptoms	<24 hours	2–14 days	Hours to weeks
Outcome	About 100% normal	80% normal; abnormal if symptoms more than 5–7 days	About 50% die; remainder with severe sequelae

*The stages in this table are a continuum reflecting the spectrum of clinical states of newborns over 36 weeks' gestational age.
Source: From Sarnat HB, Sarnat MS. Neonatal encephalopathy following fetal distress: a clinical and electroencephalographic study. *Arch Neurol* 1976;33:696–705.

VII. MULTIORGAN DYSFUNCTION. Other organ systems in addition to the brain usually exhibit evidence of asphyxial damage. In a minority of cases (<15%), the brain may be the only organ exhibiting dysfunction following asphyxia. In most cases, multiorgan dysfunction occurs as a result of systemic hypoxia-ischemia. The frequency of organ involvement in perinatal asphyxia varies among published series, depending in part on the definitions used for asphyxia and organ dysfunction.

A. The **kidney** is the most common organ to be affected in the setting of peri-natal asphyxia. The proximal tubule of the kidney is especially affected by decreased perfusion, leading to acute tubular necrosis (ATN) with oliguria and a rise in serum creatinine (Cr) (see Chapter 28).

B. **Cardiac** dysfunction is caused by transient myocardial ischemia. The elec-trocardiogram (ECG) may show ST depression in the midprecordium and T-wave inversion in the left precordium. Echocardiographic findings include decreased left ventricular contractility, especially of posterior wall; elevated ventricular end-diastolic pressures; tricuspid insufficiency; and pulmonary hypertension. In severely asphyxiated newborns, dysfunction more commonly affects the right ventricle. A fixed HR may indicate severe brainstem injury.

C. **Pulmonary** effects include increased pulmonary vascular resistance leading to PPHN, pulmonary hemorrhage, pulmonary edema due to cardiac dysfunction, and meconium aspiration.

D. **Hematologic** effects include disseminated intravascular coagulation (DIC), poor production of clotting factors due to liver dysfunction, and poor production of platelets by the bone marrow.

E. **Liver dysfunction** may be manifested by isolated elevation of hepatocellular enzymes. More extensive damage may occur, leading to DIC, inadequate glycogen stores with resultant hypoglycemia, slowed metabolism, or elimination of medications.

F. **Gastrointestinal (GI)** effects include an increased risk of bowel ischemia and necrotizing enterocolitis (see Chapter 27).

VIII. LABORATORY EVALUATION OF ASPHYXIA

A. **Cardiac evaluation.** An elevation of **serum creatine kinase myocardial bound** (CK-MB) fraction of >5% to 10% may indicate myocardial injury. Cardiac troponin I (cTnI), cardiac troponin T (cTnT), and cardiac regulatory proteins that control the calcium-mediated interaction of actin and myosin are markers of myocardial damage, and therefore, elevated levels of these proteins could support exposure to asphyxia; however, they are not currently used in clinical practice.

B. **Neurologic markers of brain injury**

1. Serum CK-BB may be increased in asphyxiated newborns within 12 hours of the insult but has not been correlated with long-term neurodevelopmental outcome. CK-BB is also expressed in placenta, lungs, GI tract, and kidneys. Other serum markers such as protein S-100, NSE, and urine markers have been measured in newborns with asphyxia and HIE.

2. In practice, serum and urine markers of brain injury are not routinely used to evaluate for the presence of brain injury or to predict outcome.

C. **Renal evaluation**

1. Blood urea nitrogen (BUN) and serum Cr may be elevated in perinatal asphyxia. Typically, elevation is noted 2 to 4 days after the insult.

2. Fractional excretion of Na^+ (FENa) or renal failure index may help confirm renal insult (see Chapter 28).

3. Urine levels of β2-microglobulin have been used as an indicator of proximal tubular dysfunction, although not routinely. This low molecular weight protein is freely filtered through the glomerulus and reabsorbed almost completely in the proximal tubule.

IX. BRAIN IMAGING

A. **Cranial sonographic** examination can demonstrate edema as loss of gray-white differentiation and small ventricles when severe but is generally insensitive for the detection of HI brain injury, particularly in the first days after birth. It may be useful to rule out large intracranial hemorrhage, particularly because this may be a contraindication to therapeutic hypothermia.

B. **CT** may be used to detect cerebral edema, hemorrhage, and eventually HI brain injury. Because of the degree of radiation exposure, CT is only indicated if imaging is urgently needed to determine clinical treatment, and neither ultrasound (US) nor MRI is available on an emergency basis.

C. **MRI.** Conventional T1- and T2-weighted MRI sequences are the best modality for determining the severity and extent of irreversible HI brain injury, but the injury is not apparent on these sequences in the first days after the HI insult, unless the injury is older than suspected or very severe. These conventional sequences are best for the detection of brain injury at least 7 to 10 days, and a scan as late as 14 days or older may be needed to show the full extent of the injury, particularly if early MRI shows less injury than suspected by clinical exam or EEG findings.

1. **Diffusion-weighted imaging (DWI)** can show abnormalities within hours of an HI insult that may be useful in the diagnosis of neonatal HIE and an early indicator of possible brain injury. However, DWI can both underestimate and overestimate the severity of HI brain injury, depending on the timing of the study. Early DWI scans will usually show restricted diffusion in brain regions affected by hypoxia-ischemia. At 7 to 10 days of age, there is pseudonormalization of diffusion, so DWI can appear normal despite the presence of HI injury. After 7 to 10 days, diffusion is usually increased in regions of HI brain injury. Hypothermia appears to delay the time to pseudonormalization of diffusion. Thus, DWI data need to be interpreted carefully within the context of the history and clinical course of the newborn with HIE.

2. **Proton magnetic resonance spectroscopy (MRS)**, also called *proton-MRS* or *H-MRS*,[1] measures the relative concentrations of various metabolites in tissue. Elevated lactate, decreased N-acetylaspartate (NAA), and alterations of the ratios of these two metabolites in relation to choline or creatine can indicate HIE and help with determining neurologic prognosis.

3. **Susceptibility-weighted imaging** may be useful for the detection of hemorrhage, including hemorrhage within areas of ischemic injury.

4. **Magnetic resonance (MR) angiography or venography** may occasionally be useful if there is suspicion of vascular anomalies, thromboembolic disease, or sinus venous thrombosis, which can occasionally be found in association with HIE.

X. **EEG** is used to both detect and monitor seizure activity and also to define abnormal background patterns such as discontinuous, burst suppression, low voltage, or isoelectric patterns. When conventional 8- or 16-channel neonatal EEG is not readily available, aEEG has been used to evaluate the background pattern, particularly when rapid assessment is needed to determine presence or severity of encephalopathy for treatment with therapeutic hypothermia. This method consists of a reduced montage with one- or two-channel EEG with parietal electrodes. Although aEEG may detect some seizures, there are data showing that aEEG detects far fewer seizures compared with conventional EEG and that the quality of aEEG interpretation depends very much on the experience and expertise of the reader.

XI. PATHOLOGIC FINDINGS OF BRAIN INJURY

A. Specific neuropathology may be seen after moderate or severe HIE.

1. Selective neuronal necrosis is the most common type of injury seen following perinatal asphyxia. It is due to differential vulnerability of specific cell types to hypoxia-ischemia; for example, neurons are more easily injured than glia. Specific regions at increased risk are the CA1 region of hippocampus, Purkinje cells of cerebellum, neurons of the thalamus and basal ganglia (particularly putamen), and brainstem nuclei. Preterm infants show predominantly cerebral white matter injury after HI, but severe HI insults can also result in subcortical and cortical neuronal injury.

2. A watershed pattern of ischemic injury occurs in boundary zones between cerebral arteries, particularly following severe hypotension. This injury reflects poor perfusion of the vulnerable periventricular border zones in the centrum semiovale and produces predominantly white matter injury, particularly in preterm newborns. In the term newborn, more severe, prolonged HI insults result in bilateral parasagittal cortical and subcortical white matter injury.

3. Focal or multifocal cortical necrosis affecting all cellular elements can result in cystic encephalomalacia and/or ulegyria (injury to cortex in depths of sulci) due to loss of perfusion in one or more vascular beds.

B. Neuropathology may reflect the type of asphyxial episode, although the precise pattern is not predictable.

1. Prolonged partial episodes of asphyxia tend to cause diffuse cerebral (especially cortical) necrosis, although there is often involvement of subcortical $\pm$ brainstem structures as well.

2. Acute total asphyxia, when relatively brief, affects primarily the brainstem, thalamus, and basal ganglia and tends to spare the cortex in large part, except for the perirolandic cortex.

3. Partial prolonged asphyxia followed by a terminal acute asphyxial event (combination) is probably present in most cases.

XII. TREATMENT

A. Perinatal management of high-risk pregnancies

1. Fetal HR abnormalities may provide supporting evidence of asphyxia, especially if accompanied by presence of thick meconium. However, they provide few data concerning duration or severity of an asphyxial event.

2. Measurement of fetal scalp pH is a better determinant of fetal oxygenation than Po_2. With intermittent hypoxia-ischemia, Po_2 may improve

transiently whereas the pH progressively falls. Fetal scalp blood lactate has been suggested as easier and more reliable than pH but has not gained wide acceptance.

3. Close monitoring of progress of labor with awareness of other signs of *in utero* distress is important.

4. The presence of a constellation of abnormal findings may indicate the need to mobilize the perinatal team for a newborn that could require immediate intervention. Alteration of delivery plans may be indicated and guidelines for intervention in cases of suspected fetal distress should be designed and placed in each medical center (see Chapter 1).

B. Delivery room management. The initial management of the HI newborn in the delivery room is described in Chapter 4.

C. Postnatal management of neurologic effects of asphyxia

1. Ventilation. CO_2 should be maintained in the normal range. Hypercapnia can cause cerebral acidosis and cerebral vasodilation. This may result in more flow to uninjured areas and relative ischemia to damaged areas ("steal phenomenon"). Excessive hypocapnia (CO_2 <25 mm Hg) decreases cerebral perfusion so should also be avoided.

2. Oxygenation. O_2 levels should be maintained in the normal range, although poor peripheral perfusion may limit the accuracy of continuous noninvasive monitoring. Hypoxemia should be treated with supplemental O_2 and/or mechanical ventilation. Hyperoxia may cause decreased CBF or exacerbate free radical damage so should be avoided.

3. Temperature. Passive cooling by turning off warming lights is an effective way to initiate therapeutic hypothermia as soon as possible after the HI insult. Hyperthermia should always be avoided.

4. Perfusion. Cardiovascular stability and adequate mean systemic arterial BP are important in order to maintain adequate cerebral perfusion pressure.

5. Maintain physiologic metabolic state
a. Hypocalcemia is a common metabolic alteration after neonatal asphyxia. It is important to maintain calcium in the normal range because hypocalcemia can compromise cardiac contractility and may cause or exacerbate seizures (see Chapter 25).
b. Hypoglycemia is often seen in asphyxiated newborns. Blood glucose level should be maintained in the normal range for term newborns. Hypoglycemia may increase CBF, exacerbate the energy deficit, and cause or exacerbate seizures. Hyperglycemia may lead to increased brain lactate, damage to cellular integrity, cerebral edema, or further disturbance in vascular autoregulation.

6. Judicious fluid management is needed, and both fluid overload and inadequate circulating volume should be avoided. Two processes predispose to fluid overload in asphyxiated newborns:
a. ATN (see Chapter 28) can result from the "diving reflex" and result in oliguria followed by polyuria.

b. Syndrome of inappropriate antidiuretic hormone (SIADH) secretion (see Chapter 23) is often seen 3 to 4 days after the HI event. It is manifested by hyponatremia and hypo-osmolarity in combination with low urine output and inappropriately concentrated urine (elevated urine specific gravity, osmolarity, and Na^+).

c. Fluid restriction may aid in minimizing cerebral edema, although the effect of fluid restriction on long-term outcome in newborns who are not in renal failure is not known.

7. **Control of seizures.** Seizures generally start within 12 hours of birth, increase in frequency, and then usually resolve within days, although seizures may persist in severe cases. Seizures caused by HIE can be extremely difficult to control and may not be possible to eliminate completely with currently available anticonvulsants. It is important to remember that seizures in HIE are often subclinical (electrographic only) and that seizures in newborns on musculoskeletal blockade may be manifested only by abrupt changes in BP, HR, and oxygenation. EEG is thus required to detect seizures and monitor the response to anticonvulsant therapy and is superior to aEEG for this purpose.[1] There is increasing evidence that seizures exacerbate brain injury,[2,3] but anticonvulsants are often incompletely effective, and it has not yet been proven that improved seizure control results in improved neurologic outcome.[4] Metabolic perturbations such as hypoglycemia, hypocalcemia, and hyponatremia that may cause or exacerbate seizure activity should be corrected.

   a. Acute anticonvulsant management

   i. **Phenobarbital** is the initial drug of choice. It is given as a loading dose of 20 mg/kg intravenous (IV). If seizures continue, additional loading doses of 5 to 10 mg/kg IV may be given as needed to control seizures. A maintenance dose of 3 to 5 mg/kg/day orally (PO) or IV divided bid should be started 12 to 24 hours after the loading dose. During loading doses of phenobarbital, the newborn needs to be monitored closely for respiratory depression. Therapeutic serum levels are 15 to 40 mg/dL. Because of a prolonged serum half-life, which may be increased by hepatic and renal dysfunction, serum levels need to be monitored and maintenance dosing adjusted accordingly.

   ii. **Phenytoin** is usually added when seizures are not controlled by phenobarbital. The loading dose is 15 to 20 mg/kg IV followed by a maintenance dose of 4 to 8 mg/kg/day divided q8h. In many centers, **fosphenytoin** is used in place of parent drug (phenytoin) because the risk of hypotension is less and extravasation has no adverse effects. Dosage is calculated and written in terms of phenytoin equivalents to avoid medication errors. Therapeutic serum level is typically 15 to 20 mg/dL, although levels in the 20 to 25 range may be effective and consideration should be given to measurement of the free phenytoin level.

   iii. **Benzodiazepines** are considered third-line drugs and include lorazepam, which can be given in doses of 0.05 to 0.1 mg/kg/dose IV. Some clinicians use midazolam boluses and IV infusions to control seizures, but there are few data regarding the safety and efficacy of this treatment.

iv. Levetiracetam has been used recently because of its availability in IV form and relative safety and efficacy for various types of childhood epilepsy. There are several published series reporting benefit in newborns but without continuous EEG monitoring to confirm efficacy, and there are few data regarding short- or long-term safety. An ongoing randomized trial may soon provide data regarding the efficacy of this drug (NCT01720667).

b. Long-term anticonvulsant management. Anticonvulsants can be weaned when the clinical exam and EEG indicate that the newborn is no longer having seizures. If a newborn is receiving more than one anticonvulsant, weaning should be in the reverse order of initiation, with phenobarbital being weaned last, unless there is strong evidence that a particular drug was more effective. There is controversy regarding when phenobarbital should be discontinued, with some favoring discontinuation shortly before discharge and some favoring continued treatment for 1 to 6 months or more. Newborns who have a higher risk of developing epilepsy in infancy or childhood are those with a large area of HI brain injury and those with a persistently epileptiform EEG.

8. Management of other target organ injury

a. Cardiac dysfunction should be managed with correction of hypoxemia, acidosis, hypocalcemia and hypoglycemia, and avoidance of volume depletion or overload. Diuretics may be less effective if concomitant renal impairment is present. Newborns will require continuous monitoring of systemic mean arterial BP, CVP (if available), and urine output. Newborns with cardiovascular compromise may require inotropic drugs such as dopamine (see Chapter 40) and may need afterload reduction (e.g., dobutamine or milrinone) to maintain BP and perfusion.

i. Arterial BP should be maintained in the normal range to support adequate systemic and cerebral perfusion.

ii. Monitoring of CVP may be helpful to assess adequacy of preload (i.e., that the newborn is not hypovolemic due to vasodilatation or third spacing); a reasonable goal is 5 to 8 mm Hg in term newborns.

b. Renal dysfunction should be monitored by measuring urine output, with serum electrolytes, paired urine/serum osmolarity, urinalysis, and urine specific gravity.

i. In the presence of oliguria or anuria, avoid fluid overload by limiting free water administration to replacement of insensible losses and urine output (~60 mL/kg/day) and consider using low-dose dopamine infusion (≤2.5 μg/kg/minute) (see Chapters 23 and 28).

ii. Volume status should be evaluated before instituting strict fluid restriction. If there is no or low urine output, a 10 to 20 mL/kg fluid challenge followed by a loop diuretic such as furosemide may be helpful.

iii. To avoid fluid overload, as well as hypoglycemia, concentrated glucose infusions delivered through a central line may be needed. Glucose levels should be monitored closely and rapid glucose boluses avoided. Infusions should be weaned slowly to avoid rebound hypoglycemia.

c. GI effects. Feeding should be withheld until BP is stable, active bowel sounds are audible, and stools are negative for blood (see Chapter 27).

d. Hematologic abnormalities (see Chapters 42 to 47). Coagulation profile should be monitored with partial thromboplastin time (PTT) and prothrombin time (PT), fibrinogen, and platelets. Abnormalities may need to be corrected with fresh frozen plasma, cryoprecipitate, and/or platelet infusions.

e. Liver function should be monitored with measurement of transaminases (ALT, AST), clotting (PT, PTT, fibrinogen), albumin, bilirubin, and ammonia. Levels of drugs that are metabolized or eliminated by the liver must be monitored.

f. Lung (see Chapters 29, 30, and 36). Management of the pulmonary effects of asphyxia depends on the specific etiology.

XIII. NEUROPROTECTIVE STRATEGIES.

A number of neuroprotective strategies have been proposed and/or are being tested in animal or clinical human trials.

A. Therapeutic hypothermia has been shown to decrease the risk of brain injury in newborns exposed to perinatal HI insult(s).[5-7] Both total body and head cooling have been shown to be safe and effective.[8-10] and are recommended for treating newborns with moderate to severe HIE.[11] We use total body cooling in large part because of the ability to perform EEG monitoring needed to detect frequent seizures (~50% of newborns with moderate to severe HIE).

1. Inclusion criteria. We offer total body cooling to newborns with HIE based on the following three criteria:

a. Postmenstrual age (PMA) ≥36 weeks, BW ≥2,000 g

b. Evidence of fetal distress or neonatal distress as evidenced by one of the following:

  i. History of acute perinatal event (e.g., placental abruption, cord prolapse, severe FHR abnormality)

  ii. pH ≤7.0 or base deficit ≥16 mmol/L in cord gas or postnatal blood gas obtained within first hour of life

  iii. 10-minute Apgar score of ≤5

  iv. Assisted ventilation initiated at birth and continued for at least 10 minutes

c. Evidence of moderate to severe neonatal encephalopathy by exam and/or aEEG as follows:

  i. Primary method for determining neonatal encephalopathy is physical exam.

  ii. If exam shows moderate or severe encephalopathy, aEEG should be performed to provide further assessment and monitoring.

  iii. In circumstances in which physical exam is unreliable (e.g., muscle relaxants), an aEEG should be performed to determine if there is encephalopathy.

  iv. Patterns on aEEG that indicate moderate or severe encephalopathy include the following, with minimum of 20 minutes recording time:

   a) Severely abnormal: upper margin <10 μV

   b) Moderately abnormal: upper margin >10 μV and lower margin <5 μV

   c) Seizures identified by aEEG

Note: A normal neurologic exam does not require confirmation by aEEG.

2. **Exclusion criteria.** Patients may be excluded from this protocol according to the judgment of the attending physicians. If an exclusion criterion is identified during therapy, the patient should be warmed according to rewarming procedure described in the following text:

   a. Presence of lethal chromosomal abnormality (e.g., trisomy 13 or 18)

   b. Presence of severe congenital anomalies (e.g., complex cyanotic congenital heart disease, major CNS anomaly)

   c. Symptomatic systemic congenital viral infection (e.g., hepatosplenomegaly, microcephaly)

   d. Symptomatic systemic congenital bacterial infection (e.g., meningitis, DIC)

   e. Significant bleeding diathesis

   f. Major intracranial hemorrhage

   Cooling should be started before 6 hours of age; therefore, early recognition is essential. The target core temperature goal during cooling is 33.5°C (33° to 34°C) with acceptable range: 32.5° to 34.5°C.

   Arterial access and central venous access should be obtained prior to initiation of therapeutic hypothermia protocol if possible. Obtaining central access in the hypothermic state can be extremely challenging due to vasoconstrictive effects.

B. There are new agents such as erythropoietin, melatonin, xenon, and stem cells that are undergoing preliminary evaluation in Phase I/II trials, but there are currently no data supporting the use of any agent besides therapeutic hypothermia for neuroprotection.

C. Agents tested in animals with few or no data in human newborns include antagonists of excitotoxic neurotransmitter receptors such as NMDA receptor blockade with ketamine or MK-801; free radical scavengers such as allopurinol, superoxide dismutase, and vitamin E; Ca^{2+}-channel blockers such as magnesium sulfate, nimodipine, nicardipine; cyclooxygenase inhibitors such as indomethacin; benzodiazepine receptor stimulation such as midazolam; and enhancers of protein synthesis such as dexamethasone.

D. **Safety monitoring of newborns during 72 hours of therapeutic hypothermia and rewarming**

   1. **Temperature**

      a. Core temperature should be monitored continuously and documented every 15 minutes until 1 hour after goal temperature of 33.5°C is achieved and then hourly. Core temperature is often measured with an esophageal temperature probe.

      b. During rewarming procedure, core temperature should be monitored continuously and documented every hour.

   2. **Respiratory status**

      a. Arterial blood gases and serum lactate should be monitored at baseline and then at 4, 8, 12, 24, 48, and 72 hours of treatment and as clinically indicated.

      b. Due to minor differences between blood gases at 33.5 compared to 37 degrees, there is no need to record the infant's core temperature on the blood gas requisitions.

3. Cardiovascular

a. Vital signs should be monitored and documented per routine.

4. Fluid, electrolyte balance, and renal/GI

a. Nothing by mouth (NPO) when passive cooling starts, typically until rewarmed to normal temperature. Glucose, serum electrolytes with calcium, BUN/Cr, and aspartate transaminase/alanine aminotransferase (AST/ALT) should be monitored at baseline, and then at 24, 48, and 72 hours of treatment, and as clinically indicated. There are some centers that are providing low-volume "trophic" or "gut priming" feeds of about 10 mL/kg/day if there are no direct contraindications such as hypotension.

b. Parenteral nutrition should generally be provided, following standard initiation and advancement guidelines, and with standard goals including protein of 3 to 3.5 g/kg/day and lipids of 3 g/kg/day. Of note, fluid restriction may limit ability to reach full goals.

c. To avoid cerebral edema in this at-risk population, goal Na level at high end of normal range. Because many of these patients have decreased urine output of multifactorial etiology, anticipating need for relative fluid restriction will assist in avoiding serum Na below 140.

d. PT/PTT, international normalized ratio (INR), fibrinogen, and platelet count should be measured daily while cooled and as clinically indicated. Coagulopathy should be treated per routine, with the exception of the platelet count which should be kept >100,000 to compensate for decreased platelet function. A hematology consult may be requested for assistance.

5. Infectious disease

a. Antibiotics should be started after complete blood count (CBC) and blood culture drawn per routine.

b. If concerns regarding renal function, change from gentamicin to cefotaxime.

6. Neurologic status

a. Neurology consult should be requested as soon as possible, wherever available.

b. aEEG or, preferably, full EEG monitoring should be initiated on admission and continued through at least the first 24 hours, and the 12-hour rewarming period, and potentially throughout the entire hypothermia protocol, particularly if there are frequent seizures. The scalp should be carefully monitored for skin breakdown given the high risk related to ischemia, hypothermia, and decreased mobility of the newborn.

c. Cranial US should be obtained as soon as possible after therapeutic hypothermia is initiated to assess for intracranial hemorrhage.

d. One or more brain MRI scans should be obtained to assess the severity and location of any HI injury. MRI scans in newborns can often be obtained without use of additional sedative medications. Brain MRI scans should be deferred if the newborn has significant cardiorespiratory instability, ongoing seizures, or any other condition in which transport and MRI considered unsafe by the medical team. MRI scans should ideally include the following:

    i. T1- and T2-weighted imaging to detect any irreversible injury or other congenital or acquired abnormalities of brain parenchyma

    ii. DWI to detect evidence of acute HI injury
    iii. Susceptibility-weighted imaging to detect hemorrhage
    iv. Proton MRS to detect lactate or other metabolites suggestive of metabolic etiology other than HIE
    v. MR venography or arteriography may be useful if there is evidence of focal venous or arterial ischemic injury suggestive of thromboembolic disease.
  e. Early brain MRI obtained within the first 1 to 5 days after birth (or after HI insult) is useful for the following:
    i. Detection of early restricted diffusion that indicates early HI injury
    ii. To assess if injury is already well established (e.g., antenatal as opposed to perinatal insult)
    iii. To establish any potential etiology of encephalopathy besides HI
    iv. To begin to assess presence/severity of any HI injury
    Note: Early scans may underestimate HI injury, depending on timing of insult and imaging.
    Late brain MRI scans are useful to detect the severity and location of HI brain injury, which is best determined by conventional T1- and T2-weighted imaging sequences at 10 to 14 days of age or older. This late brain MRI scan can be obtained as an outpatient, unsedated MRI scan if the newborn has already been discharged from the neonatal intensive care unit (NICU). Note that diffusion abnormalities detected by DWI will pseudonormalize (i.e., appear normal) at approximately 7 to 10 days following an HI insult in newborns, and following that, DWI sequences will show increased diffusion in areas of established HI injury.

  7. Pain and sedation
    a. Goal sedation level during cooling should be established and measured with a sedation tool.
    b. Sufficient sedation should be administered to optimize comfort and avoid shivering, which can increase the newborn's metabolism and temperature, thereby decreasing the efficacy of hypothermia therapy. Titrate to achieve goal sedation scores.
      At the end of 72 hours of induced hypothermia, the newborn is rewarmed at a rate of 0.5°C every 2 hours until patient reaches 36.5°C. This should take approximately 10 to 12 hours.
      If a patient is discovered to meet an exclusion criterion or undergoes a major adverse event while undergoing hypothermia treatment, rewarm according to the same procedure.

E. Controversies in administering therapeutic hypothermia

  1. Hypothermia of greater duration or depth. A question that arose following publication of the initial clinical trials of moderate hypothermia for 72 hours was whether cooling to a lower temperature and/or for a longer duration might be of greater benefit. A randomized trial addressing this question was published in 2014 and showed that neither cooling for 120 hours nor cooling to a temperature of 32°C offered additional benefit and instead showed a trend to worse outcome, with the trial being stopped early for futility.

2. **Late initiation of hypothermia.** There are data showing that hypothermia is associated with improved outcome if started at <3 to 4 hours after birth, consistent with animal data, but it is unclear if there is a benefit to hypothermia initiated >6 hours after birth. This question is being tested in an ongoing National Institute of Child Health and Human Development (NICHD)-funded trial, but in the meantime, centers such as ours do consider cooling infants beginning at 6 to 12 hours if other criteria are met.

3. **Gestational age 34 to 36 weeks.** It is currently unclear what is the lowest gestational age for which hypothermia remains both effective and safe, but some centers consider cooling newborns at 34 to 36 weeks if other criteria are met, the newborns are of normal weight, and a US can be performed early to rule out intraventricular hemorrhage, which occurs more commonly in preterm newborns.

4. **Underlying medical conditions.** There is also controversy about providing hypothermia to newborns with underlying surgical or genetic conditions. This question is unlikely to be addressed in large clinical trials so requires careful clinical consideration.

5. **Mild HIE.** Likely the greatest difficulty is deciding whether to offer hypothermia to newborns who meet some but not all of the criteria, particularly those with a mild degree of encephalopathy. Although there are some objective entry criteria such as the pH, base excess, or voltage by aEEG, other criteria are necessarily subjective, such as the determination of fetal/neonatal distress or the severity of encephalopathy by clinical exam. The threshold for which hypothermia may provide benefit without adverse effects may be somewhat different from that which has been studied in clinical trials to date. Further data are clearly needed regarding the neurologic outcome of newborns with mild HIE and the risks and benefits of hypothermia for mild HIE.

XIV. OUTCOME IN PERINATAL ASPHYXIA

A. The overall mortality rate is approximately 20%. The frequency of neurodevelopmental sequelae in surviving newborns is approximately 30%.

B. The risk of cerebral palsy (CP) in survivors of perinatal asphyxia is 5% to 10% compared to 0.2% in the general population. **Most CP is not related to perinatal asphyxia, and most perinatal asphyxia does not cause CP.**

C. Specific outcomes depend on the severity of the encephalopathy, the presence or absence of seizures, EEG results, and neuroimaging findings.

1. Severity of encephalopathy can be ascertained using the **Sarnat clinical stages of HIE** (see Table 55.1).
   a. Stage 1 or mild HIE: <1% mortality, 98% to 100% of newborns will have a normal neurologic outcome.
   b. Stage 2 or moderate HIE: 20% to 37% die or have abnormal neurodevelopmental outcomes. Prognosis can be refined by the use of EEG and MRI studies to detect the severity of encephalopathy, seizures, and the severity and location of HI brain injury. This group may benefit the most from therapeutic hypothermia.

c. Stage 3 or severe HIE: Death from effects of severe systemic asphyxia is more likely with severe HIE or from elective withdrawal of medical technology when there is severe brain injury that will result in severe neurologic disability. Survivors are likely to have one or more major neurodevelopmental disability, such as CP, intellectual disability, visual impairment, or epilepsy.

2. The presence of seizures increases a newborn's risk of CP 50- to 70-fold. Mortality and long-term morbidity are highest for seizures that begin within 12 hours of birth, are electrographic only, and/or frequent.[3]

3. Persistently low voltage activity or isoelectric background by EEG is a prognostic indicator of poor neurologic outcome. Although a transient burst suppression pattern may be associated with a good outcome, a persistent burst suppression pattern (e.g., ≥ 7 days) is associated with a high risk of death or neurodevelopmental disability. Of note, some maternal medications can transiently alter the neonatal EEG.

4. MRI adds a great deal of prognostic information to the clinical and EEG data because the pattern of HI brain injury by MRI generally correlates well with neurologic outcome when performed at the right age and interpreted by a physician with expertise in interpreting neonatal brain MRI scans. Significant injury to the cortex or subcortical nuclei is usually associated with both intellectual and motor disability, but the severity can vary considerably depending on the regions involved and severity of injury to each region. Notably, discrete lesions in the subcortical nuclei or less severe watershed pattern/parasagittal injuries can be associated with a normal cognitive outcome and only mild motor impairments. Overall, motor outcome is easier to predict than cognitive or sensory outcome, and it can be very difficult to predict which infants will have later epilepsy or feeding difficulties. Thus, these studies should be interpreted with care by physicians with experience in caring for children who had neonatal HIE.

References

1. Shellhaas RA, Soaita AI, Clancy RR. Sensitivity of amplitude-integrated electro-encephalography for neonatal seizure detection. *Pediatrics* 2007;120:770–777.

2. Wirrell EC, Armstrong EA, Osman LD, et al. Prolonged seizures exacerbate perinatal hypoxic-ischemic brain damage. *Pediatr Res* 2001;50:445–454.

3. McBride MC, Laroia N, Guillet R. Electrographic seizures in neonates correlate with poor neurodevelopmental outcome. *Neurology* 2000;55:506–513.

4. Rennie J, Boylan G. Treatment of neonatal seizures. *Arch Dis Child Fetal Neonatal Ed* 2007;92:F148–F150.

5. Gluckman PD, Wyatt JS, Azzopardi D, et al. Selective head cooling with mild systemic hypothermia after neonatal encephalopathy: multicentre randomised trial. *Lancet* 2005;365:663–670.

6. Shankaran S, Laptook AR, Ehrenkranz RA, et al. Whole-body hypothermia for neonates with hypoxic-ischemic encephalopathy. *N Engl J Med* 2005;353:1574–1584.

7. Azzopardi DV, Strohm B, Edwards AD, et al. Moderate hypothermia to treat perinatal asphyxial encephalopathy. *N Engl J Med* 2009;361:1349–1358.

8. Gunn AJ, Gluckman PD, Gunn TR. Selective head cooling in newborn infants after perinatal asphyxia: a safety study. *Pediatrics* 1998;102:885–892.

9. Eicher DJ, Wagner CL, Katikaneni LP, et al. Moderate hypothermia in neonatal encephalopathy: safety outcomes. *Pediatr Neurol* 2005;32:18–24.

10. Shankaran S, Pappas A, Laptook AR, et al. Outcomes of safety and effectiveness in a multicenter randomized, controlled trial of whole-body hypothermia for neonatal hypoxic-ischemic encephalopathy. *Pediatrics* 2008;122:e791–e798.

11. Papile LA, Baley JE, Benitz W, et al. Hypothermia and neonatal encephalopathy. *Pediatrics* 2014;133(6):1146–1150.

Suggested Readings

Bednarek N, Mathur A, Inder T, et al. Impact of therapeutic hypothermia on MRI diffusion changes in neonatal encephalopathy. *Neurology* 2012;78(18): 1420–1427.

Boylan GB, Kharoshankaya L, Wusthoff CJ. Seizures and hypothermia: importance of electroencephalographic monitoring and considerations for treatment. *Semin Fetal Neonatal Med* 2015;20(2):103–108.

Jacobs SE, Berg M, Hunt R, et al. Cooling for newborns with hypoxic ischaemic encephalopathy. *Cochrane Database Syst Rev* 2013;(1):CD003311.

Johnston MV, Trescher WH, Ishida A, et al. Neurobiology of hypoxic-ischemic injury in the developing brain. *Pediatr Res* 2001;49:735–741.

Mallard EC, Williams CE, Gunn AJ, et al. Frequent episodes of brief ischemia sensitize the fetal sheep brain to neuronal loss and induce striatal injury. *Pediatr Res* 1993;33:61–65.

Martinez-Biarge M, Diez-Sebastian J, Kapellou O, et al. Predicting motor outcome and death in term hypoxic-ischemic encephalopathy. *Neurology* 2011;76(24): 2055–2061.

Martinez-Biarge M, Diez-Sebastian J, Rutherford MA, et al. Outcomes after central grey matter injury in term perinatal hypoxic-ischaemic encephalopathy. *Early Hum Dev* 2010;86(11):675–682.

Murray DM, Boylan GB, Ryan CA, et al. Early EEG findings in hypoxic-ischemic encephalopathy predict outcomes at 2 years. *Pediatrics* 2009;124: e459–e467.

Myers RE. Four patterns of perinatal brain damage and their conditions of occurrence in primates. *Adv Neurol* 1975;10:223–234.

Nelson KB, Leviton A. How much of neonatal encephalopathy is due to birth asphyxia? *Am J Dis Child* 1991;145:1325–1331.

Sarkar S, Bhagat I, Dechert RE, et al. Predicting death despite therapeutic hypothermia in infants with hypoxic-ischaemic encephalopathy. *Arch Dis Child Fetal Neonatal Ed* 2010;95:F423–F428.

Sarnat HB, Sarnat MS. Neonatal encephalopathy following fetal distress. A clinical and electroencephalographic study. *Arch Neurol* 1976;33:696–705.

Shankaran S, Laptook AR, Pappas A, et al. Effect of depth and duration of cooling on deaths in the NICU among neonates with hypoxic ischemic encephalopathy: a randomized clinical trial. *JAMA* 2014;312(24):2629–2639.

Smit E, Liu X, Jary S, et al. Cooling neonates who do not fulfil the standard cooling criteria—short- and long-term outcomes. *Acta Paediatr* 2014;104(2):138–145.

Thoresen M, Hellström-Westas L, Liu X, et al. Effect of hypothermia on amplitude-integrated electroencephalogram in infants with asphyxia. *Pediatrics* 2010;126(1):e131–e139.

Volpe JJ. *Neurology of the Newborn*. 5th ed. Philadelphia, PA: Saunders Elsevier; 2008.

Wilkinson DJ, Thayyil S, Robertson NJ. Ethical and practical issues relating to the global use of therapeutic hypothermia for perinatal asphyxial encephalopathy. *Arch Dis Child Fetal Neonatal Ed* 2011;96:F75–F78.

56 Neonatal Seizures

Arnold J. Sansevere and Ann M. Bergin

KEY POINTS

- Neonatal seizures are usually due to an underlying injury or disorder. Treatable disorders should be sought.
- Hypoxic-ischemic encephalopathy and focal ischemia/stroke are responsible for the majority of cases of neonatal seizure.
- Neonatal seizures and their treatment may compromise respiratory and cardiovascular stability.
- A high proportion of neonatal seizures are subclinical.
- Continuous electroencephalogram (EEG) is the gold standard for detection and quantification of neonatal seizures and assessment of treatment effect.

I. **INTRODUCTION.** Seizures occur more frequently in the neonatal period than at any other time of life. Estimates of the incidence of neonatal seizures vary according to case definition, method of ascertainment and definition of the neonatal period, and range from 1 to 5/1,000 live births. In neonates, the vast majority of seizures are symptomatic of underlying disorders, although primary epileptic disorders may also present in this age group. The occurrence of seizure may be the first clinical indication of neurologic disorder.

Developmental immaturity influences many aspects of diagnosis, management, and prognosis of seizures in the newborn: (i) Clinical seizure patterns in the neonate reflect the "reduced connectivity" in the neonatal brain, with prominence of focal ictal characteristics and rarity of generalized patterns of clinical seizures. (ii) The balance of excitatory and inhibitory processes in the immature brain are weighted toward excitation with an excess of glutamatergic synapses over inhibitory (usually gamma-aminobutyric acid [GABA]-ergic) synapses. In fact, in some regions of the neonatal brain, GABA may temporarily act as an excitatory neurotransmitter via an alteration in chloride gradient and transportation in the immature brain. These developmental features may underlie the neonate's tendency to frequently recurrent seizures and may explain the poor efficacy of traditionally used GABA-ergic antiepileptic agents (phenobarbital, benzodiazepines). (iii) Systemic processes are also immature, leading to altered drug handling compared to older children. (iv) The immature brain may be more susceptible to developmental effects of anticonvulsant medications.

II. DIAGNOSIS. An epileptic seizure is a change in neurologic function (motor, sensory, experiential, or autonomic) that is associated with an abnormal synchronous discharge of cortical neurons. This abnormal electrical discharge may be recorded by electroencephalogram (EEG). At all ages, including in the newborn, paroxysmal behaviors may occur, which raise suspicion of electrical seizure but which lack correlating patterns on scalp EEG. Management of these events is difficult at any age and controversial in the newborn. For this review, only those paroxysmal events associated with an electrographic seizure pattern are considered.

Early diagnosis of neonatal seizures is important to allow (i) identification and treatment of underlying disorders, (ii) treatment to prevent additional seizures and seizure-related systemic effects such as hypoxemia and hypertension, (iii) treatment of seizures to possibly prevent seizure-related excitotoxic neuronal injury. Diagnosis of seizures in the neonate requires knowledge of the clinical patterns associated with electrographic seizures at this age and confirmation with EEG, ideally accompanied by video telemetry. The EEG usually demonstrates a rhythmic focal correlate associated with, but typically of longer duration than, the clinical event. A focus of origin and spread to adjacent areas can be seen (Fig. 56.1). The more severely encephalopathic the infant, the less the seizure pattern tends to evolve in waveform and topographic spread.

Nonepileptic paroxysmal events are common in the encephalopathic infant, and unlike seizures, lack an EEG seizure pattern. Nonepileptic events are often stimulus-evoked and may be altered or stopped by gentle restraint and/or change in position (Table 56.1).

In addition, video-EEG recordings have revealed that up to 80% of electrographic seizures in neonates lack a clinical correlate. This is particularly likely in encephalopathic newborns. This phenomenon is described as electroclinical dissociation or uncoupling. Whether subclinical electrographic seizures cause additional brain injury in the newborn is unproven to date. Recent studies have suggested that higher degrees of seizure burden and neonatal status epilepticus may impact neurologic outcome as well as mortality.

A. Common clinical seizure patterns

1. **Focal clonic seizures.** This pattern may occur unilaterally, sequentially in different limbs, or simultaneously but asynchronously. The movement is rhythmic, biphasic with a fast contraction phase, and a slower relaxation. A clinical correlate may be present for only a small portion of the total duration of the electrographic seizure. Face, upper or lower limbs, eyes, or trunk may be involved.

2. **Focal tonic seizures.** Patterns include a sustained posture of a single limb, tonic horizontal eye deviation, or asymmetric tonic truncal postures. In contrast to focal tonic events, generalized tonic movements are generally not accompanied by seizure patterns on EEG.

3. **Myoclonic seizures.** These are characterized by a rapid movement usually of flexion. Of the varieties of myoclonus occurring in the newborn, generalized myoclonus usually involving both upper limbs and less commonly the lower limbs, is most often associated with an EEG seizure pattern. Focal or multifocal myoclonic events are usually not associated with such patterns.

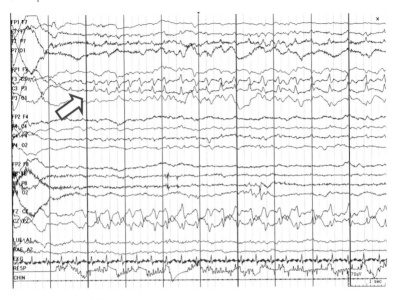

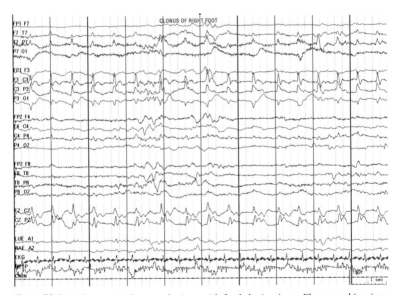

Figure 56.1. Left parasagittal neonatal seizure with focal clonic seizure. Electrographic seizure begins in the left parasagittal area (*open arrow*), and 12 seconds later, focal clonus of the right foot is noted.

Table 56.1. Differential Diagnosis of Neonatal Seizure

Paroxysmal Nonepileptic Event	History	Clinical Features	Differentiating Features
Benign neonatal sleep myoclonus Most common entity misdiagnosed as seizure in the neonate	Neonate is term, healthy, and thriving. May be present from birth to 3 months	Multifocal jerks seen in transition to and during sleep	Only present during sleep Upon wakening, the jerking ceases
Jitteriness (tremors)	May have exposure to maternal substance abuse or use of medications, metabolic disorder, hypoglycemia, perinatal insult	Stimulus sensitive, high frequency, low amplitude, and oscillatory (not jerking movement) Activated/exacerbated by arousal	Extinguishes or decreases with flexion of the extremity and gentle restraint No associated abnormal eye movements or autonomic change
Apnea of prematurity	Neonate is preterm.	Apnea and bradycardia	Apnea associated with tachycardia suggests seizure. Assess for other associated features (i.e., automatisms, oculomotor events, motor movements, etc.).

4. **Autonomic seizures.** Autonomic events such as apnea, often with associated tachycardia rather than bradycardia (particularly in term newborns), and/or pupillary dilatation. These are often also associated with hypertension.

Many newborns may have more than one seizure type. In premature infants, a wider range of clinical behaviors can be associated with electrographic seizure patterns, for instance, self-limited short periods of otherwise unexplained tachypnea, tachycardia, and other autonomic changes may represent seizures in the preterm infant, as may chewing, sucking, and cycling movements, which usually are not associated with EEG seizures in the term infant.

B. **EEG diagnosis.** Continuous electroencephalogram (cEEG), defined as >3 hours of monitoring, is considered the gold standard for the diagnosis of neonatal seizures. cEEG is particularly important given the high proportion of neonatal seizures that are subclinical (studies suggest up to 80% of neonatal seizures are electrographic only) and would go undetected without continuous monitoring due to electroclinical uncoupling or dissociation.

Including video analysis can be very helpful to correctly characterize events, preventing treatment of clinically suspicious but nonepileptic events, and avoiding misinterpretation of artifactual EEG patterns, which can be seen with suctioning, ventilation events, and physical therapy/patting.

Many neonatal intensive care units (NICUs) rely on both routine EEG and amplitude-integrated electroencephalogram (aiEEG) to evaluate cerebral function in neonates.

1. **Routine neonatal EEG** recording, typically of 1 hour duration, allows assessment of background activity, including cycling state change, developmental maturity, and sometimes, epileptic potential. Such recordings may identify patients at high risk for seizure, and especially if performed serially, are useful for prognostication. However, a typical clinical event is unlikely to be captured in such a short time. Where possible, 24-hour continuous recording is preferred.

2. **aiEEG** is a bedside technique increasingly being used by neonatologists for neuromonitoring. The background EEG activity from a limited number of electrodes (usually one to two channels, two to four electrodes) is amplified, filtered, rectified, compressed (6 cm/hour), and displayed on a semilogarithmic scale. One minute of EEG is thus represented by 1 mm of aiEEG. Electrodes are typically placed in watershed zones in the central and temporal regions. This technique allows the neonatologist to continually assess the background EEG characteristics and thereby judge the severity of encephalopathy, the improvement or deterioration over time, and response to therapies. Seizures occurring during recording of this compressed data may alter the tracing in a recognizable manner provided the seizures occur in the region of the electrodes being used for recording and are of sufficient duration. The presence of seizures may be confirmed with immediate review of raw EEG from the available one to two channels and should then be further assessed with standard EEG recording (Fig. 56.2). The sensitivity and specificity varies with the experience of the user.

III. **ETIOLOGY.** Once the presence of electrographic seizure has been identified, underlying etiologies, particularly reversible causes, must be sought. The details of the pregnancy (from point of conception to time of delivery), birth history, maternal history, and family history are most important in directing the initial evaluation. For instance, a history of traumatic delivery, with good Apgar scores in a term infant, raises the possibility of intracranial hemorrhage. The age at onset of seizure relative to the time of birth is also extremely important and may suggest likely etiologies. Hypoxic-ischemic encephalopathy (HIE), which is the single most common cause of neonatal seizures, usually causes seizures within the first 24 hours of life. Focal seizures in the setting of a well-appearing nonencephalopathic newborn raises suspicion for perinatal infarction. When seizures

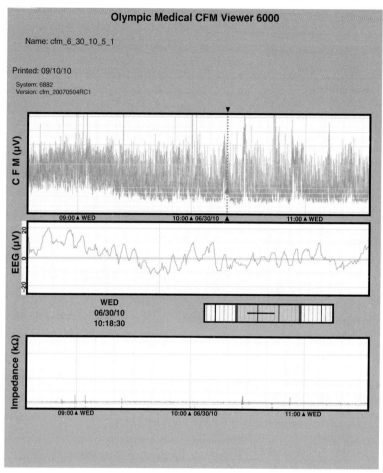

Figure 56.2. Amplitude integrated EEG.
Upper panel: Compressed EEG data with wide band of activity, occasionally with sudden elevation of lower margin—a marker for possible seizure.
Middle panel: Raw EEG at the timepoint indicated by the cursor in the upper panel. Single channel EEG with rhythmicity concerning for possible seizure. Full EEG required for confirmation.
Lower panel: Indication of electrode impedance, which is appropriately low. Patterns seen in the compressed EEG data are uninterpretable in the presence of high electrode impedance.

present after the first 48 hours of life, and particularly after a period of initial well-being, infection and biochemical disorders should be considered. Seizures occurring later (e.g., >10 days of life) are more likely to be related to disorders of calcium metabolism (now rare in the United States), cortical malformation, or neonatal epilepsy syndromes, which may be benign (e.g., benign familial neonatal seizures) or severe (e.g., early infantile epileptic encephalopathy).

Table 56.2. Etiologies of Neonatal Seizures
Hypoxic-ischemic injury   Perinatal asphyxia

Focal infarction
  Arterial
  Venous

Intracranial hemorrhage
  Intraventricular
  Parenchymal
  Subdural
  Subarachnoid

CNS infection (*Escherichia coli*, GBS, *Listeria monocytogenes*, HSV)

Malformations and other structural lesions
  Neuronal migration disorders
  Cerebral dysgenesis
  Neurocutaneous disorders, e.g., Sturge-Weber syndrome, tuberous sclerosis

Acute metabolic disorders
  Hypoglycemia
  Hypocalcemia
  Hypomagnesemia

Inborn errors of metabolism
  Aminoacidopathies
  Organic acidurias
  Peroxisomal diseases
  Mitochondrial disorders
  Disorder of glucose transport (GLUT-1 deficiency)
  Pyridoxine-dependent seizures
  Folinic acid responsive seizures

Epilepsy syndromes
  Benign familial syndromes
  Severe neonatal epileptic encephalopathies (EIEE, Ohtahara syndrome, EME)

CNS, central nervous system; GBS, group B *Streptococcus*; HSV, herpes simplex virus; GLUT-1, glucose transporter-1; EIEE, early infantile epileptic encephalopathy; EME, early myoclonic epilepsy.

Multiple possible etiologies (Table 56.2) may be identified in a neonate with seizures, such as HIE with hypoglycemia, hypocalcemia, and/or intracranial hemorrhage, and each must be treated appropriately.

A. **Specific etiologies**

1. **Hypoxic ischemic encephalopathy (HIE) (see Chapter 55).** This is the most common cause of neonatal seizures, accounting for 50% to

75% of cases. In **perinatal asphyxia**, the seizures occur in the context of a newborn who has a history of difficulty during labor and delivery with alterations of the fetal heart rate, decreased umbilical artery pH, and Apgar score <5 at 5 minutes. There is typically early suppression of the mental status, sometimes with coma and low tone, in addition to the seizures, which are usually seen within the first 12 to 24 hours. Although the insult is global, the seizures are usually focal and may be multifocal. They are typically of short duration (<1 minute) but may be very frequent and refractory, especially in the first 24 hours. Treatment is urgent and complicated in many infants by the effects of hypoxic injury to other organ systems (hepatic, pulmonary, renal, and cardiovascular). Additionally, the anticonvulsant drugs may contribute to hypotension and hypoventilation. This subpopulation is at high risk for subclinical electrographic seizures—electroclinical dissociation (incidence in this group is 22% to 65%). Where possible, prolonged EEG is invaluable in identifying ongoing subclinical seizures.

In recent years, therapeutic hypothermia has become the standard of care in neonates with suspected hypoxic injury. Therapeutic hypothermia may decrease the rate of both death and disability in neonates with hypoxic injury. It may also decrease the overall seizure burden in patients with moderate hypoxic injury. A rebound increase in seizure frequency has been documented during rewarming. Although rare, the occurrence of a first neonatal seizure during rewarming has also been described.

Perinatal stroke is the second most common cause of seizures in the newborn period accounting for up to 20% of neonatal seizures. In **focal ischemic lesions**, such as middle cerebral artery stroke, the infant usually appears well and presents with focal clonic seizures. Such arterial strokes may have occurred prior to or in early labor. Asymmetries of the motor examination are often lacking in these infants, and diagnosis may be delayed until later in their first year if they do not present with neonatal seizures. Focal electrographic seizures as well as focal attenuation of EEG background activity and focal sharp waves support the clinical suspicion for infarction.

2. **Intracranial hemorrhage (ICH).** ICH are responsible for 10% to 15% of neonatal seizures. In the term infant, primary **subarachnoid hemorrhage** (not due to extension of a deeper cerebral or intraventricular hemorrhage) is probably more common than is realized. Most are not of clinical significance and produce no symptoms. Normal delivery or deliveries with instrumentation and/or trauma may be associated with more substantial subarachnoid hemorrhages, which may present with seizures, usually on the second day of life. These infants appear clinically well between seizures and have a very good outcome. **Subdural hemorrhages** are related to large infant size, breech delivery, and instrumentation. They are due to tears in the falx, the tentorium, or superficial cerebral veins. They are often associated with underlying cerebral contusions, which may be responsible for the seizures in some cases. Presenting seizures are usually focal and occur in the first few days of life. If large, subdural hematomas may require surgical treatment making diagnosis important.

In the term infant presenting with hemorrhage, sinovenous thrombosis should be considered. In the **preterm infant, germinal matrix, intraventricular, and parenchymal hemorrhages** are the prototypic neurologic complications of premature hypoxic injury. Seizures can occur with extension of the germinal matrix hemorrhage into the adjacent hypoxic parenchyma typically after the first 3 days of life. Generalized tonic events are usually not associated with electrographic seizure patterns, reflecting instead alterations in intracranial pressure. EEG recording may confirm seizure patterns with autonomic phenomena or cycling motor movements in these premature infants and also has identified subclinical electrographic seizures in association with these hemorrhages. Seizures occurring in the setting of premature hemorrhagic lesions are not usually associated with a good outcome.

3. **Central nervous system (CNS) infection.** CNS infections account for about 5% of neonatal seizures. **Congenital intrauterine infections** such as with cytomegalovirus (CMV), toxoplasma, rubella, and herpes viruses may present early (first 2 days) with seizures in severe cases. The clinical scenario may include microcephaly; poor intrauterine growth; prematurity; and other skin, ophthalmic, and systemic findings. Meningoencephalitis, cerebral calcification, and dysgenesis (in cases of early intrauterine infection) contribute to the pathogenesis of seizures in these cases. **Postnatal sepsis**, for example, with group B *Streptococcus* or *Escherichia coli*, is often complicated by meningitis and may be associated with seizures. In this setting, the newborn has often been well for a couple of days, only to deteriorate later with seizures occurring after the first 48 to 72 hours.

4. **Acute metabolic disorders.** These rapidly remediable conditions are the focus of the initial investigations in neonatal seizures and include hypoglycemia, hypocalcemia, hypomagnesemia, and hyponatremia. They account for approximately 5% of neonatal seizures.

   a. Hypoglycemia. Even when it occurs in association with other potential causes of seizure, such as HIE, hypoglycemia should be treated (see Table 56.2). The definition of hypoglycemia is controversial, but reasonable thresholds for treatment are <40 mg/dL (<2.2 mmol/L) in the first 24 hours and <50 mg/dL (<2.8 mmol/L) after 24 hours. Most hypoglycemic infants are asymptomatic, but at any point, symptoms of neuroglycopenia should prompt immediate treatment. These are jitteriness/tremor, hypotonia, alteration of consciousness, poor feeding, apnea, and seizures. Causes of neonatal hypoglycemia include the following:

      i. Decreased glucose supply, as in the premature and small for gestational age infant

      ii. Increased utilization, such as in hyperinsulinemic states, most commonly seen in the infant of the diabetic mother. Other hyperinsulinemic states include the overgrowth syndrome Beckwith-Wiedemann syndrome, erythroblastosis, and the rare hyperinsulinemic hypoglycemia.

      iii. Disorders in which pathways of gluconeogenesis are deficient or suppressed (e.g., glycogen storage disorders, aminoacidopathies such as maple syrup urine disease, fatty acid oxidation defects)

b. Hypocalcemia. Whole blood ionized calcium (iCa) is the best measure of calcium status in ill infants. Hypocalcemia is considered present when iCa in term or premature infants >1,500 g birth weight is <4.4 mg/dL (<1.1 mmol/L) and in premature infants <1,500 g at birth, <4.0 mg/dL (<1 mmol/L). **Early-onset** hypocalcemia occurs in the first 3 days of life and is associated with prematurity, infants of diabetic mothers, intrauterine growth restriction, and perinatal asphyxia. Most is asymptomatic. Symptoms of hypocalcemia include jitteriness, stimulus-induced muscle jerks, seizures, and rarely, laryngospasm. **Late-onset** (>10 days of life) hypocalcemia can occur because of hypoparathyroidism, the feeding of high phosphate formula, DiGeorge syndrome (chromosome 22q11.2 deletion), some mitochondrial cytopathies, and hypomagnesemia. Symptomatic or persistent cases should be treated (see Table 56.2).

c. Hypomagnesemia. The most common cause is transient neonatal hypomagnesemia. It causes parathyroid hormone resistance and so causes hypocalcemia. Hypomagnesemia must be corrected before the hypocalcemia can be corrected (see Table 56.2). Levels <1.4 mg/dL (<0.6 mmol/L) are considered low.

5. **Malformations/structural lesions.** Five percent of neonatal seizures are caused by cerebral dysgenesis. **Cerebral dysgenesis** can cause seizures from the first day of life. This is most likely with the more severe disorders such as hemimegalencephaly, lissencephaly, and polymicrogyria. Seizures are often refractory to medications. Some disorders may be amenable to surgical treatments, such as hemimegalencephaly and focal polymicrogyria. In general, these infants are not encephalopathic interictally. Clues to neurocutaneous diseases may be apparent on the newborn examination—for instance, the hemangioma in the distribution of cranial nerve V1 in Sturge-Weber syndrome, which can occasionally cause seizures in the newborn period. Hypopigmented "ash-leaf" macules of tuberous sclerosis may be seen, although neonatal seizures are rare in this disorder. Neuroimaging is primary in making these diagnoses.

6. **Inborn errors of metabolism.** Although individually very rare, inborn errors of metabolism as a group cause at least 1% of cases of seizures in the newborn. Typically caused by an enzyme defect in the metabolic pathways of carbohydrates, proteins, or fat, many cause disease due to accumulation of toxic products unable to proceed along the appropriate metabolic pathways. In these disorders, infants initially appear well, due to the benefits of placental clearance of toxins until birth, and only become encephalopathic and have seizures after 2 to 3 days. Parental report of "hiccough" *in utero* may correlate with postnatal seizures and/or myoclonus. Biochemical markers for these disorders include hypoglycemia, metabolic acidosis, hyperammonemia, as well as specific patterns of alteration in amino acid or organic acid profiles. Other disorders cause disease due to a mutation-related defect in a vital function, for example, in GLUT-1 deficiency, which impairs glucose transport across the blood–brain barrier, with resulting developmental delay and seizures. This disorder illustrates the importance of identifying these disorders,

because it and some others are treatable, providing an opportunity to prevent brain injury. Diagnosis also allows reproductive counseling for later pregnancies. Among metabolic disorders, **glycine encephalopathy (nonketotic hyperglycinemia)** commonly causes myoclonic events, with or without EEG correlate, encephalopathy with depressed sensorium, respiratory compromise, and hypotonia. The EEG background often reveals a very abnormal "burst-suppression" pattern. Glycine is elevated in the cerebrospinal fluid (CSF) and usually, but not always, in plasma. The defect is in the glycine cleavage system, and because glycine is a co-agonist with the excitatory glutamate, it results in enhanced cortical excitability. In spite of efforts to block glutamate neurotransmission pharmacologically with dextromethorphan, most of these infants do very poorly. **Pyridoxine dependency**, although rare, is an important cause of neonatal seizures as treatment is available. The most common form is due to a defect in the ALDH7A1/antiquitin gene, which results in deficiency of alpha amino-adipic semialdehyde (α-AASA) dehydrogenase and accumulation of α-AASA in blood, urine, and CSF, thus providing a biologic marker for the disorder. This enzyme is involved in lysine breakdown in the brain and is believed to impact the metabolism of the neurotransmitters glutamate and GABA. Seizures present early, sometimes *in utero*, and infants are irritable. A test dose of pyridoxine 100 mg intravenous (IV), with EEG and cardiorespiratory monitoring, resulting in immediate seizure cessation and resolution of EEG abnormalities within hours, is diagnostic. Because some infants do not respond to the initial IV dose, a 3-day trial of oral pyridoxine (30 mg/kg/day) is recommended for nonresponders. If successful, supplementation is lifelong as seizures recur on withdrawal of the pyridoxine. The poorly understood disorder, **folinic acid–responsive seizures**, has recently been shown to be genetically and biochemically identical to pyridoxine dependency. Previously, this disorder, initially identified by novel peaks in CSF chromatography, was treated by supplementation with folinic acid (3 to 5 mg/kg/day). This was effective in stopping seizures in some of these cases but did not prevent severe developmental sequelae. Similarly, many patients with pyridoxine dependency, although seizure free, had long-term developmental deficits. For this reason, and based on their allelic nature, it has been suggested that patients diagnosed with either of these disorders be treated with both supplements.

7. **Epilepsy syndromes.** These syndromes are rare, together accounting for about 1% of cases of seizures in the newborn period. **Benign familial neonatal convulsions** occur in otherwise well infants on day 2 or 3 of life. Seizures may be focal clonic or tonic (usually asymmetrical). Family history should be sought because it is often unreported. Seizures resolve after a variable period, usually within 6 months. This disorder is associated with abnormality of voltage-gated potassium channels, usually KCNQ2 and less frequently KCNQ3. Developmental outcome is normal, but 5% to 15% may have later nonfebrile convulsions. **Benign infantile neonatal seizures** ("fifth day fits") present suddenly on days 4 to 6 of life, often with frequent seizures leading to status epilepticus. Seizures are initially focal clonic often with apnea. Tonic seizures are

not expected in this disorder. Seizures usually cease within 2 weeks. The etiology is unknown. More severe epilepsy syndromes are also seen, presenting in this period. These include the following:

a. Early myoclonic epilepsy (EME), often presenting in the first few days of life with focal motor seizures and myoclonus, which may be subtle and erratic and usually affects the face and limbs. Tonic seizures appear relatively late in this disorder. The seizures are very refractory to medications. The EEG is characterized by a burst-suppression pattern, which may only be seen in sleep, and, if present throughout the sleep–wake cycle, is exacerbated by sleep. This syndrome is often associated with underlying metabolic disorders, for instance, glycine encephalopathy (described earlier). Development is severely affected, and many infants die, often within their first year.

b. Early infantile epileptic encephalopathy (EIEE; Ohtahara syndrome) is also associated with very refractory epilepsy. In contrast to EME, it is characterized by early onset of tonic spasms along with focal motor seizures. Myoclonus is rare in the early stages of this disorder. It, too, is associated with a burst-suppression pattern on EEG, which is relatively invariant. Whereas EME tends to be associated with underlying metabolic disorders, EIEE is more likely to be associated with structural lesions. Developmental prognosis is also poor in this syndrome, with many evolving to a chaotic epileptiform pattern known as hypsarrhythmia on EEG and accompanied by infantile spasms. Advances in the understanding of the complex molecular genetics of epilepsy have revealed associations between the earlier disorders and abnormality in a number of genes (e.g., ARX, STXBP1, KCNQ2, SCN2A, and others). There is not a 1:1 phenotype:genotype relationship in this setting, and it may be that the same genetic disorder can be associated with either EME or EIEE, for as yet unknown pathophysiologic reasons. It is now possible, at some cost, to test arrays of genes implicated in particular clinical scenarios. The proportion of these cases for which a genetic diagnosis is possible continues to increase.

c. Malignant migrating partial seizures in infancy (Coppola syndrome) may present from the first to the tenth month of life. Focal motor seizures occur and escalate aggressively, shifting clinically and electrographically from side to side and proving highly refractory to anticonvulsant medications. Developmental status is acutely affected and prognosis for normal outcome is poor, although cases with less than devastating outcome have now been described. The etiology is unknown.

8. Other high-risk subpopulations

a. Extracorporeal membrane oxygenation (ECMO). Critically ill neonates requiring ECMO have been identified by recent guidelines as a population at high risk for seizure due to the high risk of cerebral injury during the transition to ECMO. These patients typically remain paralyzed and sedated, further masking clinical signs of seizure. There is limited data on the prevalence of seizures in neonates requiring ECMO.

b. Congenital heart disease. Neonates that undergo surgery for congenital heart disease are known to be at risk for seizure specifically in the postoperative period. Electrographic seizures have been documented to occur in 5% to 26% of this population. Studies suggest that the average time to first seizure is 20 to 22 hours into the postoperative period.

IV. INVESTIGATIONS. The approach to investigations should be individualized with an emphasis on early identification of correctable disorders. Testing is guided by a detailed history of the pregnancy, labor and delivery, and subsequent course. It should proceed in parallel with stabilization of vital functions, including supported respiration if necessary, EEG confirmation of seizures if available, and with anticonvulsant treatment of ongoing seizures. General metabolic screening and assessment for evidence of sepsis (which may include lumbar puncture and/or screening for inborn errors of metabolism) should all be considered and the approach modified by the individual case history. Neuroimaging should be considered. Cranial ultrasound examination can be accomplished at the bedside and may identify ICH, especially in the premature. However, its ability to identify convexity hemorrhages and cortical abnormalities is limited. Head computed tomography (CT) and especially brain magnetic resonance imaging (MRI) are more helpful to confirm these disorders. However, they may not be available, and if available, usually require transportation, with the risk of destabilization of ill infants and must often be deferred until after the infant is stabilized and treatment has been initiated.

V. TREATMENT. Seizures themselves and treatment with anticonvulsant medication may impair respiratory drive and the ability to maintain adequate circulation. Therefore, supportive management to ensure maintenance of adequate ventilation and perfusion is imperative (see Table 56.3 for treatment of common acute metabolic derangements; see Chapters 23 and 60).

The decision to treat neonatal seizures with anticonvulsant drugs depends on the risk of acute seizure-related respiratory or cardiac decompensation in a critically ill newborn as well as the potential for long-term seizure-related neurologic injury balanced against the potential adverse effects of anticonvulsant medications. Some newborns may not need treatment with anticonvulsant medication, for instance, those with seizures due to reversible and appropriately

Table 56.3. Initial Management of Acute Metabolic Disorders	
Hypoglycemia	Dextrose 10%, 2–3 mL/kg IV
Hypocalcemia	Calcium gluconate, 5% (50 mg/mL) 100–200 mg/kg IV; 10% (100 mg/mL) 50–100 mg/kg IV if inadequate time for dilution
Hypomagnesemia	Magnesium sulphate, 12.5% (125 mg/mL) 50–100 mg/kg IV
IV, intravenous.	

treated metabolic derangements or those with rare, short-lived events. However, in considering a decision not to treat, it is important to recognize that a significant proportion of newborns, with electroclinical seizures, have additional subclinical events. In the setting of severe neonatal encephalopathy, these events may be prolonged and refractory to treatment, and efforts to eliminate them may be limited by systemic vulnerability to the circulatory effects of anticonvulsant medications.

Adverse effects of anticonvulsants, aside from respiratory and cardiovascular suppression, are also of concern in the developing brain. In studies of normal immature animals, many anticonvulsants including phenobarbital, phenytoin, diazepam, clonazepam, valproic acid, and vigabatrin, increased the rate of apoptotic neuronal cell death, as do N-methyl-D-aspartate (NMDA) receptor antagonists. How this relates to the risk–benefit balance in human neonates with seizures is not known, and further study is required. The AMPA antagonist, topiramate, as well as levetiracetam do not appear to have this effect.

A number of factors alter the pharmacokinetics of the anticonvulsant drugs in neonates. Physiologic immaturity delays drug elimination, and asphyxial injury to the liver and kidney may further delay metabolism. Maturation of the various pathways involved in drug metabolism occurs at variable rates over the first weeks of life, and recovery from perinatal injury improves hepatic and renal function. Overall, there is a dramatic increase in the ability to eliminate the commonly used anticonvulsant drugs so that changes in dosing are required to maintain therapeutic drug levels over the first weeks of life.

When anticonvulsant treatment is indicated, phenobarbital is the drug most commonly used as first-line therapy. Other first-line options include benzodiazepines (diazepam, lorazepam) and phenytoin or, if available, its prodrug fosphenytoin. Painter et al. compared treatment with phenobarbital and phenytoin and found no difference in efficacy between the two drugs, with fewer than 50% of infants achieving control with either drug. Typical initial doses of the first-line drugs are provided in Table 56.3, and additional discussion of the individual drugs is given in the following text.

A. **Phenobarbital.** Phenobarbital affects GABA$_A$ receptors to enhance GABA-related inhibition. It may also inhibit excitatory amino acid transmission and block voltage-activated calcium currents. It is a weak acid, with low-lipid solubility. Phenobarbital is subject to protein binding, and it is the unbound (free), unionized fraction that is active. Alterations in acid–base balance in the newborn may affect efficacy of the drug for this reason. Phenobarbital is metabolized in the liver and excreted by the kidney. Its half-life is long, from 100 to 300 hours, or longer in premature infants but declines to 100 hours or less over the first weeks of life. An initial IV loading dose of 20 mg/kg may be followed by increments of 5 to 10 mg/kg IV to a total of 40 mg/kg, with higher doses associated with improved efficacy. If required, the maintenance dose should be started at 5 mg/kg/day divided twice daily. Careful monitoring of cardiac and respiratory function is required in vulnerable infants.

B. **Phenytoin/fosphenytoin.** Phenytoin acts by blockade of voltage-dependent sodium channels, probably by binding to inactivated channels and stabilizing the inactive state. This decreases the tendency of neurons to high frequency, repetitive firing and therefore their excitability. Phenytoin is a weak acid and is poorly soluble in water. High lipid solubility results in rapid entry to the brain, but it is quickly redistributed and levels decline, requiring continued administration to restore brain levels. It is protein bound, although to a lesser degree in newborns than in older children and adults. Phenytoin is metabolized in the liver and eliminated in the kidney. Its half-life varies with concentration, increasing with higher concentrations due to decreased clearance as levels increase. An IV loading dose of 20 mg/kg of phenytoin administered at no greater than 1 mg/kg/minute (to avoid cardiac arrhythmia and hypotension) is followed by a maintenance dose of 2 to 3 mg/kg/day IV divided between two and four doses. Fosphenytoin is a prodrug of phenytoin. Its advantages are its higher water solubility and lower pH, which, in addition to the lack of toxic vehicles required for its formulation, reduce local irritation of skin and blood vessels at the site of infusion. Fosphenytoin is converted to phenytoin by plasma phosphatase enzymes in neonates as in adults. Phenytoin induction of hepatic enzymes should be taken into consideration when attempting to keep additional agents in a therapeutic range.

C. **Benzodiazepines.** Diazepam, lorazepam, and midazolam, like other benzodiazepines, bind to the postsynaptic $GABA_A$ receptor to enhance GABA-activated inhibitory chloride currents. At high levels, benzodiazepines may also influence voltage-gated sodium channels and calcium channels. Benzodiazepines are lipid soluble. Differential lipid solubility confers some advantage on lorazepam, which is less lipid-soluble and therefore is not redistributed away from the brain as rapidly as diazepam. Benzodiazepines are metabolized in the liver, and the majority of the drug is excreted in the urine. The plasma half-life of both lorazepam and diazepam is approximately 30 hours and may be longer in premature and/or asphyxiated newborns. Onset of action is within minutes for both drugs, however, duration of action is longer for lorazepam (up to 24 hours). Diazepam may be more effective as a continuous infusion. Lorazepam is given IV at a dose of 0.05 to 0.1 mg/kg. Diazepam dose is 0.3 mg/kg IV. An infusion rate of 0.3 mg/kg/hour IV has been described. Midazolam is a short-acting benzodiazepine that has been used as a continuous IV infusion (0.1 to 0.4 mg/kg/hour) after an initial loading dose (0.15 mg/kg). Benzodiazepines are typically used as second- or third-line agents in neonatal seizures but may also be used as an initial treatment due to their earlier onset of action in anticipation of the effect of a concurrent dose of phenobarbital.

Upward of 90% of neonatal seizures will ultimately be controlled by the combined use of the earlier anticonvulsant medications. The natural history and evolution/resolution of underlying brain injury in the first days of neonatal life may also contribute to a reduction in seizures.

D. **Levetiracetam (Keppra).** The use of levetiracetam in the treatment of neonatal seizures continues to increase. Its IV formulation, benign side effect profile, and limited interactions make it an attractive treatment option. There are few prospective studies of its efficacy in this age group. Reported loading doses vary from 10 to 20 mg/kg to as high as 40 to 50 mg/kg.

Maintenance doses described also vary widely from 10 to 80 mg/kg/day with most providers starting at 20 mg/kg/day, whereas others suggest 40 mg/kg/day. Although twice daily dosing is usual, three-times daily dosing has been suggested. Further studies are needed to clarify the appropriate dosing regimen.

E. Topiramate. Topiramate is often used adjunctively after the acute phase of neonatal seizure for continued refractory neonatal seizures. Topiramate is thought to have neuroprotective properties. Studies of topiramate in human neonates are lacking. Appropriate dosing for neonates has not been established.

Many other drugs have been used in an attempt to control refractory cases. Support for their use is based on reports of efficacy in small, uncontrolled series. Lidocaine has been used, mostly in Europe, as an IV infusion of 4 mg/kg/hour with decreasing doses over 4 to 5 days. This drug has a narrow therapeutic range and may induce seizures at higher levels.

Orally administered anticonvulsants that have been used adjunctively include carbamazepine (10 mg/kg initially followed by 15 to 20 mg/kg/day), primidone (loading dose 15 to 25 mg/kg followed by 12 to 20 mg/kg/day), and valproic acid (three of six neonates developed hyperammonemia).

No guidelines exist as to the appropriate duration of anticonvulsant treatment for newborns with seizures, and there is wide variation in practice. There is a trend toward shorter therapy, taking into account the short-lived nature of precipitating causes, the recovery from acute HIE in many instances, and the possible detrimental effect of anticonvulsants on the immature brain. Newborns with persistent, difficult to control seizures; persistently abnormal EEG; and/or persistently abnormal neurologic examination should be considered for longer term treatment following discharge from hospital.

VI. PROGNOSIS. Advances in obstetric management and in neonatal intensive care have yielded a reduction in mortality in infants with neonatal seizures from about 40% to <20%, with <10% mortality in term infants in one recent series. Morbidity rates have changed less, partly due to increased numbers of survivors among ill premature newborns who have a greater risk of neurologic sequelae. Long-term sequelae in infants with neonatal seizures, including cerebral palsy and intellectual disabilities, still occur at a high rate of up to 30% to 35%, with postneonatal seizures occurring in up to 20%. The most important factor affecting outcome for infants with neonatal seizures is the **underlying etiology**. For instance, normal development can be expected in infants with benign idiopathic neonatal seizures and in 90% of those with primary subarachnoid hemorrhage, whereas only 50% of those with HIE, and even fewer with a brain malformation, will have normal outcome. **Gestational age** is also an important factor with increasing mortality and morbidity with increasing immaturity.

Useful clinical indicators for a good outcome include a normal neonatal neurologic exam, normal or mildly abnormal neonatal EEG background activity, and normal neuroimaging or abnormalities limited to extraparenchymal injury (Table 56.4).

Table 56.4. Anticonvulsant Drug Doses for Initial Management of Neonatal Seizures

Drug	Initial Dose	Maintenance
Phenobarbital	20 mg/kg IV Consider further 5–10 mg/kg increments to a total of 40 mg/kg.	Check drug levels—may not need further doses for many days. 5 mg/kg/day divided bid
Phenytoin	20 mg/kg IV Fosphenytoin: 20 mg PE/kg IV (see text, pp. 825–826)	5 mg/kg/day divided bid to qid
Benzodiazepines	Lorazepam: 0.05–0.1 mg/kg IV Diazepam: 0.3 mg/kg IV Midazolam: 0.15 mg/kg bolus	
Levetiracetam	20–50 mg/kg bolus (see text, pp. 826–827)	20–80 mg/kg divided bid or tid

IV, intravenous; PE, phenytoin equivalent.

Suggested Readings

Holmes GL. The long-term effects of neonatal seizures. *Clin Perinatol* 2009;36: 901–914.

Mizrahi EM, Kellaway P. Characterization and classification of neonatal seizures. *Neurology* 1987;37:1837–1844.

Painter MJ, Scher MS, Stein AD, et al. Phenobarbital compared with phenytoin for the treatment of neonatal seizures. *N Engl J Med* 1999;341(7):485–489.

Shellhaas RA, Chang T, Tsuchida T, et al. The American Clinical Neurophysiology Society's guideline on continuous electroencephalography monitoring in neonates. *J Clin Neurophysiol* 2011;28:611–617.

Silverstein FS, Jensen FE. Neonatal seizures. *Ann Neurol* 2007;62:112–120.

Tsuchida TN, Wusthoff CJ, Shellhaas RA, et al. American Clinical Neurophysiology Society standardized EEG terminology and categorization for the description of continuous EEG monitoring in neonates: report of the American Clinical Neurophysiology Society Critical Care Monitoring Committee. *J Clin Neurophysiol* 2013;30:161–173.

Volpe JJ, ed. *Neonatal Seizures in Neurology of the Newborn.* 5th ed. Philadelphia, PA: WB Saunders; 2008:203–244.

Wusthoff CJ. Diagnosing neonatal seizures and status epilepticus. *J Clin Neurophysiol* 2013;30:115–121.

Neural Tube Defects

Anne R. Hansen and Benjamin Warf

KEY POINTS

- Preoperatively, minimize bacterial colonization and tissue damage by keeping the newborn in prone position with sterile saline–moistened gauze sponge placed over the defect covered by plastic wrap.
- Administer intravenous antibiotics (ampicillin and gentamicin) to diminish the risk of meningitis, a particularly devastating complication.
- Ensure that no latex equipment is used to avoid the development of severe allergy to latex rubber due to repeated exposure in medical devices.
- Postoperatively, closely follow anterior fontanel tension, head circumference, serial cranial ultrasounds, as well as onset of feeding difficulties or stridor due to likelihood of progressive hydrocephalus following closure of the back.

I. **DEFINITIONS AND PATHOLOGY.** The central nervous system (CNS) starts as a neural tube and folds into the brain and spinal cord by a complex mechanism during early embryologic development. Failure of normal closure results in neural tube defects, one of the most serious congenital malformations in newborns. The term refers to a group of disorders that is heterogeneous with respect to embryologic timing, involvement of specific nervous system elements, clinical presentation, and prognosis.

A. Types of neural tube defects

1. **Primary neural tube defects** constitute the majority of neural tube defects and can be viewed as due to primary failure of closure of the neural tube or disruption of an already closed neural tube between 18 and 25 days' gestation. The resulting abnormality usually manifests in two anatomic lesions: an exposed (open or *aperta*) neural placode along the midline of the back caudally and rostrally and the Arnold-Chiari II (ACII) malformation (malformation of pons and medulla, with downward displacement of cerebellum, medulla, and fourth ventricle into the upper cervical region), with associated aqueductal stenosis and hydrocephalus.

a. **Myelomeningocele** is the most common primary neural tube defect. It involves a saccular outpouching of neural elements (neural placode), typically through a defect in the bone and the soft tissues of the posterior thoracic, sacral, or lumbar regions—the latter comprising 80% of lesions. Arachnoid is typically included in the sac (meningo), which contains visible neural structures (myelo), and the skin is discontinuous over the sac. Hydrocephalus occurs in around two-thirds of these children; Chiari II malformation occurs in approximately 90%, although the link between hydrocephalus and the malformation has been significantly re-evaluated in recent years, with therapeutic implications discussed in the following text. Various associated anomalies of the CNS are noted, most importantly, cerebral cortical dysplasia in up to 92% of cases.

b. Encephalocele. This defect of anterior neural tube closure is an outpouching of dura with or without brain, noted in the occipital region, in 80% of cases for North America and Europe, and less commonly in the frontal, parietal, or temporal regions. It may vary in size from a few millimeters to many centimeters.

c. Anencephaly. In the most severe form of this defect, the cranial vault and posterior occipital bone are defective, and derivatives of the neural tube are exposed, including both brain and bony tissue. The defect usually extends through the foramen magnum and involves the brainstem. It is not compatible with long-term survival. Rachischisis is a more severe form in which the spine is also involved due to nonfusion of the majority of the primary neural tube.

2. **Secondary neural tube defects.** Five percent of all neural tube defects result from abnormal development of the lower sacral or coccygeal segments during secondary neurulation. This leads to defects primarily in the lumbosacral spinal region. These heterogeneous lesions are rarely associated with hydrocephalus or the Chiari II malformation, and the skin is typically intact over the defect. Because the hindbrain abnormality of the Chiari II malformation is evident on prenatal scans, this radiographic finding is useful in distinguishing open from closed neural tube abnormalities.

   a. Meningocele is a spinal fluid-filled sac causing an outpouching of skin and dura without involvement of the neural elements aside from a commonly associated dorsal band of neurovascular tissue adherent to the sac. Meningoceles may be associated with bone and contiguous soft tissue abnormalities.

   b. Lipomeningocele is a lipomatous mass usually in the lumbar or sacral region, occasionally off the midline, typically covered with full-thickness skin. Adipose tissue frequently extends through the defect into the spine and dura and adheres extensively to a distorted spinal cord or nerve roots.

   c. Filum lipoma, **sacral agenesis/dysgenesis, diastematomyelia, myelocystocele**, all may have varying degrees of bony involvement. Although rarely as extensive as with primary neural tube defects, neurologic manifestations may be present representing distortion or abnormal development of neural structures. These lesions may be inapparent on physical examination of the child, resulting in the use of the term *occulta* to describe them.

B. **Etiologies.** The exact cause of failed neural tube closure remains unknown, and proposed etiologies for both primary and secondary neural tube defects are heterogeneous. Factors implicated include folic acid deficiency; maternal ingestion of the anticonvulsants carbamazepine and valproic acid and folic acid antagonists such as aminopterin and certain antimalarial drugs; maternal diabetes; and disruptive influences such as prenatal irradiation and maternal hyperthermia. A genetic component is supported by the fact that there is concordance for neural tube defect in monozygotic twins and an increased incidence with consanguinity and with a positive family history. Neural tube defects can occur with trisomies 13 and 18, triploidy, and Meckel syndrome (autosomal recessive syndrome of encephalocele, polydactyly, polycystic kidneys, cleft lip and palate), as well as other chromosome disorders. Although specific genes (particularly those in the folate-homocysteine pathway as well as in genes involved in planar cell polarity) have been implicated as risk factors, the genetics are likely complex and multifactorial (see Chapter 10).

C. **Epidemiology and recurrence risk.** The incidence of neural tube defects varies significantly with geography and ethnicity. In the United States, the overall frequency of neural tube defects is approximately 1 in 2,000 live births. The literature may underestimate the true prevalence because of the effects of terminating prenatally diagnosed pregnancies. A well-established increased incidence is known among individuals living in parts of Ireland and Wales and carries over to descendants of these individuals who live elsewhere in the world. This may be true also for other ethnic groups, including Sikh Indians and certain groups in Egypt. More than 95% of all neural tube defects occur to couples with no known family history. Primary neural tube defects carry an increased empiric recurrence risk of 2% to 3% for couples with one affected pregnancy, with a higher risk if more than one sibling is affected. Similarly, affected individuals have a 3% to 5% risk of having an offspring with a primary neural tube defect. Recurrence risk is strongly affected by the level of the lesion in the index case, with risks as high as 7.8% for lesions above T11. In 5% of cases, neural tube defects may be associated with uncommon disorders; some, such as Meckel syndrome, are inherited in an autosomal recessive manner, resulting in a 25% recurrence risk. Secondary neural tube defects are generally sporadic and carry no known increased recurrence risk. In counseling families for recurrence, however, it is critical to obtain a careful family history and history of drug exposure.

D. **Prevention.** Controlled, randomized clinical studies of prenatal multivitamin administration both for secondary prevention in mothers with prior affected offspring and for primary prevention in those without a prior history have shown a 50% to 70% reduced incidence of neural tube defects in women who take multivitamins for at least 3 months prior to conception and during the first month of pregnancy.[1] The Centers for Disease Control and Prevention recommends that women of childbearing age who are capable of becoming pregnant consume 0.4 mg of folic acid per day to reduce their risks of having a fetus affected with myelomeningocele or other neural tube defects. Higher doses are recommended for women with prior affected offspring. In addition, folate supplementation of enriched cereal-grain products has been mandated by the U.S. Food and Drug Administration (FDA); however, the level of folate intake from this source is not high enough to forgo additional supplementation in the large majority of women.

II. DIAGNOSIS

A. **Prenatal diagnosis.** The combination of maternal serum α-fetoprotein (AFP) determinations, prenatal ultrasonography, rapid-acquisition fetal magnetic resonance imaging (MRI) scans, and AFP and acetylcholinesterase determinations on amniotic fluid where indicated, greatly improves the ability to make a prenatal diagnosis and to distinguish from abdominal wall defects. Maternal serum AFP measurements of 2.5 multiples of the median (MoM) in the second trimester (16 to 18 weeks) have a sensitivity of 80% to 90% for myelomeningocele. The exact timing of this measurement is critical as AFP levels change throughout pregnancy. Karyotype may also be performed at the time of amniocentesis to detect associated chromosomal abnormalities. Ultrasonographic diagnosis through direct visualization of the spinal defect or through indirect signs related to Arnold-Chiari malformation has a sensitivity of >90%. The Chiari malformation is seen as a flattened cerebellum called a "banana sign" and a transient frontal bone anomaly called a "lemon sign." Ultrasound can also demonstrate the level of termination of the normal cord and placode. Prenatal MRI may define the defect more accurately. Determining the prognosis based on prenatal ultrasonography remains difficult, except in obvious cases of encephalocele or anencephaly (see Chapter 1) but an appreciation of the level of disruption can be helpful in that higher spinal levels within the thoracolumbar range portend a correspondingly higher level of neurologic deficit. Some patients with higher thoracic or cervical lesions, however, have remarkable preservation of function; often, restitution of the spinal cord below the lesion is evident by MRI in these cases.

B. **Postnatal diagnosis.** Except for some secondary neural tube defects, most neural tube defects, especially meningomyelocele, are immediately obvious at birth. Occasionally, some saccular masses, usually in the low sacrum, including sacrococcygeal teratomas, can be mistaken for a neural tube defect. Rarely, anterior sacral meningoceles can occur that are not evident at birth.

III. EVALUATION

A. **History.** Obtain a detailed family history. Ask about the occurrence of neural tube defects and other congenital anomalies or malformation syndromes. Note should be made of any of the risk factors described in the preceding text, including maternal medication use in the first trimester or maternal diabetes.

B. **Physical examination.** It is important to perform a thorough physical examination, including a neurologic examination. The following portions of the examination are likely to reveal abnormalities.

1. **Back.** Inspect the defect and note if it is leaking cerebrospinal fluid (CSF). Use a sterile nonlatex rubber glove when touching a leaking sac (in most circumstances, only the neurosurgeon needs to touch the back). Note the location, shape, and size of the defect and the thin "parchment-like" overlying skin, although it has little relation to the size of the sac. Often, the sac is deflated and has a wrinkled appearance. It is important to note the curvature of the spine and the presence of a

bony gibbus underlying the defect. For suspected closed lesions, document hemangioma, hairy patch, deep dimple, or sinus tract, if present; ultrasonography of the lower spine can show the level of the conus and presence of normal root movement in cases where this is in question.

2. **Head.** Record the head circumference and plot daily until stable postoperatively. At birth, some infants will have macrocephaly because of hydrocephalus, and still, more will develop hydrocephalus after closure of the defect on the back. Ultrasonography is useful to assess ventricular size. Assess the intracranial pressure (ICP) with the baby sitting upright by palpating the anterior fontanel and tilting the head and torso forward until the midportion of the anterior fontanel is flat. The fontanels may be quite large and the calvarial bones widely separated (see Chapter 54).

3. **Eyes.** Abnormalities in conjugate movement of the eyes are common and include esotropias, esophorias, and abducens paresis.

4. **Neurologic examination.** Observe the child's spontaneous activity and response to sensory stimuli in all extremities. Predicting ambulation and muscle strength based on the "level" of the neurologic deficit can be misleading, and very often, the anal reflex, or "wink," will be present at birth and absent postoperatively, owing to spinal shock and edema.

5. **Lower extremities.** Look for deformities (e.g., clubfeet) as well as muscle weakness and limited range of motion. Examine the thigh positions and skinfolds and perform the Ortolani and Barlow maneuvers for evidence of congenital dysplasia of the hips. With open lesions, this exam should be deferred until after the repair of the meningomyelocele. Dislocation of the hips can also be diagnosed by ultrasonography (see Chapter 58).

   Repeated neurologic examinations at periodic intervals is more helpful in predicting functional outcome than a single newborn examination. Similarly, sensory examination of the newborn can be misleading because of the potential absence of a motor response to pinprick. Carefully examine deep tendon reflexes (see Table 57.1).

6. **Bladder and kidneys.** Palpate the abdomen for evidence of bladder distension or kidney enlargement. Observe the pattern of urination and check the infant's response to the Credé maneuver to evaluate residual urine in the bladder.

C. **General newborn assessment.** Evaluate all newborns with neural tube defects for the presence of congenital heart disease (especially ventricular septal defect [VSD]), renal malformation, and structural defects of the airway, gastrointestinal tract, ribs, and hips. Although uncommon in primary neural tube defects, these can be encountered and should be considered before beginning surgical treatment or before discharge from the hospital. Other findings of associated chromosomal anomalies may be noted. In addition, plan an ophthalmologic examination and hearing evaluation during the hospitalization or following discharge.

IV. **CONSULTATION.** The care of an infant with a neural tube defect requires the coordinated efforts of a number of medical and surgical specialists as well as

Table 57.1. Correlation between Segmental Innervation; Motor, Sensory, and Sphincter Function; Reflexes; and Ambulation Potential

Lesion	Segmental Innervation	Cutaneous Sensation	Motor Function	Working Muscles	Sphincter Function	Reflex	Potential for Ambulation
Cervical/thoracic	Variable	Variable	None	None	—	—	Poor, even in full braces
Thoracolumbar	T12	Lower abdomen	None	None	—	—	
	L1	Groin	Weak hip flexion	Iliopsoas	—	—	Full braces, long-term ambulation unlikely
	L2	Anterior upper thigh	Strong hip flexion	Iliopsoas and sartorius	—	—	
Lumbar	L3	Anterior distal thigh and knee	Knee extension	Quadriceps	—	Knee jerk	—
	L4	Medial leg	Knee flexion and hip abduction	Medial hamstrings	—	Knee jerk	May ambulate with braces and crutches

Lumbosacral	L5	Lateral leg and medial knee	Foot dorsiflexion and eversion	Anterior tibial and peroneals	—	Ankle jerk	—
	S1	Sole of foot flexion	Foot plantar	Gastrocnemius, soleus, and posterior tibial	—	Ankle jerk	Ambulate with or without short leg braces
Sacral	S2	Posterior leg and thigh	Toe flexion	Flexor hallucis	Bladder and rectum	Anal wink	—
	S3	Middle of buttock	—	—	Bladder and rectum	Anal wink	Ambulate without braces
	S4	Medial buttock	—	—	Bladder and rectum	Anal wink	—

Source: From Noetzel MJ. Myelomeningocele: current concepts of management. Clin Perinatol 1989;16:311–329.

specialists in nursing, physical therapy, and social service. Some centers have a neural tube defect team to help coordinate the following specialists.

A. Specialty consultations

1. **Neurosurgery.** The initial care of the child with an open neural tube defect is predominantly neurosurgical. The neurosurgeon is responsible for assessment and surgical closure of the defect and for evaluation and treatment of elevated ICP.

2. **Neonatology/pediatrics.** A thorough evaluation before surgical procedures is important, particularly to detect other abnormalities, such as congenital cardiac anomalies that might influence surgical and anesthetic risk.

3. **Genetics.** A clinical geneticist should conduct a complete dysmorphology evaluation during the first hospitalization. Follow-up during outpatient visits should include genetic counseling.

4. **Urology.** Consult a urologist on the day of birth because of the risk of obstructive uropathy.

5. **Orthopedics.** The pediatric orthopedic surgeon is responsible for the initial assessment of musculoskeletal abnormalities and long-term management of ambulation, seating, and spine stability. Clubfeet, frequently encountered in these newborns, should be assessed and may be addressed during this hospitalization.

6. **Physical therapy.** Involve physical therapists in planning for outpatient physical therapy programs.

7. **Social service.** Arrange for a social worker familiar with the special needs of children with neural tube defects to meet the parents as early as possible. Children with meningomyelocele may require a great deal of parents' time and resources, thereby placing considerable strain on both parents and siblings.

V. MANAGEMENT

A. Fetal surgery. *In utero* repair was first performed in 1994. Observational studies have found that *in utero* repair is associated with lower rates of ventriculoperitoneal (VP) shunting and consistent reversal of hindbrain herniation. Long-term effects remain uncertain. A multicenter randomized controlled trial comparing *in utero* surgical correction with standard management found that performing prenatal surgery on fetuses with myelomeningocele may lead to better outcomes than if the surgery is performed postnatally.[2] After 12 months, the 91 infants who had prenatal surgery were 30% less likely to die or need additional surgical procedures than the 92 infants who were treated postnatally. Follow up at 2 ½ years of age revealed that those treated prenatally demonstrated improved physical development and motor function, such as unassisted walking, compared to those treated after birth. However, prenatal surgery was associated with increased risk of complications during pregnancy including premature delivery and tearing of the uterine wall from the surgical scar. When the diagnosis of myelomeningocele is made prenatally, *in utero* repair is an option that parents may consider.

B. Perinatal. Cesarean section prior to the onset of labor is the preferred mode of delivery because it decreases the likelihood of rupturing the meningeal sac and is associated with improved neurologic outcome.[3]

C. Preoperative management

1. Neurology

a. Care of placode: At birth, the very thin sac is often leaking. Keep the newborn in the prone position with a sterile saline-moistened gauze sponge placed over the defect covered by plastic wrap. This reduces bacterial contamination and tissue damage related to dehydration.

b. Chiari II: A cranial ultrasound should generally be obtained soon after birth. Chiari II malformations result from premature fusion of the posterior fossa leaving insufficient space for the cerebrum, cerebellum, and brainstem. Brainstem and portions of the cerebellum may herniate through the foramen magnum into the upper cervical spinal canal. Obstructed flow of CSF results in hydrocephalus the majority of the time.

c. Seizures: There is a 20% to 25% incidence of seizures in this population due to brain anomalies that typically accompany the Chiari II malformation, such as neuronal migration anomalies.

2. Infectious disease. Administer intravenous antibiotics (ampicillin and gentamicin) to diminish the risk of meningitis, particularly due to group B streptococci. Newborns with an open spinal defect can receive a massive inoculation of bacteria directly into the nervous system at the time of vaginal delivery or even *in utero* if the placental membranes rupture early. Meningitis is a particularly devastating complication.

3. Fluids/nutrition. Because insensible losses are minimized by covering the lesion with plastic wrap, standard maintenance fluids are generally appropriate.

4. Urologic/renal

a. Clean intermittent catheterization (CIC) is indicated to check post-void residuals until urologic and renal function are assessed.

b. If voiding pattern is abnormal, it is important to determine if the etiology is abnormal bladder emptying, renal function, or both. A serum creatinine level is useful in making this distinction.

5. Latex allergy. Because of the potential for development of a severe allergy to latex rubber due to repeated exposure in medical devices, no latex equipment should be used.

6. Surgical treatment. Open defects must be urgently closed due to the risk of infection. Infants whose defect is covered with skin and whose nervous system is therefore not at risk for bacterial contamination may undergo elective repair, typically within the first 6 months of life.

The initial neurosurgical treatment of an open meningomyelocele consists of closing the defect to prevent infection and reducing the elevated ICP. The back should be closed within the first 24 to 48 hours of life if safely possible to minimize the risk of infection. Techniques are available to rapidly close even very large cutaneous defects without skin grafting. The rare occurrence of intracranial hypertension can be initially controlled by ventricular puncture or continuous ventricular drainage. If hydrocephalus is severe from birth, it can be treated at the same time as the back closure. Because hydrocephalus often progresses following closure of the back in untreated patients, anterior fontanel tension and head circumference should be carefully monitored. Due to experience with prenatal closure and known complications with permanent shunting, increasingly, practitioners are trying to delay or avoid permanent shunting and to consider such alternatives as endoscopic third ventriculocisternostomy with choroid plexus cauterization (ETV-CPC).[4] Regardless of the planned strategy for dealing with hydrocephalus, if it becomes symptomatic, close monitoring is important.

The surgical approach varies with the precise anatomy. In brief, the translucent tissue and skin too thin to use are trimmed away around the circumference of the defect, then the placode is rolled into a more normal shape and gently held in this configuration with fine, pial sutures. The edges of what would have been dura mater are identified, isolated, and closed over the placode, then the skin is closed with the goal of attaining a well-vascularized, watertight closure.

7. **Management of hydrocephalus.** If the fluid pressure seems to put the integrity of the skin closure at risk, shunting of the ventricles (by a permanent VP shunt), or temporary external ventricular drainage, may be performed during the same operation. However, because the experience with prenatal closure has raised awareness that fewer patients need shunts than previously thought, watchful waiting in the hopes of avoiding a permanent shunt has become a more common approach. Endoscopic third ventriculostomy (ETV), sometimes accompanied by choroid plexus cauterization (CPC) is an alternative to VP shunt, creating an internal rerouting of CSF flow while decreasing CSF production. This combination of procedures may eliminate the need for shunts in about 75% of the infants with myelomeningocele requiring hydrocephalus treatment.[5–10] This has become our primary initial treatment for the majority of these patients.

D. Postoperative management

1. **Neurology**
   a. The infant must remain prone or side-lying until the wound heals. Head circumference needs to be measured daily, particularly in the infant who has not had shunt placement.
   b. MRI of the brain and spine should generally be obtained postoperatively, even if there is no clinical evidence of hydrocephalus. It is particularly valuable in assessment of the posterior fossa and syringomyelia. **Computed tomography (CT) scans** should be avoided unless no other options are available because of the relatively high radiation exposure.
   c. Sensory impairment can be associated with myelomeningocele. Strabismus is commonly associated with Chiari malformation. Hearing and vision screens may be performed prior to discharge.
   d. Seizures should be monitored, because there is a 20% to 25% incidence in this population, in part due to brain anomalies such as neuronal migration abnormalities associated with Chiari II malformations.

e. Stridor suggests vocal cord weakness that can lead to airway obstruction. This may signal the need to treat hydrocephalus or remedy treatment failure such as a shunt malfunction. If the hydrocephalus is adequately treated, surgical decompression of the posterior fossa may be indicated.

2. **Nutrition.** Feeding difficulties are commonly associated with the Chiari II malformation. Growth and nutritional status must be watched closely as well as the infant's ability to suck and swallow. Acute deterioration in feeding skills may, as with stridor, signal the need for assessing the status of hydrocephalus and, less commonly, consideration of posterior fossa decompression.

   a. Monitor daily weights and input/output.

   b. Observe for spitting, gagging, choking, nasal regurgitation, and episodes of oxygen desaturation.

3. **Urologic/renal**

   a. Obtain urine culture, urinalysis, and serum creatinine as a baseline, if not already measured preoperatively.

   b. Ultrasound of the urinary tract will detect associated renal anomalies as well as possible hydronephrosis from vesicoureteral reflux.

   c. Postvoid residuals and urodynamic studies should be performed early in the hospitalization or shortly after discharge to document the status of the bladder as well as urinary sphincter function and innervation. This study will serve as a basis for comparison later in life.

   d. Consider a voiding cystourethrogram to assess for vesicoureteral reflux if there is an abnormality seen on ultrasonographic or urodynamic study or in the setting of a rising serum creatinine level.

   e. CIC is recommended for those infants who have large postvoid residuals, evidence of significant hydronephrosis, and/or increased bladder pressure on urodynamics studies. CIC is started in the hospital and continued at discharge. Those infants who do not manifest these problems can safely be allowed to spontaneously void.

4. **Orthopedics**

   a. Obtain plain films of lower extremities if there is concern regarding clubfeet or other anomalies raised by physical exam.

   b. Obtain chest x-ray (CXR). Rib deformities are common; cardiac malformations may also be identified.

   c. Obtain plain films of spine. Abnormalities in vertebral bodies, absent or defective posterior arches, and evidence of kyphosis are common.

   d. Evidence of dysplasia of hips is common, and some children with neural tube defects are born with dislocated hips. Ultrasonographic examination of the hips can be very helpful to the orthopedic surgeon (see Chapter 58).

5. **Family and social worker**

   a. Family care providers will need to play an active role in home management. It is critical for them to understand the child's condition and the implications for home care. The involvement of multiple specialists heightens the importance of the identification of a primary care provider (pediatrician or family practitioner) to coordinate the flow of information.

b. The family stress of caring for a child with myelomeningocele cannot be underestimated. A social worker should be available for the family from the time of diagnosis. An excellent information and support resource is the Spina Bifida Association of America (available online at www.sbaa.org).

VI. PROGNOSIS

A. **Survival.** Nearly all children with neural tube defects, even those severely affected, can survive for many years, with a 78% survival rate to age 17 for those with myelomeningocele. Survival rates appear to have increased since folic acid fortification of the U.S. grain supply was started, possibly because of a general decrease in severity or location of lesions. Survival rates are significantly influenced by selection bias of prenatal diagnosis and termination of severely affected fetuses and by decisions to intervene versus to withhold aggressive medical and surgical care in the early neonatal period. Most deaths occur in the most severely affected children and are likely related to brainstem dysfunction.

B. **Long-term outcome.** There are a wide variety of medical and developmental issues associated with myelomeningocele. Children with myelomeningocele require a comprehensive multidisciplinary team of providers including neurosurgery; orthopedic surgery; urology; physiatry; gastroenterology; endocrinology; pulmonary medicine; and physical, occupational, and speech language pathology.

1. **Neurosurgical issues.** In one cohort study of myelomeningocele patients, 86% underwent VP shunt, the large majority of whom required additional shunt revision. Release of tethered cord was required in 32%, and scoliosis was diagnosed in 49%, of whom approximately half required a spinal fusion procedure.[8] The majority are affected in some way by the Chiari II malformation in the form of hydrocephalus, syringomyelia, or brainstem dysfunction. In addition to hydrocephalus, sleep apnea and dysphagia are very common in these patients.

   a. **Increased ICP** can result from evolving hydrocephalus in the unshunted child, shunt malfunction or infection in the shunted child, or failure of ETV-CPC to adequately address the problem. Beyond infancy, elevated ICP requires urgent assessment because symptoms may progress rapidly and can be fatal.[9] In the myelomeningocele population, this sometimes presents primarily as symptoms related to brainstem dysfunction or evolving syringomyelia rather than the classic symptoms of elevated ICP. Common symptoms and signs may include the following:

   i. Headache, irritability, bulging fontanel, sixth nerve palsy, paralysis of upward gaze

   ii. New onset of respiratory complications, particularly stridor from vocal cord paralysis, central and/or obstructive apnea

   iii. Worsening oromotor function, abnormal gag, and vomiting (often confused with gastroesophageal reflux)

   iv. Change in cognitive function

   These symptoms may indicate shunt malfunction but may also disappear without treatment. After insuring adequate treatment for hydrocephalus, surgical decompression of the Chiari malformation should be considered. If the symptoms persist, especially in association with cyanosis, the prognosis is poor, with risk of respiratory failure and death. Tracheostomy is occasionally necessary. Posterior fossa decompression and cervical laminectomy are surgical options but are often not successful.

b. Shunt infection should be suspected if symptoms of ICP are accompanied by fever and increased peripheral white blood cell count.

  i. A shunt tap is necessary to rule out a shunt infection.

  ii. A shunt series and brain imaging (e.g., rapid sequence MRI) may be necessary in conjunction with neurosurgical evaluation.

c. Seizures remain a risk, and families should be familiar with signs and symptoms to monitor as well as an initial treatment approach.

2. **Motor outcome.** This depends more on the level of paralysis and surgical intervention than it does on congenital hydrocephalus. In a 12-year study of adult myelomeningocele patients, one-third experienced deterioration in their ambulatory capacity over the study period. All those with lesions at the L5 neurologic levels were community ambulators, except one who was a household walker. At the L4 level, there was a slight decrease in functional ambulators. For the L3-level patients, less than one-third were still community or household ambulators at the end of the 12 years of observations.[10] Most children with neural tube defects will have a delay in motor progress, but appropriate bracing, physical therapy interventions, and monitoring and treatment of kyphosis and scoliosis can mitigate this. Factors such as obesity, frequent hospitalizations, tethering of the spinal cord, and decubitus ulcers may also contribute to reduced mobility.

3. **Intellectual outcome.** Approximately 75% of children with myelomeningocele have IQ scores >80. Many children with myelomeningocele require some sort of special education. Learning disabilities arise from challenges in language processing, visual/perceptual and fine motor deficits. A formal neurodevelopmental assessment should be obtained if any questions arise about a child's social and cognitive abilities.

An increased risk of cognitive delay is associated with high thoracic-level lesions, severe hydrocephalus at birth, development of a CNS infection early in life, intracranial hypertension, and seizures. One study found that although 37% of individuals with myelomeningocele required additional assistance with school work or attended special education classes, 85% were attending or had graduated from secondary school or college.[6]

4. **Hearing and vision** status must be formally reassessed to rule out any contribution to learning difficulties. Hearing loss has historically been a problem associated with antibiotic use in the setting of urinary tract infections but has been dramatically reduced with the advent of CIC.

5. **Urologic/renal issues**

a. Approximately 85% of children require CIC for bladder dysfunction; 80% achieve social bladder continence.

b. Urinary tract infections are common. Prophylactic antibiotics may be indicated, especially if vesicoureteral reflux is present. Amoxicillin is commonly used in newborns and young infants. Other antibiotics, such as Bactrim and nitrofurantoin, are used in older children.

6. **Growth and nutrition**. Failure to thrive is a common problem in infants and young children.

   a. Some children require gastrostomy tube placement secondary to aspiration risk or inability to take in adequate calories orally. A videofluoroscopic swallowing study can be helpful to assess risk of aspiration with oral feeds.

   b. Arm span may be a more accurate reflection of growth than height because growth below the waistline is usually disproportionately slow or distorted by lower extremity or spinal deformities.

   c. Skin fold thickness is a valuable measure of nutrition.

   d. Bowel incontinence and constipation are prominent problems. An aggressive, consistent bowel program is often required and may include laxatives, suppositories, enemas, or even antegrade colonic enemas.

7. **Orthopedic complications**

   a. Worsening scoliosis or kyphosis may cause restrictive lung disease.

   b. Osteopenia, particularly in the nonambulatory patient, increases the risk for pathologic fractures.

   c. Contractures of hips, knees and ankles, and hip dislocation are common. Treatments include physical therapy, orthotics, neuromuscular blockades, and surgeries.

   d. Decubitus ulcers may develop, especially involving pressure points such as the sacrum and ischial tuberosity and the feet, secondary to limited movement and diminished peripheral sensation. Secondary infection is an additional problem. Regular assessment of appropriate fit, padding, and positioning of wheelchairs and other seating systems minimizes ulcer risk.

8. **Endocrinopathies.** Children can develop precocious puberty as well as growth hormone deficiency, presenting as poor growth despite adequate nutrition.

9. **Rehabilitation** therapies including physical, occupational, and speech/language services are critical to optimize the health and development of a child with myelomeningocele.

   a. Initially, services should be established through state Early Intervention (EI) programs, which are mandated under the Individuals with Disabilities Education Act (IDEA). EI referral should be made early during an infant's initial hospitalization because there can be a waiting list.

   b. After age 3 years, services are provided through the public school system.

10. **Latex allergy.** Despite trying to avoid latex exposure, latex hypersensitization is seen in approximately one-third of children with neural tube defects and may be associated with life-threatening anaphylaxis. Risk is minimized by the following:

    a. Ongoing avoidance of latex containing products

    b. Avoidance of foods that may cross-react with latex, such as avocado, banana, and water chestnuts

11. **The primary care physician** plays a critical role in coordinating the care of a child with myelodysplasia. The role includes general pediatric care as well as surveillance for complications, communication with multiple subspecialists, and advocacy in school programs and the community.

References

1. Padmanabhan R. Etiology, pathogenesis and prevention of neural tube defects. *Congenit Anom* 2006;46:55–67.

2. Adzick NS, Thom EA, Spong CY, et al. A randomized trial of prenatal versus postnatal repair of myelomeningocele. *N Engl J Med* 2011;364(11):993–1004.

3. Luthy DA, Wardinsky T, Shurtleff DB, et al. Cesarean section before the onset of labor and subsequent motor function in infants with meningomyelocele diagnosed antenatally. *N Engl J Med* 1991;324:662–666.

4. Warf BC, Campbell JW. Combined endoscopic third ventriculostomy and choroid plexus cauterization as primary treatment of hydrocephalus for infants with myelomeningocele: long-term results of a prospective intent-to-treat study in 115 East African infants. *J Neurosurg Pediatr* 2008;2:310–316.

5. Warf BC. Endoscopic third ventriculostomy and choroid plexus cauterization for pediatric hydrocephalus. *Clin Neurosurg* 2007;54:78–82.

6. Warf BC. Comparison of endoscopic third ventriculostomy alone and combined with choroid plexus cauterization in infants younger than 1 year of age: a prospective study in 550 African children. *J Neurosurg* 2005;103(6 suppl):475–481.

7. Stone S, Warf BC. Combined endoscopic third ventriculostomy and choroid plexus cauterization as primary treatment for infant hydrocephalus: a prospective North American series. *J Neurosurg Pediatr* 2014;14(5):439–446.

8. Bowman RM, McLone DG, Grant JA, et al. Spina bifida outcome: a 25-year prospective. *Pediatr Neurosurg* 2001;34(3):114–120.

9. Madikians A, Conway EE Jr. Cerebrospinal fluid shunt problems in pediatric patients. *Pediatr Ann* 1997;26:613–620.

10. Esterman N. Ambulation in patients with myelomeningocele: a 12-year follow-up. *Pediatr Phys Ther* 2001;13(1):50–51.

Suggested Readings

American Academy of Pediatrics, Committee on Genetics. Folic acid for the prevention of neural tube defects. *Pediatrics* 1999;104(2, pt 1):325–327.

Bol KA, Collins JS, Kirby RS; and the National Birth Defects Prevention Network. Survival of infants with neural tube defects in the presence of folic acid fortification. *Pediatrics* 2006;117:803–813.

Czeizel AE, Dudás I. Prevention of the first occurrence of neural-tube defects by periconceptional vitamin supplementation. *N Engl J Med* 1992;327:1832–1835.

Feuchtbaum LB, Currier RJ, Riggle S, et al. Neural tube defect prevalence in California (1990–1994): eliciting patterns by type of defect and maternal race/ethnicity. *Genet Test* 1999;3:265–272.

Fletcher J, Barnes M, Dennis M. Language development in children with spina bifida. *Semin Pediatr Neurol* 2002;9(3):201–208.

Glader LJ, Elias ER, Madsen JR. Myelodysplasia. In: Hansen AR, Puder M, eds. *Manual of Neonatal Surgical Intensive Care*. 2nd ed. Shelton, CT: PMPH-USA; 2009:459–472.

Goh YI, Bollano E, Einerson TR, et al. Prenatal multivitamin supplementation and rates of congenital anomalies: a meta-analysis. *J Obstet Gynaecol Can* 2006;28:680–689.

Jobe AH. Fetal surgery for myelomeningocele. *N Engl J Med* 2002;347:230–231.

Johnson MP, Gerdes M, Rintoul N, et al. Maternal-fetal surgery for myelomeningocele: neurodevelopmental outcomes at 2 years of age. *Am J Obstet Gynecol* 2006;194:1145–1150.

Kaufman B. Neural tube defects. *Pediatr Clin North Am* 2004;51(2):389–419.

Mitchell LE, Adzick NS, Melchionne J, et al. Spina bifida. *Lancet* 2004;364(9448):1885–1895.

Oakley GP Jr. The scientific basis for eliminating folic acid-preventable spina bifida: a modern miracle from epidemiology. *Ann Epidemiol* 2009;19(4):226–230.

Shaer CM, Chescheir N, Schulkin J. Myelomeningocele: a review of the epidemiology, genetics, risk factors for conception, prenatal diagnosis, and prognosis for affected individuals. *Obstet Gynecol Surv* 2007;62(7):471–479.

Thompson DN. Postnatal management and outcome for neural tube defects including spina bifida and encephalocoeles. *Prenat Diagn* 2009;29(4):412–419.

Orthopedic Problems

James R. Kasser

KEY POINTS

- **Foot deformity**—Club feet, fixed deformity of the feet, or vertical talus at birth should be treated with exercise or casting initially.
- **Hips**—Hip instability or contracture should be recognized in the newborn with diagnostic ultrasound to document the structural abnormality.
- **Neonatal compartment syndrome**—Presents with upper extremity swelling and ulceration or bulbous skin lesion requiring emergency treatment

This chapter considers common musculoskeletal abnormalities that may be detected in the neonatal period. Consultation with an orthopedic surgeon is often required to provide definitive treatment after the initial evaluation.

I. CONGENITAL MUSCULAR TORTICOLLIS

A. **Congenital muscular torticollis (CMT)** is a disorder characterized by limited motion of the neck, asymmetry of the face and skull, and a tilted position of the head. It is usually caused by shortening of the **sternocleidomastoid (SCM) muscle** but may be secondary to muscle adaptation from an abnormal *in utero* position of the head and neck.

1. **The etiology** of the shortened SCM muscle is unclear; in many infants, it is due to an abnormal *in utero* position, and in some, it may be due to stretching of the muscle at delivery. The result of the latter is a contracture of the muscle associated with fibrosis. One hypothesis is that the SCM abnormality is secondary to a compartment syndrome occurring at the time of delivery.

2. **Clinical course.** The limitation of motion is generally minimal at birth but increases over the first few weeks. At 10 to 20 days, a mass is frequently found in the SCM muscle. This mass gradually disappears, and the muscle fibers are partially replaced by fibrous tissue, which contracts and limits head motion. Because of the limited rotation of the head, the infant rests on the ipsilateral side of the face in the prone position and on the contralateral occiput when supine. The pressure from resting on one side of the face and the opposite occipital bone contributes to the facial and skull asymmetry. The ipsilateral zygoma is depressed and the contralateral occiput flattened.

3. **Treatment.** Most infants will respond favorably to positioning the head in the direction opposite to that produced by the tight muscle. Padded bricks or sandbags can be used to help maintain the position of the head until the child is able to move actively to free the head. Passive stretching by rotating the head to the ipsilateral side and tilting it toward the contralateral side also may help. The torticollis in most infants resolves by the age of 1 year. Helmets are sometimes used to treat persistent head asymmetry after a few months of age. Patients who have asymmetry of the face and head and limited motion after 1 year should be considered for surgical release of the SCM muscle.

B. **Differential diagnosis.** Torticollis with limited motion of the neck may be due to a congenital abnormality of the cervical region of the spine. Some infants with this disorder also have a tight SCM muscle. These infants are likely to have significant limitation of motion at birth, generally not seen in CMT. Radiologic evaluation of the cervical region is necessary to make this diagnosis. Infection in the retropharyngeal area may present with torticollis. The neck mass seen in torticollis in the SCM muscle may be differentiated from other cervical lesions by ultrasound.

II. POLYDACTYLY

A. **Duplication of a digit** may range from a small cutaneous bulb to an almost perfectly formed digit. Treatment of this problem is generally surgical. Syndromes associated with polydactyly include Laurence-Moon-Biedl syndrome, chondroectodermal dysplasia, Ellis-van Creveld syndrome, and trisomy 13. Polydactyly is generally inherited in an autosomal dominant manner with variable penetrance as an isolated problem, not syndromic.

B. **Treatment**

1. The small functionless skin bulb without bone or cartilage at the ulnar border of the hand or lateral border of the foot can be ligated and allowed to develop necrosis for 24 hours. The part distal to the suture should be removed. The residual stump should have an antiseptic applied twice a day to prevent infection until healed. Do not tie off digits on the radial side of the hand (thumb) or the medial border of the foot.

2. When duplicated digits contain bone or muscle attached by more than a small bridge of skin, treatment is delayed until the patient is evaluated by an orthopedist or hand surgeon. In general, polydactyly is managed surgically in the first year of life after 6 months of age. X-rays can be delayed until necessary for definitive management.

III. FRACTURED CLAVICLE (see Chapter 6)

A. **The clavicle** is the site of the most common fracture associated with delivery.

B. **Diagnosis** is usually made soon after birth, when the infant does not move the arm on the affected side or cries when that arm is moved. There may be tenderness, swelling, or crepitance at the site. Occasionally, the bone is angulated. Diagnosis can be confirmed by radiographic examination. A "painless" fracture discovered by radiography of the chest is more likely a congenital pseudarthrosis (nonunion). All pseudarthroses occur on the right side unless associated with dextrocardia.

C. **The clinical course** is such that clavicle fractures heal without difficulty. **Treatment** consists of providing comfort for the infant. If the arm and shoulder are left unprotected, motion occurs at the fracture site when the baby is handled, causing pain. We usually pin or tape the infant's sleeve to the shirt and put a sign on the baby to remind personnel to decrease motion of the clavicle. No reduction is necessary. If the fracture appears painful, a wrap to decrease motion of the arm is useful.

IV. CONGENITAL AND INFANTILE SCOLIOSIS

A. **Congenital scoliosis** is a lateral curvature of the spine secondary to a failure either of formation of a vertebra or of segmentation. Scoliosis in the newborn may be difficult to detect; by bending the trunk laterally in the prone position, however, a difference in motion can usually be observed. Congenital scoliosis is differentiated from **infantile scoliosis**, in which no vertebral anomaly is present. Infantile scoliosis often improves spontaneously, although the condition may be progressive in infants who have a spinal curvature of >20 degrees. If the scoliosis is progressive, treatment is indicated and magnetic resonance imaging (MRI) of the spine looking for spinal cord pathology should be done. Rarely, severe congenital scoliosis may be termed *thoracic insufficiency syndrome* and be associated with pulmonary compromise.

B. **Clinical course.** Congenital scoliosis will increase in many patients. Bracing of congenital curves is usually not helpful. Body casts for correction of the deformity are beneficial, allowing growth at the chest and lungs. Surgical correction with chest expansion or limited fusion may be indicated before the curve becomes severe. Many patients with congenital curves have renal or other visceral abnormalities. Abdominal ultrasonography is used to screen all such patients.

V. DEVELOPMENTAL DISLOCATION OF THE HIP

A. **Examination and screening**

1. Most (but not all) hips that are dislocated at birth can be diagnosed by a careful physical examination (see Chapter 8).

2. The American Academy of Pediatrics Committee on Quality Improvement, Subcommittee on Developmental Dysplasia of the Hip issued a clinical practice guideline on the early detection of developmental dislocation of the hip (DDH) (Fig. 58.1).

3. Ultrasonographic examination of the hip is useful for diagnosis in high-risk cases. Ultrasonography is delayed as a screening technique until 1 month of age to avoid a high incidence of false-positive examinations.

4. X-ray examination will not lead to a diagnosis in the newborn because the femoral head is not calcified but will reveal an abnormal acetabular fossa seen with hip dysplasia.

5. The practice of triple diapers in infants with physical signs suggestive of DDH is not recommended and lacks data on effectiveness.

6. Swaddling increases the incidence of DDH.[1]

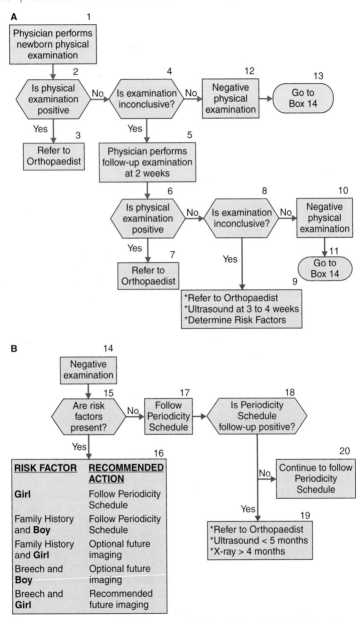

Figure 58.1. Screening for developmental hip dysplasia—clinical algorithm. (From American Academy of Pediatrics, Committee on Quality Improvement, Subcommittee on Developmental Dysplasia of the Hip. Clinical practice guideline: early detection of developmental dysplasia of the hip. *Pediatrics* 2000;105:896.)

B. **There are three types of congenital dislocations.**

1. The **classic DDH** is diagnosed by the presence of Ortolani sign. The hip is unstable and dislocates on adduction and also on extension of the femur but readily relocates when the femur is abducted in flexion. No asymmetry of the pelvis is seen. This type of dislocation is more common in females and is usually unilateral, but it may be bilateral. Hips that are unstable at birth often become stable after a few days. The infant with hips that are unstable after 5 days of life should be treated with a splint that keeps the hips flexed and abducted. The **Pavlik harness** has been used effectively to treat this group of patients, with approximately 80% success rate. Ultrasonography is used to monitor the hip during treatment as well as to confirm the initial diagnosis.

2. The **teratologic type of dislocation** occurs very early in pregnancy. The **femoral head does not relocate on flexion and abduction**; that is, Ortolani sign is not present. If the dislocation is unilateral, there may be asymmetry of the gluteal folds and asymmetric motion with limited abduction. In bilateral dislocation, the perineum is wide and the thighs give the appearance of being shorter than normal. This may be easily overlooked, however, and requires an extremely careful physical examination. Limited abduction at birth is a characteristic of this type of dislocation. Treatment of the teratologic hip dislocation is by open reduction. Exercise to decrease contracture is indicated, but use of the Pavlik harness is not beneficial.

3. The **third type of dislocation** occurs late, is unilateral, and is associated with a **congenital abduction contracture** of the contralateral hip. The abduction contracture causes a pelvic obliquity. The pelvis is lower on the side of the contracture, which is unfavorable for the contralateral hip, and the acetabulum may not develop well. After the age of 6 weeks, infants with this type of dislocation develop an apparent short leg and have asymmetric gluteal folds. Some infants will develop a dysplastic acetabulum, which may eventually allow the hip to subluxate. Treatment of the dysplasia is with the Pavlik harness, but after the age of 8 months, other methods of treatment may be necessary.

VI. **GENU RECURVATUM**, or hyperextension of the knee, is not a serious abnormality and is easily recognized and treated. It must be differentiated, however, from subluxation or dislocation of the knee, which also may present with hyperextension of the knee. The latter two abnormalities are more serious and require more extensive treatment.

A. **Congenital genu recurvatum** is secondary to *in utero* position with hyperextension of the knee. This can be treated successfully by repeated cast changes, with progressive flexion of the knee until it reaches 90 degrees of flexion. Minor degrees of recurvatum can be treated with passive stretching exercises. It may be associated with DDH.

B. All infants with **hyperextension of the knee** should have a radiographic examination to differentiate genu recurvatum **from true dislocation of the knee**. In congenital genu recurvatum, the tibial and femoral epiphyses are in proper alignment except for the hyperextension. In the subluxed knee with dislocation, the tibia is completely anterior or anterolateral to the femur. The tibia is shifted forward in relation to the femur and is frequently lateral as well.

Congenital fibrosis of the quadriceps is frequently associated with the fixed dislocated knee and open reduction is essential, as attempted treatment of the dislocated knee by stretching or by repeated cast changes is hazardous and may result in epiphyseal plate damage.

C. Treatment. Hyperextended or subluxed knees are treated with manipulation and splinting after delivery with progressive knee flexion and reduction. Fixed dislocation of the knee will require open reduction but not in the neonatal period.

VII. DEFORMITIES OF THE FEET

A. Metatarsus adductus (MTA) is a condition in which the metatarsals rest in an adducted position, but the appearance does not always reveal the severity of the condition. Whether treatment is necessary is determined by the difference in the degree of structural change in the metatarsals and tarsometatarsal joint.

1. Most infants with MTA have **positional deformities** that are probably caused by *in utero* position. The positional type of MTA is flexible, and the metatarsals can be passively corrected into abduction with little difficulty. **This condition does not need treatment.**

2. The **structural MTA** has a relatively fixed adduction deformity of the forefoot, and the metatarsals cannot be abducted passively. The etiology has not been definitely identified but is probably related to *in utero* position. This is seen more commonly in the firstborn infant and in pregnancies with oligohydramnios. Most infants with the structural types of MTA have a valgus deformity of the hindfoot. **The structural deformity needs to be treated with manipulation and immobilization in a shoe or cast** until correction occurs. Although there is no urgency to treat this condition, it is more easily corrected earlier than later and should be done before the child is of walking age but exercise only in the neonatal period.

B. Calcaneovalgus deformities result from an *in utero* position of the foot that holds the ankle dorsiflexed and abducted. At birth, the top of the foot lies up against the anterior surface of the leg. Structural changes in the bones do not seem to be present. The sequela to this deformity appears to be a valgus or pronated foot that is more severe than the typical pronated foot seen in toddlers. Whether this disorder is treated or not is variable, and no study supports either course. **Treatment consists of either exercise or application of a short leg cast** that will keep the foot plantarflexed and inverted. If the foot cannot be plantarflexed to a neutral position, casts are indicated. Casts are changed appropriately for growth and maintained until plantar flexion and inversion are equal to those of the opposite foot. Generally, the foot is held in plaster for approximately 6 to 8 weeks. Feet that remain in the calcaneovalgus position for several months may be more likely to have significant residual *pes valgus*; a fixed or rigid calcaneovalgus deformity probably represents a congenital vertical talus. It may also be related to a short tibia with posteromedial bow.

C. **Congenital clubfoot** is a deformity with a multifactorial etiology. It occurs with frequency of about 1 to 2/1,000 live births. A first-degree relative of a patient with this deformity has 20 times the risk of having a clubfoot than does the normal population. The risk in subsequent siblings is 3% to 5%. The more frequent occurrence in the firstborn and the association with oligohydramnios suggest an influence of *in utero* pressure as well. Sometimes, clubfoot is part of a syndrome. Infants with neurologic dysfunction of the feet (spina bifida) often have clubfoot.

1. **There are three and sometimes four components to the deformity.** The foot is in equinus, cavus, and varus position, with a forefoot adduction; therefore, the clubfoot is a talipes equinocavovarus with metatarsal adduction. Each of these deformities is sufficiently rigid to prevent passive correction to a neutral position by the examiner. The degree of rigidity is variable in each patient.

2. Treatment should be started early within a few days of birth. An effective method of treatment consists of manipulation and application of either tapes or plaster or fiberglass casts that are changed weekly. The Ponseti method[2] is the treatment of choice for idiopathic clubfoot in which the midfoot is sequentially corrected with casts, followed by a heel cord tenotomy to correct equinus after 6 to 8 weeks of cast correction. After tenotomy, the foot is immobilized in a corrected position for 3 weeks; braced full time for 3 months and a night bracing program is used until age 4 years. Physical therapy and splinting are used in a newborn with complex medical problems as initial management.

VIII. COMPARTMENT SYNDROME OF THE NEWBORN[3]

A. **Compartment syndrome of the newborn** is a rare condition in which a neonate presents with upper limb swelling and skin lesion evolving into compression ischemia in the hand and arm. This is a very rare but potentially devastating condition if diagnosis is delayed. At presentation, all patients have distal limb edema with a bulbous or ulcerative skin lesion varying in size from 1 cm to the entire arm. It may be associated with distal gangrene of fingertips or hand and associated with ecchymosis and swelling of the extremity.

1. **Etiology.** The exact cause of this syndrome is unknown. It is suspected that mechanical compression of the upper extremity, combined with fetal position, plays a major role in evolution of neonatal compartment syndrome. Intrauterine abnormalities or birth trauma may be related to this abnormality.

2. **Treatment.** If recognized early, treatment with emergency fasciotomy or revascularization of the limb has been beneficial. Prolonged ischemia results in scarring (known as Volkmann's ischemic contracture of muscle), nerve injury, permanent disability, and potential loss of a portion of the extremity.

References

1. Mahan ST, Kasser JR. Does swaddling influence developmental dysplasia of the hip? *Pediatrics* 2008;121(1):177–178.

2. Morcuende JA, Dolan LA, Dietz FR, et al. Radical reduction in the rate of extensive corrective surgery for clubfoot using the Ponseti method. *Pediatrics* 2004;113(2):376–380.

3. Ragland R III, Moukoko D, Ezaki M, et al. Forearm compartment syndrome in the newborn: report of 24 cases. *J Hand Surg Am* 2005;30(5):997–1003.

Suggested Readings

Cooperman DR, Thompson GH. Neonatal orthopaedics. In: Fanatoff AA, Martin RJ, eds. *Neonatal Perinatal Medicine.* 6th ed. St. Louis, MO: Mosby; 1997:1709.

Jones KL. *Smith's Recognizable Patterns of Human Malformation.* 5th ed. Philadelphia, PA: Elsevier Saunders; 1997.

Morrisey RT, Weinstein SL, eds. *Lovell and Winter's Pediatric Orthopaedics.* 6th ed. Philadelphia, PA: Lippincott Williams & Wilkins; 2006.

59 Osteopenia (Metabolic Bone Disease) of Prematurity

Steven A. Abrams

KEY POINTS

- Osteopenia remains a common problem for very preterm infants. The most common cause is inadequate dietary minerals.
- Other factors which may contribute to osteopenia include use of loop diuretics, steroids, fluid restriction, and in some cases, vitamin D deficiency.
- Prevention of osteopenia is best done by use of human milk fortifiers, specialized preterm and transitional formulas, and limiting use of calcium-losing diuretics such as furosemide.

I. GENERAL PRINCIPLES

A. Definition

1. Osteopenia is defined as postnatal bone mineralization that is inadequate to fully mineralize bones. Osteopenia occurs commonly in very low birth weight (VLBW) infants. Prior to the use of high-mineral–containing diets for premature infants, which is the current practice, significant radiographic changes were seen in about half of infants with birth weight <1,000 g.

2. The current incidence is unknown and likely closely associated with the severity of overall illness and degree of prematurity. It may still be seen in as many as half of all infants <600 g birth weight.

B. Etiology

1. **Deficiency of calcium and phosphorus are the principal causes.** Demands for rapid growth in the third trimester are met by intrauterine mineral accretion rates of approximately 120 mg of calcium and 60 mg of phosphorus/kg/day. Poor mineral intake and absorption after birth result in undermineralized new and remodeled bone.

   a. Diets low in mineral content. These diets predispose preterm newborns to metabolic bone disease.

   b. Unsupplemented human milk. In this circumstance, urinary calcium increases, suggesting a phosphorus deficiency that is greater than the calcium deficiency.

c. Excessive fluid restriction. This may lead to low mineral intake.

d. Long-term use of parenteral nutrition

e. Formulas not designed for use in preterm infants (e.g., full-term, elemental, soy-based, lactose-free). Soy-based formulas should be avoided after hospital discharge as well.

f. Furosemide therapy. This causes renal calcium wasting but is not likely the principal contributor to osteopenia for most preterm infants.

g. Long-term steroid use

2. **Vitamin D deficiency.** In mothers not supplemented with high amounts of vitamin D (e.g., >4,000 IU/day), human milk has a total vitamin D content of 25 to 50 IU/L, which is insufficient for maintaining 25-hydroxyvitamin D (25(OH)D) levels in preterm infants at >20 ng/mL. However, when vitamin D intake is adequate, even VLBW newborns can synthesize 1,25-dihydroxyvitamin D, although synthesis may be minimal in the first few weeks of life.

a. Maternal vitamin D deficiency can cause congenital rickets (uncommon) or hypocalcemia (more common).

b. Inadequate vitamin D intake or absorption produces nutritional rickets, but this is not the primary cause of osteopenia or rickets in preterm infants.

c. Vitamin D malabsorption and inadequate conversion of vitamin D to 25(OH)D can worsen osteopenia in infants with cholestatic liver disease.

d. Chronic renal failure (renal osteodystrophy)

e. Chronic use of phenytoin or phenobarbital increases 25(OH)D metabolism.

f. Hereditary pseudovitamin D deficiency: type I (abnormality or absence of 1-α-hydroxylase activity) or type II (tissue resistance to 1,25-dihydroxyvitamin D. These are extremely rare.

II. DIAGNOSIS

A. **Clinical presentation**

1. Osteopenia (characterized by bones that are undermineralized or "washed out") develops during the first postnatal weeks. Signs of rickets (epiphyseal dysplasia and skeletal deformities) usually become evident after 6 weeks postnatal age or by term-corrected gestational age. The risk of bone disease is greatest for the sickest, most premature infants.

B. **History**

1. A history of VLBW, especially <26 weeks or 800 g birth weight, and use of fluid restriction, prolonged parenteral nutrition, or long-term steroids are very common.

2. Rapid increase in alkaline phosphatase value is common.

3. A history of a fracture noticed by caregivers or incidentally on x-rays taken for other purposes may be seen.

C. **Physical examination**

1. **Clinical signs** include respiratory insufficiency or failure to wean from a ventilator; hypotonia; pain on handling due to pathologic fractures; decreased linear growth with sustained head growth; frontal bossing;

enlarged anterior fontanel and widened cranial sutures; craniotabes (posterior flattening of the skull); "rachitic rosary" (swelling of costo-chondral junctions); Harrison grooves (indentation of the ribs at the diaphragmatic insertions); and enlargement of wrists, knees, and ankles.

D. Laboratory studies

1. **Laboratory evaluation.** The earliest indications of osteopenia are often a decreased serum phosphorus concentration, typically <3.5 to 4 mg/dL (1.1 to 1.3 mmol/L), and an increased alkaline phosphatase activity. Alkaline phosphatase values >800 IU/L are worrisome, especially if combined with serum phosphorus values <4 mg/dL (1.3 mmol/L). However, it is often difficult to distinguish the normal rise in alkaline phosphatase activity associated with rapid bone mineralization from the pathologic increase related to early osteopenia. In this circumstance, decreased bone mineralization observed on a radiograph confirms the diagnosis.

   a. Serum calcium level (low, normal, or slightly elevated) is not a good indicator of the presence or severity of metabolic bone disease.

   b. Serum alkaline phosphatase level (an indicator of osteoclast activity) is often but not invariantly correlated with disease severity (>1,000 IU/L in severe rickets).

   c. Normal neonatal range of alkaline phosphatase is much higher than in adults. Values of 400 to 600 IU/L are common in VLBW infants with no evidence of osteopenia.

   d. Hepatobiliary disease also elevates alkaline phosphatase level. Determining bone isoenzymes may be helpful but is not usually clinically necessary.

   e. Solitary elevated alkaline phosphatase level rarely occurs in the absence of bone or liver disease (transient hyperphosphatasemia of infancy). This elevation can be >2,000 IU/L and persist for several months. It is not associated with any pathology, and the etiology is unknown.

   f. Serum 25(OH)D levels do not need to be routinely assessed in preterm infants. Optimal levels in infants are unknown as are functional outcomes at any level. When assessed, targets of >20 ng/mL are reasonable based on very limited evidence. There is no evidence that levels of 12 to 20 ng/mL lead to worsened osteopenia in preterm infants.

   g. An elevated serum PTH level may be indicative of osteopenia but is not commonly used as a screening tool and may be related to vitamin D status.

E. Imaging

1. **Radiographic signs** include widening of epiphyseal growth plates; cupping, fraying, and rarefaction of the metaphyses; subperiosteal new bone formation; osteopenia, particularly of the skull, spine, scapula, and ribs; and occasionally, osteoporosis or pathologic fractures.

   a. A loss of up to 40% of bone mineralization can occur without radiographic changes. Chest films may show osteopenia and sometimes rachitic changes.

   b. Wrist or knee films can be useful. Generally, if marked abnormalities are present, films should be obtained again 4 to 6 weeks later after a clinical intervention.

   c. Measurement of bone mineral content by densitometry or ultrasonography remains investigational in preterm infants.

III. TREATMENT

A. Management

1. In VLBW infants, early enteral feeding significantly enhances the establishment of full-volume enteral intake, leading to increased calcium accumulation and decreased osteopenia.

2. Mineral-fortified human milk or "premature" formulas are the appropriate diets for preterm infants weighing <1,800 to 2,000 g; their use at 120 kcal/kg/day can prevent and treat metabolic bone disease of prematurity.

3. Bone formation is dependent on a combination of adequate calcium and phosphorus availability; supplementation of either only calcium or only phosphorus alone may not be enough to prevent rickets.

4. Infants small for gestation (weighing <1,800 to 2,000 g) will usually also benefit from human milk fortification or use of premature infant formula regardless of gestational age.

5. Elemental mineral supplementation of human milk is less desirable than the use of prepackaged fortifiers containing calcium and phosphorus because of concern over medication error and potential hyperosmolarity.

6. The long-term use of specialized formulas in VLBW infants, including soy and elemental formulas, should be discouraged because they may increase the risk of osteopenia.

7. In special circumstances, including babies with radiologic evidence of rickets not responding to fortified human milk or premature formula, smaller amounts of calcium (usually up to 40 mg of elemental calcium/kg/day) and/or sodium or potassium phosphate (usually up to 20 mg of elemental phosphorus) can be provided. This is usually needed in babies whose birth weights were <800 g or who had a prolonged hospital course including long-term total parenteral nutrition (TPN), fluid restrictions, or bronchopulmonary dysplasia. Due to concerns about tolerance, it is usual to add the intravenous forms of phosphorus (sodium or potassium phosphate) orally to the diet. This may also be done when the serum phosphorus is persistently below 4.0 mg/dL, although evidence supporting this practice is lacking.

8. Ensure adequate vitamin D stores by an intake of 400 IU/day after the infant reaches about 1,500 g and full feeds. This may require giving supplemental vitamin D to both breastfed and formula-fed infants at discharge.

9. High doses of vitamin D have not been shown to have short- or long-term benefits. Some prefer to give 800 IU/day. This is unlikely to be harmful, but there is no evidence of benefit.

10. Rare defects in vitamin D metabolism may respond better to dihydrotachysterol (DHT) or calcitriol.

11. Furosemide-induced renal calcium wasting may be lessened by adding a thiazide diuretic or by alternate-day administration. Benefits of these approaches are not well established in neonates.

12. Avoid nonessential handling and vigorous chest physiotherapy in preterm infants with severely undermineralized bones. Recent data suggests that daily passive physical activity (range of motion, 5 to 10 minutes) may enhance both growth and bone mineralization.

13. Infants receiving human milk with added fortifier or premature formula should have serum calcium, phosphorus, and alkaline phosphate levels monitored periodically. Measurement of vitamin D metabolite levels and parathyroid hormone (PTH) levels are rarely useful in this setting. Once the alkaline phosphatase activity has peaked and is declining (usually to <500 to 600 IU/L), these no longer need to be measured in fully enterally fed infants if an appropriate feeding regimen is being provided.

14. Human milk fortification or the use of premature infant formula can usually be discontinued after the infant weighs approximately 1,800 to 2,000 g and is tolerating enteral feeds well. It may be continued longer for infants who are fluid restricted or have a markedly elevated alkaline phosphatase activity or radiologic evidence of osteopenia.

15. At hospital discharge, infants with birth weight <1,500 g who are formula fed may benefit from the use of a transitional formula that has calcium and phosphorus contents midrange between that of preterm formulas and formulas designed for full-term infants. Such infants may need additional vitamin D to achieve an intake of 400 IU/day.

16. Former VLBW infants discharged from hospital receiving unsupplemented mother's milk are at risk for persistent osteopenia. They, like all human milk–fed infants, should be provided vitamin D supplementation of 400 IU/day. Members of this patient population may be candidates for a follow-up measurement of serum phosphorus and alkaline phosphatase activity at 4 to 8 weeks postdischarge. Growth should also be monitored carefully.

17. Consideration should be given to the use of 2 to 3 feedings/day of a transitional formula postdischarge for otherwise human milk–fed VLBW infants to provide adequate protein as well as minerals.

Suggested Readings

Abrams SA, Hawthorne KM, Placencia JL, et al. Micronutrient requirements of high-risk infants. *Clin Perinatol* 2014;41:347–361.

Hsu HC, Levine MA. Perinatal calcium metabolism: physiology and pathophysiology. *Semin Neonatol* 2004;9:23–36.

Mimouni FB, Mandel D, Lubetsky R, et al. Calcium, phosphorus, magnesium and vitamin D requirements of the preterm infant. In: Koletzko B, Poindexter B, Uauy R, eds. *Nutritional Care of Preterm Infants: Scientific Basis and Practical Guidelines*. Basel, Switzerland: Karger; 2014:140–151.

Mitchell SM, Rogers SP, Hicks PD, et al. High frequencies of elevated alkaline phosphatase activity and rickets exist in extremely low birth weight infants despite current nutritional support. *BMC Pediatr* 2009;9:47.

Inborn Errors of Metabolism

Ayman W. El-Hattab and V. Reid Sutton

KEY POINTS

- Neonates with inborn errors of metabolism (IEMs) usually present with nonspecific signs, and early diagnosis and institution of therapy are mandatory to prevent death and ameliorate complications from many IEMs. Therefore, a high index of suspicion for IEMs should be maintained.
- After performing the initial metabolic workup, you can narrow the differential diagnosis by the following categorizations:
  - In metabolic acidosis with hyperammonemia, consider an organic acidemia (or pyruvate carboxylase deficiency if lactate is also very high).
  - In hyperammonemia with respiratory alkalosis, consider a urea cycle defect.
  - In hypoglycemia without ketosis, consider fatty acid oxidation defects.
  - In hypoglycemia with ketosis and elevated lactate, consider fructose-1,6-bisphosphatase deficiency and glycogen storage disease type I.
  - In liver failure, galactosemia and tyrosinemia type I should be evaluated.
  - In cardiomyopathy, consider glycogen storage disease type II and fatty acid oxidation defects.
- When managing acute metabolic decompensation, make sure of the following:
  - Provide adequate calories, at least 20% above what is normally needed.
  - Use insulin infusion to reverse catabolism.
  - Limit the enteral feeding restriction to 24 to 48 hours and introduce enteral feeding with the appropriate formula early (after 24 to 48 hours).

I. INTRODUCTION. Inborn errors of metabolism (IEMs) are a group of disorders each of which results from deficient activity of a single enzyme in a metabolic pathway. Although IEMs are individually rare, they are collectively common, with an overall incidence of more than 1:1,000. More than 500 IEMs have been recognized, with more than 100 of them that can present clinically in the neonatal period.

Neonates with IEMs are usually healthy at birth with signs typically developing in hours to days after birth. The signs are usually nonspecific and may include decreased activity, lethargy, poor feeding, vomiting, respiratory distress, or seizures. These signs are common to several other neonatal conditions, such as sepsis and cardiopulmonary dysfunction. Therefore, maintaining a high index of suspicion is important for early diagnosis and the institution of appropriate therapy, which are mandatory to prevent death and ameliorate complications from many IEMs.

The vast majority of IEMs are inherited in an autosomal recessive manner. Therefore, a history of parental consanguinity or a previously affected sibling should raise the suspicion of IEMs. Some IEMs, such as ornithine transcarbamylase (OTC) deficiency, are X-linked. In X-linked disorder, typically affected males have severe disease, whereas affected females are either asymptomatic or have a milder disease. So, the severely affected family member could be a maternal uncle or a brother, whereas the mildly affected member could be a mother or sister.

II. CLINICAL PRESENTATION. After an initial symptom-free period, neonates with IEMs can start deteriorating for no apparent reasons and do not respond to symptomatic therapies. The interval between birth and clinical symptoms may range from hours to weeks, depending on the enzyme deficiency. Neonates with IEMs can present with one or more of the following clinical groups:

A. **Neurologic manifestations.** Deterioration of consciousness is one of the common neonatal manifestations of IEMs that can occur due to metabolic derangements, including metabolic acidosis (see section IV), hyperammonemia (see section V), and hypoglycemia (see section VI). Neonates with these metabolic derangements typically exhibit poor feeding and decreased activity that progress to lethargy and coma. Other common neurologic manifestations of IEMs in the neonatal period are seizures (see section VII), hypotonia (see section VIII), and apnea (Table 60.1).

B. **Liver dysfunction** (see section IX). Galactosemia is the most common metabolic cause of liver disease in the neonate. Three main clinical groups of hepatic symptoms can be identified: hepatomegaly with hypoglycemia, cholestatic jaundice, and liver failure (jaundice, coagulopathy, elevated transaminases, hypoglycemia, and ascites) (Table 60.2).

C. **Cardiac dysfunction** (see section X). Some IEMs can present predominantly with cardiac diseases, including cardiomyopathy, heart failure, and arrhythmias (Table 60.3).

D. **Other manifestations.** An abnormal urine odor is present in some IEMs in which volatile metabolites accumulate (Table 60.4). Some IEMs can present with facial dysmorphism (Table 60.5), and others can present with hydrops fetalis (Table 60.6).

Table 60.1. Inborn Errors of Metabolism Associated with Neurologic Manifestations in Neonates

Deterioration in consciousness

- Metabolic acidosis
  - □ Organic acidemias
  - □ Maple syrup urine disease (MSUD)
  - □ Disorders of pyruvate metabolism
  - □ Fatty acid oxidation defects
  - □ Fructose-1,6-bisphosphatase deficiency
  - □ Glycogen storage disease type I
  - □ Mitochondrial diseases
  - □ Disorders of ketone body metabolism
- Hyperammonemia
  - □ Urea cycle disorders
  - □ Organic acidemias
  - □ Disorders of pyruvate metabolism
- Hypoglycemia
  - □ Fatty acid oxidation defects
  - □ Fructose-1,6-bisphosphatase deficiency
  - □ Glycogen storage disease type I
  - □ Organic acidemias
  - □ Mitochondrial diseases
  - □ Disorders of ketone body metabolism

Seizures

- Biotinidase deficiency
- Pyridoxine-dependent epilepsy
- Pyridoxal phosphate-responsive epilepsy
- Glycine encephalopathy
- Mitochondrial diseases

(continued)

Table 60.1. *(Continued)*
▪ Zellweger syndrome
▪ Sulfite oxidase/molybdenum cofactor deficiency
▪ Purine metabolism disorders
▪ Disorders of creatine biosynthesis and transport
▪ Neurotransmitter defects
▪ Congenital disorders of glycosylation
Hypotonia
▪ Mitochondrial diseases
▪ Zellweger syndrome
▪ Glycine encephalopathy
▪ Sulfite oxidase/molybdenum cofactor deficiency
Apnea
▪ Glycine encephalopathy
▪ MSUD
▪ Urea cycle disorders
▪ Disorders of pyruvate metabolism
▪ Fatty acid oxidation defects
▪ Mitochondrial diseases

III. **EVALUATION AND MANAGEMENT.** Early diagnosis and the institution of appropriate therapy are mandatory in IEMs to prevent death and ameliorate complications. Management of suspected IEMs should be started even before birth.

   A. **Before or during pregnancy.** When a previous sibling has a metabolic disorder or symptoms consistent with a metabolic disorder, the following steps should be taken:

   1. Clinical reports and hospital charts should be reviewed.

   2. Prenatal genetic counseling regarding the possibility of having an affected infant

   3. The parents and relatives can be screened for possible clues of an IEM.

   4. When a diagnosis is known, intrauterine diagnosis by measurement of abnormal metabolites in the amniotic fluid or by enzyme assay or DNA analysis of amniocytes or chorionic villus cells

Table 60.2. Inborn Errors of Metabolism Associated with Neonatal Hepatic Manifestations

Hepatomegaly with hypoglycemia

- Fructose-1,6-bisphosphatase deficiency
- Glycogen storage disease type I

Cholestatic jaundice

- Citrin deficiency
- Zellweger syndrome
- Alpha-1-antitrypsin deficiency
- Niemann-Pick disease type C
- Inborn errors of bile acid metabolism
- Congenital disorders of glycosylation

Liver failure

- Galactosemia
- Tyrosinemia type I
- Hereditary fructose intolerance
- Mitochondrial diseases
- Fatty acid oxidation defects

Table 60.3. Inborn Errors of Metabolism Associated with Neonatal Cardiomyopathy

Disorders of fatty acid oxidation

- Very long chain acyl-coenzyme A dehydrogenase (VLCAD) deficiency
- Long chain hydroxyacyl-coenzyme A dehydrogenase (LCHAD) deficiency
- Trifunctional protein deficiency
- Carnitine transport defect
- Carnitine–acylcarnitine translocase (CAT) deficiency
- Carnitine palmitoyltransferase II (CPT II) deficiency

Glycogen storage disease type II (Pompe disease)

Tricarboxylic acid cycle defects: α-ketoglutarate dehydrogenase deficiency

Mitochondrial diseases

Congenital disorders of glycosylations

Table 60.4. Inborn Errors of Metabolism Associated with Abnormal Urine Odor in Newborns

Inborn Error of Metabolism	Odor
Glutaric acidemia type II	Sweaty feet
Isovaleric acidemia	Sweaty feet
Maple syrup urine disease	Maple syrup
Cystinuria	Sulfur
Tyrosinemia type I	Sulfur
Hypermethioninemia	Boiled cabbage
Multiple carboxylase deficiency	Cat urine
Phenylketonuria	Mousy
Trimethylaminuria	Old fish
Dimethylglycine dehydrogenase deficiency	Old fish

Table 60.5. Inborn Errors of Metabolism Associated with Distinctive Facial Features

Disorder	Dysmorphic Features
Zellweger syndrome	Large fontanelle, prominent forehead, flat nasal bridge, epicanthal folds, hypoplastic supraorbital ridges
Pyruvate dehydrogenase deficiency	Epicanthal folds, flat nasal bridge, small nose with anteverted flared alae nasi, long philtrum
Glutaric aciduria type II	Macrocephaly, high forehead, flat nasal bridge, short nose, ear anomalies, hypospadias, rocker bottom feet
Cholesterol biosynthetic defects (Smith-Lemli-Opitz syndrome)	Epicanthal folds, flat nasal bridge, toe 2/3 syndactyly, genital abnormalities, cataracts
Congenital disorders of glycosylation	Inverted nipples, lipodystrophy, very wide variety of findings among the nearly 100 disorders
Miller syndrome (dihydroorotate dehydrogenase deficiency)	Micrognathia, cleft lip/palate, malar hypoplasia, eyelid coloboma, downslanted palpebral fissures, and absence of fifth digits

Table 60.6. Inborn Errors of Metabolism Associated with Hydrops Fetalis
Lysosomal disorders
▪ Mucopolysaccharidosis types I, IVA, and VII
▪ Sphingolipidosis: GM1 gangliosidosis, Gaucher disease, Farber disease, Niemann-Pick disease type A, multiple sulfatase deficiency
▪ Lipid storage disorders: Wolman disease, Niemann-Pick disease type C
▪ Oligosaccharidosis: galactosialidosis, sialic acid storage disease, mucolipidoses I (sialidosis), mucolipidoses II (I cell disease)
Zellweger syndrome
Glycogen storage disease type IV
Congenital disorders of glycosylation
Mitochondrial diseases
Neonatal hemochromatosis

5. Planning to deliver the baby in a facility equipped to handle potential metabolic or other complications

B. **Initial evaluation.** When an IEM is suspected in a neonate, a careful physical examination seeking any of the signs of IEM needs to be performed; nonmetabolic causes of symptoms such as infection, asphyxia, or intracranial hemorrhage need to be evaluated; and the newborn screening program should be contacted for the results of the screening and for a list of the disorders screened. Initial laboratory studies should be obtained immediately once IEMs are suspected (Table 60.7). The results of these tests can help to narrow the differential diagnosis and determine which specialized tests are required.

1. **Complete blood cell count.** Neutropenia and thrombocytopenia may be associated with a number of organic acidemias. Neutropenia may also be found with glycogen storage disease type Ib and mitochondrial diseases, such as Barth syndrome and Pearson syndrome.

2. **Electrolytes and blood gases** are required to determine whether an acidosis or alkalosis is present and, if so, whether it is respiratory or metabolic and if there is an increased anion gap. Most metabolic conditions result in acidosis in late stages as encephalopathy and circulatory disturbances progress. A persistently high anion gap metabolic acidosis with normal tissue perfusion may suggest an IEM (e.g., organic acidemia or pyruvate metabolism defects). A mild respiratory alkalosis in nonventilated babies suggests hyperammonemia. However, in late stages of hyperammonemia, vasomotor instability and collapse can cause metabolic acidosis.

3. **Glucose.** Hypoglycemia is a critical finding in some IEMs.

Table 60.7. Laboratory Studies for a Newborn Suspected of Having an Inborn Error of Metabolism

Initial Laboratory Studies
Complete blood count with differential
Serum glucose and electrolytes
Blood gases
Liver function tests and coagulation profile
Plasma ammonia
Plasma lactate
Plasma amino acids
Plasma carnitine and acylcarnitine profile
Urine reducing substances, pH, ketones
Urine organic acids
Additional Laboratory Studies Considered in Neonatal Seizures
Cerebrospinal fluid (CSF) amino acids
CSF neurotransmitters
Sulfocysteine in urine
Very long chain fatty acids

4. **Plasma ammonia level** should be determined in all neonates suspected of having an IEM. Early recognition of severe neonatal hyperammonemia is crucial because irreversible damage can occur within hours.

5. **Plasma lactate level.** A high plasma lactate can be secondary to hypoxia, cardiac disease, infection, or seizures, whereas primary lactic acidosis may be caused by disorders of gluconeogenesis, pyruvate metabolism, and mitochondrial diseases. Some IEM (fatty acid oxidation disorders, organic acidemias, and urea cycle disorders [UCDs]) may also be associated with a secondary lactic acidosis. Persistent increase of plasma lactate above 3 mmol/L in a neonate who did not suffer from asphyxia and who has no evidence of other organ failure should lead to further investigation for an IEM. Specimens for lactate measurement should be obtained from a central line or through an arterial stick because use of tourniquet during venous sampling may result in a spurious increase in lactate.

6. **Liver function tests.** Some IEMs are associated with liver dysfunction.

7. **Urine for reducing substances, pH, and ketones.** Reducing substances are tested by the Clinitest reaction that detects excess excretion of galactose and glucose but not fructose. A positive reaction with the Clinitest should be investigated further with the Clinistix reaction (glucose oxidase) that is specific for glucose. Reducing substances in urine can be used as screening for galactosemia; however, this test is not very reliable because of high false-positive and false-negative rates. Urine pH <5 is expected in cases of metabolic acidosis associated with IEM; otherwise, renal tubular acidosis is a consideration. In neonates, the presence of ketonuria is always abnormal and an important sign of metabolic disease.

8. **Plasma amino acid analysis.** Plasma amino acid analysis is indicated for any infant suspected of having IEM. Recognition of patterns of abnormalities is important in the interpretation of the results.

9. **Urine organic acid analysis** is indicated for patients with unexplained metabolic acidosis, seizures, hyperammonemia, hypoglycemia, and/or ketonuria.

10. **Plasma carnitine and acylcarnitine profile.** Carnitine transports long-chain fatty acids across the inner mitochondrial membrane. An elevation of carnitine esters may be seen in fatty acid oxidation defects (FODs), organic acidemias, and ketosis. In addition to patients with inherited disorders of carnitine uptake, low carnitine levels are common in preterm infants and neonates receiving total parenteral nutrition (TPN) without adequate carnitine supplementation. Several metabolic diseases may cause secondary carnitine deficiency.

C. **Management of acute metabolic decompensation.** Several IEMs can present with acute metabolic decompensation during the neonatal period, such as urea cycle defects and organic acidemias. The principles of managing acute metabolic decompensation are as follows:

1. **Decrease production of the toxic intermediates** by holding enteral intake for 24 to 48 hours and suppressing catabolism. Reversal of catabolism and promotion of anabolism can be achieved by the following:
   a. Providing adequate caloric intake
   b. Administering insulin. Insulin is a potent anabolic hormone and can be administered as a continuous infusion (0.05 to 0.1 unit/kg/hour) with adjusting the intravenous (IV) glucose to maintain a normal blood glucose.
   c. Providing adequate hydration and treating infections aggressively
   d. Introducing enteral feeding as early as possible. The period of enteral feed restriction should not exceed 24 to 48 hours; after that, a special formula appropriate for the suspected IEM should be introduced if there are no contraindications for enteral feeding.

2. **Elimination of toxic metabolites** by the following:
   a. IV hydration, which can promote renal excretion of toxins
   b. The use of specific medications that create alternative pathways. For example, carnitine can bind organic acid metabolites and enhance their excretion in urine in organic acidemias. Another example is

sodium benzoate, which is used in glycine encephalopathy and urea cycle defects, because it binds to glycine-forming hippurate, which is excreted in urine.

c. Hemodialysis/hemofiltration may be employed in cases of unresponsive hyperammonemia (>500 mg/dL) in urea cycle defects and hyperleucinemia in maple syrup urine disease (MSUD).

3. Correction of metabolic acidosis. If the infant is acidotic (pH <7.22) or the bicarbonate level is <14 mEq/L, sodium bicarbonate can be given at dose of 1 to 2 mEq/kg as a bolus followed by a continuous infusion. If hypernatremia is a problem, potassium acetate can be used in the maintenance fluid.

4. Correction of hypoglycemia (see Chapter 24)

5. Calories. Provided calories during a period of decompensation, in order to support anabolism, should be at least 20% greater than that needed for ordinary maintenance. Adequate calories can be achieved parenterally by IV glucose and intralipid and enterally by giving protein-free formula or special formula appropriate for the IEM. One must remember that withholding natural protein from the diet also eliminates this source of calories, which should be replaced using other dietary or nutritional (nonnitrogenous) sources.

6. Lipids. To supply extra calories, the neonate can be supplied with lipids in the form of oral medium-chain triglycerides (MCTs) or parenteral intralipid. However, before feeding MCT, it is very important to be certain that the infant does not have a medium-chain acylcoenzyme A dehydrogenase (MCAD) deficiency; otherwise, this could provoke a very severe metabolic reaction.

7. Protein. All natural protein should be withheld for 24 hours while the patient is acutely ill. Afterward, amino acid supplementation may be very beneficial in facilitating clinical improvement by promoting anabolism, but it should be implemented only under the supervision of a physician/dietitian with expertise in IEMs. Special parenteral amino acid solutions and specialized formulas are available for many disorders when individuals with IEMs require prolonged parenteral nutrition.

8. L-Carnitine. Free carnitine levels are low in organic acidemias because of increased esterification with organic acid metabolites. Carnitine supplementation (100 to 300 mg/kg/day) may facilitate excretion of these metabolites. Diarrhea is the primary adverse effect of oral carnitine.

9. Antibiotics. For certain organic acidemias (propionic acidemia [PA] and methylmalonic acidemia [MMA]), gut bacteria are a significant source of organic acid synthesis (propionic acid). Eradicating the gut flora with a short course of a broad-spectrum antibiotic (e.g., neomycin, metronidazole) enterally may speed the recovery of a patient in acute metabolic decompensation.

10. Cofactor supplementation. Pharmacologic doses of appropriate cofactors may be useful in cases of vitamin-responsive enzyme deficiencies, e.g., thiamine in MSUD.

11. Treatment of precipitating factors. Infection should be treated as per usual protocols. Excess protein ingestion should be discontinued.

D. Monitoring the patient. Neonates with IEMs should be monitored closely for any mental status changes, overall fluid balance, evidence of bleeding (if thrombocytopenic), and symptoms of infection (if neutropenic). Biochemical parameters need to be followed including electrolytes, glucose, ammonia, blood gases, complete blood cell count, and urine for ketones.

E. Recovery and initiation of feeding

1. The neonate should be kept nothing by mouth (NPO) until his or her mental status is more stable. Anorexia, nausea, and vomiting during the acute metabolic decompensation period make significant oral intake unlikely.

2. If the neonate is not significantly neurologically compromised, consideration should be given to providing the neonate (orally or by nasogastric/gastric tube) with a modified formula preparation containing all but the offending amino acids. When the neonate is able to take oral feedings, a specific diet must be used. The diet will be individualized for each child and his or her metabolic defect, e.g., in galactosemia, the infant should be fed a lactose-free formula.

F. Long-term management. Several IEMs require dietary restrictions (e.g., leucine-restricted diet in isovaleric acidemia [IVA]). If hypoglycemia occurs, then frequent feeding and the use of uncooked cornstarch are advised. Cofactors are used in vitamin-responsive IEMs (e.g., pyridoxine in pyridoxine-dependent epilepsy). Examples of other oral medications used in chronic management of IEMs are carnitine for organic acidemias, sodium benzoate for urea cycle defects, and nitisinone (NTCB) in tyrosinemia type I.

IV. INBORN ERROR OF METABOLISM WITH METABOLIC ACIDOSIS.

Metabolic acidosis with a high anion gap is an important laboratory feature of many IEM including MSUD, organic acidurias, fatty acid oxidation disorders, disorders of pyruvate metabolism, glycogen storage diseases, and mitochondrial diseases (Table 60.1). The presence or absence of ketosis in metabolic acidosis can distinguish certain groups of disorders from each other (Fig. 60.1).

A. Maple syrup urine disease

1. An autosomal recessive disorder due to deficiency of branched-chain α-ketoacid dehydrogenase (Fig. 60.2)

2. Manifestations. Severe form of MSUD presents during the first week of life with poor feeding, vomiting, irritability, ketosis, lethargy, seizures, hypertonicity, opisthotonus, coma, and maple syrup odor of urine and cerumen (Table 60.4).

3. Diagnosis. MSUD can be diagnosed biochemically by the identification of increased plasma levels of branched-chain amino acids (leucine, isoleucine, alloisoleucine, and valine with perturbation of the normal 1:2:3 ratio of isoleucine:leucine:valine) and the presence of branched-chain keto- and hydroxyacids in urine organic acid analysis. Leucine

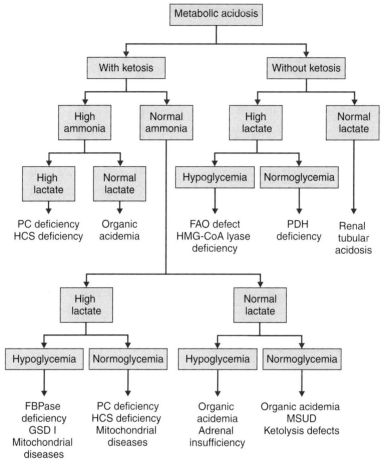

Figure 60.1. Approach to neonatal metabolic acidosis. Note that although a significant elevation in lactate is more associated with mitochondrial diseases and pyruvate metabolism disorders, milder lactate elevations can be seen in organic acidemias and MSUD. FAO, fatty acid oxidation; FBPase, fructose-1,6-bisphosphatase deficiency; GSD I, glycogen storage disease type I; HMG-CoA, 3-hydroxy-3-methylglutaryl coenzyme A; MSUD, maple syrup urine disease; PC, pyruvate carboxylase; HCS, holocarboxylase synthetase; PDH, pyruvate dehydrogenase.

is the primary neurotoxic metabolite. Most newborn screening programs include MSUD. Enzyme assay and molecular genetic tests are available.

4. **Management.** Management of acute presentation includes holding protein intake and suppressing catabolism with glucose and insulin infusions. Isoleucine and valine supplementation (20 to 120 mg/kg/day) and

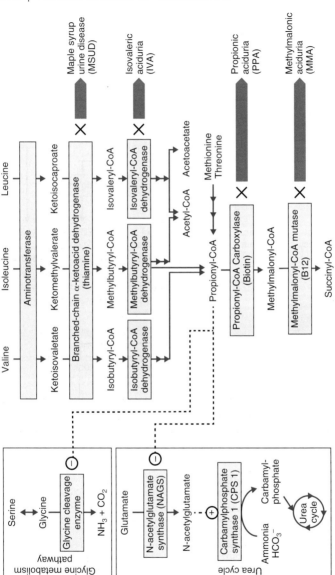

Figure 60.2. Branched-chain amino acid metabolism and enzyme defects associated with inborn errors of metabolism. Note that propionic acid inhibits glycine cleavage enzyme and N-acetylglutamate synthetase resulting in elevated glycine and hyperammonemia in propionic and methylmalonic acidemias. ⊖, negative effect/inhibition; ⊕, positive effect/acceleration.

adequate caloric intake also are needed. Hemodialysis/hemofiltration may be considered for rapid correction of hyperleucinemia. Thiamine (10 mg/kg/day) trial for 4 weeks can be considered. Long-term management requires a branched-chain amino acid–restricted diet.

B. Organic acidemias

1. Organic acidemias are autosomal recessive disorders that are characterized by the excretion of organic acids in urine. The most commonly encountered organic acidemias in the neonatal period, IVA, PA, and MMA, result from enzymatic defects in the branched-chain amino acid metabolism (Fig. 60.2).

2. **Manifestations.** Organic acidemias can present in the neonatal period with lethargy, poor feeding, vomiting, truncal hypotonia with limb hypertonia, myoclonic jerks, hypothermia, cerebral edema, coma, multiorgan failure, and unusual odor (Table 60.4).

3. **Diagnosis.** Laboratory test usually reveal high anion gap metabolic acidosis and occasionally hyperammonemia, hyperglycinemia, hypoglycemia, neutropenia, thrombocytopenia, pancytopenia, and elevated transaminases. The specific diagnosis can be reached by performing urine organic acid analysis and serum acylcarnitine profile (Table 60.8). Enzyme assays and molecular genetic tests are available for confirmation. Newborn screening programs that have expanded metabolic screening can detect IVA, PA, and MMA.

4. **Management.** Management of acute decompensation includes holding protein intake, suppressing catabolism with glucose and insulin infusions, correcting acidosis with sodium bicarbonate infusion, and administering

Table 60.8. Biochemical Diagnosis of Organic Acidemias

Organic Acidemias	Enzymes	Urine Organic Acid Analysis	Plasma Acylcarnitine Profile
Propionic acidemia (PPA)	Propionyl-CoA carboxylase	Elevated 3-hydroxypropionic acid, methylcitric acid, and propionyl glycine	Elevated propionylcarnitine (C3)
Methylmalonic acidemia (MMA)	Methylmalonyl-CoA mutase	Elevated methylmalonic, and methylcitric acids	Elevated propionylcarnitine (C3)
Isovaleric acidemia (IVA)	Isovaleryl-CoA dehydrogenase	Elevated 3-hydroxy-isovaleric acid and isovalerylglycine	Elevated pentanoyl carnitine (C5)

CoA, coenzyme A.

carnitine (100 to 300 mg/kg/day IV) to enhance the excretion of organic acids in urine. Hemodialysis may be considered if these measures fail. Chronic treatment includes oral carnitine and dietary restrictions. A diet low in amino acids producing propionic acid (isoleucine, valine, methionine, and threonine) is used for PA and MMA, and a leucine-restricted diet is used for IVA. Vitamin B_{12} (adenosylcobalamin) is a cofactor for methylmalonyl-coenzyme A (CoA) mutase, and hydroxocobalamin injection (1 mg daily) can be given as a trial in MMA. Glycine (150 to 250 mg/kg/day) enhances the excretion of isovaleric acid in urine and should be used in IVA.

C. **Defects of pyruvate metabolism** can present with severe neonatal metabolic acidosis with elevated lactate and include pyruvate dehydrogenase (PDH), pyruvate carboxylase (PC), and holocarboxylase synthetase (HCS) deficiencies (Fig. 60.3).

1. **Pyruvate dehydrogenase deficiency**

   a. PDH deficiency is usually inherited in an X-linked manner with the most severe illness in male infants.

   b. Manifestations. Neonates with PDH deficiency typically present with severe lactic acidosis, hypotonia, feeding difficulties, apnea, seizures, lethargy, coma, brain changes (cerebral atrophy, hydrocephaly, corpus callosum agenesis, cystic lesions, gliosis, and hypomyelination), and distinctive facial features (Table 60.5).

   c. Diagnosis. Very high lactate in various body fluids is suggestive of the diagnosis. The diagnosis is confirmed by enzyme studies and molecular genetic testing.

   d. Management. The prognosis is very poor, and treatment is generally not effective. Acidosis correction with bicarbonate and hydration with glucose infusion are needed during the acute presentation. However, excess administration of glucose may worsen the acidosis, and a ketogenic diet (where ~80% of caloric intake is from fat) may reduce the lactic acidosis. Thiamin, a cofactor for PDH, can be used (10 mg/kg/day).

2. **Pyruvate carboxylase deficiency**

   a. PC deficiency is an autosomal recessive disorder.

   b. Manifestations. Neonates with severe form of PC deficiency present with severe neonatal lactic acidosis, lethargy, coma, seizures, and hypotonia

   c. Diagnosis. Lactic acidosis, ketosis, hyperammonemia, hypercitrullinemia, and low aspartate are suggestive of the diagnosis. The diagnosis is confirmed by enzyme studies and molecular genetic testing.

   d. Management. The prognosis is poor, and treatment is generally not effective. Correction of acidosis with bicarbonate and hydration with glucose infusion are needed during the acute presentation. Biotin is a cofactor for PC and can be given (5 to 20 mg/day).

3. **Holocarboxylase synthetase deficiency**

   a. HCS deficiency (multiple carboxylase deficiency) is an autosomal recessive disorder due to deficiency of HCS enzyme that catalyzes the binding of biotin with the inactive apocarboxylases, leading to carboxylase activation. Deficiency of this enzyme causes

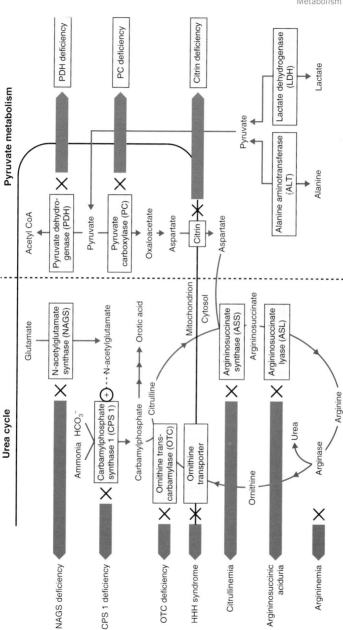

Figure 60.3. Metabolic pathways for urea cycle and pyruvate with the related inborn errors of metabolism. HHH, hyperornithinemia-hyperammonemia-homocitrullinuria.

malfunction of all carboxylases including propionyl-CoA, acetyl-CoA, 3-methylcrotonyl-CoA, and PCs.

b. Manifestations. Affected infants become symptomatic in the first few weeks of life with respiratory distress, hypotonia, seizures, vomiting, and failure to thrive. Skin manifestations include generalized erythematous rash with exfoliation and alopecia totalis. These infants may also have an immunodeficiency manifested by a decrease in the number of T cells.

c. Diagnosis. The biochemical profile for HCS deficiency includes lactic acidosis, ketosis, hyperammonemia, and urine organic acids showing methylcrotonylglycine and 3-hydroxyisovaleric, 3-hydroxypropionic, and methylcitric acids. Enzyme studies and molecular genetic studies are available. Many individuals are identified by newborn screening through elevation of hydroxypentanoylcarnitine and/or propionylcarnitine.

d. Management. Almost all affected infants respond to treatment with very large dose of biotin (10 to 40 mg/day), although in some affected infants, the response may be only partial.

V. INBORN ERROR OF METABOLISM WITH HYPERAMMONEMIA. It is essential to measure ammonia in every sick neonate, whenever an IEM or septic workup is considered. Early recognition of severe neonatal hyperammonemia is crucial because irreversible damage can occur within hours. Hyperammonemia can be caused by IEMs or acquired disorders (Table 60.9). Hyperammonemia is the principal presentation for most UCDs. However, hyperammonemia with ketoacidosis suggests an underlying organic acidemia. Therefore, the presence of respiratory alkalosis or metabolic acidosis can help in distinguishing UCDs from organic acidemias, respectively (Fig. 60.4). Transient hyperammonemia of the newborn (THN) can be seen in premature neonates with respiratory distress; plasma glutamine is typically normal in THN in contrast to UCDs where glutamine is elevated.

A. Urea cycle disorders

1. UCDs are among the most common IEMs. Most UCDs are inherited as autosomal recessive conditions, with the exception of the X-linked disorder OTC deficiency. UCDs result from defects in urea cycle enzymes leading to the accumulation of ammonia and urea cycle intermediates (Fig. 60.3).

2. **Manifestations.** UCDs can present at any age. Neonates with severe forms of UCDs typically present with rapidly progressive symptoms appear between 48 and 72 hours of life after a short, symptom-free interval. These symptoms include poor feeding, vomiting, lethargy, hypotonia, hypothermia, and hyperventilation. Affected neonates may also develop seizures, apnea, coma, and increased intracranial pressure unless hyperammonemia is diagnosed and treated promptly.

3. **Diagnosis.** In neonatal-onset UCDs, ammonia levels are usually higher than 300 μmol/L and are often in the range of 500 to 1,500 μmol/L. Respiratory alkalosis secondary to hyperventilation (ammonia stimulates the respiratory center) is an important initial clue for

Table 60.9. Differential Diagnosis of Hyperammonemia

Inborn Errors of Metabolism

- Urea cycle enzyme defects
  - □ N-Acetylglutamate synthase (NAGS) deficiency
  - □ Carbamoyl phosphate synthase 1 (CPS 1) deficiency
  - □ Ornithine transcarbamoylase (OTC) deficiency
  - □ Argininosuccinate synthase (ASS) deficiency (citrullinemia)
  - □ Argininosuccinate lyase (ASL) deficiency (argininosuccinic aciduria)
  - □ Arginase deficiency
- Transport defects of urea cycle intermediates
  - □ Mitochondrial ornithine transporter (HHH syndrome)
  - □ Aspartate–glutamate shuttle (citrin) deficiency
  - □ Lysinuric protein intolerance
- Organic acidemias
  - □ Propionic acidemia
  - □ Methylmalonic acidemia
  - □ Isovaleric acidemia
- Pyruvate carboxylase deficiency
- Fatty acid oxidation disorders
  - □ Very long chain acyl-coenzyme A dehydrogenase (VLCAD) deficiency
  - □ Carnitine transport defect
- Tyrosinemia type I
- Galactosemia
- Ornithine aminotransferase deficiency
- Hyperinsulinism-hyperammonemia syndrome
- Mitochondrial respirator chain defects

(continued)

Table 60.9. Differential Diagnosis of Hyperammonemia *(Continued)*

Acquired Disorders
▪ Transient hyperammonemia of the newborn
▪ Disorders of the liver and biliary tract
☐ Herpes simplex virus infection
☐ Biliary atresia
☐ Liver failure
☐ Vascular bypass of the liver (portosystemic shunt)
▪ Severe systemic neonatal illness
☐ Neonates sepsis
☐ Infection with urease-positive bacteria (with urinary tract stasis)
☐ Reye syndrome
▪ Medications (valproic acid, cyclophosphamide, 5-pentanoic acid, asparaginase)
▪ Technical
☐ Inappropriate sample (e.g., capillary blood)
☐ Sample not immediately analyzed
HHH, hyperornithinemia-hyperammonemia-homocitrullinuria.

the diagnosis of a UCD. Other laboratory abnormalities may include low blood urea nitrogen (BUN), mild/modestly elevated liver transaminases, and coagulopathy. Plasma amino acid analysis and urinary orotic acid can help in reaching the diagnosis (Fig. 60.4). The diagnosis is confirmed by enzyme assay and/or molecular genetic testing. Newborn screening programs that have expanded metabolic screening typically detect citrullinemia, argininosuccinic aciduria, and argininemia but *not* OTC or carbamoyl-phosphate synthetase (CPS) deficiencies.

4. **Acute management.** Prompt correction of hyperammonemia is critical to minimize neurologic injury:

a. Decreasing the production of ammonia from protein intake and breakdown. Suppression of catabolism can be achieved through the use of glucose infusion, insulin infusion, and intralipid administration. Protein intake can be completely restricted for 24 to 48 hours, followed by introducing an essential amino acid formula to maintain the appropriate levels of essential amino acids, which is necessary to reverse the catabolic state.

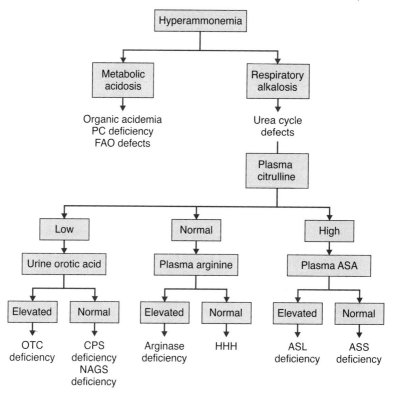

Figure 60.4. Approach to the investigation of neonatal hyperammonemia. FAO, fatty acid oxidation; PC, pyruvate carboxylase; OTC, ornithine transcarbamylase; CPS, carbamyl phosphate synthetase; NAGS, N-acetyl glutamate synthase; HHH, hyperornithinemia-hyperammonemia-homocitrullinuria; ASA, argininosuccinic acid; ASL, argininosuccinic acid lyase; ASS, argininosuccinic acid synthetase.

b. Removing ammonia. IV ammonia-scavenging drugs (Ammonul) should be started for ammonia levels above 300 μmol/L. Ammonul (sodium benzoate 100 mg/mL and sodium phenylacetate 100 mg/mL) is given as loading dose of 2.5 mL/kg in 25 mL/kg of 10% dextrose solution over a 60- to 120-minute period followed by the same dose over 24 hours as maintenance infusion. L-arginine hydrochloride is used with Ammonul as loading and maintenance as well. The L-arginine doses are 200 mg/kg for loading and similar dose for maintenance in CPS and OTC deficiencies and 600 mg/kg in argininosuccinate synthase (ASS) and argininosuccinate lyase (ASL) deficiencies. L-arginine hydrochloride is not used in arginase deficiency. A repeat loading dose of Ammonul can be given in neonates with severe illness not sooner than 24 hours of the first loading dose. Iatrogenic hypernatremia may be seen due to the high sodium load from Ammonul. Oral citrulline (170 mg/kg/day) should be given for OTC and CPS deficiencies. Hemodialysis/hemofiltration is the only method for rapid removal of ammonia from blood and should be considered if ammonia is very high (>500 mmol/L). However, while preparing for dialysis, the glucose, insulin, and ammonia scavenger therapy should be maintained. Hemodialysis is preferred over peritoneal dialysis because it is much more effective at removing ammonia.

    c. Reduce the risk for neurologic damage by avoiding fluid overload and treating seizures that can be subclinical.

  5. Long-term management. Maintenance therapy includes the following:

    a. Protein-restricted diet. After the patient is stabilized, enteral feeding should be started in consultation with a dietitian with expertise in managing UCDs. In general, infants require 1.2 to 2.0 g protein/kg with half of the required protein provided from essential amino acids formula and half from regular infant formula.

    b. Oral ammonia scavenger medications include sodium benzoate (250 to 400 mg/kg/day), sodium phenylbutyrate (250 to 500 mg/kg/day), and glycerol phenylbutyrate (Ravicti) (4.5 to 11.2 mL/M^2/day divided tid).

    c. Replacement of arginine (200 to 600 mg/kg/day for ASS and ASL deficiencies) and citrulline (100 to 200 mg/kg/day for OTC and CPS deficiencies)

    d. Carbamyl glutamate (Carbaglu) is a synthetic analogue for N-acetylglutamate, which is the natural activator of CPS. Therefore, Carbaglu may be effective in N-acetylglutamate synthase (NAGS) deficiency and can be tried in individuals with CPS deficiency.

    e. In children with severe types of UCDs, liver transplantation can be considered.

VI. INBORN ERROR OF METABOLISM WITH HYPOGLYCEMIA.
Hypoglycemia is a frequent finding in neonates. The suspicion of an IEM should be raised if it is severe and persistent without any other etiology (see Chapter 24). The presence or absence of ketosis can help in guiding the diagnostic workup (Fig. 60.5).

  A. Defects of fatty acid oxidation. FODs can present in neonatal period with hypoketotic hypoglycemia. The diagnosis is based on the abnormalities found in acylcarnitine profile (Table 60.10), enzyme studies, and molecular genetic testing. Expanded newborn screening programs detect most FODs.

    1. Long-chain FODs include very long chain acyl-coenzyme A dehydrogenase (VLCAD), long chain hydroxyacyl-coenzyme A dehydrogenase (LCHAD), trifunctional protein (TFP), and carnitine palmitoyltransferase (CPT2) deficiencies.

      a. Manifestations. Infants with the severe forms typically present in the first months of life with cardiomyopathy, arrhythmias, hypotonia, hepatomegaly, and hypoglycemia.

      b. Management. Hypoglycemia should be treated with glucose infusion and avoided by frequent feeding. Diet restrictions with a low-fat formula

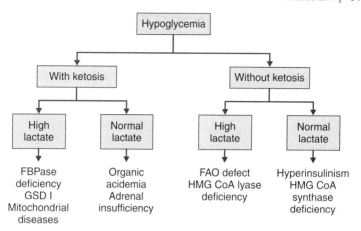

Figure 60.5. Approach to persistent hypoglycemia in the newborn with suspected inborn errors of metabolism. FAO, fatty acid oxidation; FBPase, fructose-1,6-bisphosphatase; GSD I, glycogen storage disease type I; HMG CoA, 3-hydroxy-3-methylglutaryl coenzyme A.

and supplemental MCTs should be initiated early. Cardiac dysfunction is reversible with early intensive supportive care and diet modification.

2. **MCAD deficiency**
   a. Manifestations. Infants with MCAD deficiency usually present between ages 3 and 24 months with hypoketotic hypoglycemia, vomiting, hepatomegaly elevated hepatic transaminases, lethargy, and seizures. Sudden and unexplained death can be the first manifestation of MCAD deficiency.
   b. Management. Hypoglycemia should be treated with glucose infusion and avoided by frequent feeding. Uncooked cornstarch also can be used to prevent the hypoglycemia.

B. **Disorders of ketone body metabolism.** Ketone bodies (acetoacetate and β-hydroxybutyrates) are important fuel for many tissues during fasting. Ketone bodies are synthesized via the enzymes 3-hydroxy-3-methylglutaryl coenzyme A (HMG-CoA) synthase and lyase, whereas succinyl-coenzyme A oxoacid coenzyme A transferase (SCOT) and β-ketothiolase catabolize ketone bodies (Fig. 60.6). Disorders of ketone body synthesis (ketogenesis) typically with hypoketotic hypoglycemia. On the other hand, disorders of ketone body degradation (ketolysis) present with recurrent episodes of severe ketoacidosis.

1. **HMG-CoA synthase deficiency**
   a. Manifestations. HMG-CoA synthase deficiency can present in infancy with hypoketotic hypoglycemia precipitated by acute illness. Blood lactate and ammonia concentrations were normal, and urine was negative for ketone bodies.

Table 60.10. Acylcarnitine Profile in Fatty Acid Oxidation Defects

Fatty Acid Oxidation Defect	Acylcarnitine Profile
Very long chain acyl-CoA dehydrogenase (VLCAD) deficiency	Elevated: C16 (hexadecanoylcarnitine) C14 (tertadecanoylcarnitine) C14:1 (tetradecenoylcarnitine) C12 (dodecanoylcarnitine)
Medium-chain acyl-CoA dehydrogenase (MCAD) deficiency	Elevated: C6 (hexanoylcarnitine) C8 (octanoylcarnitine) C10 (decanoylcarnitine) C10:1 (decenoylcarnitine)
Short chain acyl-CoA dehydrogenase (SCAD) deficiency	Elevated: C4 (butyrylcarnitine)
Long chain hydroxyacyl-CoA dehydrogenase (LCHAD) deficiency	Elevated: C14OH (hydroxytetradecenoylcarnitine) C16OH (hydroxyhexadecanoylcarnitine) C18OH (hydroxystearoylcarnitine) C18:1OH (hydroxyoleylcarnitine)
Carnitine palmitoyltransferase I (CPTI) deficiency	Elevated total carnitine Decreased: C16 (hexadecanoylcarnitine) C18 (octadecanoylcarnitine) C18:1 (octadecenoylcarnitine)
Carnitine palmitoyltransferase II (CPTII) deficiency	Decreased total carnitine Elevated: C16 (hexadecanoylcarnitine) C18:1 (octadecenoylcarnitine)
Carnitine transport defect	Decreased total carnitine
CoA, coenzyme A.	

    b. Diagnosis. Urine organic acid analysis shows dicarboxylic aciduria without ketosis. The diagnosis can be confirmed molecularly by genetic testing.
    c. Management. Hypoglycemia should be treated with glucose infusion and avoided by frequent feeding.

  2. HMG-CoA lyase deficiency
    a. Manifestations. Some affected individuals with HMG-CoA lyase present during the first week of life with vomiting, hypotonia, lethargy, hepatomegaly, hypoketotic hypoglycemia, abnormal liver function tests, elevated lactate, acidosis, and hyperammonemia.

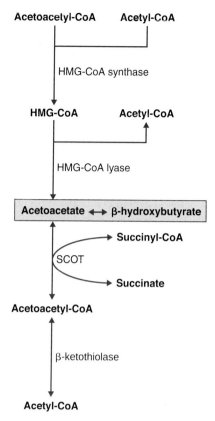

Figure 60.6. Ketone bodies (acetoacetate and β-hydroxybutyrates) synthesis and degradation. HMG-CoA. 3-hydroxy-3-methylglutaryl coenzyme A; SCOT, succinyl-coenzyme A oxoacid coenzyme A transferase.

b. Diagnosis. Urine organic acid analysis shows 3-hydroxy-3-methylglutarate (HMG) and methylglutaconate. The diagnosis can be confirmed molecularly by genetic testing. Expanded newborn screening detects this condition.

c. Management. Hypoglycemia should be treated with glucose infusion and acidosis by sodium bicarbonate infusion. Carnitine is also used. Long-term management include avoid fasting, carnitine, and low-fat protein-restricted diet.

C. **Fructose-1,6-bisphosphatase deficiency.** Deficiency of fructose-1,6-bisphosphatase (FBPase), a key enzyme in gluconeogenesis, impairs the formation of glucose.

1. **Manifestations.** Infants with FBPase deficiency can present during the first week of life with lactic acidosis, hypoglycemia, ketosis, hepatomegaly, seizures, irritability, lethargy, hypotonia, apnea, and coma.

2. **Diagnosis.** Diagnosis is confirmed by enzyme assay and molecular genetic testing.

3. **Management.** The acute presentation can be treated with glucose infusion and bicarbonate to control hypoglycemia and acidosis. Maintenance therapy aims at avoiding fasting by frequent feeding and uncooked starch use. Restriction of fructose and sucrose is also recommended.

D. **Glycogen storage disease type I (GSD I).** GSD I is caused by the deficiency of glucose-6-phosphatase (G6Pase) activity.

1. **Manifestations.** Some neonates with GSD I present with severe hypoglycemia; however, the common age of presentation is 3 to 4 months with hypoglycemia, lactic acidosis, hepatomegaly, hyperuricemia, hyperlipidemia, growth failure, and hypoglycemic seizures. Hypoglycemia and lactic acidosis can develop after a short fast (2 to 4 hours).

2. **Diagnosis.** Diagnosis can be confirmed by enzyme assay and molecular genetic testing.

3. **Management.** The acute presentation should be treated with glucose infusion and bicarbonate to control the hypoglycemia and the acidosis. Maintenance therapy aims to maintain normal glucose levels by frequent feeding, the use of uncooked starch, and intragastric continuous feeding if needed. The diet should be low in fat, sucrose, and fructose and high in complex carbohydrate.

VII. INBORN ERROR OF METABOLISM WITH NEONATAL SEIZURES. The possibility of IEMs should always be considered in neonates with unexplained and refractory seizures (Table 60.1).

A. **Biotinidase deficiency**

1. Biotinidase is essential for the recycling of the vitamin biotin, which is a cofactor for several essential carboxylase enzymes.

2. **Manifestations.** Untreated children with profound biotinidase deficiency usually present between ages 1 week and 10 years with seizures, hypotonia, metabolic acidosis, elevated lactate, hyperammonemia, and cutaneous symptoms, including skin rash, alopecia, and recurrent viral or fungal infections.

3. **Diagnosis.** The diagnosis is established by assessing the biotinidase enzyme activity in blood. Molecular genetic test can also be performed. Newborn screening detects biotinidase deficiency.

4. **Management.** Acute metabolic decompensation can be treated by glucose and sodium bicarbonate infusions. Symptoms typically improve with biotin (5 to 10 mg oral daily) treatment. Children with biotinidase deficiency who are diagnosed before developing symptoms (e.g., by newborn screening) and who are treated with biotin do not develop any manifestations.

B. **Pyridoxine-dependent epilepsy**

1. Pyridoxine-dependent epilepsy is an autosomal recessive disorder that occurs due to the deficiency of the enzyme antiquitin in the lysine

metabolism pathway. Antiquitin functions as a piperideine-6-carboxylate (P6C)/α-aminoadipic semialdehyde (AASA) dehydrogenase; therefore, its deficiency results in the accumulation of AASA and P6C. The latter binds and inactivates pyridoxal phosphate, which is a cofactor in neurotransmitters metabolism.

2. Manifestations. Newborns with pyridoxine-dependent epilepsy present soon after birth with irritability, lethargy, hypotonia, poor feeding, and seizures that are typically prolonged with recurrent episodes of status epilepticus.

3. Diagnosis. The diagnosis is established clinically by showing a response to pyridoxine. Administering 100 mg of pyridoxine IV while monitoring the electroencephalogram (EEG) can result in cessation of the clinical seizures with corresponding EEG changes generally over a period of several minutes; however, delayed responses have been described. If a clinical response is not demonstrated, the dose can be repeated up to 500 mg. Oral pyridoxine (30 mg/kg/day) can result in cessation of the seizures within 3 to 5 days. The diagnosis can be confirmed biochemically by demonstrating high levels of pipecolic acid, ASAA, and P6C and by molecular genetic testing.

4. Management. In general, seizures are controlled with 50 to 100 mg of pyridoxine daily.

C. Pyridoxal phosphate-responsive epilepsy

1. Pyridoxal phosphate-responsive epilepsy is an autosomal recessive disorder that results from deficiency of pyridox(am)ine phosphate oxidase (PNPO), an enzyme that interconverts the phosphorylated forms of pyridoxine and pyridoxamine to the biologically active pyridoxal phosphate.

2. Manifestations. Neonates with pyridoxal phosphate-responsive epilepsy typically present during the first day of life with lethargy, hypotonia, and refractory seizures that are not responsive to pyridoxine.

3. Diagnosis. Diagnosis is established by the demonstration of cessation of seizures with pyridoxal phosphate administration (50 mg orally) with corresponding EEG changes usually within an hour. Glycine and threonine are elevated in plasma and cerebrospinal fluid (CSF), whereas monoamine metabolites and pyridoxal phosphate are low in CSF. Molecular genetic testing is available.

4. Management. Seizures can usually be controlled with pyridoxal phosphate 30 to 50 mg/kg/day divided in four doses.

D. Glycine encephalopathy (nonketotic hyperglycinemia)

1. Glycine encephalopathy is an autosomal recessive disorder that occurs due to the deficiency of glycine cleavage enzyme system resulting in defective glycine degradation and glycine accumulation in tissues.

2. Manifestations. Individuals with neonatal form of glycine encephalopathy present with lethargy, hypotonia, poor feeding, seizures, and apnea within a few days of birth. EEG shows a characteristic burst-suppression pattern. Many infants die within a few weeks of life, typically from apnea; survivors develop profound psychomotor retardation. In transient glycine encephalopathy, which is secondary to the immaturity of glycine cleavage enzymes, laboratory and clinical abnormalities return to normal by 2 to 8 weeks of age.

3. Diagnosis. Biochemical diagnosis is based on the demonstration of elevated plasma glycine levels and the CSF-to-plasma glycine ratio (samples of plasma and CSF should be obtained around the same time for accurate calculation of the ratio). Enzyme assay and molecular genetic testing can be used to confirm the diagnosis.

4. Management. There is no known effective treatment for glycine encephalopathy. Sodium benzoate (250 to 750 mg/kg/day) can be used to reduce glycine levels. The N-methyl-D-aspartate (NMDA) receptor antagonists dextromethorphan, memantine, ketamine, and felbamate can be used in an attempt to block the neuroexcitatory effects of glycine on NMDA receptors and possibly improve seizure control. However, these treatments have been of limited benefit to the ultimate neurodevelopmental outcome.

E. Sulfite oxidase deficiency and molybdenum cofactor deficiency

1. Sulfite oxidase deficiency is an autosomal recessive disorder due to deficiency of sulfite oxidase enzyme. Molybdenum is a cofactor for both sulfite oxidase and xanthine oxidase.

2. Manifestations. Sulfite oxidase and molybdenum cofactor deficiencies can present with neonatal seizures, lethargy, microcephaly, and progressive psychomotor retardation.

3. Diagnosis. The biochemical diagnosis is established by the demonstration of elevated sulfocysteine in urine and decreased homocysteine and cysteine in plasma. In addition, serum uric acid is low in molybdenum cofactor deficiency. Enzyme studies and molecular genetic testing are available for diagnosis confirmation.

4. Management. There is no known effective treatment.

F. Purine metabolism disorders. Purine nucleotides are essential cellular constituents, which intervene in energy transfer, metabolic regulation, and synthesis of DNA and RNA. Some disorders of purine metabolism can present with neonatal seizures.

1. Adenylosuccinate lyase deficiency. Adenylosuccinate lyase (ADSL) catalyzes two steps in purine synthesis the conversion of succinylaminoimidazole carboxamide ribotide (SAICAR) to AICAR and that of adenylosuccinate (S-AMP) to AMP.

a. Manifestations. ADSL can present in intractable seizures starting within the first days to weeks of life. Other manifestations include hypotonia, microcephaly, psychomotor retardation, and brain atrophy, hypomyelination, and cerebellar atrophy in brain imaging.

b. Diagnosis. Biochemical diagnosis is based on the presence of SAICAR and succinyladenosine in CSF and urine. Diagnosis can be confirmed by enzyme assay and molecular genetic testing.

c. Management. There is no known effective treatment.

VIII. INBORN ERROR OF METABOLISM WITH HYPOTONIA.
Hypotonia is a common symptom in sick neonates. Some IEMs can present predominantly as hypotonia in the neonatal period (Table 60.1).

A. Mitochondrial diseases

1. The principal function of mitochondria is to produce adenosine triphosphate (ATP) from the oxidation of fatty acids and sugars through the electron transport chain. Therefore, tissues that are more dependent on aerobic metabolism, such as brain, muscle, and heart, are more likely to be affected in these disorders.

2. **Manifestations.** Manifestations of mitochondrial diseases can start at any age. Neonates with mitochondrial diseases can present with apnea, lethargy, coma, seizures, hypotonia, spasticity, muscle weakness and atrophy, cardiomyopathy, renal tubulopathy, hepatomegaly, liver dysfunction or failure, lactic acidosis, hypoglycemia, anemia, neutropenia, and pancytopenia. Some infants with mitochondrial diseases display a cluster of clinical features that fall into a discrete clinical syndrome (Table 60.11); however, there is often considerable clinical variability, and many affected individuals do not fit into one particular syndrome.

3. **Diagnosis.** The diagnosis of mitochondrial disorders can be challenging. Biochemical abnormalities in mitochondrial diseases may include lactic acidosis, ketosis, and elevated tricarboxylic acid cycle intermediates in urine organic acid analysis. The histology of affected muscles in older individuals may show ragged red fibers that represent peripheral and intermyofibrillar accumulation of abnormal mitochondria, but this finding is rare in neonates and young children. The enzymatic activity of respiratory chain complexes can be assessed on skeletal muscle, skin fibroblast, or liver tissue, but this may be nondiagnostic. Molecular testing for mitochondrial DNA content and sequencing for mitochondrial DNA and known mitochondrial-related nuclear DNA genes is the preferred mode of testing due to limitations of biochemical and histologic analyses.

4. **Management.** Currently, there are no satisfactory therapies available for the vast majority of mitochondrial disorders. Treatment remains largely symptomatic and does not significantly alter the course of the disease.

B. Zellweger syndrome

1. Zellweger syndrome is a disorder of peroxisomal biogenesis. Peroxisomes are cell organelles that possess anabolic and catabolic functions, including synthesizing plasmalogens, which are important constituents of cell membranes and myelin, β-oxidation of very long chain fatty acids (VLCFAs), oxidation of phytanic acid, and formation of bile acids.

2. **Manifestations.** Neonates with Zellweger syndrome typically present with severe weakness and hypotonia, poor feeding, widely split sutures, seizures, hepatomegaly, jaundice, elevated transaminases, short proximal limbs, stippled epiphyses, and distinctive facial features (Table 60.5).

Table 60.11. Mitochondrial Syndromes Associated with Neonatal Presentation

Barth syndrome

- Hypertrophic cardiomyopathy
- Skeletal myopathy
- Neutropenia
- Affects male individuals (X-linked)

Pearson syndrome

- Sideroblastic anemia
- Neutropenia
- Thrombocytopenia
- Exocrine pancreatic dysfunction
- Renal tubulopathy

Hepatocerebral mitochondrial DNA depletion syndromes

- Hepatic dysfunction or failure
- Hypotonia
- Seizures
- Lactic acidosis
- Hypoglycemia

Transient infantile liver failure due to mitochondrial translation defect (*TRMU* mutation)

- Hepatic dysfunction or failure
- Hepatomegaly
- Poor feeding and vomiting
- Lactic acidosis
- Hypotonia
- Liver functions return to normal after 3 to 4 months

3. Diagnosis. Biochemical abnormalities include elevated phytanic acid and VLCFAs and low plasmalogens. Many proteins are involved in peroxisomal biogenesis. Therefore, complementation analyses allow the determination of which protein is defective, and molecular genetic analysis for the responsible gene can be performed for molecular confirmation.

4. Management. There is no effective treatment, and management is largely symptomatic.

IX. INBORN ERROR OF METABOLISM WITH LIVER DYSFUNCTION. Several IEMs can have hepatic manifestations in the neonatal period (Table 60.2). Galactosemia is the most common metabolic cause of liver disease in neonates. Some mitochondrial diseases can present with hepatopathy in neonatal period (Table 60.11).

A. **Galactosemia** (see Chapter 26)

1. Galactosemia is an autosomal recessive disease due to deficiency of galactose-1-phosphate uridyltransferase (GALT) which functions in the catabolic pathway of galactose.

2. **Manifestations.** Typical symptoms of galactosemia in the newborn develop after ingestion of lactose (glucose–galactose disaccharide) through a standard lactose-containing formulas or breast milk. Clinical manifestations include vomiting, diarrhea, feeding difficulties, failure to thrive, hypoglycemia, jaundice, hepatomegaly, elevated transaminases, coagulopathy, ascites, liver failure, renal tubulopathy, lethargy, irritability, seizures, cataracts, and increased risk of *Escherichia coli* neonatal sepsis.

3. **Diagnosis.** The biochemical profile of galactosemia includes elevated galactose in plasma, galactose-1-phosphate in red blood cells, and galactitol in urine. Diagnosis is confirmed by enzyme assay and molecular genetic testing. All newborn screening programs screen for galactosemia.

4. **Management.** Lactose-free formula should be started during the first 3 to 10 days of life for optimal results.

B. **Hereditary fructose intolerance**

1. Hereditary fructose intolerance is an autosomal recessive disorder due to deficiency of fructose-1,6-biphosphate aldolase (aldolase B) which in part of the catabolic pathway of fructose.

2. **Manifestations.** Clinical manifestations develop when the neonate is exposed to fructose from the sucrose (glucose–fructose disaccharide) in soy-based formulas or later at weaning when the infant is exposed to fructose from fruits and vegetables. Early manifestations include vomiting, hypoglycemia, irritability, seizures, lethargy, coma, hepatomegaly, jaundice, elevated transaminases, coagulopathy, edema, ascites, liver failure, and renal tubulopathy.

3. **Diagnosis.** Diagnosis is established by enzyme assay and molecular genetic testing.

4. **Management.** Management is based on elimination of sucrose, fructose, and sorbitol from the diet.

C. **Tyrosinemia type I**

1. Tyrosinemia type I is an autosomal recessive disorder due to deficiency of fumarylacetoacetate hydrolase, which functions in the catalytic pathway of tyrosine.

2. **Manifestations.** Tyrosinemia type I can present in early infancy with vomiting, diarrhea, hypoglycemia, septicemia, hepatomegaly, elevated transaminases, jaundice, coagulopathy, ascites, liver failure, renal tubulopathy, and abnormal odor (Table 60.4).

3. **Diagnosis.** Biochemical abnormalities include elevated urine succinylacetone and tyrosine metabolites (p-hydroxyphenylpyruvate, p-hydroxyphenyllactate, and p-hydroxyphenylacetate) and elevated plasma tyrosine and methionine. Serum α-fetoprotein is markedly elevated. Diagnosis can be confirmed by enzyme assay and molecular genetic testing. Newborn screening programs may screen for tyrosine and/or succinylacetone in the bloodspot to diagnose tyrosinemia; however, many cases may be missed when the screening uses tyrosine alone.

4. **Management.** NTCB (1 to 2 mg/kg/day divided in two doses) and tyrosine-restricted diet are effective at preventing symptoms if instituted early in life.

D. **Neonatal intrahepatic cholestasis caused by citrin deficiency**

1. Neonatal intrahepatic cholestasis caused by citrin deficiency (NICCD) is an autosomal recessive disorder due to deficiency of citrin which is a mitochondrial aspartate–glutamate carrier (Fig. 60.3).

2. **Manifestations.** NICCD can present in the neonatal period with transient intrahepatic cholestasis, prolonged jaundice, hepatomegaly, elevated transaminases, hypoproteinemia, coagulopathy, growth failure, hemolytic anemia, and hypoglycemia. NICCD is generally not severe, and most symptoms disappear by age 1 year with appropriate treatment.

3. **Diagnosis.** Biochemical abnormalities include elevated plasma citrulline, arginine, methionine, tyrosine lysine, and increased threonine:serine ratio. Molecular genetic testing is available. Elevated citrulline on newborn screening may lead to the diagnosis.

4. **Management.** Management includes the supplementation of fat-soluble vitamins and the use of lactose-free formula and high MCTs. Subsequently, a diet rich in lipids and protein and low in carbohydrates is recommended.

X. INBORN ERROR OF METABOLISM WITH CARDIOMYOPATHY. Some metabolic disorders can present predominantly with cardiomyopathy (Table 60.3).

A. **Glycogen storage disease type II (Pompe disease)**

1. Glycogen storage disease type II (GSD II) is caused by the deficiency of the lysosomal enzyme acid α-glucosidase (GAA, acid maltase). The enzyme defect results in the accumulation of glycogen within the lysosomes in different organs.

2. **Manifestations.** Infants with the classic infantile-onset GSD II typically present in the first 2 months of life with hypotonia, muscle weakness,

hepatomegaly, hypertrophic cardiomyopathy, feeding difficulties, failure to thrive, macroglossia, respiratory distress, and hearing loss.

3. **Diagnosis.** Nonspecific tests supporting the diagnosis include elevated serum creatinine kinase level and urinary oligosaccharides. The diagnosis is confirmed by enzyme assay and molecular genetic testing.

4. **Management.** Enzyme replacement therapy using alglucosidase alfa (Myozyme) should be initiated as soon as the diagnosis is established. The response to enzyme replacement therapy is better for those in whom the therapy is initiated before age 6 months and before the need for ventilatory assistance.

XI. POSTMORTEM DIAGNOSIS.
If an infant is dying or has died of what may be a metabolic disease, it is important to make a specific diagnosis in order to help the parents with genetic counseling for future reproductive planning. Sometimes, families that will not permit a full autopsy will allow the collection of some premortem or immediately postmortem specimens that may help in diagnosis. Specimens that should be collected include the following:

A. **Blood**, both clotted and heparinized. The specimen should be centrifuged and the plasma frozen. Lymphocytes may be saved for culture.

B. **Urine**, frozen

C. **Cerebrospinal fluid**, frozen

D. **Skin biopsy** for fibroblast culture to be used for DNA analysis or enzyme assay. Two samples should be taken from a well-perfused area in the torso. The skin should be well cleaned, but any residual cleaning solution should be washed off with sterile water. The skin can be placed briefly in sterile saline until special media are available.

E. **Liver and/or muscle biopsy samples**, both premortem samples and generous-size postmortem samples, should be flash-frozen to preserve enzyme integrity as well as tissue histology.

F. **Others.** Depending on the nature of the disease, other tissues such as cardiac muscle, brain, and kidney should be preserved. Photographs can be taken as well as a full skeletal radiologic screening for infants with dysmorphic features. A full autopsy should be done if permitted.

XII. ROUTINE NEWBORN SCREENING.
Each state in the United States mandates the disorders evaluated in its own newborn screening program. Recent advances have enabled tandem mass spectrometry (MS/MS) to be applied to the newborn screening specimen. This technique is currently being used in all states to offer screening for many treatable IEMs. A list of what each state screens for may be found on the individual state governmental website or in aggregate on the national newborn screening and genetic resource center website (http://genes-r-us.uthscsa.edu/). Very useful information for follow-up of newborn screening ("ACT Sheets") and for confirmation of a disorder identified by newborn screening ("Algorithms") is available on the website of the American College of Medical Genetics: http://www.acmg.net/resources/policies/ACT/condition-analyte-links.htm. Table 60.12 includes the newborn screen analytes and the suspected diagnoses with each analyte.

Table 60.12. Newborn Screen Primary Analytes and the Suspected Diagnoses

Analyte	Condition
Biotinidase enzyme	Biotinidase deficiency
Elevated galactose and/or deficient GALT enzyme	Classical galactosemia
Elevated galactose and normal GALT	Galactokinase deficiency Galactose epimerase deficiency
C0	Carnitine transport defect
C0; C0/C16 + C18	Carnitine palmitoyltransferase I (CPT I) deficiency
C3	Methylmalonic acidemias Propionic acidemia
C3DC	Malonic acidemia
C4	Short chain acyl-CoA dehydrogenase (SCAD) deficiency Ethylmalonic encephalopathy Isobutyryl-CoA dehydrogenase deficiency
C4OH	Medium/short chain hydroxyacyl-CoA dehydrogenase (M/SCHAD) deficiency
C4, C5	Glutaric acidemia 2 Ethylmalonic encephalopathy
C5	Isovaleric acidemia Short/branched-chain acyl-CoA dehydrogenase deficiency
C5DC	Glutaric acidemia type I
C5OH	Beta-ketothiolase deficiency Biotinidase deficiency Holocarboxylase deficiency HMG-CoA lyase deficiency Methylcrotonyl-CoA carboxylase (MCC) deficiency
C8, C6, C10	Medium-chain acyl-CoA dehydrogenase (MCAD) deficiency
C14:1	Very long chain acyl-CoA dehydrogenase (VLCAD) deficiency
C16 and/or C18:1	Carnitine palmitoyltransferase II (CPT II) deficiency
	(continued)

Table 60.12. *(Continued)*

Analyte	Condition
C16OH ± C18:1-OH	Long chain hydroxyacyl-CoA dehydrogenase (LCHAD) deficiency Trifunctional protein (TFP) deficiency
Arginine	Argininemia
Citrulline	Argininosuccinate lyase deficiency (argininosuccinic aciduria) Argininosuccinate synthetase deficiency (citrullinemia I) Citrin deficiency (citrullinemia II) Pyruvate carboxylase deficiency
Methionine	Homocystinuria Hypermethioninemia Glycine N-methyltransferase (GNMT) deficiency Adenosylhomocysteine hydrolase deficiency
Leucine	Maple syrup urine disease (MSUD) Hydroxyprolinuria
Phenylalanine	Phenylketonuria (PKU) Biopterin cofactor metabolism defect
Elevated tyrosine and normal succinylacetone	Tyrosinemia II Tyrosinemia III
Tyrosine normal/elevated and succinylacetone elevated	Tyrosinemia I

GALT, galactose-1-phosphate uridyltransferase; DC, dicarboxylic; CoA, coenzyme A; HMG-CoA, 3-hydroxy-3-methylglutaryl coenzyme A.

Suggested Readings

Ah Mew N, Lanpher BC, Gropman A, et al. Urea cycle disorders overview. In: Pagon RA, Adam MP, Ardinger HH, et al, eds. *GeneReviews*. Seattle, WA: University of Washington; 1993–2016. http://www.ncbi.nlm.nih.gov/books/NBK1217/. Accessed March 31, 2016.

Chinnery PF. Mitochondrial disorders overview. In: Pagon RA, Adam MP, Ardinger HH, et al, eds. *GeneReviews*. Seattle, WA: University of Washington; 1993–2016. http://www.ncbi.nlm.nih.gov/books/NBK1224/. Accessed March 31, 2016.

Seashore MR. The organic acidemias: an overview. In: Pagon RA, Adam MP, Ardinger HH, et al, eds. *GeneReviews*. Seattle, WA: University of Washington; 1993–2016. http://www.ncbi.nlm.nih.gov/books/NBK1134/. Accessed March 31, 2016.

61

Thyroid Disorders

Ari J. Wassner and Mandy Brown Belfort

KEY POINTS

- Fetal and neonatal hyperthyroidism occurs in approximately 1% to 2% of infants born to mothers with Graves' disease.
- Women with preexisting hypothyroidism who are treated appropriately typically deliver healthy infants.
- Congenital hypothyroidism is one of the most common preventable causes of intellectual disability.
- Neonatal hyperthyroidism is uncommon (accounting for ~1% of hyperthyroidism in children) and is almost always transient.

I. **THYROID PHYSIOLOGY IN PREGNANCY.** Multiple changes occur in maternal thyroid physiology during normal pregnancy.

   A. **Increased iodine clearance.** Starting early in pregnancy, increased renal blood flow and glomerular filtration lead to increased clearance of iodine from maternal plasma. Iodine is also transported across the placenta to enable iodothyronine synthesis by the fetal thyroid gland, which begins after the first trimester. These processes increase the maternal dietary requirement for iodine but have little impact on maternal plasma iodine concentration or on maternal or fetal thyroid function in iodine-sufficient regions such as the United States. In contrast, in regions with insufficient iodine intake, increased iodine clearance and transplacental transfer may lead to decreased thyroxine (T_4), increased thyroid-stimulating hormone (TSH), and increased thyroid gland volume in both mother and fetus. To ensure adequate intake, supplementation with 150 µg of iodine per day is recommended for all pregnant and lactating women; of note, many prenatal vitamins lack iodine.

   B. **Human chorionic gonadotropin (hCG) has weak intrinsic TSH-like activity.** The high circulating level of hCG in the first trimester leads to a slight, transient increase in free T_4 accompanied by partial suppression of TSH that resolve by approximately the 14th week of gestation.

   C. **Increased thyroxine-binding globulin (TBG) levels** occur early in pregnancy. TBG doubles by midgestation and then plateaus at a high level. This rise in TBG results largely from diminished hepatic clearance of TBG due to increased estrogen-stimulated sialylation of the TBG protein. Estrogen also stimulates TBG synthesis in the liver.

D. **Increased total triiodothyronine (T_3) and T_4 levels** occur early in gestation due to rapidly increasing TBG levels (see section I.C). Free T_4 levels rise much less than total T_4 in early pregnancy (see section I.B), then decline progressively in the second and third trimesters. This physiologic decline is minimal (<10%) in iodine-sufficient regions but may be more pronounced in regions with borderline or deficient iodine intake. Assays that directly measure free T_4 may be affected by changes in TBG and should be used to monitor maternal thyroid function only if assay-specific and trimester-specific normal ranges are available; otherwise, an assay of total T_4 should be used.

E. **TSH levels decline in the first trimester** in the setting of elevated levels of hCG (see section I.B) and may transiently fall below the normal range for nonpregnant women in approximately 20% of healthy pregnancies. After the first trimester, TSH levels return to the normal, nonpregnant range.

F. **The negative feedback control mechanisms of the hypothalamic-pituitary-thyroid (HPT) axis** remain intact throughout pregnancy.

G. **Placental metabolism and transplacental passage.** Iodine and thyrotropin-releasing hormone (TRH) freely cross the placenta. The placenta is also permeable to antithyroid drugs and to TSH receptor-stimulating and -blocking immunoglobulin G (IgG) antibodies, but it is impermeable to TSH. T_4 crosses the placenta in limited amounts due to inactivation by the placental enzyme type 3 deiodinase (D3), which converts T_4 to inactive reverse T_3. T_3 is similarly inactivated by placental D3 and has minimal transplacental passage. In the setting of fetal hypothyroxinemia, maternal-fetal transfer of T_4 is increased, particularly in the second and third trimesters, which helps protect the developing fetus from the effects of fetal hypothyroidism.

II. MATERNAL HYPERTHYROIDISM. Hyperthyroidism complicates 0.1% to 1% of pregnancies.

A. **Graves' disease** accounts for ≥85% of clinical hyperthyroidism in pregnancy. Hyperemesis gravidarum is associated with transient subclinical or mild hyperthyroidism that may be due to the TSH-like effects of hCG and typically resolves without treatment.

B. **Signs and symptoms of hyperthyroidism** may include tachycardia, palpitations, increased appetite, tremor, anxiety, and fatigue. The presence of goiter, ophthalmopathy, or myxedema suggests Graves' disease.

C. **Poorly controlled maternal hyperthyroidism is associated with serious pregnancy complications** including spontaneous abortion, preterm delivery, intrauterine growth restriction, fetal demise, preeclampsia, placental abruption, thyroid storm, and congestive heart failure.

D. **Treatment** of maternal hyperthyroidism substantially reduces the risk of associated maternal and fetal complications.

1. **Antithyroid drugs** are indicated for the treatment of **moderate-to-severe hyperthyroidism**. In the first trimester, propylthiouracil (PTU) rather than methimazole (MMI) is recommended due to possible teratogenic effects of MMI, which has been associated with aplasia cutis

congenita, tracheoesophageal fistula, and choanal atresia. Although PTU has also been associated with congenital malformations such as face/neck cysts and urinary tract abnormalities, these are less common and generally less severe than those caused by MMI, and PTU remains the drug of choice in the first trimester. However, because PTU can cause severe maternal liver dysfunction, in the second trimester, PTU should be switched to MMI. Both MMI and PTU cross the placenta, and the fetus is more sensitive than the mother to the effects of antithyroid drugs, so fetal hypothyroidism and goiter can occur even with doses in the therapeutic range for the mother. Clinicians should use the lowest possible dose and monitor closely, aiming to maintain T_4 levels in the high-normal range and TSH levels in the low-normal or suppressed range. **Mild hyperthyroidism** can be monitored without treatment.

2. **β-Adrenergic blocking agents** such as propranolol may be useful in controlling hypermetabolic symptoms; however, long-term use should be avoided due to potential neonatal morbidities including hypotension, bradycardia, and impaired response to hypoglycemia.

3. **Surgical thyroidectomy** may be needed to control hyperthyroidism in women who cannot take antithyroid drugs due to allergy or agranulocytosis or in cases of maternal nonadherence to medical therapy. If thyroidectomy is necessary, it should be performed during the second trimester if possible, rather than in the first or third trimesters when risks to the fetus are higher.

4. **Iodine** given at a pharmacologic dose is generally contraindicated because prolonged administration can cause fetal hypothyroidism and goiter. However, a short course of iodine in preparation for thyroidectomy appears to be safe, and clinicians may also use iodine in selected cases in which antithyroid drugs cannot be used. **Radioactive iodine (RAI)** is contraindicated during pregnancy.

E. **Fetal and neonatal hyperthyroidism** occurs in approximately 1% to 2% of infants born to mothers with Graves' disease. In these cases, hyperthyroidism results from transplacental passage of TSH receptor-stimulating antibodies. High levels of these antibodies in maternal serum during the third trimester are predictive of fetal and neonatal hyperthyroidism, as is a maternal history of having a prior child with the condition. All pregnant women with Graves' disease should be monitored for fetal hyperthyroidism through serial measurement of fetal heart rate as well as prenatal ultrasound to assess for fetal goiter and to monitor fetal growth. Fetal hyperthyroidism can be treated by administration of antithyroid drugs to the mother, but excessive treatment can suppress the fetal thyroid gland and cause hypothyroidism.

F. **Fetal and neonatal hypothyroidism in maternal Graves' disease.** Fetal exposure to MMI or PTU can cause transient hypothyroidism that resolves rapidly and usually does not require treatment (see section VI.A.2.a). In mothers with a history of Graves' disease, transplacental passage of TSH receptor-blocking antibodies may cause fetal hypothyroidism (see section VI.A.2.e). A rare neonatal outcome of maternal Graves' disease is transient central hypothyroidism, which may be due to pituitary suppression from prolonged intrauterine hyperthyroidism.

G. **Infants of mothers with Graves' disease** can present with thyrotoxicosis or hypothyroidism in the newborn period and require close monitoring after birth (see section VII).

III. MATERNAL HYPOTHYROIDISM. Maternal hypothyroidism in pregnancy can be overt (0.3% to 0.5% of pregnancies) or subclinical (2% to 2.5% of pregnancies).

A. **The most common cause of maternal hypothyroidism** in iodine-sufficient regions is chronic autoimmune thyroiditis. Other causes include previous treatment of Graves' disease or thyroid cancer with surgical thyroidectomy or radioiodine ablation, drug- or radiation-induced hypothyroidism, congenital hypothyroidism (CH), and pituitary dysfunction. Chronic autoimmune thyroiditis is more common in patients with type 1 diabetes mellitus. Occasionally, mothers with a prior history of Graves' disease become hypothyroid due to the development of TSH receptor-blocking antibodies.

B. **Signs and symptoms of hypothyroidism in pregnancy** include weight gain, cold intolerance, dry skin, weakness, fatigue, and constipation. These may go unnoticed in the setting of pregnancy, particularly if hypothyroidism is mild.

C. **Unrecognized or untreated hypothyroidism** is associated with spontaneous abortion and maternal complications of pregnancy including anemia, preeclampsia, postpartum hemorrhage, placental abruption, and need for cesarean delivery. Associated adverse fetal and neonatal outcomes include preterm birth, intrauterine growth restriction, congenital anomalies, fetal distress in labor, and fetal and perinatal death. However, these complications are avoided with adequate treatment of hypothyroidism, ideally from early in pregnancy. **Affected fetuses may experience neurodevelopmental impairments, particularly if both the fetus and the mother are hypothyroid during gestation** (e.g., iodine deficiency, TSH receptor-blocking antibodies).

D. **Women with preexisting hypothyroidism who are treated appropriately typically deliver healthy infants.** Such patients should increase their usual L-thyroxine dose by 25% to 30% immediately upon missing a menstrual period or obtaining a positive result on a pregnancy test. Thyroid function tests should be measured as soon as pregnancy is confirmed, every 4 weeks during the first half of pregnancy, at least once between 26 and 32 weeks' gestation, and 4 weeks after any L-thyroxine dose change. The TSH level should be maintained in trimester-specific normal ranges of 0.1 to 2.5 mU/L in the first trimester, 0.2 to 3 mU/L in the second trimester, and 0.3 to 3 mU/L in the third trimester. Achieving this goal often requires an L-thyroxine dose of 20% to 50% higher than in the nonpregnant state.

E. **Routine thyroid function testing in pregnancy** is currently recommended only for women at high risk for hypothyroidism, including those who are symptomatic; older than 30 years; live in an iodine-deficient area; have a family or personal history of thyroid disease; or have a history of thyroperoxidase (TPO) antibodies, type 1 diabetes, neck irradiation, morbid obesity, infertility, miscarriage, or preterm delivery. Because this strategy detects only two-thirds of women with hypothyroidism, many authors advocate universal screening in early pregnancy, but this has not been shown to improve outcomes, and this topic remains controversial.

F. **TSH receptor-blocking antibodies** cross the placenta and may cause fetal and transient neonatal hypothyroidism (see section VI.A.2.e).

IV. FETAL AND NEONATAL GOITER

A. **Fetal ultrasound** by an experienced ultrasonographer is an excellent tool for intrauterine diagnosis and monitoring of fetal goiter.

B. **Maternal Graves' disease is the most common cause of fetal and neonatal goiter**, which results most often from fetal hypothyroidism due to MMI or PTU even when given at relatively low doses. Fetal and neonatal goiter can also result from fetal hyperthyroidism due to TSH receptor-stimulating antibodies. TSH receptor antibodies can be present both in women with active Graves' disease and in women previously treated for Graves' disease with surgical thyroidectomy or RAI ablation. Maternal history and serum antibody testing is usually diagnostic. Rarely, cord blood sampling is necessary to determine where fetal goiter is due to MMI- or PTU-induced fetal hypothyroidism or to fetal hyperthyroidism induced by TSH receptor-stimulating antibodies. After delivery, neonates exposed *in utero* to PTU or MMI eliminate the drug rapidly. Thyroid function tests usually normalize by 1 week of age, and treatment is not required.

C. **Other causes of fetal and neonatal goiter** include fetal disorders of thyroid hormonogenesis (usually inherited), excessive maternal iodine ingestion, and maternal iodine deficiency. All of these conditions are associated with fetal or neonatal hypothyroidism, and goiter resolves after normalization of the serum TSH concentration with L-thyroxine treatment.

D. **Fetal goiter due to hypothyroidism is usually treated with maternal L-thyroxine administration.** Rarely, treatment with intra-amniotic injections of L-thyroxine is used during the third trimester to reduce the size of a fetal goiter when needed to **prevent complications of tracheal/esophageal compression** including polyhydramnios, lung hypoplasia, and airway compromise at birth.

V. THYROID PHYSIOLOGY IN THE FETUS AND NEWBORN

A. The **fetal HPT axis** develops relatively independent of the mother due to the high placental expression of D3, which inactivates most of the T_4 and T_3 presented from the maternal circulation (see section I.G).

B. **Thyroid embryogenesis** is complete by 10 to 12 weeks' gestation by which time the fetal thyroid gland starts to concentrate iodine and synthesize and to secrete T_3 and T_4. Concentrations of T_4 and TBG increase gradually throughout gestation. Circulating T_3 levels remains low, although T_3 levels in the brain and pituitary are considerably higher due to local expression of type 2 deiodinase (D2), which converts T_4 to the active thyroid hormone, T_3. In the setting of fetal hypothyroidism, upregulation of D2 activity in the brain maintains the local T_3 concentration, allowing normal development to proceed.

C. TSH from the fetal pituitary gland increases beginning in midgestation. The **negative feedback mechanism of the HPT axis** starts to mature by 26 weeks' gestation. Circulating levels of TRH are high in the fetus relative to the mother, although the physiologic significance of this is unclear.

D. **Exogenous iodine suppresses thyroid hormone synthesis**, a property known as the Wolff-Chaikoff effect. However, the ability of the thyroid gland to escape from the suppressive effect of an iodine load does not mature until 36 to 40 weeks' gestation. Thus, premature infants are more susceptible than term infants to iodine-induced hypothyroidism.

E. **Neonatal physiology.** Within 30 minutes after delivery, there is a dramatic surge in serum TSH, with peak levels as high as 80 mU/L at 6 hours of life. TSH then declines rapidly over 24 hours, then more slowly over the first week of life. The TSH surge causes marked stimulation of the neonatal thyroid gland, leading to sharp increases in serum T_3 and T_4 levels, which peak within 24 hours of life and then slowly decline.

F. In the preterm infant, the pattern of postnatal thyroid hormone changes is similar to that seen in the term infant, but the TSH surge is less marked and the resulting T_4 and T_3 increases are blunted. In very preterm infants (<31 weeks' gestation), no TSH surge occurs, and circulating T_4 may fall rather than rise over the first 7 to 10 days. Thyroid hormone levels in umbilical cord blood are related to gestational age and birth weight (Table 61.1).

VI. CONGENITAL HYPOTHYROIDISM

A. CH is one of the **most common preventable causes of intellectual disability**. The incidence of CH varies globally. In the United States, the incidence is approximately 1/2,500 and appears to be rising. CH is more common among Hispanic (1/1,600) and Asian Indian (1/1,757) infants but less common among non-Hispanic black infants (1/11,000). The female-to-male ratio is 2:1. CH is also more common in infants with trisomy 21, congenital heart disease, and other congenital malformations including cleft palate and renal, skeletal, or gastrointestinal anomalies. CH may be permanent or transient. Hypothyroxinemia with delayed TSH rise can be caused by permanent or transient conditions.

1. Causes of **permanent CH** (see Table 61.2)
   a. **Thyroid dysgenesis.** Abnormal thyroid gland development is the cause of permanent CH in about 70% of cases. Thyroid dysgenesis includes agenesis, hypoplasia, and ectopy (failure to descend normally into the neck). It is almost always sporadic with no increased risk to subsequent siblings. Rarely, thyroid dysgenesis is associated with a mutation in one of the transcription factors necessary for thyroid gland development (*PAX8*, *FOXE1*, *NKX2.1*, *NKX2.5*). Clinically, infants with thyroid dysgenesis have no goiter, low total and free T_4 levels, elevated TSH, and normal TBG. The serum concentration of thyroglobulin (TG) reflects the amount of thyroid tissue present and is low in cases of thyroid agenesis or hypoplasia. Ultrasound confirms the presence or absence of a normally located thyroid gland, whereas scintigraphy with RAI or pertechnetate (^{99m}Tc) can locate a normally placed or ectopic gland that is able to concentrate iodine.

Table 61.1. Thyroid Hormone Reference Ranges (*M* ± *SD*) for Full-Term and Preterm Neonates

Gestational Age (Weeks)	Age			
	Birth	7 Days	14 Days	28 Days
Total T$_4$ (µg/dL)				
23–27	5.4 ± 2.0	4.0 ± 1.8	4.7 ± 2.6	6.1 ± 2.3
28–30	6.3 ± 2.0	6.3 ± 2.1	6.6 ± 2.3	7.5 ± 2.3
31–34	7.6 ± 2.3	9.4 ± 3.4	9.1 ± 3.6	8.9 ± 3.0
≥37	9.2 ± 1.9	12.7 ± 2.9	10.7 ± 1.4	9.7 ± 2.2
Free T$_4$ (ng/dL)				
23–27	1.3 ± 0.4	1.5 ± 0.6	1.4 ± 0.5	1.5 ± 0.4
28–30	1.4 ± 0.4	1.8 ± 0.7	1.6 ± 0.4	1.7 ± 0.4
31–34	1.5 ± 0.3	2.1 ± 0.6	2.0 ± 0.4	1.9 ± 0.5
≥37	1.4 ± 0.4	2.7 ± 0.6	2.0 ± 0.3	1.6 ± 0.3
Total T$_3$ (ng/dL)				
23–27	19.5 ± 14.9	32.6 ± 20.2	41.0 ± 24.7	63.1 ± 27.3
28–30	28.6 ± 20.8	56.0 ± 24.1	72.3 ± 28.0	87.2 ± 31.2
31–34	35.2 ± 23.4	91.8 ± 35.8	109.4 ± 41.0	119.8 ± 40.1
≥37	59.9 ± 34.5	147.8 ± 50.1	167.3 ± 31.2	175.8 ± 31.9
TSH (mU/L)				
23–27	6.8 ± 2.9	3.5 ± 2.6	3.9 ± 2.7	3.8 ± 4.7
28–30	7.0 ± 3.7	3.6 ± 2.5	4.9 ± 11.2	3.6 ± 2.5
31–34	7.9 ± 5.2	3.6 ± 4.8	3.8 ± 9.3	3.5 ± 3.4
≥37	6.7 ± 4.8	2.6 ± 1.8	2.5 ± 2.0	1.8 ± 0.9
TBG (mg/dL)				
23–27	0.19 ± 0.06	0.17 ± 0.04	0.19 ± 0.05	0.23 ± 0.06
28–30	0.20 ± 0.05	0.20 ± 0.05	0.21 ± 0.05	0.22 ± 0.06
31–34	0.24 ± 0.08	0.24 ± 0.08	0.23 ± 0.08	0.23 ± 0.08
≥37	0.29 ± 0.06	0.34 ± 0.11	0.28 ± 0.04	0.27 ± 0.07

TSH, thyroid-stimulating hormone; TBG, thyroxine-binding globulin.
Source: Adapted from Williams FL, Simpson J, Delahunty C, et al. Developmental trends in cord and postpartum serum thyroid hormones in preterm infants. *J Clin Endocrinol Metab* 2004;89(11):5314–5320.

Table 61.2. Interpretation of Thyroid Function Tests and Imaging Results in Congenital Hypothyroidism and Related Disorders

Cause of Hypothyroidism	Total T$_4$	Free T$_4$	TSH	TG	Thyroid Imaging	Treatment	Comments
Permanent							
Dysgenesis	↓	↓	↑	↓	Absent, small, or ectopic	Yes	Almost always sporadic
Dyshormonogenesis	↓	↓	↑	*	Normal or large	Yes	Usually autosomal recessive
TSH resistance	Normal or ↓	Normal or ↓	↑	↓	Normal or small	Depends on severity	Autosomal dominant or recessive
Central hypothyroidism	↓	↓	Normal or ↓	↓	Normal	Yes	Not detected on primary TSH NB screen; usually have other pituitary hormone deficiencies
Transient							
Maternal antithyroid medication (MMI, PTU)	↓	↓	↑	Normal or ↑	Normal or large	Not usually	Resolves within 1 week
TSH receptor-blocking antibodies	↓	↓	↑	↓	Normal or small	Yes	Usually resolves within 2–3 months

(continued)

Table 61.2. Interpretation of Thyroid Function Tests and Imaging Results in Congenital Hypothyroidism and Related Disorders *(Continued)*

Cause of Hypothyroidism	Total T$_4$	Free T$_4$	TSH	TG	Thyroid Imaging	Treatment	Comments
Transient							
Hypothyroxinemia of prematurity	↓	↓	Normal	Normal	Normal	Controversial	Some physicians treat infants <27 weeks' gestation
Iodine deficiency	↓	↓	↑	↑	Normal or large	Yes[†]	↓Urinary iodine
Iodine excess	↓	↓	↑	↑	Normal or large	Yes	↑Urinary iodine; infants <36 weeks' gestation most susceptible
TBG deficiency	↓	Normal	Normal	Normal	Normal	No	—
Liver hemangioma	↓	↓	↑	↑	Normal	Yes	Rare, usually presents after newborn period May require high doses of L-thyroxine ± T$_3$

*Absent or ↓ in TG synthetic defect, ↑ in other forms of dyshormonogenesis.
[†]Treat with iodine, not L-thyroxine.
TSH, thyroid-stimulating hormone; TG, thyroglobulin; NB, newborn; MMI, methimazole; PTU, propylthiouracil; TBG, thyroxine-binding globulin.

b. Defects in thyroid hormone synthesis and secretion (thyroid dyshormonogenesis) are responsible for most of the remaining 30% of permanent CH cases. Most are recessive and carry a 25% recurrence risk in subsequent siblings. The most common defect is abnormal TPO activity, which results in impaired organification of iodine. Additional defects affect other key steps in thyroid hormone synthesis such as TG synthesis, iodine trapping, hydrogen peroxide generation, and iodotyrosine deiodination. **Pendred syndrome** is an important cause of sensorineural deafness associated with goiter due to a mild organification defect; however, hypothyroidism rarely occurs in the newborn period. In thyroid dyshormonogenesis, goiter may be present. Total and free T_4 levels are low, TSH is elevated, and TBG is normal. Defects in TG synthesis can be distinguished from other abnormalities in thyroid hormone formation by measurement of serum TG, which is low in TG synthetic defects and high in other forms of dyshormonogenesis. Unlike in thyroid dysgenesis, thyroid imaging typically reveals a normally placed thyroid gland that may be normal or large in size.

c. TSH resistance is usually caused by mutations in the TSH receptor. Rarely, it is due to a loss-of-function mutation in the stimulatory G_s subunit that links TSH binding to TSH receptor action (Albright hereditary osteodystrophy). In TSH resistance, the thyroid gland is small. T_4 is normal or low, and TSH is elevated with the severity of hypothyroidism depending on the degree of TSH resistance.

d. Central (hypothalamic-pituitary) hypothyroidism is less common than primary hypothyroidism. Although previously thought to be rare, this condition may be more common than generally appreciated, with an incidence of 1/25,000 to 1/16,000. Affected infants usually have other pituitary hormone deficits and may have signs of pituitary dysfunction such as hypoglycemia, microphallus, and midline facial abnormalities. Septo-optic dysplasia is an important cause of central hypothyroidism. Goiter is not present. Total and free T_4 are low, TSH is low or inappropriately normal, and TBG is normal. If central hypothyroidism is suspected, cortisol and growth hormone levels should be measured and magnetic resonance imaging performed to visualize the hypothalamus and pituitary. Failure to identify associated pituitary-hypothalamic defects, particularly adrenocorticotropic and growth hormone deficiencies, may lead to substantial morbidity or mortality.

2. Causes of **transient CH** (see Table 61.2)

   a. Antithyroid drugs. As discussed in section IV.B, intrauterine exposure to MMI or PTU can cause transient hypothyroidism that typically resolves within 1 week and does not require treatment. The elimination half-life of MMI is 4 to 6 hours and that of PTU is 1.5 to 5 hours.

   b. Iodine excess. Neonates may be exposed to excess iodine in the perinatal or neonatal period. Preterm infants are particularly susceptible to the thyroid-suppressing effects of excess iodine (see section V.D), such as from topical antiseptic solutions (e.g., povidone iodine), radiographic contrast solutions, and medications (e.g., amiodarone). Iodine is excreted into breast milk and can be excessive in mothers who ingest large amounts of seaweed (e.g., in Korea). In infants with hypothyroidism due to iodine excess, goiter may be present, T_4 is low, and TSH is elevated.

RAI and ^{99m}Tc uptake are blocked by excess iodine, and ultrasound shows a normally positioned thyroid gland that may be enlarged.

c. Iodine deficiency is the most common cause of transient hypothyroidism worldwide, particularly in preterm infants but is less common in the United States, a generally iodine-sufficient region. Preterm infants who are not exposed to iodine-containing skin cleansers (e.g., povidone iodine) may be at risk for iodine deficiency due to the low iodine content of their diet including parenteral nutrition, many standard preterm formulas and caloric supplements, and some breast milk (e.g., of women with inadequate dietary iodine intake).

d. Transient hypothyroxinemia of prematurity is most common in infants born before 31 weeks' gestation. Etiologic factors include hypothalamic-pituitary immaturity (particularly in infants <27 weeks' gestation), acute illness, and medications (e.g., dopamine, steroids). T_4 is low, usually with total T_4 more affected than free T_4. Unlike in primary hypothyroidism, TSH is inappropriately normal rather than elevated.

Observational studies in premature infants have demonstrated an association of transient hypothyroxinemia with adverse short- and long-term outcomes, including neonatal death, intraventricular hemorrhage, periventricular leukomalacia, cerebral palsy, intellectual impairment, and school failure. However, randomized trials of L-thyroxine supplementation have failed to show a beneficial effect, so the extent to which low T_4 levels directly cause these adverse outcomes is unclear. Treatment is controversial but, if given, may be most beneficial to infants born before 27 weeks' gestation.

e. TSH receptor-blocking antibodies account for 1% to 2% of all cases of CH and occur in 1/180,000 live births, typically in the setting of maternal autoimmune thyroid disease. These IgG antibodies cross the placenta and persist in the neonatal circulation with a half-life of approximately 2 weeks. TSH receptor-blocking and -stimulating antibodies may be present simultaneously, and their relative proportions may change over time. Neonatal hypothyroidism typically persists for 2 to 3 months and depends on the initial titer and the potency of the receptor-blocking activity. In these infants, goiter is not present. T_4 is low, TSH is elevated, and TBG is normal. High concentrations of TSH receptor-blocking antibodies can be measured in maternal and neonatal serum. Uptake is low or absent on thyroid scintigraphy, but a normally placed thyroid gland is visible by ultrasound.

f. Large liver hemangiomas can be associated with severe, refractory primary hypothyroidism due to massive expression of thyroid hormone-inactivating D3 by the hemangioma. Infants typically present after the newborn period as the hemangioma enlarges. Large doses of L-thyroxine, and occasionally addition of T_3, are required for treatment. Hypothyroidism resolves over time as the hemangioma regresses.

3. **Hypothyroxinemia with delayed TSH elevation (atypical CH)** is often due to recovery from sick euthyroid syndrome but needs to be distinguished from transient hypothyroidism and from a mild form of permanent CH. This condition is most common among extremely low birth weight infants (<1,000 g, reported incidence 1/58), very low birth

weight infants (<1,500 g, reported incidence 1/95), and in other critically ill newborns including those with congenital heart disease. Monozygotic twins discordant for CH can present with delayed TSH rise because mixing of fetal blood before birth allows the normal twin's thyroid to compensate for CH in the affected twin. Delayed TSH elevation may be missed on the initial newborn screen, particularly in programs using TSH as the primary screen (see section VI.B.1). Some screening programs require repeat testing at 2 to 6 weeks of age for infants at high risk for delayed TSH elevation, and a few programs require repeat testing for all infants.

B. Diagnosis. Over 95% of newborns with CH are asymptomatic at birth, but universal newborn screening permits early diagnosis and treatment, resulting in optimal neurodevelopmental outcome. In the United States, 1,600 cases of intellectual disability per year are prevented by newborn screening for CH.

  1. **Newborn screening for CH** is routine in most developed countries but is not yet performed in many developing countries. Screening is mandated by law in the United States, but specific screening protocols and cutoff values vary by state. Some programs measure TSH as the primary screen, whereas others measure T_4 as the primary screen, followed by TSH when T_4 is low. Each approach has advantages and disadvantages. A few states measure both T_4 and TSH in the initial screen for all newborns, or for a subset of high-risk newborns, which is an ideal but expensive strategy.

  2. In Massachusetts, the screening protocol is to measure T_4, followed by TSH measurement in infants whose T_4 is ≤13 µg/dL or in the lowest 10% of the set of samples run together. Additionally, TSH is measured in all cases for infants in the neonatal intensive care unit (NICU), infants weighing <1,500 g, infants with a family history or clinical signs of hypothyroidism, or if a previous specimen was unsatisfactory (e.g., collected too early, incorrect technique). The TSH level is considered elevated if it is ≥25 mU/L for infants <24 hours of age, ≥20 mU/L for infants 24 to 96 hours of age, and ≥15 mU/L for infants >96 hours of age. Infants with abnormal screening test results should be evaluated urgently in consultation with a pediatric endocrinologist (see section VI.B.5 and Fig. 61.1).

  3. A **filter paper blood spot specimen** should be sent from all newborns, ideally between 48 and 72 hours of age, although often, this timing is not feasible due to the early discharge of many healthy newborns. For infants discharged prior to 48 hours of age, a specimen should be sent prior to discharge. Infants tested and discharged before 24 hours of age should be retested at 48 to72 hours to minimize the risk of false-negative results. For infants transferred to another hospital, the receiving hospital should send a specimen if it cannot be confirmed that the hospital of birth sent one. For infants <1,500 g birth weight, repeat specimens should be sent at 2, 6, and 10 weeks of age due to the risk of delayed TSH elevation (see section VI.A.3).

  4. **If clinical signs of hypothyroidism** are present (e.g., constipation, hypothermia, poor tone, mottled skin, prolonged jaundice, poor feeding, large tongue, open posterior fontanel), thyroid function tests should be sent immediately, **even if the initial screen was normal**. Rarely, screening programs miss cases of CH as a result of early discharge, improper or no

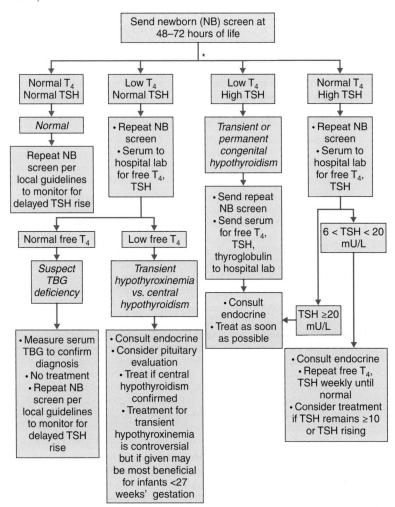

Figure 61.1. Suggested approach to follow-up of newborn screening for hypothyroidism in the hospitalized preterm infant. *In the United States, screening protocols and cutoff values vary slightly by state. TSH, thyroid-stimulating hormone; TBG, thyroxine-binding globulin. (Modified from Brodsky D, Ouellette MA, eds. *Primary Care of the Premature Infant*. Philadelphia, PA: Elsevier Saunders; 2008.)

specimen collection (e.g., hospital transfers, home births, sick or premature neonates), laboratory error, delayed TSH elevation, or human error in reporting results. Primary TSH screening programs may miss infants with central (pituitary) hypothyroidism. Acquired hypothyroidism (e.g., due to postnatal excess iodine exposure) will also be missed on newborn screening.

5. **Follow-up of newborn screening for CH** in hospitalized preterm infants is outlined in Figure 61.1. Screening protocols and cutoffs for T_4 and TSH levels vary by screening program (see section VI.B.2).

a. Any infant with abnormal screening results should be evaluated without delay. Consultation with a pediatric endocrinologist is recommended. Maternal and family history should be reviewed and a physical examination performed. Thyroid function tests should be repeated on a serum sample within 24 hours. Most infants with an initial TSH level >50 mU/L have a permanent form of CH. If the initial TSH is 20 to 40 mU/L, the CH may be transient. If it is not possible to see the patient promptly, therapy should be initiated as soon as the diagnosis is confirmed. If total T_4 is low but the TSH level is not elevated, a serum-free T4 level should be measured to exclude TBG deficiency. Patients with TBG deficiency generally have normal free T_4 levels and are almost always male (the condition is X-linked); this diagnosis should be confirmed by measurement of a serum TBG level. If both total T4 and free T4 are low but TSH is not elevated, central hypothyroidism or transient hypothyroxinemia of prematurity should be suspected. In such cases, consultation with an endocrinologist may be helpful to guide diagnostic evaluation and treatment.

b. Measurement of serum **TG level** and **thyroid ultrasound and/or thyroid scintigraphy with RAI or ^{99m}Tc** can help differentiate thyroid dysgenesis from defects in thyroid hormone synthesis, and conditions that may be transient from those likely to be permanent. These tests are not necessary if transient hypothyroxinemia of prematurity is suspected (see section VI.A.2.d). Thyroid scintigraphy is useful to detect dysgenetic or ectopic thyroid tissue as long as the serum TSH level is >30 mU/L at the time of scintigraphy. **Treatment should not be delayed to perform thyroid scintigraphy.** If scintigraphy cannot be performed within 5 days of diagnosis, it should be deferred until the child is 3 years old, at which time thyroid hormone replacement can be safely discontinued for a brief period. Unlike thyroid scintigraphy, ultrasound can be performed at any time, irrespective of the TSH concentration.

c. Bone age may be helpful in assessing the severity and duration of intrauterine hypothyroidism but does not usually alter management and is performed infrequently.

C. **Treatment and monitoring.** Optimal neurodevelopmental outcome depends on early, adequate treatment of CH.

1. For **infants with suspected transient or permanent CH**, L-thyroxine should be initiated at **10 to 15 µg/kg/day**, with higher doses used for infants with the lowest T_4 and highest TSH levels. The goal of treatment is to normalize thyroid hormone levels as soon as possible to achieve goals of total T_4 10 to 16 µg/dL, free T_4 1.4 to 2.3 ng/dL, and TSH 0.5 to 5 mU/L. Ideally, the T_4 level will normalize within 1 week and the TSH level within 2 weeks of starting therapy. Repeat T_4 and TSH measurements should be performed 1 week after starting therapy, every 1 to 2 weeks until thyroid hormone levels have normalized, 2 to 4 weeks after any dose change, and every 1 to 2 months in the first year of life. Nonadherence to treatment can have serious, permanent

neurodevelopmental consequences for the infant and should always be considered when thyroid function tests fail to normalize with treatment.

2. **L-thyroxine** tablets should be crushed and fed directly to the infant, or mixed in a small amount of juice, water, or breast milk. Soy-based formulas, ferrous sulfate, calcium supplements, and fiber interfere with absorption should be administered at least 2 hours apart from the L-thyroxine dose. There are no commercially available liquid preparations of L-thyroxine in the United States.

3. For **preterm infants suspected of having transient hypothyroxinemia of prematurity**, treatment decisions are complicated by incomplete data on the risks and benefits of treatment. Although most observational studies have found an association in preterm infants between low serum T_4 concentration with increased morbidity and mortality, a recent study showed, in contrast, that higher free T4 levels are associated with poorer developmental outcomes. Moreover, randomized trials have failed to demonstrate a short- or long-term benefit of routine L-thyroxine supplementation for all premature infants. Some physicians prefer to treat infants <27 weeks' gestation due to presumed hypothalamic-pituitary immaturity, but this practice is controversial. Infants with serum TSH levels persistently between 10 and 20 mU/L, or with a rising TSH level, are usually also treated. The starting dose of L-thyroxine is **8 µg/kg/day**, lower than the usual starting dose for CH.

4. For infants with **suspected transient CH**, a brief **trial off medication can be attempted at 3 years of age** after thyroid hormone-dependent brain development is complete. Usually, in infants with transient hypothyroidism, the dose required to maintain normal thyroid function does not increase with age as it generally does in permanent CH.

D. **Prognosis.** With prompt diagnosis and treatment, the neurodevelopmental outcome is excellent for infants with CH. Subtle defects in visuospatial processing, memory, and sensorimotor function have been reported, particularly in infants with severe CH, but the clinical significance of these differences is controversial. In contrast, infants in whom diagnosis is delayed may have substantial cognitive and behavioral defects ranging from mild to severe, depending on the severity of the CH and the length of delay in starting treatment.

VII. **NEONATAL HYPERTHYROIDISM** is uncommon (accounting for <1% of hyperthyroidism in children) and is almost always transient. Most newborns with hyperthyroidism are born to mothers with Graves' disease. Rarely, permanent hyperthyroidism can be caused by an activating mutation of the TSH receptor, a condition that is usually inherited in autosomal dominant fashion and may require thyroid gland removal or ablation.

A. **Incidence.** The overall incidence of neonatal hyperthyroidism is about 1/25,000. Of infants born to mothers with Graves' disease, 1% to 5% develop hyperthyroidism.

B. **Pathogenesis.** Most neonatal hyperthyroidism result from transplacentally acquired maternal TSH receptor-stimulating antibodies. Rarely, both TSH receptor-stimulating and -blocking antibodies may be present simultaneously. In such cases, infants may present initially with hypothyroidism due to the potent blocking antibodies; hyperthyroidism may emerge later due to the more rapid clearance of blocking antibodies compared to stimulating antibodies. More commonly, neonatal hyperthyroidism may follow initial hypothyroidism caused by transplacental passage of MMI or PTU, which are typically cleared within the first week of life.

C. **Neonatal hyperthyroidism** usually occurs in the setting of active maternal Graves' disease but may also occur in infants of mothers with Graves' disease who have previously undergone surgical thyroidectomy or RAI ablation. These mothers are no longer hyperthyroid but may continue to produce TSH receptor autoantibodies. High maternal serum levels of TSH receptor-stimulating antibodies increase the risk of hyperthyroidism in the newborn, but precise values differ depending on the sensitivity of the assay used.

D. **Clinical findings.** Neonatal thyrotoxicosis usually presents toward the end of the first week of life as maternal antithyroid medication is cleared from the newborn's circulation but can occur earlier. Clinical manifestations include prematurity, intrauterine growth restriction, tachycardia, irritability, poor weight gain, goiter, prominent eyes, hypertension, and craniosynostosis. Arrhythmias and congestive heart failure can be life threatening. Rarely, neonatal thyrotoxicosis can present with signs and symptoms suggestive of congenital viral infection, including hepatosplenomegaly, petechiae, fulminant hepatic failure, and coagulopathy. Diagnosis is based on maternal history of Graves' disease, high titers of TSH receptor-stimulating antibodies, elevation of total and free T_4 levels, and suppression of TSH.

E. **Treatment**

1. **MMI** (0.5 to 1 mg/kg/day in three divided doses) is used to treat neonatal thyrotoxicosis. PTU (5 to 10 mg/kg/day in three divided doses) is also effective but is not recommended as first-line therapy due to the risk of hepatotoxicity.

2. For severe hyperthyroidism, an **iodine preparation** can be used to block the release of thyroxine immediately. Lugol's solution (potassium iodide 100 mg/mL and iodine 50 mg/mL) or SSKI (potassium iodide 1 g/mL) can be given at a dose of 1 drop three times per day for 10 to 14 days.

3. **β-Blockade** with propranolol (2 mg/kg/day in three divided doses) is used to control tachycardia. If congestive heart failure develops, β-blockade should be discontinued and treatment with digoxin considered in consultation with a cardiologist.

4. Additional therapy for severe cases may include **prednisolone** (1 to 2 mg/kg/day).

5. **Supportive care** maintains adequate oxygenation, fluid balance, calorie and nutrient intake for growth, and temperature regulation.

6. **Treatment course.** Thyroid function tests (free T_4, total T_3, and TSH) are repeated every few days initially, and the dose of antithyroid drug is adjusted to maintain levels within the normal range. Treatment is usually required for 2 to 3 months but may be needed longer. Once control is achieved, the infant can be discharged with close follow-up. Iodine solutions are given for 10 to 14 days. Infants are weaned off β-blockade as indicated by the heart rate, and then the dose of antithyroid drug is tapered as allowed by the T_4 level and clinical symptoms.

F. **Prognosis.** Delayed diagnosis and inadequate treatment are associated with serious long-term consequences, including craniosynostosis, failure to thrive, developmental delay, and hyperactivity. Older case series report a 10% to 20% mortality rate, but with early diagnosis and proper treatment, most newborns improve rapidly, and therapy can be withdrawn within 2 to 3 months. Rarely, persistent central hypothyroidism may occur as a result of exposure of the fetal hypothalamus and pituitary to high thyroid hormone levels at a critical period in development.

VIII. MATERNAL THYROID MEDICATIONS AND BREASTFEEDING

A. **MMI** and **PTU** are excreted into breast milk but only in small amounts. Breastfeeding is considered safe for mothers taking doses of MMI under 30 mg per day or of PTU under 300 mg. MMI is preferred over PTU in breastfeeding women due to the risk of hepatotoxicity from PTU.

B. **Propranolol** is excreted into breast milk only in very small amounts. It is generally considered safe to breastfeed while taking propranolol without any special precautions.

C. **L-thyroxine** is transferred minimally to breast milk, similarly to endogenous T_4 in euthyroid women. Thus, breastfeeding is safe for women taking L-thyroxine replacement.

D. **Iodine** is excreted into the breast milk, and **the iodine status of the exclusively breastfed infant is dependent on the iodine status of the mother**. Even in regions considered iodine-sufficient, such as the United States, pregnant and lactating women should take 150 µg daily of supplemental iodine. Of note, many prenatal vitamins do not contain iodine. Preterm infants are particularly susceptible to the thyroid-suppressive effects of excess iodine, which can lead to subclinical or overt hypothyroidism. Excess iodine in the mother can come from the diet (e.g., seaweed) or from exposure to iodine-containing topical antiseptic agents (such as povidone iodine) used during labor and delivery.

Suggested Readings

Brown RS. Disorders of the thyroid gland in infancy, childhood, and adolescence. http://www.thyroidmanager.org. Updated March 2012.

Léger J, Olivieri A, Donaldson M, et al. European Society for Paediatric Endocrinology consensus guidelines on screening, diagnosis, and management of congenital hypothyroidism. *J Clin Endocrinol Metab* 2014;99: 363–384.

National Newborn Screening and Global Resource Center. Newborn screening. http://genes-r-us.uthscsa.edu/resources/newborn/newborn_menu.htm. Accessed June 29, 2015.

Rose SR, Brown RS, Foley T, et al. Update of newborn screening and therapy for congenital hypothyroidism. *Pediatrics* 2006;117:2290–2303.

Stagnaro-Green A, Abalovich M, Alexander E, et al. Guidelines of the American Thyroid Association for the diagnosis and management of thyroid disease during pregnancy and postpartum. *Thyroid* 2011;21:1081–1125.

62 Neonatal Effects of Maternal Diabetes

Terri Gorman

KEY POINTS

- The majority of infants of diabetic mothers are born to women with gestational diabetes, with pregestational type 2 diabetes rates now eclipsing type 1.
- Pregestational diabetes has a strong association with congenital abnormalities, perinatal mortality, and prematurity with rates linked to periconception glycemic control.
- Frequent neonatal morbidities associated with diabetes in pregnancy include macrosomia, postnatal hypoglycemia, prematurity, and birth trauma.
- Prenatal hyperglycemia exposure leads to increased neonatal metabolic complications including obesity, impaired glucose metabolism, and potential decrements in neurodevelopmental outcomes later in life.

I. **BACKGROUND.** Diabetes in pregnancy is associated with increased risks of fetal, neonatal, and lifelong complications in the offspring. Although the adverse effects of diabetes and hyperglycemia in pregnancy have been noted for hundreds of years, the modern history of classification of diabetes in pregnancy began in 1949 with Priscilla White's classification of maternal diabetes, ranging from gestational diabetes to long-standing insulin-dependent diabetes with systemic complications (Table 62.1). Most importantly, White highlighted the relationship between maternal end-organ disease and poor perinatal outcomes. In 1952, Jorgen Pedersen advanced the study of diabetes in pregnant women and their offspring by proposing a mechanism of maternal hyperglycemia leading to fetal hyperinsulinism, explaining many of the neonatal complications. Efforts since have led to improved prenatal monitoring and management of diabetes in pregnancy, reducing the incidence of adverse perinatal outcomes. However, as the incidence of obesity and type 2 diabetes climbs, and as we grow to further understand the long-term metabolic impact of exposure to obesity and diabetes in the developing fetus, we are entering a new era that will require vigilance for both mothers and their offspring.

II. **CLASSIFICATION OF DIABETES IN PREGNANCY.** Pregnancy itself is characterized by increased insulin resistance as gestation progresses with peak insulin resistance during the third trimester. A state of relative insulin resistance

Table 62.1. White Classification of Maternal Diabetes

Gestational diabetes (GD):	Diabetes not known to be present before pregnancy
	Abnormal glucose tolerance test in pregnancy
GD diet	Euglycemia maintained by diet alone
GD insulin	Diet alone insufficient; insulin required
Class A:	Chemical diabetes; glucose intolerance before pregnancy; treated by diet alone; rarely seen
	Prediabetes; history of large babies >4 kg or unexplained stillbirths after 28 weeks
Class B:	Insulin-dependent; onset after 20 years of age; duration <10 years
Class C:	C_1: Onset at 10–19 years of age
	C_2: Duration 10–19 years
Class D:	D_1: Onset before 10 years of age
	D_2: Duration 20 years
	D_3: Calcification of vessels of the leg (macrovascular disease)
	D_4: Benign retinopathy (microvascular disease)
	D_5: Hypertension (not preeclampsia)
Class F:	Nephropathy with >500 mg/day of proteinuria
Class R:	Proliferative retinopathy or vitreous hemorrhage
Class RF:	Criteria for both classes R and F coexist
Class G:	Many reproductive failures
Class H:	Clinical evidence of arteriosclerotic heart disease
Class T:	Prior renal transplantation

Note: All classes below A require insulin. Classes R, F, RF, H, and T have no criteria for age of onset or duration of disease but usually occur in long-term diabetes.
Source: Modified from Hare JW. Gestational diabetes. In: *Diabetes Complicating Pregnancy: The Joslin Clinic Method*. New York, NY: Alan R. Liss; 1989.

occurs during pregnancy as a result of the actions of various placental hormones including human placental lactogen, progesterone, prolactin, placental growth hormone, and cortisol. Whereas hormones of pregnancy allow an environment for normal development of the fetus, the pregnant state leaves a narrower margin of error in which women's propensity for carbohydrate intolerance can become apparent. This chapter will review the effects of both diabetes mellitus (DM) diagnosed before conception (pregestational diabetes) and diabetes diagnosed during pregnancy, most specifically diagnosed in the second to third trimester (gestational diabetes mellitus [GDM]).

A. **Pregestational diabetes.** Pregestational diabetes is present in 1% to 2% of all pregnancies and 13% to 21% of diabetes in pregnancy. This includes women with type 1 diabetes and type 2 diabetes that have been diagnosed and treated prior to conception. Type 2 pregestational diabetes mellitus (PGDM) is now more common than type 1 as obesity prevalence and its associations climb. Type 1 DM is typically diagnosed early in life and is characterized by relative or absolute insulin deficiency. Type 2 DM is typically diagnosed later in life and is associated with obesity and peripheral insulin resistance.

Poor early glycemic control correlates with adverse maternal and neonatal outcomes including preeclampsia, macrosomia, fetal congenital anomalies, prematurity, and perinatal mortality. Monitoring glucose control and glycosylated hemoglobin (Hgb A1C) levels is very important to improve maternal and neonatal outcomes. Therefore, preconception counseling should be an important part of maternal management for all women with preexisting DM. Unfortunately, less than one-third of women with type 1 or 2 DM actively seek preconceptual counseling. The impacts of PGDM should be discussed during routine gynecologic or primary care visits.

Obstetrical management of women with PGDM includes controlling blood glucoses with a goal of near-normal glucose control (fasting glucose ≤95 mg/dL, 1-hour postprandial glucose ≤140 mg/dL, and 2-hour postprandial glucose ≤120 mg/dL). Most women with PGDM will already be receiving insulin therapy, and insulin requirements will increase from the first to third trimester.

Although women with type 2 DM tend to have milder disturbances in glucose, in general, neonatal outcomes are similar to those with type 1 DM, whereas women with type 1 DM are more likely to have pregestational microvascular complications, increased risk of hyper- and hypoglycemia, as well as diabetic ketoacidosis, which is more likely to lead to fetal growth restriction.

1. **Maternal complications.** Obstetric complications of pregestational diabetes include miscarriage, preeclampsia, gestational hypertension, polyhydramnios, preterm delivery, and increased risk of requiring a cesarean section. Preterm delivery is not typically associated with preterm labor but rather with signs of fetal distress such as growth restriction or maternal hypertension necessitating preterm delivery.

2. **Congenital malformations.** Congenital malformations occur two- to fourfold higher in pregestational diabetes, with incidence for type 1 DM 2.9% to 7.5% of offspring and for type 2 DM 2.1% to 12.3% of offspring. Hyperglycemia during organogenesis (weeks 5 to 8 of gestation) reflected by an increase in Hgb A1C levels correlates directly with frequency of anomalies. The rate of congenital anomalies in nondiabetic women with Hgb A1C of 5.5% is 2%; this number rises to 2.7% at Hgb A1C 6.2%, 4% with Hgb A1C 7.6%, and up to 20% with Hgb A1C ≥14%. With good glycemic control, the rate of congenital malformations in pregestational diabetes can fall to approximate levels

of nondiabetic mothers, and a 30% reduction in risk can occur for every 1% lowering of Hgb A1C.

Congenital anomalies in order of prevalence include congenital heart disease, central nervous system (CNS) defects, urogenital defects, limb defects, orofacial clefts, and rarely, yet highly associated with DM, sacral agenesis/caudal dysplasia (15% to 25% of all cases result from DM). Most prevalent cardiac defects include tetralogy of Fallot, transposition of the great arteries, septal defects, and anomalous pulmonary venous return. CNS defects include anencephaly, spina bifida, encephalocele, hydrocephaly, and anotia/microtia.

3. **Intrauterine growth restriction (IUGR).** Although macrosomia is a risk of DM, a poor intrauterine environment can also lead to growth restriction. In pregnant women with pregestational diabetes plus preexisting hypertension or microvascular complications, there is a 6- to 10-fold higher risk relative to those without vascular disease of having a fetus with growth restriction.

4. **Further complications.** The earlier discussed complications are much more specifically associated with pregestational diabetes. Other complications that overlap with diabetic fetopathy that occurs due to glycemic derangements later in the pregnancy will be addressed later in this chapter.

B. **GDM.** GDM is defined as any carbohydrate intolerance first diagnosed during pregnancy. This does not exclude the possibility of some undiagnosed pregestational diabetes. GDM prevalence has been increasing in association with societal increase in obesity and is directly related to the prevalence of type 2 DM in a given population. GDM currently complicates up to 14% of all pregnancies and accounts for the vast majority of all cases of diabetes in pregnancy. Furthermore, 15% to 50% of women diagnosed with GDM will go on to be diagnosed with type 2 DM later in life. Thus, all women with GDM will be screened postpartum for persistent glucose intolerance.

1. **Screening and diagnosis.** Appropriate screening and diagnosis are crucial first steps to minimize the risks of GDM to the mother and infant. Risk factors for GDM should be screened at the first prenatal visit (Table 62.2). Women at risk for undiagnosed type 2 DM typically warrant screening on the first prenatal visit for potential preexisting glucose intolerance. Screening for all women is by glucose challenge at 24 to 28 weeks. Such screening was first developed by O'Sullivan and Mahan in 1950 with criteria established in 1964. Subsequent modifications have been made to the initial criteria, and controversies exist in the determination of exact thresholds for diabetic screening and diagnosis.

Currently, in the United States, most women are screened using a two-step method. The first step is a nonfasting 50-g oral glucose load with a 1-hour postprandial cutoff of either ≤140 mg/dL or ≤130 mg/dL. The cutoffs based on work by Carpenter and Coustan between 130 and 140 mg/dL demonstrate improved sensitivity compared to using the 130-mg/dL limit. It is most important to know your local obstetrical practices in interpreting the prenatal evaluation. For those above the cutoff, the second step is a 100-g oral glucose load after a 12-hour fast, with 1-, 2-, and 3-hour postload glucoses.

Table 62.2. Risk Factors for Gestational Diabetes Mellitus

Advanced maternal age
Maternal obesity
High parity
Previous delivery of a macrosomic infant
Family history of type 2 DM
Maternal short stature
Polycystic ovarian syndrome
Prior GDM
Prior neonatal death
Prior cesarean section
Previous stillbirth or congenital malformations
High blood pressure during pregnancy
Multiple pregnancy
DM, diabetes mellitus; GDM, gestational diabetes mellitus.

The Hyperglycemia and Adverse Pregnancy Outcome (HAPO) study published in 2008 was the first to link increasing 1- and 2-hour postprandial plasma glucoses with birth weight >90%, primary cesarean section, neonatal hypoglycemia, preterm delivery, shoulder dystocia, neonatal intensive care admission, hyperbilirubinemia, and preeclampsia. Subsequently, the International Association of Diabetes and Pregnancy Study Groups (IADPSG) developed recommendations based on the HAPO study to establish a one-step screening for all women. Their recommendation entailed a fasting 75-g glucose load with 1- and 2-hour postload glucose evaluation. A one-step screening process is relatively standard across the world with support from the World Health Organization (WHO) and the American Diabetes Association (ADA). However, a 2013 National Institutes of Health (NIH) Consensus Development Conference evaluated the current data and supported the continued use of a two-step tiered approach to diagnosis, citing concerns that transition to the current one-step method would certainly increase the diagnosis of GDM with all of its associated costs of increased monitoring and intervention but with unclear benefits to maternal and neonatal outcomes. Thus, the majority of pregnancies in the United States are evaluated by the two-step method. It is important to understand the local obstetrical screening and diagnostic practices for consistency of care from pre- to postnatal.

2. Treatment. Standard GDM management has aimed at tight control of maternal glucose levels to diminish the potential for fetal hyperinsulinemia. This can be achieved in three ways, escalating as the clinical scenario dictates, from diet control to oral antidiabetic agents to insulin therapy. Appropriate dietary management includes carefully calculated total daily caloric intake based on body mass index (BMI) as well as managing the dietary components of carbohydrates, protein, and fat to optimize appropriate weight gain during pregnancy. Previously, oral antidiabetic agents were felt to be contraindicated due to concern for fetal anomalies. However, careful studies have shown that glyburide and metformin are safe to use and can assist in achieving targeted glycemic control. Insulin and oral antidiabetic agents have equivalent efficacy in achieving target glucoses. Glyburide is a sulfonylurea that binds to pancreatic beta cell adenosine triphosphate calcium channel receptors to increase insulin secretion and sensitivity of peripheral tissues. Metformin is a biguanide that inhibits hepatic gluconeogenesis and glucose absorption and stimulated glucose uptake in peripheral tissues. These oral antidiabetics are now becoming the therapy of choice in women with GDM for whom diet alone cannot achieve glycemic targets. Obstetrical decision making regarding use of oral hypoglycemic agents depends on gestational age, glycemic control, and fetal growth patterns on ultrasound. Approximately 15% of GDM women will require oral antidiabetic agents or insulin to achieve glycemic control. Although multiple decision factors must go into considering insulin use for GDM, fetal abdominal circumference >70% after 29 to 30 weeks' gestation is an indication for the need for insulin therapy.

III. **MATERNAL MANAGEMENT AND DELIVERY.** Maternal prenatal management is vital to outcomes both for the mother and infant and typically will include the following objectives:

A. Close follow-up with obstetrician every 1 to 2 weeks during the first and second trimesters and weekly from 28 to 30 weeks onward with close attention to glucose management

B. Consultation with a registered dietitian and potentially maternal-fetal medicine and endocrinology based on local referral practices as well as disease severity

C. Routine level 2 ultrasound at 16 to 18 weeks with specific attention paid to potential for congenital anomalies in the presentational diabetic as well as an ultrasound in the late second to early third trimester as indicated by clinical glucose control both for estimation of fetal growth as well as to evaluate for fetal cardiac hypertrophy

D. Nonstress testing, biophysical profile evaluation, and contraction stress testing, especially in women with poor glycemic control, is recommended by the American College of Obstetricians and Gynecologists (ACOG).

E. Well-controlled DM should be managed expectantly with the majority delivering on or after 39 weeks' gestation. However, expected management is not recommended beyond the due date, and women with DM are good candidates for induction at 40 weeks. Induction of labor for suspected macrosomia has not been found to reduce birth trauma but may increase rates of cesarean section.

F. Cesarean delivery should be considered if the estimated fetal weight is >4,500 g in women with diabetes.

IV. FETAL AND NEONATAL EFFECTS OF MATERNAL DIABETES MELLITUS

A. Fetal effects of maternal DM. In the first trimester, thus primarily in women with pregestational diabetes, maternal hyperglycemia will cause a diabetic embryopathy resulting in congenital anomalies outlined earlier and increased risk of spontaneous abortion.

Maternal hyperglycemia in the second and third trimesters will result in a diabetic fetopathy characterized by fetal hyperglycemia, hyperinsulinemia, and macrosomia. Chronic fetal hyperinsulinemia causes increased metabolic rates in the fetus that lead to increased oxygen consumption. The oxygen needs may not be met by the placenta flow leading to fetal hypoxemia. This contributes to increased mortality, metabolic acidosis, and increased erythropoiesis in the fetus. Increased erythropoietin synthesis causes polycythemia and increased catecholamine production. Increased catecholamines contribute to fetal hypertension and cardiac hypertrophy. Also, polycythemia will cause redistribution of iron stores from developing organs to the red blood cell (RBC) mass which can affect cardiac and neurodevelopment.

Hyperinsulinemia has been linked to impaired lung maturation, increasing the risk for respiratory distress in the newborn. Hyperinsulinemia will also cause overgrowth of insulin-sensitive tissues including the heart, liver, muscle, and subcutaneous fat, leading to macrosomia with truncal asymmetry in which there is a disproportionate ratio of the shoulder-to-head or abdomen-to-head ratio (ponderal index). This increases the risk of shoulder dystocia, brachial plexus injury, fractures, and neonatal depression due to difficulty of extraction. One cohort series demonstrated that, due to increased ponderal index, obstetrical and neonatal outcomes were worse in infants of diabetic mothers (IDMs) who are large for gestational age (LGA) relative to infants of nondiabetic mothers who are LGA.

B. Neonatal effects of maternal DM. As explained by the *in utero* mechanisms earlier, the neonatal effects of DM include the following:

1. **Mortality.** IDMs are at increased risk for intrauterine fetal demise or postnatal mortality.
   a. For women with PGDM, the risk of spontaneous abortion, intrauterine demise, and perinatal mortality rises as her early conception Hgb A1C rises above 6. In women with type 1 DM, mortality is largely attributable to complications of prematurity and congenital anomalies. For those with type 2 DM, mortality is attributable to stillbirths, birth asphyxia or hypoxic ischemic encephalopathy, and intra-amniotic infections.
   b. For women with GDM, mortality is more often attributable to intrauterine fetal demise in the setting of poor glycemic control.

2. **Prematurity.** Thirty-six percent of IDMs are born at <38 weeks' gestation, with just over half being born late preterm at 34 to 37 weeks, with the remainder born at <34 weeks. The majority of prematurity is associated with maternal complications of hypertension or preeclampsia or with fetal IUGR leading to preterm delivery. In the recent past, more infants were electively induced prior to 39 weeks due to concern for macrosomia. But with obstetrical efforts to curtail unnecessary late preterm and early term inductions, the incidence of late preterm IDMs is expected to fall.

3. **Large for gestational age.** A large for gestation infant is defined as having a birth weight >90th percentile for gestational age and occurs in 36% to 47% of IDMs, relative to 7% to 9% of infants of nondiabetic women. Due to the distribution of size in IDMs, they have a threefold increased risk of shoulder dystocia and 10-fold increase in brachial plexus injury.

4. **Respiratory distress** occurs in approximately 30% to 40% of IDMs. This can be partially accounted for by increased rates of prematurity, but IDMs are more likely to develop respiratory distress syndrome (RDS) at any given gestational age as hyperinsulinemia interferes with glucocorticoid induction of surfactant synthesis. This can lead to increased rates of both RDS and pneumothorax due to less compliant lungs in larger infants. Transient tachypnea of the newborn (TTN) occurs 2 to 3 times more frequently in IDMs, with both increased rates of cesarean section and inherent reduced fluid clearance.

5. **Hypoglycemia** occurs in approximately 25% of IDMs, partly, but not completely, dependent on glycemic control prenatally and peridelivery. Even in rigorously controlled type 1 DM women, 14% of their infants experience hypoglycemia after birth. As Pederson noted in 1952 in his hyperglycemia hyperinsulinism hypothesis, maternal hyperglycemia is perpetuated through the placenta to fetal hyperglycemia, which causes hypertrophy of the fetal pancreatic islet tissue with hypersecretion of insulin in a fetal attempt to lower the plasma glucose. At birth, the maternal glucose supply is abruptly discontinued with clamping of the umbilical cord, but the infant cannot acutely decrease the insulin secretion, leading to neonatal hypoglycemia. Onset of hypoglycemia is typically within the first few hours after birth and lasts 2 to 4 days as neonatal insulin levels adjust. These infants frequently need intravenous (IV) glucose supplementation to maintain normal plasma glucose levels. Routine testing of insulin levels is not necessary in the majority of IDMs as the level is known to be initially elevated but will fall appropriately over time. Hence, supportive care and close prefeed glucose monitoring are standard for IDMs. Infants requiring glucose infusion rates (GIRs) exceeding 8 to 10 mg/kg/minute beyond the first week of life require further evaluation of their hypoglycemia, including testing of insulin and cortisol during a period of relative hypoglycemia. Severe, prolonged symptomatic hypoglycemia can result in permanent neurologic injury; thus, timely screening and intervention is important to long-term outcomes (see Chapter 24).

6. **Hypocalcemia.** Defined as total serum calcium <7 μg/dL (1.8 mmol/L) or ionized calcium <4 mg/dL (1 mmol/L), hypocalcemia occurs in 5% to 30% of IDMs. The calcium nadir typically occurs between 24 and 72 hours of life. For the majority of term infants who are feeding well, the hypocalcemia is asymptomatic and resolves with oral feeding. Thus, routine screening is not necessary for all IDMs. However, evaluation should occur in all infants with jitteriness, respiratory distress or apnea, seizures, neonatal depression, suspected infection, or prematurity (see Chapter 25). For the ill infant for whom enteral supplementation is not possible, calcium can be administered as an IV bolus, typically 200 mg/kg of calcium gluconate or via continuous infusion of IV fluids with calcium.

7. **Hypomagnesemia.** Defined as serum magnesium concentration <1.5 mg/dL (0.75 mmol/L), hypomagnesemia occurs in up to 40% of IDMs within the first 72 hours of life. Contributing factors include maternal hypomagnesemia related to urinary losses and prematurity. With the increased use of maternal magnesium predelivery for neuroprotection in the preterm population, hypomagnesemia is now less common. As with hypocalcemia, it is typically transient, asymptomatic, and does not require therapy. However, any infant screened for hypocalcemia should also be screened for hypomagnesemia. Hypomagnesemia can reduce parathyroid hormone (PTH) secretion and responsiveness, which in turn will exacerbate hypocalcemia until the hypomagnesemia is corrected.

8. **Hyperbilirubinemia** occurs in approximately 25% of IDMs. Contributing factors include prematurity, macrosomia, and polycythemia. All IDMs should undergo routine screening for jaundice either with transcutaneous or blood testing, with phototherapy as indicated (see Chapter 26).

9. **Polycythemia**, defined as a central venous hematocrit $>65\%$, occurs in 5% of IDMs. In one series, 17% of IDMs had hematocrits $>60\%$. Polycythemia is due to increased erythropoietin resulting from chronic fetal hypoxemia. A smaller contributing factor may be transfusion of placental blood with maternal or fetal distress around the time of delivery.

   Polycythemia can be associated with hyperviscosity which can cause vascular sludging, ischemia, and infarction of vital organs. This may explain the increased incidence of renal vein thrombosis (RVT) seen in IDMs. As such, infants of poorly controlled DM should have screening of a central venous hematocrit within 12 hours of birth. Routine hematocrits are not necessary for all IDMs due to the lower incidence, but infants should be screened if maternal control was known to be poor, if the infant is notably macrosomic, or if the infant has other clinical signs such as deeply ruddy appearance or early signs of jaundice.

10. **RVT** may occur *in utero* or postpartum due to polycythemia and hyperviscosity. Postnatal presentation includes hematuria, flank mass, hypertension, or embolic phenomena. Whereas half of RVT

is associated with prematurity and with central venous lines, IDMs account for almost 15% of cases.

11. **Small left colon syndrome** is a rare form of bowel obstruction highly associated with maternal DM. Forty percent to 50% of all cases of small left colon syndrome occur in IDMs. As presentation is typically abdominal distention with inability to pass stool, an alternated differential diagnosis includes Hirschsprung disease. Infants with small left colon syndrome have appropriate ganglion cells in the rectum, but the left colon, past the splenic flexure, is small in caliber. Diagnosis is by hyperosmotic contrast enema, which will often also result in evacuation of the colon. These can often be treated conservatively with enemas.

12. **Hypertrophic cardiomyopathy** is characterized by thickening of the intraventricular septum and/or ventricular walls, with a reduction in size of the ventricular chambers of the heart. Hypertrophic cardiomyopathy occurs with increased frequency in PGDM and GDM but has been shown to be more prevalent in pregestational diabetes (as high as 40% in one series) even in the setting of strict glycemic control. The hypertrophy can be detected in late second to early third trimester; thus, careful ultrasound screening or fetal echocardiography with concentration on ventricular size is recommended. Fetal hyperinsulinism triggers an increase in fat and protein synthesis, leading to hypertrophied and disorganized cardiac myocytes. The structural hypertrophy can lead to obstruction of left ventricular outflow. Although most infants with hypertrophic cardiomyopathy are asymptomatic, 5% to 10% may present with respiratory distress, signs of heart failure, or poor cardiac output. The standard for diagnosis is echocardiography, which should be reserved for symptomatic infants or those with notable intraventricular hypertrophy on prenatal ultrasound. For those infants with outflow tract obstruction, supportive care includes increasing ventricular filling by IV fluid administration and propranolol to slow the heart rate to allow better ventricular filling. Inotropes are likely to worsen the outflow obstruction by decreasing the ventricular size, so they should generally be avoided. Most infants will improve with supportive care within 2 to 3 weeks of birth, and most echocardiographic hypertrophy will resolve within 6 to 12 months.

    Less commonly, IDMs may develop a congestive cardiomyopathy with more diffuse hypertrophy related to perinatal hypoxemia or metabolic derangements such as hypoglycemia or hypocalcemia that lead to a poorly contractile heart. Supportive care and correction of metabolic derangements can reverse the congestive cardiomyopathy.

13. **Poor feeding** is a significant issue especially in poorly controlled IDMs, leading to prolonged hospital stays and interruption of parental infant bonding. Poor feeding can be related to prematurity or respiratory distress associated with IDM; however, it is often present in the absence of other complicating factors. In a series of 150 IDMs at Brigham and Women's Hospital, 37% of IDMs experienced poor feeding.

V. NEONATAL MANAGEMENT OF IDMs. Just as the prenatal management of a pregnancy complicated by DM is a combined effort of obstetricians, maternal fetal medicine specialists, endocrinologists, and dietitians, so must the neonatal management of the IDM be a multidisciplinary effort. Excellent communication of prenatally diagnosed anomalies as well as prenatally predicted complications from the obstetric provider to the pediatric team is imperative. Additional consultation from a neonatologist and other pediatric subspecialists may be warranted prenatally or once the infant has been born to aid in postnatal management. A balance must be made to provide appropriate screening and evaluation while promoting infant maternal bonding.

A. **Delivery room care.** Proper assessment of the need for neonatal resuscitation should be made based on gestational age, predicted birth weight, prenatally diagnosed congenital anomalies, mode of delivery, and any complications of labor. The appropriate Neonatal Resuscitation Program (NRP)-trained team should be in attendance to provide care specifically to the infant. The initial evaluation immediately after birth will determine the need for further interventions. If the infant does not require resuscitative measures, the infant should have timely skin-to-skin care and initiation of breastfeeding in the delivery room.

Any infant with cyanosis in the delivery room should have pulse oximetry evaluation with specific attention to the cardiovascular and respiratory systems given the infant's risk of RDS, TTN, congenital heart disease, and hypertrophic cardiomyopathy.

B. **Postdelivery management.** IDMs are at increased risk for postnatal hypoglycemia and should have systematic evaluation of serum glucose measurements. Infants should feed soon after birth either breast milk or formula, with preference for breastfeeding, with bedside glucose monitoring within the first 1 to 2 hours of life. Prior practices of feeding glucose water were found to actually increase insulin release and, therefore, is not recommended. The Committee on the Fetus and Newborn provide guidance in their 2011 clinical report on target glucoses in the newborn. Target glucose within the first 24 hours of life is ≥45 mg/dL prior to routine feedings. Prefeed glucoses should be followed through the first 36 hours of life with feeding established and normalized glucose levels.

Any infant with lethargy, respiratory distress, jitteriness, apnea, or seizures should have immediate bedside glucose testing as a subset of IDMs will require immediate and aggressive treatment of hypoglycemia. Any low bedside testing should also have serum glucose samples run by the laboratory for confirmation, but such confirmation should not delay timely treatment of hypoglycemia. For infants with glucose <25 mg/dL or with persistent glucose <40 mg/dL despite adequate feeding within the first 4 hours of life, or <35 mg/dL or persistent <45 mg/dL after feeding in the first 24 hours of life, warrant administration of IV glucose. Initial boluses of dextrose 10% in water ($D_{10}W$) 2 mL/kg (200 mg/kg) should be administered to bring the glucose into the 40 to 50 mg/dL range. Then a continuous infusion of $D_{10}W$ should be initiated. An infusion of 60 mL/kg/day of $D_{10}W$ will result in a GIR of approximately 4 mg/kg/minute, and a $D_{10}W$ infusion rate of 100 mL/kg/day will result in a GIR of approximately 7 mg/kg/minute. Of those requiring IV glucose infusion, a small subset will require a GIR in excess of 8 to 10 mg/kg/minute, necessitating placement of a central catheter, typically an umbilical venous catheter, to maintain euglycemia (see Chapter 24).

Following transition from the delivery room, ongoing evaluation of the IDM should include screening for hyperbilirubinemia, polycythemia, hypocalcemia, and hypomagnesemia as indicated. Venous hematocrit should be obtained within the first 12 hours of life for those at risk. Heightened attention to the potential for jaundice should include close clinical monitoring of bilirubin by either bedside transcutaneous bilirubin screening or serum screening. Many units routinely screen all infants at 36 hours of life with a transcutaneous bilirubinometer, with earlier screening if jaundice is noted. For infants who fall into the high or high intermediate risk zone on the bilirubin nomogram, a serum bilirubin is sent for confirmation, and phototherapy is initiated when indicated.

VI. LONG-TERM EFFECTS.
Prenatal exposure to hyperglycemia has been shown to increase longer term metabolic and neurodevelopmental outcomes in the offspring of women with DM.

A. **Metabolic syndrome** is classified as a combination of obesity, hypertension, dyslipidemia, and glucose intolerance. This syndrome was originally described in Pima Indians, a population with high rates of gestational diabetes. In the offspring of these women with GDM, 45% developed type 2 DM by their mid-20s and more than two-thirds by their mid-30s. The increased risk persisted despite accounting for paternal diabetes (factoring in genetic risk), the offspring's BMI, and age of onset of DM in parents, pointing to contribution from the intrauterine environment. Metabolic syndrome has now been shown to have increased incidence in infants who were LGA at birth or born to women with gestational diabetes. Risk of metabolic syndrome was found in a population-based study out of Denmark to be 4 times greater in offspring of GDM women and 2.5 times for offspring of PGDM.

B. **Obesity.** Multiple studies have shown an association between DM and obesity in the offspring. Although the macrosomia at birth often resolves within the first year of life, later in childhood, IDMs whose mothers had type 1 or 2 DM tend to have higher BMIs than controls. Offspring of women with gestational diabetes have also been shown to have a higher BMI, a higher risk of being overweight, and higher fasting insulin levels relative to offspring of nondiabetic women. Overall, the risk of being overweight is approximately twofold for offspring of women with pregestational and gestational DM.

C. **Diabetes.** IDMs have an increased risk of developing diabetes later in life. Type 1 and type 2 DM are both known to be influenced by genetics, with type 1 diabetes occurring 4 times more often in offspring of women with type 1 DM. The lifetime risk of an offspring of a type 2 DM is 5 to 10 times higher than age- and weight-matched controls without a family history. The *in utero* environment has also been shown to contribute to impaired glucose tolerance later in life, with the presence of glucose intolerance correlating with elevated amniotic fluid insulin concentrations during pregnancy.

D. Impaired neurodevelopmental outcomes. Poor maternal glycemic control can adversely affect the developing brain. However, it is important to note that neurodevelopmental outcomes of the well-controlled DM are similar to those of infants of nondiabetic mothers.

Increasing Hgb A1C levels are associated with decreasing head circumference and decreased intellectual performance at 3 years of age. Another study correlated decrements in psychomotor development at 6 to 9 years, with elevated maternal ketone concentrations during the second and third trimesters.

Suggested Readings

American College of Obstetricians and Gynecologists. ACOG Practice Bulletin No. 60: pregestational diabetes milletus. *Obstet Gynecol* 2005;105:675–685.

American College of Obstetricians and Gynecologists. ACOG Practice Bulletin No. 137: gestational diabetes mellitus. *Obstet Gynecol* 2013;122:406–416.

Ashwal E, Hod M. Gestational diabetes mellitus: where are we now? *Clin Chim Acta* 2015;451(pt A):14–20.

HAPO Study Cooperative Research Group. Hyperglycemia and adverse pregnancy outcomes. *N Engl J Med* 2008;358(19):1991–2002.

Nold JL, Georgieff MK. Infants of diabetic mothers. *Pediatr Clin North Am* 2004;51:619–637.

63

Disorders of Sex Development

Jonathan M. Swartz and Yee-Ming Chan

KEY POINTS

- Disorders of sex development (DSD) are a heterogeneous group of disorders broadly defined by atypical development of genetic, gonadal, and/or anatomic sex. DSD frequently present in the newborn period with ambiguous genitalia and/or other issues.
- The rapid evaluation of infants with genital ambiguity is critical to identify and, if necessary, treat salt-wasting congenital adrenal hyperplasia, which is potentially life-threatening.
- The main goal of sex assignment in children with DSD is to attempt to match the child's future gender identity. This is a challenging, imperfect, and humbling endeavor.

I. **DEFINITION AND NOMENCLATURE.** The term *disorders of sex development* (DSD) was introduced to replace older terms such as *ambiguous genitalia*, *pseudohermaphroditism*, and *intersex* to denote atypical development of genetic, gonadal, and/or anatomic sex (Table 63.1). Examples of DSD presenting in the newborn period include infants with the following findings:

A. Ambiguous genitalia

B. A penis and bilaterally nonpalpable testes (cryptorchidism)

C. Unilateral cryptorchidism with hypospadias

D. Severe penoscrotal, scrotal, or perineal hypospadias, with or without microphallus, even if the testes are descended.

E. Apparently female appearance with enlarged clitoris (clitoromegaly) and/or inguinal hernia(s) or palpable gonad(s)

F. Asymmetry of in size, pigmentation, or rugation of labioscrotal folds

G. Discordance of external genitalia with prenatal karyotype

Because internal genital anatomy, karyotype, and sex assignment cannot be determined from a baby's external appearance, a thorough evaluation is required. The evaluation must be expedited because of the possibility of salt-wasting congenital adrenal hyperplasia (CAH), which can be life-threatening within the first week of life as well as the urgency felt by most parents in assigning a sex of rearing.

Table 63.1. Revised Nomenclature	
Previous	**Proposed**
Intersex	DSD
Male pseudohermaphrodite	46,XY DSD
Undervirilization of an XY male	46,XY DSD
Undermasculinization of an XY male	46,XY DSD
Female pseudohermaphrodite	46,XX DSD
Virilization of an XX female	46,XX DSD
Masculinization of an XX female	46,XX DSD
True hermaphrodite	Ovotesticular DSD
XX male or XX sex reversal	46,XX testicular DSD
XY sex reversal	46,XY complete gonadal dysgenesis

DSD, disorder of sex development.
Source: From Hughes IA, Houk C, Ahmed SF, et al; for the Lawson Wilkins Pediatric Endocrine Society/European Society for Paediatric Endocrinology Consensus Group. Consensus statement on management of intersex disorders. *Arch Dis Child* 2006;91(7):554–563.

II. IMMEDIATE POSTNATAL CONSIDERATIONS PRIOR TO SEX ASSIGNMENT.
Although a rapid decision about sex assignment is essential for the parents' peace of mind, care must be taken to avoid drawing premature conclusions. Until a sex assignment is made, gender-specific names, pronouns, or other references should be avoided. Prompt consultation with a pediatric endocrinologist will facilitate the evaluation, and most causes of DSD can be identified in 2 to 4 days, although some cases may take 1 to 2 weeks or longer. The physician should examine the infant's genitalia in the presence of the parents and then discuss with them the process of genital development, that their child's genitalia are incompletely or variably formed, and that further tests will be required before a decision can be made regarding the infant's sex. Circumcision is contraindicated until a determination is made concerning the need for surgical reconstruction.

III. NORMAL SEX DEVELOPMENT.
The process of gonadal differentiation and genital development is depicted in Figure 63.1. In general, early structures will develop down the female pathway unless specific factors are present that direct development down the male pathway.

A. **Genetic sex** refers to the sex chromosome complement.

B. **Gonadal sex.** Undifferentiated gonads develop in the bilateral genital ridges around 6 weeks of gestation and begin to differentiate by 7 weeks. *SRY*, which encodes the primary testis-determining transcription factor on the

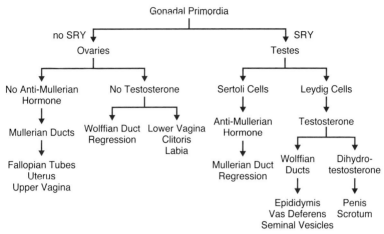

Figure 63.1. The process of gonadal, internal genital, and external genital differentiation. (From Holm IA. Ambiguous genitalia in the newborn. In: Emans SJ, Laufer M, Goldstein D, eds. *Pediatric and Adolescent Gynecology*. Philadelphia, PA: Lippincott Williams & Wilkins; 1998:53.)

short arm of the Y chromosome, promotes the gonads to develop into testes. Several other genes can also promote testicular and/or ovarian development, including *NR5A1* (*SF1*), *NR0B1* (*DAX1*), *SOX3*, *SOX9*, *WNT4*, and *RSPO1*.

C. **Anatomic sex** refers to the external and internal genitalia. The testis secretes two hormones critical for male genital formation: Anti-müllerian hormone (AMH, also called müllerian inhibiting substance or factor, MIS or MIF) is produced by Sertoli cells, and testosterone is produced by Leydig cells.

1. **Internal genitalia.** AMH causes regression of the müllerian ducts that would otherwise become the uterus, fallopian tubes, cervix, and upper vagina. Testosterone prevents the regression of the wolffian ducts and promotes their development into the vas deferens, seminal vesicles, and epididymis. Müllerian duct regression and wolffian duct development require high *local* concentrations of AMH and testosterone, respectively. Failure of a testis to develop on one side may result in ipsilateral retention of müllerian structures and regression of wolffian structures.

2. **External genitalia.** The enzyme 5α-reductase, present in high concentration in genital skin, converts testosterone to dihydrotestosterone (DHT). DHT is the primary hormone responsible for masculinizing the external genitalia, including the genital tubercle and labioscrotal folds, which form the penis and scrotum, respectively. In the absence of DHT, these undifferentiated structures develop into the clitoris and labia. Testicular descent from the abdomen to the inguinal ring requires insulin-like peptide 3 (INSL3), and descent from the inguinal ring into the scrotum requires testosterone. This generally occurs in the last 6 weeks of gestation.

Formation of normal male internal and external genitalia under the influence of testosterone and DHT requires functional androgen receptors in the target tissues.

D. Time course. The timeline of fetal sexual differentiation is depicted in Figure 63.2 and Table 63.2.

1. **First trimester.** Testicular synthesis of testosterone is stimulated by activation of the luteinizing hormone (LH) receptor by human chorionic gonadotropin (hCG) produced by the placenta. The first trimester is the only period during which the labioscrotal folds are susceptible to fusion. If a 46,XX fetus is exposed to excess androgens during the first trimester, the clitoris and labioscrotal folds will virilize and may appear indistinguishable from a normal male penis and scrotum, although the latter will be empty.

2. **Second and third trimesters.** Testicular androgen production is stimulated by LH from the fetal pituitary and is responsible for penile growth, scrotal maturation (rugation, pigmentation, and thinning), and final testicular descent. High intrauterine concentrations of testosterone may influence brain development, possibly affecting later behavior, sexual orientation, and gender identity.

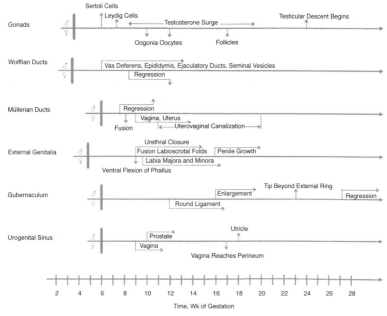

Figure 63.2. Timelines for six aspects of sex differentiation. (Adapted from White PC, Speiser PW. Congenital adrenal hyperplasia due to 21-hydroxylase deficiency. *Endocr Rev* 2000;21[3]:245–291. Adapted from Barthold JS, Gonzalez R. Intersex states. In: Gonzalez ET, Bauer SB, eds. *Pediatric Urology Practice*. Philadelphia, PA: Lippincott Williams & Wilkins; 1999:547–578.)

Table 63.2. Timetable of Sex Development	
Days after Conception	**Events of Sex Development**
19	Primordial germ cells migrate to the genital ridge
40	Genital ridge forms an undifferentiated gonad
44	Müllerian ducts appear; testes develop
62	Anti-müllerian hormone (from testes) becomes active
71	Testosterone synthesis begins (induced by placental hCG)
72	Fusion of the labioscrotal swellings
73	Closure of the median raphe
74	Closure of the urethral groove
77	Müllerian regression is complete
hCG, human chorionic gonadotropin.	

IV. NURSERY EVALUATION OF A NEWBORN WITH SUSPECTED DISORDERS OF SEX DEVELOPMENT

A. **History**

1. **Maternal drug exposure** during pregnancy, such as to androgens (e.g., testosterone, danazol), drugs that interfere with androgen synthesis or action (e.g., finasteride, spironolactone), or antiseizure medications (e.g., phenytoin, trimethadione)

2. **Maternal virilization** during pregnancy due to poorly controlled maternal CAH, a virilizing adrenal or ovarian tumor, or placental aromatase deficiency

3. **Placental insufficiency.** First-trimester synthesis of testosterone in the fetal testis is dependent on placental hCG due to its activation of the LH receptor.

4. **Prenatal findings** of genital ambiguity; sex chromosome mosaicism; a karyotype discordant with phenotypic sex; or potential DSD-associated conditions, such as oligohydramnios, renal anomalies (genitourinary malformations), or skeletal abnormalities (campomelic dysplasia)

5. **Family history** of CAH, hypospadias, cryptorchidism, infertility, pubertal delay, corrective genital surgery, genetic syndromes, or consanguinity. Death of a male family member from vomiting or dehydration in early infancy may suggest undiagnosed CAH.

B. **Physical examination**

1. **External genitalia.** The examiner should note the stretched penile length, width of the corpora, engorgement, presence of chordee (abnormal downward curvature of the penis), position of the urethral orifice,

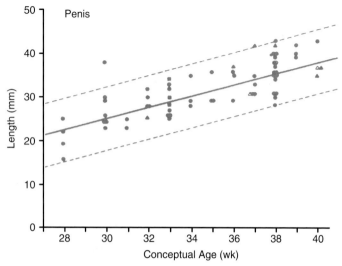

Figure 63.3. Stretched penile length of normal premature and full-term babies *(closed circles)*, showing lines of mean ±2 standard deviations. Superimposed are data for two small-for-gestational-age infants *(open triangles)*, seven large for gestational age infants *(closed triangles)*, and four twins *(closed boxes)*, all of whom are in the normal range. (From Feldman KW, Smith DW. Fetal phallic growth and penile standards for newborn male infants. *J Pediatr* 1975;86:395.)

presence of a vaginal opening, and pigmentation and symmetry of the scrotum or labioscrotal folds. The normal full-term male infant has a penile length of at least 2.5 cm, measured stretched from the pubic ramus to the tip of the glans (Fig. 63.3), and usually 1 cm or more in width. The normal full-term female infant has a clitoris <1 cm in length and <0.5 cm in width. Posterior fusion of the labioscrotal folds is assessed by determining the **anogenital ratio**, which is the distance between the anus and the posterior fourchette divided by the distance between the anus and the base of the phallus. An anogenital ratio >0.5 indicates first-trimester androgen exposure.

2. **Gonadal size, position, and descent** should be carefully noted. A gonad below the inguinal ligament is usually a testis (normal or dysgenetic) but may be an ovotestis or even a uterus herniating into the inguinal canal. Abnormal genital development with bilateral nonpalpable gonads should raise immediate concern for salt-wasting CAH.

3. **Associated anomalies** should be noted. Additional features may indicate a more generalized disorder, although such features may not be present at birth. Denys-Drash syndrome (Wilms tumor and/or diffuse glomerulosclerosis) or WAGR (**W**ilms tumor, **A**niridia, **G**enitourinary anomalies, and mental **R**etardation) syndrome, both due to mutations

of *WT1* (11p13), can cause DSD in 46,XY infants. A few examples of other conditions associated with DSD include Smith-Lemli-Opitz, Robinow, Antley–Bixler, and Goldenhar syndromes; campomelic dysplasia (*SOX9* mutations); and trisomy 13.

C. Diagnostic tests

1. **Laboratory tests** are tailored to the differential diagnosis.

   a. Chromosome analysis on peripheral blood can be performed by karyotype within 48 hours in many centers and sometimes more rapidly by **fluorescent *in situ* hybridization (FISH)**. Although a standard karyotype may show 46,XX, FISH for *SRY* may reveal that it has been translocated to an X chromosome or an autosome. Any abnormal karyotype detected prenatally should be confirmed immediately after birth.

   b. First-line testing in addition to a karyotype should include a 17-hydroxyprogesterone (part of newborn screens in all U.S. states), LH, and testosterone to be drawn after 48 hours of life. Baseline labs can also include serum electrolytes, blood urea nitrogen (BUN), and creatinine, with electrolytes followed frequently to look for evidence of salt wasting.

   c. Other tests such as plasma renin activity, follicle-stimulating hormone (FSH), AMH, or other adrenal precursors and hormones may be indicated in certain circumstances.

   d. Targeted genetic testing and/or chromosomal microarray may be indicated to look for specific causes of DSD. *SRY, SOX9, WT1, NR5A1* (formerly called *SF1*), and *NR0B1* (formerly called *DAX1*) are a few examples of genes with variants known to be associated with DSD. Duplications in enhancer regions of *SOX9* and *SOX3* have been reported in 46,XX males. With the input of geneticists, testing may be appropriate in many cases of DSD. Some institutions have started to use whole-exome sequencing to aid in the diagnosis of DSD cases. Cost, insurance coverage, and incomplete knowledge of the genetics of DSD remain limiting factors with this approach.

2. **Pelvic ultrasonography**, especially when the bladder is full, can determine whether a uterus is present. However, this determination can be difficult and may require an experienced ultrasonographer. Testes can often be visualized by ultrasound, but ovaries are less likely to be identified. Given the association between urologic and genital malformations, ultrasonographic evaluation should include the kidneys, ureters, and bladder. Adrenal hyperplasia can often be found in babies with CAH but is not diagnostic. Magnetic resonance imaging (MRI) may be needed to locate intra-abdominal testes or to confirm the presence of a uterus when ultrasonography is indeterminate.

3. **Voiding cystourethrogram (VCUG) or genitogram** may reveal a vagina with a cervix at its apex (indicating the presence of a uterus) or a utricle (a müllerian duct remnant). It may also reveal the presence of abnormal connections between the urinary and genital tracts (e.g., urogenital sinus).

   Table 63.3 summarizes causes, and Figure 63.4 describes an approach to patients with DSD.

Table 63.3. Causes of Disorders of Sex Development

Disorder	Phenotype		Karyotype
	External Genitalia	Gonads	
Disorders of gonadal differentiation			
Ovotesticular DSD	Variable	Ovarian and testicular tissue	46,XX; 46,XY; 46,XX/ 46,XY; others
Mixed gonadal dysgenesis	Variable	Streak gonad and dysgenetic testis	45,X/46,XY; 46,XYp-; others
46,XY complete gonadal dysgenesis	Female or ambiguous	Dysgenetic testes or streak gonads	46,XY
46,XX testicular DSD	Male or ambiguous	Testes	46,XX
Other 46,XX DSD (masculinization of the genetic female)			
Congenital adrenal hyperplasia			
21α-hydroxylase deficiency	Ambiguous	Ovaries	46,XX
11β-hydroxylase deficiency	Ambiguous	Ovaries	46,XX
3β-hydroxysteroid dehydrogenase deficiency	Ambiguous	Ovaries	46,XX
Placental aromatase deficiency	Ambiguous	Ovaries	46,XX
Maternal androgen excess	Ambiguous	Ovaries	46,XX
Other 46,XY DSD (incomplete masculinization of the genetic male)			
Testicular unresponsiveness to hCG and LH (LH receptor mutation)	Female or ambiguous	Testes	46,XY

(continued)

Table 63.3. *(Continued)*

| Disorder | Phenotype | | Karyotype |
	External Genitalia	Gonads	
Disorders of testosterone/ dihydrotestosterone synthesis			
Steroidogenic acute regulatory protein deficiency	Female or ambiguous	Testes	46,XY
Side-chain cleavage enzyme deficiency	Female or ambiguous	Testes	46,XY
17α-hydroxylase/ 17,20-lyase deficiency	Female or ambiguous	Testes	46,XY
3β-hydroxysteroid dehydrogenase deficiency	Ambiguous	Testes	46,XY
17β-hydroxysteroid dehydrogenase deficiency	Ambiguous	Testes	46,XY
5α-reductase deficiency	Ambiguous	Testes	46,XY
End-organ resistance to testosterone			
Complete androgen insensitivity syndrome	Female	Testes	46,XY
Partial androgen insensitivity syndrome	Ambiguous	Testes	46,XY
Testicular regression syndrome ("vanishing testes syndrome")	Male	Absent gonads	46,XY

DSD, disorder of sex development; hCG, human chorionic gonadotropin; LH, luteinizing hormone.
Source: Modified from Wolfsdorf JI, Muglia L. Endocrine disorders. In: Graef JW, ed. *Manual of Pediatric Therapeutics*. Philadelphia, PA: Lippincott-Raven; 1997:381–413.

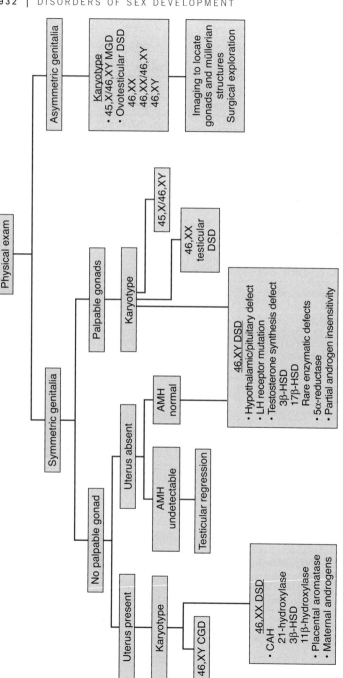

Figure 63.4. Algorithm for the evaluation of disorders of sex development (DSDs). MGD, mixed gonadal dysgenesis; AMH, anti-müllerian hormone; CGD, complete gonadal dysgenesis; CAH, congenital adrenal hyperplasia; LH, luteinizing hormone; 3β-HSD, 3β-hydroxysteroid dehydrogenase; 17β-HSD, 17β-hydroxysteroid dehydrogenase.

V. GONADAL DIFFERENTIATION DISORDERS

A. Mixed gonadal dysgenesis (MGD). The hallmark of MGD is the presence of a testis on one side of the body and either a streak gonad or dysgenetic gonad on the other side. This disorder is most often due to a 45,X/46,XY mosaic karyotype. Often, the Y chromosome is abnormal, or Y chromosome material may be translocated to an autosome.

1. Physical findings. The combination of asymmetric external genitalia and one palpable testis in the labioscrotal fold is often MGD. However, 45,X/46,XY mosaicism can result in an appearance of the external genitalia ranging from normal male to normal female. In fact, 90% of 45,X/46,XY infants diagnosed prenatally appear phenotypically male at birth. In patients with MGD, each gonad governs the differentiation of the ipsilateral internal genital structures. A fallopian tube and uterus are frequently present on the side of the streak/dysgenetic gonad, and these structures can herniate into the labioscrotal fold. Children with MGD may have features similar to Turner syndrome such as webbed neck, lymphedema, short stature, renal abnormalities, and cardiac defects (e.g., coarctation of the aorta).

2. Management. If AMH is measurable, or if hCG stimulation testing causes a significant rise in serum testosterone indicative of testicular tissue, the testis should be sought by imaging and/or surgery. See section VIII for discussion of sex assignment. Streak gonads and some dysgenetic testes should be removed in infancy because germ cell tumors may arise in up to 30% of these children, sometimes within the first few years of life. All children with MGD should be evaluated by a pediatric endocrinologist because many will have poor linear growth and are candidates for growth hormone therapy.

B. 46,XY gonadal dysgenesis. 46,XY complete gonadal dysgenesis (CGD) is also called Swyer syndrome. Infants with 46,XY CGD fail to masculinize due to a failure of testicular differentiation, which can be a result of abnormal functioning of *SRY* or factors that regulate or are regulated by *SRY*. Bilateral streak gonads are typically present, and internal genital structures are female due to inadequate production of AMH and testosterone. The external genitalia usually appear female, but clitoromegaly may occur if "gonadal" hilus cells secrete testosterone. These patients are usually raised female and may not be diagnosed until they fail to initiate puberty and exhibit high gonadotropins consistent with gonadal failure. Up to 30% of patients with 46,XY CGD may develop germ cell tumors, so their streak gonads should be removed in infancy.

Partial gonadal dysgenesis occurs when there is partial but incomplete testicular differentiation, leading to inadequate production of testosterone and/or AMH, and in turn leading to varying degrees of external virilization and müllerian regression. The tumor risk is also elevated in these cases, but there remains a lack of consensus regarding the degree of tumor risk and whether close monitoring is adequate if the gonad has a scrotal location and can be evaluated by physical exam and ultrasound.

C. 46,XX testicular DSD. These individuals usually appear phenotypically male, but 20% have ambiguous genitalia. At puberty, they may produce insufficient testosterone and can resemble patients with Klinefelter syndrome (small testes, azoospermia, disproportionately long limbs, gynecomastia). Cryptic mosaicism with a Y chromosome-bearing cell line or translocation of *SRY* to the X chromosome or an autosome is frequently responsible. In *SRY*-negative individuals, duplication of *SOX9* (17q24) may be detected by FISH. Additional genes have been reportedly associated with testicular or ovotesticular DSD including *SOX3*, *WNT4*, and *RSPO1*.

D. Ovotesticular DSD. The chromosomal complement in this rare condition is variable: Seventy percent of patients are 46,XX; <10% are 46,XY; and the remainder show mosaicism with a Y chromosome-containing cell line (most commonly 46,XX/46,XY).

1. **Physical findings.** The external genitalia may appear normal or may show partial labioscrotal fusion, asymmetric labioscrotal folds, or hypospadias. Whether the internal structures contain wolffian or müllerian elements depends on the local presence of testosterone and AMH on that side of the abdomen.

2. **Evaluation.** An hCG stimulation test that produces a rise in serum testosterone confirms the presence of Leydig cells, whereas a measurable AMH level indicates the presence of Sertoli cells.

3. **Diagnosis** is based on the histology of the gonads, which by definition contain both testicular and ovarian tissue. Laparoscopy, gonadal biopsy, or both may be required for diagnosis.

4. **Management.** Dysgenetic gonadal tissue that contains a Y chromosome should be assessed further by exam and/or imaging. The rate of tumors in ovotestes is lower than with gonadal dysgenesis but is still elevated from normal testicular tissue. Beyond the tumor risk, hormone production in puberty can be troubling. Girls with intact ovotestes may experience virilization, and boys may undergo breast development. Ideally, this should be carefully addressed by the medical team, family, and patient prior to the onset of puberty. For details of sex assignment, see section VIII.

VI. OTHER 46,XX DSD. The infant has undergone virilization due to exposure to excess androgens, which can be of adrenal or gonadal origin (or rarely, maternal or exogenous origin).

A. CAH. The most common DSD presenting in the neonatal period is a 46,XX infant with CAH. The most common form of CAH (>90%) is deficiency of 21-hydroxylase (21-OHase in Fig. 63.5) caused by mutations in *CYP21A2*. Virilization may occur in rarer forms of CAH due to deficiency of 11β-hydroxylase (11-OHase, encoded by *CYP11B1*) or 3β-hydroxysteroid dehydrogenase (3β-HSD, encoded by *HSD3B2*). Individuals with CAH typically do not have testicular tissue and therefore usually have normally developed müllerian structures and no wolffian structures.

1. **Epidemiology.** The incidence of 21-OHase deficiency is 1:16,000 births based on data from worldwide newborn screening programs. Patients with salt wasting outnumber those with "simple virilizing" CAH by 3:1. The male:female sex ratio is 1:1. Whereas females are easily detected at birth due to abnormal genital development, males

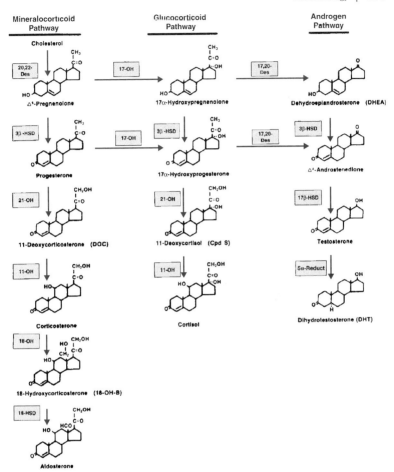

Figure 63.5. Pathways of steroid biosynthesis. (From Esoterix, Calabasas Hills, CA.)

have normal genitalia and may be missed on clinical exam (although hyperpigmentation of the scrotum can be a clue).

2. **Diagnosis.** In the United States, all state newborn screening programs include screening for 21-OHase deficiency. Blood spots are obtained on filter paper, ideally between 48 and 72 hours of age, and 17-hydroxyprogesterone (17-OHP) is measured. Normal values must be determined for each individual screening program because they depend on the filter paper thickness and the immunoassay used. The 17-OHP is elevated on newborn screening in 99% of infants with salt-wasting or simple virilizing 21-OHase deficiency.

   a. **False-positive results.** Obtaining a blood sample before 48 hours of age can cause a false-positive result. Because normal values for 17-OHP are inversely related to gestational age and birth weight, false-positive results can also occur in premature and low birth weight infants as well as in infants who are acutely ill.

b. False-negative results. Prenatal administration of steroids (e.g., betamethasone) may suppress 17-OHP levels and cause false-negative results; newborns who received such medications should be rescreened after 3 to 5 days.

c. Rapid evaluation of suspected 21-OHase deficiency is critical to avert salt-wasting crisis. Clinical suspicion or abnormal newborn screening results should be confirmed immediately by measurement of serum 17-OHP. An adrenocorticotropic hormone (ACTH) level may aid diagnosis, and measurement of plasma renin activity and aldosterone may help differentiate between salt-wasting and simple virilizing forms. Serum electrolytes should be monitored at least every other day until salt wasting is confirmed or ruled out.

d. Rare forms of CAH. In an infant with 11-OHase deficiency, levels of 11-deoxycortisol and 11-deoxycorticosterone are elevated and can cause hypertension. An infant with 3β-HSD deficiency may have mildly elevated 17-OHP on newborn screen; 17-hydroxypregnenolone and the 17-hydroxypregnenolone-to-cortisol ratio are markedly elevated in these infants.

e. Newborn screening may not detect infants with mild simple virilizing 21-OHase deficiency. Therefore, in a virilized 46,XX female suspected of having a form of CAH, or who has equivocal 17-OHP levels, an **ACTH stimulation test** may be necessary to demonstrate the adrenal enzyme defect (Fig. 63.5).

3. **Management.** In an infant suspected of 21-OHase deficiency, treatment should be started as soon as the laboratory tests mentioned have been obtained.

a. Glucocorticoids. Hydrocortisone 20 mg/m^2/day, divided into dosing every 8 hours, should be given to all infants suspected of 21-OHase deficiency.

$$\text{Body surface area (m}^2) = \sqrt{\frac{\text{Length (cm)} \times \text{Weight (kg)}}{3{,}600}}$$

b. Mineralocorticoids. In cases of salt-wasting CAH, fludrocortisone acetate (Florinef) 0.1 to 0.2 mg daily should be given. Salt-wasting crises usually develop between the 5th and 14th day of life but can occur as late as 1 month and may occur even in affected infants whose virilization is not severe. Weight, fluid balance, and electrolytes must be monitored closely, with blood samples at least every 2 days during the first few weeks of life to detect hyponatremia or hyperkalemia. If salt wasting occurs, salt loss should be replaced initially with intravenous normal saline with glucose added. Salt wasting due to aldosterone deficiency typically requires replacement of about 8 mEq/kg/day of sodium. Once the infant is stabilized, NaCl 1 to 2 g daily, divided into dosing every 6 hours, should be added to the formula (each gram of NaCl contains 17 mEq of sodium).

B. **Maternal hyperandrogenic conditions.** Maternal CAH, virilizing tumors of the adrenal or ovary, or exposure to androgenic medications during pregnancy must be severe to overcome placental aromatase, which protects the fetus from androgens by converting them to estrogens.

C. **Placental aromatase deficiency.** The hallmark of this rare disorder is that both mother and infant are virilized due to an inability to convert androgens to estrogens.

D. **Cytochrome P450 oxidoreductase (POR) deficiency.** Mutations in the *POR* gene lead to a form of CAH. This disorder of steroidogenesis affects multiple microsomal P450 enzymes involved in steroid hormone synthesis including *CYP21A2* (21-OHase), *CYP17A1* (17α-OHase and 17,20 lyase), and *CYP19A1* (aromatase). Patients may have positive newborn screens with elevated 17-OH progesterone levels and may also present with maternal virilization during pregnancy.

E. See section V for discussion of 46,XX ovotesticular and testicular DSD.

VII. OTHER 46,XY DSD.

Evaluation of the infant with 46,XY DSD is complex, and early consultation with a pediatric endocrinologist will help direct the evaluation. Nevertheless, only 20% to 50% of children with 46,XY DSD will receive a definitive diagnosis. Even if genetic testing demonstrates Y chromosome material, the parents should not be told hastily that a male sex assignment is appropriate.

A. **Disorders of testicular development.** Impaired testicular function can be due to unresponsiveness to hCG and LH (LH/hCG receptor mutation). Gonadal dysgenesis and ovotesticular DSD are discussed in section V.

B. **Defects in androgen synthesis or action.** These individuals typically have no müllerian structures because AMH is produced normally.

1. **Enzymatic defects in testosterone synthesis** include deficiency of 17β-hydroxysteroid dehydrogenase type 3 (17β-HSD in Fig. 63.5, encoded by *HSD17B3*), 3β-hydroxysteroid dehydrogenase (3β-HSD, encoded by *HSD3B2*), 17α-hydroxylase/17,20-lyase (17-OHase or *CYP17*), isolated 17,20-lyase (17,20 Des in Fig. 63.5), or very rarely side-chain cleavage enzyme (20,22 Des or *CYP11A1*) or steroidogenic acute regulatory protein (StAR).

2. **Defect in testosterone metabolism.** Patients with 5α-reductase type 2 (*SRD5A2*) deficiency have impaired conversion of testosterone to DHT. Although generally uncommon, this defect has a higher prevalence in the Dominican Republic and the Middle East. DHT can also be produced by an alternative, "backdoor" pathway that starts with 17-hydroxyprogesterone. Mutations in enzymes in this backdoor pathway have also been reported in 46,XY DSD.

3. **End-organ resistance** to testosterone and DHT is caused by mutations of the androgen receptor. Such mutations are X-linked. The degree of resistance is variable, leading to a clinical spectrum from partial androgen insensitivity syndrome (PAIS) to complete androgen insensitivity syndrome (CAIS).

C. **Environmental disorders.** Maternal drug ingestion of antiandrogens (e.g., spironolactone) and 5α-reductase inhibitors (e.g., finasteride) can cause ambiguous genitalia. Maternal phenytoin exposure has been associated with ambiguous genitalia in rare cases.

D. **Evaluation** focuses on establishing the presence or absence of testes and their ability to produce androgens.

1. **Presence of testes.** If testes are not palpable, their presence should be determined by imaging and/or AMH level (see sections VII.F and VII.G).

2. **Laboratory evaluation** is focused on determining whether the cause of undervirilization is due to a defect in gonadal development or testosterone synthesis, metabolism, or action. Blood samples should be obtained for measurement of electrolytes, FSH, LH, testosterone, DHT, androstenedione, 17-hydroxyprogesterone, 17-hydroxypregnenolone, cortisol, and AMH. Serum electrolytes may reveal hyponatremia and hyperkalemia in 3β-HSD deficiency. Measurement of 11-deoxycorticosterone and plasma renin activity may help define the type of enzyme deficiency.

3. An **hCG stimulation test** may be necessary if the above results do not lead to a diagnosis.
   a. **Technique.** The hCG is given intramuscularly daily or every 2 days for a total of three doses. Androstenedione, testosterone, and DHT concentrations are measured before the first dose and 24 hours after the final dose of hCG.
   b. **Interpretation.** Inability to increase the testosterone level in response to hCG is characteristic of testicular dysgenesis, LH-receptor mutations, gestational loss of testicular tissue, or an enzymatic defect in testosterone synthesis. An elevated testosterone:DHT ratio (>20:1) after hCG stimulation suggests 5α-reductase deficiency, whereas a low testosterone:androstenedione ratio (<0.8:1) suggests 17β-HSD deficiency.

4. An **ACTH stimulation test** may be necessary to define defects in earlier enzymatic steps of testosterone synthesis that also affect cortisol synthesis, such as deficiencies of 3β-HSD, side-chain cleavage enzyme, StAR, or 17-OHase, which result in CAH (Fig. 63.5). The former three deficiencies are associated with salt wasting; 17-OHase deficiency is associated with salt retention and hypertension, although these are often not present in the newborn period.

5. **Androgen insensitivity syndrome.** If the initial laboratory tests show high levels of testosterone, and the testosterone-to-androstenedione and testosterone-to-DHT ratios are normal, the infant may have **PAIS**.
   a. **Further evaluation** may include monthly administration of 25 to 50 mg of intramuscular depot testosterone for 3 months. Failure of the stretched penile length to increase by 1.5 cm supports the diagnosis of PAIS.

b. Genetic studies of the androgen receptor will detect mutations in some but not necessarily all clinical cases of PAIS.

c. Newborns with **CAIS** have normal-appearing female external genitalia (including the lower third of the vagina) and absent müllerian and wolffian structures. They may be identified by an antepartum 46,XY karyotype or by the presence of an apparent inguinal hernia that proves to be a testis. More often, they present in late puberty with primary amenorrhea.

E. **Microphallus** (<2.5 cm in a full-term infant) with or without cryptorchidism has many causes in addition to those mentioned earlier, including hypothalamic-pituitary disorders of gonadotropin production such as Kallmann syndrome, holoprosencephaly, optic nerve hypoplasia (also referred to as septo-optic dysplasia), and other causes of multiple pituitary hormone deficiencies. Growth hormone deficiency can also be associated with microphallus. Infants with panhypopituitarism often have neonatal hypoglycemia and direct hyperbilirubinemia. Among the many other conditions associated with microphallus are CHARGE syndrome; trisomy 21; and Prader-Willi, Robinow, Klinefelter, Carpenter, Meckel-Gruber, Noonan, de Lange, Fanconi, and fetal hydantoin syndromes. Treatment with testosterone enanthate or cypionate 25 to 50 mg intramuscularly given monthly for 3 months may substantially increase penile length in these patients.

F. **Bilateral cryptorchidism.** Bilateral cryptorchidism at birth occurs in 3:1,000 infants, most of whom are premature. By 1 month of life, the testes are still undescended in 1:1,000 infants.

1. **Imaging.** Either ultrasonography or MRI may reveal inguinal or intra-abdominal testes, although MRI is more sensitive for locating the latter.

2. **Laboratory evaluation.** If testicular tissue cannot be found by exam or imaging, levels of serum FSH, LH, testosterone, and AMH should be measured. The testosterone and gonadotropins rise shortly after birth (usually by 72 hours) and are present at pubertal levels until approximately 6 months of age in boys.

   a. Elevated serum gonadotropins with a low testosterone concentration suggests absent or nonfunctioning testes.

   b. Undetectable serum **AMH** is indicative of bilateral anorchia rather than undescended testes (see section VII.G in the following text).

3. **Management.** A urologist should be consulted, and if surgery is indicated, orchidopexy should be performed by 1 year of life. If intra-abdominal testes cannot be brought into the scrotum, removal should be considered because of the 3- to 10-fold increased risk of potentially malignant tumors in cryptorchid testes.

4. **Persistent müllerian duct syndrome (PMDS)** in 46,XY infants is caused by defects in AMH or its receptor. Cryptorchidism is common in infants with PMDS, who otherwise have normal male genitalia but retain a uterus and fallopian tubes.

5. **Other conditions** associated with cryptorchidism include trisomy 21; neural tube defects; renal and urinary tract malformations; and numerous syndromes including Prader-Willi, Bardet-Biedl, Aarskog, Cockayne, Fanconi, Noonan, Klinefelter, and fetal hydantoin syndromes.

    6. The presence of any of the following physical findings also merits evaluation for a DSD:

      a. Unilateral cryptorchidism with hypospadias, especially proximal (e.g., perineoscrotal or penile) hypospadias

      b. Unilateral cryptorchidism with microphallus

G. Use of AMH measurements. The hCG stimulation test is used to assess the presence and function of testicular tissue, specifically Leydig cells, but can be cumbersome and expensive and occasionally requires protracted dosing to stimulate a refractory testis. AMH is an alternative marker of the presence of testicular tissue, specifically Sertoli cells. AMH is produced in a sexually dimorphic manner. Starting at birth, AMH from Sertoli cells rises to a peak of 115 ng/mL at 6 months of age and then declines during adolescence to an adult male level of 4 ng/mL. In contrast, granulosa cells of the ovary do not make significant amounts of AMH until puberty, when levels in girls also reach approximately 4 ng/mL. Thus, measuring AMH in an infant can distinguish whether testicular tissue is present or absent. AMH in the normal or detectable range has a 100% positive predictive value for the presence of testicular tissue; the predictive value for anorchia is 94% if AMH is undetectable.

VIII. ISSUES OF SEX ASSIGNMENT. Today, most providers agree that the primary goal in sex assignment is to attempt to match the child's future gender identity, but this is a challenging, imperfect, and humbling endeavor. Several factors influence gender identity, including chromosomal sex and fetal (and possibly neonatal) exposure to androgens (the degree of which is inferred from the appearance of the external genitalia), as well as sex of rearing itself, but there are undoubtedly other, currently unknown factors that affect the formation of gender identity. Only in cases of complete androgen insensitivity and 46,XY CGD can sex assignment (as female) be done with confidence.

    Other factors to be considered in sex assignment include prospects for fertility and considerations for genitoplasty. In the past, a primary criterion for male sex assignment was a penile size deemed to be adequate for sexual function. The 46,XY infants born with little or no penile tissue had traditionally been assigned a female sex and surgically and hormonally feminized by means of genitoplasty and gonadectomy early in life and estrogen treatment at the age of puberty. This practice is no longer routine.

    Likewise, under debate is the issue of sex assignment in the most severely virilized 46,XX newborns with CAH who have completely fused labioscrotal folds and a penile urethra. A minority opinion recommends male sex assignment and gonadectomy, thereby eliminating the need for feminizing genitoplasty. Nevertheless, many geneticists and endocrinologists and existing guidelines continue to recommend female sex assignment to preserve fertility.

    Another subject of controversy is whether and when to perform other gonadal and/or genital surgeries, such as clitoral reduction in virilized infants being raised female or gonadectomy in infants with CAIS. Whereas some adults with DSD view their genital surgery as mutilation, many parents prefer surgery so that their child's genitalia appear more consistent with the assigned sex. One-stage surgical procedures that preserve the neurovascular bundle can be done in infancy and are much improved compared to the clitorectomies routinely performed several decades ago, but there is increasing reluctance to irreversibly remove structures when future gender identity is uncertain. Nevertheless, there is general consensus on the importance of removing a dysgenetic abdominal gonad that contains Y chromosome material because of the high risk of gonadoblastoma.

Parents require a thorough explanation of their child's condition as laboratory and imaging data become available. They should participate with the interdisciplinary team in decision making during assessment of the options for medical and surgical therapy and of the prospects for gender identity, genital appearance, sexual functioning, and fertility. The full medical team should include a pediatrician/neonatologist, pediatric endocrinologist, pediatric surgeon and/or pediatric urologist, geneticist, and counselor experienced in dealing with DSD. Finally, long-term, unbiased studies of gender identity, sexual functioning, and surgical outcomes in individuals born with various forms of DSD are needed to provide insight into the difficult task of sex assignment for these infants.

Suggested Readings

American Academy of Pediatrics Committee on Genetics. Evaluation of the newborn with developmental anomalies of the external genitalia. *Pediatrics* 2000;106:138–142.

Anhalt H, Neely K, Hintz RL. Ambiguous genitalia. *Pediatr Rev* 1996;17:213–220.

Arboleda VA, Sandberg DE, Vilain E. DSDs: genetics, underlying pathologies and psychosexual differentiation. *Nat Rev Endocrinol* 2014;10(10):603–615.

Hughes IA, Houk C, Ahmed SF, et al; for the Lawson Wilkins Pediatric Endocrine Society/European Society for Paediatric Endocrinology Consensus Group. Consensus statement on management of intersex disorders. *Arch Dis Child* 2006;91(7):554–563.

Ono M, Harley VR. Disorders of sex development: new genes, new concepts. *Nat Rev Endocrinol* 2013;9(2):79–91.

White PC, Speiser PW. Congenital adrenal hyperplasia due to 21-hydroxylase deficiency. *Endocr Rev* 2000;21:245–291.

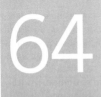

64

Surgical Emergencies in the Newborn

Steven A. Ringer and Anne R. Hansen

I. POTENTIAL SURGICAL CONDITIONS PRESENTING IN THE FETUS

A. **Polyhydramnios** (amniotic fluid volume >2 L) occurs in 1 in 1,000 births.

1. Gastrointestinal (GI) obstruction (including esophageal atresia [EA]) is the most frequent surgical cause of polyhydramnios.

2. Other causes of polyhydramnios include abdominal wall defects (omphalocele and gastroschisis), anencephaly, diaphragmatic hernia (DH), maternal diabetes with consequent fetal hyperglycemia and glucosuria and other conditions impairing the ability of the fetus to concentrate urine, tight nuchal cord and other causes of impaired fetal swallowing, and fetal death.

3. All women with suspected polyhydramnios should have an ultrasonographic examination. In experienced hands, this is the study of choice for the diagnosis of intestinal obstruction, abdominal wall defects, DH, as well as abnormalities leading to an inability of the fetus to swallow.

4. If intestinal obstruction is diagnosed antenatally and there is no concern for dystocia, vaginal delivery is acceptable. Pediatric surgical consultation should be obtained before delivery.

B. **Oligohydramnios** is associated with amniotic fluid leak, intrauterine growth restriction, postmaturity, fetal distress, and renal dysgenesis or agenesis (Potter syndrome; see Chapter 28). If the duration of oligohydramnios is prolonged, it is important to anticipate respiratory compromise in these infants, as adequate amniotic fluid volume is generally necessary for normal pulmonary development, particularly during the second trimester of gestation. Severity of pulmonary hypoplasia correlates with degree and duration of oligohydramnios.

C. **Meconium peritonitis** can be diagnosed prenatally by ultrasonography, typically seen as areas of calcification scattered throughout the abdomen. Postnatally, calcifications are confirmed by plain film of the abdomen. It is usually due to antenatal perforation of the intestinal tract; thus, this diagnosis should prompt an evaluation for a congenital lesion causing intestinal obstruction, either anatomic or functional (see section IV.A).

D. **Fetal ascites** is usually associated with urinary tract anomalies (e.g., lower urinary tract obstruction due to posterior urethral valves). Other possible causes include hemolytic disease of the newborn, any severe anemia (e.g., α-thalassemia), peritonitis, thoracic duct obstruction, cardiac disease, hepatic or portal vein obstruction, hepatitis, and congenital infection (e.g., TORCH infections; see Chapters 48 to 53) as well as other causes of hydrops fetalis (see Chapter 26). After birth, ascites may be seen in congenital nephrotic syndrome. Accurate prenatal ultrasonography is important in light of the potential for fetal surgery to minimize renal parenchymal injury by decompressing either the bladder or a hydronephrotic kidney (see Chapters 1 and 28).

E. **Dystocia** may result from fetal hydrocephalus, intestinal obstruction, abdominal wall defect, genitourinary anomalies, or fetal ascites (see section I.D).

F. **Fetal surgery.** The potential for surgical intervention during fetal life continues to develop. It depends heavily on the availability of precise prenatal diagnostic techniques and experience in accurately characterizing disorders including the use of ultrasonography and fast magnetic resonance imaging (MRI).

Advances in obstetric and anesthesia management have also contributed to the feasibility of performing *in utero* procedures. The mother must be carefully managed through what is often a long and unpredictable anesthesia course. Medications that reduce uterine irritability have been developed that maximally ensure that the uterus can be maintained without contractions during and after the procedure. The criteria for consideration of a procedure include the following:

1. **Ethical considerations** are important, including balancing both the potential risk and benefit to the fetus with the potential pain or harm to the mother as well as the impact on the family as a whole.

2. **Technical feasibility**

3. **Severity of fetal condition.** Initially, most cases dealt with conditions that were life threatening either because they caused death *in utero* or the inability to survive postnatal life if born unrepaired. Currently, some cases are considered when a condition is not life threatening but is severe and either the condition itself is progressive (such as the growth of a large tumor partially obstructing the fetal airway) or the consequences of the condition worsen progressively (such as worsening hydrops due to a large teratoma).

4. **Necessary resources.** The care of the mother, fetus, and potential baby during surgery, in the immediate postoperative period and after birth, must all be available in seamless proximity to the institution where the surgery is performed.

Fetal surgery has been successfully used for removal of an enlarging chest mass, such as an adenomatoid malformation of the lung or a bronchopulmonary sequestration. Mass lesions, such as sacrococcygeal teratoma, when diagnosed *in utero*, have been treated with excision or by fetoscopically guided laser ablation of the feeder vessels, resulting in involution, but this type of intervention is only considered when the lesion is causing life-threatening complications, such as fetal hydrops. Progressive fetal urethral obstruction has been ameliorated by the use of shunts or fulguration of posterior urethral valves. Similar fetoscopic laser ablation of connecting vessels has been used successfully in the treatment of twin–twin transfusion syndrome (TTTS) or twin reversed arterial perfusion (TRAP).

Fetal surgical correction of meningomyelocele is a rapidly evolving area of endeavor. A multicenter randomized controlled trial comparing *in utero* surgical correction with standard management found that performing prenatal surgery may lead to better outcomes than postnatal surgery. After 12 months, the 91 infants who had prenatal surgery were 30% less likely to die or need additional surgical procedures than the 92 infants who were treated postnatally. At 2.5-year follow-up, those treated prenatally showed improved physical development and motor function, such as unassisted walking, compared to those treated after birth. However, prenatal surgery was associated with increased risk of complications during pregnancy including premature delivery and tearing of the uterine wall from the surgical scar. Long-term effects of this approach remain uncertain. When the diagnosis of myelomeningocele is made prenatally, *in utero* repair is an option that parents may consider.

Successful fetal procedures that we are currently performing include ***ex utero* intrapartum treatment** (EXIT) procedures for complex airway obstructions and complex congenital DH, aortic valve dilation for critical aortic stenosis, atrial septostomy, or stent placement for intact atrial septum with hypoplastic left heart syndrome, vascular photocoagulation for TTTS or TRAP syndrome, and percutaneous bladder shunt for bladder outlet obstruction. Indications for fetal intervention continue to evolve and change.

II. POSTNATAL SURGICAL DISORDERS: DIAGNOSIS BY PRESENTING SYMPTOM

A. **Respiratory distress** (see sections III.B and III.C; Chapters 29 to 39). Although most etiologies of respiratory distress are treated medically, some respiratory disorders do require surgical therapies.

1. Choanal atresia (see section III.C.1)

2. Laryngotracheal clefts (see section III.C.3)

3. Tracheal agenesis

4. EA with or without tracheoesophageal fistula (TEF) (see section III.A)

5. Congenital lobar emphysema

6. Cystic adenomatoid malformation of the lung, pulmonary sequestration

7. DH (see section III.B)

8. Biliary tracheobronchial communication (extremely rare)

B. Scaphoid abdomen

1. DH (see section III.B)

2. EA without TEF (see section III.A)

C. Excessive mucus and salivation. EA with or without TEF (see section III.A)

D. Abdominal distention can be due to ascites, pneumoperitoneum, or intestinal obstruction (mechanical or functional).

1. Pneumoperitoneum. Any perforation of the bowel may cause pneumoperitoneum (see Chapter 27).

a. Any portion of the GI tract can potentially perforate for a variety of reasons including poor bowel wall integrity (e.g., necrotizing enterocolitis or localized ischemia of the stomach or small bowel associated with some medications such as indomethacin) and excessive pressure (e.g., obstruction, TEF, or instrumentation [i.e., with a nasogastric tube]). Perforated stomach is associated with large amounts of free intra-abdominal air. Active GI air leak requires urgent surgical closure. It may be necessary to aspirate air from the abdominal cavity to relieve respiratory distress before definitive surgical repair.

b. Air from a pulmonary air leak may dissect into the peritoneal cavity of infants receiving mechanical ventilation. Treatment of pneumoperitoneum transmitted from pulmonary air leak should focus on managing the pulmonary air leak.

2. Intestinal obstruction

a. EA with TEF (see section III.A) can present as abdominal distension. Obstruction of proximal bowel (e.g., complete duodenal atresia) typically results in rapid distension of the left upper quadrant. Obstruction of distal bowel causes more generalized distension, varying with location of obstruction.

b. Obstruction may be suspected when the progression of the air column through the gut is slowed or halted. Normally, when assessed by plain radiographs, air is seen 1 hour after birth at a point past the stomach and into the upper jejunum; 3 hours after birth, it is at the cecum; 8 to 12 hours after birth, it is at the rectosigmoid. This progression is slower in the premature infant.

E. Vomiting. The causes of vomiting can be differentiated by the presence or absence of bile.

1. Bilious emesis. The presence of bile-stained vomit in the newborn should be treated as a life-threatening emergency, with at least 20% of such infants requiring emergency surgical intervention after evaluation. Surgical consultation should be obtained immediately. Unless the infant is clinically unstable, a contrast study of the upper gastrointestinal (UGI) tract should be obtained as quickly as possible.

Intestinal obstruction may result from malrotation with or without midgut volvulus; duodenal, jejunal, ileal, or colonic atresias; annular pancreas; Hirschsprung disease; aberrant superior mesenteric artery; preduodenal portal vein; peritoneal bands; persistent omphalomesenteric duct; or duodenal duplication.

Bile-stained emesis is occasionally seen in infants without intestinal obstruction who have decreased motility (see section II.E.2.c). In these cases, the bile-stained vomiting will only occur one or two times and will present without abdominal distention. However, a nonsurgical condition is a diagnosis of exclusion; bilious emesis is malrotation until proven otherwise.

2. Nonbilious emesis
   a. Feeding excessive volume
   b. Milk (human or formula) intolerance
   c. Decreased motility
      i. Prematurity
      ii. Antenatal exposure to $MgSO_4$ or ante-, pre-, or postnatal exposure to narcotics
      iii. Sepsis with ileus
      iv. Central nervous system (CNS) lesion
   d. Lesion above ampulla of Vater
      i. Pyloric stenosis
      ii. Upper duodenal stenosis
      iii. Annular pancreas (rare)

F. Failure to pass meconium can occur in sick and/or premature babies with decreased bowel motility. It also may be the result of the following disorders:

   1. Imperforate anus

   2. Microcolon

   3. Mucous plug

   4. Other causes of intestinal obstruction

G. Failure to develop transitional stools after the passage of meconium

   1. Volvulus, other intestinal obstruction

   2. Malrotation

H. Hematemesis or hematochezia

   1. Nonsurgical conditions. Many patients with hematemesis, and most patients with **hematochezia** (bloody stools), have a nonsurgical condition. Differential diagnosis includes the following:
   a. Milk intolerance/allergy (usually cow's milk protein allergy)
   b. Instrumentation (e.g., nasogastric tube, endotracheal tube)
   c. Swallowed maternal blood
      i. Maternal blood is sometimes swallowed by the newborn during labor and delivery. This can be diagnosed by an Apt test performed on blood aspirated from the infant's stomach (see section XI.G).
      ii. In breastfed infants, either micro- or macroscopic blood noted several days after birth in either emesis or stool may be due to swallowed blood during breastfeeding in setting of cracked maternal nipples.

Inspecting the mother's breasts or expressed milk is usually diagnostic. If not, aspirate the contents of the baby's stomach after a feeding and send the recently swallowed milk for an Apt test.

d. Coagulation disorders including disseminated intravascular coagulation (DIC), lack of postnatal vitamin K injection (see Chapter 43)

2. Surgical conditions resulting in hematemesis and bloody stool
a. Necrotizing enterocolitis (most frequent cause of hematemesis and bloody stool in premature infants; see Chapter 27)
b. Gastric or duodenal ulcers (due to stress, steroid therapy)
c. GI obstruction: late sign, concerning for threatened or necrotic bowel
d. Volvulus
e. Intussusception
f. Polyps, hemangiomas
g. Meckel diverticulum
h. Duplications of the small intestine
i. Cirsoid aneurysm

I. Abdominal masses (see section VIII)

1. Genitourinary anomalies including distended bladder (see section VII and Chapter 28)

2. Hepatosplenomegaly: may be confused with other masses; requires medical evaluation

3. Tumors (see section VII)

J. Birth trauma (see Chapter 6)

1. Fractured clavicle/humerus (see Chapter 58)

2. Intracranial hemorrhage (see Chapter 54)

3. Lacerated solid organs—liver, spleen

4. Spinal cord transection with quadriplegia

III. LESIONS CAUSING RESPIRATORY DISTRESS

A. EA and TEF. At least 85% of infants with EA also have TEF. Pure EA and TEF with proximal TEF may be suspected on prenatal ultrasonography by the absence of a stomach bubble.

1. Postnatal presentation depends on the presence or absence as well as location of a TEF.
a. Infants often present with excessive salivation and vomiting soon after feedings. They may develop respiratory distress due to the following:
  i. Airway obstruction by excess secretions
  ii. Aspiration of saliva and milk
  iii. Compromised pulmonary capacity due to diaphragmatic elevation secondary to abdominal distension
  iv. Reflux of gastric contents up the distal esophagus into the lungs through the fistula
b. If there is no fistula, or if it connects the trachea to the esophagus proximal to the atresia, no GI gas will be seen on x-ray examination, and the abdomen will be scaphoid.

c. TEF without EA (H-type fistula) is extremely rare and usually presents after the neonatal period. The diagnosis is suggested by a history of frequent pneumonias or respiratory distress temporally related to meals.

2. **Diagnosis**

a. EA itself is diagnosed by the inability to pass a catheter from the mouth or nose into the stomach. The catheter is inserted into the esophagus until resistance is met. Air is then injected into the catheter while listening (for lack of air) over the stomach. The diagnosis is confirmed by x-ray studies showing the catheter coiled in the upper esophageal pouch. Plain x-ray films may demonstrate a distended blind upper esophageal pouch filled with air that is unable to progress into the stomach. (The plain films may also show associated cardiac or vertebral anomalies of the cervical or upper thoracic region of the spine.)

b. H-type fistula. This disorder can often be demonstrated with administration of nonionic water-soluble contrast medium (Omnipaque) during cinefluoroscopy. The definitive examination is combined fiberoptic bronchoscopy and esophagoscopy with passage of a fine balloon catheter from the trachea into the esophagus. The H-type fistula is usually high in the trachea (cervical area).

3. **Associated issues and anomalies.** Babies with TEF and EA are often of low birth weight. Approximately 20% of these babies are premature (five times the normal incidence), and another 20% are small for gestational age (eight times the normal incidence). Other anomalies may be present, including chromosomal abnormalities and the VACTERL association: **V**ertebral defects, imperforate **A**nus, **C**ardiac defects, **TE**F with EA, **R**enal dysplasia or defects and **L**imb anomalies.

4. **Management.** Preoperative management focuses on minimizing the risk of aspiration and avoiding gaseous distension of the GI tract with positive pressure crossing from the trachea into the esophagus.

a. A multiple end-hole suction catheter (Replogle or Vygon) should be placed in the proximal pouch and put to continuous suction immediately after the diagnosis is made.

b. The head of the bed should be elevated 30 degrees to diminish reflux of gastric contents into the fistula and aspiration of oral secretions that may accumulate in the proximal esophageal pouch.

c. If possible, mechanical ventilation of these babies should be avoided until the fistula is controlled because the positive pressure may cause severe abdominal distension compromising respiratory function. If intubation is required, the case should be considered an emergency. Guidelines for intubation are the same as for other types of respiratory distress. The endotracheal tube should be advanced to just above the carina in the hopes of obstructing airflow through the fistula. Most commonly, the fistula connects to the trachea near the carina. Care must be taken to avoid accidental intubation of the fistula. Optimally, if mechanical ventilation is required, it should be done using a relatively high rate and low pressure to minimize GI distention. Heavy sedation should be avoided because it compromises patient's spontaneous respiratory effort which generates negative intrathoracic pressure, minimizing passage of air through the fistula into the esophagus.

d. Surgical therapy usually involves immediate placement of a gastrostomy tube. If the patient is of adequate size and stability, the fistula is divided, and if possible, the proximal and distal ends of the esophagus are anastomosed primarily.

e. Coincident prematurity or the presence of associated defects may make it advisable to delay primary repair. Mechanical ventilation and nutritional management may be difficult in these infants because of the TEF. These patients need careful nursing care to prevent aspiration and gastrostomy with G-tube feedings to allow growth until repair is possible. In some cases, the fistula can be divided, with deferral of definitive repair.

f. If the infant has cardiac disease that requires surgery, it is usually best to repair the fistula first. If not, the postoperative ventilatory management can be very difficult.

g. Patients with long-gap EA can be extremely challenging to manage. We have developed a referral center for such patients who are treated with innovative esophageal growth induction techniques that can allow for primary repairs thereby avoiding the need for gastric, colonic, or jejunal interposition.

B. Diaphragmatic hernia

1. **Anatomy.** The most common site is the left hemithorax, with the defect in the diaphragm being posterior (foramen of Bochdalek) in 70% of infants. It can also occur on the right, with either an anterior or a posterior defect. Bilateral DH is extremely rare.

2. **Incidence** occurs in approximately 1 in 4,000 live births. Fifty percent of these hernias are associated with other malformations, especially cardiac, neural tube, intestinal, skeletal, and renal defects. DH has been associated with trisomies 13 and 18 and 45,XO and has been reported as part of Goldenhar, Beckwith-Wiedemann, Pierre Robin, Wolf-Hirschhorn syndrome (4p deletion); Pallister-Killian syndrome (tetrasomy 12p); Fryns syndrome; Goltz-Gorlin syndrome; and congenital Rubella syndrome. In rare cases, DH is familial.

3. **Symptoms.** Infants with large DHs usually present at birth with cyanosis, respiratory distress, a scaphoid abdomen, decreased or absent breath sounds on the side of the hernia, and heart sounds displaced to the side opposite the hernia. Small hernias, right-sided hernias, sac-type hernias, and substernal hernias of Morgagni may have a more subtle and/or later presentation, manifested as feeding problems and mild respiratory distress. Associated structural malformations include congenital heart disease (CHD), neural tube defects, skeletal anomalies, intestinal atresias, and renal anomalies.

4. **Diagnosis**
   a. Prenatal diagnosis. DHs often occur after the routine 16-week prenatal ultrasonography; therefore, many of these cases are not diagnosed prenatally. The development of polyhydramnios should prompt a later fetal ultrasonography that will detect DH. Diagnosis earlier in gestation may correlate with a poorer prognosis due to severity of condition. The prognostic advantage of prenatal diagnosis is that it generally leads to delivery in a center equipped to optimize chances for survival. If delivery

before term is likely, fetal lung maturity should be assessed to evaluate the need for maternal betamethasone therapy (see Chapter 33). Presence of liver in the thorax correlates with increased severity and poorer prognosis. Percent predictive lung volume (PPLV) measures relative lung volumes by MRI. We have found this biometric parameter quite useful in predicting the risk of morbidity and mortality. The lower the PPLV, the higher the risk. Lung-to-head ratio (LHR) can also be measured prenatally and in skilled hands can help predict severity of involvement. In our institution, there are no reported survivors with an LHR <1. An LHR >1.4 has a 100% survival rate, and an LHR between 1 and 1.4 has a 38% survival rate with a high need for extracorporeal membrane oxygenation (ECMO). We continue to search for additional methods to accurately predict the postnatal course of fetuses found to have congenital DH.

b. Postnatal diagnosis. The diagnosis is made or confirmed by radiograph. Because of the possibility of marked cardiothymic shift, a radiopaque marker should be placed on one side of the chest to aid interpretation of the x-ray film.

c. Differential diagnosis. Diaphragmatic eventration, congenital cystic adenomatoid malformation (CCAM), pulmonary sequestration, bronchogenic cyst

5. **Treatment**

a. Severe cases that have been diagnosed before birth may be best managed with delivery by the EXIT procedure, with immediate institution of ECMO (see Chapter 39). This requires a multidisciplinary team consisting of obstetricians, specialized anesthesiologists, surgeons, neonatologists, nurses, respiratory therapists, and ECMO technicians to be assembled at a specialized center. The fetus is partially delivered from the mother, and initial interventions are completed including intubation and ventilation.

A decision is then made whether delivery should be completed at that point, and further care continued as detailed in (see sections III.B.5.b and c). If the fetal condition does not improve upon intubation or if the DH is known to be severe, the EXIT procedure may be used as a bridge to immediate initiation of ECMO before umbilical blood flow ceases. Portable ECMO equipment brought to the operating room is then used during transport to the intensive care unit or during subsequent surgery on the delivered newborn.

b. Intubation. All infants with known DH should be intubated immediately after delivery or at the time of postnatal diagnosis. Bag-and-mask ventilation is contraindicated. Immediately after intubation, a large sump nasogastric tube should be inserted and attached to **continuous** suction. Care must be taken with assisted ventilation to keep inspiratory pressures low to avoid damage or rupture of the contralateral lung. Peripheral venous and arterial lines are preferable, as umbilical lines may need to be removed during surgery. However, if umbilical lines are the only practical access, these should be placed initially. Heavy sedation should be avoided as spontaneous respiratory effort enables the use of the pressure support mode of ventilation which we have found to induce the least barotrauma.

c. Preoperative management is focused on avoiding barotrauma and minimizing pulmonary hypertension. Permissive hypercapnia is the preferred respiratory approach, although the optimal mode of ventilation remains controversial, including the role for high-frequency ventilation. Avoidance of hypoxia and acidosis will aid in minimizing pulmonary hypertension. Inhaled nitric oxide has not been shown to reduce the need for ECMO, but its role in reducing right heart strain may be beneficial. The role of exogenous surfactant remains controversial.

6. **Surgical repair** is through either the abdomen or the chest, with reduction of intestine into the abdominal cavity.

7. **Mortality and prognosis**
   a. Mortality from DHs is largely related to associated defects, especially pulmonary hypoplasia and CHD. Our local survival is now >90% for infants without associated CHD. Repair of the defect itself is relatively straightforward; the underlying pulmonary hypoplasia and pulmonary hypertension are largely responsible for overall mortality (see Chapter 36).
   b. Prognosis. Factors associated with better prognosis include herniation of bowel into chest after second trimester, absence of liver herniation, and absence of coexisting anomalies, especially cardiac. Early oxygen tension (Po_2) and carbon dioxide tension (Pco_2) are predictive of prognosis. In addition, the later the onset of postnatal symptoms, the higher the survival rate.

C. **Other mechanical causes for respiratory distress**

1. **Choanal atresia.** Bilateral atresia presents in the delivery room as respiratory distress that resolves with crying, during which breathing is oral, rather than the usual obligate nasal breathing of infants less than approximately 4 months of age. An oral airway is effective initial treatment. Definitive therapy includes opening a hole through the bony plate, which can be accomplished with a laser in some settings.

2. **Robin anomaly** (Pierre Robin syndrome) consists of a hypoplastic mandible associated with a secondary U-shaped midline cleft palate. Often, the tongue occludes the airway causing obstruction. Prone positioning or forcibly pulling the tongue forward will relieve the obstruction. These infants may need mechanical ventilation with continuous positive airway pressure if relatively mild, or with intubation if more severe. If the infant can be supported for a few days, he or she will sometimes adapt, and aggressive procedures can be avoided. In some cases, a lip tongue adhesion or mandibular distraction can avoid the need for tracheostomy or enable earlier decannulation. A specialized feeder (Breck) facilitates PO feeding the infant, but sometimes, a gastrostomy is necessary. Severely affected babies will require tracheostomy and gastrostomy.

3. **Laryngotracheal clefts.** The length of the cleft determines the symptoms. The diagnosis is made by direct bronchoscopy under anesthesia. Very ill newborns should undergo immediate bronchoscopy without contrast studies.

4. **Laryngeal web occluding the larynx.** Perforation of the web by a stiff endotracheal tube or bronchoscopy instrument may be lifesaving.

5. **Tracheal agenesis.** This rare lesion is suspected when a tube cannot be passed down the trachea. The infant ventilates by way of bronchi coming off the esophagus. Diagnosis is by direct bronchoscopy should time permit. Prognosis is poor as tracheal reconstruction is difficult.

6. **Congenital lobar emphysema** may be due to a malformation, a cyst in the bronchus, or a mucous or meconium plug in the bronchus. These lesions cause air trapping, compression of surrounding structures, and respiratory distress. There may be a primary malformation of the lobe (polyalveolar lobe). Overdistension from mechanical ventilation may cause lobar emphysema. Extrinsic pressure on a bronchus can also cause obstruction. Lower lobes are generally relatively spared. Diagnosis is by chest x-ray.

   a. High-frequency ventilation may enable the lobar emphysema to recover (see Chapter 29).

   b. Selective intubation. After consultation with a surgeon, selective intubation of the opposite bronchus may be attempted in an effort to decompress the emphysematous lobe if overinflation is thought to be the cause. It should generally be viewed as a temporizing therapy and should not be employed for more than a few hours. Many infants will not tolerate this procedure due to both overdistension of the ventilated lung and profound ventilation–perfusion ($\dot{V}/\dot{Q}$) mismatch; therefore, it must be carefully considered and monitored. Rarely, selective intubation is successful and the lobar emphysema does not recur. Much more commonly, even if the selective intubation is initially helpful, the infant goes on to develop recurrence and progression of the emphysema and further respiratory compromise. Occasionally, selective suctioning of the bronchus on the side of the emphysema may remove obstructing mucus or meconium.

   c. Bronchoscopy, resection. If the infant is symptomatic and conservative measures fail, bronchoscopy should be performed to remove any obstructing material or rupture a bronchogenic cyst. If this procedure fails, surgical resection of the involved lobe should be considered.

7. **Cystic pulmonary airway malformation (CPAM) and pulmonary sequestration** may be confused with a DH. Respiratory distress is related to the effect of the mass on the uninvolved lung. This malformation can cause shifting of the mediastinal structures.

8. **Vascular rings.** The symptomatology of vascular rings is related to the anatomy of the ring. Both respiratory (stridor) and GI (vomiting, difficulty swallowing) symptoms may occur. Barium swallow radiography may be diagnostic. MRI can be useful to more clearly delineate the anatomy, especially in the setting of double aortic arch. An echocardiogram may be necessary to rule out intracardiac anomalies. Bronchoscopy can be helpful if tracheal stenosis is suspected.

IV. LESIONS CAUSING INTESTINAL OBSTRUCTION. The most critical lesion
to rule out is malrotation with midgut volvulus. All patients with suspected intestinal obstruction should have a nasogastric sump catheter placed to continuous

suction without delay. Any infant with a GI obstruction is at increased risk for exacerbated hyperbilirubinemia due to increased enterohepatic circulation.

A. Congenital mechanical obstruction

1. Intrinsic types include areas of atresia or stenosis, meconium ileus (most commonly associated with cystic fibrosis [CF]), small left colon syndrome, cysts within the lumen of the bowel, and imperforate anus.

2. Extrinsic forms of congenital mechanical obstruction include congenital peritoneal bands with or without malrotation, annular pancreas, duplications of the intestine, aberrant vessels (usually the mesenteric artery or preduodenal portal vein), hydrometrocolpos, and obstructing bands (persistent omphalomesenteric duct).

B. Acquired mechanical obstruction

1. Malrotation with volvulus

2. Strictures secondary to necrotizing enterocolitis

3. Peritoneal adhesions
   a. After meconium peritonitis
   b. After abdominal surgery
   c. Idiopathic

4. Incarcerated inguinal hernia (relatively common in premature infants)

5. Hypertrophic pyloric stenosis

6. Mesenteric thrombosis

7. Intussusception; unusual in neonatal period

C. Functional intestinal obstruction constitutes the major cause of intestinal obstruction seen in the neonatal unit.

1. Immature bowel motility

2. Defective innervation (Hirschsprung disease) or other intrinsic defects in the bowel wall

3. Paralytic ileus
   a. Induced by medications
      i. Narcotics (pre- or postnatal exposure)
      ii. Hypermagnesemia usually due to prenatal exposure to magnesium sulfate
   b. Septic ileus

4. Meconium ileus, 90% of cases associated with CF

5. Meconium and mucous plugs

6. Formation of abnormal intestinal concretions not associated with CF

7. Endocrine disorders (e.g., hypothyroidism)

D. The more **common etiologies** of GI obstruction warrant more detailed discussion.

1. Duodenal atresia. Seventy percent of cases have other associated malformations, including Down syndrome, cardiovascular anomalies, and

such GI anomalies as annular pancreas, EA, malrotation of the small intestine, other small-bowel atresias, and imperforate anus.

a. There may be a history of polyhydramnios.

b. It is commonly diagnosed prenatally by ultrasonography.

c. Vomiting of bile-stained material usually begins a few hours after birth.

d. Abdominal distention is limited to the upper abdomen.

e. The infant may pass meconium in the first 24 hours of life and then bowel movements cease.

f. The diagnosis is suggested if aspiration of the stomach yields >30 mL of gastric contents before feeding.

g. A plain radiograph of the abdomen will show air in the stomach and upper part of the abdomen ("double bubble") with no air in the small or large bowel. Contrast radiographs of the upper intestine are not mandatory.

h. Preoperative management includes decompression with nasogastric suction.

i. Antibiotics should be started until perinatal sepsis evaluation is complete and then consider tailoring to prophylactic antibiotics until definitive repair given likelihood of fistula from intestinal to urinary tract.

2. Jejunal and ileal atresias. Most are the result of intrauterine vascular accidents, but as many as 15% to 30% are associated with CF; these patients should therefore be screened (see section IV.D.3.b).

3. Meconium ileus is a frequent cause of meconium peritonitis. Unlike most other etiologies of obstruction in which flat and upright x-ray films will demonstrate fluid levels, in cases of nonperforated meconium ileus, the distended bowel may be granular in appearance or may show tiny bubbles mixed with meconium.

a. No meconium will pass through the rectum, even after digital stimulation.

b. Ninety percent of babies with meconium ileus have CF. Blood sample or cheek brushing for DNA analysis can be used to screen for CF if newborn or antenatal screening has not been performed. If the results are negative or equivocal or if the baby weighs >2 kg and is older than 2 weeks ideally (but certainly older than 3 days), a sweat test should be performed. Sweat tests on babies who are younger or smaller risk both false-positive results due to the high NaCl content of the sweat of newborn babies and false-negative or uninterpretable results when an adequate volume of sweat cannot be obtained.

c. Decompression with continuous nasogastric suction will minimize further distention. Contrast enemas with water-soluble agents can be both diagnostic and therapeutic. Diluted (1:3 to 1:4) diatrizoate meglumine (Gastrografin) is still used by some radiologists, but more commonly, diatrizoate sodium (Hypaque) is employed. Because these contrast agents are hypertonic, the baby should start the procedure well hydrated, and careful attention should be paid to fluid balance after the procedure. If the diagnosis is certain and the neonate stable, repeat therapeutic enemas may be administered in an effort to relieve the impaction.

d. Surgical therapy is required if the contrast enema fails to relieve the obstruction.

e. Microcolon distal to the atresia will generally dilate spontaneously with use.

4. **Imperforate anus.** Fifty percent have anomalies including those in the VACTERL association. Infants with imperforate anus may pass meconium if a rectovaginal or rectourinary fistula exists. A fistula is present in 80% to 90% of affected males and 95% of females. It may take 24 hours for the fistula to become evident. The presence or absence of a visible fistula at the perineum is the critical distinction in the diagnosis and management of imperforate anus. Of note, in order to prevent urinary tract infections, prophylactic antibiotics should be considered until the fistula can be definitively repaired.

a. Perineal fistula. Meconium may be visualized on the perineum. It may be found in the rugal folds or scrotum in boys and in the vagina in girls. This fistula may be dilated to allow passage of meconium to temporarily relieve intestinal obstruction. When the infant is beyond the newborn period, the imperforate anus can generally be primarily repaired.

b. No perineal fistula present. There may be a fistula that enters the urinary tract or, for girls, the vagina. The presence of meconium particles in the urine is diagnostic of a rectovesicular fistula. Vaginal examination with a nasal speculum or cystoscope may reveal a fistula. A cystogram may show a fistula and document the level of the distal rectum, which can also be defined by ultrasonography. A temporary colostomy may be necessary in neonates with an imperforate anus without a perineal fistula. Primary repair of these infants without a colostomy is now being performed at some institutions.

5. **Volvulus with or without malrotation of the bowel**

a. Malrotation may be associated with other GI abnormalities such as DH, annular pancreas, and bowel atresias and is always seen with omphalocele.

b. If this condition develops during fetal life, it may cause the appearance of a large midabdominal calcific shadow on x-ray examination; this results from calcification of meconium in the segment of necrotic bowel.

c. After birth, there is a sudden onset of bilious vomiting in an infant who has passed some normal stools. Malrotation, as the cause of intestinal obstruction, is a surgical emergency because intestinal viability is at stake. **Bilious emesis equals malrotation until proven otherwise.**

d. If the level of obstruction is high, there may not be much abdominal distension.

e. Signs of shock and sepsis are often present.

f. A radiograph of the abdomen will often show a dilated small bowel, although a normal radiograph does not rule out malrotation, which can be intermittent.

g. If a malrotation is present, barium enema may show failure of barium to pass beyond the transverse colon or may show the cecum in an abnormal position.

h. The test of choice is an UGI series, specifically looking for an absent or abnormal position of the ligament of Treitz that confirms the diagnosis of malrotation.

6. **Meconium and mucous plug syndrome** is seen in infants who are premature or sick (see section II.F), and those with functional immaturity of the bowel with a small left colon, as seen in infants of diabetic mothers or those with Hirschsprung disease (see section IV.D.7). CF should also be ruled out. Treatment may simply consist of a glycerin suppository, warm half-normal saline enemas (5 to 10 mL/kg), and rectal stimulation with a soft rubber catheter. More typically, and if these maneuvers are unsuccessful, a contrast enema with a hyperosmolar contrast material may be both diagnostic and therapeutic. A normal stooling pattern should follow evacuation of a plug.

7. **Hirschsprung disease** should be suspected in any newborn who fails to pass meconium spontaneously by 24 to 48 hours after birth and who develops distension relieved by rectal stimulation. This is especially so if the infant is neither premature nor born to a diabetic mother. The diagnosis should be considered until future development shows sustained normal bowel function.

   a. When the diagnosis is suspected, every effort should be made to rule the condition in or out. If the diagnosis is considered but seems very unlikely, parents taking the newborn home must specifically understand the importance of immediately reporting any obstipation, diarrhea, poor feeding, distention, lethargy, or fever. Development of a toxic megacolon may be fatal.

   b. Contrast enema frequently does not show the characteristic transition zone in the newborn, but a follow-up radiograph 24 hours after the initial study may reveal retained contrast material.

   c. Rectal biopsy is obtained to confirm the diagnosis. If suspicion is relatively low, a suction biopsy is useful, as presence of ganglion cells in the submucosal zone rules out the diagnosis. If the index of suspicion is high, or the suction biopsy is positive, formal full-thickness rectal biopsy is the definitive method for diagnosis. Absence of ganglion cells and hypertrophic nonmyelinated axons is diagnostic. Histochemical tests of biopsy specimens show an increase in acetylcholine.

   d. Obstipation can be relieved by gentle rectal irrigations with warm saline solution. If the patient has a barium enema, gentle rectal saline washes are helpful in removing trapped air and barium. Once the abdomen is decompressed, feedings may be offered.

   e. Babies require surgical intervention when the diagnosis is made. A primary pull-through procedure is usually possible for correction, avoiding the need for a colostomy. In many institutions, colostomy is the standard, and it is always indicated when there is enterocolitis or adequate decompression cannot be achieved. Definitive repair is postponed until the infant is of adequate size and stability.

   f. Even after the aganglionic segment is removed, the bowel that remains is not completely normal. These patients remain at risk for constipation, encopresis, and even life-threatening enterocolitis.

8. **Pyloric stenosis** typically presents with nonbilious vomiting, classically in a firstborn boy, after the age of 2 to 3 weeks, but it has been reported in the first week of life. Radiographic examination will show

a large stomach with little or no gas below the duodenum. Often, the pyloric mass, or "olive," cannot be felt in the newborn. The infant may have associated jaundice and hematemesis. Diagnosis can usually be confirmed by ultrasonography, which limits the need for a UGI series and the consequent radiation exposure.

   9. **Annular pancreas** may be nonobstructing but associated with duodenal atresia or stenosis. It presents as a high intestinal obstruction.

   10. **Hydrometrocolpos.** In this rare condition, a membrane across the vagina prevents fluid drainage and the consequent accumulation causes distension of the uterus and vagina.
      a. The hymen bulges.
      b. Accumulated secretions in the uterus may cause intestinal obstruction by bowel compression.
      c. This intestinal obstruction may, in turn, cause meconium peritonitis or hydronephrosis.
      d. Edema and cyanosis of the legs may be observed.
      e. If hydrometrocolpos is not diagnosed at birth, the secretions will decrease, the bulging will disappear, and the diagnosis will be delayed until puberty.

V. OTHER GASTROINTESTINAL SURGICAL CONDITIONS

   A. **Omphalocele.** The sac may be intact or ruptured. The diagnosis is often made by prenatal ultrasonography. Cesarean section may prevent rupture of the sac but is not specifically indicated unless the defect is large (>5 cm) or contains liver.

   1. **Intact sac.** Emergency treatment includes the following:
      a. Provide continuous nasogastric sump suction.
      b. It is preferable to encase intestinal contents in a bowel bag (e.g., Vi-Drape Isolation Bag) as it is the least abrasive. Otherwise, cover the sac with warm saline-soaked gauze and then wrap the sac on abdomen with Kling gauze and cover with plastic wrap to support the intestinal viscera on the abdominal wall, taking great caution to ensure no kinking of the mesenteric blood supply.
      c. Do not attempt to reduce the sac because this can rupture it, interfere with venous return from the sac, or cause respiratory compromise.
      d. Bowel viability may be compromised with a small abdominal wall defect and an obstructed segment of eviscerated intestine. In these circumstances, with surgical consultation, it may be necessary before transfer, to enlarge the defect by incising the abdomen cephalad or caudad to relieve the strangulated viscera.
      e. Keep the baby warm, including thoroughly wrapping in warm blankets to prevent heat loss.
      f. Place a reliable intravenous line in an upper extremity.
      g. Monitor temperature, pH, and electrolytes.
      h. Start broad-spectrum antibiotics (ampicillin and gentamicin).
      i. Obtain a surgical consultation; definitive surgical therapy should be delayed until the baby is stabilized. In the presence of other more serious

abnormalities (respiratory or cardiac), definitive care can be postponed as long as the sac remains intact.

2. Ruptured sac. As in the preceding text for intact sac, except surgery is more emergent.

3. As up to 80% will have associated anomalies, physical examination should include a careful search for phenotypic features of chromosomal defects as well as CHD, genitourinary defects such as cloacal exstrophy, craniofacial, musculoskeletal, vertebral, or limb anomalies. The Beckwith-Wiedemann syndrome includes (typically small) omphalocele, macroglossia, hemihypertrophy, and hypoglycemia.

B. Gastroschisis, by definition, contains no sac, and the intestine is eviscerated.

1. For uncomplicated gastroschisis, there is no advantage to a specific route of delivery, but a cesarean section is recommended for large lesions or those in which the liver is exposed. Preoperative management as per omphalocele with ruptured sac (see section V.A.2).

2. Obtain immediate surgical consultation.

3. About 12% of these infants will have other GI anomalies, including volvulus, atresias, intestinal stenosis, or perforation.

4. Unlike omphalocele, gastroschisis is not commonly associated with anomalies unrelated to the GI tract.

C. Appendicitis is extremely rare in newborns. Its presentation may be that of pneumoperitoneum. The appendix usually perforates before the diagnosis is made; therefore, the baby may present with intestinal obstruction, sepsis, or even DIC related to the intra-abdominal infection. Rule out Hirschsprung disease.

VI. RENAL DISORDERS (see Chapter 28)

A. Genitourinary abnormalities. First void should be noted in all infants. Approximately 90% of babies void in the first 24 hours of life and 99% within the first 48 hours of life. Genitourinary abnormalities should be suspected in babies with abdominal distention, ascites, flank masses, persistently distended bladder, bacteriuria, pyuria, or poor growth. Male infants exhibiting these symptoms should be observed for the normal forceful voiding pattern.

1. Posterior urethral valves may cause obstruction.

2. Renal vein thrombosis should be considered in the setting of hematuria with a flank mass. It is more common among infants of diabetic mothers.

a. Renal ultrasonography will initially show a large kidney on the side of the thrombosis. Kidney will return to normal size over ensuing weeks to months.

b. Doppler ultrasonography will show diminished or absent blood flow to involved kidney.

c. Current treatment in most centers starts with medical support in the hope of avoiding surgery. Heparin is generally not indicated, but its use has been advocated by some (see Chapters 28 and 44).

3. Exstrophy of the bladder. Ranges from an epispadias to complete extrusion of the bladder onto the abdominal wall. Most centers attempt bladder turn in within the first 48 hours of life.

a. Preoperative management

i. Protect the exposed bladder mucosa by covering with clear plastic wrap.

ii. Transport the infant to a facility for definitive care as soon as possible.

iii. Start prophylactic antibiotics with choice of agent and dose appropriate for estimated renal function.

iv. Provide adequate hydration in setting of increased insensible losses; monitor lytes and renal function.

v. Obtain renal ultrasonography.

b. Intraoperative management. Surgical management of an exstrophied bladder includes turn-in of the bladder to preserve bladder function. The symphysis pubis is approximated. For males, the penis is lengthened. Iliac osteotomies are not necessary if repair is accomplished within 48 hours. No attempt is made to make the bladder continent at this initial procedure.

4. Cloacal exstrophy is a complex GI and genitourinary anomaly that includes vesicointestinal fissure, omphalocele, exstrophied bladder, hypoplastic colon, imperforate anus, absence of vagina in females, and microphallus in males.

a. Preoperative management

i. Gender assignment. It is surgically easier to create a phenotypic female, regardless of genotype. Understanding of the long-term psychological effects of this practice has made this decision extremely controversial, and no one approach is correct for all patients. Endocrine consultation is critical when deciding phenotypic gender assignment (see Chapter 63), and decisions should be made only after a collaborative discussion including the parents, urologist, surgeon, endocrinologist, neonatologist, and appropriate counselors.

ii. Nasogastric suction relieves partial intestinal obstruction. The infant excretes stool through a vesicointestinal fissure that is often partially obstructed.

iii. A series of complex operations is required in stages to achieve the most satisfactory results.

b. Surgical management

i. The focus is first on separating the GI from the genitourinary tract. The hemibladders are sewn together and closed. A colostomy is created, and the omphalocele is closed.

ii. Later stages focus on bladder reconstruction, often requiring augmentation using intestine or stomach.

iii. Subsequent procedures are designed to reduce the number of stomas and create genitalia, although this remains controversial.

VII. TUMORS

A. Teratomas are the most common tumor in the neonatal period. Although they are most commonly found in the sacrococcygeal area, they can arise anywhere, including the retroperitoneal area or the ovaries. Approximately

10% contain malignant elements. Prenatal diagnosis is often made by ultrasonography. The possibility of dystocia or airway compromise should be considered prenatally. Masses compromising the airway have been successfully managed by the EXIT procedure (see section III.B.5.a) with establishment of an airway before complete delivery of the baby.

After delivery, evaluation may include rectal examination, ultrasonography, computed tomography (CT), MRI, as well as serum α-fetoprotein and β-human chorionic gonadotropin measurement. Calcifications are often seen on plain radiographs. Excessive heat loss and platelet trapping are possible complications.

B. Neuroblastoma is the most common malignant neonatal tumor, accounting for approximately 50% of cases, although the overall incidence is rare. It is irregular, stony hard, and ranges in size from minute to massive. There are many sites of origin; the adrenal–retroperitoneal area is the most common. On rare occasions, this tumor can cause hypertension or diarrhea by the release of tumor by-products, especially catecholamines or vasointestinal peptides. Serum levels of catecholamines and their metabolites should be measured. Calcifications can often be seen on plain radiographs. Ultrasonography is the most useful diagnostic test. Prenatal diagnosis by ultrasonography is associated with improved prognosis. Of note, many neuroblastomas diagnosed prenatally resolve spontaneously before birth.

C. Wilms tumor is the second most common malignant tumor in the newborn. It presents as a smooth flat mass and may be bilateral. One should palpate gently to avoid rupture. Ultrasonography is the most useful diagnostic test.

D. Hemangiomas are the most common tumor of infancy, although they rarely present in the neonate. Precursors such as bumps or telangiectasia may be seen in newborns. They may occur anywhere on the body, including within solid organs or the GI tract. The incidence is unknown, but estimated as high as 4% to 5% in Caucasian newborns, and most are benign. Other tumors such as lymphangiomas, hepatoblastomas, hepatomas, hamartomas, and nephromas and sarcoma botryoides may be seen in newborns, but they are extremely rare.

VIII. ABDOMINAL MASSES

A. Renal masses (see section VI and Chapter 28) are the most common etiology: polycystic kidneys, multicystic dysplastic kidney, hydronephrosis, and renal vein thrombosis.

B. Other causes of abdominal masses include tumors (see section VII), adrenal hemorrhage, ovarian tumor or cysts, pancreatic cyst, choledochal cyst, hydrometrocolpos, mesenteric or omental cyst, intestinal duplications, and hepatosplenomegaly.

IX. INGUINAL HERNIA is found in 5% of premature infants with birth weight <1,500 g and as many as 30% of infants with birth weight <1,000 g. It is more common in small for gestational age infants and male infants. In females, the ovary is often in the sac.

A. Surgical repair. Inguinal hernia repair is the most common operation performed on prematurely born infants. In general, hernias in this patient population can be repaired shortly before discharge home if they are easily reducible and cause no other problems.

1. **Repair before discharge.** Often, the hernia repair is arranged prior to hospital discharge to avoid the risk of incarceration at home. In a term infant, repair should be scheduled when the diagnosis is made. For stable premature infants, repair is usually delayed until just prior to discharge. An incarcerated hernia can usually be reduced with sedation, steady firm pressure, and elevation of the feet. If a hernia has been incarcerated, it should be repaired as soon as the edema has resolved. The operation may be difficult and should be performed by an experienced pediatric surgeon. The use of spinal anesthesia has simplified the postoperative care of the infants with respiratory problems. As these infants often develop postoperative apnea, they should be monitored in hospital for at least 24 hours after surgery.

2. **Repair after discharge.** Infants with significant pulmonary disease, such as bronchopulmonary dysplasia, are often best repaired at a later time when their respiratory status has improved. We have occasionally had well-instructed parents bring their babies home and then have them readmitted later for repair. The risks and benefits of this option must be weighed carefully because there is a real risk of the hernia incarcerating at home.

X. SCROTAL SWELLING

A. Differential diagnosis includes the following:

1. **Testicular torsion.** Approximately 70% of the cases of testicular torsion that are diagnosed in the newborn period actually occur prenatally. In the newborn, testicular torsion is generally extravaginal (the twist occurs outside the tunica vaginalis) and is caused by an incomplete attachment of the gubernaculum to the testis, allowing torsion and infarction.

   a. **Diagnosis is made by physical examination.** The testicle is generally nontender, firm, indurated, and swollen with a slightly bluish or dusky cast of the affected side of the scrotum. If the torsion is acute, rather than long-standing, it will be extremely tender to palpation. The testicle can have a transverse lie or be high-riding. The overlying skin, limited to the scrotum itself, may be erythematous or edematous. Transillumination is negative, and the cremasteric reflex is absent. Ultrasonography employing Doppler flow studies can be helpful if available, but testing should not delay referral for surgery if there is a possibility that the torsion is recent.

   b. **Treatment.** In the vast majority of cases, the torsed testicle is already necrotic at birth; therefore, surgical intervention will not salvage the testicle. However, if there is *any possibility* that the torsion occurred recently, and the infant is otherwise healthy, emergency surgical exploration and detorsion should be performed within 4 to 6 hours. This may result in salvage of the torsed testicle. Because there have been reports of bilateral testicular torsion, surgical exploration should include contralateral orchiopexy. Even if emergency exploration is not indicated because of definitive evidence of chronicity of torsion, exploration should be performed on a nonemergent basis to rule out a tumor with clinical and imaging findings identical to testicular torsion.

c. Prognosis. Testicular protheses are available. Oligospermia has been reported after unilateral testicular torsion.

2. **Hydrocele** is the most common cause of scrotal swelling in the newborn, affecting as many as 2% of infants. Hydrocele forms when fluid remains within the processus vaginalis as the testicle descends into the scrotum during normal development. The fluid may be loculated (noncommunicating) in which case the swelling remains unchanged, or there may be a communication allowing the collected fluid volume (and hydrocele size) to vary over time.

3. **Incarcerated hernia**

4. **Trauma/scrotal hematoma.** Most commonly secondary to breech delivery. This is generally bilateral and may present with hematocele, scrotal swelling, and ecchymoses. Typically, transillumination is negative. Resolution is usually spontaneous, but severe cases may require surgical exploration, evacuation of the hematocele, and repair of the testes.

5. **Torsion of the testicular appendage.** Swelling is usually less marked and may present on palpation or as a blue dot on the scrotum. The cremasteric reflexes are preserved, and Doppler flow ultrasonography may be helpful in ruling out testicular torsion. No treatment is needed.

6. **Spontaneous idiopathic scrotal hemorrhage.** Most common in large for gestational age (LGA) infants. Distinguishable from torsion by the appearance of a small but distinct ecchymosis over the superficial inguinal ring.

7. **Tumor.** These are usually nontender, solid, and firm. Transillumination is negative.

XI. **COMMON TESTS** used in the diagnosis of surgical conditions include the following:

A. **Abdominal x-ray examinations.** A flat plate radiograph of the abdomen kidney-ureter-bladder (KUB) is sufficient for assessing intraluminal gas patterns and mucosal thickness. A left lateral decubitus or cross-table lateral radiograph is obtained to ascertain the presence of free air in the abdomen.

1. Contrast enema may be diagnostic in suspected cases of Hirschsprung disease. It may reveal microcolon in the infant with complete obstruction of the small intestine and may show a narrow segment in the sigmoid in the infant with meconium plug syndrome due to functional immaturity.

2. UGI series with diatrizoate meglumine may be used to demonstrate obstructions of the UGI tract.

3. In patients with suspected malrotation, a combination of contrast studies may be necessary, starting with an UGI contrast study. In combination with air or contrast media, an UGI series will determine the presence or absence of the normally placed ligament of Treitz. A contrast enema may show malposition of the cecum but will not always rule out malrotation. Neonates with intestinal obstruction presumed secondary to malrotation require urgent surgery to relieve possible volvulus of the midgut.

B. Ultrasonography is the preferred method of evaluating abdominal masses in the newborn. It is useful for defining the presence of masses, together with their size, shape, and consistency.

C. MRI is useful to better define the anatomy and location of masses.

D. CT is a modality that is used with decreasing frequency due to large radiation exposure. It is an excellent modality to evaluate abdominal masses as well as their relation to other organs. Contrast enhancement can outline the intestine, blood vessels, kidneys, ureter, and bladder.

E. Intravenous pyelogram (IVP) should be restricted to evaluating genitourinary anatomy if other modalities (ultrasonography and contrast CT) are not available. The IVP dye is poorly concentrated in the newborn.

F. Radionuclide scan of the kidneys can aid in determining function. This is especially useful in assessing complex genitourinary anomalies and in evaluating the contribution of each kidney to renal function.

G. **The Apt test** differentiates maternal from fetal blood. A small amount of bloody material is mixed with 5 mL of water and centrifuged. One part 0.25N sodium hydroxide is added to five parts of the pink supernatant. The fluid remains pink in the presence of fetal blood but rapidly becomes brown if maternal blood is present. The test is useful only if the sample is not contaminated by pigmented material (e.g., meconium/stool).

H. Screening for CF is usually done by measuring immunoreactive trypsin from Guthrie spots. More definitive genetic testing can be performed on DNA sampling obtained from blood or cheek brush sampling. When the test result is negative but clinical suspicion remains high, a sweat test should be done. Ideally, the baby should be older than 2 weeks (certainly older than 3 days) and weigh >2 kg to avoid both false-positive results due to the relatively high chloride content of newborn infants' sweat as well as false-negative or be uninterpretable results if <100 mg of sweat can be collected. It may be necessary to repeat the test when the infant is 3 to 4 weeks old if an adequate volume of sweat cannot be collected.

XII. PREOPERATIVE MANAGEMENT BY PRESENTING SYMPTOM

A. **Vomiting without distention**

1. The mechanics of feeding the baby should be observed. Rapid feeding, intake of excessive volume, and lack of burping are all causes of nonbilious vomiting without distension.

2. Functional and mechanical causes must be ruled out. Often, a history, physical examination, and observation of feedings are sufficient. An abdominal x-ray may be useful.

3. If the baby's general condition is good, feedings of dextrose water should be attempted. If this is tolerated, milk should be tried again. If vomiting recurs and there is a family history of milk allergy, blood in the stool, or elevated percentage of eosinophils on the complete blood count (CBC), consider a trial of non–cow's milk-based formula (e.g., elemental). In order for the mother to continue breastfeeding, she should remove cow's milk protein from her diet for approximately 1 week prior to reintroducing her breast milk.

B. **Nonbilious vomiting with distension.** An overall assessment of the well-versus-sick appearance of the baby as well as the degree of the abdominal distension is critical in determining the evaluation and management of nonbilious vomiting and distension. In general, there should be a low threshold to assess for mechanical and functional obstruction, starting with history, physical examination, abdominal radiographs, $+/-$ contrast studies depending on the clinical presentation. If no source of obstruction is identified, many babies with nonbilious vomiting and mild distension respond to a combination of glycerin suppositories, half-strength saline enemas (5 mL/kg body weight), and rectal stimulation with a soft rubber catheter. Limited feedings, stimulation to the rectum, and care for the general condition of the baby will solve most of these problems.

C. **Bilious vomiting and abdominal distension**

1. Immediately arrange for appropriate diagnostic evaluation (generally UGI series) to rule out malrotation with midgut volvulus.

2. **Enteral feedings should be discontinued.** Continuous gastric decompression with a sump catheter is mandatory if intestinal obstruction is suspected. All infants with presumed intestinal obstruction should be transported with a nasogastric suction catheter in place, attached to a catheter-tip syringe for continuous aspiration of gastric contents. Failure to decompress the stomach could lead to gastric rupture, aspiration, or respiratory compromise secondary to excessive diaphragmatic convexity into the thorax. This is especially important in infants who are to be transported by air because loss of cabin pressure would create a high-risk setting for the rupture of an inadequately drained viscous.

3. Shock, dehydration, and electrolyte imbalance should be prevented or treated if present (see Chapters 23 and 40).

4. Broad-spectrum antibiotics (ampicillin and gentamicin) should be initiated if there is suspicion of volvulus or any question about bowel integrity. Clindamycin should be added, or ampicillin and gentamicin should be substituted with piperacillin and tazobactam (Zosyn) if perforation is high risk or documented.

5. Studies that should be performed include the following:
   a. Monitoring of oxygen saturation, blood pressure, and urine output
   b. Blood tests as follows:
      i. CBC with differential and blood culture
      ii. Electrolytes
      iii. Blood gases and pH
      iv. Clotting studies (e.g., prothrombin time, partial thromboplastin time)
   c. Contrast study (start with UGI) to rule out malrotation

D. **Masses.** The following steps may be taken to determine the etiology of abdominal masses:

1. CBC with differential

2. Determination of the level of catecholamines and their metabolites

3. Urinalysis

4. X-ray examination of the chest and abdomen with the infant supine and upright

5. Abdominal ultrasonography

6. Contrast-enhanced CT

7. MRI

8. Angiography; venous and arterial

9. Surgical consultation

XIII. GENERAL INTRAOPERATIVE MANAGEMENT

A. **Monitoring devices**

1. Temperature probe

2. Electrocardiogram (ECG) and/or CVR monitor

3. Pulse oximetry responds rapidly to changes in patient condition but is subject to artifacts.

4. Transcutaneous Po_2 (see Chapter 30) is helpful if pulse oximetry is unavailable but can be inaccurate in the setting of anesthetic agents that dilate skin vessels.

5. Arterial cannula to monitor blood gases and pressure

B. **Well-functioning intravenous line.** Babies with omphalocele or gastroschisis should have the intravenous line in the upper extremities, neck, or scalp.

C. **Maintenance of body temperature**

1. Warmed operating room

2. Humidified, warmed anesthetic agents

3. Warmed blood and other fluids used intraoperatively

4. Cover exposed parts of the baby, especially the head (with a hat).

D. **Fluid replacement**

1. Replace loss of >15% of total blood volume with warmed packed red blood cells.

2. Replace ascites loss with normal saline mL/mL to maintain normal blood pressure.

3. The neonate loses approximately 5 mL of fluid per kilogram for each hour that the intestine is exposed. This should generally be replaced by Ringer lactate.

E. Anesthetic management of the neonate is reviewed in Chapter 70.

F. Postoperative pain management is discussed in Chapter 70.

G. Postoperatively, the newborn fluid requirement must be monitored closely, including replacement of estimated losses due to bowel edema as well as losses through drains.

Suggested Readings

Achildi O, Grewal H. Congenital anomalies of the esophagus. *Otolaryngol Clin North Am* 2007;40:219–244.

Adzick NS, Thom EA, Spong CY, et al; for the MOMS Investigators. A randomized trial of prenatal versus postnatal repair of myelomeningocele. *N Engl J Med* 2011;364(11):993–1004.

American Academy of Pediatrics, Committee on Bioethics. Fetal therapy: ethical considerations. *Pediatrics* 1999;103:1061–1063.

Chandler JC, Gauderer MW. The neonate with an abdominal mass. *Pediatr Clin North Am* 2004;51:979–997.

Cohen AR, Couto J, Cummings JJ, et al; for the MMC Maternal-Fetal Management Task Force. Position statement on fetal myelomeningocele repair. *Am J Obstet Gynecol* 2014;210(2):107–111.

Desai AA, Ostlie DJ, Juang D. Optimal timing of congenital diaphragmatic hernia repair in infants on extracorporeal membrane oxygenation. *Semin Pediatr Surg* 2015;24(1):17–19.

Glick RD, Hicks MJ, Nuchtern JG, et al. Renal tumors in infants less than 6 months of age. *J Pediatr Surg* 2004;39:522–525.

Grivell RM, Andersen C, Dodd JM. Prenatal versus postnatal repair procedures for spina bifida for improving infant and maternal outcomes. *Cochrane Database Syst Rev* 2014;(10):CD008825.

Hansen A, Puder M. *Manual of Surgical Neonatal Intensive Care*. 3rd ed. Shelton, CT: People's Medical Publishing House—USA; 2016.

Irish MS, Pearl RH, Caty MG, et al. The approach to common abdominal diagnosis in infants and children. *Pediatr Clin North Am* 1998;45(4):729–772.

Keckler SJ, St. Peter SD, Valusek PA, et al. VACTERL anomalies in patients with esophageal atresia: an updated delineation of the spectrum and review of the literature. *Pediatr Surg Int* 2007;4:309–313.

Kunisaki SM, Barnewolt CE, Estroff JA, et al. Ex utero intrapartum treatment with extracorporeal membrane oxygenation for severe congenital diaphragmatic hernia. *J Pediatr Surg* 2007;42:98–104.

Nuchtern JG. Perinatal neuroblastoma. *Semin Pediatr Surg* 2006;15:10–16.

Sheldon CA. The pediatric genitourinary examination: inguinal, urethral, and genital diseases. *Pediatr Clin North Am* 2001;48:1339–1380.

Skin Care
Caryn E. Douma, Denise Casey, and Arin K. Greene

KEY POINTS
- Primary treatment of intravenous extravasation injuries is elevation of the area.
- Hot or cold packs should not be applied to an extravasation site.
- Evidence proving the efficacy of antidotes for extravasation injuries does not exist.
- Intravenous extravasation rarely causes significant morbidity if skin loss occurs; it heals secondarily with local wound care.

I. **INTRODUCTION.** The skin performs a vital role in the newborn period. It provides a protective barrier that assists in the prevention of infection, facilitates thermoregulation, and helps control insensible water loss and electrolyte balance. Other functions include tactile sensation and protection against toxins. The neonatal intensive care unit (NICU) environment presents numerous challenges to maintaining skin integrity. Routine care practices including bathing, application of monitoring devices, intravenous (IV) catheter insertion and removal, tape application, and exposure to potentially toxic substances disrupt normal barrier function and predispose both premature and term newborns to skin injury. This chapter will describe developmental newborn aspects of skin integrity, skin care practices in the immediate newborn period, and common skin disorders.

II. **ANATOMY.** The two layers of the skin are the epidermis and dermis. The epidermis is the outermost layer providing the first line of protection against injury. It performs a critical barrier function, retaining heat and fluid and providing protection from infection and environmental toxins. Its structural development has generally occurred by 24 weeks' gestation, but epidermal barrier function is not complete until after birth. Maturation typically takes 2 to 4 weeks following exposure to the extrauterine environment. The epidermis is composed primarily of keratinocytes, which mature to form the stratum corneum. The dermis is composed of collagen and elastin fibers that provide elasticity and connect the dermis to the epidermis. Blood vessels, nerves, sweat glands, and hair follicles are another integral part of the dermis. The subcutaneous layer, composed of fatty connective tissue, provides insulation, protection, and calorie storage.

The premature infant has significantly fewer layers of stratum corneum than term infants and adults, which can be seen by the translucent, ruddy appearance of their skin. Infants born at <30 weeks may have <2 to 3 layers of stratum corneum compared with 10 to 20 in adults and term newborns. The maturation of the stratum corneum is accelerated following premature birth and improved barrier function, and skin integrity is generally present within 10 to 14 days. Other differences in skin integrity in premature infants include decreased cohesion between the epidermis and dermis, less collagen, and a marked increase in transepidermal water loss.

III. **SKIN CARE PRACTICES.** Routine assessment, identification, and avoidance of harmful exposures combined with early treatment can eliminate or minimize neonatal skin injury. The identification of potential risk factors for injury and the development of skin care policies and guidelines are an essential part of providing care to both premature and term newborns.

An evidence-based neonatal skin care guideline was created through the collaboration of the National Association of Neonatal Nurses (NANN) and the Association of Women's Health, Obstetric and Neonatal Nurses (AWHONN)[1] in an effort to provide clinical practice recommendations for practitioners caring for newborns from birth to 28 days of age. This guideline provides a comprehensive reference for developing unit-based skin care policies.

A. **Assessment**
1. Daily inspection and assessment of all skin surfaces is an essential part of neonatal skin care. The utilization of a validated skin care assessment tool provides a standardized method to perform the assessment and develop appropriate treatment plans. A widely used tool is the Neonatal Skin Condition Score (NSCS) developed and validated as part of the AWHONN/NANN skin care guideline (Table 65.1).
2. Identification of risk factors
   a. Prematurity
   b. Use of monitoring equipment
   c. Adhesives used to secure central and peripheral access lines, endotracheal tubes
   d. Edema
   e. Immobility secondary to extracorporeal membrane oxygenation (ECMO), muscle relaxant, high-frequency ventilation, which can cause pressure necrosis
   f. Use of high-risk medications including vasopressors and vesicants (calcium, sodium bicarbonate)
   g. Devices with potential for thermal injury such as radiant warmers. Temperature of any product in contact with the skin should not be higher than 41°C/105°F.
3. Avoidance of practices with potential to cause injury

B. **Bathing**
1. Initial bath should be delayed until 2 to 4 hours after admission when temperature has been stabilized to prevent risk of hypothermia. Provide a controlled environment using warming lights and warm blankets. Bathing is often deferred for the first 24 hours in infants <36 weeks' gestation.
2. Use mild, nonalkaline, preservative-free soap. Avoid the use of dyes or perfumes.

Table 65.1. Association of Women's Health, Obstetric and Neonatal Nurses Neonatal Skin Condition Score

Dryness
1 = Normal, no sign of dry skin
2 = Dry skin, visible scaling
3 = Very dry skin, cracking/fissures
Erythema
1 = No evidence of erythema
2 = Visible erythema, <50% body surface
3 = Visible erythema, ≥50% body surface
Breakdown
1 = None evident
2 = Small, localized areas
3 = Extensive

Note: Perfect score = 3, and worst score = 9.
Source: From Association of Women's Health, Obstetric and Neonatal Nurses. *Evidence-Based Clinical Practice Guideline: Neonatal Skin Care.* 2nd ed. Washington, DC: Association of Women's Health, Obstetric and Neonatal Nurses; 2007.

3. Daily bathing is not indicated. Generally, two to three times per week is sufficient. Warm sterile water is sufficient for premature infants during the first few weeks of life.

C. **Adhesives**

1. Minimize use of adhesives and tape.

2. Use nonadhesive products in conjunction with transparent dressings and double-backed tape to secure IV catheters.

3. Avoid use of adhesive bonding agents that can be absorbed easily through the skin.

4. Pectin barriers should be applied to skin before application of adhesives when securing umbilical lines, endotracheal tubes, feeding tubes, nasal cannulas, and urine bags. Remove carefully using soft gauze or cotton balls soaked in warm water.

5. Use warm sterile water to remove adhesives from the skin to prevent epidermal stripping.

6. Adhesive removers contain hydrocarbon derivatives or petroleum distillates that can result in toxicity in the preterm and term infants.

D. Cord care

1. Clean umbilical cord area with mild soap and water during first bath. Keep clean and dry. Wipe gently with water if area becomes soiled with stool or urine.

2. Routine application of alcohol is not recommended and may delay cord separation.

3. The routine use of antibiotic ointments and creams are not recommended.

4. Assess for signs of swelling or redness at base of cord.

E. Humidity

1. Consider the use of humidification for infants <32 weeks' gestation and/or <1,200 g to decrease transepidermal water loss, maintain skin integrity, decrease fluid requirements, and minimize electrolyte imbalance. Humidification is typically used for 10 to 14 days of life until the epidermis matures.

2. Recommended relative humidity (RH) is typically set between 60% and 80% dependent on the clinical situation.

3. Humidification requires a gradual wean over a few days. Decrease RH levels by 5% to 10% every 12 hours until reaching 30% and then discontinue. Monitor temperature closely during this time and adjust isolette temperature as necessary to maintain euthermia.

4. Strict equipment cleaning protocols must be in place during humidification (i.e., changing out isolette, humidification chamber, linen changes, etc.).

F. Circumcision care

1. Maintain dressing with petroleum gauze for the first 24 hours.

2. After dressing is removed, clean site with water and dry gently for the first few days.

G. Disinfectants

1. **Generally**, use alcohol or chlorhexidine as primary disinfectants prior to procedures. In preterm infants, use sterile water to remove residual disinfectant following the procedure to avoid the risk of chemical burns. Current recommendation for chlorhexidine is to use with caution in infants <2 months of age. There is no data to support use in the premature infant, but it is widely used in NICUs across the country. Povidone-iodine is no longer used due to the side effect of altering thyroid function in premature infants due to their permeable skin and increased risk of systemic absorption.

H. Emollients

1. Emollients are used to prevent and treat skin breakdown and dryness.

2. Emollients should not be used routinely in extremely premature infants because their use may increase the risk of systemic infection.

3. Single-use or patient-specific containers should be used to minimize risk of contamination.

4. Product should not contain perfumes, dyes, or preservatives.

IV. WOUND CARE. Wounds acquired in the immediate newborn period are most commonly related to surgical procedures, trauma, or excoriation. Skin care protocols and careful attention to positioning can prevent many of the common wounds requiring treatment. Epidermal stripping is common and can be avoided by minimizing adhesive use and applying protective barriers. Routine assessment and prompt treatment maximizes healing.

A. Common causes of neonatal wounds

1. Surgical procedures

2. Trauma

3. Pressure necrosis

4. IV extravasation

5. Prolonged contact with moisture or chemicals

6. Skin excoriation

B. Three phases of wound healing

1. Inflammatory phase begins with hemostasis and leads to inflammation. This phase removes necrotic tissue, debris, and bacteria from the wound.

2. Proliferative phase is characterized by collagen production, increase in wound strength, creation of new capillaries, and epithelization.

3. Remodeling phase includes collagen remodeling, increase in wound strength, and wound contraction.

C. Treatment. Accurate assessment followed by immediate, effective treatment promotes wound healing and prevents further damage. Individualized, multidisciplinary care plans should be developed and implemented considering the etiology, type of wound, and the gestational age of the infant. Optimal wound treatment is achieved through proper assessment, cleansing, and dressing choice. Multiple wound care products are currently available to optimize healing and prevent further injury.

1. Wound assessment

a. Assess wound for location, color, depth, size, odor, and exudates along with characterizing tissue type covering the wound base and description of surrounding skin in order to provide consistent, objective documentation.

2. Wound cleansing

a. Avoid the use of antiseptics in open wounds. Sterile normal saline (NS) is the preferred cleanser to remove debris and devitalized tissue, using gentle friction or irrigation. Moistening the wound every 4 to 6 hours until the wound surface is clear facilitates the healing process.

b. A full-thickness wound is not sterile and does not require sterile saline, and so forth to clean (tap water with baby shampoo is often preferred).

c. Clinical signs of infection (erythema, induration, and/or drainage) may require culture and treatment with local or systemic antibiotics.

3. Common wound dressings and products

   a. A full-thickness wound is very unlikely to become infected as long as it is "open" and allowed to drain without occlusive dressings.

   b. Occlusive, nonadherent dressings provide a moist environment to promote healing and protect the site from further injury. These dressings should only be considered for partial-thickness wounds involving only the epidermis and/or dermis. Occlusive dressings should not be used for full-thickness wounds through the dermis.

   c. Gauze

   d. Foam dressings

   e. Hydrocolloids

   f. Hydrogels

   g. Barrier creams

V. IV EXTRAVASATION. IV extravasation injuries can be minimized with frequent site assessment and prompt intervention.

A. Prevention

   1. Assess and document appearance of peripheral IV sites hourly.

   2. Peripheral IV infusions should not exceed 12.5% dextrose concentrations.

   3. Use central access whenever possible for vasopressors and other high-risk medications.

B. Treatment

   1. When an infiltration or extravasation occurs, stop the infusion and attempt to aspirate fluid, if possible. Elevate the extremity above the heart to facilitate venous return of the fluid and DO NOT apply heat or cold because further tissue damage may occur. Pharmacologic intervention should be administered as soon as possible but no later than 12 to 24 hours from time of injury if applicable.

   2. Convincing evidence that antidotes improve outcomes for extravasation injuries does not exist. Although health care providers and patients feel better "doing something" when an iatrogenic injury occurs, often the best management is "active nonintervention." The added volume of an antidote administered to an injured area theoretically may worsen the injury from pressure necrosis. In addition, by the time the extravasation is appreciated, the antidote is ordered, the drug arrives at the bedside, and a health care provider has injected it, the effects of the extravasation have worn off. For example, vasoconstriction from epinephrine lasts 60 minutes, and its effects are likely resolved by the time an antidote has been administered. Although the plastic surgery service at our institution does not advocate for the use of antidotes, the two most commonly used are briefly described in the following text.

   a. Hyaluronidase has been used in an effort to facilitate subcutaneous diffusion of an extravasate (i.e., parenteral nutrition). Administer as a solution diluted to 1 mL in NS. Refer to hospital formulary for concentration and dilution guidelines. Inject 0.2 mL subcutaneously in five separate sites around the leading edge of the infiltrate using a 25G or 27G needle. Change the needle after each skin entry.

b. Phentolamine has been used to treat injury caused by extravasation of vasoconstrictive agents such as dopamine, epinephrine, or dobutamine. Use a 0.5 to 1 mg/mL solution of phentolamine diluted in NS. Consult hospital formulary for dosage. Inject 0.2 mL subcutaneously in five separate sites around the leading edge of the infiltrate using 25G or 27G needle. Change the needle after each skin entry.

3. Consider consultation with plastic surgery for severe injury.

VI. COMMON SKIN LESIONS. Transient cutaneous lesions are common in the neonatal period. Among the most common are the following:

A. Erythema toxicum

1. Scattering of macules, papules, and even some vesicles or small white or yellow pustules, which usually occur on the trunk but also frequently appear on the extremities and face. It occurs in up to 70% of term newborns; occurs rarely in premature infants.

2. Unknown etiology

3. Vesicle contents when smeared and stained with Wright stain will show a predominance of eosinophils.

4. No treatment necessary

B. Incontinence-associated dermatitis

1. Common skin disorder in infants and children most often affecting the groin, buttocks, perineum, and anal area. It is multifactorial, most often caused by friction or exposure to urine and feces, sensitivity to chemicals contained in detergent, clothing, or diapers. The damp environment increases the skin pH, leading to impaired barrier function and skin breakdown.

2. Prevention is the best treatment, including frequent diaper changes, keeping diaper area clean with warm water, and applying barrier products if needed. Vaseline can be used preventatively to intact skin. If signs of incontinence-associated dermatitis (IAD) are present (redness, excoriation, bleeding), start treatment with barrier products. Cleanse skin with water or pH-balanced cleanser and soft cloths. Reassess ointment regimen every 48 hours; if no improvement, consider alternate regimens. Start with application of thin creams to provide a skin barrier, and if skin is not responding, move to thick pastes. If candidal rash present, use antifungal ointment or powder first and then apply barrier cream. Consider astringent and oatmeal baths to dry out and soothe irritated skin. Dab or gently wipe off excess stool and reapply barrier cream with each diaper change. Remove all barrier products at least once daily to assess skin.

3. Use of powder is not recommended due to the risk of inhalation.

C. Milia

1. Multiple pearly white or pale yellow papules or cysts mainly found on the nose, chin, and forehead in term infants

2. Consists of epidermal cysts up to 1 mm in diameter that develop in connection with the pilosebaceous follicle

a. Disappears within the first few weeks requiring no treatment

D. Sebaceous gland hyperplasia

1. Similar to milia with smaller, more numerous lesions primarily confined to the nose, upper lip, and chin

2. Rarely occurs in preterm infants

3. Related to maternal androgen stimulation

4. Disappears within the first few weeks

E. Infection

1. Infections caused by bacterial (especially staphylococcal, *Pseudomonas*, *Listeria*), viral (herpes simplex), or fungal (e.g., candidal) organisms; may also cause vesicular, bullous, or other skin manifestations

VII. VASCULAR ABNORMALITIES. Vascular anomalies occur in up to 40% of newborns.

A. Infantile hemangiomas. Affect 5% of infants within the first few weeks of life. Premature infants have a higher incidence, especially those born at <1,000 g. Intervention is only required in the rare instance when the hemangioma interferes with vital functions. Management options for problematic lesions in infancy include topical timolol, intralesional triamcinolone, oral prednisolone, or oral propranolol. Lesions grow for the first 5 months of age and then begin to regress at 12 months of age. They improve until 3.5 years of age, and some may leave a deformity requiring intervention in childhood.

B. Fading capillary stains. The most common vascular lesion found in the newborn, occurring in 30% to 40% of infants. Also called "angel's kiss" or "stork bite." They are flat, pink macular lesions on the forehead, upper eyelid, nasolabial area, glabella, or nape of the neck. Most resolve by 2 years of age.

C. Capillary malformation (port-wine stain). Pink lesion that can affect any area of integument. The lesion is a vascular malformation of dilated capillaries that do not involute. The association of capillary malformation in the region of the first branch of the trigeminal nerve with cortical lesions of the brain and ocular abnormalities is known as the Sturge-Weber syndrome.

D. Disorders of lymphatic vessels

1. Microcystic lymphatic malformation ("lymphangioma")

2. Macrocystic lymphatic malformation ("cystic hygroma")

3. Lymphedema

VIII. PIGMENTATION ABNORMALITIES. Pigmentary lesions may be present at birth and are most often benign. Some of the most common are briefly described

in the subsequent text. A diffuse pattern of hyperpigmentation presenting in the newborn period is unusual and may indicate a variety of hereditary, nutritional, or metabolic disorders. Hypopigmentation presenting in a diffuse pattern may be linked to endocrine, metabolic, or genetic disease.

A. Mongolian spots. Benign pigmented lesions found in 70% to 90% of Black, Hispanic, and Asian infants. The lesions may be small or large or grayish blue or bluish black in color. Caused by the increased presence of melanocytes, most commonly found in the lumbosacral region

B. Café au lait spots. Flat, brown, round, or oval lesions with smooth edges occurring in 10% of normal infants. Usually of little or no significance, but they may indicate neurofibromatosis if larger than 4 to 6 cm or >6 are present.

C. Albinism. Most commonly an autosomal recessive condition involving abnormal melanin synthesis leading to a deficiency in pigment production. The only effective treatment is protection from light.

D. Piebaldism (partial albinism). Autosomal dominant disorder present at birth characterized by off-white macules (depigmented lesions with hyperpigmented borders) on the scalp and forehead, trunk, and extremities. The hair may be involved as well. A white "forelock," as in Waardenburg syndrome, is a feature of this disorder.

E. Junctional nevi. Brown or black, flat or slightly raised lesions present at birth occurring at the junction of the dermis and epidermis. They are benign lesions requiring no treatment.

F. Compound nevi. Larger than junctional nevi, involving the dermis and epidermis. Removal is recommended to decrease possibility of later progression to malignant melanoma.

G. Giant hairy nevi. Present at birth, they may involve 20% to 30% of the body surface, with other pigmentary abnormalities frequently present. Brown to black and leathery in appearance, also known as bathing trunk nevi, they have a large amount of hair and may include central nervous system involvement. Surgical removal is indicated for cosmetic reasons and because they can progress to malignant melanoma.

IX. DEVELOPMENTAL ABNORMALITIES OF THE SKIN

A. Skin dimples and sinuses can occur on any part of the body, but they are most common over bony prominences such as the scapula, knee joint, and hip. They may be simple depressions in the skin of no pathologic significance or actual sinus tracts connecting to deeper structures.

  1. A pilonidal dimple or sinus may occur in the sacral area. A sinus that is deep but does not communicate with the underlying structures is usually insignificant.

  2. Some deep sinuses connect to the central nervous system. Occasionally, a dimple, sometimes accompanied by a nevus or hemangioma, may signify an underlying spinal disorder. These usually require neuroimaging scans for diagnosis.

3. Dermal sinuses or cysts along the cheek or jawline or extending into the neck may represent remnants of the branchial cleft structures of the early embryo.

4. A preauricular sinus is the most common and may be unilateral or bilateral. It appears in the most anterior upper portion of the tragus of the external ear. They rarely cause problems in the newborn period but may require later excision due to infection.

B. Small skin tags can occur on the chest wall near the breast and are of no significance.

C. Aplasia cutis (congenital absence of the skin) occurs most frequently in the midline of the posterior part of the scalp. Treatment involves protection from trauma and infection. Other malformations may be associated, including trisomy 13.

X. OTHER SKIN DISORDERS. Complete identification and description of all dermatologic disorders is beyond the scope of this chapter. Several of the more common developmental and hereditary disorders are mentioned in the following text.

A. Scaling disorders

1. Most common causes of scaling in neonatal period are related to desquamation found in postmature and dysmature infants. The condition is time-limited and transient without long-term consequences.

2. Less common scaling disorders that occur within the first month of life include harlequin ichthyosis, collodion baby, X-linked ichthyosis, bullous ichthyosis, and others.

B. Vesicobullous eruptions

1. Epidermolysis bullosa is a group of genetic disorders characterized by lesions that appear at birth or within the first few weeks. Severity of symptoms ranges from simple, nonscarring bullae to more severe forms with large numerous lesions that result in scarring, contractions, and loss of large areas of epidermis. Specific diagnosis requires skin biopsy. Prevention of infection and protection of fragile skin surfaces is the goal of treatment.

Reference

1. Association of Women's Health, Obstetric and Neonatal Nurses. *Evidence-Based Clinical Practice Guideline: Neonatal Skin Care*. 3rd ed. Washington, DC: Association of Women's Health, Obstetric and Neonatal Nurses; 2013.

Suggested Readings

Doellman D, Hadaway L, Bowe-Geddes L, et al. Infiltration and extravasation: update on prevention and management. *J Infus Nurs* 2009;32(4):203–211.

Eichenfield LF, Frieden IJ, Esterly NB, eds. *Textbook of Neonatal Dermatology*. 2nd ed. Philadelphia, PA: Saunders Elsevier; 2008.

McNichol L, Lund C, Rosen T, et al. Medical adhesives and patient safety: state of the science: consensus statements for the assessment, prevention, and treatment of adhesive-related skin injuries. *J Wound Ostomy Continence Nurs* 2013;40(4):365–380.

Tamma PD, Aucott SW, Milstone AM. Chlorhexidine use in the neonatal intensive care unit: results from a national survey. *Infect Control Hosp Epidemiol* 2010;31(8):846–849.

Vascular Anomalies

Javier A. Couto, Steven J. Fishman, and
Arin K. Greene

KEY POINTS

- Vascular anomalies are relatively common, affecting approximately 5% of the population.
- There are two broad types of vascular anomalies: tumors and malformations.
- Despite improved treatments for vascular anomalies, many lesions continue to cause significant morbidity and are not curable.

I. **INTRODUCTION.** Vascular anomalies affect approximately 5% of the population and can involve any component of the vasculature. The field is confusing because different lesions may look similar and terminology is difficult. Vascular anomalies are classified based on their clinical behavior and cellular characteristics (Table 66.1). The International Society for the Study of Vascular Anomalies (ISSVA) has recently released an expanded classification. Ninety percent of lesions can be diagnosed by history and physical examination. There are two broad types of vascular anomalies: tumors and malformations. Tumors typically arise postnatally and demonstrate endothelial proliferation. There are four major lesions: (i) infantile hemangioma, (ii) congenital hemangioma, (iii) kaposiform hemangioendothelioma, and (iv) pyogenic granuloma (Fig. 66.1). Vascular malformations are errors in vascular development, are present at birth, and have minimal endothelial turnover. There are four major categories: (i) capillary malformation, (ii) lymphatic malformation, (iii) venous malformation, and (iv) arteriovenous malformation (Fig. 66.2).

II. **VASCULAR TUMORS**

A. **Infantile hemangioma.** Infantile hemangioma (IH) is the most common tumor of infancy, affecting 4% to 5% of infants. IH is more frequent in premature children and in females. The median age of appearance is 2 weeks. IH is red when it involves the superficial dermis and can appear bluish if it is located beneath the skin. IH grows faster than the child during the first 9 months of age (proliferating phase); 80% of its size is achieved by 3.2 ($\pm$1.7) months. The majority of IH are small, harmless lesions that can be monitored under the watchful eye of a pediatrician. However, a minority of proliferating IH can cause significant deformity or complications. Infants with five or more small (<5 mm) tumors are more likely to have IH of the liver, although the risk is low (~16%). After 12 months, the tumor begins

Table 66.1. Classification of Vascular Anomalies

Tumors	Malformations		Overgrowth Syndromes
	Slow-Flow	Fast-Flow	
Infantile hemangioma	Capillary malformation	Arteriovenous malformation	CLOVES
Congenital hemangioma	Lymphatic malformation		Klippel-Trenaunay
Kaposiform hemangioendothelioma	Venous malformation		Parkes Weber
Pyogenic granuloma			Sturge-Weber

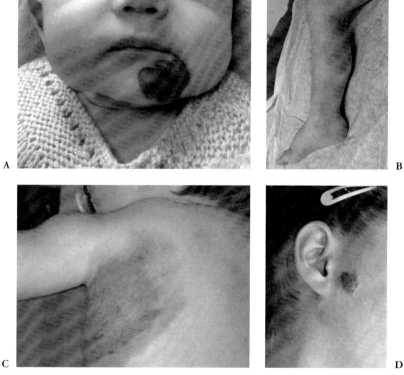

Figure 66.1. Examples of the four major types of vascular tumors. **A:** Infantile hemangioma. **B:** Congenital hemangioma. **C:** Kaposiform hemangioendothelioma. **D:** Pyogenic granuloma.

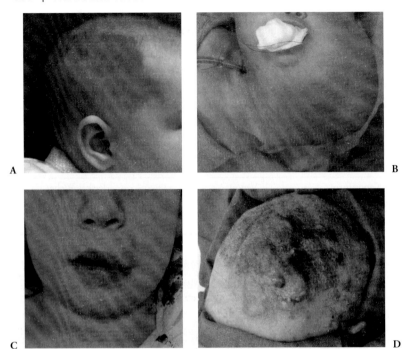

Figure 66.2. Examples of the four major types of vascular malformations. **A:** Capillary malformation. **B:** Lymphatic malformation. **C:** Venous malformation. **D:** Arteriovenous malformation.

to regress (involuting phase). Involution ceases in most of children by age 4 years (involuted phase). After involution, one-half of children will have a residual deformity.

Most IHs are simply observed. To protect against ulceration, IH should be kept moist with hydrated petroleum during the proliferative phase. If ulceration develops, the wound is washed gently with soap and water at least twice daily. Small, superficial areas are managed by the application of topical antibiotic ointment and occasionally with a petroleum gauze barrier. Large, deep ulcers require damp-to-dry dressing changes. Bleeding from an ulcerated IH is usually minor and is treated by applying direct pressure. Ulcerations will heal with local wound care within 2 to 3 weeks.

A diffuse hemangioma replacing hepatic parenchyma necessitates thyroid-stimulating hormone (TSH) monitoring to prevent potentially devastating and irreversible effects on neurologic function. Hypothyroidism results from the expression of a deiodinase by the hemangioma which cleaves iodine from thyroid hormone and inactivates it. Massive intravenous thyroid replacement may be necessary until the hemangioma regresses. In contrast to diffuse hepatic hemangioma, a large single hemangioma in the liver is often a rapidly involuting congenital hemangioma and does not require intervention. Similarly, multiple small hepatic hemangioma do not cause morbidity unless significant shunting is present.

1. **Topical pharmacotherapy.** Topical corticosteroid is relatively ineffective, especially if IH involves the deep dermis and subcutis. Although lightening may occur, if there is deep component, it will not be affected. Adverse effects include hypopigmentation, cutaneous atrophy, and even adrenal suppression. Topical timolol may be effective for superficial lesions but will not affect hemangiomas with a subcutaneous component.

2. **Intralesional corticosteroid.** Problematic IHs that are well localized and <3 cm in diameter are best managed by intralesional corticosteroid. Triamcinolone (not to exceed 3 mg/kg) will stop the growth of the lesion; two-thirds will decrease in size. The corticosteroid lasts 2 to 3 weeks, and thus, infants may require two to three injections during the proliferative phase.

3. **Systemic pharmacotherapy.** Problematic IH that is larger than 3 cm in diameter is managed by oral prednisolone or propranolol. Prednisolone has been used to treat IH for >40 years and has proven to be very safe and effective. Patients are given 3 mg/kg/day for 1 month; the drug is then tapered slowly by volume (0.5 mL every 2 to 4 weeks) until it is discontinued between 10 and 12 months of age when the tumor is no longer proliferating. All tumors will stabilize in growth, and 88% will become smaller. Twenty percent of infants will develop a cushingoid appearance that resolves during tapering of therapy. Approximately 12% of infants treated after 3 months of age exhibit decreased gain in height but return to their pretreatment growth curve by 24 months of age.

   Propranolol has largely replaced corticosteroid use in recent years. Dosing typically is 2 mg/kg/day. Approximately 90% of tumors will stop growing or regress. Risks (<3%) include bronchospasm, bradycardia, hypotension, hypoglycemia, seizures, and hyperkalemia. Preterm infants and those <3 months of age are more likely to have adverse events. Patients usually have cardiology consultation; electrocardiogram; echocardiogram; glucose/electrolyte measurements; and frequent blood pressure, heart rate, and respiratory examinations. Inpatient initiation of treatment is used for premature or infants <3 months of age. Potential contraindications include asthma, glucose abnormalities, heart disease, hypotension, bradycardia, PHACES association.

4. **Laser therapy.** Pulsed-dye laser generally is not indicated for a proliferating IH. The laser only affects the superficial portion of the tumor. Although lightening may occur, the mass is not affected. Patients have an increased risk of skin atrophy, ulceration, pain, bleeding, scarring, and hypopigmentation. Pulsed-dye laser is effective during the involuted phase to fade residual telangiectasias.

5. **Resection.** Resection of IH typically is not recommended during the early growth phase. The tumor is highly vascular, and there is a risk for blood loss, iatrogenic injury, and an inferior outcome, compared to excising residual tissue after the tumor has regressed. It is preferable to intervene surgically between 3 and 4 years of age. During this period, the IH will no longer improve significantly, and the procedure is performed

before the child's long-term memory and self-esteem begin to form at about 4 years of age.

B. Congenital hemangioma. Congenital hemangiomas are fully grown at birth and do not have postnatal growth. They are red violaceous with a peripheral pale halo. Lesions are more common in the extremities, have an equal sex distribution, and have an average diameter of 5 cm. There are two forms: *rapidly involuting congenital hemangioma* (RICH) and *noninvoluting congenital hemangioma* (NICH). RICH involutes rapidly after birth, and 50% of lesions have completed regression by 7 months of age; the remaining tumors are fully involuted by 14 months. NICH, in contrast, does not regress; it remains unchanged with persistent fast-flow.

RICH usually does not require resection in infancy because it regresses so quickly. Rarely, surgical removal may be necessary to control hemorrhage from ulceration or high-output congestive heart failure caused by progressive flow through the tumor. After involution, RICH may leave behind atrophic skin and subcutaneous tissue. NICH is rarely problematic in infancy and is observed until the diagnosis is clear; resection may be indicated to improve the appearance of the area.

C. Kaposiform hemangioendothelioma. Kaposiform hemangioendothelioma (KHE) is a rare vascular neoplasm that does not metastasize. KHE is present at birth in 50% of patients; has an equal sex distribution; and affects the head/neck (40%), trunk (30%), or an extremity (30%). The tumor is often >5 cm in dimensions and appears as a flat, reddish-purple, edematous lesion. Seventy percent of patients have Kasabach-Merritt phenomenon (KMP) (thrombocytopenia <25,000/mm^3, petechiae, bleeding). KHE partially regresses after 2 years of age, although it usually persists long term causing chronic pain and stiffness.

Most lesions are extensive, involving multiple tissues, and well beyond the limits of resection. Vincristine is first-line therapy; the response rate is 90%. KHE does not respond as well to second-line drugs, interferon (50%), or corticosteroid (10%). Recently, patients have been treated with sirolimus as first-line therapy with good efficacy. Thrombocytopenia is not significantly improved with platelet transfusion which should be avoided unless there is active bleeding or a surgical procedure is planned. By 2 years of age, the tumor usually has undergone partial involution and the platelet count normalizes.

D. Pyogenic granuloma. Pyogenic granuloma (PG) is a solitary, red papule that grows rapidly on a stalk. It is small, with an average diameter of 6.5 mm; the mean age of onset is 6.7 years. PG is commonly complicated by bleeding and ulceration. The lesion involves the skin or mucous membranes. It is distributed on the head or neck (62%), trunk (19%), upper extremity (13%), or lower extremity (5%). In the head and neck region, affected sites include cheek (29%), oral cavity (14%), scalp (11%), forehead (10%), eyelid (9%), or lips (9%).

PGs require intervention to control likely ulceration and bleeding. Numerous methods have been described: curettage, shave excision, laser therapy, and excision. Because the lesion extends into the reticular dermis, it may be out of the reach of the pulse-dye laser, cautery, or shave excision.

Consequently, these modalities have a recurrence rate of approximately 50%. Full-thickness excision is definitive treatment.

III. VASCULAR MALFORMATIONS

A. **Capillary malformation.** Capillary malformation was previously referred to as "port-wine stain." The lesion is obvious at birth, and the pink-purple skin discoloration can cause psychosocial distress. Over time, the lesion darkens and the soft tissue and bone may enlarge underneath the stain. This birthmark referred to as an "angel kiss" or "stork bite," present in one-half of Caucasian newborns, is located on the forehead, eyelids, nose, upper lip, or posterior neck. This lesion is a fading capillary stain; no treatment is necessary because it lightens over the first 2 years of life.

The mainstay of treatment is pulse-dye laser. Intervention during infancy or early childhood is recommended because superior lightening of the lesion is achieved. Pulse-dye laser is less effective for capillary malformations that have progressed to a dark color with cutaneous thickening. Surgical procedures are indicated to correct overgrowth caused by the malformation.

B. **Lymphatic malformation.** Lymphatic malformation is defined by the size of its channels: macrocystic, microcystic, or combined. The most commonly affected sites are the neck and axilla. Lymphatic malformation can cause infection, bleeding, and psychosocial morbidity. Macrocystic lesions contain cysts large enough to be accessed by a needle (typically ≥5 mm) and are amenable to sclerotherapy. Microcystic lesions have cysts that are too small to be cannulated by a needle (usually <5 mm) and thus cannot be treated by sclerotherapy. Approximately one-half of lymphatic malformations are not purely macrocystic or microcystic; they contain both macrocysts and microcysts. Small, superficial lymphatic malformations do not require further diagnostic evaluation. Large or deep lesions are evaluated by magnetic resonance imaging (MRI).

Lymphatic malformation is benign, and thus, intervention is not mandatory. Small, asymptomatic lesions may be observed. First-line management for a large or problematic macrocystic/combined lymphatic malformation is sclerotherapy. Generally, sclerotherapy gives superior results and has lower morbidity compared to resection. Resection of a macrocystic lymphatic malformation is indicated if sclerotherapy is no longer possible or if excision may be curative because the lesion is small. Symptomatic microcystic lesions are managed by resection which is typically subtotal. Sirolimus recently has shown efficacy for very problematic microcystic lymphatic malformations.

C. **Venous malformation.** Lesions are blue, soft, and compressible. Hard calcified phleboliths may be palpable. Lesions cause psychosocial morbidity as well as pain secondary to congestion, thrombosis, and phlebolith formation. Patients with venous malformations are not at risk for thromboembolism unless a large phlebectatic vein is connected to the deep venous system. Small, superficial venous malformations do not require further diagnostic workup. Large or deep lesions are evaluated by MRI.

Individuals with recurrent discomfort are given low-dose daily aspirin to prevent phlebothrombosis. Intervention is reserved for symptomatic lesions or asymptomatic phlebectatic areas at risk for thromboembolism. If possible, intervention should be postponed until after 12 months of age when the risk of anesthesia is lowest. Therapy for lesions causing a visible deformity should be considered before 4 years of age to limit psychological morbidity. Sclerotherapy typically is first-line treatment and is generally safer and more effective than resection. Resection of a venous malformation should be considered for small lesions that can be completely removed or for persistent symptoms after completion of sclerotherapy.

D. Arteriovenous malformation. Arteriovenous malformation has an absent capillary bed which causes shunting of blood directly from the arterial to venous circulation through a fistula (direct connection of an artery to a vein) or nidus (abnormal channels bridging the feeding artery to the draining veins). Lesions have a pink-red cutaneous stain, are warm, and can have palpable pulsations. Patients are at risk for disfigurement, destruction of tissues, pain, ulceration, bleeding, and congestive heart failure. Handheld Doppler examination shows fast flow. MRI is usually obtained to confirm the diagnosis and determine the extent of the lesion. An angiogram is obtained if the diagnosis remains unclear following ultrasound and MRI or if embolization is planned.

Because the lesion is often diffuse and involves multiple tissue planes, cure is rare. An asymptomatic arteriovenous malformation should be observed unless it can be removed for possible cure with minimal morbidity. Embolization is generally first-line therapy for a symptomatic lesion. Embolization is generally not curative, and most arteriovenous malformations will reexpand following treatment.

Resection of an arteriovenous malformation has a lower recurrence rate than embolization. Indications for resection include (i) a well-localized lesion, (ii) correction of a focal deformity, or (iii) a symptomatic arteriovenous malformation that has failed embolization. When excision is planned, preoperative embolization will facilitate the procedure by minimizing blood loss. Excision should be carried out 24 to 72 hours after embolization, before recanalization restores blood flow to the lesion.

Suggested Readings

Chang LC, Haggstrom AN, Drolet BA, et al. Growth characteristics of infantile hemangiomas: implications for management. *Pediatrics* 2008;122:360–367.

Couto RA, Maclellan RA, Zurakowski D, et al. Infantile hemangioma: clinical assessment of the involuting phase and implications for management. *Plast Reconstr Surg* 2012;130:619–624.

Drolet BA, Frommelt PC, Chamlin SL, et al. Initiation and use of propranolol for infantile hemangioma: report of a consensus conference. *Pediatrics* 2013;131:128–140.

Greene AK, Couto RA. Oral prednisolone for infantile hemangioma: efficacy and safety using a standardized treatment protocol. *Plast Reconstr Surg* 2011;128:743–752.

Greene AK, Liu AS, Mulliken JB, et al. Vascular anomalies in 5,621 patients: guidelines for referral. *J Pediatr Surg* 2011;46:1784–1789.

Hassanein AH, Mulliken JB, Fishman SJ, et al. Evaluation of terminology for vascular anomalies in current literature. *Plast Reconstr Surg* 2011;127:347–351.

International Society for the Study of Vascular Anomalies. http://www.issva.org. Accessed June 10, 2015.

Mulliken JB, Glowacki J. Hemangiomas and vascular malformations in infants and children: a classification based on endothelial characteristics. *Plast Reconstr Surg* 1982;69:412–422.

Wassef M, Blei F, Adams D, et al. Vascular anomalies classification: recommendations from the International Society for the Study of Vascular Anomalies. *Pediatrics* 2015;136(1):e203–e214.

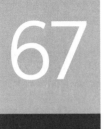

67 Retinopathy of Prematurity

Kristen T. Leeman and Deborah K. VanderVeen

KEY POINTS

- Retinopathy of prematurity (ROP) typically develops in premature infants weighing <1,500 g and/or <30 weeks' gestation at birth. Other risk factors include prolonged or labile oxygen exposure and increased illness severity.
- The risk for ROP increases with decreasing gestational age.
- The timing of first screening by an ophthalmologist is critical and based on postnatal gestational age.

GENERAL PRINCIPLES

I. DEFINITION. Retinopathy of prematurity (ROP) is a multifactorial vasoproliferative retinal disorder that increases in incidence with decreasing gestational age. Approximately 65% of infants with a birth weight <1,250 g and 80% of those with a birth weight <1,000 g will develop some degree of ROP.

II. PATHOGENESIS

A. Normal development. After the sclera and choroid have developed, retinal elements, including nerve fibers, ganglion cells, and photoreceptors, migrate from the optic disc at the posterior pole of the eye and move toward the periphery. The photoreceptors have progressed 80% of the distance to their resting place at the ora serrata by 28 weeks' gestation. Before the retinal vessels develop, the avascular retina receives its oxygen supply by diffusion across the retina from the choroidal vessels. The retinal vessels, which arise from the spindle cells of the adventitia of the hyaloid vessels at the optic disc, begin to migrate outward at 16 weeks' gestation. Migration is complete by 36 weeks on the nasal side and by 40 weeks on the temporal side.

B. Possible mechanisms of injury. Clinical observations suggest that the onset of ROP consists of two stages:

1. The **first stage** involves an initial insult or insults, such as hyperoxia, hypoxia, or hypotension, at a critical point in retinal vascularization that results in vasoconstriction and decreased blood flow to the developing retina, with a subsequent arrest in vascular development. The relative hyperoxia after birth is hypothesized to downregulate the production of growth factors, such as vascular endothelial growth factor (VEGF), that are essential for the normal development of the retinal vessels.

2. During the **second stage**, neovascularization occurs. This aberrant retinal vessel growth is thought to be driven by excess angiogenic factors (such as VEGF) upregulated by the hypoxic avascular retina. New vessels grow within the retina and into the vitreous. These vessels are permeable; therefore, hemorrhage and edema can occur. Extensive and severe extraretinal fibrovascular proliferation can lead to retinal detachment and abnormal retinal function. In most affected infants, however, the disease process is mild and regresses spontaneously.

C. Risk factors. ROP has been consistently associated with low gestational age, low birth weight, and prolonged oxygen exposure. In addition, potential or confirmed risk factors include lability in oxygen requirement as well as markers of neonatal illness severity, such as mechanical ventilation, systemic infection, blood transfusion, intraventricular hemorrhage, and poor postnatal weight gain.

III. DIAGNOSIS

A. Screening. Because no extraocular signs or symptoms indicate developing ROP, timely and regular retinal examination is necessary. The timing of the occurrence of ROP is related to the maturity of retinal vessels and therefore to postnatal age. In the Cryotherapy for Retinopathy of Prematurity (CRYO-ROP) study, for infants <1,250 g, the median postnatal ages at the onset of stage 1 ROP, prethreshold disease, and threshold disease were 34, 36, and 37 weeks, respectively. At the time of the first examination, 17% of infants had ROP, and prethreshold ROP has been reported as early as 29 weeks' gestational age. These findings led to the current screening recommendations outlined in the following text. Because ROP that meets treatment criteria may be reached after discharge from the neonatal intensive care unit (NICU), all preterm infants who meet screening criteria and are discharged before they show resolution of the ROP or have mature retinal vasculature must continue to have ophthalmologic examinations on an outpatient basis.

B. Diagnosis. ROP is diagnosed by retinal examination with indirect ophthalmoscopy; this should be performed by an ophthalmologist with expertise in ROP screening. The current recommendation is to screen all infants with a birth weight <1,500 g or gestational age <30 weeks. Infants who are born after 30 weeks' gestational age may be considered for screening if they have been ill (e.g., those who have had severe respiratory distress syndrome, hypotension requiring pressor support, or surgery in the first several weeks of life). Because the timing of ROP is related to postnatal age, infants who are born at <26 weeks' gestation are examined at the postnatal age of 6 to 8 weeks, those born at 27 to 28 weeks at the postnatal age of 5 weeks, those born at 29 to 30 weeks at the postnatal age of 4 weeks, and those >30 weeks at the postnatal age of 3 weeks. Patients are examined every 2 weeks until their vessels have grown out to the ora serrata and the retina is considered mature. If ROP is diagnosed, the frequency of examination depends on the severity and rapidity of progression of the disease.

Digital imaging may be used as an alternative to indirect ophthalmoscopy, and telescreening for ROP has been shown to be a valid alternative to detect significant ROP.

IV. CLASSIFICATION AND DEFINITIONS

A. **Classification.** The International Classification of Retinopathy of Prematurity (ICROP) is used to classify ROP. This classification system consists of four components (see Fig. 67.1).

1. **Location** refers to how far the developing retinal blood vessels have progressed. The retina is divided into three concentric circles or zones.
   a. Zone 1 consists of an imaginary circle with the optic nerve at the center and a radius of twice the distance from the optic nerve to the macula.
   b. Zone 2 extends from the edge of zone 1 to the ora serrata on the nasal side of the eye and approximately half the distance to the ora serrata on the temporal side.
   c. Zone 3 consists of the outer crescent-shaped area extending from zone 2 out to the ora serrata temporally.

2. Severity refers to the **stage** of disease.
   a. Stage 1. A demarcation line appears as a thin white line that separates the normal retina from the undeveloped avascular retina.
   b. Stage 2. A ridge of fibrovascular tissue with height and width replaces the line of stage 1. It extends inward from the plane of the retina.
   c. Stage 3. The ridge has extraretinal fibrovascular proliferation. Abnormal blood vessels and fibrous tissue develop on the edge of the ridge and extend into the vitreous.
   d. Stage 4. Partial retinal detachment may result when fibrovascular tissue pulls on the retina. Stage 4A is partial detachment not involving the macula so that there is still a chance for good vision. Stage 4B is partial detachment that involves the macula, thereby limiting the likelihood of good vision in that eye.
   e. Stage 5. Complete retinal detachment occurs. The retina assumes a funnel-shaped appearance and is described as either open or closed in the anterior and posterior regions.

3. **Extent** refers to the circumferential location of disease and is reported as clock hours in the appropriate zone.

4. **Plus disease** is an additional designation that refers to the presence of vascular dilatation and tortuosity of the posterior retinal vessels in at least two quadrants. This indicates a more severe degree of ROP and may also be associated with iris vascular engorgement, pupillary rigidity, and vitreous haze. **Preplus disease** describes vascular abnormalities of the posterior pole (mild venous dilatation or arterial tortuosity) that are present but are insufficient for the diagnosis of plus disease.

B. **Definitions**

1. **Aggressive posterior ROP** is an uncommon, rapidly progressing, severe form of ROP characterized by its posterior location (usually zone 1) and prominence of plus disease out of proportion to the peripheral retinopathy.

Children's Hospital Boston

OPHTHALMOLOGIC CONSULTATION FOR RETINOPATHY OF PREMATURITY (ROP)

Gestational age (weeks) _____ Birth weight _____ gm

Date of exam _____ Adjusted age (weeks) _____

Ophthalmologist _____ MD
                         (PRINT NAME)

USE PLATE OR PRINT

NAME _____
              LAST   FIRST

DATE _____ DIV _____

MED. REC. NO. _____

EXAMINATION:

☐ Pertinent record reviewed

Extended Ophthalmoscopy

Right Eye   **Left Eye**

Penlight examination (both eyes)

☐ External   ☐ Anterior chamber
☐ Lids   ☐ Iris
☐ Conjunctiva   ☐ Lens
☐ Cornea   ☐ _____

COMMENTS: _____

_____

_____

Right eye	Other findings (mark with an "X")	Left eye
	Dilatation/Tortuosity	
☐	Mild	☐
☐	Moderate	☐
☐	Severe	☐
_____	Iris vessel dilatation	_____
_____	Pupil rigidity	_____
_____	Vitreous haze	_____
_____	Hemorrhages	_____

Neovascular tufts posterior to ridge

_____   _____

Neovascular cylinders posterior to ridge

_____   _____

	Right eye	Summary diagnosis	Left eye
	_____	Mature retina	_____
	_____	Immature, no ROP	_____
	Zone		Zone

ROP

Stage	Zone	Number of clock hours	Stage	Zone	Number of clock hours

Other: _____

_____

_____

Plan: Repeat exam in: _____

Examined by: _____ , M.D.
                    (Signature)

Physician I.D. #

03241 25/pkg 05/06

Figure 67.1. Sample of form for ophthalmologic consultation. (*Source*: Boston Children's Hospital, Ophthalmology Department.)

Stage 3 ROP may appear as a flat, intraretinal network of neovascularization. When untreated, this type of ROP usually progresses to stage 5.

2. Threshold ROP is present if 5 or more contiguous or 8 cumulative clock hours (30-degree sectors) of stage 3 with plus disease in either zone 1 or 2 are present. This is the level of ROP at which the risk of blindness is predicted to be at least 50% and at which the CRYO-ROP study showed that the risk of blindness could be reduced to approximately 25% with appropriate treatment.

3. Prethreshold ROP is any ROP in zone 1 less than threshold ROP, and in zone 2, stage 2 ROP with plus disease, stage 3 without plus disease, or stage 3 with plus disease but fewer than the requisite clock hours that define threshold ROP.

    a. Type 1 prethreshold ROP includes the following:

        i. In zone 1, any ROP and plus disease or stage 3 with or without plus disease

        ii. In zone 2, stage 2 or 3 ROP with plus disease

    b. Type 2 prethreshold ROP includes the following:

        i. In zone 1, stage 1 or 2 ROP, without plus disease

        ii. In zone 2, stage 3 ROP without plus disease

V. TIMING OF TREATMENT

A. Current recommendations are to consider treatment for eyes with **type 1 prethreshold ROP** based on the Early Treatment for ROP (ETROP) randomized trial that showed a significant benefit for treatment of eyes with type 1 ROP.

B. Close observation is currently recommended for **type 2 prethreshold ROP**. Treatment should be considered for an eye with type 2 ROP when progression to type 1 status or threshold ROP occurs. Approximately 15% of type 2 eyes progress to type 1 ROP.

VI. PROGNOSIS

A. Short-term prognosis. Risk factors for ROP requiring treatment include posterior location (zone 1 or posterior zone 2), presence of ROP on the first properly timed examination, increasing severity of stage, circumferential involvement, the presence of plus disease, and rapid progression of disease. Most infants with stage 1 or 2 ROP will experience spontaneous regression. If prethreshold ROP develops, about 77% of type 2 eyes regress without treatment, but only 32% of eyes with type 1 regress spontaneously. In ETROP, treatment for type 1 ROP (compared to conventional timing at threshold) reduced unfavorable visual outcomes from 33% to 25%. Unfortunately, only 35% of patients maintained visual acuity at 6 years of age of 20/40 or better, suggesting more work to prevent development of ROP is needed. Any zone 3 disease has an excellent prognosis for complete recovery.

B. Long-term prognosis. Infants with significant ROP have an increased risk of myopia, anisometropia, astigmatism, strabismus, amblyopia, late retinal detachment, and glaucoma. **Cicatricial disease** refers to residual scarring in the retina and may be associated with retinal detachment years later.

The prognosis for stage 4 ROP depends on the involvement of the macula; the chance for good vision is greater when the macula is not involved. Once the retina has detached, the prognosis for good vision is poor even with surgical reattachment, although some useful vision may be preserved. All premature infants who meet screening criteria regardless of the diagnosis of ROP are at risk for long-term vision problems, from either ocular or neurologic abnormalities. We recommend a follow-up evaluation by an ophthalmologist with expertise in neonatal sequelae at approximately 1 year of age or sooner if ocular or visual abnormalities have been noted.

VII. PREVENTION. Currently, no proven methods are available to prevent ROP. Multiple large clinical trials to prevent ROP have been performed evaluating the use of prophylactic vitamin E therapy, reduction in exposure to bright light, and administration of penicillamine, but none of these have shown clear benefit. Nonrandomized studies have suggested that lower or more tightly regulated oxygen saturation limits early on in the neonatal course may reduce the severity of ROP without adverse effects on mortality, bronchopulmonary dysplasia, or neurologic sequelae. In the SUPPORT study, preterm infants under 28 weeks' gestation who were randomized to lower oxygen ranges had lower rates of retinopathy but higher rates of mortality. Several other multicenter randomized trials to formally test this hypothesis are currently underway.

VIII. TREATMENT

A. **Laser therapy.** Laser photocoagulation therapy for ROP is the preferred initial treatment in most centers. Laser treatment is delivered through an indirect ophthalmoscope and is applied to the avascular retina anterior to the ridge of extraretinal fibrovascular proliferation for 360 degrees. An average of 1,000 spots are placed in each eye, but the number may range from a few hundred to approximately 2,000. Both argon and diode laser photocoagulation have been successfully used in infants with severe ROP. The procedure can be performed in the NICU and usually can be performed with local anesthesia and sedation, avoiding the possible adverse effects of general anesthesia. Clinical observations and comparative studies suggest that laser therapy is at least as effective as cryotherapy in achieving favorable visual outcomes. The development of cataracts, glaucoma, or anterior segment ischemia following laser surgery or cryotherapy have been reported.

B. **Cryotherapy.** A cryoprobe is applied to the external surface of the sclera, and areas peripheral to the ridge of the ROP are frozen until the entire anterior avascular retina has been treated. Approximately 35 to 75 applications are made in each eye. The procedure is usually done under general anesthesia. Cryotherapy causes more inflammation and requires more analgesia than laser therapy but may be necessary in special cases, such as when there is poor pupillary dilation or vitreous hemorrhage, both of which prevent adequate delivery of laser therapy.

C. **Anti-VEGF therapy.** Intravitreal injection of VEGF inhibitors has been offered for ROP treatment in many centers, particularly for cases of zone 1 or aggressive posterior ROP, as salvage treatment after laser therapy or in conjunction with vitreoretinal surgery. Although use of these agents for

ROP treatment is off-label, at least two randomized trials and multiple small case series have shown the efficacy of this treatment. However, some concerns remain about dosing and safety because systemic absorption may result in reduced VEGF and vascularization of other organ systems. The ocular safety profile is reasonably good, although endophthalmitis is a rare but potentially devastating complication. Some benefits of intravitreal injection include potentially less stress for the infant (because the procedure time is short and only requires topical anesthesia); less destruction of the retina (because laser and cryotherapy are ablative procedures); and long-term, lower rates of very severe myopia.

D. Retinal reattachment. Once the macula detaches in stage 4B or 5 ROP, retinal surgery may be performed in an attempt to reattach the retina. Vitrectomy with or without lensectomy, and membrane peeling if necessary, is performed to remove tractional forces causing the retinal detachment. A scleral buckling procedure may be useful for more peripheral detachments, with drainage of subretinal fluid for effusional detachments. Repeat operations for redetachment of the retina are common. Even if the retina can be successfully attached, with rare exception, the visual outcome is in the range of legal blindness. Despite the measurement of low visual acuity, children find any amount of vision useful, and untreated stage 5 ROP eventually leads to no light perception vision. The achievement of even minimal vision can result in a large difference in a child's overall quality of life.

Suggested Readings

American Academy of Pediatrics Section on Ophthalmology, American Academy of Ophthalmology, American Association for Pediatric Ophthalmology and Strabismus. Screening examination of premature infants for retinopathy of prematurity. *Pediatrics* 2006;117:572–576.

Early Treatment for Retinopathy of Prematurity Cooperative Group. Final visual acuity results in the early treatment for retinopathy of prematurity study. *Arch Ophthalmol* 2010;128(6):663–671.

Early Treatment for Retinopathy of Prematurity Cooperative Group. Revised indications for the treatment of retinopathy of prematurity: results of the early treatment for retinopathy of prematurity randomized trial. *Arch Ophthalmol* 2003;121(12):1684–1694.

International Committee for the Classification of Retinopathy of Prematurity. The International Classification of Retinopathy of Prematurity revisited. *Arch Ophthalmol* 2005;123(7):991–999.

Mintz-Hittner HA, Kennedy KA, Chuang AZ; for the BEAT-ROP Cooperative Group. Efficacy of intravitreal bevacizumab for stage 3+ retinopathy of prematurity. *N Engl J Med* 2011;364(7):603–615.

Quinn GE, Ying GS, Daniel E, et al; for the e-ROP Cooperative Group. Validity of a telemedicine system for the evaluation of acute-phase retinopathy of prematurity. *JAMA Ophthalmol* 2014;132(10):1178–1184.

SUPPORT Study Group of the Eunice Kennedy Shriver NICHD Neonatal Research Network. Target ranges of oxygen saturation in extremely preterm infants. *N Engl J Med* 2010;362(21):1959–1969.

68 Hearing Loss in Neonatal Intensive Care Unit Graduates

Jane E. Stewart, Jennifer Bentley, and Aimee Knorr

KEY POINTS

- 1-3-6: screened before 1 month, diagnosis before 3 months, habilitation/treatment before 6 months
- Neonatal intensive care unit (NICU) graduates at increased risk for hearing loss
- Even mild and unilateral hearing losses can cause significant delays.
- Children with risk factors should be monitored by an audiologist.
- The earlier habilitation starts, the better the child's chance of achieving age-appropriate language and communication skills.

I. **DEFINITION.** Neonatal intensive care unit (NICU) graduates have an increased risk of developing hearing loss. When undetected, hearing loss can delay language, communication, and cognitive development. Hearing loss falls into four major categories:

A. **Sensorineural loss** is the result of abnormal development or damage to the cochlear hair cells (sensory end organ) or auditory nerve.

B. **Conductive loss** is the result of interference in the transmission of sound from the external auditory canal to the inner ear. The most common cause of conductive hearing loss is fluid in the middle ear or middle ear effusion. Less common are anatomic causes such as microtia, canal stenosis, or stapes fixation that often occur in infants with craniofacial malformations.

C. **Auditory dyssynchrony or auditory neuropathy** is a rare type of hearing loss accounting for only 10% of children diagnosed with severe permanent hearing loss. The inner ear or cochlea appears to receive sounds normally; however, the transfer of the signal from the cochlea to the auditory nerve is abnormal. The etiology of this disorder is not well understood; however, babies who have a history of extreme prematurity, hypoxia, severe hyperbilirubinemia, and immune disorders are at increased risk. In approximately 40% of cases, there is a genetic basis for their auditory dyssynchrony.

D. **Central hearing loss** occurs despite an intact auditory canal and inner ear and normal neurosensory pathways because of abnormal auditory processing at higher levels of the central nervous system.

II. INCIDENCE. The overall incidence of severe congenital hearing loss is 1 to 3 per 1,000 live births. However, 20 to 40 per 1,000 infants surviving neonatal intensive care have some degree of sensorineural hearing loss.

III. ETIOLOGY

A. Genetic. Approximately 50% of congenital hearing loss is thought to be of genetic origin (30% syndromic and 70% nonsyndromic). Of the nonsyndromic, 75% to 85% are autosomal recessive, 15% to 24% autosomal dominant, and 1% to 2% X-linked. The most common genetic cause of nonsyndromic autosomal recessive hearing loss is a mutation in the **connexin 26 (Cx26) gene**, located on chromosome 13q11–12 (at least 90 deletions have been associated with hearing loss). The carrier rate for a Cx26 mutation is 3%, and it causes approximately 20% to 30% of all congenital hearing loss. Deletion of the **mitochondrial gene** 12SrRNA, A1555G, is associated with a predisposition for hearing loss after exposure to aminoglycoside antibiotics. Approximately 30% of infants with hearing loss have other associated medical problems that are part of a **syndrome**. More than 400 syndromes are known to include hearing loss (e.g., Robin sequence, Usher, Waardenburg syndrome, neurofibromatosis type 2, branchio-oto-renal syndrome, trisomy 21). To see a full review of the genetics of hearing, please see Smith et al.[1]

B. Nongenetic. In approximately 25% of childhood hearing loss, a nongenetic cause is identified. Hearing loss is thought to be secondary to injury to the developing auditory system in the intrapartum or perinatal period. This injury may result from infection, hypoxia, ischemia, metabolic disease, hyperbilirubinemia, or ototoxic medication. Preterm infants and infants who require newborn intensive care or a special care nursery are often exposed to these factors.

1. **Cytomegalovirus (CMV)** congenital infection is the most common cause of nonhereditary sensorineural hearing loss. Approximately 1% of all infants are born with CMV infection in this country. Of these (~40,000 infants per year), 10% have clinical signs of infection at birth (small for gestational age, hepatosplenomegaly, jaundice, thrombocytopenia, neutropenia, intracranial calcifications, or skin rash), and 50% to 60% of these infants develop hearing loss. Although most (90%) infants born with CMV infection have no clinical signs of infection, hearing loss still develops in 10% to 15% of these infants, and it is often progressive. Some promising new data indicate that treatment with the antiviral agent valganciclovir given orally for 6 months after birth is associated with improved long-term hearing function as well as improved neurodevelopmental outcomes at 2 years of life. Prompt diagnosis of congenital CMV is essential to determine if the infant is a possible candidate for treatment; ideally, treatment is initiated within 1 month after birth. Screening for CMV with urine or saliva in all babies who fail their newborn hearing screen has been implemented by some hospitals to facilitate making this diagnosis. Educating women on strategies to avoid CMV exposure during pregnancy is equally important.

C. Risk factors. The Joint Committee on Infant Hearing (JCIH) listed the following risk indicators associated with permanent congenital, progressive, or delayed-onset hearing loss in their 2007 Position Statement:

1. Caregiver concern* regarding hearing, speech, language, or developmental delay

2. Family history of permanent childhood hearing loss

3. Neonatal intensive care of >5 days or any of the following regardless of length of stay: extracorporeal membrane oxygenation (ECMO),* assisted ventilation, exposure to ototoxic medications (gentamicin, tobramycin) or loop diuretics (furosemide), and hyperbilirubinemia that requires exchange transfusion (some centers use a level of ≥20 mg/dL as a general guideline for risk)

4. *In utero* infections such as CMV,* herpes, rubella, syphilis, and toxoplasmosis

5. Craniofacial anomalies, including those that involve the pinna, ear canal, ear tags, ear pits, and temporal bone anomalies

6. Physical findings, such as a white forelock, that are associated with a syndrome known to include a sensorineural or permanent conductive hearing loss

7. Syndromes associated with progressive or late-onset hearing loss such as neurofibromatosis, osteopetrosis, and Usher syndrome. Other frequently identified syndromes include Waardenburg, Alport, Pendred, and Jervell and Lange-Neilsen.

8. Neurodegenerative disorders,* such as Hunter syndrome, or sensory motor neuropathies, such as Friedreich ataxia and Charcot-Marie-Tooth syndrome

9. Culture-positive postnatal infections associated with sensorineural hearing loss,* including bacterial and viral (especially herpes viruses and varicella) meningitis

10. Head trauma, especially basal skull/temporal bone fractures that require hospitalization

11. Chemotherapy*

12. Recurrent or persistent otitis media for at least 3 months

All infants with one or more risk factors should have ongoing developmentally appropriate hearing screening and at least one diagnostic audiology assessment by 24 to 30 months (the current recommendation of the JCIH). Risk factors that are highly associated with late-onset hearing loss or progressive hearing loss such as congenital CMV or treatment with ECMO warrant earlier and more frequent follow-up.

The JCIH risk factor recommendations are currently being updated. One additional high-risk group is those infants with hypoxic-ischemic encephalopathy meeting criteria for therapeutic hypothermia in whom the incidence of permanent hearing loss has been reported to be 6% to 10%.

---

*Greater concern for delayed hearing loss.

D. Detection. Universal newborn hearing screening is recommended to detect hearing loss as early as possible. The JCIH and the American Academy of Pediatrics (AAP) endorse a goal of testing 100% of infants during their hospital birth admission. The percentage of infants screened in this country prior to 1 month of age has increased from 46.5% in 1999 to 97.2% in 2013.

IV. SCREENING TESTS. The currently acceptable methods for physiologic hearing screening in newborns are auditory brainstem response (ABR) and evoked otoacoustic emissions (EOAEs). A threshold of ≥35 dB has been established as a cutoff for an abnormal screen, which prompts further testing.

A. ABRs measure the electroencephalographic waves generated by the auditory system in response to clicks through three electrodes placed on the infant's scalp. The characteristic waveform recorded from the electrodes becomes more well defined with increasing postnatal age. ABR is reliable after 34 weeks' postnatal age. The automated version of ABR allows this test to be performed quickly and easily by trained hospital staff. Although the otoacoustic emission (OAE) is acceptable for routine screening of low-risk infants, the AAP recommends the ABR over the OAE in high-risk infants including NICU patients and graduates. This is because the ABR tests the auditory pathway beyond the cochlea and picks up neural hearing loss including auditory dyssynchrony.

B. EOAEs. This records acoustic "feedback" from the cochlea through the ossicles to the tympanic membrane and ear canal following a click or tone burst stimulus. EOAE is even quicker to perform than ABR. However, EOAE is more likely to be affected by debris or fluid in the external and middle ear, resulting in higher referral rates. Furthermore, EOAE is unable to detect some forms of sensorineural hearing loss including auditory dyssynchrony. EOAE is often combined with automated ABR in a two-step screening system.

V. FOLLOW-UP TESTING. Follow-up testing of infants who fail their newborn screen is critical. Despite the high success in screening of newborns (97%), currently, 32% of infants who fail their initial screen are lost to follow-up. Family issues associated with poor follow-up include age of mother, insurance status, poverty level, and lack of family education regarding screening.[2] Loss to follow-up also varies geographically. Newborns born at home or in more remote areas are more likely to miss or forgo hearing screening and follow-up services.

Infants who fail the screen should have a diagnostic ABR performed by a pediatric audiology specialist within 3 weeks of their initial test. The diagnostic testing format should include measures to rule out or identify auditory dyssynchrony, sensorineural, or conductive hearing loss. Testing should include a full diagnostic frequency-specific ABR to measure hearing thresholds, EOAEs, and evaluation of middle ear function (tympanometry using a 1000-Hz probe tone). Observation of the infant's behavioral response to sound and parental report of emerging communication and auditory behaviors should also be included.

A. Definitions of the degree and severity of hearing loss are listed in Table 68.1.

B. Infants who have risk factors for progressive or delayed-onset sensorineural and/or conductive hearing loss require continued surveillance, even if the initial newborn screening results are normal.

Table 68.1. Degree and Severity of Hearing Loss	
Degree of Hearing Loss	**Hearing Loss Range (dB HL)**
Normal	−10 to 15
Slight	16 to 25
Mild	26 to 40
Moderate	41 to 55
Moderately severe	56 to 70
Severe	71 to 90
Profound	91+

Source: Clark JG. Uses and abuses of hearing loss classification. *ASHA* 1981;23:493–500.

C. Infants with **mild or unilateral hearing loss** should also be monitored closely with repeat audiology evaluations and provided with early intervention services because they are at increased risk for both progressive hearing loss and delayed and abnormal development of language and communication skills.

D. All infants should be monitored by their primary care providers for normal hearing and language development.

VI. MEDICAL EVALUATION. An infant diagnosed with true hearing loss should have the following additional evaluations:

A. Complete evaluation should be performed by an otolaryngologist or otologist who has experience with infants. Referral for radiologic imaging with computed tomography (CT) or magnetic resonance imaging (MRI) should occur when needed.

B. Genetic evaluation and counseling should be provided for all infants with true hearing loss.

C. Examination should be performed by a pediatric ophthalmologist to detect eye abnormalities that may be associated with hearing loss.

D. Developmental pediatrics, neurology, cardiology, and nephrology referral should be made as indicated.

VII. HABILITATION/TREATMENT. Infants with true hearing loss, regardless of degree of loss or laterality, should be referred for early intervention services to enhance the child's acquisition of developmentally appropriate language skills. This should include therapy from speech and language pathologists, audiologists, and special educators. For infants who are appropriate candidates for personal amplification systems (hearing aid, bone-anchored hearing aid—BAHA), if parents consent, the child should be fitted as soon as possible. Children with severe to profound bilateral hearing loss may be candidates for cochlear implants by the end of the first year of age. Another option currently in clinical trials for children with profound hearing loss who have exhausted all other alternatives is the auditory brainstem implant.

Families who do not choose personal amplification systems may use American Sign Language (ASL) or Signing Exact English (SEE) for their child's primary language. Because it may take up to 1 year for an infant to be eligible for implants, many families opt to incorporate both oral and manual languages into their child's repertoire. Auditory perception and speech production develop similarly in both children who learn oral and manual modes of communication together and those who focus only on oral.

There are also a number of assistive listening devices available to help in classrooms, homes, and public venues. Frequency modulation, infrared, and inductive loop systems allow for minimization of background noise and can help override poor acoustics.

Early intervention resources and information for parents to make decisions regarding communication choices should be provided as promptly as possible.

VIII. PROGNOSIS. The prognosis depends largely on the extent of hearing loss, the time of diagnosis and treatment, as well as the presence of syndromes or other congenital anomalies. For optimal auditory brain development, normal maturation of the central auditory pathways depends on the early maximizing of auditory input. The earlier habilitation starts, the better the child's chance of achieving age-appropriate language and communication skills. Fitting of hearing aids by the age of 6 months has been associated with improved speech outcomes. Language and communication outcomes for children receiving early cochlear implants and the accompanying intensive multidisciplinary team therapy are also very promising. Initiation of early intervention services before 3 months of age has been associated with improved cognitive developmental outcomes at 3 years. Family involvement is also critical to success. Early identification, together with early intervention and an actively involved family, result in higher level language outcomes at age 5 years.

References

1. Smith RJH, Shearer AE, Hildebrand MS, et al. Deafness and hereditary hearing loss overview. In: Pagon RA, Adam MP, Ardinger HH, et al, eds. *GeneReviews*. Seattle, WA: University of Washington; 1999.

2. American Speech-Language-Hearing Association. *Loss to Follow-Up in Early Hearing Detection and Intervention*. Rockville, MD: American Speech-Language-Hearing Association; 2008.

Suggested Readings

American Academy of Pediatrics, Joint Committee on Infant Hearing. Year 2007 Position Statement: principles and guidelines for early hearing detection and intervention programs. *Pediatrics* 2007;120:898–921.

Grosse S, Ross D, Dollard S. Congenital cytomegalovirus (CMV) infection as a cause of permanent bilateral hearing loss: a quantitative assessment. *J Clin Virol* 2008;41:57–62.

Harlor AD Jr, Bower C; and the Committee on Practice and Ambulatory Medicine, Section on Otolaryngology—Head and Neck Surgery. Clinical report—hearing assessment in infants and children: recommendations beyond neonatal screening. *Pediatrics* 2009;124:1252–1263.

Joint Committee on Infant Hearing. Supplement to the JCIH 2007 Position Statement: principles and guidelines for early intervention that a child is deaf or hard of hearing. *Pediatrics* 2013;131:e1324–e1349.

Kaye CI; and the American Academy of Pediatrics Committee on Genetics. Newborn screening fact sheets. *Pediatrics* 2006;118:e934–e963.

Kral A, O'Donoghue GM. Profound deafness in childhood. *N Engl J Med* 2010;363:1438–1450.

Morton CC, Nance WE. Newborn hearing screening—a silent revolution. *N Engl J Med* 2006;354:2151–2164.

Weichbold V, Nekahm-Heis D, Welzl-Mueller K. Universal newborn hearing screening and postnatal hearing loss. *Pediatrics* 2006;117(4):e631–e636.

Online Resources

American Academy of Audiology. **http://www.audiology.org**. Accessed July 5, 2016.

American Speech-Language-Hearing Association. **http://www.asha.org**. Accessed July 5, 2016.

Better Hearing Institute. **http://www.betterhearing.org/**. Accessed July 5, 2016.

Boystown National Research Center. **http://www.babyhearing.org**. Accessed July 5, 2016.

Center for Disease Control and Prevention. **http://www.cdc.gov/ncbddd/hearingloss/index.html**. Accessed July 5, 2016.

Hands & Voices. **http://www.handsandvoices.org/**. Accessed July 5, 2016.

Harvard Medical School Center for Hereditary Deafness. **http://hearing.harvard.edu**. Accessed July 5, 2016.

Laurent Clerc National Deaf Education Center, Gallaudet University. **http://www.gallaudet.edu/clerc-center.html**. Accessed July 5, 2016.

Marion Downs National Center for Infant Hearing. **http://www.mariondowns.com**. Accessed July 5, 2016.

National Association of the Deaf: **http://www.nad.org**. Accessed July 5, 2016.

National Center for Hearing Assessment and Management. **http://www.infanthearing.org/**. Accessed July 5, 2016.

Common Neonatal Procedures

Steven A. Ringer

KEY POINTS

- The benefit of a procedure must be balanced against the impact on patient stability and the risk of complications.
- Procedures are often painful or uncomfortable, and care should be taken to ensure adequate environmental and medical support to minimize these effects.
- All procedures, no matter how invasive, should be done with strict attention to safety, infection control, and clear and complete documentation.

Invasive procedures are a necessary but potentially risk-laden part of newborn intensive care. To provide maximum benefit, these techniques must be performed in a manner that both accomplishes the task at hand and maintains the patient's general well-being.

I. GENERAL PRINCIPLES

A. **Consideration of alternatives.** For each procedure, all alternatives should be considered and risk–benefit ratios evaluated. Many procedures involve the placement of indwelling devices made of plastic. Polyvinylchloride-based devices leach a plasticizer, Di(2-ethylhexyl)-phthalate (DEHP), which may be toxic over long-term exposure. Alternatives exist, and devices that are DEHP-free should be used for procedures on neonates whenever possible.

B. **Infection control.** For any procedure, care should be taken to ensure antisepsis. The optimal agent to use for an infant is not clear; chlorhexidine (for patients with mature skin) and alcohol are common choices. It is important to avoid chemical burns caused by iodine solution by carefully cleaning the skin with sterile water after the solution has dried. For extremely preterm infants (<28 weeks), alcohol can also cause a chemical burn and should be washed off with sterile water as mentioned earlier.

C. **Monitoring and homeostasis.** Ideally, the operator should delegate another care provider to be responsible for the ongoing monitoring and management of the patient during a procedure. This person's primary focus should be on the patient rather than the procedure being performed. They must assess cardiorespiratory and thermoregulatory stability throughout the procedure and apply interventions when needed. Continuous cardiorespiratory monitoring can be accomplished through a combination of invasive (e.g., arterial blood pressure monitoring) or noninvasive (e.g., oximeter) techniques. For sterile procedures, a particularly important function is ensuring the integrity of the sterile field.

This monitoring can most effectively be standardized through the use of a procedure checklist so that the monitoring caregiver can ensure that each step is appropriately completed and documented by signoff on the part of all providers at the conclusion of the procedure.

D. Pain control. Treatment of procedure-associated discomfort can be accomplished with pharmacologic or nonpharmacologic approaches (see Chapter 70). The potential negative impact of any medication on the patient's cardiorespiratory status should be considered. Oral sucrose (e.g., 24% solution, 0.2 to 0.4 mL/kg) is very effective in reducing pain of minor procedures including blood drawing. It can also be used as adjunctive therapy for more painful procedures when the patient can tolerate oral medication. Either morphine or fentanyl is commonly administered before beginning potentially painful procedures. The use of neonatal pain scales to assess the need for medication is recommended.

E. Informing the family. Other than during true emergencies, we notify parents of the need for invasive procedures in their child's care before we perform them. We discuss the indications for and possible complications of each procedure. In addition, alternative procedures, when available, are also discussed. Informed consent should be obtained for procedures with a significant degree of invasiveness or risk.

F. Precautions. The operator should use universal precautions, including wearing gloves, impermeable gowns, barriers, and eye protection, to prevent exposure to blood and bodily fluids that may be contaminated with infectious agents.

G. Time out and checklist. Before beginning any procedure, the entire team should take a "time out" or "safety pause" to ascertain that the correct procedure is to be performed on the correct patient and, if appropriate, on the correct side (e.g., thoracostomy tube). This pause should be incorporated into a complete checklist that includes all the steps of the procedure. Use of such a list helps ensure that a key step or assessment is not inadvertently omitted.

H. Education and supervision. Individuals should be trained in the conduct of procedures before performing the procedure on patients. This training should include a discussion of indications, possible complications and their treatment, alternatives, and the techniques to be used. For some procedures, there are mannequins or other options for simulation training, which also offer the opportunity to refine team skills. Experienced operators should be available at all times to provide further guidance and needed assistance.

I. Documentation. Careful documentation of procedures enhances patient care. For example, noting difficulties encountered at intubation or the size and insertion depth of an endotracheal tube (ETT) provides important information if the procedure must be repeated. We routinely write notes after all procedures, including unsuccessful attempts. We document the date and time, indications, performance of the time out, monitoring, premedication for pain control, the techniques used, difficulties encountered, complications (if any), and results of any laboratory tests performed.

II. BLOOD DRAWING. The preparations for withdrawing blood depend somewhat on the studies that are required.

A. Capillary blood is drawn when there is not a need for large volume of blood.

    1. Applicable blood studies include hematocrit, blood glucose (using glucometers or other point-of-care testing methods), bilirubin levels, electrolyte determinations, and occasionally blood gas studies.

    2. Techniques
      a. The extremity to be used should be warmed to increase peripheral blood flow.
      b. The skin should be cleaned carefully with an antiseptic such as alcohol or povidone-iodine before puncture to avoid infection of soft tissue or underlying bone.
      c. Capillary punctures of the foot should be performed on the lateral side of the sole of the heel, avoiding previous sites if possible.
      d. Spring-loaded lancets minimize pain while ensuring a puncture adequate for obtaining blood. The blood should flow freely, with minimal or no squeezing. This will ensure the most accurate determination of laboratory values.

B. Venous blood for blood chemistry studies, blood cultures, and other laboratory studies can be obtained from a peripheral vein of adequate caliber to enable access and withdrawal of blood. The **antecubital and saphenous veins are often promising sites**. For blood cultures, the area should be cleaned with an alcohol or iodine-containing solution; if the position of the needle is directed by using a sterile gloved finger, the finger should be cleaned in the same way. A new sterile needle should be used to insert the blood into the culture bottles.

C. Arterial blood may be needed for blood gases, some metabolic studies, and when the volume of blood needed would be difficult to obtain from a peripheral vein and no indwelling catheter is available. **Arterial punctures** usually involve the radial artery or posterior tibial artery. Rarely, the potential risk of brachial artery puncture may be justified when no other site is available. Radial artery punctures are most easily done using a 25G to 23G butterfly needle, and transillumination often aids in locating the vessel. Traditionally, an Allen test is performed to ensure collateral perfusion. (Recently, it has become controversial whether or not the Allen test should be considered standard of care, especially regarding the interpretation of an abnormal test.) The radial artery is identified and entered with the bevel of the needle facing up and at a 15-degree angle against the direction of flow. If blood is not obtained immediately during insertion, the needle may be advanced until the artery is transfixed and then slowly withdrawn until blood flow occurs.

D. Catheter blood samples

1. Umbilical artery or radial artery catheters are often used for repetitive blood samples, especially for blood gas studies.

2. Techniques

a. A needleless system for blood sampling from arterial catheters should be used. Specific techniques for use vary with the product, and the manufacturer's guidelines should be followed.

b. For blood gas studies, a 1-mL preheparinized syringe, or a standard 1-mL syringe rinsed with 0.5 mL of heparin, is used to withdraw the sample. The rate of sample withdrawal should be limited to 1.5 mL/minute to avoid altering downstream arterial perfusion.

c. The catheter must be adequately cleared of infusate before withdrawing samples to avoid false readings. After the sample is drawn, blood should be cleared from the catheter by infusing a small volume of heparinized saline-flushing solution.

III. INTRAVENOUS THERAPY.
The insertion and management of intravenous catheters require great care. As in older infants, hand veins are used most often, but veins in the foot, ankle, and scalp can be used. Transillumination of an extremity can help identify a vein, and newer devices that enhance the detection of veins may be even more useful.

IV. BLADDER CATHETERIZATION

A. A sterile technique is crucial. Careful cleaning with an antiseptic such as alcohol or an iodine solution over the prepubic region is essential.

B. Technique. The urethral meatus is identified, and a small gauge (3 French to 5 French) silicone catheter is gently advanced into the bladder, with care taken to keep the distal end of the catheter sterile until the urine sample is collected. Resistance to insertion should be minimal. If obstruction is sensed, it is usually best to abort the procedure and consult urology as indicated.

V. LUMBAR PUNCTURE

A. Technique

1. The infant should be placed in the lateral decubitus position or in the sitting position with legs straightened. The assistant should hold the infant firmly at the shoulders and buttocks so that the lower part of the spine is curved. Neck flexion should be avoided so as not to compromise the airway.

2. A sterile field is prepared and draped with towels, and the skin of the back cleansed with antiseptic solution. Chlorhexidine should not be used on the skin prior to a lumbar puncture (LP) as it is specifically not intended to be introduced into the central nervous system.

3. A 22G to 24G spinal needle with a stylet should be used. Avoid the use of a nonstylet needle, such as a 25G butterfly needle, as this may introduce skin tissue into the subarachnoid space.

4. The needle is inserted in the midline into the space between the fourth and fifth lumbar spinous processes and angled slightly superior to follow the intervertebral space. The needle is advanced gradually in the direction of the umbilicus, and the stylet is withdrawn frequently to detect the presence of spinal fluid. In infants, the insertion distance is only a few millimeters. Usually a slight "pop" is felt as the needle enters the subarachnoid space.

5. The cerebrospinal fluid (CSF) is collected into three or four tubes, each with a volume of 0.5 to 1.0 mL.

B. **Examination of the spinal fluid.** CSF should be inspected immediately for turbidity and color. In many newborns, normal CSF may be mildly xanthochromic, but it should always be clear.

1. **Tube 1.** Glucose and protein determinations should be obtained.

2. **Tube 2.** Cell count and differential should be determined from the unspun fluid.

3. **Tube 3.** Culture and sensitivity studies should be obtained.

4. **Tube 4.** The cells in this tube also should be counted if the fluid is bloody. The fluid can be sent for other tests (such as polymerase chain reaction amplification for herpes simplex virus [HSV], etc.).

C. **Information obtainable**

1. When the CSF is collected in three or four separate containers, a red blood cell (RBC) count can be measured on the second and last tubes to see if there is a decrease in the number of RBCs per cubic millimeter between the first and last specimens. In fluid obtained from a traumatic tap, the final tube may have fewer RBCs than the second; more equal numbers suggest the possibility of an intracranial hemorrhage, but the sensitivity and specificity of this finding are low. The presence of blood may be due to either the technical difficulty of obtaining a sample from a small patient or the small amount of partuitional bleeding that can normally result from birth.

2. **White blood cell (WBC) count.** The normal number of WBCs per cubic millimeter in newborns is a matter of some controversy, and different practitioners may accept different numbers of cells as normal, including the presence of some polymorphonuclear cells. Data obtained from infants in a neonatal intensive care unit (NICU) have shown that the upper limit (95th percentile) of CSF WBC count is 12 cells/μL in preterm infants and 14 cells/μL in term infants. If there is contamination of the CSF sample with RBCs, there is no reliable method to "correct" the WBC. In infants with proven meningitis, higher WBC counts are generally seen when the infection is caused by gram-negative organisms rather than in group B streptococcal disease; as many as 50% of the latter group will have 100 WBCs/mm^3 or less. Because of the overlap between normal infants and those with meningitis, the

Table 69.1. Cerebrospinal Fluid Examination in High-risk Neonates without Meningitis

Determination	Term	Preterm
White blood cell count (cells/mL)		
No. of infants	87	30
Mean	8.2	9.0
Median	5	6
Standard deviation	7.1	8.2
Range	0–32	0–29
±2 Standard deviations	0–22.4	0–25.4
Percentage of polymorphonuclear cells	61.3%	57.2%
Protein (mg/dL)		
No. of infants	35	17
Mean	90	115
Range	20–170	65–150
Glucose (mg/dL)		
No. of infants	51	23
Mean	52	50
Range	34–119	24–63
Glucose in cerebrospinal fluid divided by blood glucose (%)		
No. of infants	51	23
Mean	81	74
Range	44–248	55–105

Source: From Sarff LD, Platt LH, McCracken GH Jr. Cerebrospinal fluid evaluation in neonates: comparison of high-risk neonates with and without meningitis. *J Pediatr* 1976;88(3):473–477.

presence of polymorphonuclear leukocytes in CSF deserves careful attention. Ultimately, the diagnosis depends on culture results and clinical course.

3. Data on **glucose and protein levels** in CSF from high-risk newborns are shown in Table 69.1. Normally, the CSF glucose level is approximately

80% of the blood glucose level for term infants and 75% for preterm infants. If the blood glucose level is high or low, there is a 4- to 6-hour equilibration period with the CSF glucose.

The normal level of CSF protein in newborns may vary over a wide range. CSF protein levels are higher in preterm infants (upper limit 209 mg/dL) than in term infants (159 mg/dL), and this declines with increasing postnatal age. The level of CSF protein in the premature infant appears to be related to the degree of prematurity.

No single parameter can be used to rule out or rule in meningitis. Meningitis may occur in the absence of positive blood cultures (see Chapter 49).

VI. INTUBATION

A. **Endotracheal intubation.** In most cases, an infant can be adequately ventilated by bag and mask so that endotracheal intubation can be performed as a controlled procedure.

1. **Tube size and length.** The correct tube size (see Chapter 4) and insertion depth can be estimated from the infant's weight as well as by several other methods based on weight and gestational age. For insertion depth of oral ETTs, the most common rule is wt (kg) + 6 cm. A simple estimation for very premature infants is the naso-tragus distance + 1 cm. It is most important to remember that all of these methods are estimates, and insertion depth must be confirmed by physical examination and radiograph if the tube is to remain in place.

2. **Route.** Contradictory data exist over whether oral or nasal endotracheal intubation is preferred. Oral ETTs can cause a palatal groove, and nasal ETTs can cause asymmetry of the nares. In most circumstances, local practice should guide this selection with two exceptions. First, oral intubation should be performed in all emergent situations because it is generally easier and quicker than nasal intubation. Second, oral intubation is preferable when significant coagulopathy or thrombocytopenia exists. Generally, a functioning ETT should not be electively changed simply to provide an alternate route.

3. **Technique**

a. **The patient should be adequately ventilated using bag and mask** to ensure that the patient has normal oxygen saturations (appropriate for gestational age) before laryngoscopy. Laryngoscopy and intubation of an active, unmedicated patient is more uncomfortable for the patient and more difficult for the operator, and the risk of complications may be increased. Whenever possible, the patient should be premedicated either with a narcotic +/− a short-acting benzodiazepine or by using a modified rapid sequence with atropine and a muscle relaxant unless the patient's condition is a contraindication (see Chapter 70).

b. Throughout the intubation procedure, **observation of the patient and monitoring of the heart rate are mandatory**. Pulse oximetry should also be used when available. Electronic monitoring with an audible pulse rate enables the team to be aware of the heart rate throughout the procedure. If bradycardia is observed, especially if accompanied by hypoxia, the procedure should be stopped and the baby ventilated with bag and mask. An anesthesia bag attached to the tube adapter can deliver oxygen to the pharynx during the procedure. Alternatively, free-flow oxygen at 5 L/minute can be given from a tube placed 1/2 inch from the infant's mouth.

c. The baby's neck should be slightly extended (the "sniffing" position) with the baby's body aligned straight. The operator should stand looking down the midline of the body.

d. The **laryngoscope** is held between the thumb and first finger of the left hand, with the second and third fingers holding the baby's chin and stabilizing the head.

e. The **laryngoscope blade** is passed into the right side of the mouth and then to the midline, sweeping the tongue up and out of the way. The blade tip should be advanced into the vallecula and the handle of the laryngoscope raised to an angle of approximately 60 degrees relative to the bed. The blade should then be lifted while maintaining the same angle, with care being taken not to rock or lever the laryngoscope blade. Visualization of the vocal cords may be improved by providing cricoid pressure by pushing down slightly on the larynx with the fourth or fifth finger of the left hand (or having an assistant do it) to displace the trachea posteriorly.

f. The **ETT** is held with the right hand and inserted between the vocal cords to the appropriate estimated depth. During nasotracheal intubation, the tube can be guided by small Macgill-type forceps or by moving the baby's head slightly. If a finger of the operator or an assistant is used to gently press down over the trachea, the tube can be felt passing through.

g. The anatomic structures of the larynx and pharynx have different appearances. The esophagus is a horizontal posterior muscular slit. The glottis, in contrast, consists of an anterior triangular opening formed by the vocal cords meeting anteriorly at the apex. This orifice lies directly beneath the epiglottis, which is lifted away by gentle upward traction with the laryngoscope.

h. The **tube position** is checked by auscultation of the chest to ensure equal aeration of both lungs and observation of chest movement with positive-pressure inflation. The tube will usually "steam up" if it is correctly placed in the trachea, and the baby should show improved oxygenation, but an end-tidal CO_2 monitor is recommended to confirm the intratracheal position of the tube. If air entry is poor over the left side of the chest, the tube should be pulled back until it becomes equal to the right side.

4. Once correct position is ascertained, the tube should be held against lips/nose or the palate with one finger, until it can be taped securely in place; the position of the tube should be confirmed by radiograph when possible.

5. Increasingly, video laryngoscopes are being used for intubation of neonates. These devices offer the possibility of concurrent observation of tube placement by another observer and easier or more reliable tube insertion. Among the available devices, each has its particular limitations in terms of size or design.

6. **Commonly observed errors during intubation**

a. Focus is placed on the procedure and not the patient.

b. The baby's neck is hyperextended. This displaces the cords anteriorly and obscures visualization or makes the passing of the ETT difficult.

c. Excessive pressure is placed on the infant's upper gum by the laryngoscope blade. This occurs when the tip of the laryngoscope blade is tilted or rocked upward instead of traction being exerted parallel to the baby.

d. The tube is inserted too far and the position not assessed, resulting in intubation of the right main stem bronchus.

7. **Laryngeal mask airway.** Occasionally, it is not possible for a team to successfully insert an ETT despite multiple attempts, or the length of ventilatory support is anticipated to be very short. In the former case, a laryngeal mask airway can be a life-saving alternative to provide rescue ventilation until a more stable airway can be established. The size 1 laryngeal mask is appropriate and recommended for infants weighing 1.5 to 5 kg, although there are reports of its successful use in preterm babies as small as 0.8 kg.

The laryngeal mask may be especially useful during the initial resuscitation after birth especially when a person skilled in intubation is not readily available. Current versions are not however designed to be used for tracheal suctioning or instillation of surfactant.

VII. THORACENTESIS AND CHEST TUBE PLACEMENT (see Chapter 38)

VIII. VASCULAR CATHETERIZATION (see Figs. 69.1 and 69.2 for diagrams of the newborn venous and arterial systems)

A. **Types of catheters**

1. **Umbilical artery catheters (UACs)** are used (i) for frequent monitoring of arterial blood gases, (ii) as a stable route for infusion of some parenteral fluids, and (iii) for continuous monitoring of arterial blood pressure.

2. **Peripheral artery catheters** are used when frequent blood gas monitoring is still required and a UAC is contraindicated, cannot be placed, or is removed because of complications. Peripheral artery catheters must not be used to infuse alimentation solution or medications. They require that motion of the infant's arm be kept restricted.

3. **Umbilical vein catheters (UVCs)** (when passed through the ductus venous and near the right atrium) are used for monitoring of central venous pressure and infusion of fluids. Low UVCs can be used for exchange transfusion and as emergency vascular access for infusion of fluid, blood, or medications until alternate access can be obtained.

4. **Central venous catheters**, used largely for prolonged parenteral nutrition or antibiotics, or for pressor administration and occasionally to monitor central venous pressure, can be placed percutaneously through the saphenous, subclavian, basilic, or external jugular vein.

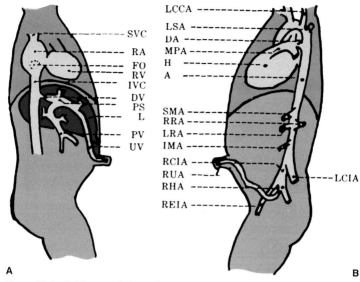

Figure 69.1. A: Diagram of the newborn umbilical venous system. SVC, superior vena cava; RA, right atrium; FO, foramen ovale; RV, right ventricle; IVC, inferior vena cava; DV, ductus venosus; PS, portal sinus; L, liver; PV, portal vein; UV, umbilical vein. **B:** Diagram of the newborn arterial system, including the umbilical artery. LCCA, left common carotid artery; LSA, left subclavian artery; DA, ductus arteriosus; MPA, main pulmonary artery; H, heart; A, aorta; SMA, superior mesenteric artery; RRA, right renal artery; LRA, left renal artery; IMA, inferior mesenteric artery; LCIA, left common iliac artery; RCIA, right common iliac artery; RUA, right umbilical artery; RHA, right hypogastric artery; REIA, right external iliac artery. (From Kitterman JA, Phibbs RH, Tooley WH. Catheterization of umbilical vessels in newborn infants. *Pediatr Clin North Am* 1970;17:898.)

B. Umbilical artery catheterization

1. **Guidelines.** In general, only seriously ill infants should have a UAC placed. If only a few blood gas measurements are anticipated, peripheral arterial punctures should be performed together with noninvasive oxygen monitoring, and a peripheral intravenous route should be used for fluids and medications.

2. **Technique**

   a. Sterile technique is used. Before preparing cord and skin, make external measurements to determine how far the catheter will be inserted (see Figs. 69.2 to 69.4). For a "high" UAC, the distance is usually (umbilicus-to-shoulder) +2 cm plus the length of the stump. In a high setting, the catheter tip is placed between the 8th and 10th thoracic vertebrae; in a low setting, the tip is between the third and fourth lumbar vertebrae.

   b. The cord stump is suspended with forceps. It and the surrounding area are washed carefully with an antiseptic solution as discussed

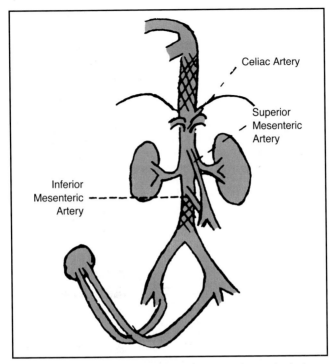

Figure 69.2. Localization of umbilical artery catheters. The cross-hatched areas represent sites in which complications are least likely. Either site may be used for placement of the catheter tip.

in section I.B earlier, with care taken to avoid potential burns from these solutions by cleaning the skin with sterile water (including the back and trunk). Following this, the abdomen is draped with sterile towels.

c. Umbilical (twill) tape should be placed as a simple tie around the base of the cord itself. In unusual circumstances, it is necessary to place the tape on the umbilical skin itself. If this is done, care must be taken to loosen the tie after the procedure. The tape is used to gently constrict the cord to prevent bleeding. The cord stump is then cut cleanly with a scalpel to a length of 1.0 to 1.5 cm.

d. The cord is stabilized with a forceps or hemostat, and the two arteries are identified.

e. The open tip of an iris forceps is inserted into an arterial lumen and gently used to **dilate the vessel**, and then the closed tip is inserted into the lumen of an artery to a depth of 0.5 cm. Tension on the forceps tip is released, and the forceps is left in place to dilate the vessel for approximately 1 minute. This pause may be the most critical step for ensuring successful insertion of the catheter.

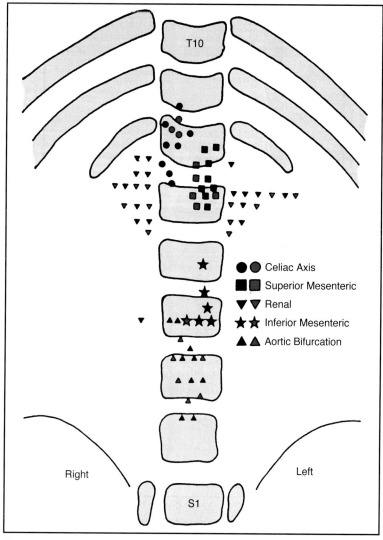

Figure 69.3. Distribution of the major aortic branches found in 15 infants by aortography as correlated with the vertebral bodies. Filled symbols represent infants with cardiac or renal anomalies (or both); open symbols represent those without either disorder. Major landmarks appear at the following vertebral levels: diaphragm, T12 interspace; celiac artery, T12; superior mesenteric artery, L1 interspace; renal artery, L1; inferior mesenteric artery, L3; aortic bifurcation, L4. (From Phelps DL, Lachman RS, Leake RD, et al. The radiologic localization of the major aortic tributaries in the newborn infant. *J Pediatr* 1972;81:336–339.)

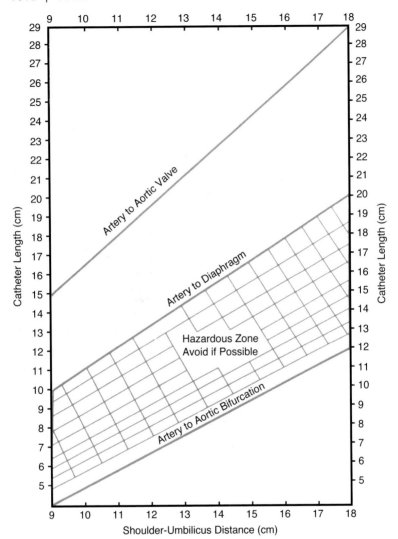

Figure 69.4. Distance from shoulder to umbilicus measured from above the lateral end of the clavicle to the umbilicus, as compared with the length of umbilical artery catheter needed to reach the designated level. (From Dunn PM. Localization of the umbilical catheter by postmortem measurement. *Arch Dis Child* 1969;41:69.)

 f. The forceps is withdrawn, and a sterile saline–filled 3.5F or 5F single-lumen umbilical vessel catheter with an end hole is threaded into the artery. The smaller catheter is generally used for infants weighing <1,500 g. A slightly increased resistance will be felt as the catheter passes through the base of the cord (near the cord tie) and as it navigates the umbilical artery–femoral artery junction. The following problems with umbilical artery catheterization may occur.

    i. The catheter will not pass into the abdominal aorta. Sometimes, a double-catheter technique will allow successful cannulation in this situation, especially if the first catheter has made a false track and is no longer in the lumen of the umbilical artery. Leave the original catheter in place and gently pass a second catheter alongside it.

    ii. The catheter may pass into the lower aorta but then loop caudad into the contralateral iliac artery or out one of the arteries to the buttocks. There may be difficulty advancing the catheter, and cyanosis or blanching of the leg or buttocks may occur. This happens more frequently when a small catheter (3.5 French) is placed in a large baby. Sometimes, using a larger, stiffer catheter (5 French) will allow the catheter to advance up the aorta. Alternatively, retracting the catheter into the umbilical artery, rotating it, and readvancing it into the aorta may result in aortic placement. If this fails, the catheter should be removed, and placement attempted through the other umbilical artery. Sometimes, the catheter goes up the aorta and then loops back on itself. This also happens more frequently when a small catheter is used in a large baby. The catheter may also enter any of the vessels coming off the aorta. If the catheter cannot be advanced to the desired position, the tip should be pulled to a low position or the catheter removed.

    iii. There is persistent cyanosis, blanching, or poor distal extremity perfusion. This may be improved by warming the contralateral leg, but if there is no improvement, the catheter should be removed. **Hematuria** is also an indication for catheter removal.

  g. When the catheter is advanced, the appropriate distance and placement should be confirmed by radiographic examination.

  h. The catheter should be fixed in place with a purse-string suture using silk thread and a tape bridge added for further stability (see Chapter 65).

3. Catheter removal

  a. The UAC should be removed when any one of the following criteria is met:

    i. The infant improves such that continuous monitoring and frequent blood drawings are no longer necessary.

    ii. A maximum dwell time of 7 days is recommended by the Centers for Disease Control and Prevention (CDC) to reduce infectious and thrombotic complications.

    iii. Complications are noted.

  b. Method of catheter removal. The catheter is removed slowly over a period of 30 to 60 seconds, allowing the umbilical artery to constrict at its proximal end while the catheter is still occluding the distal end. This usually prevents profuse bleeding. Old sutures should be removed. If bleeding should occur despite this method, pressure should be held at the stump of the umbilical artery until the bleeding ceases. This may take several minutes.

4. Complications associated with umbilical artery catheterization. Significant morbidity can be associated with complications of umbilical artery catheterization. These complications are mainly due to vascular accidents, including thromboembolic phenomena to the kidney, bowel, legs, or rarely, the spinal cord. These may manifest as hematuria; hypertension; signs of necrotizing enterocolitis or bowel infarction; and cyanosis or blanching of the skin of the back, buttocks, or legs. Other potential complications include infection, disseminated intravascular coagulation, and vessel perforation. All these complications are indications for catheter removal. Close observation of the skin, monitoring of the urine for hematuria, measuring blood pressure, and following the platelet count may give clues to complications.

a. Blanching of a leg following catheter placement is the most common complication noted clinically. Although this often occurs transiently, it deserves careful attention. One technique that may reverse this finding is to warm the opposite leg. If the vasospasm resolves, the catheter may be left in place. If there is no improvement, the catheter should be removed.

b. Thrombi. We perform Doppler ultrasonographic examination of the aorta and renal vessels in infants in whom we are concerned about vascular complications. If thrombi are observed, the catheter is removed.

If there are small thrombi without symptoms or with increased blood pressure alone, after catheter removal, we follow resolution of the thrombi by ultrasonographic examination and treat hypertension if necessary (see Chapter 28). If there are signs of emboli or loss of pulses, or coagulopathy, and no intracranial hemorrhage is present, we consider heparinization, maintaining the partial thromboplastin time (PTT) at double the control value. Published data to guide practice are limited. If there is a large clot with impairment of perfusion, we consider the use of fibrinolytic agents (see Chapter 44). Surgical treatment of thrombosis is not generally effective.

5. **Other considerations**

   a. Use of heparin for anticoagulation to prevent clotting. Whether the use of heparin in the infusate decreases the incidence of thrombotic complications is not known. We use dilute heparin 0.5 unit/mL of infusate.

   b. Positioning of the catheter tip. Little helpful information convincingly supports the choice between high and low placement of UACs. Renal complications and emboli to the bowel may be more common with catheter tips placed high (T8–T10), whereas catheters placed low (L3–L4) are associated with complications such as cyanosis and blanching of the leg, which are easier to observe. No difference between the high- and low-position groups was seen in the rate of complications requiring catheter removal.

   c. Indwelling time. The incidence of complications associated with umbilical artery catheterization appears to be directly related to the length of time the catheter is left in place. The need for the catheter should be reassessed daily, and the catheter should be removed as soon as possible.

6. **Infection and use of antibiotics.** We do not use prophylactic antibiotics for placement of UACs. In infants with indwelling UACs, after appropriate cultures have been obtained, we treat with antibiotics that include coverage of coagulase-negative *Staphylococcus* whenever infection is suspected.

C. **Umbilical vein catheterization** (see Figs. 69.1 and 69.5)

1. **Indications.** In critically ill and extremely premature infants, we use high-lying UVC to infuse vasopressors and as the primary route of venous access in the first several days after birth.

We use low-lying umbilical vein catheterization for exchange transfusions and emergency vascular access; in the latter case, the venous

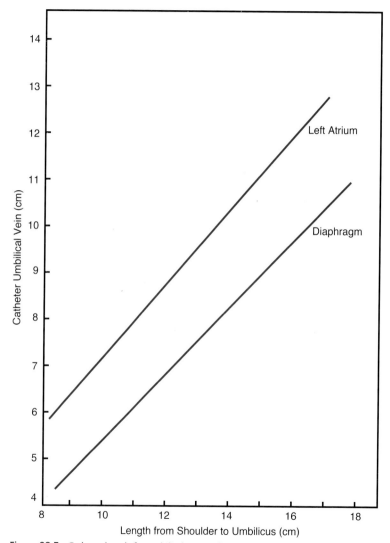

Figure 69.5. Catheter length for umbilical vein catheterization. The catheter tip should be placed between the diaphragm and the left atrium. (From Dunn PM. Localization of the umbilical catheter by post-mortem measurements. *Arch Dis Child* 1966;41:69.)

catheter may be used as a peripheral intravenous catheter until peripheral or central venous access can be obtained.

2. Technique

a. The site is prepared as for umbilical artery catheterization after determining the appropriate length of catheter to be inserted (see Fig. 69.5).

b. Any clots seen are removed with a forceps, and the umbilical vein is gently dilated as with the umbilical artery in section VIII.C.

c. The catheter (3.5 French or 5 French) is prepared by filling the lumen with heparinized saline solution, 1 unit/mL of saline solution through an attached syringe. The catheter should never be left open to the atmosphere because negative intrathoracic pressure could cause an air embolism.

d. The catheter is inserted while gentle traction is exerted on the cord. Once the catheter is in the vein, one should try to slide the catheter cephalad just under the skin, where the vein runs very superficially. If the catheter is being placed for emergency vascular access or for an exchange transfusion, it should be advanced only as far as is necessary to establish good blood flow (usually 2 to 5 cm). If the catheter is being used for continuous infusion or to monitor central venous pressure, it should be advanced through the ductus venosus into the inferior vena cava and its position verified by x-ray.

e. Only isotonic solutions should be infused until the position of the catheter is verified by x-ray studies. If the catheter tip is in the inferior vena cava, hypertonic solutions may be infused.

f. If no other access is available, catheters may be left in place for up to 10 days, after which the increased risk of infectious or other complications is excessive. In very low birth weight infants, our practice is to change access to a peripherally placed central venous catheter by 10 days whenever possible.

D. Multiple-lumen catheters for umbilical venous catheterization

1. Indications. Placement of a double- or triple-lumen catheter into the umbilical vein provides additional venous access for administration of incompatible solutions (e.g., those containing vasopressor agents, sodium bicarbonate, or calcium). The use of a multiple-lumen catheter significantly reduces the need for multiple peripheral intravenous catheters and skin punctures and is often preferred in very low birth weight infants. The disadvantage is that infusions must be maintained through lumens that are no longer needed, which can alter the ability to provide full nutritional support or appropriately adjust fluid therapy.

2. Technique

a. Direct placement. Multiple-lumen catheters are inserted according to the same procedure as single-lumen catheters described earlier. The increased pliability of many of the multiple-lumen catheters makes inadvertent passage into the hepatic veins more likely.

b. Modified Seldinger technique. In patients with an indwelling single-lumen catheter, a wire exchange technique may be used to change to a multiple-lumen catheter. Although this method decreases the probability of catheter loss during exchange, it entails the risks of wire passage including cardiac dysrhythmias and perforation and should be attempted only by those familiar with the Seldinger technique.

   3. Usage. Where possible, infusions that should not be interrupted (e.g., vasopressors) are placed in the proximal lumen to allow measurement of central venous pressure from the distal port.

E. Percutaneous radial artery catheterization. Placement of an indwelling radial artery catheter is a useful alternative to umbilical artery catheterization to monitor blood gas levels and blood pressure.

   1. Advantages
   a. If umbilical artery cannot be cannulated or arterial access needed after UAC must be removed
   b. Reflection of preductal flow (if the right radial artery is used)
   c. Avoidance of thrombosis of major vessels, which is sometimes associated with umbilical vessel catheterization

   2. Risks are usually small if the procedure is performed carefully but include arterial occlusion and subsequent impaired tissue perfusion, inadvertent injection of a solution that is potentially injurious to the artery, infection, or air embolus.

   3. Equipment required includes a 22G or 24G intravenous cannula with stylet, a T-connector, heparinized saline flushing solution (0.5 to 1.0 unit of heparin per milliliter of solution), and an infusion pump.

   4. Method of catheterization
   a. As noted, it is controversial whether or not the Allen test should be considered standard of care, especially regarding the interpretation of an abnormal test. We continue to recommend that the adequacy of the ulnar collateral flow to the hand must be assessed before catheterizing the radial artery. The radial and ulnar arteries should be simultaneously compressed, and the ulnar artery should then be released. The degree of flushing of the blanched hand should be noted. If the entire hand becomes flushed while the radial artery is occluded, the ulnar circulation is adequate.
   b. The hand may be secured on an arm board with the wrist extended, leaving all fingertips exposed, to observe color changes.
   c. The wrist is prepared with an antiseptic such as alcohol, chlorhexidine, or an iodine-containing solution. The site of maximum arterial pulsation is palpated.
   d. The intravenous cannula is inserted through the skin at an angle <30 degrees to horizontal and is slowly advanced into the artery. Transillumination may help delineate the vessel and its course. If the artery is entered as the catheter is advanced, the stylet is removed and the catheter is advanced in the artery. If there is no blood return, the artery may be transfixed. The stylet is then removed, and the catheter is slowly withdrawn until blood flow occurs, and then it is advanced into the vessel.

   5. Caution. Only heparinized saline solution (0.45% to 0.9%) is infused into the catheter. The minimum infusion rate is 0.8 mL/hour; the maximum is 2 mL/hour.

F. **Percutaneous central venous catheterization** is useful for long-term venous access for intravenous fluids, particularly parenteral nutrition.

1. The central venous catheter is inserted into a **peripheral vein and advanced into the central circulation**. This is the primary method of central venous access. We recommend establishing a specialized team of nurses and/or physicians who are responsible for placing these lines.

a. **The equipment** required includes sterile towels, a 1.1 French or 1.9 French silicone or double-lumen polyurethane catheter cut to the appropriate length, a splittable introducer needle, and iris forceps.

b. **Technique.** Careful attention to sterile technique is required. The operator should be assisted by another caregiver who can obtain additional equipment as needed, ensure integrity of the sterile field, and monitor the progress of the procedure using a specific step-by-step checklist for the procedure. The infant is sedated and placed supine. An appropriate vein of entry is selected. This may be a basilic, greater saphenous, or external jugular vein. The cephalic vein should be avoided because central placement is more difficult. The site is prepared with an antiseptic solution such as chlorhexidine (for infants with mature skin) or alcohol, and the introducer needle is inserted into the vein until blood flows freely. The silicone catheter is inserted through the needle with forceps and is slowly advanced the predetermined distance for central venous positioning. The introducer needle is removed, the extra catheter length is coiled on the skin near the insertion site, and the site is covered with transparent surgical covering. The catheter tip is positioned at the junction of the vena cava and right atrium, as confirmed by radiography. Especially with the smaller gauge catheters, visualization is best accomplished by an oblique radiograph, to separate the catheter position from that of the cardiothymic silhouette. It is important to position the infant with their arms oriented as during usual care so that tip position is not altered (raising the arm can cause the tip to shift). Some physicians inject a small amount of isotonic contrast material to make visualization easier.

c. **Complications** include hemorrhage during insertion, infection, and thrombosis of the catheter, but these are unusual. Some babies will develop a thrombophlebitis, usually within 24 hours of catheter placement. If the tip of the catheter is in the right atrium, a rare but potentially lethal complication is pericardial tamponade. Early diagnosis and treatment by pericardiocentesis is critical. Care must be taken when flushing or infusing to minimize the pressure on the catheter, which could cause catheter rupture. By using a larger syringe (10 mL), infusion pressure is reduced over that obtained with a smaller (3 mL) syringe.

2. **Subclavian vein catheterization** may occasionally be useful in infants weighing >1,200 g, although in general, a surgically placed central venous catheter is preferred when other access cannot be established. Operators should receive specific training in this procedure before performing it.

IX. ABDOMINAL PARACENTESIS FOR REMOVAL OF ASCITIC FLUID

A. **Indications**

1. Therapeutic indications include respiratory distress resulting from abdominal distension (e.g., hydropic infants, infants with urinary ascites)

for which removal of ascitic fluid will ameliorate respiratory symptoms. In addition, interference with urine production or lower extremity perfusion resulting from increased intra-abdominal pressure may be improved by paracentesis.

    2. Diagnostic indications include the evaluation of suspected peritonitis.

B. Technique

    1. The equipment needed includes an 18G to 22G intravenous catheter, three-way stopcock, and a 10- to 50-mL syringe.

    2. The lower abdomen is prepared with antiseptic such as alcohol or povidone-iodine solution, and the area is draped. If the bladder is distended, it is drained with manual pressure or a urinary catheter. A local anesthetic such as 1% lidocaine (Xylocaine) is infiltrated into the subcutaneous tissues when possible. A syringe is attached to the catheter, and then it is inserted just lateral to the rectus sheath (about 1.5 cm lateral to the midline) about one-third of the distance between the umbilicus and the symphysis pubis: A midline entry is also acceptable. As the catheter is inserted through the abdominal wall, the syringe is aspirated. The catheter is advanced approximately 1 cm until the resistance of passing through the abdominal wall diminishes or fluid is obtained. Five to 10 mL of fluid is removed for diagnostic paracentesis, whereas 10 to 20 mL/kg should be removed for therapeutic effects. The catheter is removed and the site bandaged. Ultrasound guidance can be useful, especially in situations when the volume of intraperitoneal fluid is minimal enough that there is concern that the fluid may be difficult to locate or that an abdominal viscus could accidentally be punctured during the procedure.

C. Potential complications

    1. Cardiovascular effects, including tachycardia, hypotension, and decreased cardiac output, may result from rapid redistribution of intravascular fluid to the peritoneal space following removal of large amounts of ascites.

    2. Bladder or intestinal aspiration occurs more frequently in the presence of a dilated bladder or bowel. These puncture sites usually heal spontaneously and without significant clinical findings.

X. PERICARDIOCENTESIS

A. Indications

    1. If a pericardial effusion is suspected based on physical examination (muffled heart sounds, sinus tachycardia, narrow pulse pressure, and signs of diminished cardiac output), chest radiograph (cardiomegaly [not always present], evidence of cardiac failure), or in situations of pulseless electrical activity with no other explanation, emergency drainage may be necessary. Sudden cardiorespiratory decompensation when a central line is in place, especially if the tip is in or near the right atrium, should prompt serious consideration of pericardial effusion with tamponade physiology.

2. In most cases, even significant effusions produce little or no symptoms or signs. Diagnosis may be suspected based on physical exam, vital sign, and radiographic findings and should be confirmed by ultrasonographic examination before drainage is attempted if time permits.

B. Technique

1. The patient should be prepared and the area cleaned with antiseptic solution according to standard sterile technique. This should include the subxiphoid area extending up over the left anterior chest.

2. If time permits, the procedure should be performed with ultrasonographic guidance; however, this potentially life-saving intervention often cannot be delayed.

3. Drainage is typically done using a 22G or 24G intravenous catheter. The catheter is inserted, just below the xiphoid process and just to the left of midline (to avoid puncturing the right atrium), and angled toward the left shoulder. The catheter is advanced forward until the pericardial sac is entered, while monitoring for arrhythmias that can signal needle advancement into the myocardium. The introducer trochar can then be removed, and a syringe and connecting tube is attached, and the fluid is aspirated as the catheter is advanced. Once no further fluid can be aspirated, the catheter is removed and the entry site covered with occlusive gauge and transparent dressing.

C. Potential complications

Cardiac puncture, pneumopericardium, pneumothorax, or transient dysrhythmias may occur. Ultrasonographic guidance may lower the risk of these complications.

Suggested Readings

Barone JE, Madlinger RV. Should an Allen test be performed before radial artery cannulation? *J Trauma* 2006;61(2):468–470.

Fletcher MA, McDonald MG, Avery GB, eds. *Atlas of Procedures in Neonatology.* Philadelphia, PA: Lippincott Williams & Wilkins; 1994.

Garges HP, Moody MA, Cotten CM, et al. Neonatal meningitis: what is the correlation among cerebrospinal fluid cultures, blood cultures, and cerebrospinal fluid parameters? *Pediatrics* 2006;117:1094–1100.

Garland JS, Henrickson K, Maki DG. The 2002 Hospital Infection Control Practices Advisory Committee Centers for Disease Control and Prevention guideline for prevention of intravascular device-related infection. *Pediatrics* 2002;110:1009–1013.

Green R, Hauser R, Calafat AM, et al. Use of di(2-ethylhexyl) phthalate–containing medical products and urinary levels of mono(2-ethylhexyl) phthalate in neonatal intensive care unit infants. *Environ Health Perspect* 2005;113(9): 1222–1225.

Latini G. Potential hazards of exposure to di-(2-ethylhexyl)-phthalate in babies. A review. *Biol Neonate* 2000;78:269–276.

Martín-Ancel A, García-Alix A, Salas S, et al. Cerebrospinal fluid leucocyte counts in healthy neonates. *Arch Dis Child Fetal Neonatal Ed* 2006;91(5):F357–F358.

Pronovost P, Needham D, Berenholtz S, et al. An intervention to decrease catheter-related bloodstream infections in the ICU. *N Engl J Med* 2006;355: 2725–2732.

Srinivasan L, Shah SS, Padula MA, et al. Cerebrospinal fluid reference ranges in term and preterm infants in the neonatal intensive care unit. *J Pediatr* 2012;161:729–734.

Wang TC, Kuo LL, Lee CY. Utilizing nasal-tragus length to estimate optimal endotracheal tube depth for neonates in Taiwan. *Indian J Pediatr* 2011; 78(3):296–300.

70 Preventing and Treating Pain and Stress Among Infants in the Newborn Intensive Care Unit

Carol Turnage Spruill and Michelle A. LaBrecque

KEY POINTS

- Pain and the effects of analgesia can be assessed using validated instruments.
- Lack of physical and behavioral responses to a painful condition or stimulus does not indicate an absence of pain.
- Pain treatment is selected based on the type, location, intensity, and duration of the pain stimulus.
- Nonpharmacologic interventions are used alone or as an adjunct to pharmacologic therapy.
- Monitoring for adverse effects of opioids and benzodiazepines such as respiratory depression and hypotension are an essential part of safe pain control.

I. BACKGROUND. Recognition that both premature and full-term infants experience pain has led to increasing appreciation of the prevalent problem of undertreatment of stress and pain of hospitalized infants. Both humanitarian considerations and scientific principles favor improved management strategies to prevent pain and stress whenever possible and, when discomfort is unavoidable, to provide prompt and appropriate treatment. Optimal pain management should be individualized and requires an understanding of developmental analgesic pharmacology, neonatal physiology, pain assessment, and techniques for providing pain relief.

  A. **Fetal and neonatal physiologic responses to pain.** There is considerable maturation of peripheral, spinal, and supraspinal neurologic pathways necessary for nociception by late in the second trimester. By 20 weeks' gestation, cutaneous sensory nerve terminals are present in all body areas and a full complement of cortical neurons is present within the central nervous system. Research using near-infrared spectroscopy (NIRS) shows a specific pattern of activation of the somatosensory cortex in preterm infants after noxious stimulation suggesting that painful stimuli reach the cerebral cortex.

Peripheral sensory fibers have larger, more overlapping receptive fields and inhibitory cortical descending pathways such as the dorsolateral funiculus that modulate pain postnatally, suggesting that neonates and young infants have hyperresponsiveness to pain.

Infants exhibit predictable pain response patterns with respect to stress hormone levels, changes in heart rate, blood pressure, and oxygen saturation. Although the fetus is capable of mounting a stress response beginning at approximately 23 weeks' gestation, physiologic parameters are nonspecific and are not necessarily reliable indicators of pain, particularly among critically ill neonates who may be hemodynamically unstable, septic, or mechanically ventilated. As a result, pain assessment tools in infants are composite scales that typically combine physiologic parameters with observed distress behaviors. Behavioral and physiologic responses are less reliable among infants exposed to chronic or persistent noxious stimuli.

B. **Medical and developmental outcomes**

1. **Neonatal medical and surgical outcomes.** Neonatal responses to pain may worsen compromised physiologic states such as hypoxia, hypercarbia, acidosis, hyperglycemia, respiratory dyssynchrony, and pneumothorax. Changes in intrathoracic pressure due to diaphragmatic splinting and vagal responses produced in response to pain following invasive procedures precipitate hypoxemic events and alterations in oxygen delivery and cerebral blood flow. Early studies of surgical responses showed a more stable intraoperative course and improved postoperative recovery among infants who received perioperative analgesia and anesthesia.

2. **Neurodevelopmental outcomes.** There is evidence that infants have the ability to form implicit memory of pain and that there are negative behavioral consequences of untreated pain. Behavioral and neurologic studies suggest that preterm infants who experience numerous painful procedures and noxious stimuli are less responsive to painful stimuli at 18 months corrected age. Neonatal males who were circumcised with little or no analgesia showed significantly increased pain responses when immunized at 2, 4, and 6 months of age compared to infant males who were not circumcised or who received adequate analgesia. Evidence suggests that neonatal pain and stress influence neurodevelopment and affect later perceptions of painful stimuli and behavioral responses and that prevention and control of pain are likely to benefit infants. Newborns undergoing cardiac surgery for patent ductus arteriosus (PDA) ligation who receive less opioid analgesia experienced a significantly greater stress response and more postoperative morbidities compared to infants receiving adequate opioid analgesia.

   There are few large randomized clinical trials of pain management in neonates. One such trial (NEOPAIN trial) evaluated preemptive analgesia with morphine infusion up to 14 days among ventilated preterm infants and showed no difference overall in the primary composite outcome (i.e., neonatal death, severe intraventricular hemorrhage [IVH], or periventricular leukomalacia) between placebo and preemptive morphine-treated groups. Concerns were raised, however, when post hoc analyses revealed an increased risk of severe IVH among morphine infusion–treated infants in the subgroup born at 27 to 29 weeks of gestation.

Subsequent analyses suggested the adverse outcomes were limited to infants who were hypotensive before morphine therapy was initiated. These data indicate that treatment with prophylactic morphine infusion should be limited to infants who are normotensive. There is limited data on the long-term consequences of opioid analgesia in infants, and preliminary studies show mixed results. The potential risk associated with morphine use as indicated in the NEOPAIN trial must be weighed against the known risk of untreated pain in the neonatal population, including increased sensitivity to subsequent painful stimuli and potential negative effects in neurodevelopment. Animal research suggests morphine may be either neuroprotective or neurotoxic depending on the presence or absence of pain, but how that translates to newborns is unknown. Further research is needed to identify safe and effective options for pain management in term and preterm infants.

II. COMMITTEE ON THE FETUS AND NEWBORN OF THE AMERICAN ACADEMY OF PEDIATRICS PRINCIPLES OF PREVENTION AND MANAGEMENT OF NEONATAL PAIN AND STRESS

A. Neuroanatomic components and neuroendocrine systems of the neonate are sufficiently developed to allow transmission of painful stimuli.

B. Exposure to prolonged or severe pain may increase neonatal morbidity.

C. Infants who have experienced pain during the neonatal period may respond differently to subsequent painful events.

D. Severity of pain and effects of analgesia can be assessed in the neonate using validated instruments.

E. Newborn infants usually are not easily comforted when analgesia is needed.

F. A lack of behavioral responses (including crying and movement) does not necessarily indicate the absence of pain.

G. The pain intensity of the anticipated painful procedure from venipuncture to abdominal surgery differs dramatically. Careful thought and planning help the health care team develop an appropriate pain management plan before a painful event.

III. EVALUATING NEONATAL PAIN AND STRESS. A number of validated and reliable scales of pain assessment are available. Behavioral indicators (e.g., facial expression, crying, and body/extremity movement) as well as physiologic indicators (e.g., tachycardia or bradycardia, hypertension, tachypnea or apnea, oxygen desaturation, palmar sweating, vagal signs) are useful in assessing an infant's level of comfort or discomfort. Biochemical markers for pain and stress such as plasma cortisol or catecholamine levels are not typically used in the clinical setting but may be useful for research.

Physiologic responses to painful stimuli include release of circulating catecholamines, heart rate acceleration, blood pressure increase, and a rise in intracranial pressure. Because the stress response of the immature fetus or preterm infant is less robust than that of the more mature infant or child, gestational age and postmenstrual age (PMA) must be considered when evaluating the pain response. Among preterm infants experiencing pain, a change in vital signs associated with the stress response (e.g., tachycardia, hypertension) and agitation are not consistently evident. Even among infants with an intact response to pain, a painful stimulus that persists for hours or days exhausts sympathetic nervous system output and obscures the clinician's ability to objectively assess the infant's level of discomfort.

Changes in vital signs are not specific to pain and may be unreliable when used alone to identify pain. Changes in facial activity and heart rate are the most sensitive measures of pain observed in term and preterm infants. By 25 to 26 weeks, the facial expression is the same as for children/adults. Before that, various facial components of a grimace may be observed separately, such as eye squeeze. The Premature Infant Pain Profile (PIPP) scores the facial components separately to capture the premature infant who may be limited in the ability to produce and sustain a full grimace.

A. Assessment of pain and stress in the newborn

1. Newborns should be assessed for pain routinely (at least every 4 to 6 hours and before and after invasive procedures) by caregivers who are trained to assess pain using multidimensional tools. The pain scales used should help guide caregivers to provide effective pain relief. Because small variations in scoring points can result in under- or overtreatment, the proficiency of individual caregivers using the chosen pain scale should be reassessed periodically to maintain reliability in assessing pain.

2. Selecting the most appropriate tool for evaluating neonatal pain is essential to its management. Physicians, nurses, and parents express different perceptions of pain cues when presented with the same infant pain responses. A caregiver's bias can influence both judgment and action when they are evaluating and treating pain. A pain scoring tool with appropriate age range, acceptable psychometric properties, clinical utility, and feasibility may reduce bias even though none is perfect. Many tools exist, and a few of the more common ones are shown in Table 70.1.

3. Documentation of pain is essential. In general, pain scores that are documented along with vital signs can be monitored most easily for trends and subtle patterns so that pain, unrelieved pain, or opioid tolerance can be identified early.

4. Because no pain tool is completely accurate in identifying all types of pain in every infant, other patient data must be included in the assessment of pain. Pain that is persistent or prolonged, associated with end-of-life care, or influenced by medications cannot be reliably measured using current pain instruments.

B. Critically ill infants. Pain responses are influenced by the PMA and behavioral state of an infant. Most pain scales that have been tested used acute pain for the stimulus (heel stick), and very few tools that measure acute prolonged or chronic pain have been adequately tested. Critically ill infants may not be able to exhibit indicators of pain due to their illness acuity. Few scales include parameters of nonresponse that may be present when an infant is severely ill or extremely premature. A lack of response does not mean an infant is not in pain. The caregiver must base treatment decisions on other data such as type of disease, health status, pain risk factors, maturity, invasive measures (i.e., chest tubes), medications that blunt response, and

Table 70.1. Summary of Neonatal Pain Assessment Tools

Pain Assessment Tool	Gestational Age/ Post-conceptional Age	Physiologic Components	Behavioral Components	Type of Pain	Adjusts for Prematurity	Scale Metric
PIPP (Premature Infant Pain Profile)[1]	28–40 wk	Heart rate, oxygen saturation	Alertness, brow bulge, eye squeeze, nasolabial furrow	Procedural and Postoperative	Yes	0 to 21
CRIES (Cries, Requires Oxygen, Increased Vital Signs, Expression, Sleeplessness)[2]	32–56 wk	Blood pressure, heart rate, oxygen saturation	Cry, expression, sleeplessness	Postoperative	No	0 to 10
NIPS (Neonatal Infant Pain Scale)[3]	28–38 wk	Breathing pattern	Facial expression, cry, arms, legs, alertness	Procedural	No	0 to 7
COMFORT (and COMFORTneo)[4,5]	0–3 y (COMFORTneo: 24–42 wk)	Respiratory response, blood pressure, heart rate	Alertness, agitation, physical movements, muscle tone, facial tension	Postoperative (COMFORTneo: prolonged)	No	8 to 40
NFCS (Neonatal Facial Coding System)[6]	25 wk to Term	None	Brow bulge, eye squeeze, nasolabial furrow, open lips, stretch mouth (vertical and horizontal), lip purse, taut tongue, chin quiver	Procedural	No	0 to 10

N-PASS (Neonatal Pain, Agitation, and Sedation Scale)[7]	0–100 d	Heart rate, respiratory rate, blood pressure, oxygen saturation	Crying/irritability, behavior state, facial expression, extremities/tone	Acute and prolonged pain Also assesses sedation	Yes	Pain: 0 to 10 Sedation −10 to 0
EDIN (Échelle de la Douleur Inconfort Noveau-Né – Neonatal Pain and Discomfort Scale)[8]	25–36 wk	None	Facial activity, body movements, quality of sleep, quality of contact with nurses, consolability	Prolonged	No	0 to 15
BPSN (Bernese Pain Scale for Neonates)[9]	27–41 wk	Respiratory pattern, heart rate, oxygen saturation	Alertness, duration of cry, time to calm, skin color, brow bulge with eye squeeze, posture	Procedural	No	0 to 27

[1]Stevens B, Johnston C, Petryshen P, et al. Premature infant pain profile: development and initial validation. *Clin J Pain* 1996;12:13–22.

[2]Krechel SW, Bildner J, CRIES: a new neonatal postoperative pain measurement score. Initial testing of validity and reliability. *Paediatr Anaesth* 1995;5:53–61.

[3]Lawrence J, Alcock D, McGrath P, et al. The development of a tool to assess neonatal pain. *Neonatal Netw* 1993;12:59–66.

[4]van Dijk M, Roofthooft DW, Anand KJ, et al. Taking up the challenge of measuring prolonged pain in (premature) neonates: the COMFORTneo scale seems promising. *Clin J Pain* 2009;25:607–616.

[5]van Dijk M, de Boer JB, Koot HM, et al. The reliability and validity of the COMFORT scale as a postoperative pain instrument in 0 to 3-year-old infants. *Pain* 2000;84:367–377.

[6]Grunau RV, Craig KD. Facial activity as a measure of neonatal pain expression. *Adv Pain Res Ther* 1990;15:147–155.

[7]Hummel P, Puchalski M, Creech SD, et al. Clinical reliability and validity of the N-PASS: Neonatal Pain, Agitation and Sedation Scale with prolonged pain. *J Perinatol* 2008;28:55–60.

[8]Debillon T, Zupan V, Ravault N, et al. Development and initial validation of the EDIN scale, a new tool for assessing prolonged pain in preterm infants. *Arch Dis Child Fetal Neonatal Ed* 2001;85:F36–F41.

[9]Cignacco E, Mueller R, Hamers JP, et al. Pain assessment in the neonate using the Bernese Pain Scale for Neonates. *Early Hum Dev* 2004;78:125–131.

Source: Reprinted with permission from Maxwell LG, Malavolta CP; Fraga MV. Assessment of pain in the neonate. *Clin Perinatol* 2013;40:457–469.

scheduled painful procedures. Existing pain instruments do not account for the extremely premature infant whose immature physiologic and behavioral responses are challenging to interpret. Infants with neurologic impairment can mount a similar pain response to healthy term infants, although the intensity of that response may be diminished. The pain response can be increased in individual infants based on prior pain history and handling before a painful event.

C. **Chronic or prolonged pain.** Physiologic and behavioral indicators can be markedly different when pain is prolonged. Infants may become passive with few or no body movements, little or no facial expression, less heart rate and respiratory variation, and consequently, lower oxygen consumption. Caregivers may erroneously interpret these findings to indicate that these infants are not feeling pain due to their lack of physiologic or behavioral responses. Quality and duration of sleep, feeding, quality of interactions, and consolability combined with risk factors for pain may be more indicative of persistent pain. A promising tool for assessment of prolonged pain in preterm infants is the EDIN (Échelle Douleur Inconfort Nouveau-Né, Neonatal Pain and Discomfort Scale), although psychometric evaluation is incomplete. There is evidence that repetitive and/or prolonged exposure to pain may increase the pain response (hyperalgesia) to future painful stimulation and may even result in pain sensation from nonpainful stimuli (allodynia).

IV. MANAGEMENT: PAIN PREVENTION AND TREATMENT. Attention to

the intensity of diagnostic, therapeutic, or surgical procedures commonly performed in the neonatal intensive care unit (NICU) is fundamental to the development of strategies appropriate for mild, moderate, or severe pain levels. This should include consideration of the history, clinical status, and PMA of the patient. A summary of painful skin-breaking procedures (Table 70.2) illustrates some options available for management of pain.

Caregivers often underuse nonpharmacologic measures for pain relief. When used appropriately, these approaches to pain relief have been shown to be effective and can also be used as an adjunct to pharmacologic treatment of pain.

A. **Environmental modification.** Painful or stressful procedures should be reviewed daily in order to decrease redundant or unwarranted blood sampling. Combining painful procedures with nonurgent, routine care or prior handling may intensify the pain experience.

1. **Light** should be shielded from an infant's eyes especially when procedural lights are used or the infant is positioned where light is directed toward the face.

2. **Sound** often occurs at levels and frequencies that disturb rest and sleep in neonatal patients. Efforts are made to minimize sound levels to promote a restful environment in the unit and around the bedside.

3. **Positioning** infants comfortably is a skill all caregivers regardless of discipline need to acquire. It is even more important when risk factors for pain are present. The use of supportive positioning aids may be needed to assist positions of comfort and enhance the effects of other forms of pain management.

Table 70.2. Summary of Procedures and Recommendations for Pain Relief

Skin-Breaking Procedures*,†	Proposed Interventions	Comments
Heel stick	Use nonpharmacologic measures + mechanical lance, squeezing the heel is the most painful phase	Venipuncture is more efficient, less painful; local anesthetics, acetaminophen, heel warming do not reduce heel stick pain
Venipuncture	Nonpharmacologic measures, use topical local anesthetics	Required less time & less resampling than heel stick
Arterial puncture	Nonpharmacologic measures, use topical and subcutaneous local anesthetics	More painful than venipuncture
IV cannulation	Nonpharmacologic measures, use topical local anesthetics	—
Central line placement	Nonpharmacologic measures, use topical local anesthetics, consider low-dose opioids or deep sedation based on clinical factors	Some centers prefer using general anesthesia
Finger stick	Nonpharmacologic measures and use mechanical device	Venipuncture is more efficient, less painful; local anesthetics, acetaminophen, or warming may not reduce finger stick pain
Subcutaneous injection	Avoid if possible, use nonpharmacologic measures and topical local anesthetics if procedure cannot be avoided	—
Intramuscular injection	Avoid if possible, use nonpharmacologic measures and topical local anesthetics if procedure cannot be avoided	—
Lumbar puncture	Nonpharmacologic measures and topical local anesthetic, lidocaine infiltration, careful positioning	Use IV analgesia/sedation, if patients are intubated and ventilated

(continued)

Table 70.2. Summary of Procedures and Recommendations for Pain Relief *(Continued)*

Skin-Breaking Procedures*,†	Proposed Interventions	Comments
Peripheral arterial line	Nonpharmacologic measures and topical local anesthetic, lidocaine infiltration, consider IV opioids	—
Circumcision	Nonpharmacologic measures and topical local anesthetic, lidocaine infiltration, IV/PO acetaminophen before and after procedure	Lidocaine infiltration for distal, ring, or dorsal penile nerve blocks (DPNB); liposomal lidocaine is more effective than DPNB
Suprapubic bladder aspiration	Nonpharmacologic measures and topical local anesthetic, lidocaine infiltration, consider IV fentanyl (0.5–1.0 mcg/kg)	—
Arterial or venous cutdown	Nonpharmacologic measures and topical local anesthetic, lidocaine infiltration, IV fentanyl (1–2 mcg/kg), consider deep sedation	Most arterial or venous cutdowns can be avoided, consider referral to interventional radiology
Peripherally inserted central catheter (PICC)	Nonpharmacologic measures and topical local anesthetic, lidocaine infiltration, consider IV fentanyl (1 mcg/kg) or IV ketamine (1 mg/kg)	Some centers prefer using deep sedation or general anesthesia
ECMO Cannulation	Propofol 2–4 mg/kg, ketamine 1–2 mg/kg, fentanyl 1–3 mcg/kg, muscle relaxant as needed	—
Tracheal intubation (eg, for mechanical ventilation)	Give fentanyl (1 mcg/kg) or morphine (10–30 mcg/kg), with midazolam (50–100 mcg/kg), ketamine (1 mg/kg) use muscle relaxant only if experienced clinician, consider atropine	Superiority of one drug regimen over another has not been investigated
Gastric tube insertion	Nonpharmacologic measures, consider local anesthetic gel	Perform rapidly, use lubricant, avoid injury

(continued)

Table 70.2. *(Continued)*

Skin-Breaking Procedures*,†	Proposed Interventions	Comments
Chest physiotherapy	Gentle positioning, fentanyl (1 mcg/kg) if a chest tube is present	Avoid areas of injured or inflamed skin, areas with indwelling drains or catheters
Removal of IV catheter	Solvent swab, consider nonpharmacologic measures	—
Wound treatment	Nonpharmacologic measures, use topical local anesthetics, consider low-dose opioids, or deep sedation based on extent of injury	See also "Dressing change"
Umbilical catheterization	Nonpharmacologic measures, IV acetaminophen (10 mg/kg), avoid sutures to the skin	Cord tissue is not innervated, but avoid injury to skin
Bladder compression	Consider nonpharmacologic measures or IV acetaminophen (10 mg/kg) if severe or prolonged	—
Tracheal extubation	Use solvent swab for tape, consider nonpharmacologic measures	—
Dressing change	Nonpharmacologic measures and topical local anesthetic, consider deep sedation if extensive	—

*Nonpharmacologic measures include pacifier, oral sucrose, swaddling, skin-to-skin contact with mother.
†The frequency of procedures can be reduced without sacrificing the quality of neonatal intensive care.
Source: Reprinted with permission from Hall RW, Anand KJS. Pain management in newborns. *Clin Perinatol* 2014;41(4):895–924.

4. **Facilitated tucking** or "hand swaddling" consists of placing a hand on a baby's head or back and feet keeping extremities flexed and contained close to the trunk where an infant is not restricted but can push against the gentle containment, moving as needed. This technique has been successful in relieving the pain of endotracheal suctioning and heel stick.

5. **Skin-to-skin (STS) holding** or kangaroo care is when an infant is placed on a parent's chest inside the clothes, clad only in a diaper and hat usually with a warm blanket laid over the infant. Enzymes and

hormones that are released during STS chemically elevate the pain threshold resulting in better tolerance of painful procedures and a decreased crying response. For both STS and facilitated tucking, the analgesic effect remains only as long as an infant is held.

Multisensory stimulation, massage, and music therapy may have potential for pain management. These interventions need much more investigation to understand how they work and if they are more or less effective and safe than other options.

B. **Nonpharmacologic interventions** also consist of taste-mediated analgesia frequently combined with environmental, hand containment or facilitated tucking, nonnutritive sucking, and STS holding.

1. **Sweet-tasting solutions** (sucrose or glucose) given orally 2 minutes before and again just prior to a painful procedure decreases the pain response in infants up to 12 months of age (Fig. 70.1). For repetitive painful procedures, taste-mediated analgesia is more effective than environmental modification alone.

   a. For procedures that last longer than 5 minutes, repeated dosing should be considered.

   b. Optimal dosing of sweet-tasting solutions has not been established. Long-term outcomes from repeated dosing of sweet solutions in early infancy and in preterm infants are not known. A Cochrane Review recently presented concerns regarding repeated sucrose dosing or use in extremely premature or critically ill neonates due to limited data on long-term outcomes.

   c. Sweet-tasting solutions must be given on the tongue where taste buds for sweet taste are concentrated. They are not effective if given by nasogastric tube.

   d. They are even more effective when combined with other nonpharmacologic strategies such as nonnutritive sucking (e.g., gloved finger or pacifier).

2. **Breastfeeding** is an effective pain intervention strategy decreasing both crying time and pain reaction. This may be due to the sweetness of breast milk or the combined effects of STS holding, smell, touch, containment, and general sensory ambiance.

   a. An additional advantage of this approach is that mothers have an active role in alleviating their infants' pain.

   b. Breast milk alone as an analgesic is inconclusive with some reports concluding that it may be as effective as sucrose but others that it is only as effective as water for pain management.

3. **Nonnutritive sucking** is more effective when used in conjunction with glucose or sucrose administration. As long as the infant is sucking, the analgesic properties are maintained.

V. PHARMACOLOGIC TREATMENT OF PROCEDURE-RELATED PAIN

A. **Analgesia for minimally invasive procedures**

1. Topical anesthetics such as lidocaine-prilocaine (EMLA) are safe and effective as a topical anesthetic for certain procedures such as venipuncture, venous cannulation, and lumbar puncture but are ineffective for

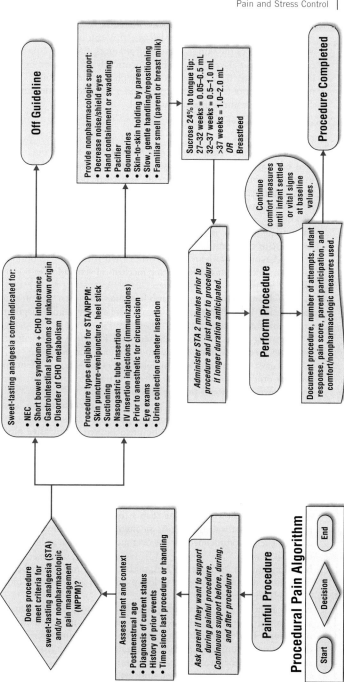

Figure 70.1. Procedural pain algorithm for minor procedures. NEC, necrotizing enterocolitis; CHO, carbohydrates.

heel-stick blood draws. Topical agents should be used with caution and repeated doses should be limited because they can be toxic when used over large areas of the skin in substantial amounts. EMLA is contraindicated in infants <1 year of age who concurrently take methemoglobin-inducing agents (i.e., sulfas, acetaminophen, phenobarbital). New topical anesthetics (e.g., 4% tetracaine and 4% liposomal lidocaine) are faster acting but not as effective as EMLA.

B. **Analgesia for invasive procedures**

   1. General principles

      a. Pain prevention versus treatment: Opioid analgesia given on a scheduled basis as a preventative measure results in a lower total dose and improved pain control compared with "as needed" dosing.

      b. Prematurity: Pain should be assumed and treatment initiated in the immature acutely ill infant who may be incapable of mounting a stress response to signal discomfort. The inability of the infant to mount an appropriate response is especially relevant when the infant is extremely immature or the painful stimulus is severe and/or prolonged.

      c. The American Academy of Pediatrics (AAP) does not recommend routine opioid administration during mechanical ventilation of preterm infants.

      d. Opioids and sedatives (e.g., benzodiazepines) are often used in treating critically ill newborns undergoing invasive or very painful diagnostic or therapeutic procedures.

      e. Alleviating pain is the most important goal. Therefore, treatment with analgesics is recommended over sedation without analgesia.

      f. The most commonly used opioids are morphine and fentanyl; however, others are used including sufentanil, tramadol, and short-acting opioids such as alfentanil and remifentanil.

      g. For most invasive procedures, pharmacologic **premedication** is recommended. Except in instances of emergency intubation when it may not be feasible, newborns should be premedicated for invasive procedures. Examples of procedures for which premedication is indicated include elective intubation, chest tube insertion or removal, peripheral arterial catheter placement, laser surgery, and circumcision.

   2. **Intubation** (see Intubation Sedation Guidelines)

      a. The AAP recommends medication with fentanyl 1 to 3 µg/kg. Fentanyl must be infused slowly (no faster than 1 µg/kg/minute) to avoid complications of chest wall rigidity. As an alternative to fentanyl, remifentanil has been recommended for use over morphine when a short-acting opioid is desired.

      b. Among infants >35 weeks' PMA, midazolam 0.1 mg/kg may be used in addition to opioid analgesia to lessen agitation and potential movement-related trauma.

      c. The addition of a short-acting muscle relaxant given after analgesia administration may decrease the procedure duration and number of attempts needed, thereby decreasing the potential for severe oxygen desaturation. Before adding a short-acting muscle relaxant (rocuronium, succinylcholine) for intubation, airway control and the ability to perform effective bag-and-mask ventilation must be assured.

3. During mechanical ventilation

a. The AAP guideline on pain management does not recommend routine continuous opioid infusions for mechanically ventilated newborns because of concern about short-term adverse effects and lack of data on long-term outcomes.

b. If analgesia is needed, medication with fentanyl 0.5 to 2 μg/kg or morphine 0.02 to 0.1 mg/kg can be given as a continuous infusion or intermittently every 4 hours.

4. Circumcision

a. Pretreatment includes both oral (24%) sucrose analgesia and acetaminophen 15 mg/kg and, for the procedure, dorsal penile block or ring block with a maximum 0.5% lidocaine dose of 0.5 mL/kg.

b. Developmental positioning of the upper extremities using a blanket and restraining only the lower limbs may decrease the stress of medical immobilization.

c. Following the procedure, an infant may benefit from acetaminophen 10 mg/kg every 6 hours for 24 hours (total dose not to exceed 40 mg/kg).

5. Chest drains

a. Analgesia for chest-drain insertion comprises all of the following:
  i. General nonpharmacologic measures
  ii. Systemic analgesia with a rapidly acting opiate such as fentanyl
  iii. Slow infiltration of the skin site with a local anesthetic before incision unless there is life-threatening instability

b. Indwelling chest drains
  i. Discomfort from indwelling chest drains varies. Pain management with general nonpharmacologic measures, acetaminophen, and opioids is individualized based on infant's pain assessment.

c. Analgesia for chest drain removal comprises the following:
  i. General nonpharmacologic measures (especially positioning/swaddling)
  ii. Short-acting, rapid onset systemic analgesia

6. Ophthalmology procedures

a. Data show anesthetic drops, sucrose, and containment reduce the pain response to eye exams for retinopathy of prematurity.

b. There are no data on the effects of bright lighting following dilatation for eye exams. A thoughtful approach to minimize discomfort after an exam may be to decrease lighting or shield the infant's eyes from light for 4 to 6 hours.

c. Retinal surgery should be considered major surgery, and effective opiate-based pain relief should be provided.

7. Postoperative analgesia.
Tissue injury, which occurs during all forms of surgery, elicits profound physiologic responses. The more marked these responses, the greater the morbidities. Thus, minimizing the endocrine and metabolic responses to surgery by decreasing pain has been shown to significantly improve outcomes after neonatal surgery. Anticipation and planning for pain management is essential to the success of any pain management program. Information aids the planning process and includes PMA, acuity, comorbidities, type of procedure or surgery,

and respiratory support along with standard handoff communication to reduce variation in pain management.

a. Health care facilities providing surgery for neonates should establish a protocol for pain management in collaboration with anesthesia, surgery, neonatology, nursing, and pharmacy. Sufficient anesthesia and analgesia is provided to prevent intraoperative pain and stress responses and adequately control postoperative pain.

b. Improving pain management and outcomes in the neonate requires a team approach and a coordinated multidimensional strategy of pain reduction. A postoperative pain algorithm guides practice and provides a standard of care for most infants during the postoperative period (Fig. 70.2). Factors considered in developing a postoperative pain management plan include the following:

   i. Pain history and previous opioid/sedative use

   ii. Severity of procedure (invasiveness, anesthesia time, and amount of tissue manipulation)

   iii. Airway management postoperatively (expected extended intubation, short-term intubation, or not intubated)

   iv. Desired level of sedation postoperatively

c. The goal of postoperative pain management is preventive analgesia rather than trying to "catch up" after pain has begun. Central sensitization is induced by noxious inputs, and the administration of analgesic drugs immediately postoperatively (prior to "awakening" from general anesthesia) may prevent the spinal and supraspinal hyperexcitability caused by acute pain, resulting in decreased analgesic use.

d. Opioids are the basis for postoperative analgesia after moderate/major surgery in the absence of regional anesthesia. During the immediate postoperative period, opioids are most effective when scheduled at regular intervals or continuously; data is limited which offers more benefit. As needed (PRN) dosing can lead to a delay in treatment, a missed dose, or fluctuating drug levels that do not provide adequate pain relief. Morphine and fentanyl provide a similar degree of analgesia. Morphine has greater sedative effect, less risk of chest wall rigidity, and produces less tolerance yet carries a greater risk of hypotension. Fentanyl has faster onset; shorter duration of action; and has less of an effect on gastrointestinal (GI) motility, hemodynamics, and urinary retention.

e. Elimination of opioids may be influenced by enterohepatic recirculation and elevated plasma concentrations; therefore, monitoring for side effects should be maintained for several hours after opioids are discontinued.

f. Acetaminophen is often used as an adjunct to regional anesthetics and opioids for postoperative pain management. Acetaminophen has been shown to provide effective analgesia as an adjunct to regional anesthesia or opioid therapy and decrease cumulative opioid exposure in postoperative neonates. Acetaminophen can be administered immediately after surgery as an adjunct when indicated. Acetaminophen is not recommended if PMA <28 weeks due to inadequate pharmacokinetic data for appropriate dosage calculation. Acetaminophen should be used with caution in patients with hepatic impairment; lower doses or an alternative therapy

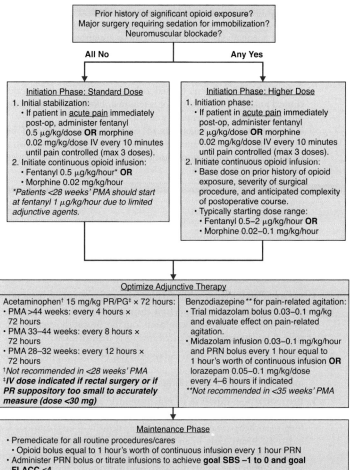

Figure 70.2. Postoperative pain management algorithm for moderate/major surgery. post-op, postoperation; IV, intravenous; PMA, postmenstrual age; PR, per rectum; PG, per gastric; PRN, as needed; SBS, state behavior scale; FLACC, faces, legs, activity, cry, consolability scale.

may be indicated. Rectal administration route is avoided in patients following anorectal procedures; alternatively, the enteral route may be used in adequate GI motility. Intravenous acetaminophen is used when both rectal and enteral routes are not optimal. The administration of acetaminophen for procedural pain management has not been established as effective.

g. Postoperative analgesia is used as long as pain assessment scales and clinical judgment indicate that it is required. Dosing intervals or dosages can be weaned if pain remains well controlled.

h. Nonpharmacologic methods of pain management should be optimized in addition to minimizing noxious stimuli. Using distraction techniques and other nonpharmacologic measures helps to decrease anxiety.

C. Benzodiazepines and other sedatives are often given in conjunction with pain medication.

1. Sedatives (i.e., benzodiazepines) do not provide analgesia but may be given to manage agitation related to other factors such as mechanical ventilation.

2. Sedatives postoperatively can be administered in combination with analgesia to reduce opioid requirements and associated adverse effects.

3. Sedatives and opioids with sedative properties (fentanyl, MSO4) may cause respiratory depression, and their use should be restricted to settings where respiratory depression can be promptly recognized and treated by clinicians experienced in airway management.

4. Caution should be used in administering benzodiazepines in patients <35 weeks' PMA due to the potential for neurotoxicity including the induction of myoclonic jerking movements.

5. Benzodiazepine exposure in rodent models extends cortical apoptosis, alters developing γ-aminobutyric acid (**GABA**) receptors, and results in long-term behavioral and cognitive impairment. Thus, cautious use of sedatives during early brain development is recommended. Additional studies on the use of midazolam infusions in preterm neonates have shown conflicting results on neurologic outcomes. Due to these results, the use of midazolam infusions in preterm neonates cannot currently be recommended.

D. Naloxone for reversal of opioid side effects. Naloxone (Narcan) is used to treat the side effects of excessive opioid, most commonly respiratory depression, although pruritus and emesis may also occur in newborns. Pruritus in an infant may appear as agitation and increased movement in an attempt to alleviate symptoms. In an infant receiving opioid analgesia, carefully dosed naloxone can be used to reverse the adverse effects without exacerbating pain. If the infant's clinical status permits, one approach is to titrate administration of naloxone, giving it in increments of 0.05 mg/kg until the side effects are reversed. Of note, to reverse the adverse effect of chest wall and laryngeal rigidity, airway management equipment and a neuromuscular blocker agent must be immediately available in case severe hypoxemia and the inability to ventilate are not immediately reversed by naloxone administration.

E. **Opioid tolerance.** Prolonged opioid administration may lead to tolerance; pain behaviors recur, sleep is disrupted, and an infant may exhibit a high-pitched cry or tremors during handling. Infants are not able to interact with their parent or caregiver as they did when pain was well controlled. In this case, there is a need to increase the dose, typically in increments of 10% to 20%, to relieve symptoms.

F. **Opioid and sedative weaning.** Prolonged use of opioids and sedatives can result in iatrogenic physical dependence. Opioids and sedatives are weaned with a goal to avoid both excess exposure to these medications and unsafe symptoms of withdrawal (see Chapter 12). Long-term effects of exposure to these agents on neonatal neurodevelopment are not fully understood.

Neonates exposed to continuous or higher doses of opioids for >5 days are at increased risk for opioid withdrawal; therefore, weaning rather than abrupt discontinuation is recommended. Opioid withdrawal is more prevalent and may occur earlier in infants receiving fentanyl compared to morphine. An overall opioid and sedative weaning plan should be developed and individualized prior to implementation. Factors considered in developing an opioid and sedative weaning plan include the following:

1. Length of opioid and sedative exposure

2. History of previous opioid and sedative exposure and weans

3. Patient stability and ability to tolerate symptoms of withdrawal

4. Enteral feeds

5. Intravenous access

Opioids and sedatives are weaned by a percentage of the original dose the patient is on when weaning begins, typically in 10% increments. For example, a patient receiving morphine 0.2 mg/kg/hour would wean by 10% or 0.02 mg/kg at each wean. The weaning frequency is tailored to the individual patient; every 8 to 12 hours for moderate length of exposure and every 24 to 48 hours for longer lengths of exposure. This strategy continues throughout weaning unless symptoms of withdrawal or a change in condition occur. Weaning is further individualized by using a withdrawal assessment tool such as the Finnegan Neonatal Abstinence Scoring System to monitor symptoms and guide the frequency of weaning and potential need for rescue doses.

Nonpharmacologic comfort methods are essential in addition to minimizing noxious stimuli. Removing noxious environmental stressors, protecting sleep, swaddling, and rocking have been used to support infants undergoing withdrawal. In general, feeding should be encouraged, and continuous feedings may be considered if bolus feeds are not tolerated. Withdrawal assessment is continued until opioids and/or sedatives have been discontinued for a minimum of 72 hours and there is no evidence of withdrawal symptoms.

G. **Epidural analgesia** is the administration of analgesics and local anesthetic agents into the epidural space as a single or intermittent bolus or continuous infusion. Advantages of epidural anesthesia and postoperative analgesia in preterm and term neonates are effective analgesia at lower doses of systemic opioids and earlier extubation. This may be a better option than general anesthesia for former preterm infants with chronic lung disease because it decreases the need for intubation during surgical procedures such as hernia repair or ileostomy takedown/repair. In some institutions, a pain service manages patients with epidural analgesia and is responsible for the continuous infusion and any bolus requirements until the epidural is discontinued. Postoperative complications include accidental injection of local anesthetic agents into the intravascular system, venous air embolism, local or systemic infection, and meningitis. Cardiorespiratory monitoring and assessment of the infant's respiratory status, sensory responses, pain behaviors, integrity of dressing, urine output, and any changes in pump settings or additional bolus requirements are essential.

VI. CONCLUSION.

Research on the safety and efficacy of current and new medications is ongoing in the search for better pain management with less potential for undesirable effects. Teamwork with anticipatory planning before painful, invasive procedures optimizes timely, effective pain management (Tables 70.3 and 70.4).

Table 70.3. Opioids

Drug	Advantages	Disadvantages
Morphine	Potent pain relief Better ventilator synchrony Sedation Hypnosis Muscle relaxation Inexpensive	Respiratory depression Arterial hypotension Constipation, nausea Urinary retention Central nervous system depression Tolerance, dependence Long-term outcomes not studied Prolonged ventilator use
Fentanyl	Fast acting Less hypotension	Respiratory depression Short half-life Quick tolerance and dependence Chest wall rigidity Inadequately studied
Remifentanil	Fast acting Degraded in the plasma Unaffected by liver metabolism	—

Source: Reprinted with permission from Hall RW, Anand KJS. Pain management in newborns. *Clin Perinatol* 2014;41(4):895–924.

Table 70.4. Benzodiazepines

Drug	Advantages	Disadvantages
Benzodiazepines	Better ventilator synchrony Antianxiety Sedation Hypnosis Muscle relaxation Amnesia Anticonvulsant	No pain relief Arterial hypotension Respiratory depression Constipation, nausea Urinary retention Myoclonus Seizures Central nervous system depression Tolerance, dependence Alters bilirubin metabolism Propylene glycol and benzyl alcohol exposure
Midazolam	Most studied benzodiazepine Quickly metabolized	Short acting Benzyl alcohol exposure
Lorazepam	Longer acting Better anticonvulsant	More myoclonus reported Propylene glycol exposure
Diazepam	—	Not recommended in the neonate

Source: Reprinted with permission from Hall RW, Anand KJ. Pain management in newborns. *Clin Perinatol* 2014;41(4):895–924.

Suggested Readings

American Academy of Pediatrics Committee on Fetus and Newborn, Section on Anesthesiology and Pain Medicine. Prevention and management of procedural pain in the neonate: an update. *Pediatrics* 2016;137(2):1–13.

Anand KJ, Stevens BJ, McGrath PJ, eds. *Pain in Neonates and Infants.* 3rd ed. Edinburgh, United Kingdom: Elsevier; 2007.

Hall RW, Anand KJ. Pain management in newborns. *Clin Perinatol* 2014;41(4):895–924.

Kumar P, Denson SE, Mancuso T; for the American Academy of Pediatrics Committee on Fetus and Newborn, Section on Anesthesiology and Pain Medicine. Premedication for nonemergency endotracheal intubation in the neonate. *Pediatrics* 2010;125(3):608–615.

McGrath P, Stevens BJ, Walker S, et al, eds. *Oxford Textbook of Paediatric Pain.* Oxford, United Kingdom: Oxford University Press; 2014.

McPherson C, Grunau RE. Neonatal pain control and neurologic effects of anesthetics and sedatives in preterm infants. *Clin Perinatol* 2014;41(1):209–227.

Stevens B, Yamada J, Lee GY, et al. Sucrose for analgesia in newborn infants under-going painful procedures. *Cochrane Database Syst Rev* 2013;(1):CD001069.

Walden M, Gibbins S. *Pain Assessment and Management: Guideline for Practice.* 3rd ed. Glenview, IL: National Association of Neonatal Nurses; 2012.

Walden M, Spruill CT. Pain assessment in the newborn. In: Tappero EP, Honeyfield ME, eds. *Physical Assessment of the Newborn: A Comprehensive Approach to the Art of Physical Examination.* 5th ed. Petaluma, CA: NICU Ink; 2015:239–254.

Index

Note: Page numbers followed by an "*f*" denote figures; those followed by a "*t*" denote tables. Page numbers preceded by "A*" indicate online appendix pages.

A

abdominal catastrophes, surgical, 358
abdominal distention, 945, 964, 1018–1019
abdominal examination, 99–100
abdominal imaging, 962–963
abdominal injuries, 74
abdominal masses, 371, 372*t*, 947, 964–965
abdominal paracentesis, 1018–1019
abortion, spontaneous, 135
abrasions, 75
abstinence syndrome. *See* neonatal abstinence
     syndrome
acardia, 136
ACE inhibitors, 394*t*, A*1116*t*
acetaminophen, 1036–1038, A*1043, A*1100*t*
acetazolamide, 776–777
acid–base disorders, 305–306. *See also specific types*
   in congenital heart disease, 532
   in inborn errors of metabolism, 867, 868–874,
      869*f,* 870*f*
acid–base regulation, renal, 369–370
acidemias, organic, 871–872, 871*t*
acidosis
   fetal, in perinatal asphyxia, 790
   metabolic, 305–306, 306*t,* 385, 867, 868–874,
      869*f,* 870*f*
   in pulmonary hemorrhage, 480
   renal tubular, 398–399
Acinetobacter baumannii, 706
acquired heart disease, 562
ACTH stimulation test, 935*f,* 936, 938
acute bilirubin encephalopathy (ABE), 344,
      349–350
acute kidney injury, neonatal, 381–386
   complication management in, 384–386
   criteria for, 381, 381*t*
   etiology of, 382–383*t*
   evaluation for, 383–384, 384*t*
   management of, 384
acyclovir, 653, A*1043–1044, A*1043*t,* A*1112*t*
acylcarnitine, 866, 878, 880*t*
additive solution units, RBC, 578–579, 579*t*
adenosine, 573, A*1044
adenovirus, 59
adenylosuccinate lyase deficiency, 884
adhesives, 969
adrenal hemorrhage, 74
afterload-reducing agents, 564–565
age, gestational, 1, 78–79
age, maternal, 76, 132, 136
air embolism, 482, 490
air leak, 482–490
   in mechanical ventilation, 412*t,* 416–417, 418
   in meconium aspiration, 466
   in neonatal resuscitation, 48

   in respiratory distress syndrome, 441–442, 444
   surgery for, 945
air transports, 205, 212–213
air travel, BPD and, 194
AKI. *See* acute kidney injury
Alagille syndrome, 524*t*
albinism, 975
albumin, 336, A*1044–1045, A*1045*t*
albumin solutions, 300
albuterol, A*1045
alcohol, 144*t*
alkalosis, metabolic, 306, 307*t,* 311
allergic colitis, 358
α-fetoprotein (AFP), 2, 832
alprostadil, A*1045–1046
ambiguous genitalia, 117, 923, 930–931*t,* 933, 938
amblyopia, 195
ambulance regulations, 207
AMH. *See* anti-müllerian hormone
amikacin, 746, 748, 752*t,* A*1046–1047, A*1046*t,*
      A*1109*t*
amino acids, 261–262, 866
ammonia, plasma level of, 865, 874–878
amniocentesis, 5, 56, 133
amnioinfusion, 12, 463
amnion, multiple birth, 131, 132
amoxicillin, A*1047
amphotericin B, 712, A*1111*t*
amphotericin-B deoxycholate, A*1047–1048
amphotericin-B lipid complex, A*1048
amphotericin-B liposomal, A*1048–1049
ampicillin, A*1049, A*1049*t*
amplitude-integrated electroencephalogram
      (aiEEG), 816, 817*f*
anaerobic bacterial infections, 709
analgesia
   maternal, fetal effects of, A*1100*t*
   neonatal, 1032–1040
   neonatal postoperative, 1035–1038, 1037*f*
androgen defects, 937–938
androgen insensitivity syndrome, 937, 938–939
anemia, 195, 613–623
   classification of, 618*t*
   diagnostic approach in newborn, 617–619
   etiology in neonate, 615–617
   prophylaxis against, 622–623
   therapy for, 619–623
   transfusion for, 619–622, 620*t*
anencephaly, 87, 830
anesthesia
   carbon dioxide monitoring in, 424
   fetal effects of, A*1101–1104*t*
aneuploidy, 2–4, 18, 124*t*
angel's kiss, 974, 980*f,* 983
anion gap, 305–306, 306*t,* 868

Intubation Sedation Guidelines

(See Chapter 70 and Appendix A)

Name: _____
Completed by: _____

Weight: _____ kg
Date: _____

Medication	Dose	Patient-Specific Dose	Duration of Effect	Comments
Analgesic Medications				
Fentanyl	IV: 1–3 µg/kg/dose		30–60 minutes	Infuse over 2–5 minutes. May cause chest wall rigidity with rapid infusion Neuromuscular blocking agent if suspect chest wall rigidity Antidotes: naloxone
Morphine	IV: 0.05–0.1 mg/kg/dose		2–4 hours	Infuse over 5 minutes. Use with caution in patients with hypotension.
Sedative Medications				
Midazolam (Versed)	IV: 0.05–0.1 mg/kg May be given IM: 0.1 mg/kg Intranasal: 0.2–0.3 mg/kg (5 mg/mL conc.)		1–4 hours	Infuse over 2–5 minutes. Do not use if <35 weeks' postmenstrual age. Use 5 mg/mL concentration for intranasal administration. Antidote: flumazenil
Short-Acting Neuromuscular Blocking Agents—Only Use if Able to Provide Adequate Facial/Mask PPV				
Rocuronium	IV: 0.6–1.2 mg/kg/dose		20–40 minutes (peak effect 30–60 seconds)	Rapid IV push Antidote: neostigmine
Succinylcholine	IV: 2 mg/kg/dose May be given IM		4–6 minutes (peak effect 30–60 seconds)	Always administer atropine first (see dose below). Rapid IV push Do not repeat dose. Do not use in patients with history of musculoskeletal disease, hyperkalemia, renal dysfunction, or trauma.
Anticholinergic Medication				
Atropine	IV: 0.02 mg/kg/dose		4–6 hours	Infuse over 1 minute. No further minimum weight or dose

ETT size: _____

Distance from tip of tube to ☐ nares ☐ lip _____

CCS0120